the calorie carb & fat bible

The UK's Most Comprehensive Calorie Counter

the calorie, carb & fat bible 2004

© Weight Loss Resources 2004

Published by
Weight Loss Resources
Remus House
Peterborough
PE2 9JX

ISBN 1 904512 01 1

Authors
Dr Jeremy Sims MB BS FRIPH FRSH
Tracey Walton

Editor: Pat Wilson
Design & Layout: Joanne Readshaw

Printed and bound in Great Britain by
Antony Rowe Ltd, Chippenham, Wiltshire SN14 6LH

Contents

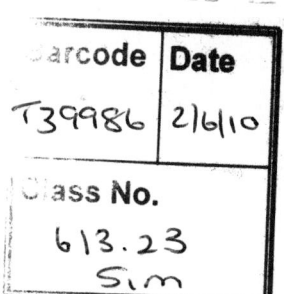

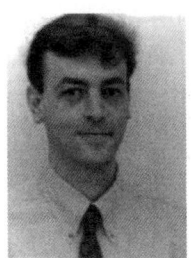

INTRODUCTION

Losing Weight:
Taking Control & Winning

How do we achieve sustainable and ongoing success in our weight loss efforts?

"Success breeds success". So goes that well-known adage. That incredible tendency for small successes to lead on to even greater ones. We attain small goals and feel empowered to move on to even greater achievements. It can be true in many areas of our lives. And it can be just as applicable in our personal weight management efforts. We lose a few pounds, reach an early goal we have set ourselves, and we feel our confidence grow. We feel spurred on to our next weight goal. We have a growing sense of control.

But hey, wait up! I hear you cry. That doesn't sound like me. Yes I can lose a few pounds, feel great for a while, and then before I know it my confidence is blown sky high when next week I'm stuck at the same weight. Or, what about when I reach a healthier weight and then put it all back on again after a few months. You know, I'm not at all sure about all this success breeds success business.

And therein lies the problem, or to be more precise problems, for so many of us. How do we achieve sustainable and ongoing success in our weight loss efforts? And, then, having attained our ultimate goal of a healthier weight, how do we ensure it lasts? How do we ensure we maintain this healthy weight not just tomorrow, or next month, or next year even… but for a lifetime.

In recent years there has been much research attempting to find the answers to just these questions. How do the successful weight losers amongst us manage to lose their weight and then keep it off? What are the possible secrets that such individuals can reveal to the rest of us?

Research in this area has provided in depth information about the most effective strategies for weight control

Many of the people in these studies have been dubbed "maintainers"- they have been able to lose weight successfully and then remain stable at their goal weight for the long term. These are the "winners" in the weight battles. Is it possible to learn from these individuals and use the knowledge gleaned to benefit others? Indeed we can. And what has been learnt has been invaluable.

Copying the positive actions of others is a proven technique, for success in achieving a goal. Who better to copy in our weight loss endeavours than those who have gone before us and triumphed? Research in this area has provided in depth information about the most effective strategies for weight control – both effective weight loss and maintenance. This information has highlighted many key factors common to most, if not all, successful weight losers:

The Secrets of Successful Weight Losers

1. They always eat a healthy breakfast which sets them up for the day, and boosts metabolism.

2. They maintain a low fat diet but never cut out fats altogether. They understand that all fats are not the same when it comes to health and are careful about saturated fat.

3. They never deny themselves the foods they enjoy – even those "naughties" – but ensure that they limit these foods.

4. They eat regular meals throughout the day – breakfast, lunch and dinner. They never skip meals. Also they always ensure that they eat a broad range of foods including plenty of fruit and veg.

5. They don't eat too many snacks, and they tend to choose healthy options.

6. They never deny themselves the opportunity to eat out but are very careful about consuming fast food.

7. They are regular monitors of what they eat. They have good knowledge of such essentials as calorie counting and the nutritional contents of food e.g. the saturated fat content.

8. They check their weight regularly but never go overboard. Once weekly is considered sufficient by most.

9. They maintain an active lifestyle. Many exercise for at least thirty minutes each day.

10. They are careful to lose weight gradually, in a healthy way. They set themselves small and achievable goals as steps towards their ultimate healthier weight.

11. They never berate themselves or feel guilty about lapses in their weight management programme. They have developed a self-belief that they can easily get back on track. They practice what is known as flexible restraint: they follow their programme but allow themselves the flexibility for occasional favourite foods or the enjoyment of a meal out.

We can easily conclude that these individuals have really taken control of their weight and, by following their example, you can take control of yours. But in order to do so you may also need change certain practices, attitudes and beliefs.

Never Rush Your Weight Loss

Muscle is the great calorie burning apparatus of the body, helping to set your metabolism

We live in a fast track world with seemingly fast track expectations. But trying to rush weight loss always fails. It simply does not work. Consider this: it may have taken you years to accumulate your extra weight. To expect that you can lose this weight in a matter of a few weeks is totally unrealistic. Research has shown that in general it is very difficult to lose more than 1-2 lbs of body fat weight per week – your body is highly protective of its fat stores and does not give them up readily.

When we crash diet we lose not just body fat but also water, glucose stores and protein. And the latter, in the form of muscle, you do not want to lose. Muscle is the great calorie burning apparatus of the body, helping to set your metabolism. As you lose muscle you also lose this calorie-burning capacity, removing one of the important factors in weight control.

Healthy weight loss should be gradual and careful. A steady weight loss of one or two pounds per week is best – ensuring body fat loss whilst retaining as much muscle weight as possible. You will also find it easier to stick to a steady weight loss programme with readily achievable weight loss goals.

Set Yourself Realistic & Achievable Goals

Successful weight losers are honest with themselves and set themselves readily achievable weight loss goals. They know that setting unrealistic goals is sure-fire way of demotivating themselves.

Learn from these experts and set yourself small steps to your own ultimate goal. These should be steps that you know with all confidence that you can achieve. Do go easy on yourself and likewise make your goals easy. For instance, as mentioned above, aim for one or two pounds weight reduction per week or, if you like, 5% of your weight in three months. Each small step will lead you further along the path to your ultimate goal of a healthier weight. And what's more you will find that the path is a far less arduous one than you ever expected it to be.

Visualize The New You

Before starting out on a weight loss programme try to sit down and visualize your new life as a slimmer, healthier you. Find somewhere quiet, where you cannot be disturbed. Sit in a comfortable chair and close your eyes. In your mind's eye see yourself as the slimmer you. How does it feel? How much more confident are you? What will you be doing in your new life? See yourself not only achieving a new healthier weight but also achieving all those ambitions which you have been storing up but have not felt confident enough to attempt.

Hold onto this image of the new you and, as you continue on your path to losing weight, take time to revisit it at regular intervals. The image will help you to stay focused and to boost your determination when things may not be going as well as you might hope.

Go Easy On Yourself

Weight loss should not be an ordeal. It should not be about denial, deprivation, and suffering. Look back at the key characteristics of our successful weight losers. Note that they never allow themselves to feel guilty about mistakes or lapses. They never deny themselves those little goodies that make our lives a happy experience. They still eat out and enjoy restaurant food. And they still lose weight and reach their goal weight. If they can do it without suffering and self-reproach then so can you.

Successful weight losers are smart with food. They ensure that they don't overindulge on the those "naughty" foods but they certainly don't remove them from their lives altogether. Everything in moderation.

By denying ourselves completely of the things we enjoy it is very easy to slip into feelings of deprivation. This can easily become self-loathing when we break down and binge on what we have denied ourselves, resulting in a big blow to our self-confidence and motivation. The answer is never to deny yourself, just moderate. You'll find your weight loss efforts a whole lot more gratifying.

Before closing this introduction to the latest edition of *The Calorie, Carb & Fat Bible* I'd like to spotlight some further observations of successful weight losers.

First of all, most will have devised their own weight loss programme. They will have taken time to arm themselves with information from a variety of sources and will have taken those aspects which fit their lifestyles and motivations. In short they have tailored a weight management programme to meet their personal needs. Remember no one programme will suit all. Take time to develop your personal weight loss strategy – this book is a great start.

Secondly, very few successful weight losers get it right first time. Like all of us they make mistakes; they suffer lapses; and they fail – very often more than once. However, what is highly important is that they never give up. They dust themselves off and learn from their mistakes – and try not to make the same errors twice.

You too must never see yourself as a failure if you have not achieved a goal or a desired weight. These are positive learning opportunities and as such your knowledge and personal understanding will have been invaluably reinforced. Learn from your mistakes or lapses, understand why these occurred, so that you can utilise this understanding to march on to success the next time.

Thirdly, and finally, because they have been careful and lost weight gradually, the new practices and attitudes they have acquired have become a lasting and rewarding part of their lives. Thus proving after all, that in weight management, success really can breed success when you take control.

Dr Jeremy Sims
MB BS FRIPH FRSH

Using this Book to Lose Weight

You only need to eat or drink a sausage roll and a can of cola more than you need each day to create and store a pound of fat in a week

THE CALORIE BALANCE CONCEPT

Calories Consumed

greater than calories expended	= weight gain
equal to calories expended	= weight maintenance
less than calories expended	= weight loss

Making sure that calories consumed are less than calories expended is the best, if not the only, way to lose weight. After all, we put on weight by doing the exact opposite – eating a little more than we need each day, and becoming less active as each year passes.

You only need to eat or drink 500 calories (a sausage roll and a can of cola) more than you need each day to create and store a pound of fat in a week – 2 stones in just over six months. It's no wonder people say that excess weight tends to 'creep up on you'.

The good news is that the reverse is true. Eat 500 calories less than you need each day and you will lose a pound a week; a stone in 3 months, 2 stones in six months. If you combine this calorie cutting strategy with some exercise or activity that gets you moving, you'll lose weight more quickly.

How Much Weight To Lose

Use the body mass index chart and information on pages 16-17, to determine what is the right weight for you, and set a goal. You may find it helpful to set milestone goals of a stone, or half a stone, to measure your progress by; giving your confidence and motivation a boost as you go along. (Half a stone is the equivalent of 14 (½lb/250g) packs of butter!)

How Fast to Lose It

A pound a week is probably the best rate of loss for achieving sustained, healthy, permanent weight loss. If you have more than a couple of stones to lose, you could start out at 1½ – 2lb a week and see how you get on. If you begin to find this level too restrictive, slow your rate of loss down a bit – it's better to keep going at a pound a week than to give up because trying to lose 2lb a week is making you miserable! The following words may help you to keep your goal in perspective:

Never give up on a goal because of the time it will take to achieve it – the time will pass anyway.

How Many Calories

Use the calorie tables on pages 18-19 to find out how many calories you need to consume each day to maintain your current weight. Then subtract the 'calorie deficit' required to lose weight at your chosen rate, from the table below. This will give you a daily calorie allowance.

Rate of Loss	Calorie Deficit
½lb a week	250
1lb a week	500
1½lb a week	750
2lb a week	1000

Keep Track

Write down everything you eat and drink in a day – be as accurate as possible on serving sizes. Use the photocopiable Food and Exercise Diary on page 21 to help you keep track.

To start with, eat as you normally would for a few days. This will help you to see opportunities for cutting calories by substituting one food or drink item for another, and/or cutting portion sizes of high calorie foods, or eating them less often. Slowly introduce changes to your diet to bring your consumption within your chosen calorie allowance. Exercising will help you lose weight - not only does it burn extra calories (see page 20) but it will help you burn and maintain muscle tissue - which burns more calories, in the background, even when you are at rest.

Progressing

Each time you lose half a stone – celebrate! Treat yourself to a little luxury – something new to wear, a little pampering or some other (non-food!) treat. Review how well you've done, and set yourself up to lose the next half a stone by calculating a new calorie allowance based on your new weight.

Maintaining the Loss

I lost nearly three stones in just under a year of calorie counting. I reached my goal weight in February 2001, and have had no problem in keeping to that weight. The great thing about calorie counting is that you learn so much about what you eat, and make such important changes to your eating and drinking habits as you go along, that its difficult to go back to your old ways. The couple of times I have put on a pound or two, for example after a holiday, I've spent a few days calorie counting and got right back where I want to be. You can do it too – best of luck!

Tracey Walton
Founder www.weightlossresources.co.uk

Eating Healthily

Many people are unsure of what healthy eating means

As well as helping you to lose weight, a healthy and varied diet can also reduce the risk of a number of diseases including cancer, heart disease, stroke, osteoporosis and diabetes.

Many people are unsure of what healthy eating means - not surprising when you consider the variety of, often conflicting, advice given. The following guidelines are based on the UK Government's 'Balance of Good Health' and apply to most people over the age of 5. People under medical supervision or with special dietary requirements may have different needs and should check with their doctor.

The Balance of Good Health

Fruit & Vegetables
Eat at least 5 servings a day

This includes frozen, canned, dried and pure juices as well as fresh. Also included in this group are beans, including baked beans, pulses and lentils. The key for good health is to choose a wide variety - aiming for five different portions per day. A portion is approximately 80g, e.g. one medium apple or two medium plums.

Bread, Other Cereals & Potatoes
Eat 5 portions daily - about one third of of food intake

This group includes breakfast cereals, pasta, rice, noodles, oats and other cereals as well as bread and potatoes. You should aim to include at least one food from this group at each meal.

Milk & Dairy Foods
2-3 servings daily

Milk, cheese, yoghurt and fromage frais are included in this group, but not butter, eggs and cream. Serving sizes in this group vary, depending on how concentrated the food is, e.g. 1 serving of milk is 200ml, a serving of yoghurt is 150g and a serving of cheese is 30g.

Meat Fish & Alternatives
2-3 servings daily

This group includes eggs, poultry, and meat and fish products such as beefburgers and fishcakes. Some of these products can be high in fat - so it's best to choose lower fat versions of products, and trim visible fat from meat and poultry. Alternatives are non-meat sources of protein such as nuts, tofu, mycoprotein, textured vegetable protein (TVP) and kidney beans.

Food Containing Fat & Foods Containing Sugar
Eat in small quantities, 0-3 servings daily

These are foods high in fat and/or sugar. Butter, margarine, oil, mayonnaise, cream, crisps and fried foods are high in fat. Soft drinks, sweets and jam are high in sugar. Cakes, chocolate, biscuits, pastries and ice-cream are high in both. It is essential to include a small amount of fat in your diet, but most people need to eat less. The emphasis should be on unsaturated fat e.g. olive, sunflower and corn oil, rather than saturated fat which tends to come from animal products, cakes, biscuits and pastries.

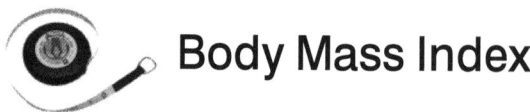

Body Mass Index

Body Mass Index is a number calculated from an individual's weight and height, that is used to determine whether a person is within, or outside of, a normal weight range. Use the Body Mass Index Chart to look up your BMI, and use the table below to see what range you fall into.

BMI	
Less than 20	Under Weight
20-25	Normal Weight
25-30	Over Weight
30-40	Obese
Over 40	Severely Obese

The spread from 20-25 shows that what is normal covers quite a big range. This is because 'normal' weight for height covers both men and women, and people of different shapes and body composition. A man would normally be expected to have a higher BMI than a woman of the same height, because men tend to have more muscle than women (women naturally have more fat) and muscle weighs more per square inch than fat. For the same reason a slim, muscular woman will have a higher BMI (i.e. weigh more) than a slim, not very muscular woman of the same height.

What's the Right Weight for You?

As a general rule women, unless they are very strong and muscular, will tend to look at their best at the lower end of the normal range, men around the middle to top of the range. 'Ideal weight' is a very individual thing, probably the best thing to do is set a goal within the normal range as described above and, as you get closer to it, adjust to a level at which you feel at your best.

BODY MASS INDEX CHART

	HEIGHT IN FEET / INCHES														
	4'6	4'8	4'10	5'0	5'2	5'4	5'6	5'8	5'10	6'0	6'2	6'4	6'6	6'8	6'10
6st 7	22.0	20.5	19.1	17.8	16.7	15.7	14.7	13.9	13.1	12.4	11.7	11.1	10.6	10.0	9.5
7st 0	23.7	22.1	20.6	19.2	18.0	16.9	15.9	15.0	14.1	13.3	12.6	12.0	11.4	10.8	10.3
7st 7	25.4	23.6	22.0	20.6	19.3	18.1	17.0	16.0	15.1	14.3	13.5	12.8	12.2	11.6	11.0
8st 0	27.1	25.2	23.5	22.0	20.6	19.3	18.1	17.1	16.1	15.2	14.4	13.7	13.0	12.3	11.8
8st 7	28.8	26.8	25.0	23.3	21.8	20.5	19.3	18.2	17.1	16.2	15.3	14.5	13.8	13.1	12.5
9st 0	30.5	28.4	26.4	24.7	23.1	21.7	20.4	19.2	18.1	17.2	16.2	15.4	14.6	13.9	13.2
9st 7	32.2	29.9	27.9	26.1	24.4	22.9	21.5	20.3	19.2	18.1	17.1	16.2	15.4	14.7	14.0
10st 0	33.9	31.5	29.4	27.4	25.7	24.1	22.7	21.4	20.2	19.1	18.0	17.1	16.2	15.4	14.7
10st 7	35.6	33.1	30.8	28.8	27.0	25.3	23.8	22.4	21.2	20.0	18.9	18.0	17.0	16.2	15.4
11st 0	37.3	34.7	32.3	30.2	28.3	26.5	24.9	23.5	22.2	21.0	19.8	18.8	17.9	17.0	16.2
11st 7	39.0	36.2	33.8	31.6	29.6	27.7	26.1	24.6	23.2	21.9	20.7	19.7	18.7	17.8	16.9
12st 0	40.7	37.8	35.2	32.9	30.8	28.9	27.2	25.6	24.2	22.9	21.6	20.5	19.5	18.5	17.6
12st 7	42.3	39.4	36.7	34.3	32.1	30.1	28.3	26.7	25.2	23.8	22.5	21.4	20.3	19.3	18.4
13st 0	44.0	41.0	38.2	35.7	33.4	31.4	29.5	27.8	26.2	24.8	23.5	22.2	21.1	20.1	19.1
13st 7	45.7	42.5	39.6	37.0	34.7	32.6	30.6	28.8	27.2	25.7	24.4	23.1	21.9	20.8	19.8
14st 0	47.4	44.1	41.1	38.4	36.0	33.8	31.7	29.9	28.2	26.7	25.3	23.9	22.7	21.6	20.6
14st 7	49.1	45.7	42.6	39.8	37.3	35.0	32.9	31.0	29.2	27.6	26.2	24.8	23.5	22.4	21.3
15st 0	50.8	47.3	44.0	41.2	38.5	36.2	34.0	32.0	30.2	28.6	27.1	25.7	24.4	23.2	22.0
15st 7	52.5	48.8	45.5	42.5	39.8	37.4	35.2	33.1	31.2	29.5	28.0	26.5	25.2	23.9	22.8
16st 0	54.2	50.4	47.0	43.9	41.1	38.6	36.3	34.2	32.3	30.5	28.9	27.4	26.0	24.7	23.5
16st 7	55.9	52.0	48.5	45.3	42.4	39.8	37.4	35.2	33.3	31.4	29.8	28.2	26.8	25.5	24.2
17st 0	57.6	53.6	49.9	46.6	43.7	41.0	38.6	36.3	34.3	32.4	30.7	29.1	27.6	26.2	25.0
17st 7	59.3	55.1	51.4	48.0	45.0	42.2	39.7	37.4	35.3	33.3	31.6	29.9	28.4	27.0	25.7
18st 0	61.0	56.7	52.9	49.4	46.3	43.4	40.8	38.5	36.3	34.3	32.5	30.8	29.2	27.8	26.4
18st 7	62.7	58.3	54.3	50.8	47.5	44.6	42.0	39.5	37.3	35.3	33.4	31.6	30.0	28.6	27.2
19st 0	64.4	59.9	55.8	52.1	48.8	45.8	43.1	40.6	38.3	36.2	34.3	32.5	30.8	29.3	27.9
19st 7	66.1	61.4	57.3	53.5	50.1	47.0	44.2	41.7	39.3	37.2	35.2	33.3	31.7	30.1	28.6
20st 0	67.8	63.0	58.7	54.9	51.4	48.2	45.4	42.7	40.3	38.1	36.1	34.2	32.5	30.9	29.4
20st 7	69.4	64.6	60.2	56.3	52.7	49.4	46.5	43.8	41.3	39.1	37.0	35.1	33.3	31.6	30.1
21st 0	71.1	66.2	61.7	57.6	54.0	50.6	47.6	44.9	42.3	40.0	37.9	35.9	34.1	32.4	30.9
21st 7	72.8	67.7	63.1	59.0	55.3	51.9	48.8	45.9	43.3	41.0	38.8	36.8	34.9	33.2	31.6
22st 0	74.5	69.3	64.6	60.4	56.5	53.1	49.9	47.0	44.4	41.9	39.7	37.6	35.7	34.0	32.3
22st 7	76.2	70.9	66.1	61.7	57.8	54.3	51.0	48.1	45.4	42.9	40.6	38.5	36.5	34.7	33.1
23st 0	77.9	72.5	67.5	63.1	59.1	55.5	52.2	49.1	46.4	43.8	41.5	39.3	37.3	35.5	33.8
23st 7	79.6	74.0	69.0	64.5	60.4	56.7	53.3	50.2	47.4	44.8	42.4	40.2	38.2	36.3	34.5
24st 0	81.3	75.6	70.5	65.9	61.7	57.9	54.4	51.3	48.4	45.7	43.3	41.0	39.0	37.0	35.3
24st 7	83.0	77.2	71.9	67.2	63.0	59.1	55.6	52.3	49.4	46.7	44.2	41.9	39.8	37.8	36.0
25st 0	84.7	78.8	73.4	68.6	64.2	60.3	56.7	53.4	50.4	47.6	45.1	42.8	40.6	38.6	36.7
25st 7	86.4	80.3	74.9	70.0	65.5	61.5	57.8	54.5	51.4	48.6	46.0	43.6	41.4	39.4	37.5
26st 0	88.1	81.9	76.3	71.3	66.8	62.7	59.0	55.5	52.4	49.5	46.9	44.5	42.2	40.1	38.2
26st 7	89.8	83.5	77.8	72.7	68.1	63.9	60.1	56.6	53.4	50.5	47.8	45.3	43.0	40.9	38.9
27st 0	91.5	85.1	79.3	74.1	69.4	65.1	61.2	57.7	54.4	51.5	48.7	46.2	43.8	41.7	39.7
27st 7	93.2	86.6	80.8	75.5	70.7	66.3	62.4	58.7	55.4	52.4	49.6	47.0	44.7	42.4	40.4
28st 0	94.9	88.2	82.2	76.8	72.0	67.5	63.5	59.8	56.4	53.4	50.5	47.9	45.5	43.2	41.1
28st 7	96.5	89.8	83.7	78.2	73.2	68.7	64.6	60.9	57.5	54.3	51.4	48.7	46.3	44.0	41.9
29st 0	98.2	91.4	85.2	79.6	74.5	69.9	65.8	62.0	58.5	55.3	52.3	49.6	47.1	44.8	42.6
29st 7	99.9	92.9	86.6	80.9	75.8	71.1	66.9	63.0	59.5	56.2	53.2	50.5	47.9	45.5	43.3

WEIGHT IN STONES / LBS

CALORIES REQUIRED TO MAINTAIN WEIGHT
ADULT MALES

AGE / ACTIVITY LEVEL

WEIGHT IN STONES / LBS	VERY SEDENTARY			MODERATELY SEDENTARY			MODERATELY ACTIVE			VERY ACTIVE		
	<30	30-60	60+	<30	30-60	60+	<30	30-60	60+	<30	30-60	60+
9st 0	1856	1827	1502	2010	1979	1627	2320	2284	1878	2784	2741	2254
9st 7	1913	1871	1547	2072	2026	1676	2391	2338	1933	2870	2806	2320
10st 0	1970	1914	1591	2134	2074	1724	2463	2393	1989	2955	2871	2387
10st 7	2027	1958	1636	2196	2121	1772	2534	2447	2045	3041	2937	2454
11st 0	2084	2001	1680	2258	2168	1820	2605	2502	2100	3127	3002	2520
11st 7	2141	2045	1724	2320	2215	1868	2677	2556	2156	3212	3067	2587
12st 0	2199	2088	1769	2382	2262	1916	2748	2611	2211	3298	3133	2654
12st 7	2256	2132	1813	2444	2310	1965	2820	2665	2267	3384	3198	2720
13st 0	2313	2175	1858	2506	2357	2013	2891	2719	2322	3470	3263	2787
13st 7	2370	2219	1902	2568	2404	2061	2963	2774	2378	3555	3329	2854
14st 0	2427	2262	1947	2630	2451	2109	3034	2828	2434	3641	3394	2920
14st 7	2484	2306	1991	2691	2498	2157	3106	2883	2489	3727	3459	2987
15st 0	2542	2350	2036	2753	2545	2205	3177	2937	2545	3813	3525	3054
15st 7	2599	2393	2080	2815	2593	2253	3248	2992	2600	3898	3590	3120
16st 0	2656	2437	2125	2877	2640	2302	3320	3046	2656	3984	3655	3187
16st 7	2713	2480	2169	2939	2687	2350	3391	3100	2711	4070	3721	3254
17st 0	2770	2524	2213	3001	2734	2398	3463	3155	2767	4155	3786	3320
17st 7	2827	2567	2258	3063	2781	2446	3534	3209	2823	4241	3851	3387
18st 0	2884	2611	2302	3125	2828	2494	3606	3264	2878	4327	3917	3454
18st 7	2942	2654	2347	3187	2876	2542	3677	3318	2934	4413	3982	3520
19st 0	2999	2698	2391	3249	2923	2591	3749	3373	2989	4498	4047	3587
19st 7	3056	2741	2436	3311	2970	2639	3820	3427	3045	4584	4112	3654
20st 0	3113	2785	2480	3373	3017	2687	3891	3481	3100	4670	4178	3721
20st 7	3170	2829	2525	3434	3064	2735	3963	3536	3156	4756	4243	3787
21st 0	3227	2872	2569	3496	3112	2783	4034	3590	3211	4841	4308	3854
21st 7	3285	2916	2614	3558	3159	2831	4106	3645	3267	4927	4374	3921
22st 0	3342	2959	2658	3620	3206	2880	4177	3699	3323	5013	4439	3987
22st 7	3399	3003	2702	3682	3253	2928	4249	3754	3378	5098	4504	4054
23st 0	3456	3046	2747	3744	3300	2976	4320	3808	3434	5184	4570	4121
23st 7	3513	3090	2791	3806	3347	3024	4392	3862	3489	5270	4635	4187
24st 0	3570	3133	2836	3868	3395	3072	4463	3917	3545	5356	4700	4254
24st 7	3627	3177	2880	3930	3442	3120	4534	3971	3600	5441	4766	4321
25st 0	3685	3220	2925	3992	3489	3168	4606	4026	3656	5527	4831	4387
25st 7	3742	3264	2969	4054	3536	3217	4677	4080	3712	5613	4896	4454
26st 0	3799	3308	3014	4116	3583	3265	4749	4135	3767	5699	4962	4521
26st 7	3856	3351	3058	4177	3630	3313	4820	4189	3823	5784	5027	4587
27st 0	3913	3395	3103	4239	3678	3361	4892	4243	3878	5870	5092	4654
27st 7	3970	3438	3147	4301	3725	3409	4963	4298	3934	5956	5158	4721
28st 0	4028	3482	3191	4363	3772	3457	5035	4352	3989	6042	5223	4787
28st 7	4085	3525	3236	4425	3819	3506	5106	4407	4045	6127	5288	4854
29st 0	4142	3569	3280	4487	3866	3554	5177	4461	4101	6213	5354	4921
29st 7	4199	3612	3325	4549	3913	3602	5249	4516	4156	6299	5419	4987
30st 0	4256	3656	3369	4611	3961	3650	5320	4570	4212	6384	5484	5054

CALORIES REQUIRED TO MAINTAIN WEIGHT
ADULT FEMALES

AGE / ACTIVITY LEVEL

WEIGHT IN STONES / LBS	VERY SEDENTARY			MODERATELY SEDENTARY			MODERATELY ACTIVE			VERY ACTIVE		
	<30	30-60	60+	<30	30-60	60+	<30	30-60	60+	<30	30-60	60+
7st 7	1425	1473	1304	1544	1596	1412	1781	1841	1630	2138	2210	1956
8st 0	1481	1504	1338	1605	1629	1450	1852	1880	1673	2222	2256	2008
8st 7	1537	1535	1373	1666	1663	1487	1922	1919	1716	2306	2302	2059
9st 0	1594	1566	1407	1726	1696	1524	1992	1957	1759	2391	2349	2111
9st 7	1650	1596	1442	1787	1729	1562	2062	1996	1802	2475	2395	2163
10st 0	1706	1627	1476	1848	1763	1599	2133	2034	1845	2559	2441	2214
10st 7	1762	1658	1511	1909	1796	1637	2203	2073	1888	2644	2487	2266
11st 0	1819	1689	1545	1970	1830	1674	2273	2111	1931	2728	2534	2318
11st 7	1875	1720	1580	2031	1863	1711	2344	2150	1975	2813	2580	2370
12st 0	1931	1751	1614	2092	1897	1749	2414	2188	2018	2897	2626	2421
12st 7	1987	1781	1648	2153	1930	1786	2484	2227	2061	2981	2672	2473
13st 0	2044	1812	1683	2214	1963	1823	2555	2266	2104	3066	2719	2525
13st 7	2100	1843	1717	2275	1997	1861	2625	2304	2147	3150	2765	2576
14st 0	2156	1874	1752	2336	2030	1898	2695	2343	2190	3234	2811	2628
14st 7	2212	1905	1786	2397	2064	1935	2766	2381	2233	3319	2858	2680
15st 0	2269	1936	1821	2458	2097	1973	2836	2420	2276	3403	2904	2732
15st 7	2325	1967	1855	2519	2130	2010	2906	2458	2319	3488	2950	2783
16st 0	2381	1997	1890	2580	2164	2047	2976	2497	2362	3572	2996	2835
16st 7	2437	2028	1924	2640	2197	2085	3047	2535	2405	3656	3043	2887
17st 0	2494	2059	1959	2701	2231	2122	3117	2574	2449	3741	3089	2938
17st 7	2550	2090	1993	2762	2264	2159	3187	2613	2492	3825	3135	2990
18st 0	2606	2121	2028	2823	2298	2197	3258	2651	2535	3909	3181	3042
18st 7	2662	2152	2062	2884	2331	2234	3328	2690	2578	3994	3228	3093
19st 0	2719	2182	2097	2945	2364	2271	3398	2728	2621	4078	3274	3145
19st 7	2775	2213	2131	3006	2398	2309	3469	2767	2664	4162	3320	3197
20st 0	2831	2244	2166	3067	2431	2346	3539	2805	2707	4247	3366	3249
20st 7	2887	2275	2200	3128	2465	2383	3609	2844	2750	4331	3413	3300
21st 0	2944	2306	2235	3189	2498	2421	3680	2882	2793	4416	3459	3352
21st 7	3000	2337	2269	3250	2531	2458	3750	2921	2836	4500	3505	3404
22st 0	3056	2368	2303	3311	2565	2495	3820	2960	2879	4584	3552	3455
22st 7	3112	2398	2338	3372	2598	2533	3890	2998	2923	4669	3598	3507
23st 0	3169	2429	2372	3433	2632	2570	3961	3037	2966	4753	3644	3559
23st 7	3225	2460	2407	3494	2665	2608	4031	3075	3009	4837	3690	3611
24st 0	3281	2491	2441	3554	2699	2645	4101	3114	3052	4922	3737	3662
24st 7	3337	2522	2476	3615	2732	2682	4172	3152	3095	5006	3783	3714
25st 0	3394	2553	2510	3676	2765	2720	4242	3191	3138	5091	3829	3766
25st 7	3450	2583	2545	3737	2799	2757	4312	3229	3181	5175	3875	3817
26st 0	3506	2614	2579	3798	2832	2794	4383	3268	3224	5259	3922	3869
26st 7	3562	2645	2614	3859	2866	2832	4453	3307	3267	5344	3968	3921
27st 0	3618	2676	2648	3920	2899	2869	4523	3345	3310	5428	4014	3973
27st 7	3675	2707	2683	3981	2932	2906	4594	3384	3353	5512	4060	4024
28st 0	3731	2738	2717	4042	2966	2944	4664	3422	3397	5597	4107	4076
28st 7	3787	2768	2752	4103	2999	2981	4734	3461	3440	5681	4153	4128

Calories Burned in Exercise

This table shows the approximate number of extra* calories that would be burned in a five minute period of exercise activity.

Activity	Calories Burned in 5 Minutes
Aerobics, Low Impact	25
Badminton, Recreational	17
Cross Trainer	30
Cycling, Recreational, 5mph	17
Dancing, Modern, Moderate	13
Fencing	24
Gardening, Weeding	19
Hill Walking, Up and Down, Recreational	22
Jogging	30
Kick Boxing	30
Netball Playing	23
Rebounding	18
Roller Skating	30
Rowing Machine, Moderate	30
Running, 7.5mph	48
Situps, Continuous	17
Skiing, Moderate	30
Skipping, Moderate	30
Squash Playing	39
Tennis Playing, Recreational	26
Toning Exercises	17
Trampolining	17
Volleyball, Recreational	10
Walking, Uphill, 15% Gradient, Moderate	43
Walking Up and Down Stairs, Moderate	34
Walking, 4mph	24
Weight Training, Moderate	12
Yoga	13

*Extra calories are those in addition to your normal daily calorie needs.

Food and Exercise Diary

DATE:

[/ /]

DAILY CALORIE ALLOWANCE [   ] **A**

FOOD/DRINK CONSUMED	SERVING SIZE	CALORIES

TOTAL CALORIES CONSUMED [   ] **B**

EXERCISE/ACTIVITY	NO. MINS	CALORIES

CALORIES USED IN EXERCISE [   ] **C**

CALORIE BALANCE [   ] **D**

You are aiming for your Calorie Balance (Box D) to be as close to zero as possible - ie. you consume the number of calories you need.

Your Daily Calorie Allowance (Box A) should be set to lose 1-2lb a week, or maintain weight, depending on your goals.

Daily Calorie Allowance (A) *plus* Extra Calories used in Exercise (C) *minus* Total Calories Consumed (B) *equals* Calorie Balance (D)

$A + C - B = D$

Food Information

Nutritional Information

Calorie values are given per serving, plus calorie and nutrition values per 100g of product. This makes it easy to compare the proportions of fat, protein, carbohydrate and fibre in each food.

The values given are for uncooked, unprepared foods unless otherwise stated.

Finding Foods

The Calorie, Carb & Fat Bible has a new, improved format for this edition. Most foods are grouped together by type, and then put in to alphabetical order. This makes it easy to compare different brands, and will help you to find lower calorie and/or fat alternatives where they are available.

This format also makes it easier to locate foods. Foods are categorised by their main characteristics so, for example, if it is bread, ciabatta or white sliced, you'll find it under "Bread".

There are, however, some foods which are not so easy to categorise, especially combination foods like ready meals. The following pointers will help you to find your way around the book until you get to know it a little better.

FILLED ROLLS AND SANDWICHES - Bagels, baguettes, etc which are filled are listed as "Bagels (filled)" etc. Sandwiches are under "Sandwiches".

Serving sizes vary greatly from person to person...it's very important to be accurate.

CURRIES - Popular types of curry, like Balti or Jalfrezi, are listed under their individual types. Unspecified or lesser known types are listed under their main ingredient.

BURGERS - All burgers, including chicken-type sandwiches from fast-food outlets, are listed under "Burgers".

CHIPS & FRIES - Are listed seperately, depending on the name of the particular brand. All other types of potato are listed under "Potatoes".

SWEETS & CHOCOLATES - Well-known brands, eg. Aero, Mars Bar, are listed under their brand names. Others are listed under "Chocolate" (for bars) and "Chocolates" (for individual sweets).

READY MEALS - Popular types of dishes are listed under their type, eg. "Chow Mein", "Casserole", "Hot Pot", etc. Others are listed by their main ingredient, eg. "Cicken With", "Chicken In", etc.

Serving Sizes

Many ready-meal type foods are given with calories for the full pack size, so that an individual serving can be worked out by estimating the proportion of the pack that has been consumed. For example, if you have eaten a quarter of a packaged pasta dish, divide the calorie value given for the whole pack by 4 to determine the number of calories you have consumed. Where serving sizes are not appropriate, or unknown, values are given per 1oz/28g. Serving sizes vary greatly from person to person and, if you are trying to lose weight, it's very important to be accurate – especially with foods that are very high in calories such as those that contain a fair amount of fat, sugar, cream, cheese, alcohol etc.

Food Data

Nutrition information for basic (non-branded) foods is from The Composition of Foods 5th Edition (1991) Reproduced under licence from the Controller of Her Majesty's Stationery Office.

Nutrition information for branded goods is from details supplied by retailers and manufacturers, and researched by Weight Loss Resources staff from packaging information. Calorie and nutrition data for all food and drink items are typical values.

The publishers gratefully acknowledge all the manufacturers and retailers who have provided information on their products. All product names, trademarks or registered trademarks belong to their respective owners and are used only for the purpose of identifying products.

Caution

The information in The Calorie, Carb and Fat Bible is intended as an aid to weight loss and weight maintenance, and is not medical advice. If you suffer from, or think you may suffer from a medical condition you should consult your doctor before starting a weight loss and/or exercise regime, If you start exercising after a period of relative inactivity, you should start slowly and consult your doctor if you experience pain, distress or other symptons.

Abbreviations

kcal	kilocalories / calories
prot	protein
carb	carbohydrate
sm	small
med	medium
lge	large

tsp	teaspoon
tbsp	tablespoon
dtsp	desertspoon

Brand Abbreviations

Asda
Good for You .... GFY
SmartPrice .... SP
Healthy Choice .... HC

Marks & Spencer .... M&S
Count on Us .... COU
Steam Cuisine .... SC
Food to Go .... FTG

Morrisons
Better For You .... BFY

Safeway
Eat Smart .... ES
Healthy Choice .... HC

Sainsbury's
Be Good to Yourself .... BGTY
Way to Five .... WTF
Taste the Difference .... TTD
Blue Parrot Cafe .... BPC

Somerfield
Good Intentions .... GI
So Good .... SG
Healthy Selection .... HS

Tesco
Healthy Eating .... HE
Healthy Living .... HL

Waitrose
Perfectly Balanced .... PB
Food Explorers .... FE

McVities
Go Ahead .... GA

Northern Bites
Calorie Conscious CC

New Covent Garden Soup Co.
New Covent Garden Soup
Company .... NCGSC

	Measure INFO/WEIGHT	per Measure KCAL	Nutrition Values per 100g / 100ml				
			KCAL	PROT	CARB	FAT	FIBRE
ACKEE,							
Canned, Drained	1oz/28g	42	151	2.9	0.8	15.2	0.0
ADVOCAAT, Average	1 Shot/25ml	65	260	4.7	28.4	6.3	0.0
AERO,							
Creamy White Centre, Nestle	1 Bar/46g	244	530	7.6	57.4	30.0	0.0
Honeycomb, Nestle*	1 Serving/40g	199	497	5.9	62.2	25.0	0.0
Minis, Nestle*	1 Bar/11g	57	518	7.6	57.2	28.8	0.0
Mint, Nestle*	1 Bar/48g	252	526	6.5	60.2	28.8	0.0
Nestle*	1 Bar/46g	238	518	7.6	57.2	28.8	0.0
ALCOPOPS, (Calculated Estimate)	1fl oz/30ml	22	73	0.3	5.0	0.0	0.0
ALFALFA SPROUTS, Raw	1oz/28g	7	24	4.0	0.4	0.7	1.7
ALLSPICE, Powder	1 Tsp/3g	8	263	6.1	50.5	8.7	0.0
ALMONDS,							
Average	6 Whole/10g	61	612	21.1	6.9	55.8	7.4
Blanched, Waitrose*	1 Pack/100g	588	588	24.9	7.3	51.0	10.0
Flaked, Tesco*	1 Tbsp/7g	43	614	21.1	6.9	55.8	7.4
Ground, Nature's Harvest, Holland & Barrett*	1oz/28g	176	630	25.4	6.5	55.8	7.4
Ground, Sainsbury's*	1 Tbsp/20g	123	614	25.4	2.6	55.8	7.4
Ground, Tesco*	1 Serving/10g	61	614	21.1	6.9	55.8	7.4
Nature's Haverst*	5 Nuts/10g	63	630	25.4	5.5	55.8	7.4
Organic Shelled, Waitrose*	1oz/28g	176	630	25.4	6.5	55.8	7.4
Roasted, Sweet Smoke, KP*	1oz/28g	172	616	24.7	8.8	53.6	7.1
Sainsbury's*	1 Nut/1g	6	612	21.1	6.9	55.8	7.4
Smoked, Sainsbury's*	1 Serving/40g	264	660	26.0	9.0	57.8	7.5
Toasted, Flaked, Morrisons*	1 Serving/10g	65	652	25.2	4.4	59.3	6.1
Whole Blanched, Asda*	1 Serving/25g	158	632	25.0	7.0	56.0	7.0
Whole, Organic, Crazy Jack*	1 Portion/20g	115	573	25.0	19.0	50.0	13.0
Whole, Organic, Evernat*	1oz/28g	172	614	21.1	6.9	55.8	7.4
Yoghurt Coated, Holland & Barrett*	1 Pack/100g	536	536	10.9	45.3	37.0	2.8
ALOO TIKKI, Mini, Indian Snack Selection, Sainsbury's*	1 Tikki/17.9g	34	190	4.4	27.6	6.9	3.2
ALOO WADA, Mini, Indian Snack Selection, Sainsbury's*	1 Wada/19.6g	36	179	5.9	27.9	4.9	3.4
ALPHABITES, Bird's Eye*	9 Bites/56g	75	134	2.0	19.5	5.3	1.4
ANCHOVIES,							
Canned in Oil, Drained	1 Anchovy/3g	8	280	25.2	0.0	19.9	0.0
Fillets, Flat, John West*	1 Can/50g	113	226	25.0	0.1	14.0	0.0
Fillets, Marinated, Waitrose*	1 Serving/5g	9	177	22.0	2.0	9.0	0.0
In Olive Oil, John West*	1oz/28g	63	226	25.0	0.0	14.0	0.0
In Olive Oil, Sainsbury's*	1 Serving/10g	19	185	23.7	0.1	10.0	0.1
Salted, Finest, Tesco*	1 Serving/10g	9	93	18.2	0.0	2.2	0.0
ANGEL DELIGHT,							
Banana Flavour, Kraft*	1 Sachet/59g	289	490	2.5	72.0	21.0	0.0
Banana Toffee Flavour, No Added Sugar, Kraft*	1 Sachet/59g	292	495	4.8	58.5	26.5	0.0
Butterscotch Flavour, Kraft*	1 Sachet/59g	280	475	2.4	73.5	19.0	0.0
Chocolate Flavour With Topples, Kraft*	1 Sachet/59g	274	465	5.0	67.0	20.0	0.5
Chocolate Flavour, Kraft*	1 Sachet/59g	268	455	3.7	69.5	18.0	0.4
Chocolate Flavour, No Added Sugar, Kraft*	1 Sachet/59g	266	450	6.3	56.5	22.0	0.0
Forest Fruit Flavour, Kraft*	1 Sachet/59g	289	490	2.5	71.5	21.5	0.0
Raspberry Flavour, Kraft*	1 Sachet/59g	289	490	2.5	72.0	21.0	0.0
Raspberry Flavour, No Added Sugar, Kraft*	1 Sachet/59g	292	495	4.8	59.5	26.0	0.0
Strawberry Flavour With Topples, Kraft*	1 Sachet/59g	266	450	2.8	74.5	14.0	0.0
Strawberry Flavour, Kraft*	1 Sachet/59g	286	485	2.5	71.0	21.0	0.0
Strawberry Flavour, No Added Sugar, Kraft*	1 Sachet/59g	289	490	4.8	59.0	26.5	0.0
Tangerine Flavour, No Added Sugar, Kraft*	1 Sachet/59g	292	495	4.8	58.0	27.0	0.9
Toffee Flavour, Kraft*	1 Sachet/59g	283	480	2.6	70.0	21.0	0.0

A

INFO/WEIGHT	Measure	per Measure KCAL	Nutrition Values per 100g / 100ml				
			KCAL	PROT	CARB	FAT	FIBRE
ANGEL DELIGHT,							
Vanilla Ice Cream Flavour, Kraft*	1 Sachet/59g	289	490	2.5	71.5	21.5	0.0
Vanilla Ice Cream Flavour, No Added Sugar, Kraft*	1 Sachet/59g	295	500	4.8	59.5	27.0	0.0
ANGEL HAIR, Pasta, Sainsbury's*	1 Serving/100g	357	357	12.3	73.1	1.7	2.5
ANTIPASTO,							
Artichoke, Sainsbury's*	1 Serving/50g	68	135	2.0	3.6	12.5	2.3
Mixed Mushroom, Sainsbury's*	¼ Jar/72g	70	97	2.7	1.4	9.0	3.7
Mixed Pepper, Sainsbury's*	½ Jar/145g	183	126	1.5	11.0	8.4	1.8
Seafood, Drained, Sainsbury's*	½ Jar/84g	150	178	14.3	4.1	11.6	1.4
Sun Dried Tomato, Sainsbury's*	1 Tomato/5g	12	232	4.7	15.5	16.8	6.6
Wild Mushroom, Sainsbury's*	1 Serving/100g	97	97	2.7	1.4	9.0	3.7
APPLE &,							
Blackcurrant Juice Drink, No Added Sugar, Asda*	1 Glass/250ml	13	5	0.0	1.0	0.0	0.0
Blackcurrant Juice Drink, With Sweeteners, Aldi*	1 Glass/200ml	5	2	0.0	0.2	0.0	0.0
Cranberry Juice, Copella*	1 Glass/250ml	113	45	0.2	9.2	0.0	0.0
Elderflower Juice, Copella*	1 Glass/250ml	108	43	0.4	10.2	0.1	0.0
Grape, Snack, Blue Parrot Cafe, Sainsbury's*	1 Pack/80g	42	53	0.4	12.5	0.1	2.1
Mango, Juice, Pressed, Tesco*	1 Glass/200ml	102	51	0.3	12.0	0.0	0.1
Mango Juice, Marks & Spencer*	1 Bottle/250ml	138	55	0.3	13.0	0.0	0.0
Mango Juice, Pressed, Marks & Spencer*	1 Bottle/250ml	138	55	0.3	13.0	0.0	0.3
Mango Juice, Sainsbury's*	1 Glass/200ml	108	54	0.3	12.6	0.1	0.1
Raspberry Juice, Pressed, Safeway*	1 Glass/200ml	96	48	0.4	10.9	0.0	0.3
Strawberry Juice, 100% Pure, BPC, Sainsbury's*	1 Glass/200ml	82	41	0.3	9.4	0.1	0.2
APPLE JUICE,							
Chilled, Asda*	1 Glass/200ml	98	49	0.1	12.0	0.0	0.0
Copella*	1 Glass/250ml	110	44	0.4	10.3	0.1	0.0
Del Monte*	1 Carton/200ml	94	47	0.3	10.8	0.0	0.0
English Cox, Marks & Spencer*	1 Glass/200ml	98	49	0.2	11.6	0.0	0.0
English, Somerfield*	1 Glass/200ml	188	94	0.0	23.0	0.0	0.0
Freshly Pressed, Copella*	1 Glass/200ml	88	44	0.4	10.3	0.1	0.0
Freshly pressed, Johnsons*	1 Glass/250ml	120	48	0.1	11.8	0.0	0.0
Lightly Sparkling, Organic, Sainsbury's*	1 Can/330ml	155	47	0.1	10.7	0.1	0.1
Marks & Spencer*	1 Bottle/250ml	130	52	0.2	12.2	0.0	0.0
Organic, Evernat*	1 Glass/200ml	92	46	0.0	11.0	0.1	0.2
Organic, Marks & Spencer*	1 Carton/250ml	100	40	0.5	8.9	0.1	0.1
Organic, Tesco*	1 Glass/250ml	118	47	0.0	11.3	0.0	0.0
Pressed Cloudy, Tesco*	1 Glass/220ml	110	50	0.3	11.7	0.0	0.0
Pressed, 100%, Sainsbury's*	1 Bottle/250ml	120	48	0.2	11.7	0.1	0.3
Pressed, Marks & Spencer*	1 Carton/250ml	113	45	0.3	10.5	0.0	0.1
Pressed, Sainsbury's*	1 Glass/200ml	100	50	0.2	11.8	0.1	0.2
Pure, Boots*	1 Carton/250ml	120	48	0.1	12.0	0.0	0.0
Pure, Princes*	1 Sm Glass/150ml	66	44	0.1	10.4	0.1	0.0
Pure, Sainsbury's*	1 Glass/200ml	90	45	0.1	11.0	0.1	0.1
Pure, SmartPrice, Asda*	1 Glass/200ml	88	44	0.1	10.0	0.1	0.0
Pure, Somerfield*	1 Glass/200ml	94	47	0.0	12.0	0.0	0.0
Pure, Sunpride*	1 Carton/200ml	88	44	0.1	10.2	0.0	0.0
Pure, Tesco*	1 Glass/200ml	94	47	0.1	11.1	0.0	0.0
Pure, Waitrose*	1 Glass/200ml	92	46	0.1	11.0	0.0	0.0
Sparkling, Somerfield*	1 Glass/200ml	112	56	0.0	14.0	0.0	0.0
Value, Tesco*	1 Glass/200ml	86	43	0.1	10.4	0.0	0.0
With Mango Puree, Safeway*	1 Glass/150ml	80	53	0.3	12.6	0.0	0.0
APPLE JUICE DRINK,							
Healthy Eating, Tesco*	1 Glass/100ml	30	30	0.1	7.0	0.1	0.0
No Added Sugar, Asda*	1 Glass/200ml	10	5	0.0	1.0	0.0	0.0

INFO/WEIGHT	per Measure KCAL	KCAL	PROT	CARB	FAT	FIBRE
APPLES,						
Bites, Fresh, Sainsbury's*	1 Pack/118g	58	49	0.3	11.6	0.1	1.8
Braeburn, Fresh, Sainsbury's*	1 Apple/100g	49	49	0.4	11.6	0.1	1.8
Braeburn, Safeway*	1 Serving/100g	49	49	0.4	11.6	0.1	1.8
Braeburn, Tesco*	1 Apple/65g	30	46	0.3	10.8	0.2	1.7
Cooking, Baked With Sugar, Flesh Only	1 Serving/140g	109	78	0.5	20.1	0.1	1.7
Cooking, Raw, Peeled	1oz/28g	10	35	0.3	8.9	0.1	1.6
Cooking, Stewed With Sugar	1 Serving/140g	104	74	0.3	19.1	0.1	1.2
Cooking, Stewed Without Sugar	1 Serving/140g	46	33	0.3	8.1	0.1	1.5
Cooking, Weighed With Skin & Core	1oz/28g	7	26	0.2	6.4	0.1	1.1
Cox, Waitrose*	1 Pack/200g	100	50	0.4	11.8	0.1	2.7
Dessert, Organic, Tesco*	1 Apple/150g	81	54	0.3	13.0	0.1	1.9
Eating, Average, Raw	1 Med Apple/112g	53	47	0.4	11.8	0.1	1.8
Eating, Average, Raw, Peeled	1 Med Apple/102g	46	45	0.4	11.2	0.1	1.6
Eating, Dried	1oz/28g	67	238	2.0	60.1	0.5	9.7
Empire, Tesco*	1 Apple/100g	50	50	0.4	11.8	0.1	1.8
English Cox, Sainsbury's*	1 Apple/108g	53	49	0.4	11.6	0.1	1.8
Gala, Organic, Tesco*	1 Apple/152g	70	46	0.3	10.8	0.2	1.7
Gala, Safeway*	1 Apple/100g	49	49	0.4	11.6	0.1	1.8
Gala, Tesco*	1 Med Apple/115g	58	50	0.3	11.5	0.1	1.7
Golden Delicious, Sainsbury's*	1 Apple/100g	49	49	0.4	11.6	0.1	1.8
Golden Delicious, Tesco*	1 Apple/100g	46	46	0.3	10.8	0.2	1.7
Granny Smith, Sainsbury's*	1 Med Apple/130g	64	49	0.4	11.6	0.1	1.8
Granny Smith, Tesco*	1 Sm Apple/75g	36	48	0.3	11.5	0.1	1.7
Granny Smith, Waitrose*	1 Apple/125g	63	50	0.4	11.8	0.1	2.7
Pink Lady, Sainsbury's*	1 Apple/125g	61	49	0.4	11.6	0.1	1.8
Royal Gala, Organic, Waitrose*	1 Apple/125g	63	50	0.4	11.8	0.1	0.0
Royal Gala, Sainsbury's*	1 Med Apple/140g	69	49	0.4	11.6	0.1	1.8
Rubinette, Tesco*	1 Apple/123g	62	50	0.4	11.8	0.1	1.8
Slices, Canned, Asda*	1 Can/200g	78	39	0.7	9.0	0.0	2.5
Slices, John West*	1oz/28g	6	21	0.1	5.0	0.0	1.4
Slices, Sainsbury's*	1 Bag/120g	59	49	0.3	11.6	0.1	1.8
Small & Sweet, Garden Gang, Asda*	1oz/28g	15	55	0.4	12.0	0.1	1.8
Stewed, Sainsbury's*	¼ Can/100g	71	71	0.2	17.4	0.0	1.2
Wedges, Shapers, Boots*	1 Pack/120g	59	49	0.3	11.7	0.1	1.8
APPLETISE, Schweppes*	1 Glass/200ml	98	49	0.0	11.8	0.0	0.0
APRICOTS,						
Breakfast, Sainsbury's*	½ Can/149.0g	152	102	0.5	24.0	0.4	107.0
Canned, In Juice	1oz/28g	10	34	0.5	8.4	0.1	0.9
Canned, In Syrup	1oz/28g	18	63	0.4	16.1	0.1	0.9
Dried	1oz/28g	53	188	4.8	43.4	0.7	7.7
Dried Fruits, Ready to Eat, Sainsbury's*	1 Serving/75g	124	165	3.9	36.0	0.6	6.3
Dried, Garden Gang, Asda*	1 Pack/50g	74	147	3.4	31.0	0.5	5.0
Dried, Nature's Harvest*	4 Apricots/25g	40	158	4.0	36.6	0.6	6.3
Dried, Organic, Crazy Jack*	1 Serving/100g	180	180	4.4	40.0	0.6	0.0
Dried, Organic, Waitrose*	1oz/28g	50	179	4.3	39.1	0.6	6.9
Dried, Ready To Eat, Tesco*	1 Serving/28g	47	167	4.0	36.5	0.6	6.3
Dried, Ready To Eat, Whitworth's*	1 Pack/87g	144	165	3.9	36.0	0.6	6.3
Dried, Ready to Eat, Asda*	1 Serving/25g	36	142	3.4	31.0	0.3	5.0
Dried, Safeway*	1 Pack/250g	518	207	2.2	48.7	0.4	6.3
Dried, Shapers, Boots*	1 Pack/50g	83	165	3.9	36.0	0.6	6.3
Dried, Sundora*	1 Serving/50g	83	165	3.9	36.0	0.6	6.3
Dried, Vanilla, Ready to Eat Fruit, Sainsbury's*	1/3 Pack/85g	131	154	2.4	40.3	0.1	4.9
Dried, Waitrose*	½ Pack/125g	209	167	4.0	36.5	0.6	6.3

A

A

INFO/WEIGHT	Measure	per Measure KCAL	Nutrition Values per 100g / 100ml				
			KCAL	PROT	CARB	FAT	FIBRE
APRICOTS,							
Garland Tangy, Tesco*	1 Serving/50g	100	199	4.8	43.4	0.7	7.7
Halves in Fruit Juice, Waitrose*	1 Sm Can/221g	75	34	0.5	8.0	0.0	0.9
Halves, Healthy Choice, Asda*	1 Can/411g	140	34	0.5	8.0	0.0	0.9
Halves, In Fresh Juice, Sainsbury's*	½ Can/120g	49	41	0.5	9.4	0.1	1.2
Halves, In Fruit Juice, Sainsbury's*	½ Can/206g	103	50	0.4	11.5	0.1	1.2
Halves, In Grape Juice, Tesco*	1oz/28g	13	46	0.5	10.0	0.1	0.9
In Fruit Juice, John West*	1oz/28g	11	38	0.5	9.0	0.0	1.0
Raw, Fresh	1 Med Apricot/40g	12	31	0.9	7.2	0.1	1.7
Raw, Safeway*	1 Fruit/125g	51	41	1.4	8.6	0.1	1.2
Raw, Weighed With Stones	1 Apricot/40g	12	29	0.8	6.6	0.1	1.6
Soft Dried, Blue Parrot Cafe, Sainsbury's*	1 Sm Pack/50g	111	222	3.5	51.2	0.4	8.7
Soft, Snack Pack, Marks & Spencer*	1 Pack/50g	108	215	1.8	51.3	0.2	3.9
ARCHERS*,							
Peach Aqua, Schnapps, Archers (Calculated Estimate)	1 Bottle/275ml	206	75	0.3	5.1	0.0	0.0
Peach Snapps, (Calculated Estimate)	1 Shot/35ml	91	260	0.0	0.0	0.0	0.0
ARTICHOKE,							
Hearts, Chargrilled in Olive Oil, TTD, Sainsbury's*	¼ Jar/73g	150	205	1.0	3.4	20.8	0.0
Hearts, Drained, Sainsbury's*	½ Can/117g	34	29	2.0	4.9	0.1	2.3
Hearts, In Brine, Tesco*	1 Serving/70g	22	31	1.8	6.0	0.0	2.0
Hearts, Marinated & Grilled, Waitrose*	1 Serving/50g	57	114	3.0	3.0	10.0	3.0
Raw, Fresh	1oz/28g	13	47	3.3	10.5	0.2	5.4
ASPARAGUS,							
Boiled in Salted Water	5 Spears/125g	33	26	3.4	1.4	0.8	1.4
Canned, Re-Heated, Drained	1oz/28g	7	24	3.4	1.5	0.5	2.9
Raw, Fresh	1oz/28g	7	25	2.9	2.0	0.6	1.7
Spears, Asda*	1 Serving/100g	26	26	3.4	1.4	0.8	2.0
Spears, Green Giant*	1 Can/250g	40	16	2.1	2.0	0.0	1.2
Tips, Tesco*	1 Serving/100g	25	25	2.9	2.0	0.6	1.7
AUBERGINE,							
Baked Topped, Marks & Spencer*	1 Serving/150g	165	110	2.4	7.4	7.7	0.9
Fried in Blended Oil	1oz/28g	85	302	1.2	2.8	31.9	2.3
Fried in Butter	1oz/28g	85	302	1.2	2.8	31.9	2.3
Marinated & Grilled, Waitrose*	½ Pack/100g	106	106	1.0	3.0	10.0	2.0
Parmigiana, Marks & Spencer*	1 Pack/350g	333	95	4.6	7.6	5.3	1.1
Raw, Fresh	1 Sm/120g	18	15	0.9	2.2	0.4	2.0
AUTHENTIC MIX,							
Bacon & Mushroom Taglietelle, Schwartz*	1 Pack/33g	115	349	8.1	77.5	0.7	0.0
Bombay Potatoes, Schwartz*	1 Pack/33g	110	332	15.3	61.7	2.7	0.2
Cajun Chicken, Schwartz*	1 Pack/38g	112	294	6.6	61.5	2.4	0.0
Chicken & White Wine, Schwartz*	½ Pack/35g	113	322	10.3	65.2	2.2	0.3
Chicken Balti, Schwartz*	1oz/28g	91	324	13.5	54.4	5.8	0.0
Chilli Con Carne, Schwartz*	1 Pack/40.9g	126	308	8.2	64.6	1.9	0.5
Creamy Tikka Masala, Schwartz*	1oz/28g	97	346	13.7	63.6	4.1	0.2
For Spagetti Bolognese, Schwartz*	1 Pack/40g	122	306	10.5	63.0	1.3	0.0
For Spaghetti Carbonara, Schwartz*	½ Pack/16g	70	436	9.5	56.0	19.3	0.3
Hot Chili Con Carne, Schwartz*	1 Pack/41g	126	308	10.6	61.8	0.8	0.2
Lamb Casserole, Schwartz*	1 Pack/35g	116	332	7.7	68.0	3.3	1.3
Lasagne, Schwartz*	1 Pack/36g	113	313	6.6	70.1	0.7	0.3
Mexican Chili Chicken, Schwartz*	1 Pack/35g	113	322	8.8	64.2	3.3	0.4
Thai Lemon Chicken, Schwartz*	1 Serving/10g	37	365	3.6	78.3	4.2	0.0
Thai Red Curry, Schwartz*	1 Serving/20g	70	349	5.7	70.2	5.0	0.7
Tuna Napolitana, Schwartz*	1 Serving/30g	107	357	10.3	49.7	13.0	0.3
AVOCADO, Average	1 Med /145g	276	190	1.9	1.9	19.5	3.4

	Measure	per Measure		Nutrition Values per 100g / 100ml			
	INFO/WEIGHT	KCAL	KCAL	PROT	CARB	FAT	FIBRE
BACARDI,							
37.5% Volume	1 Shot/25ml	52	207	0.0	0.0	0.0	0.0
Breezer (Calculated Estimate)	1 Bottle/275ml	198	72	0.3	5.0	0.0	0.0
BACON,							
Back, Dry-Cured, Grilled	1 Rasher/25g	64	257	28.4	0.0	15.9	0.0
Back, Dry-Fried	1 Rasher/25g	74	295	24.2	0.0	22.0	0.0
Back, Drycure, Asda*	1 Rasher/32g	61	192	19.7	0.8	12.2	0.0
Back, Extra Trim, Balanced Lifestyle, Aldi*	1 Rasher/33g	53	160	17.4	0.2	10.0	1.0
Back, Fat Trimmed, Grilled	1 Rasher/23g	49	214	25.7	0.0	12.3	0.0
Back, Fat Trimmed, Raw	1 Rasher/28g	38	136	18.8	0.0	6.7	0.0
Back, Grilled	1 Rasher/25g	72	287	23.2	0.0	21.6	0.0
Back, Grilled Crispy	1 Rasher/25g	78	313	36.0	0.0	18.8	0.0
Back, Lean & Fat, Fried	1 Rasher/25g	116	465	24.9	0.0	40.6	0.0
Back, Microwaved	1 Rasher/25g	77	307	24.2	0.0	23.3	0.0
Back, Rapid Rasher, Danepak*	1 Rasher/19g	51	268	24.0	2.3	18.1	0.0
Back, Rashers, Danepack*	1 Rasher/25g	61	242	15.5	0.0	20.0	0.0
Back, Raw	1 Rasher/26g	56	215	16.5	0.0	16.5	0.0
Back, Reduced Salt, Grilled	1 Rasher/25g	71	282	24.1	0.0	20.6	0.0
Back, Rindless, No Fat	1 Rasher/30g	73	243	18.4	0.0	17.8	0.0
Back, Smoked Back, Rindless, Co-Op*	1 Rasher/30g	75	250	18.0	0.0	20.0	0.0
Back, Smoked British, Rindless, Waitrose*	1 Rasher/29g	59	203	17.0	0.0	15.0	0.0
Back, Smoked Medallion, Sainsbury's*	2 Rashers/28g	40	143	29.9	0.0	2.2	0.0
Back, Smoked, Dry Cure, TTD, Sainsbury's*	1 Rasher/54g	144	267	31.8	0.1	15.5	0.1
Back, Smoked, Grilled	1 Rasher/25g	73	293	23.4	0.0	22.1	0.0
Back, Smoked, Maple Cure, TTD, Sainsbury's*	1 Rasher/31g	70	225	24.0	0.8	14.0	0.7
Back, Smoked, Rindless, Asda*	1 Slice/28g	77	275	23.0	0.7	20.0	0.0
Back, Smoked, Rindless, Rouch Foods*	1 Rasher/37.5g	92	243	18.4	0.0	17.8	0.0
Back, Smoked, Rindless, Somerfield*	1 Rasher/30g	74	246	31.0	0.0	14.0	0.0
Back, Smoked, Sainsbury's*	1 Rasher/30g	85	282	26.3	0.1	19.6	0.1
Back, Sweetcure, Grilled	1 Rasher/25g	65	258	23.8	1.6	17.4	0.0
Back, Tendersweet, Grilled	1 Rasher/25g	53	213	26.4	0.0	11.9	0.0
Back, Unsmoked, Asda*	1 Serving/100g	317	317	25.0	0.3	24.0	0.0
Back, Unsmoked, Co-Op*	3 Rashers/50g	80	160	17.0	0.0	10.0	0.0
Back, Unsmoked, Danepak*	1 Rasher/25g	61	242	15.5	0.0	20.0	0.0
Back, Unsmoked, Danish, Sainsbury's*	1 Rasher/17g	43	255	25.9	0.0	16.8	0.0
Back, Unsmoked, Extra Trimmed, Asda*	1 Rasher/27g	67	248	26.0	0.0	16.0	0.0
Back, Unsmoked, Good for You, Asda*	1 Av Rasher/28g	30	107	21.0	0.0	2.5	0.0
Back, Unsmoked, Rindless, Co-Op*	1 Rasher/50g	108	215	17.0	0.0	17.0	0.0
Back, Unsmoked, Rindless, Grilled, Asda*	1 Rasher/38g	108	284	26.0	0.0	20.0	0.0
Back, Unsmoked, Rindless, Plumrose*	1 Rasher/33g	80	242	15.5	0.0	20.0	0.0
Back, Unsmoked, Rindless, Somerfield*	1 Rasher/30g	74	246	31.0	0.0	14.0	0.0
Back, Unsmoked, Rindless, Waitrose*	1 Rasher/25g	62	246	23.6	0.0	17.0	0.0
Back, Unsmoked, Sainsbury's*	1 Rasher/20g	56	282	26.3	0.1	19.6	0.1
Back, Unsmoked, Tendersweet, TTD, Sainsbury's*	1 Rasher/21g	60	288	33.2	0.9	16.8	0.1
Back, Unsmoked, Reduced Salt, Rindless, Tesco*	1 Serving/113g	220	195	17.2	0.0	14.0	0.0
Chops, BBQ Sainsbury's*	1 Chop/78g	184	236	21.2	4.6	14.8	0.1
Chops, Marks & Spencer*	1 Chop/103g	232	225	15.9	0.0	18.0	0.0
Chops, Reduced Salt, Somerfield*	1 Chop/68g	165	243	22.2	0.0	17.1	0.0
Chops, Smoked, Asda*	1oz/28g	56	199	28.7	0.0	9.4	0.0
Chops, in Cheese Sauce, Tesco*	1 Serving/185g	311	168	16.3	5.6	8.9	1.5
Collar Joint, Lean & Fat, Boiled	1oz/28g	91	325	20.4	0.0	27.0	0.0
Collar Joint, Lean & Fat, Raw	1oz/28g	89	319	14.6	0.0	28.9	0.0
Collar Joint, Lean Only, Boiled	1oz/28g	53	191	26.0	0.0	9.7	0.0
Crispy Smoked, Cooked, Safeway*	1 Rasher/25g	113	450	51.7	3.0	25.7	0.0

B

INFO/WEIGHT	Measure	per Measure KCAL	Nutrition Values per 100g / 100ml				
			KCAL	PROT	CARB	FAT	FIBRE
BACON,							
Crispy Strips, Unsmoked, Marks & Spencer*	1 Serving/25g	121	485	55.6	0.4	29.2	0.0
Diced, Below 5% Fat, Healthy Choice, Asda*	1oz/28g	28	101	19.0	1.0	2.3	0.9
Extra Lean, Marks & Spencer*	1 Rasher/30g	33	110	20.2	0.0	3.4	0.0
Fat Only, Cooked, Average	1oz/28g	194	692	9.3	0.0	72.8	0.0
Fat Only, Raw, Average	1oz/28g	209	747	4.8	0.0	80.9	0.0
Gammon Rasher, Lean Only, Grilled	1oz/28g	48	172	31.4	0.0	5.2	0.0
Lean & Low, Danepak*	1 Serving/26g	44	171	18.3	0.0	10.9	0.0
Lean Only, Fried, Average	1 Rasher/25g	83	332	32.8	0.0	22.3	0.0
Lean Only, Grilled, Average	1 Rasher/25g	73	292	30.5	0.0	18.9	0.0
Lean Only, Raw, Average	1oz/28g	41	147	20.2	0.0	7.4	0.0
Loin Rashers, Unsmoked, Less Than 3% Fat, Safeway*	1 Rasher/25g	22	87	19.6	0.0	0.9	0.0
Loin Steaks, Grilled	1 Serving/120g	229	191	25.9	0.0	9.7	0.0
Maple Cure, Medallions, So Good, Somerfield*	1 Slice/25g	42	168	30.7	2.5	3.9	0.0
Middle, Fried	1 Rasher/40g	140	350	23.4	0.0	28.5	0.0
Middle, Grilled	1 Rasher/40g	123	307	24.8	0.0	23.1	0.0
Middle, Raw	1 Rasher/43g	104	241	15.2	0.0	20.0	0.0
Organic, Marks & Spencer*	1oz/28g	67	240	18.3	2.1	17.9	0.3
Quorn*	1 Rasher/30g	42	141	13.5	8.1	6.1	3.0
Rasher, Streaky, Sainsbury's*	1 Rasher/14g	49	353	19.7	1.0	30.0	0.0
Rashers, COU, Marks & Spencer*	1 Pack/20g	72	360	9.4	77.5	2.9	3.5
Rashers, Lite, Tulip*	1 Rasher/26g	44	171	18.3	0.0	10.9	0.0
Rashers, Smoked Rindless, Healthy Eating, Tesco*	1 Rasher/20g	21	106	19.8	0.0	3.0	0.0
Rashers, Smoked, Safeway*	1 Serving/100g	144	144	33.3	0.0	1.2	0.0
Rashers, Smoked, Wall's*	1 Rasher/30g	56	188	16.2	0.5	13.5	0.0
Rashers, Streaky, Fried	1 Rasher/20g	67	335	23.8	0.0	26.6	0.0
Rashers, Unsmoked, Rindless, Healthy Eating, Tesco*	1 Rasher/20g	21	106	19.8	0.0	3.0	0.0
Rashers, Unsmoked, Wall's*	1 Rasher/25g	47	188	16.2	0.5	13.5	0.0
Rindless, Smoked, Danish, Healthy Eating, Tesco*	1 Rasher/20g	21	106	19.8	0.0	3.0	0.0
Smoked Medallions, BGTY, Sainsbury's*	1 Rasher/18g	26	143	29.9	0.8	2.2	0.1
Smoked, Back, Reduced Salt, Sainsbury's*	1 Rasher/20.3g	49	246	22.2	0.1	17.1	0.6
Smoked, Medallion Rashers, Lidl*	1 Rasher/28g	41	147	28.4	0.2	3.6	0.1
Smoked, Rindless, Back, Safeway*	1 Rasher/30g	73	243	18.4	0.0	17.8	0.0
Smoky, Heat 'n' Eat, Thin Sliced, Asda*	1 Slice/50g	81	161	18.7	1.7	8.8	0.5
Streaky, Grilled	1 Rasher/20g	67	337	23.8	0.0	26.9	0.0
Streaky, Raw	1 Rasher/23g	63	276	15.8	0.0	23.6	0.0
Streaky, Smoked, Extra Trimmed, Asda*	1 Rasher/25g	74	297	27.0	0.0	21.0	0.0
Streaky, Unsmoked, Extra Trimmed, Asda*	1 Rasher/25g	74	297	27.0	0.0	21.0	0.0
Unsmoked, Dry Cure, Marks & Spencer*	1 Rasher/32g	48	151	22.2	4.7	4.8	0.0
Unsmoked, Low Fat, Marks & Spencer*	1oz/28g	31	112	20.2	0.0	3.4	0.0
Unsmoked, Streaky Rashers, Marks & Spencer*	1 Rasher/13g	33	250	16.8	0.0	20.2	0.0
Vegetarian, Rashers, Tesco*	1 Rasher/20g	47	237	19.9	14.5	11.0	6.0
Vegetarian, Realeat*	2 Rashers/35.7g	99	275	28.0	26.6	6.2	1.7
BACON BITS,							
Smoked, Sainsbury's*	1 Pack/250g	585	234	18.4	0.1	17.8	0.1
Smoked, Somerfield*	1oz/28g	75	269	24.0	0.0	19.0	0.0
BAGEL,							
Cheese & Jalapeno, Starbucks*	1 Bagel/115g	292	254	10.8	45.8	3.1	1.5
Chicken, Lemon & Watercress, Safeway*	1 Pack/153g	329	215	12.8	28.2	4.1	0.0
Ham & Pesto, COU, Marks & Spencer*	1 Pack/173g	260	150	11.1	23.5	1.4	1.7
Smoked Salmon & Soft Cheese, Shapers, Boots*	1 Pack/158g	344	218	12.0	29.0	6.0	0.9
Soft Cheese & Smoked Salmon, American, Sainsbury's*	1 Bagel/130.9g	356	272	8.3	31.8	12.4	1.7
Tuna & Sweetcorn Relish, Safeway*	1 Bagel/162g	284	175	11.5	26.2	2.7	0.0
Tuna Salad, BGTY, Sainsbury's*	1 Bagel/170g	325	191	10.4	26.0	4.2	1.0

	Measure INFO/WEIGHT	per Measure KCAL	Nutrition Values per 100g / 100ml				
			KCAL	PROT	CARB	FAT	FIBRE
BAGEL,							
Turkey, Pastrami & American Mustard, Shapers, Boots*	1 Bagel/146g	296	203	11.0	32.0	3.4	1.4
BAGUETTE,							
All Day Breakfast, Darwins Deli*	1 Serving/184g	498	271	13.4	31.9	11.7	0.0
Cheese, Mixed, & Spring Onion, Asda*	1 Pack/190g	629	331	9.5	32.1	18.3	1.3
Cheese, Tomato & Basil, Asda*	¼ Bread/42g	138	329	10.0	40.8	14.0	1.3
Chicken & Mayonnaise, Asda*	1 Pack/190g	407	214	9.7	30.5	8.7	1.3
Chicken & Stuffing, Hot, Sainsbury's*	1 Baguette/227g	543	239	13.7	29.6	7.2	0.0
Chicken Tikka, Asda*	1 Pack/190g	439	231	10.4	32.8	9.4	1.3
Chicken Tikka, Hot, Sainsburys*	1 Pack/190g	386	203	8.5	28.4	6.1	0.0
Egg & Tomato, Breakfast, Pret A Manger*	1 Av Pack/230g	281	122	5.4	15.9	5.3	2.5
Egg & Tomato, Oldfields*	1 Pack/198g	416	210	8.7	27.0	7.6	0.0
Ham & Cheese, Snack 'n' Go, Sainsbury's*	1 Baguette/178g	381	215	12.6	29.6	5.1	1.9
Ham & Greve, Pret A Manger*	1 Av Pack/350g	535	153	9.8	16.1	5.4	1.2
Prawn Mayonnaise, Asda*	1 Pack/190g	399	210	9.1	32.5	4.9	1.3
Prawn, French, Shell*	1 Baguette/63g	171	272	9.7	32.4	11.5	0.0
Salmon & Egg, Pret A Manger*	1 Av Pack/230g	349	152	7.2	15.3	6.9	1.5
Steak & Onion, Snack 'n' Go, Sainsbury's*	1 Baguette/177g	396	225	14.3	30.6	5.0	2.2
Tuna Mayo, Pret A Manger*	1 Av Pack/230g	535	233	10.8	25.0	10.0	1.7
Tuna Melt, Sainsbury's*	1 Serving/204g	373	183	11.3	25.8	3.9	0.0
Turkey & Ham, Asda*	1 Baguette/360g	774	215	11.6	30.7	5.1	1.3
BAILEYS*, Irish Cream, Original	1 Glass/37g	130	350	3.2	20.0	15.7	0.0
BAKE,							
Bean & Pasta, Asda*	1 Pack/450g	599	133	5.0	17.0	5.0	1.7
Broccoli & Three Cheese, Marks & Spencer*	1 Serving/225g	315	140	6.3	6.3	9.7	1.8
Cauliflower & Broccoli Bake, Tesco*	½ Pack/250g	178	71	2.8	5.8	4.1	1.0
Cheese & Spinach, Tesco*	1 Serving/140g	258	184	4.8	22.4	8.3	1.6
Chicken & Mushroom, COU, Marks & Spencer*	1 Serving/360g	324	90	7.3	10.3	2.3	1.1
Chicken Arrabbbiata, Marks & Spencer*	1 Pack/450g	540	120	7.6	16.0	3.0	2.0
Chicken, Broccoli & Mushroom, Safeway*	1 Serving/175g	425	243	8.9	22.4	13.1	3.0
Cod & Prawn, COU, Marks & Spencer*	1 Pack/400g	320	80	6.5	8.8	2.0	1.0
Roast Onion & Potato, COU, Marks & Spencer*	1 Pack/450g	338	75	1.9	13.6	1.3	1.5
Roast Potato, Cheese & Onion, Asda*	½ Pack/200g	288	144	4.2	14.0	8.0	1.1
BAKING POWDER, Average	1 Tsp/2g	3	163	5.2	37.8	0.0	0.0
BALTI,							
Chicken & Potato Wedges, Healthy Living, Tesco*	1 Pack/450g	387	86	6.0	10.8	2.1	1.1
Chicken & Naan Bread, Somerfield*	1 Pack/335g	489	146	10.0	16.0	5.0	0.0
Chicken & Rice, Good Choice, Iceland*	1 Pack/400g	440	110	5.2	18.1	1.9	0.7
Chicken & Rice, Patak's*	1 Pack/370g	440	119	6.1	16.7	3.5	1.7
Chicken Rice, COU, Marks & Spencer*	1 Pack/400g	360	90	7.5	12.5	0.9	1.0
Chicken Tikka, Finest, Tesco*	½ Pack/200g	280	140	15.8	1.1	8.6	3.2
Chicken Tikka, Tesco*	1 Pack/350g	466	133	11.1	6.4	7.0	0.7
Chicken Tikka, Weight Watchers*	1 Pack/320g	224	70	4.8	10.2	1.1	0.6
Chicken With Naan Bread, Perfectly Balanced, Waitrose*	1 Pack/375g	450	120	12.1	9.7	3.6	2.8
Chicken With Naan Bread, Sharwood's*	1 Pack/375g	540	144	6.5	15.4	6.3	2.2
Chicken With Rice, Weight Watchers*	1 Pack/329g	253	77	4.8	10.7	1.7	0.5
Chicken, BGTY, Sainsbury's*	1 Pack/400g	356	89	5.1	15.8	0.6	0.7
Chicken, Blue Parrot Cafe, Sainsbury's*	1 Can/400g	308	77	8.9	4.6	2.5	0.8
Chicken, Finest Ceylon, Tesco*	1 Pack/400g	588	147	14.4	0.9	9.5	5.0
Chicken, Iceland*	1 Pack/544g	740	136	12.0	5.7	7.2	1.6
Chicken, Indian Takeaway, Iceland*	1 Pack/402.2g	362	90	7.8	4.0	4.8	0.7
Chicken, Marks & Spencer*	1 Pack/350g	350	100	10.8	3.9	4.8	1.3
Chicken, Ready Meals, Marks & Spencer*	1oz/28g	34	120	10.2	4.7	6.5	1.6
Chicken, Sainsbury's*	1 Serving/200g	230	115	12.8	4.2	5.2	3.5

	Measure INFO/WEIGHT	per Measure KCAL	Nutrition Values per 100g / 100ml				
			KCAL	PROT	CARB	FAT	FIBRE
BALTI,							
Chicken, Takeaway, Sainsbury's*	1 Pack/400g	404	101	10.4	4.8	4.5	1.4
Chicken, Tesco*	1 Pack/460g	662	144	6.1	17.4	5.6	1.6
Chicken, Tin, Sainsbury's*	1 Serving/200g	168	84	9.4	4.0	3.4	1.0
Chicken, With Pilau Rice, Asda*	1 Pack/504g	625	124	5.0	15.0	4.9	1.2
Chunky Vegetable, Aldi*	1 Can/400g	404	101	1.5	9.3	6.4	1.4
Lamb With Rice & Naan, Iceland*	1 Pack/460g	1904	414	14.7	65.3	10.4	3.2
Prawn, Budgens*	1 Pack/350g	375	107	5.6	5.2	7.1	1.3
Vegetable & Rice, Tesco*	1 Pack/450g	378	84	2.0	15.6	1.6	1.3
Vegetable With Naan Bread & Raita, Eat Smart, Safeway*	1 Pack/371g	315	85	3.8	12.5	1.9	3.1
Vegetable With Naan Bread, PB, Waitrose*	1 Pack/375g	304	81	3.5	10.0	3.0	4.3
Vegetable, Asda*	½ Can/200g	206	103	2.2	10.0	6.0	2.5
Vegetable, Good For You, Asda*	1 Pack/450g	324	72	1.9	14.0	0.9	1.5
Vegetable, Indian Meal for 2, Finest, Tesco*	½ Pack/150g	144	96	1.6	6.1	7.2	2.9
BAMBOO SHOOTS,							
Canned, Drained	1oz/28g	3	11	1.5	0.7	0.2	1.7
Sliced, Asda*	1 Sm Can/120g	8	7	0.7	1.2	0.0	0.2
Sliced, In Water, Sainsbury's*	1 Serving/8g	1	7	0.6	1.0	0.1	0.2
BANANA,							
Average, Fresh, Raw, Without Skin	1 Med/118g	112	95	1.2	23.2	0.3	1.1
Chips	1oz/28g	143	511	1.0	59.9	31.4	1.7
Junior, Tesco*	1 Serving/100g	100	100	3.5	23.3	0.3	0.0
Organic, Tesco*	1 Banana/110g	110	100	1.2	23.2	0.3	1.1
BANANA CHIPS,							
Garden Gang, Asda*	1 Pack/30g	157	523	1.0	60.0	31.0	1.7
BANGERS & MASH,							
Co-Op*	1 Pack/300g	375	125	4.0	13.0	6.0	0.8
Meal for One, Marks & Spencer*	1 Pack/370g	481	130	4.7	9.5	7.9	1.1
Morrisons*	1 Pack/300g	306	102	3.0	12.3	4.9	0.8
BARS,							
AM, Cereal, Apple, McVitie's*	1 Bar/40g	160	400	4.3	65.5	13.5	3.0
AM, Cereal, Apricot, McVitie's*	1 Bar/30g	146	486	6.5	68.8	20.5	0.5
AM, Cereal, Berry, McVitie's*	1 Bar/30g	146	486	6.5	68.8	20.5	0.5
AM, Cereal, Fruit & Nut, McVitie's*	1 Bar/35g	167	477	6.6	64.9	21.4	3.4
AM, Cereal, Grapefruit, McVitie's*	1 Bar/35g	136	389	5.1	70.9	9.4	3.1
AM, Cereal, Orange Marmalade, McVitie's*	1 Bar/40g	151	378	4.5	53.3	18.0	1.8
AM, Cereal, Raisin & Nut, McVitie's*	1 Bar/35.1g	148	422	6.4	62.1	16.4	2.4
AM, Cereal, Strawberry, McVitie's*	1 Bar/34.9g	138	395	5.7	70.5	10.1	2.7
AM, Muesli Fingers, McVitie's*	1 Bar/35g	154	440	6.0	59.8	19.6	3.1
All Day Breakfast, Weight Watchers*	1 Bar/50g	179	358	6.8	72.2	4.6	3.2
Almond, Apricot & Mango, Marks & Spencer*	1 Bar/50g	205	410	8.9	60.2	14.9	5.0
Alpen* Apple & Blackberry With Yoghurt, Weetabix*	1 Bar/29g	122	421	5.7	73.0	11.8	0.0
Alpen*, Fruit & Nut With Milk Chocolate, Weetabix*	1 Bar/29g	125	431	7.0	68.0	14.5	0.0
Alpen*, Fruit & Nut, Weetabix*	1 Bar/28g	110	394	6.5	71.2	9.2	0.0
Alpen*, Strawberry With Yoghurt, Weetabix	1 Bar/29g	123	425	5.6	73.5	12.1	0.0
Alpini, Continental Chocolate, Thorntons*	1 Bar/35.6g	194	539	7.0	55.1	32.2	2.1
Apple & Cinnamon, Breakfast Snack, Tesco*	1 Bar/38g	139	365	4.3	58.8	12.5	2.0
Apple & Cinnamon, Chewy, GFY, Asda*	1 Bar/27g	95	351	6.0	74.0	3.4	8.0
Apple & Raisin, Snack, Traidcraft, Geobar*	1 Bar/35g	127	362	3.3	76.4	4.8	2.3
Apple & Raspberry, Chewy & Crisp, Tesco*	1 Bar/27.0g	123	456	3.4	66.8	19.5	2.8
Apple, Traidcraft, Geobar*	1 Bar/35.1g	132	376	5.3	69.0	8.8	3.5
Apricot & Almond, Chewy & Crisp, Tesco*	1 Bar/27g	122	452	6.2	60.0	20.8	2.6
Apricot & Coconut, Chewy & Crisp, Sainsbury's*	1 Bar/27g	123	457	5.2	58.8	22.3	4.0
Apricot & Raisin, Thorntons*	1 Bar/40g	185	462	8.0	46.0	27.3	3.5

BARS,	Measure INFO/WEIGHT	per Measure KCAL	Nutrition Values per 100g / 100ml KCAL	PROT	CARB	FAT	FIBRE
Apricot, Oat Snack, Waitrose*	1 Bar/27g	121	447	4.9	65.2	18.5	2.4
Banana, Fruit Break, Lyme Regis Foods*	1 Bar/42g	162	385	9.0	51.9	15.7	3.9
Biscuit & Raisin, Reduced Fat, Tesco*	1 Bar/21g	85	406	4.9	68.5	12.5	1.8
Blue Riband, Double Choc, Nestle*	1 Bar/22g	113	513	5.1	63.1	26.7	1.1
Blue Riband, Nestle*	1 Bar/21.1g	108	516	5.2	64.0	26.6	0.0
Blueberrry, Fruit & Grain, Asda*	1 Bar/37g	123	332	3.3	64.0	7.0	2.7
Breakaway, Nestle*	1oz/28g	145	519	6.6	57.4	29.2	2.0
Brunch, Cranberry & Orange, Cadbury's*	1 Bar/35g	154	440	6.2	67.9	15.9	0.0
Brunch, Hazelnut, Cadbury's*	1 Bar/35g	163	465	7.1	61.0	21.6	0.0
Brunch, Raisin, Cadbury's*	1 Bar/35g	151	430	5.8	66.9	15.8	0.0
Cappuccino Coll, Marks & Spencer*	1 Bar/35g	185	529	6.0	50.0	35.0	1.0
Caramel Crisp, Go Ahead, McVities*	1 Bar/33g	141	428	4.8	75.1	12.0	0.8
Caramel, Asda*	1 Bar/29.5g	152	508	8.0	56.0	28.0	2.4
Caramelised Nut & Raisin Crunch, TTD, Sainsbury's*	1 Bar/50g	206	412	8.3	64.4	13.5	5.3
Cereal & More, Marks & Spencer*	1 Bar/40g	154	385	20.0	58.2	7.8	2.9
Cereal, Apple & Cinnamonr, Fruit 'n' Grain, Asda*	1 Bar/37g	131	353	4.5	68.0	7.0	2.9
Cereal, Apple & Raisin, Harvest, Quaker*	1 Bar/22g	87	396	5.0	70.0	11.5	4.0
Cereal, Apple & Raspberry, Chewy & Crisp, Tesco*	1 Bar/27g	123	456	3.3	66.7	19.6	3.0
Cereal, Apple & Raspberry, Waitrose*	1 Bar/25g	90	359	5.0	77.1	3.4	4.6
Cereal, Apple & Sultana, Go Ahead, McVitie's*	1 Bar/35g	137	392	4.1	77.6	7.2	1.8
Cereal, Apple, Chewy, BGTY, Sainsbury's*	1 Bar/25g	85	340	4.8	76.0	2.0	2.0
Cereal, Apricot & Yoghurt, Shapers, Boots*	1 Bar/27g	99	366	3.7	75.0	5.7	3.3
Cereal, Apricot Fruit & Cereal, Organic, Organix*	1 Bar/30g	122	408	7.2	55.3	20.4	6.2
Cereal, Apricot Yoghurt, COU, Marks & Spencer*	1 Bar/25g	90	360	6.1	76.6	2.5	2.9
Cereal, Apricot, Organic, Evernat*	1oz/28g	101	360	5.6	64.9	8.7	7.2
Cereal, Apricot, Perfectly Balanced, Waitrose*	1 Bar/25g	89	356	4.9	76.9	3.2	3.8
Cereal, Balance With Fruit, Sainsbury's*	1 Bar/25g	100	401	5.8	75.2	8.6	1.9
Cereal, Balance, Orco*	1 Bar/21g	81	388	5.3	78.2	6.0	0.0
Cereal, Benefit With Fruit, Harvest Morn*	1 Bar/27g	108	401	5.8	75.2	8.6	1.9
Cereal, Berry & Cream, COU, Marks & Spencer*	1 Bar/20g	72	360	5.3	79.7	2.3	3.1
Cereal, Blueberry Flavour, Breakfast, Sweet Mornings*	1 Bar/38g	152	399	4.5	66.0	13.0	2.5
Cereal, Chewy & Crisp With Choc Chips, Tesco*	1 Bar/27g	125	463	9.2	54.0	23.4	3.8
Cereal, Chewy & Crisp With Roasted Nuts, Tesco*	1 Bar/27g	127	471	9.3	57.0	22.9	2.5
Cereal, Chewy Apple, Fruitus*	1 Bar/34.9g	132	378	5.4	64.8	10.8	5.4
Cereal, Chocolate & Orange, Tesco*	1 Bar/25g	96	384	4.0	77.7	6.3	1.9
Cereal, Chocolate & Raisin, Seeds of Change*	1 Bar/29g	109	375	4.6	69.8	8.5	0.0
Cereal, Chocolate Milk, Kellogg's*	1 Bar/26.7g	122	450	9.0	67.0	16.0	1.5
Cereal, Coconut Muesli, Kellogg's*	1 Bar/25g	108	430	5.0	65.0	17.0	5.0
Cereal, Cranberrry & Blackcurrant, Healthy Living, Tesco*	1 Bar/25g	79	316	5.5	68.2	2.3	8.6
Cereal, Cranberry & Orange, BGTY, Sainsbury's*	1 Bar/26g	93	358	2.7	75.8	4.9	2.3
Cereal, Cranberry & Orange, Weight Watchers*	1 Bar/28g	102	365	4.5	77.6	4.1	2.3
Cereal, Cranberry, Eat Smart, Safeway*	1 Bar/25g	86	345	4.7	75.7	2.3	3.9
Cereal, Cranberry, Waitrose*	1 Bar/25g	91	363	4.5	78.3	3.5	2.9
Cereal, Dark Chocolate, Le Noir, Orco*	1 Bar/21g	95	451	7.3	69.9	15.8	0.0
Cereal, Frosties & Milk, Kellogg's*	1 Bar/27g	122	450	10.0	68.0	16.0	1.0
Cereal, Fruit & Fibre, Asda*	1 Bar/28g	111	398	6.0	71.0	10.0	3.8
Cereal, Fruit & Fibre, Harvest Morn*	1 Bar/29g	114	392	6.5	69.1	10.0	4.1
Cereal, Fruit & Fibre, Sainsbury's*	1 Bar/28g	111	397	5.7	70.9	10.1	3.8
Cereal, Fruit & Nut Break, Jordans*	1 Bar/37g	135	374	7.0	63.2	10.4	8.1
Cereal, Ginger, Waitrose*	1 Bar/25g	92	367	4.9	79.3	3.3	3.3
Cereal, Golden Grahams, Nestle*	1 Bar/25g	106	425	6.5	68.8	13.7	0.0
Cereal, Granola, Starbucks*	1 Bar/90g	324	360	8.0	38.6	21.3	4.8
Cereal, Hazelnut & Pistachio, Go Ahead, McVitie's*	1 Bar/35g	147	419	5.4	68.3	13.8	2.3

BARS,

Measure INFO/WEIGHT	per Measure KCAL	Nutrition Values per 100g / 100ml				
		KCAL	PROT	CARB	FAT	FIBRE
Cereal, Hazelnut & Sultana, Organic, Seeds of Change*	1 Bar/36g	143	396	5.6	64.5	12.7	0.0
Cereal, Hazelnuts & Raisins, Organic, Tesco*	1 Bar/30g	144	481	7.2	50.3	27.9	3.8
Cereal, Honey, Sultana & Sesame, COU, Marks & Spencer*	1 Bar/20g	70	350	4.8	81.7	2.1	3.4
Cereal, Lemon & Sultana, Eat Smart, Safeway*	1 Bar/25g	89	355	4.2	78.4	2.2	2.6
Cereal, Lemon, Marks & Spencer*	1 Bar/25g	90	360	4.1	79.0	2.8	2.8
Cereal, Maple, Healthy Living, Tesco*	1 Bar/25g	93	372	5.5	76.6	4.9	2.0
Cereal, Milk Chocolate, Weetos*	1 Bar/20g	88	440	6.0	71.0	14.5	0.0
Cereal, Mixed Berry, Go Ahead, McVitie's*	1 Bar/35g	134	383	4.6	77.1	6.3	3.1
Cereal, Muesli Break, Breakfast in a Bar, Jordans*	1 Bar/46g	178	387	5.9	66.6	10.8	4.3
Cereal, Muncho Chocolate & Coconut, Orco*	1 Bar/21g	93	441	5.0	71.4	15.0	0.0
Cereal, Nesquik, Nestle*	1 Bar/25g	108	433	6.2	68.7	14.9	0.0
Cereal, Nuts & Raisins, Organic, Evernat*	1oz/28g	108	385	6.5	62.2	12.3	6.8
Cereal, Nutty, Sainsbury's*	1 Bar/25.1g	114	454	6.8	61.8	20.0	2.3
Cereal, Orange & Grapefruit, Healthy Eating, Tesco*	1 Bar/24.9g	90	361	4.1	79.9	2.8	2.2
Cereal, Orange, Lyme Regis Foods*	1 Bar/35g	132	377	4.6	73.4	9.5	5.2
Cereal, Pure Points, Weight Watchers*	1 Bar/50g	179	358	6.8	72.2	4.6	3.2
Cereal, Raisin & Nut Snack Bar, Benecol*	1 Bar/25g	98	390	3.9	68.5	11.1	2.0
Cereal, Rice Krispies & Milk, Kellogg's*	1 Bar/20g	84	421	7.0	70.0	13.0	0.3
Cereal, Roast Hazelnut, Organic, Jordans*	1 Bar/33g	150	455	8.0	56.7	21.8	7.8
Cereal, Roasted Peanut, Weight Watchers*	1 Bar/26g	104	400	9.5	66.1	10.8	2.8
Cereal, Strawberry, BGTY, Sainsbury's*	1 Bar/26g	100	385	3.8	82.0	4.6	5.2
Cereal, Strawberry, Fruit 'n' Grain, Asda*	1 Bar/37g	128	346	3.5	64.9	8.1	3.0
Cereal, Sultana & Honey, Jordans*	1 Bar/36g	130	361	6.0	65.9	8.2	9.2
Cereal, White Choc Chip, Harvest*	1 Bar/22g	94	425	6.0	67.0	15.5	3.5
Cereal, White Chocolate Muesli, Kellogg's*	1 Bar/25g	110	440	5.0	70.0	16.0	2.0
Cereal, With Pink Grapefruit, Chewy, Sainsbury's*	1 Bar/25g	86	344	5.2	76.4	2.0	2.4
Cheerios Cereal & Milk Bar, Nestle*	1 Bar/24g	98	407	7.6	64.5	13.2	0.0
Choc Chip & Nut, Chewy & Crisps, Sainsbury's*	1 Bar/27.1g	129	476	8.8	51.8	26.0	4.4
Chocolate & Orange, Crispy, Free From, Sainsbury's**	1 Bar/30g	132	440	4.8	68.2	16.2	1.2
Chocolate & Orange, Oat Snack, FE, Waitrose*	1 Bar/27g	112	416	5.4	67.0	14.0	1.8
Chocolate & Orange, Shapers, Boots*	1 Bar/26g	98	378	4.2	73.0	13.0	1.5
Chocolate & Raisin Oat Snack, Waitrose*	1 Bar/27g	112	416	5.4	67.2	14.0	2.1
Chocolate & Raisin, Shapers, Boots*	1 Bar/27g	95	353	4.7	76.0	9.1	2.7
Chocolate & Raspberry, COU, Marks & Spencer*	1 Bar/25g	90	360	5.4	78.2	2.7	3.2
Chocolate Brownie, Big Softies, To Go, Fox's*	1 Bar/25g	87	348	5.5	74.9	2.9	0.0
Chocolate Heaven, Ainsley Harriott*	1 Bar/27.1g	147	543	7.0	56.0	32.0	2.5
Chocolate, Apricot & Raisin, Crispy, Sainsbury's*	1 Bar/30g	122	408	3.3	70.9	12.4	0.7
Chocolate, Crisp, Weight Watchers*	1 Bar/25g	92	369	5.4	75.1	10.2	0.8
Chocolate, Crispy, Sainsbury's*	1 Bar/24g	107	446	3.6	68.8	17.4	0.8
Chocolate, Digestive, Farmfoods*	1 Bar/21g	104	495	6.7	63.6	23.8	2.3
Chocolate, Milk Fimbles, Kinnerton*	1 Bar/12.1g	65	539	5.8	57.0	31.8	1.9
Chocolate, Milk, Diabetic, Thorntons*	½ Bar/37g	174	470	7.3	43.0	33.1	2.2
Chocolate, Toffee Pecan, Marks & Spencer*	1 Bar/36g	179	498	4.9	58.3	27.3	0.7
Chocolate, Traidcraft, Geobar*	1 Bar/35g	126	360	5.2	72.6	5.4	4.8
Club, Fruit, Jacob's*	1 Biscuit/25g	124	496	5.6	62.2	25.0	2.3
Club, Milk Chocolate, Jacob's*	1 Biscuit/24g	123	511	5.8	62.6	26.4	2.0
Club, Mint, Jacob's*	1 Biscuit/24g	124	517	5.6	62.5	27.2	1.7
Club, Orange, Jacob's*	1 Biscuit/24g	125	519	5.6	62.2	27.6	1.7
Coco Pops & Milk Bar, Kellogg's*	1 Bar/20g	90	450	8.0	69.0	16.0	1.0
Coconut Chocolate Crisp, Weight Watchers*	1 Bar/25g	89	356	3.6	71.2	10.4	3.2
Coconut, Mueslix, Kellogg's*	1 Bar/25g	108	430	5.0	65.0	17.0	5.0
Cookie, Apple Crumble, COU, Marks & Spencer*	1 Bar/27g	90	335	5.8	72.6	2.6	2.3
Cookie, Oreo, Nabisco*	1 Bar/35g	180	514	2.0	66.0	29.0	0.0

BARS,	Measure INFO/WEIGHT	per Measure KCAL	Nutrition Values per 100g / 100ml				
			KCAL	PROT	CARB	FAT	FIBRE
Cookies & Cream, Myoplex*	1 Bar/100g	250	250	29.0	20.0	6.0	2.0
Cool Coconut, Tesco*	1 Bar/25g	121	484	3.9	60.4	25.2	2.8
Corn Flakes & Chocolate Milk, Kellogg's*	1 Bar/40g	176	440	9.0	68.0	15.0	1.5
Cranberry & Raisin, Snack, Traidcraft*	1 Bar/35g	131	374	3.7	72.6	8.0	2.3
Cranberry, Perfectly Balanced, Waitrose*	1 Bar/25g	91	363	4.5	78.3	3.5	2.9
Crazy Caramel, Tesco*	1 Treat Bar/20g	94	469	4.1	66.0	21.0	1.1
Creme Brulee Chocolate, Marks & Spencer*	1 Bar/36g	178	495	4.4	54.0	29.2	0.4
Crispy Caramel, Shapers, Boots*	1 Bar/24g	96	400	3.9	67.0	17.0	0.4
Crispy Orange, Reduced Fat, Tesco*	1 Bar/22g	95	431	3.6	75.5	12.7	0.6
Crunchy Caramel, Tesco*	1 Bar/21g	98	467	4.6	56.0	25.0	1.4
Crunchy, Honey & Almond, Jordans*	1 Bar/33g	153	465	8.8	56.1	22.8	5.8
Crunchy, Maple & Pecan, Jordans*	1 Bar/33g	153	464	7.7	56.8	22.9	6.5
Dark, Chocolate, Diabetic, Thorntons*	1 Bar/75g	345	460	5.4	28.5	35.8	8.1
Date & Fruit, Lyme Regis Foods*	1 Bar/42g	169	402	7.3	58.2	15.5	8.9
Date & Walnut, Eat Natural*	1 Bar/50g	220	440	8.0	57.2	20.0	0.0
Digestive, Milk Chocolate, Marks & Spencer*	1 Bar/23g	117	510	6.6	64.6	25.1	1.9
Digestive, Milk Chocolate, McVitie's*	1 Bar/23g	118	511	6.6	64.6	25.1	1.9
Digestive, Milk Chocolate, Value, Tesco*	1 Bar/24g	119	495	6.7	63.6	23.8	0.0
Double Caramel, Go Ahead, McVitie's*	1 Cake/32g	97	302	4.0	65.3	4.4	0.7
Double Caramel, Good For You, Asda*	1 Bar/40g	92	231	5.0	47.0	2.6	0.0
Double Chocolate, Shapers, Boots*	1 Bar/23g	95	413	4.8	73.9	10.9	1.3
Double Cream Chocolate, Nestle*	1 Bar/47g	250	531	8.5	54.8	30.9	0.0
Fruit & Nut Crisp, Go Ahead, McVitie's*	1 Bar/23.0g	99	430	5.3	71.3	13.7	1.7
Fruit & Nut, Eat Natural*	1 Bar/50g	112	223	5.8	24.9	11.2	2.2
Fruit 'n Fibre, Kellogg's*	1 Bar/25g	96	383	4.5	72.0	9.0	4.5
Fruitsome, Citrus, Rowntree's*	1 Bar/35g	140	400	4.1	65.1	13.7	2.3
Fruity Cereal Bar, Free From, Sainsbury's*	1 Bar/25.1g	100	399	4.4	72.3	10.2	2.6
Fruity Cereal, Go, Soreen*	1 Bar/40g	133	332	5.5	68.1	4.2	0.0
Frusli, Absolutely Apricot, Jordans*	1 Bar/33g	120	365	5.0	63.8	10.0	6.3
Frusli, Blueberry Burst, Jordans*	1 Bar/33g	133	402	4.8	68.8	11.9	4.6
Frusli, Cranberry & Apple, Jordans*	1 Bar/34g	131	385	5.1	68.9	9.9	5.8
Frusli, Raisin & Hazelnut, Jordans*	1 Bar/34g	145	426	6.3	61.3	17.3	3.9
Frusli, Tangy Citrus, Jordans*	1 Bar/33g	130	393	4.1	70.4	10.5	4.3
Frusli, Wild Berries, Jordans*	1 Bar/33g	128	387	4.6	75.2	7.5	3.3
Fudge, Cake, Cadbury's*	1 Pack/52.4g	218	420	5.7	60.3	17.6	0.0
Ginger Oat, Snack, Waitrose*	1 Bar/27.0g	119	441	4.8	63.5	18.6	2.2
Ginger, Perfectly Balanced, Waitrose*	1 Bar/25g	92	367	4.9	79.3	3.3	3.3
Gold Bar, McVitie's*	1 Bar/23g	121	524	6.0	64.6	26.8	0.6
Gold, McVitie's*	1 Bar/45g	232	516	6.4	65.0	25.6	0.6
Granola, Nature Valley*	1 Bar/42g	180	429	9.5	69.0	14.3	4.8
Harvest Chewy, Apple & Raisin, Quaker*	1 Bar/22g	89	405	5.5	68.0	12.0	3.0
Harvest Chewy, Choc Chip, Quaker*	1 Bar/22g	94	426	6.0	64.0	16.0	3.0
Harvest Chewy, Toffee, Quaker*	1 Bar/22g	94	427	5.0	68.2	15.0	3.2
Harvest Chewy, White Chocolate Chip, Quaker*	1 Bar/92g	392	426	6.0	66.0	14.0	3.0
Honey, Natural, Trail Mix, Kallo*	1 Bar/40g	196	490	15.7	40.9	33.2	5.7
Italian Tiramisu, Marks & Spencer*	1 Bar/35g	184	527	6.3	49.1	34.0	0.8
K-Time, Honey Nut Crunch, Kellogg's*	1 Bar/33.4g	126	382	5.0	82.7	2.5	1.8
K-Time, Mixed Berry, Kellogg's*	1 Bar/28g	104	372	4.9	80.1	2.2	3.8
Lemon, Sicilian, Continental, Thorntons*	1 Bar/40g	201	502	4.1	55.4	29.3	0.4
Milk Chocolate Chip & Hazelnut, Snack, Benecol*	1 Bar/25g	99	395	4.7	64.5	13.1	2.5
Milk Chocolate Coated Orange Flavour, Energy, Boots*	1 Bar/70g	274	391	5.2	70.0	10.0	2.8
Milk Chocolate Whirls, Asda*	1 Bar/26g	116	447	3.7	72.0	16.0	0.8
Milk Chocolate, Mueslix, Kellogg's*	1 Bar/25g	110	440	6.0	63.0	18.0	2.0

B

	Measure INFO/WEIGHT	per Measure KCAL	Nutrition Values per 100g / 100ml				
			KCAL	PROT	CARB	FAT	FIBRE
BARS,							
Milk Chocolate, Sandwich, SmartPrice, Asda*	1 Bar/25g	132	528	6.0	63.0	28.0	0.0
Mixed Nut Feast, Eat Natural*	1 Bar/50g	324	648	22.0	40.0	46.0	1.0
Muesli, The Cookie Coach Company*	1 Bar/75g	289	385	6.8	65.1	11.1	0.0
Muffin, Cadbury's*	1 Bar/68g	270	403	5.6	38.0	25.4	0.0
Nuts & Choc Chip, Asda*	1 Bar/27g	127	471	8.0	58.0	23.0	2.8
Nutty Nougat Caramel, Tesco*	1 Bar/20g	99	493	8.5	54.0	27.0	2.4
Oat Crunchy, Blueberry & Cranberry, Waitrose*	1 Bar/60g	262	437	8.0	67.0	15.2	7.4
Oats, Raisins, Honet & Apricots, Traidcraft, Geobar*	1 Bar/35g	132	376	5.3	69.0	8.8	3.5
Orange Crunch, Go Ahead, McVitie's*	1 Bar/23g	99	430	4.1	78.0	12.8	0.8
Orange Truffle, Marks & Spencer*	1 Bar/33g	177	535	6.6	55.6	31.9	1.4
Pecan Apricot & Peach, Marks & Spencer*	1 Bar/50g	255	510	9.3	38.2	35.5	4.9
Penguin, Chukka, McVitie's*	1 Bar/28g	135	481	6.1	65.1	21.8	0.0
Penguin, McVitie's*	1 Bar/25g	133	532	5.4	65.0	27.8	1.5
Penguin, Mint, McVitie's*	1 Bar/25g	133	531	5.4	65.0	27.7	1.5
Penguin, Orange, McVitie's*	1 Bar/25g	133	531	5.4	65.0	27.7	1.5
Penguin, Snack, McVitie's*	1 Bar/24g	121	504	5.2	54.6	29.5	0.0
Raisin & Hazelnut, Weight Watchers*	1 Bar/24g	95	396	5.0	71.3	10.0	2.9
Raisin & Oatmeal, Breakfast, Tesco*	1 Bar/37.5g	135	355	5.6	56.8	11.7	2.9
Rice Crisp With Honey, Go Ahead, McVitie's*	1 Bar/21.9g	91	415	4.1	76.1	10.5	0.8
Rice Krispies, Kellogg's*	1 Bar/20g	92	460	9.0	66.0	18.0	0.5
Roasted Nut, Chewy & Crisp, Sainsbury's*	1 Bar/27g	120	446	10.1	46.6	24.3	3.9
Rocky, Caramel, Fox's*	1 Bar/24g	111	461	6.7	61.3	21.0	0.8
Smarties, Nestle*	1 Bar/45g	235	522	6.6	61.2	27.9	0.5
Snack, Chocolate & Hazelnut, Benecol*	1 Bar/25g	99	397	4.7	64.5	13.1	2.5
Special K, Kellogg's*	1 Bar/24g	94	390	7.0	75.0	7.0	1.0
Special K, Peach & Apricot, Kellogg's*	1 Bar/23g	92	400	7.0	77.0	7.0	2.0
Strawberry, Organic, Seeds of Change*	1 Bar/26.2g	101	390	5.4	75.7	7.3	0.0
Strawberry, Shapers, Boots*	1 Bar/22g	82	374	2.5	79.0	12.0	0.2
Sultana & Honey, Breakfast, Jordans*	1 Bar/36.7g	134	361	6.0	65.9	8.2	9.2
Three Musketeer, Candy, Mars*	1 Bar/60.4g	258	430	3.3	76.2	13.2	1.7
Toffee & Banana, Chewy, Good for You!, Asda*	1 Bar/27.3g	98	362	6.0	76.0	3.8	6.0
Toffee & Banana, Weight Watchers*	1 Bar/18g	67	372	6.1	77.2	3.9	1.7
Toffee Apple, Chewy, Eat Smart, Safeway*	1 Bar/25g	89	355	4.0	78.3	2.8	2.9
Toffee Crisp, Nestle*	1 Bar/26g	129	497	4.5	62.1	25.6	0.0
Tracker, Breakfast Banana, Mars*	1 Bar/37g	176	476	4.7	63.3	22.6	9.4
Tracker, Chocolate Chip, Mars*	1 Bar/37g	188	509	8.6	55.8	27.9	0.0
Tracker, Roasted Nut, Mars*	1 Bar/27g	139	515	9.8	53.5	29.1	0.0
Tracker, Strawberry, Mars*	1 Bar/27g	129	479	4.7	63.6	22.8	0.0
Tracker, Yoghurt, Mars*	1 Bar/27g	133	491	6.3	64.2	23.2	0.0
Trophy, Organic, Four Seeds, Village Bakery*	1 Bar/42.6g	175	410	9.6	58.5	15.3	5.6
Tropical Fruit Breakfast, Asda*	1 Bar/28g	101	361	6.0	75.0	4.1	4.4
Turkish Delight, Co-Op*	1 Bar/53g	207	390	2.0	78.0	8.0	0.1
Vanilla Fudge, Diabetic, Thorntons*	1 Bar/34g	156	460	3.3	69.2	18.8	0.6
Very Berry, Cookie, Big Softies, Fox's*	1 Bar/26.2g	85	325	5.7	69.7	2.5	2.5
Viennese, Continental, Thorntons*	1 Bar/38g	207	545	4.4	59.3	34.7	0.6
White Chocolate, Mueslix, Kellogg's*	1 Bar/25g	110	440	5.0	70.0	16.0	2.0
Wild & Whippy, Tesco*	1 Treat Bar/17.5g	80	447	3.7	72.0	16.0	0.8
Yoghurt Coated Almond & Apricot, Eat Natural*	1 Bar/50g	278	556	9.4	55.4	33.8	0.0
BASIL,							
Dried, Ground	1 Tsp/1.4g	3	251	14.4	43.2	4.0	0.0
Fresh	1 Tbsp/5.3g	2	40	3.1	5.1	0.8	0.0
BASS,							
Sea, Farmed, Asda*	1oz/28g	29	105	20.5	0.0	2.5	0.0

	Measure INFO/WEIGHT	per Measure KCAL	Nutrition Values per 100g / 100ml				
			KCAL	PROT	CARB	FAT	FIBRE
BASS,							
Sea, Raw	1oz/28g	28	100	19.3	0.0	2.5	0.0
BATON, Chicken & Bacon, Tesco*	1 Pack/201g	511	254	9.4	24.7	13.1	1.7
BATTER MIX,							
For Pancakes & Yorkshire Puddings, McDougalls*	1 Pancake/38g	83	218	6.3	24.8	10.4	1.9
For Yorkshire Puddings & Pancakes, Morrisons*	1 Pudding/30g	43	143	6.4	23.1	2.8	4.1
For Yorkshire Puddings & Pancakes, Tesco*	1 Serving/17g	61	359	12.3	74.4	1.4	7.7
Pancakes, Sainsbury's*	1 Pancake/63g	96	152	6.5	27.4	1.8	3.1
SmartPrice, Asda*	1 Pack/128g	421	329	11.0	69.0	1.0	3.3
Somerfield*	1 Pancake/100g	179	179	6.6	28.2	4.4	2.2
Tesco*	1 Pack/130g	467	359	12.3	74.4	1.4	7.7
Value, Tesco*	½ Pack/64g	92	143	6.4	23.1	2.8	4.1
BAY LEAVES, Dried	1oz/28g	88	313	7.6	48.6	8.4	0.0
BEAN & PEA MIX, Marks & Spencer*	1oz/28g	13	48	4.2	6.5	0.5	6.1
BEAN MIX, Waitrose*	1 Serving/75g	269	358	22.1	60.3	3.1	19.5
BEAN SPROUTS,							
Amoy*	1oz/28g	6	21	1.9	3.2	0.1	0.0
Asda*	¼ Can/52g	12	23	1.8	3.4	0.2	2.7
Chinese, Sainsbury's*	1 Serving/150g	92	61	1.8	0.7	5.7	1.0
Cooked, Safeway*	½ Pack/150g	93	62	1.9	2.4	5.0	0.9
Mung, Canned, Drained	1 Serving/90g	9	10	1.6	0.8	0.1	0.7
Mung, Raw	1oz/28g	9	31	2.9	4.0	0.5	1.5
Mung, Stir-Fried in Blended Oil	1 Serving/90g	65	72	1.9	2.5	6.1	0.9
Raw	1oz/28g	9	32	2.9	4.0	0.5	1.5
Sainsbury's*	1 Serving/55g	12	21	1.9	3.2	0.1	0.4
Tesco*	1 Serving/100g	32	32	2.9	4.0	0.5	1.5
BEANFEAST,							
Bolognese, Batchelors*	1 Serving/65g	196	302	23.9	39.0	5.6	13.5
Mexican Chilli, Batchelors*	1 Serving/65g	203	312	24.3	42.7	4.9	13.6
Savoury Mince, Batchelors*	1 Serving/65g	205	316	24.7	39.5	6.6	12.7
BEANS, ADUKI,							
Dried, Boiled in Unsalted Water	1 Tbsp/30g	37	123	9.3	22.5	0.2	5.5
Dried, Raw	1 Tbsp/30g	82	272	19.9	50.1	0.5	11.1
BEANS, BAKED,							
& Jumbo Sausages, Asda*	1 Serving/210g	317	151	7.0	15.0	7.0	2.6
& Sausage In Tomato Sauce, SmartPrice Asda*	½ Can/203g	256	126	5.0	13.0	6.0	0.0
& Sausage, Asda*	½ Can/205g	252	123	6.0	16.0	3.9	3.0
& Sausage, Good For You, Asda*	1 Serving/217g	178	82	4.7	10.0	2.6	1.8
& Vegetarian Sausages, In Tomato Sauce, Tesco*	1 Can/420g	538	128	6.7	13.6	3.4	2.7
Aldi*	1 Serving/200g	166	83	4.9	14.3	0.7	3.4
American, Heinz*	1 Serving/130g	140	108	4.6	20.8	0.4	3.8
Barbecue, Heinz*	½ Can/100g	82	82	4.9	14.9	0.3	4.0
Canned in Tomato Sauce	1oz/28g	23	81	4.8	15.1	0.6	3.5
Canned in Tomato Sauce, Reduced Sugar	1oz/28g	21	74	5.4	12.8	0.6	3.8
Cheezy, Heinz*	1oz/28g	53	189	11.6	24.5	4.9	6.2
Corale, Aldi*	½ Can/220g	183	83	4.9	14.3	0.7	3.4
Crosse & Blackwell*	1 Can/420g	353	84	4.6	15.8	0.3	3.5
Economy, Sainsbury's*	½ Can/211g	137	65	3.9	12.0	0.2	3.1
Hacendado*	1 Can/212g	170	80	6.0	13.0	0.4	0.0
Healthy Choice, Asda*	1oz/28g	16	58	2.9	11.0	0.2	2.6
Healthy Choice, Safeway*	1 Can/220g	205	93	4.7	17.3	0.5	3.7
Healthy Living, Tesco*	1 Sm Can/220g	84	38	2.3	6.9	0.1	1.6
In Tomato Sauce, Asda*	1 Serving/100g	77	77	4.6	14.0	0.3	3.7
In Tomato Sauce, Bettabuy, Morrisons*	1 Can/210g	164	78	4.2	14.7	0.3	3.2

B

	Measure INFO/WEIGHT	per Measure KCAL	Nutrition Values per 100g / 100ml				
			KCAL	PROT	CARB	FAT	FIBRE
BEANS, BAKED,							
In Tomato Sauce, Everyday Saving, Aldi*	1 Can/425g	340	80	4.6	14.2	0.5	0.0
In Tomato Sauce, Healthy Balance, Heinz*	½ Can/207g	139	67	4.6	11.7	0.2	3.7
In Tomato Sauce, Healthy Eating, Tesco*	1 Can/420g	353	84	5.1	15.1	0.3	3.6
In Tomato Sauce, Healthy Selection, Somerfield*	1 Can/220g	125	57	3.0	11.0	0.0	0.0
In Tomato Sauce, Healthy, HP*	1 Can/420g	266	63	4.4	11.0	0.2	3.7
In Tomato Sauce, Heinz*	½ Can/207g	155	75	4.7	13.6	0.2	3.7
In Tomato Sauce, HP*	1 Sm Can/215g	183	85	4.7	15.0	0.7	3.7
In Tomato Sauce, Morrisons*	1 Can/420g	294	70	2.9	14.0	0.2	0.0
In Tomato Sauce, Organic, Sainsbury's*	½ Can/210g	204	97	5.1	18.0	0.5	3.5
In Tomato Sauce, Princes*	½ Can/212g	180	85	4.7	15.5	0.5	4.6
In Tomato Sauce, Safeway*	½ Can/209g	211	101	4.7	19.3	0.5	3.7
In Tomato Sauce, Tesco*	1 Can/210g	179	85	4.6	15.9	0.3	3.5
In Tomato Sauce, Waitrose*	½ Can/210g	170	81	4.2	14.8	0.6	3.3
In Tomato Sauce, Weight Watchers*	½ Can/207g	137	66	4.7	11.3	0.2	3.7
In Tomato Sauce, With Sugar & Sweetener, Asda*	1 Can/420g	307	73	4.6	13.0	0.3	3.7
Marks & Spencer*	1oz/28g	23	81	5.0	19.2	0.4	3.7
Organic, Heinz*	½ Can/207g	157	76	4.9	13.7	0.2	3.9
Reduced Salt & Sugar, Safeway*	½ Can/210g	195	93	4.7	17.3	0.5	3.7
Reduced Sugar & Salt, Co-Op*	½ Can/210g	126	60	3.0	12.0	0.2	3.0
Reduced Sugar & Salt, Sainsbury's*	½ Can/210g	158	75	4.9	13.0	0.4	5.2
Reduced Sugar & Salt, Tesco*	1 Can/420g	353	84	5.1	15.1	0.3	3.6
Reduced Sugar & Salt, Waitrose*	½ Can/220g	150	68	5.0	11.5	0.2	3.7
Sainsbury's*	½ Can/210g	179	85	4.9	15.5	0.4	5.2
Savers, Morrisons*	1 Can/420g	302	72	3.9	13.5	0.3	0.0
Small, Heinz*	1 Can/200g	146	73	4.6	13.1	0.2	3.6
SmartPrice, Asda*	1 Serving/100g	69	69	2.9	14.0	0.2	3.7
Value, Tesco*	1 Can/420g	328	78	4.5	16.6	0.3	3.5
With Pork Sausages, Heinz*	½ Can/207g	184	89	5.5	11.2	2.5	2.6
With Pork Sausages, Tesco*	1 Can/220g	279	127	5.7	14.9	3.1	2.9
With Tomato Sauce, Oven, Asda*	1 Serving/150g	104	69	2.9	14.0	0.2	3.7
With Vegetable Sausages, Heinz*	1 Can/200g	212	106	6.1	12.2	3.6	2.9
BEANS, BLACKEYE							
Asda*	1 Can/172g	203	118	8.1	19.6	0.8	3.1
Dried, Raw	1oz/28g	87	311	23.5	54.1	1.6	8.2
Dried, Sainsbury's*	1 Serving/100g	71	71	6.0	11.2	0.0	6.4
Safeway*	½ Can/117g	142	121	8.8	19.9	0.7	3.5
Sainsbury's*	1 Can/235g	284	121	8.8	19.9	0.7	3.5
Tesco*	1 Can/175g	207	118	8.1	19.6	0.8	3.1
BEANS, BORLOTTI,							
Canned	1oz/28g	29	103	7.4	17.4	0.4	4.7
Canned, Drained, Sainsbury's	1oz/28g	29	103	7.4	17.4	0.4	4.7
Tesco*	1oz/28g	29	103	8.1	16.0	0.7	4.6
BEANS, BROAD,							
Boiled in Unsalted Water	1oz/28g	13	48	5.1	5.6	0.8	5.4
Canned, Re-Heated, Drained	1oz/28g	24	87	8.3	12.7	0.7	5.2
Dried, Raw	1oz/28g	69	245	26.1	32.5	2.1	27.6
Farmfoods*	1oz/28g	13	48	6.0	6.0	0.0	7.3
Freshly Frozen, Iceland*	1 Serving/100g	81	81	7.9	11.7	0.6	6.5
Frozen, Great Value, Asda*	1 Serving/100g	81	81	8.0	11.0	0.6	6.0
Marks & Spencer*	1oz/28g	27	98	8.8	13.8	0.8	7.3
Raw	1oz/28g	17	59	5.7	7.2	1.0	6.1
Sainsbury's*	1 Serving/90g	72	80	7.9	10.7	0.6	6.5
Young & Tender, Sainsbury's*	½ Can/47g	42	90	8.3	12.7	0.7	5.2

B

	Measure INFO/WEIGHT	per Measure KCAL	Nutrition Values per 100g / 100ml				
			KCAL	PROT	CARB	FAT	FIBRE
BEANS, BUTTER,							
Batchelors*	1 Can/130g	108	83	6.0	13.9	0.4	4.8
Canned, Re-Heated, Drained	1oz/28g	22	77	5.9	13.0	0.5	4.6
Dried, Boiled in Unsalted Water	1oz/28g	29	103	7.1	18.4	0.6	5.2
Dried, Raw	1oz/28g	81	290	19.1	52.9	1.7	16.0
Sainsbury's*	1oz/28g	31	109	7.3	18.9	0.6	5.2
Salted Sweetened Water, Safeway*	1 Can/109g	87	80	5.9	13.0	0.5	4.6
Tesco*	1oz/28g	20	72	5.9	11.0	0.5	4.6
Waitrose*	1 Can/130g	104	80	5.9	13.0	0.5	4.6
Water, Added Sugar & Salt, Somerfield*	1 Can/220g	176	80	5.9	13.0	0.5	4.6
Water, Salt & Sugar Added, Asda*	½ Can/116g	89	77	6.0	12.0	0.5	4.6
BEANS, CANNELLINI,							
Asda*	1 Serving/175g	152	87	7.0	14.0	0.3	6.0
Canned, Drained, Sainsbury's*	1oz/28g	24	84	6.8	13.5	0.3	6.0
Dried, Sainsbury's*	1 Pack/250g	243	97	6.8	16.6	0.5	7.4
Tesco*	1 Can/175g	193	110	7.7	17.5	1.0	5.0
BEANS, CHILLI,							
Asda*	½ Can/142.5g	114	80	4.8	14.0	0.5	3.7
Mexican, Tesco*	1 Can/420g	370	88	5.7	13.6	1.2	5.0
Tesco*	1 Can/215g	249	116	5.5	22.0	0.7	5.0
BEANS, CURRIED, Heinz*	½ Can/100g	103	103	4.9	17.9	1.3	4.0
BEANS, DWARF, Sainsbury's*	1oz/28g	7	25	1.9	3.1	0.5	2.2
BEANS, FLAGEOLET,							
Sainsbury's*	½ Can/133g	132	99	6.8	16.9	0.5	1.8
Tesco*	1 Can/175g	180	103	7.5	15.7	1.1	5.9
Waitrose*	1 Can/265g	193	73	6.7	10.6	0.4	1.9
BEANS, FRENCH,							
Boiled in Unsalted Water	1oz/28g	6	22	1.8	2.9	0.5	2.4
Canned, Re-Heated, Drained	1oz/28g	6	22	1.5	4.1	0.1	2.6
Raw	1oz/28g	7	24	1.9	3.2	0.5	2.2
BEANS, GREEN,							
Cut, Asda*	1 Can/170g	41	24	1.5	3.8	0.3	2.6
Cut, Hartley's*	1 Can/225g	41	18	1.7	2.9	0.0	1.8
Cut, Iceland*	1 Serving/28g	7	25	1.7	4.7	0.1	4.1
Cut, In Salted Water, Morrisons*	1 Serving/150g	32	21	1.5	3.8	0.0	0.0
Cut, Organic, Waitrose*	1oz/28g	7	24	1.9	3.2	0.5	2.2
Egyptian, Tesco*	1 Serving/50g	13	25	1.9	3.2	0.5	2.2
Fine, Sainsbury's*	1 Serving/120g	30	25	3.2	1.9	0.5	2.2
Fine, Tesco*	1 Serving/45g	11	25	1.9	3.2	0.5	2.2
Fresh, Sliced, Tesco*	1 Serving/100g	25	25	1.7	4.4	0.1	4.1
Safeway*	1 Serving/100g	25	25	1.9	3.1	0.5	0.0
Sliced, Boiled, Sainsbury's*	1oz/28g	7	25	1.7	4.4	0.1	4.1
Sliced, Farmfoods*	1 Serving/100g	25	25	1.7	4.4	0.1	4.1
Sliced, Frozen, Asda*	1 Serving/50g	13	25	1.7	4.4	0.1	4.1
Sliced, Frozen, Basics, Somerfield*	1oz/28g	6	20	2.0	3.0	0.0	0.0
Sliced, Frozen, Tesco*	1 Serving/75g	18	24	1.9	3.0	0.5	2.2
Very Fine, Whole, Frozen, Tesco*	1 Serving/75g	17	23	1.7	3.0	0.5	2.2
Whole In Salted Water, Tesco*	½ Can/110g	14	13	1.0	1.6	0.3	1.3
Whole, Asda*	1oz/28g	7	24	1.5	3.8	0.3	2.6
Whole, Very Fine, Organic, Iceland*	1oz/28g	7	25	1.7	4.7	0.1	4.1
BEANS, HARICOT,							
Dried, Boiled in Unsalted Water	1oz/28g	27	95	6.6	17.2	0.5	6.1
Dried, Raw	1oz/28g	80	286	21.4	49.7	1.6	17.0
BEANS, KIDNEY							

INFO/WEIGHT	Measure per Measure KCAL	Nutrition Values per 100g / 100ml				
		KCAL	PROT	CARB	FAT	FIBRE
BEANS, KIDNEY,						
Organic, Sainsbury's*	1 Can/200g 198	99	8.4	15.9	0.5	6.7
Red, Added Sugar & Salt, Sweet Harvest, Aldi*	1 Can/240g 250	104	6.9	17.8	0.6	6.2
Red, Asda*	1oz/28g 32	113	8.4	18.8	0.5	6.7
Red, Batchelors*	1 Can/130g 118	91	8.1	13.5	0.5	6.4
Red, Canned, Drained	1 Can/240g 240	100	6.9	17.8	0.6	6.2
Red, Dried, Boiled in Unsalted Water	1oz/28g 29	103	8.4	17.4	0.5	6.7
Red, Dried, Raw	1oz/28g 74	266	22.1	44.1	1.4	15.7
Red, Economy, Sainsbury's*	1oz/28g 29	105	8.2	17.0	0.5	8.2
Red, In Chilli Sauce, Sainsbury's*	1 Can/420g 340	81	5.1	14.3	0.4	4.3
Red, In Salted Water, Safeway*	1 Can/130g 135	104	6.9	17.8	0.6	6.2
Red, In Salted Water, Sweet Harvest, Aldi*	1 Can/255g 258	101	8.3	15.5	0.6	0.0
Red, In Water, Morrisons*	1 Sm Can/130g 121	93	7.1	14.8	0.6	5.7
Red, In Water, Organic, Sainsbury's*	½ Can/120g 119	99	8.4	15.9	0.5	6.7
Red, In Water, Sainsbury's*	½ Can/119g 129	108	8.4	17.4	0.5	6.7
Red, In Water, Somerfield*	1 Can/220g 264	120	9.0	20.0	1.0	0.0
Red, In Water, Tesco*	1 Can/420g 391	93	6.9	15.0	0.6	6.2
Red, Sugar & Salt Added, Sainsbury's*	½ Can/120g 136	113	8.4	18.8	0.5	6.7
Red, Waitrose*	½ Can/90g 82	91	7.1	14.8	0.4	5.7
BEANS, MIXED,						
Hot & Spicy, Tesco*	1 Serving/78g 61	78	5.0	13.3	0.5	3.9
In Spicy Pepper Sauce, Sainsbury's*	½ Can/210g 187	89	4.7	15.3	1.0	3.2
In a Mild Chilli Sauce, Sainsbury's*	½ Can/208g 162	78	5.2	13.5	0.3	5.2
Italian Style, Tesco*	1 Can/300g 237	79	6.0	12.1	0.7	3.9
Safeway*	½ Can/210.1g 187	89	4.7	15.3	1.0	3.2
Tesco*	1 Can/300g 330	110	7.7	17.6	1.0	5.3
BEANS, MUNG,						
Whole, Dried, Boiled in Unsalted Water	1oz/28g 25	91	7.6	15.3	0.4	3.0
Whole, Dried, Raw	1oz/28g 78	279	23.9	46.3	1.1	10.0
BEANS, PINTO,						
Dried, Boiled in Unsalted Water	1oz/28g 38	137	8.9	23.9	0.7	0.0
Dried, Raw	1oz/28g 92	327	21.1	57.1	1.6	0.0
In Water, Sugar & Salt Added, Sainsbury's*	½ Can/118g 124	105	7.7	17.5	0.7	5.0
Re-fried Beans	1oz/28g 30	107	6.2	15.3	1.1	0.0
BEANS, REFRIED, Old El Paso*	1 Serving/100g 83	83	5.0	13.5	1.0	0.0
BEANS, RUNNER						
& Carrots, Marks & Spencer*	1 Serving/240g 60	25	1.0	4.8	0.1	2.1
Boiled in Unsalted Water	1oz/28g 5	18	1.2	2.3	0.5	1.9
Fresh, Sainsbury's*	½ Pack/87g 17	19	1.2	2.3	0.5	1.9
Raw	1oz/28g 6	22	1.6	3.2	0.4	2.0
Sliced, Marks & Spencer*	1oz/28g 6	22	1.6	3.1	0.4	2.0
BEANS, SOYA,						
Dried, Boiled in Unsalted Water	1oz/28g 39	141	14.0	5.1	7.3	6.1
Dried, Raw	1oz/28g 104	370	35.9	15.8	18.6	15.7
GMO Free, Organic, Evernat*	1oz/28g 104	370	32.5	15.0	18.0	23.5
BEANS, SPICY, Refried, Discovery*	1 Serving/215g 146	68	4.2	11.9	0.4	3.5
BEANS, STRINGLESS, Somerfield*	1 Serving/50g 12	23	1.6	3.2	0.4	2.0
BEEF,						
Braised & Veg With Mashed Potato, Sainsbury's*	1 Pack/453g 331	73	6.5	8.9	1.3	1.2
Braised, Sainsbury's*	1 Serving/250g 240	96	13.3	5.4	2.4	0.8
Brisket, Raw, Lean	1oz/28g 39	139	21.1	0.0	6.1	0.0
Brisket, Raw, Lean & Fat	1oz/28g 61	218	18.4	0.0	16.0	0.0
Cantonese, Sainsbury's*	½ Pack/175g 200	114	5.5	20.1	1.3	0.5
Casserole, Diced, Lean, Sainsbury's*	1 Serving/100g 136	136	22.5	0.0	5.1	0.0

BEEF,

INFO/WEIGHT	per Measure KCAL	KCAL	PROT	CARB	FAT	FIBRE
Casserole, Diced, Less Than 10% Fat, Asda*	1 Pack/227g	275	121	24.0	0.0	2.8	0.0
Casserole, Steak, BGTY, Sainsbury's*	1 Serving/100g	122	122	22.6	0.1	3.5	0.1
Collops With Whisky, Sainsbury's*	1 Pack/450g	513	114	8.0	4.1	7.3	1.2
Cooked, Tesco*	1 Slice/13g	14	105	19.6	1.3	2.4	0.0
Cooked, With Added Water, Sainsbury's*	1 Serving/20g	21	103	19.3	1.1	2.4	0.5
Diced, Lean, Safeway*	1 Serving/167g	200	120	21.1	0.0	4.0	0.0
Fillet, Steak, Marks & Spencer*	1 Steak/150g	233	155	20.9	0.0	7.9	0.0
Flank, Pot-Roasted, Lean	1oz/28g	71	253	31.8	0.0	14.0	0.0
Flank, Pot-Roasted, Lean & Fat	1oz/28g	87	309	27.1	0.0	22.3	0.0
Flank, Raw, Lean	1oz/28g	49	175	22.7	0.0	9.3	0.0
Flank, Raw, Lean & Fat	1oz/28g	74	266	19.7	0.0	20.8	0.0
Fore Rib, Bone In, Asda*	1oz/28g	40	142	21.9	0.1	6.0	0.4
Fore-Rib, Raw, Lean	1oz/28g	41	145	21.5	0.0	6.5	0.0
Fore-Rib, Raw, Lean & Fat	1oz/28g	71	253	18.8	0.0	19.8	0.0
Fore-Rib, Roasted, Lean	1oz/28g	66	236	33.3	0.0	11.4	0.0
Fore-Rib, Roasted, Lean & Fat	1oz/28g	84	300	29.1	0.0	20.4	0.0
Hot & Sour With Garlic Rice, BGTY, Sainsbury's*	1 Pack/400g	428	107	5.9	17.0	1.7	0.6
In Ale Gravy, Chunky, Bird's Eye*	1 Pack/340g	272	80	7.4	8.3	2.0	1.5
In Gravy, Sliced, Sainsbury's*	1 Serving/125g	100	80	13.5	3.3	2.3	0.3
Joint, Sirloin, Roasted, Lean	1oz/28g	53	188	32.4	0.0	6.5	0.0
Joint, Sirloin, Roasted, Lean & Fat	1oz/28g	65	233	29.8	0.0	12.6	0.0
Mince, 5% Fat, GFY, Asda*	1 Serving/227g	279	123	24.0	0.0	3.0	0.0
Mince, 5%, Co-Op	1 Serving/112g	150	134	20.5	0.0	5.4	0.0
Mince, 90% Lean, Marks & Spencer*	1 Serving/100g	175	175	21.9	0.0	9.6	0.0
Mince, British, Tesco*	½ Pack/120g	278	232	18.9	0.0	17.4	0.0
Mince, British, Value, Tesco*	1 Serving/125g	396	317	16.3	0.0	27.4	0.0
Mince, Extra Lean, Frozen, Morrisons*	1oz/28g	41	145	21.0	0.0	6.9	0.0
Mince, Extra Lean, Raw	1oz/28g	49	174	21.9	0.0	9.6	0.0
Mince, Extra Lean, Sainsbury's*	1oz/28g	49	174	21.9	0.1	9.6	0.1
Mince, Extra Lean, Stewed	1oz/28g	50	177	24.7	0.0	8.7	0.0
Mince, Farmfoods*	1oz/28g	62	221	18.8	0.0	16.2	0.0
Mince, Healthy Eating, Tesco*	1 Serving/250g	310	124	20.9	0.0	4.5	0.0
Mince, Lean, Tesco*	1oz/28g	50	178	19.7	0.0	11.0	0.0
Mince, Marks & Spencer*	1oz/28g	37	133	16.0	3.0	7.0	0.1
Mince, Organic, Sainsbury's*	1 Serving/125g	321	257	18.2	0.0	20.5	0.0
Mince, Organic, Tesco*	1 Pack/400g	928	232	18.9	0.0	17.4	0.0
Mince, Raw	1oz/28g	63	225	19.7	0.0	16.2	0.0
Mince, Scotch, Extra Lean, Sainsbury's*	1oz/28g	49	174	21.9	0.1	9.6	0.1
Mince, Steak, 95% Fat Free, BGTY, Sainsbury's*	1oz/28g	35	124	21.3	0.1	4.3	0.1
Mince, Steak, Extra Lean, Lidl*	1 Serving/100g	134	134	20.9	0.0	7.0	0.0
Mince, Steak, Frozen, Asda*	1 Serving/125g	200	160	22.0	0.0	8.0	0.0
Mince, Steak, Frozen, Healthy Living, Tesco*	¼ Pack/125g	185	148	20.4	0.0	7.4	0.0
Mince, Steak, Healthy Eating, Tesco*	1 Pack/500g	620	124	20.9	0.0	4.5	0.0
Mince, Steak, Lean, Co-Op*	1 Serving/125g	231	185	21.0	0.0	11.0	0.0
Mince, Steak, Lean, Asda*	1 Serving/150g	246	164	23.0	0.0	8.0	0.0
Mince, Steak, Lean, Less Than 10% Fat, Asda*	1oz/28g	44	158	22.5	0.0	7.5	0.0
Mince, Steak, Lean, Somerfield*	1 Serving/100g	153	153	22.6	0.0	6.5	0.0
Mince, Steak, Lean, Tesco*	1oz/28g	50	178	19.7	0.0	11.0	0.0
Mince, Steak, Somerfield*	1oz/28g	64	229	23.0	0.0	15.0	0.0
Mince, Steak, Super Lean, Less Than 5% Fat, Asda*	1oz/28g	33	119	22.0	0.0	3.6	0.0
Mince, Steak, Tesco*	1 Serving/125g	155	124	20.9	0.0	4.5	0.0
Mince, Stewed	1oz/28g	59	209	21.8	0.0	13.5	0.0
Mince, Traditional, Raw, TTD, Sainsbury's*	1oz/28g	63	225	19.7	0.0	16.2	0.0

	Measure INFO/WEIGHT	per Measure KCAL	Nutrition Values per 100g / 100ml				
			KCAL	PROT	CARB	FAT	FIBRE
BEEF,							
Minced, & Yorkshire Pudding, Sainsbury's*	1 Pack/350g	375	107	8.4	10.7	3.4	1.1
Patties, Oriental, Perfectly Balanced, Waitrose*	½ Pack/200g	238	119	9.6	13.8	2.8	1.2
Peppered, Carvery, Morrisons*	1 Serving/25g	36	143	23.4	0.1	5.4	1.0
Peppered, Fresh, Marks & Spencer*	1oz/28g	38	135	11.4	1.7	9.2	0.6
Peppered, Steak, Sainsbury's*	1 Steak/155g	246	159	25.8	4.4	4.2	0.4
Peppered, Thin Slices, Sainsbury's*	1 Slice/20g	22	108	19.7	2.2	2.3	1.4
Potted, Yorkshire, Sutherland*	1 Serving/10g	20	199	17.2	1.1	14.0	0.0
Rib Eye, Asda*	1oz/28g	49	174	26.1	1.3	7.2	0.4
Roast Silverside, Wafer Thin, Safeway*	1 Slice/15g	25	165	30.4	0.0	4.5	0.0
Roast Topside, Safeway*	1 Pack/113g	138	122	23.1	0.0	3.2	0.0
Roast, Cooked, Asda*	1 Serving/100g	110	110	20.0	0.1	3.0	0.0
Roast, Finest, Tesco*	1 Serving/50g	77	153	32.3	0.0	2.3	0.0
Roast, Organic, Waitrose*	1 Pack/70g	88	125	26.8	0.3	1.8	0.0
Roast, Scottish, Marks & Spencer*	1oz/28g	36	130	26.3	0.0	2.8	0.0
Roast, Scottish, Topside, Wafer Thin, Marks & Spencer*	1 Serving/28g	35	125	24.3	0.4	3.2	0.0
Roast, Slices, Sainsbury's*	1 Slice/28.3g	34	120	24.4	0.1	2.4	0.5
Roast, Slices, Waitrose*	1 Slice/20g	26	132	24.0	0.0	4.0	0.0
Roast, TTD, Sainsbury's*	1oz/28g	52	185	32.6	1.4	5.4	0.5
Roast, Tesco*	1 Slice/25g	31	125	22.4	0.0	3.9	0.0
Roast, Thin Sliced, Asda*	1 Slice/10g	9	92	17.0	2.1	1.7	0.8
Salt, American Style, Safeway*	1 Serving/70g	67	95	19.0	0.7	1.7	0.0
Salt, Safeway*	1oz/28g	29	105	18.4	1.3	2.9	0.0
Salt, Slices, American Style, Tesco*	1 Slice/7g	8	108	19.9	0.7	2.8	0.3
Salted, Dried, Raw	1oz/28g	70	250	55.4	0.0	1.5	0.0
Salted, Fat Removed, Raw	1oz/28g	33	119	27.1	0.0	0.4	0.0
Shin, Asda*	1oz/28g	50	178	32.7	1.4	4.6	0.4
Silverside, Joint, British, Healthy Eating, Tesco*	1 Serving/200g	214	107	21.0	0.0	2.6	0.0
Silverside, Pot Roasted, Lean	1oz/28g	54	193	34.0	0.0	6.3	0.0
Silverside, Pot-Roasted, Lean & Fat	1oz/28g	69	247	31.0	0.0	13.7	0.0
Silverside, Raw, Lean	1oz/28g	38	134	23.8	0.0	4.3	0.0
Silverside, Raw, Lean & Fat	1oz/28g	60	215	20.4	0.0	14.8	0.0
Silverside, Salted, Boiled, Lean	1oz/28g	52	184	30.4	0.0	6.9	0.0
Silverside, Salted, Boiled, Lean & Fat	1oz/28g	63	224	27.9	0.0	12.5	0.0
Silverside, Salted, Raw, Lean	1oz/28g	39	140	19.2	0.0	7.0	0.0
Silverside, Salted, Raw, Lean & Fat	1oz/28g	64	227	16.3	0.0	18.0	0.0
Slices in Gravy, Tesco*	1 Serving/200g	158	79	11.9	2.6	2.3	0.6
Steak, Braising, Braised, Lean	1oz/28g	63	225	34.4	0.0	9.7	0.0
Steak, Braising, Braised, Lean & Fat	1oz/28g	69	246	32.9	0.0	12.7	0.0
Steak, Braising, Raw, Lean	1oz/28g	39	139	21.8	0.0	5.7	0.0
Steak, Braising, Raw, Lean & Fat	1oz/28g	45	160	20.7	0.0	8.6	0.0
Steak, Cubed, Healthy Eating, Tesco*	1 Serving/142g	142	100	22.7	0.0	1.0	0.0
Steak, Fillet, Fried, Lean	1oz/28g	52	184	28.2	0.0	7.9	0.0
Steak, Fillet, Fried, Lean & Fat	1oz/28g	54	192	28.0	0.0	8.9	0.0
Steak, Fillet, Grilled, Lean	1oz/28g	53	188	29.1	0.0	8.0	0.0
Steak, Fillet, Grilled, Lean & Fat	1oz/28g	56	200	28.7	0.0	9.5	0.0
Steak, Fillet, Raw, Lean	1oz/28g	39	140	21.2	0.0	6.1	0.0
Steak, Fillet, Raw, Lean & Fat	1oz/28g	43	155	20.9	0.0	7.9	0.0
Steak, Fillet, Somerfield*	1oz/28g	51	182	29.0	0.0	7.0	0.0
Steak, Frying, 3.6% Fat, Healthy Choice, Asda*	1oz/28g	33	119	21.6	0.0	3.6	0.0
Steak, Frying, Good For You, Asda*	1 Serving/145g	178	123	24.0	0.0	3.0	0.0
Steak, Frying, Prime, Healthy Choice, Safeway*	1 Steak/110g	114	104	21.5	0.0	2.0	0.0
Steak, Frying, Quick Cook, Grilled, Asda*	1 Serving/100g	133	133	22.0	0.0	5.0	0.0
Steak, Ground, Scottish, Finest, Tesco*	1 Serving/100g	161	161	19.4	0.0	9.3	0.0

BEEF,

	Measure INFO/WEIGHT	per Measure KCAL	Nutrition Values per 100g / 100ml				
			KCAL	PROT	CARB	FAT	FIBRE
Steak, Medallion, Healthy Choice, Asda*	1 Medallion/100g	163	163	36.1	0.0	2.1	0.0
Steak, Rump, Barbecued, Lean	1oz/28g	49	176	31.2	0.0	5.7	0.0
Steak, Rump, Barbecued, Lean & Fat	1oz/28g	57	203	29.5	0.0	9.4	0.0
Steak, Rump, Fried, Lean	1oz/28g	51	183	30.9	0.0	6.6	0.0
Steak, Rump, Fried, Lean & Fat	1oz/28g	64	228	28.4	0.0	12.7	0.0
Steak, Rump, Grilled, Lean	1oz/28g	50	177	31.0	0.0	5.9	0.0
Steak, Rump, Grilled, Lean & Fat	1oz/28g	61	218	27.3	0.0	12.1	0.0
Steak, Rump, Healthy Living, Tesco*	1 Serving/250g	328	131	23.4	0.0	4.2	0.0
Steak, Rump, Marinated Strips, Asda*	1oz/28g	66	235	17.6	0.1	18.3	0.1
Steak, Rump, Raw, Lean	1oz/28g	35	125	22.0	0.0	4.1	0.0
Steak, Rump, Raw, Lean & Fat	1oz/28g	49	174	20.7	0.0	10.1	0.0
Steak, Rump, Seared, Marks & Spencer*	1oz/28g	63	225	19.6	2.9	14.9	0.1
Steak, Sirloin, Fried, Lean	1oz/28g	53	189	28.8	0.0	8.2	0.0
Steak, Sirloin, Fried, Lean & Fat	1oz/28g	65	233	26.8	0.0	14.0	0.0
Steak, Sirloin, Grilled, Medium-Rare, Lean	1oz/28g	49	176	26.6	0.0	7.7	0.0
Steak, Sirloin, Grilled, Medium-Rare, Lean & Fat	1oz/28g	60	213	24.8	0.0	12.6	0.0
Steak, Sirloin, Grilled, Rare, Lean	1oz/28g	46	166	26.4	0.0	6.7	0.0
Steak, Sirloin, Grilled, Rare, Lean & Fat	1oz/28g	60	216	25.1	0.0	12.8	0.0
Steak, Sirloin, Grilled, Well-Done, Lean	1oz/28g	63	225	33.9	0.0	9.9	0.0
Steak, Sirloin, Grilled, Well-Done, Lean & Fat	1oz/28g	72	257	31.8	0.0	14.4	0.0
Steak, Sirloin, Raw, Lean	1oz/28g	38	135	23.5	0.0	4.5	0.0
Steak, Sirloin, Raw, Lean & Fat	1oz/28g	56	201	21.6	0.0	12.7	0.0
Steak, Tender, British, Healthy Eating, Tesco*	½ Pack/150g	173	115	20.3	0.0	3.7	0.0
Steak, Thin Sliced, Marks & Spencer*	1 Serving/100g	115	115	23.0	0.0	2.7	0.0
Steak, Top Rump, Asda*	1 Steak/62g	184	302	35.0	0.0	18.0	0.0
Steak, Top Rump, Grilled, Iceland*	1 Steak/57.6g	172	297	34.6	0.0	17.6	0.0
Steaks, Peppered With Garlic Butter, Asda*	1 Serving/100g	227	227	35.0	1.6	9.0	0.5
Stewed Steak, & Onions With Gravy, John West*	½ Can/205g	269	131	14.0	3.0	7.0	0.0
Stewed Steak, SmartPrice, Asda*	1 Serving/205g	230	112	14.0	2.8	5.0	0.0
Stewed Steak, With Gravy, John West*	1oz/28g	37	131	16.5	5.0	5.0	0.0
Stewing Steak, Casserole, Sainsbury's*	1 Serving/100g	146	146	22.1	0.1	6.4	0.1
Stewing Steak, Raw, Lean	1oz/28g	34	122	22.6	0.0	3.5	0.0
Stewing Steak, Raw, Lean & Fat	1oz/28g	41	146	22.1	0.0	6.4	0.0
Stewing Steak, Stewed, Lean	1oz/28g	52	185	32.0	0.0	6.3	0.0
Stewing Steak, Stewed, Lean & Fat	1oz/28g	57	203	29.2	0.0	9.6	0.0
Strips, Stir Fry, Fresh, Heathy Living, Tesco*	1 Serving/125g	138	110	23.1	0.0	2.0	0.6
Szechuan, Sizzling Hot Spicy, Oriental Express*	1 Pack/400g	380	95	6.4	13.2	1.9	2.0
Topside Joint, Somerfield*	1oz/28g	60	214	27.0	0.0	12.0	0.0
Topside, Oven Roast, Scottish, Asda*	1 Slice/25g	35	138	24.0	1.4	4.0	0.1
Topside, Peppered Roast, Sainsbury's*	1 Slice/16g	20	122	23.2	0.3	3.1	0.1
Topside, Raw, Lean	1oz/28g	32	116	23.0	0.0	2.7	0.0
Topside, Raw, Lean & Fat	1oz/28g	55	198	20.4	0.0	12.9	0.0
Topside, Roasted, Medium-Rare, Lean	1oz/28g	49	175	32.2	0.0	5.1	0.0
Topside, Roasted, Medium-Rare, Lean & Fat	1oz/28g	62	222	29.9	0.0	11.4	0.0
Topside, Roasted, Well-Done, Lean	1oz/28g	57	202	36.2	0.0	6.3	0.0
Topside, Roasted, Well-Done, Lean & Fat	1oz/28g	68	244	32.8	0.0	12.5	0.0
Wafer Thin, Finest, Tesco*	1 Pack/100g	162	162	30.4	0.0	4.5	0.0
Wafer Thin, Roast, Asda*	1 Serving/50g	52	104	20.0	0.3	2.5	0.0
Wafer Thin, Roast, Iceland*	1 Serving/30g	31	102	19.6	0.3	2.5	0.0
Wafer Thin, Tesco*	1 Serving/50g	53	105	19.6	1.3	2.4	0.0
BEEF & GRAVY, Lean Roast, Bird's Eye*	1 Portion/114g	111	97	13.3	3.0	3.5	0.1
BEEF BORDELAISE, Sainsbury's*	1 Pack/400.8g	525	131	8.7	9.7	6.4	1.0
BEEF BOURGUIGNON, Finest, Tesco*	1 Serving/300g	351	117	15.5	3.5	4.5	1.2

	Measure INFO/WEIGHT	per Measure KCAL	Nutrition Values per 100g / 100ml				
			KCAL	PROT	CARB	FAT	FIBRE
BEEF BRAISED							
& Vegetables With Mashed Potato, BGTY, Sainsbury's*	1 Pack/453g	331	73	6.5	8.9	1.3	1.2
With Parsnip Mash, Eat Smart, Safeway*	1 Pack/400g	300	75	7.4	7.6	1.6	1.8
BEEF BRAISED STEAK							
& Ale With Baby Onions, Marks & Spencer*	1 Serving/220g	253	115	14.3	6.5	3.8	1.2
& Cabbage, COU, Marks & Spencer*	1 Pack/380g	323	85	8.3	6.7	2.6	1.9
& Carrots, Mini Favourites, Marks & Spencer*	1 Serving/200g	140	70	8.0	4.2	2.5	1.3
& Mash, Good For You, Asda*	1 Pack/400g	260	65	3.4	11.0	0.8	0.7
& Mash, Good Intentions, Somerfield*	1 Pack/400g	396	99	7.4	10.5	3.0	0.5
& Mustard Mash, Healthy Eating, Tesco*	1 Pack/450g	392	87	7.4	9.5	2.1	0.7
& Red Wine With Vegetable Mash, Healthy Living, Tesco*	1 Pack/500g	360	72	5.1	6.9	2.7	1.2
COU, Marks & Spencer*	½ Pack/225g	180	80	11.9	3.6	2.2	0.7
BEEF CHASSEUR,							
& Potato Mash, BGTY, Sainsbury's*	1 Pack/450g	468	104	8.8	11.0	2.8	0.7
& Potato Mash, New, BGTY, Sainsbury's*	1 Pack/452g	411	91	7.6	9.6	2.5	0.8
BEEF ESCALOPE,							
GFY, Asda*	1 Serving/170g	209	123	24.0	0.0	3.0	0.0
Healthy Choice, Asda*	1 Escalope/100g	163	163	36.1	0.0	2.1	0.0
Marks & Spencer*	½ Pack/220g	275	125	12.5	3.5	6.8	1.2
BEEF GRILL STEAK,							
Aberdeen Angus, Waitrose*	1 Steak/170g	354	208	20.0	1.0	13.8	0.0
Bird's Eye*	1 Steak/66g	205	310	16.2	3.6	25.6	0.1
Black Pepper, Tesco*	1 Serving/87g	261	300	16.2	8.6	22.3	0.0
Iceland*	1 Grillsteak/93g	322	346	24.7	0.8	27.1	0.0
Mighty, Bird's Eye*	1 Serving/134g	420	313	20.9	5.0	23.1	0.1
Peppered, Asda*	1 Serving/170g	386	227	22.2	5.7	12.8	0.6
Peppered, Sainsbury's*	1 Serving/172g	378	220	21.2	5.1	12.7	0.2
Ross*	1 Grillsteak/61g	182	298	15.2	2.0	25.5	0.3
BEEF IN,							
Black Bean Sauce, Marks & Spencer*	1 Pack/350g	350	100	7.8	9.1	3.4	1.1
Bourbon, Leek & Chive Creamed Potatoes, TTD, Sainsbury's*	½ Pack/400g	520	130	10.0	8.8	6.1	0.8
Burgundy Red Wine, GFY, Asda*	1 Pack/405g	348	86	8.0	9.0	2.0	1.1
Madras Sauce, BGTY, Sainsbury's*	1 Can/400g	344	86	9.5	4.0	3.6	0.9
Oriental Sauce, Lean Cuisine, Findus*	1 Pack/350g	420	120	4.5	20.0	2.5	1.5
Red Wine Sauce, Marks & Spencer*	1oz/28g	34	120	13.2	3.6	5.9	0.3
Red Wine With Mashed Potato, Healthy Living, Tesco*	1 Pack/400g	288	72	3.4	10.2	1.9	1.7
Red Wine With Spinach Mash, Waitrose*	1 Pack/400g	304	76	6.7	9.6	1.2	1.3
BEEF MINCED,							
Vegetables & Gravy, Bird's Eye*	1 Pack/178g	155	87	9.1	5.1	3.4	0.6
With Onions, Co-Op*	½ Can/196g	274	140	12.0	4.0	8.0	0.9
BEEF ROAST,							
Dinner, Bird's Eye*	1 Pack/283g	297	105	8.2	10.8	3.2	0.0
Dinner, Iceland*	1 Serving/340g	354	104	8.5	9.1	3.7	1.6
Dinner, New, Bird's Eye*	1 Pack/340g	374	110	8.4	11.1	3.6	1.4
BEEF STEAK, & Chips, Healthy Eating, Tesco*	1 Pack/450g	473	105	6.3	13.8	2.7	0.5
BEEF WELLINGTON,							
Extra Special, Asda*	1 Serving/218.4g	604	277	11.0	20.0	17.0	0.9
Finest, Tesco*	1/3 Pack/216g	525	243	13.0	12.3	15.7	1.5
Marks & Spencer*	1oz/28g	76	270	10.7	17.5	18.3	1.4
Sainsbury's*	1 Wellington/175g	473	270	14.7	18.0	15.5	0.4
BEEF WITH,							
Honey & Black Pepper, Waitrose*	1 Pack/350g	326	93	9.1	9.4	2.1	1.8
Oyster Sauce, Ooodles Of Noodles, Oriental Express*	1 Pack/425g	378	89	4.9	14.2	1.3	1.5
Vegetable Rice, Hot & Sour, COU, Marks & Spencer*	1 Pack/400g	360	90	5.5	14.4	1.4	0.6

	Measure INFO/WEIGHT	per Measure KCAL	Nutrition Values per 100g / 100ml				
			KCAL	PROT	CARB	FAT	FIBRE
BEER,							
Bitter, Canned	1 Can/440ml	141	32	0.3	2.3	0.0	0.0
Bitter, Draught	1 Pint/568ml	182	32	0.3	2.3	0.0	0.0
Bitter, Keg	1 Pint/568ml	176	31	0.3	2.3	0.0	0.0
Bitter, Low Alcohol	1 Pint/568ml	74	13	0.2	2.1	0.0	0.0
Brown Ale, Bottled	1 Bottle/330ml	99	30	0.3	3.0	0.0	0.0
Extra Light, Sleeman Breweries*	1 Bottle/341ml	90	26	0.0	0.7	0.0	0.0
Ginger, Classic, Schweppes*	1 Can/330ml	115	35	0.0	8.4	0.0	0.0
Ginger, Diet, Sainsbury's*	1 Glass/200ml	2	1	0.0	0.1	0.0	0.0
Ginger, Light, Waitrose*	1 Glass/250ml	3	1	0.0	0.0	0.1	0.1
Ginger, Old Jamaica, Light, DG	1 Glass/200ml	6	3	0.1	0.1	0.1	0.0
Ginger, Sainsbury's*	1 Can/330ml	178	54	0.0	13.0	0.0	0.0
Ginger, Traditional Style, Tesco*	1 Can/330ml	218	66	0.0	16.1	0.0	0.0
Guinness, Stout	1 Pint/568ml	170	30	0.4	1.5	0.0	0.0
Mackeson, Stout	1 Pint/568ml	204	36	0.4	4.6	0.0	0.0
Mild, Draught	1 Pint/568ml	136	24	0.2	1.6	0.0	0.0
Ultra, Michelob*	1 Bottle/275ml	88	32	0.0	0.9	0.0	0.0
Weissbier, Alcohol Free, Erdinger*	1 Bottle/500ml	125	25	0.4	5.3	0.0	0.0
Wheat, Tesco*	1 Bottle/500ml	155	31	0.5	0.4	0.0	0.0
BEETROOT,							
Baby, Baxters*	1 Jar/340g	102	30	1.5	6.0	0.0	1.2
Baby, In Sweet Vinegar, Sainsbury's*	1 Serving/50g	30	60	1.3	12.9	0.1	1.1
Baby, In Vinegar, Sainsbury's*	1oz/28g	12	42	1.6	7.5	0.1	1.8
Baby, Marks & Spencer*	1 Pack/255g	115	45	2.3	9.5	0.1	1.9
Baby, Pickled, Budgens*	1oz/28g	8	30	1.4	6.0	0.1	0.0
Baby, Whole, Tesco*	1oz/28g	8	28	1.4	4.4	0.1	1.8
Boiled In Salted Water	1oz/28g	13	46	2.3	9.5	0.1	1.9
Cocktail, Sainsbury's*	1 Serving/50g	44	87	0.9	20.7	0.1	1.5
Cooked, In Vinegar, Safeway*	1 Serving/79g	36	46	2.3	9.0	0.1	0.0
Cooked, Organic, Waitrose*	1 Serving/65g	31	48	2.3	9.5	0.1	1.9
Cooked, Sainsbury's*	1 Serving/250g	120	48	2.3	9.4	0.1	1.9
Crinkle Cut, Baxters*	1 Slice/10g	3	30	1.5	6.0	0.0	1.2
Crinkle Cut, Cooked In Vinegar, Sainsbury's*	1oz/28g	12	43	1.5	8.8	0.2	1.9
Dipped In Malt Vinegar, Traditional Cooked, Tesco*	1 Pack/250g	138	55	0.9	12.0	0.1	1.6
In Natural Juices, Tesco*	1 Serving/50g	24	48	2.3	9.4	0.1	1.9
In Sweet Vinegar, Asda*	1 Serving/100g	50	50	1.1	11.0	0.2	1.8
Marks & Spencer*	1oz/28g	12	44	1.8	9.9	0.0	2.5
Organic, Cooked, Marks & Spencer*	1 Serving/100g	55	55	1.1	11.9	0.1	0.9
Pickled, Baxters*	1 Serving/60g	18	30	1.5	6.0	0.0	0.0
Pickled, Drained	1oz/28g	8	28	1.2	5.6	0.2	1.7
Pickled, Sliced, Better For You, Morrisons*	1 Serving/25g	7	28	1.2	5.6	0.2	0.0
Pickled, Sliced, Organic, Haywards*	1 Serving/25g	8	31	1.1	6.3	0.0	0.0
Raw	1oz/28g	10	36	1.7	7.6	0.1	1.9
Sliced, Baxters*	1 Slice/10g	3	30	1.5	6.0	0.0	1.2
Sliced, in Malt Vinegar, Asda*	1 Serving/28g	9	32	1.6	6.4	0.1	1.7
Sliced, in Sweet Vinegar, Sainsburys*	1 Serving/50g	25	50	1.2	11.4	0.1	1.4
Sliced,Tesco*	1 Serving/100g	25	25	1.4	4.4	0.1	1.8
BHAJI,							
Aubergine & Potato	1oz/28g	36	130	2.0	12.0	8.8	1.7
Bhajia Selection, Occasions, Sainsbury's*	1 Serving/15g	32	211	4.8	19.7	12.6	0.0
Cabbage & Pea With Vegetable Oil	1oz/28g	50	178	3.3	9.2	14.7	3.4
Cauliflower	1oz/28g	60	214	4.0	4.0	20.5	2.0
Mushroom	1oz/28g	46	166	1.7	4.4	16.1	1.3
Mushroom, Marks & Spencer*	1 Pack/225g	293	130	3.6	5.1	10.4	3.9

B

	Measure INFO/WEIGHT	per Measure KCAL	Nutrition Values per 100g / 100ml				
			KCAL	PROT	CARB	FAT	FIBRE
BHAJI,							
Okra, Bangladeshi With Butter Ghee	1oz/28g	27	95	2.5	7.6	6.4	3.2
Onion, Asda*	1 Mini Bhaji/49g	96	196	6.0	20.0	10.0	2.0
Onion, Indian Meal For One, Tesco*	1 Bhaji/100g	204	204	5.5	29.2	7.3	1.3
Onion, Indian Starter Selection, Marks & Spencer*	1 Bhaji/22g	65	295	5.7	15.8	23.3	2.8
Onion, Mini, Indian Snack Selection, Sainsbury's*	1 Bhaji/21.8g	46	211	4.8	19.7	12.6	3.2
Onion, Mini, Morrisons*	1 Bhaji/18g	58	320	5.7	36.3	16.8	3.2
Onion, Mini, Sainsbury's*	1 Serving/22g	43	196	5.9	18.7	10.8	3.4
Onion, Mini, Tesco*	1 Serving/23g	48	210	7.3	26.7	8.2	1.3
Onion, Mini, Waitrose*	1 Bhaji/21g	51	243	5.0	13.9	18.6	4.2
Onion, Morrisons*	1 Bhaji/50g	111	222	5.7	20.3	13.1	3.5
Onion, Safeway*	1 Bhaji/23g	40	175	5.7	20.3	7.5	3.5
Onion, Sainsbury's*	1 Bhaji/33g	75	226	6.0	31.7	8.3	1.1
Onion, Somerfield*	1 Bhaji/15g	39	262	5.0	15.0	20.0	0.0
Onion, Waitrose*	1 Bhaji/45g	100	223	5.6	17.7	14.4	4.3
Potato & Onion	1oz/28g	45	160	2.1	16.6	10.1	1.6
Potato, Onion & Mushroom	1oz/28g	58	208	2.0	12.0	17.5	1.5
Potato, Spinach & Cauliflower	1oz/28g	47	169	2.2	7.1	15.1	1.4
Spinach	1oz/28g	23	83	3.3	2.6	6.8	2.4
Spinach & Potato	1oz/28g	53	191	3.7	13.4	14.1	2.3
Turnip & Onion	1oz/28g	36	128	1.3	7.1	10.9	2.2
Vegetable With Vegetable Oil	1oz/28g	59	212	2.1	10.1	18.5	2.4
BHUNA,							
Chicken Tikka, Tesco*	1 Pack/350g	462	132	11.4	4.5	7.6	0.5
Prawn, Co-Op*	1 Pack/400g	300	75	3.0	6.0	4.0	1.0
BIERWURST,							
German, Sainsbury's*	1 Slice/10g	25	250	14.1	1.1	21.0	0.1
Waitrose*	1 Serving/28g	71	255	14.8	0.8	21.4	0.0
BILBERRIES, Fresh, Raw	1oz/28g	8	30	0.6	6.9	0.2	1.8
BIRYANI,							
Chicken Tikka With Basmati Rice, Sharwood's*	1 Pack/373g	481	129	6.3	16.2	4.3	0.9
Chicken Tikka, BGTY, Sainsbury's*	1 Pack/450g	491	109	9.7	13.2	1.9	1.3
Chicken Tikka, Easy Steam, BGTY, Sainsbury's*	1 Pack/400g	432	108	7.5	17.8	0.7	0.4
Chicken Tikka, Northern Indian, Sainsbury's*	1 Pack/450g	698	155	9.4	16.5	5.7	1.2
Chicken, Easy Steam, Healthy Living, Tesco	1 Pack/400g	424	106	7.0	15.5	1.8	0.6
Chicken, Healthy Eating, Tesco*	1 Pack/370g	289	78	8.5	10.0	0.5	0.4
Chicken, Marks & Spencer*	1 Pack/400g	800	200	7.8	19.8	10.1	1.2
Chicken, Rice Bowl, Eat Smart, Safeway*	1 Pack/300g	255	85	5.5	11.3	1.6	2.4
Chicken, Tesco*	1 Pack/500g	640	128	6.0	15.0	4.9	0.6
Chicken, Waitrose*	1 Pack/450g	657	146	10.1	15.4	4.9	1.6
Chicken, Weight Watchers*	1 Pack/330g	300	91	6.0	14.2	1.1	0.6
Vegetable & Rice, Patak's*	1 Pack/370g	481	130	2.5	18.8	5.5	0.7
Vegetable & Rice, Sainsbury's*	½ Pack/125.0g	229	183	4.4	32.4	4.0	0.7
Vegetable With Curry, Budgens*	1 Serving/250g	378	151	3.4	22.9	5.1	1.5
Vegetable, Healthy Living, Tesco*	1 Pack/450g	455	101	2.7	17.9	2.1	1.6
Vegetable, Sainsbury's*	1 Serving/225g	329	146	2.4	16.3	7.9	1.1
Vegetable, Waitrose*	1 Pack/450g	486	108	2.8	15.2	4.0	2.2
BISCUITS,							
Abbey Crunch, McVitie's*	1 Biscuit/9g	43	477	6.0	72.8	17.9	2.5
Abernethy, Simmers*	2 Biscuits/12.4g	59	490	5.7	69.2	21.9	0.0
Ace Milk Chocolate, McVitie's*	1 Biscuit/24g	122	510	6.1	66.2	24.5	1.6
After Eight, Nestle*	1 Biscuit/5g	26	525	6.5	62.6	27.7	1.5
All Butter Viennese, Marks & Spencer*	1 Biscuit/7g	40	571	7.1	71.4	31.4	1.4
All Butter, Asda*	1 Biscuit/9g	44	487	6.0	64.0	23.0	1.9

BISCUITS,	Measure INFO/WEIGHT	per Measure KCAL	Nutrition Values per 100g / 100ml				
			KCAL	PROT	CARB	FAT	FIBRE
All Butter, Tesco*	1 Biscuit/9g	44	486	6.3	63.5	23.0	1.9
Almond Fingers, Tesco*	1 Finger/46g	180	391	6.2	58.4	14.7	1.0
Almond Thins, Sainsbury's*	1 Biscuit/3g	13	430	7.0	80.3	9.0	1.0
Almond, Cantuccini*	1 Biscuit/8g	39	483	10.0	70.0	17.0	0.0
Amaretti, Doria*	1 Biscuit/4g	17	433	6.0	84.8	7.8	0.0
Amaretti, Sainsbury's*	1 Biscuit/6g	27	450	6.5	80.5	11.3	1.1
Animal Bites, Cadbury's*	1 Pack/25g	120	480	7.1	69.8	19.0	0.0
Animals, Might Minis, Cadbury's*	1 Biscuit/2.1g	10	480	6.5	68.5	20.1	0.0
Animals, Milk Chocolate, Cadbury's*	1 Biscuit/19g	94	493	6.6	69.8	20.9	0.0
Animals, Mini Packs, Cadburys*	1 Pack/25g	123	491	6.7	70.7	20.2	0.0
Apple Crumble, Officially Low Fat, Fox's*	1 Biscuit/23.3g	84	365	5.4	80.4	2.4	2.5
Apple Strudel, Big Softies, Fox's*	1 Biscuit/23g	80	348	5.3	77.0	1.6	2.8
Apricot, Low Fat, Marks & Spencer*	1 Biscuit/23g	79	343	6.1	69.6	4.4	7.8
Arrowroot, Thin, Crawfords*	1 Biscuit/7.4g	33	473	7.4	76.7	15.2	2.2
BN Chocolate Flavour, McVitie's*	1 Biscuit/18g	83	460	6.6	71.0	16.7	2.6
BN Strawberry Flavour, McVitie's*	1 Biscuit/18g	71	395	5.6	78.0	6.8	0.0
BN Vanilla Flavour, McVitie's*	1 Biscuit/18g	85	470	5.9	74.0	16.6	1.2
Belgian Chocolate, Selection, Finest, Tesco*	1 Biscuit/10g	52	515	6.0	62.0	27.0	3.0
Bisc & Bounty, Masterfoods*	1 Bar/25g	132	526	4.8	52.3	33.0	0.0
Bisc & M&M's, Masterfoods*	1 Biscuit/25g	132	527	5.8	59.2	29.6	0.0
Bisc & Mars, Masterfoods*	1 Bar/27g	141	523	5.3	61.4	28.5	0.0
Bisc & Twix, Masterfoods*	1 Bar/27g	140	520	5.2	61.1	28.3	0.0
Biscotti, Starbucks*	1 Biscuit/27g	100	370	7.4	55.6	14.8	0.0
Blackcurrant With Wheat Bran, Bisca*	4 Biscuits/30g	126	420	6.0	72.0	12.0	5.5
Boasters, Hazelnut & Choc Chip, McVitie's*	1 Biscuit/16g	88	549	7.0	55.5	33.3	2.4
Bourbon Creams, Asda*	1 Biscuit/14g	70	485	6.0	68.0	21.0	2.2
Bourbon Creams, Crawfords*	1 Biscuit/12g	59	495	5.9	71.2	20.7	2.2
Bourbon Creams, Sainsbury's*	1 Biscuit/13g	60	476	5.7	70.4	19.1	1.7
Bourbon Creams, Tesco*	1 Biscuit/14g	68	485	5.6	67.8	21.3	2.2
Brandy Snaps	1oz/28g	122	437	2.5	64.0	20.3	0.8
Brandy Snaps, All Butter, Fox's*	1 Biscuit/12g	54	452	2.7	79.5	13.9	0.9
Butter Crinkle Crunch, Fox's*	1 Biscuit/11g	51	464	6.2	69.4	18.0	0.0
Butter Puffs, McVitie's*	1 Biscuit/10g	52	523	10.4	60.7	26.5	2.5
Cantuccini, Sainsbury's*	1 Biscuit/8g	35	440	10.4	63.1	16.2	4.4
Caramel Crunch, Go Ahead, McVitie's*	1 Bar/24g	106	440	4.7	76.6	13.8	0.8
Caramel Log, Tunnock's*	1 Biscuit/25g	118	472	4.2	64.3	24.0	0.0
Caramel Shortcake, Aulds*	1 Slice/58g	286	493	4.4	52.9	29.7	0.8
Caramel Shortcake, Boots*	1 Piece/70g	317	453	4.8	59.0	22.0	1.0
Caramel Shortcake, Mr Kipling*	1 Shortcake/36g	178	508	4.2	58.1	28.8	0.0
Caramel Shortcake, Tesco*	1 Shortcake/45g	217	482	4.6	57.8	25.8	0.5
Caramelised, Lotus*	1 Biscuit/9g	44	488	5.0	72.0	20.0	0.8
Caramels, Milk Chocolate, McVitie's*	1 Serving/17g	81	478	5.6	65.8	21.4	1.8
Cherry Bakewell, Fox's*	1 Biscuit/24.3g	84	350	5.8	72.5	3.1	2.3
Chocolate Caramel Crunch, Go Ahead, McVitie's*	1 Biscuit/24g	106	443	4.8	76.8	14.1	0.8
Chocolate Fingers, Caramel, Cadbury's*	1 Finger/8g	39	490	5.8	63.2	23.8	0.0
Chocolate Fingers, Milk, Cadbury's*	1 Biscuit/6g	30	526	6.9	64.2	26.8	0.0
Chocolate Fingers, Milk, Extra Crunchy, Cadbury's*	1 Biscuit/5g	25	505	6.6	66.2	23.6	0.0
Chocolate Fingers, Plain, Cadbury's*	1 Biscuit/6g	30	508	6.2	60.6	26.8	0.0
Chocolate Fingers, White, Cadbury's*	1 Biscuit/6g	30	530	6.7	62.4	28.2	0.0
Chocolate Kimberley, Jacob's*	1 Biscuit/20g	86	428	3.9	64.4	17.2	1.1
Chocolate Orange, Thick Milk, Marks & Spencer*	1 Biscuit/13g	68	520	7.1	59.7	28.1	1.1
Chocolate Teddy, Arnotts*	1 Biscuit/16.7g	81	478	6.6	69.3	19.2	2.0
Chocolate Viennese Sandwich, Fox's*	1 Biscuit/14g	76	542	6.9	57.4	31.6	1.6

BISCUITS,	Measure INFO/WEIGHT	per Measure KCAL	Nutrition Values per 100g / 100ml				
			KCAL	PROT	CARB	FAT	FIBRE
Chocolinis, Milk Chocolate, Go Ahead, McVitie's*	1 Biscuit/12g	56	466	7.7	77.2	14.0	2.0
Chocolinis, Plain Chocolate, McVitie's*	1 Biscuit/12g	56	468	6.9	77.0	14.7	2.6
Classic Creams, Fox's*	1 Biscuit/14g	72	516	4.4	65.2	25.8	1.7
Classic, Fox's*	1 Biscuit/9g	43	480	4.6	68.6	20.8	2.2
Classic, Milk Chocolate, Fox's*	1 Biscuit/13g	67	517	6.1	64.9	24.0	1.6
Coconut Crinkle, Sainsbury's*	1 Biscuit/11g	54	500	6.4	59.6	26.2	3.7
Coconut Macaroon, Tesco*	1 Macaroon/30g	134	448	5.5	63.7	19.0	1.6
Coconut Rings, Tesco*	1 Biscuit/9g	44	485	6.2	66.1	21.7	2.6
Continental Chocolate, Parkwood, Aldi*	1 Biscuit/13g	65	499	7.5	62.5	24.3	2.6
Cranberry With Hip & Honey, Bisca*	4 Biscuits/30g	123	410	6.5	69.0	12.0	6.5
Crunchy Caramel, Tesco*	1 Bar/21g	98	467	4.8	56.2	25.2	1.4
Curls, Marks & Spencer*	1 Curl/8g	43	540	5.0	63.8	30.0	1.3
Custard Creams, 25% Less Fat, Tesco*	1 Biscuit/12.5g	61	473	5.8	72.2	17.9	1.2
Custard Creams, BGTY, Sainsbury's*	1 Biscuit/12g	57	473	5.8	72.2	17.9	1.2
Custard Creams, Crawfords*	1 Biscuit/11g	57	517	5.9	69.2	24.1	1.5
Custard Creams, Good For You, Asda*	1 Biscuit/25g	119	474	6.0	72.0	18.0	1.2
Custard Creams, Jacob's*	1 Biscuit/16g	77	481	5.3	68.0	20.9	1.6
Custard Creams, Sainsbury's*	1 Cream/13g	64	496	6.0	67.3	22.6	1.6
Custard Creams, SmartPrice, Asda*	1 Biscuit/12.6g	63	486	6.0	69.0	21.0	1.6
Custard Creams, Somerfield*	1 Biscuit/11g	57	514	6.1	69.7	23.4	1.6
Custard Creams, Tesco*	1 Biscuit/12g	61	509	6.1	65.0	25.0	1.5
Custard Creams, Waitrose*	1 Biscuit/11.9g	62	514	5.5	70.4	23.4	1.6
Dark Chocolate All Butter, Marks & Spencer*	1 Biscuit/15g	72	480	6.9	52.4	27.2	11.4
Dark Chocolate Ginger, Marks & Spencer*	1 Biscuit/13.1g	64	495	5.6	68.2	22.3	1.6
Digestive, 25% Less Fat, Asda*	1 Biscuit/16g	73	455	7.3	69.8	16.3	2.6
Digestive, 25% Less Fat, Tesco*	1 Biscuit/14g	65	462	7.3	71.0	16.5	3.8
Digestive, BGTY, Sainsbury's*	1 Biscuit/15g	70	468	7.4	71.0	17.2	3.8
Digestive, Caramels, Milk Chocolate, McVitie's*	1 Biscuit/16g	76	477	5.6	65.7	21.4	1.8
Digestive, Caramels, Plain Chocolate, McVitie's*	1 Biscuit/17g	82	481	5.7	65.5	22.1	2.1
Digestive, Chocolate	1 Biscuit/ 17g	84	493	6.8	66.5	24.1	2.2
Digestive, Chocolate Chip, Co-Op*	1 Biscuit/14g	69	490	6.0	65.0	23.0	3.0
Digestive, Chocolate Chip, Waitrose*	1 Biscuit/15g	71	473	5.6	62.9	22.1	2.3
Digestive, Cracker Selection, Tesco*	1 Biscuit/12g	56	464	7.1	65.2	19.4	4.3
Digestive, Crawfords*	1 Biscuit/12g	58	484	7.1	68.8	20.0	3.4
Digestive, Creams, McVitie's*	1 Biscuit/12g	60	502	5.6	68.2	23.0	2.1
Digestive, Plain Chocolate, Organic, Doves Farm*	1 Biscuit/13g	56	428	5.8	51.4	22.1	6.4
Digestive, Economy, Sainsbury's*	1 Biscuit/13g	65	498	6.8	66.3	22.8	3.3
Digestive, Finger, Sainsbury's*	1 Finger/8g	39	482	6.8	63.6	22.2	3.2
Digestive, Good For You, Asda*	1 Biscuit/14g	65	461	6.0	71.0	17.0	3.6
Digestive, Hovis, Jacob's*	1 Biscuit/12g	56	469	7.8	66.0	19.3	2.9
Digestive, Jacob's*	1 Biscuit/14g	67	479	6.6	65.7	21.1	3.4
Digestive, Light, McVitie's*	1 Biscuit/15g	70	466	7.3	72.9	16.2	3.0
Digestive, McVitie's*	1 Biscuit/15g	74	495	7.0	67.6	21.9	2.8
Digestive, Milk Chocolate Homewheat, McVitie's*	1 Biscuit/17g	86	505	6.8	65.8	23.9	2.3
Digestive, Milk Chocolate, 25% Less Fat, Tesco*	1 Biscuit/17g	79	466	7.4	69.0	17.8	2.6
Digestive, Milk Chocolate, BGTY, Sainsbury's*	1 Biscuit/17g	77	480	7.4	72.5	17.8	2.6
Digestive, Milk Chocolate, Budgens*	1 Biscuit/12.7g	66	511	6.8	66.4	24.2	2.4
Digestive, Milk Chocolate, Good For You, Asda*	1 Biscuit/17g	79	466	7.0	69.0	18.0	2.6
Digestive, Milk Chocolate, Marks & Spencer*	1 Biscuit/17g	89	522	6.4	65.3	26.1	2.1
Digestive, Milk Chocolate, Mini, McVitie's*	1 Bag/40g	206	516	6.5	65.7	25.3	2.3
Digestive, Milk Chocolate, Safeway*	1 Biscuit/17g	86	504	7.0	61.5	25.5	2.2
Digestive, Milk Chocolate, Sainsbury's*	1 Biscuit/17g	87	511	6.9	65.9	24.5	2.5
Digestive, Milk Chocolate, Somerfield*	1 Biscuit/17g	87	513	7.0	67.0	24.0	0.0

BISCUITS,

INFO/WEIGHT	Measure	per Measure KCAL	KCAL	PROT	CARB	FAT	FIBRE
Digestive, Milk Chocolate, Tesco*	1 Biscuit/17g	85	499	6.9	63.7	24.1	2.4
Digestive, Mini Milk Chocolate, Tesco*	1 Pack/30g	153	510	6.6	59.8	27.1	1.8
Digestive, Munch Bites, McVitie's*	1 Pack/40g	205	513	6.5	64.5	25.5	2.0
Digestive, Organic, Waitrose*	1 Biscuit/12.6g	63	485	6.8	60.8	23.8	5.8
Digestive, Plain	1 Biscuit/14g	66	471	6.3	68.6	20.9	2.2
Digestive, Plain Chocolate Homewheat, McVitie's*	1 Biscuit/17g	86	507	6.1	65.6	24.4	2.8
Digestive, Plain Chocolate, BGTY, Sainsbury's*	1 Biscuit/17g	81	478	6.8	72.6	17.8	3.1
Digestive, Plain Chocolate, Tesco*	1 Biscuit/17g	85	499	6.2	63.5	24.4	2.8
Digestive, Reduced Fat, McVitie's*	1 Biscuit/15g	70	467	7.1	72.8	16.3	3.4
Digestive, Reduced Fat, Safeway*	1 Biscuit/14g	66	469	6.5	73.4	22.9	2.8
Digestive, SmartPrice, Asda*	1 Biscuit/15g	71	474	7.0	62.0	22.0	5.0
Digestive, Sweetmeal, Sainsbury's*	1 Biscuit/14g	72	498	6.0	66.4	23.1	3.3
Digestive, Sweetmeal, Tesco	1 Biscuit/18g	80	444	8.4	70.0	14.5	3.1
Echo, Fox's*	1 Bar/25g	128	510	7.8	59.5	26.7	1.2
Florentines, Sainsbury's*	1 Florentine/8g	40	506	10.0	47.2	30.8	7.0
Fruit Shortcake, Asda*	1 Biscuit/10g	45	445	6.0	67.0	17.0	4.6
Fruit Shortcake, McVitie's*	1 Biscuit/8g	39	483	5.9	69.6	20.1	2.1
Fruit Shortcake, Sainsbury's*	1 Biscuit/8g	39	483	5.9	69.6	20.1	2.1
Fruit Shortcake, Tesco*	1 Biscuit/9g	43	473	5.8	70.1	18.8	1.9
Fruit Shorties, Parkside, Aldi*	1 Biscuit/26g	120	461	6.4	69.1	17.7	2.1
Fruity Iced, Blue Parrot Cafe, Sainsbury's*	1 Pack/20g	83	415	6.0	82.0	7.0	1.1
Fruity Oat, Doves Farm*	1 Biscuit/16.7g	80	471	7.6	62.7	21.1	4.0
Fudge Flavour Choc Chip, Go Eat*	1 Biscuit/14.9g	77	510	6.5	59.2	27.4	1.7
Garibaldi, Crawfords*	1 Biscuit/10g	40	397	5.1	70.8	10.4	2.6
Garibaldi, Sainsbury's*	1 Biscuit/9g	35	389	5.7	67.1	10.9	3.3
Garibaldi, Tesco*	1 Section/10g	40	397	5.1	70.8	10.4	2.6
Ginger Crinkle, Sainsbury's*	1 Biscuit/11g	53	486	6.2	63.8	22.9	2.9
Ginger Crunch Creams, Fox's*	1 Biscuit/14g	73	518	4.6	64.8	26.7	0.0
Ginger Nuts, Asda*	1 Biscuit/10g	45	447	5.0	73.0	15.0	0.0
Ginger Nuts, McVitie's*	1 Biscuit/12g	57	473	5.6	75.3	16.6	1.7
Ginger Nuts, Milk Chocolate, McVitie's*	1 Biscuit/14g	68	489	5.8	71.8	19.9	1.5
Ginger Nuts, Tesco*	1 Biscuit/11g	49	447	5.5	73.3	14.6	1.7
Ginger Snap, BGTY, Sainsbury's*	1 Biscuit/12g	51	427	6.5	78.2	9.8	1.8
Ginger Snap, Fox's*	1 Biscuit/8g	35	443	4.6	77.1	12.8	1.5
Ginger Snap, Marks & Spencer*	1 Biscuit/8g	36	445	5.4	76.7	12.9	1.5
Ginger Snap, Sainsbury's*	1 Biscuit/10g	46	461	5.5	76.9	14.6	1.7
Ginger Snap, Starbucks*	1 Biscuit/21g	89	426	7.9	73.1	11.3	0.0
Ginger Thins, Asda*	1 Biscuit/5g	23	462	6.0	73.0	16.0	1.9
Ginger, Safeway*	1 Biscuit/12g	55	456	5.9	73.9	15.3	1.7
Ginger, Traditional, Fox's*	1 Biscuit/8.2g	32	404	4.4	70.1	11.7	1.4
Gingered, Duchy Original*	1 Biscuit/15.7g	76	472	6.0	64.8	21.0	2.5
Gingernut	1 Biscuit/11g	50	456	5.6	79.1	15.2	1.4
Golden Crunch Creams, Fox's*	1 Biscuit/13g	66	511	4.3	65.6	25.7	1.2
Golden Crunch, Go Ahead, McVitie's*	1 Biscuit/9g	38	419	7.7	75.2	9.7	2.1
Golden Shortie, Jacob's*	1 Biscuit/11g	54	492	6.0	64.9	23.2	0.0
Golden Syrup, McVitie's*	1 Biscuit/12.4g	61	508	5.1	67.3	24.2	2.2
Happy Faces, Jacob's*	1 Biscuit/16g	78	485	4.8	66.1	22.3	1.6
Hazelnut Meringue, Sainsbury's*	1 Biscuit/6g	24	404	5.0	43.0	23.5	1.1
Hob Nobs Munch Bites, McVitie's*	1 Pack/40g	203	508	6.8	63.4	25.2	2.8
Hob Nobs, Chocolate Creams, McVitie's*	1 Biscuit/12g	60	503	6.7	60.3	26.1	4.0
Hob Nobs, McVitie's*	1 Biscuit/14g	68	485	7.7	63.6	22.1	4.7
Hob Nobs, Milk Chocolate, McVitie's*	1 Biscuit/16g	79	496	7.3	63.0	24.0	3.7
Hob Nobs, Plain Chocolate, McVitie's*	1 Biscuit/16.2g	80	498	6.7	63.3	24.3	4.2

BISCUITS,

	Measure INFO/WEIGHT	per Measure KCAL	Nutrition Values per 100g / 100ml				
			KCAL	PROT	CARB	FAT	FIBRE
Hob Nobs, Vanilla Creams, McVitie's*	1 Biscuit/12g	60	501	6.1	62.3	25.2	3.6
Honey & Oatmeal, Walkers*	1 Biscuit/34g	158	465	6.7	64.1	22.4	3.8
Iced Gems, Jacob's*	1 Portion/30g	117	390	5.2	85.2	3.1	1.5
Jaffa Viennese, Marks & Spencer*	1 Biscuit/17.2g	79	465	5.9	61.1	21.7	0.9
Jam Rings, Crawfords*	1 Biscuit/12g	56	470	5.5	73.0	17.2	1.9
Jam Sandwich Creams, Marks & Spencer*	1 Serving/15g	70	465	4.8	61.3	22.3	1.1
Jammie Dodgers, Burton's*	1 Biscuit/19g	85	448	4.8	68.8	16.7	1.7
Jammie Dodgers, Mini, Burton's	1 Biscuit/29g	123	424	6.5	74.3	13.2	0.0
Jestives, Fruit & Nut, Cadbury's*	1 Biscuit/17g	85	500	6.7	60.7	25.6	0.0
Jestives, Milk Chocolate, Cadbury's*	1 Biscuit/17g	86	506	6.4	64.4	24.8	0.0
Lemon Curd Sandwich, Fox's*	1 Biscuit/14g	69	494	4.7	66.2	23.4	1.3
Lemon Puff, Jacob's*	1 Biscuit/13g	69	533	4.3	58.8	31.2	2.8
Lemon Thins, Sainsbury's*	1 Biscuit/10g	47	468	5.6	72.3	17.3	1.7
Lincoln, McVitie's*	1 Biscuit/8g	41	514	6.3	69.0	23.6	2.0
Lincoln, Sainsbury's*	1 Biscuit/8g	40	479	7.2	66.1	20.6	2.1
Malted Milk, Asda*	1 Biscuit/8g	39	490	7.0	66.0	22.0	2.0
Malted Milk, Milk Chocolate, Asda*	1 Biscuit/11g	56	509	7.0	64.0	25.0	1.7
Malted Milk, Sainsbury's*	1 Biscuit/8g	40	488	7.1	65.5	21.9	2.0
Malted Milk, Tesco*	1 Biscuit/8g	39	488	7.2	65.6	21.9	2.0
Marie, Crawfords*	1 Biscuit/7g	33	475	7.5	76.3	15.5	2.3
Milk Chocolate, All Butter, Marks & Spencer*	1 Biscuit/14g	70	500	7.5	58.3	26.4	4.6
Milk Chocolate, Tesco*	1 Biscuit/25.3g	134	535	6.4	62.1	29.0	1.8
Mini Assortment, Marks & Spencer*	4 Biscuits/10g	48	480	6.1	63.9	22.5	2.8
Mint, Plain Chocolate, Tesco*	1 Biscuit/25.3g	135	538	5.1	63.0	29.5	1.7
Morning Coffee, Spar*	1 Biscuit/5g	24	471	7.6	77.5	14.5	2.4
Morning Coffee, Tesco*	1 Biscuit/4.8g	23	450	7.6	72.3	14.5	2.4
Nice, Asda*	1 Biscuit/8g	38	480	6.0	68.0	21.0	2.4
Nice, Fox's*	1 Biscuit/8g	38	474	5.9	65.9	20.4	3.8
Nice, Jacob's*	1 Biscuit/7g	33	471	6.1	68.5	19.2	1.8
Nice, Sainsbury's*	1 Biscuit/8g	34	485	6.5	68.0	20.8	2.4
Nice, Tesco*	1 Biscuit/8g	39	485	6.5	68.0	20.8	2.4
Nice, Value, Tesco*	1 Biscuit/5g	24	489	6.9	64.6	22.6	2.4
Oat & Wholemeal, Crawfords*	1 Biscuit/14g	67	482	7.7	64.2	21.6	4.8
Oat Crunchies, Weight Watchers*	1 Biscuit/23g	103	449	7.2	65.3	17.7	6.1
Oat, Santiveri*	1 Biscuit/5.4g	21	428	10.0	58.8	17.0	7.0
Oaten, Organic, Duchy Originals*	1 Biscuit/16g	71	441	9.8	62.3	16.9	5.3
Oatmeal Crunch, Jacob's*	1 Biscuit/8g	37	458	6.8	65.9	18.6	3.6
Orange Milk Chocolate Sandwich, Farmfoods*	1 Biscuit/26g	131	503	6.1	65.7	24.1	1.4
Orange Munchy Bites, Blue Riband, Nestle*	1 Box/125g	653	522	5.2	61.4	27.9	2.0
Parmesan Cheese, Sainsbury's*	3 Biscuits/10g	53	553	14.7	56.4	29.9	1.8
Party Rings, Fox's*	1 Biscuit/6g	27	453	4.3	77.8	13.8	1.3
Petit Beurre, Stella*	1 Biscuit/6g	26	440	9.0	73.0	15.0	0.0
Puffin Chocolate, Asda*	1 Biscuit/25.0g	133	533	5.0	63.0	29.0	0.0
Raisin & Honey, Doves Farm*	1 Biscuit/16.6g	85	501	4.7	59.5	27.1	4.2
Rich Tea Creams, Fox's*	1 Biscuit/11.4g	50	456	5.3	62.7	20.4	1.4
Rich Tea Finger, Marks & Spencer*	1 Biscuit/5g	24	471	7.4	77.9	14.4	0.4
Rich Tea Finger, Tesco*	1 Biscuit/5g	23	451	7.4	72.9	14.4	2.3
Rich Tea, 25% Less Fat, Tesco*	1 Biscuit/10g	44	435	7.1	77.0	11.0	1.3
Rich Tea, Asda*	1 Biscuit/10g	45	447	7.0	71.0	15.0	2.3
Rich Tea, BGTY, Sainsbury's*	1 Biscuit/10g	39	430	7.8	75.9	10.6	2.4
Rich Tea, Balanced Lifestyle, Parkwood, Aldi*	1 Biscuit/10g	42	421	7.3	75.5	10.0	2.1
Rich Tea, Economy, Sainsbury's*	1 Biscuit/8g	33	470	7.8	77.5	14.3	2.4
Rich Tea, Marks & Spencer*	1 Biscuit/10g	46	460	6.9	71.6	15.7	2.4

BISCUITS	Measure INFO/WEIGHT	per Measure KCAL	KCAL	PROT	CARB	FAT	FIBRE
			Nutrition Values per 100g / 100ml				
Rich Tea, McVitie's*	1 Biscuit/8.3g	38	475	7.5	76.3	15.5	2.3
Rich Tea, Milk Chocolate, Sainsbury's*	1 Biscuit/13.1g	66	504	6.3	68.5	22.7	2.1
Rich Tea, Plain Chocolate, Sainsbury's*	1 Biscuit/13g	65	497	6.6	66.0	23.0	2.6
Rich Tea, Reduced Fat, Marks & Spencer*	1 Biscuit/10g	43	430	7.8	75.9	10.6	2.4
Rich Tea, Safeway*	1 Biscuit/10g	45	454	7.4	71.5	15.4	2.3
Rich Tea, Sainsbury's*	1 Biscuit/10g	45	454	7.5	71.4	15.4	2.3
Rich Tea, Tesco*	1 Biscuit/10g	45	454	7.4	71.5	15.4	2.3
Rich Tea, Value, Tesco*	1 Biscuit/7.8g	37	462	7.4	70.2	16.8	2.2
Riva Milk, McVitie's*	1 Biscuit/25.2g	135	540	6.4	57.7	31.5	1.6
Rolo, Nestle*	1 Biscuit/22g	109	494	5.5	62.0	24.9	0.7
Rosemary & Raisin, Marks & Spencer*	1 Biscuit/7.1g	34	490	5.1	62.5	24.1	1.8
Savoury, Gluten, Wheat & Dairy Free, Sainsbury's*	1 Biscuit/16.5g	75	467	11.7	65.1	17.7	2.4
Savoury, Organic, Marks & Spencer*	1 Biscuit/7g	28	395	7.0	58.4	14.6	8.7
Shortbread, Organic, Waitrose*	1 Biscuit/12.5g	64	495	5.8	63.0	24.4	1.8
Shortcake, Asda*	1 Biscuit/14g	73	518	5.0	66.0	26.0	2.0
Shortcake, Crawfords*	1 Biscuit/10.3g	52	518	6.4	68.1	24.4	2.0
Shortcake, Dairy Milk Chocolate, Cadbury's*	1 Bar/49g	252	515	7.5	59.2	27.5	0.0
Shortcake, Dutch, Marks & Spencer*	1 Biscuit/16g	90	563	6.3	60.6	31.9	1.3
Shortcake, Extremely Chocolatey, Marks & Spencer*	1 Biscuit/23g	120	522	7.8	60.0	28.7	0.9
Shortcake, Farmfoods*	1 Biscuit/11g	56	506	6.9	63.1	25.1	1.9
Shortcake, Jacob's*	1 Biscuit/10g	49	485	6.7	65.6	21.8	2.0
Shortcake, Organic, Waitrose*	1 Biscuit/13g	64	495	5.8	63.0	24.4	1.8
Shortcake, Sainsbury's*	1 Biscuit/11g	53	484	7.2	66.6	21.0	2.0
Shortcake, Snack, Cadbury's*	1 Biscuit/8g	42	525	7.0	64.2	26.6	0.0
Shortcake, Value, Tesco*	1 Biscuit/10g	48	484	7.3	66.6	21.0	2.1
Shortcake, Waitrose*	1 Biscuit/13g	67	512	6.0	68.1	24.0	1.9
Shorties, Cadbury's*	1 Biscuit/15g	77	511	6.5	67.3	24.0	0.0
Shorties, Sainsbury's*	1 Biscuit/10g	50	500	6.4	69.8	21.8	2.0
Sports, Fox's*	1 Biscuit/7.1g	30	434	6.1	61.5	18.8	1.8
St Clements Big Softies, Fox's*	1 Biscuit/14g	50	355	6.0	75.2	2.1	3.3
Strawberry Mallows, Go Ahead, McVitie's*	1 Biscuit/18g	69	385	4.3	70.6	9.5	0.9
Strawberry, Cream Tease, McVitie's*	1 Biscuit/19g	97	510	4.8	65.9	25.2	1.2
Summer Fruits, Big Softies, Fox's	1 Bar/25g	89	356	5.9	77.8	2.6	0.0
Tangy Jaffa Viennese, Creations, Fox's*	1 Biscuit/17g	76	447	5.0	63.5	19.2	0.9
Taxi, McVitie's*	1 Biscuit/26.5g	131	504	4.2	63.3	26.0	0.7
Toffee Apple Flavoured, Officially Low Fat, Fox's*	1 Bar/25.7g	91	350	5.6	75.9	2.6	2.4
Toffee Chip Crinkle Crunch, Fox's*	1 Biscuit/11g	51	460	4.6	69.6	18.2	0.0
Treacle Crunch Creams, Fox's*	1 Biscuit/13g	65	502	4.5	65.3	24.8	1.4
Triple Chocolate, Fox's*	1 Biscuits/20.9g	100	478	5.7	57.3	25.1	2.5
Twix Fingers, Master Foods*	1 Pack/30g	148	494	4.6	64.8	24.1	0.0
Viennese Finger, Mr Kipling*	1 Finger/32g	167	523	4.3	54.9	31.8	0.0
Viennese Whirl, Fox's*	1 Biscuit/25g	130	518	6.7	60.1	27.8	0.0
Viscount* Mint	1 Biscuit/16g	83	521	4.8	62.7	27.9	1.3
Water	1oz/28g	123	440	10.8	75.8	12.5	3.1
Water, Carr's*	1 Biscuit/8g	35	436	9.3	76.7	9.2	0.0
Water, High Bake, Jacob's*	1 Biscuit/5.3g	21	414	10.5	76.4	7.4	3.0
Water, High Bake, Sainsbury's*	1 Biscuit/5g	21	412	9.8	76.3	7.5	3.2
Water, High Bake, Tesco*	3 Biscuits/16g	64	401	10.5	73.1	7.4	3.0
Water, High Bake, Waitrose*	1 Cracker/6g	24	408	10.3	75.0	7.4	2.6
Water, Table, Large, Carr's*	1 Biscuit/8g	35	434	10.3	79.1	7.6	3.2
BITES,							
Bacon Rice, Asda*	1 Pack/30g	136	452	7.0	70.0	16.0	0.4
Bacon, Crispy, Shapers, Boots*	1 Bag/23g	99	431	8.0	66.0	15.0	3.0

B

	Measure INFO/WEIGHT	per Measure KCAL	Nutrition Values per 100g / 100ml KCAL	PROT	CARB	FAT	FIBRE
BITES,							
Cheese & Ham, Sainsbury's*	1 Pack/21g	65	309	9.7	14.4	23.6	1.0
Chicken Tikka , Roast, Asda*	1 Pack/250g	485	194	21.0	5.0	10.0	1.0
Chicken Tikka, Marks & Spencer*	1 Serving/50g	95	190	19.9	3.8	10.5	3.2
Chicken, Roasted, Bird's Eye*	5 Bites/80g	160	200	15.0	3.4	13.8	0.1
Mexican Chicken, Somerfield*	1 Pack/227g	508	224	26.0	15.0	7.0	0.0
Southern Fried Chicken, Tesco*	1 Pack/300g	720	240	18.1	16.9	11.1	2.1
BITTER LEMON,							
Diet, Asda*	1 Glass/200ml	4	2	0.0	0.3	0.0	0.0
Low Calorie, Tesco*	1 Glass/200ml	6	3	0.0	0.8	0.0	0.0
Sainsbury's*	1 Glass/250ml	45	18	0.1	4.4	0.1	0.1
BLACK GRAM, Urad Gram, Dried, Raw	1oz/28g	77	275	24.9	40.8	1.4	0.0
BLACK PUDDING,							
Asda*	1oz/28g	66	235	8.0	17.0	15.0	1.6
Farmfoods*	1 Slice/44g	136	309	11.7	20.2	20.1	0.7
Grilled, As Instruction, Sainsbury's*	1 Serving/100g	351	351	9.7	25.0	23.6	0.0
Scottish, Sliced, Somerfield*	1 Slice/50g	129	257	14.0	14.0	16.0	0.0
BLACKBERRIES,							
Fresh, Raw	1oz/28g	7	25	0.9	5.1	0.2	3.1
In Fruit Juice, Asda*	½ Can/145g	46	32	0.6	7.0	0.2	1.8
In Fruit Juice, John West*	1oz/28g	11	39	0.7	9.0	0.0	0.0
In Fruit Juice, Safeway*	1 Serving/210g	69	33	0.6	7.1	0.2	1.8
In Fruit Juice, Sainsbury's*	1 Serving/115g	46	40	0.6	8.6	0.4	1.5
BLACKCURRANTS,							
Fresh, Raw	1oz/28g	8	28	0.9	6.6	0.0	3.6
In Fruit Juice, Asda*	1oz/28g	10	34	0.6	8.0	0.0	2.2
In Fruit Juice, John West*	1 Serving/30g	10	34	0.6	7.9	0.5	1.0
In Fruit Juice, Sainsbury's*	1 Can/290g	119	41	0.7	9.2	0.1	3.3
Stewed With Sugar	1oz/28g	16	58	0.7	15.0	0.0	2.8
Stewed Without Sugar	1oz/28g	7	24	0.8	5.6	0.0	3.1
BLUEBERRIES,							
Fresh, Tesco*	1 Serving/125g	40	32	0.6	6.9	0.2	1.8
BOILED SWEETS,							
Average	1oz/28g	92	327	0.0	87.1	0.0	0.0
Blackcurrant & Liquorice, Co-Op*	1 Sweet/8g	32	405	0.9	91.0	5.0	0.0
Clear Fruits, Sainsbury's*	1 Sweet/7g	26	372	0.1	92.9	0.0	0.0
Cough Sweets, Fundays, Bassett's*	1oz/28g	107	383	0.0	94.9	0.0	0.0
Fruit Drops, Co-Op*	1 Sweet/6g	24	395	0.2	98.0	0.0	0.0
Fruit Rocks, Assorted, Marks & Spencer*	1oz/28g	107	381	0.0	95.2	0.0	0.0
Fruit Sherbets, Assorted, Marks & Spencer*	1 Sweet/8g	34	425	0.0	89.7	7.3	0.0
Lockets, Mars*	1 Pack/43g	165	383	0.0	95.8	0.0	0.0
Pear Drops, Marks & Spencer*	1oz/28g	109	390	0.0	96.9	0.0	0.0
BOK CHOY, Tesco*	1 Serving/100g	11	11	1.0	1.4	0.2	1.2
BOLOGNESE,							
Beef, Asda*	1 Pack/392g	412	105	8.0	7.0	5.0	0.0
Extra Meaty, Marks & Spencer*	1oz/28g	31	110	9.0	4.8	6.1	0.3
Fusilli, Ready Meals, Marks & Spencer*	1oz/28g	38	135	7.0	13.1	6.2	1.0
Meat Free, Asda*	1 Serving/229g	179	78	6.0	11.0	1.1	0.6
Meatless, Granose*	1 Pack/400g	400	100	8.0	8.0	4.0	0.0
Medaglione, Rich Red Wine, Waitrose*	1 Serving/125g	253	202	11.6	29.6	4.1	3.1
Penne, BGTY, Sainsbury's*	1 Pack/400g	428	107	7.2	16.0	1.6	0.9
Penne, Heinz*	1 Pack/300g	213	71	3.8	11.8	0.9	0.6
Ravioli, Beef, Asda*	1 Serving/125g	206	165	7.0	28.0	2.8	1.2
Vegetarian, Marks & Spencer*	1 Pack/360g	360	100	4.5	12.5	3.5	2.1

	Measure INFO/WEIGHT	per Measure KCAL	Nutrition Values per 100g / 100ml				
			KCAL	PROT	CARB	FAT	FIBRE
BOLOGNESE SHELLS,							
BGTY, Sainsbury's*	1 Can/400g	340	85	5.0	11.8	2.0	0.7
Italiana, Weight Watchers*	1 Can/395g	284	72	5.3	9.8	1.3	0.8
Ready Meals, Marks & Spencer*	1 Pack/390g	585	150	7.8	11.4	8.3	0.9
BOMBAY ALOO, Marks & Spencer*	1oz/28g	20	70	1.8	9.5	2.7	2.0
BOMBAY MIX,							
Average	1oz/28g	141	503	18.8	35.1	32.9	6.2
Tesco*	1 Serving/100g	502	502	13.4	40.3	31.9	5.6
BON BONS,							
Apple, Lemon & Strawberry, Co-Op*	¼ Bag/50g	203	405	1.0	88.0	5.0	0.0
Bassett's*	5 Bonbons/200g	834	417	1.1	85.4	7.5	0.0
BOOST,							
Cadbury's*	1 Bar/55g	297	540	5.9	62.3	29.3	0.0
Treat Size, Cadbury's*	1 Bar/24.3g	128	535	5.3	59.6	30.5	0.0
With Glucose & Guarana, Cadbury's*	1 Bar/61g	323	530	5.8	60.3	29.6	0.0
With Glucose, Cadbury's*	1 Bar/61g	326	535	5.3	59.6	30.5	0.0
BOUILLON,							
Beef, Benedicta*	1floz/30ml	22	73	7.5	9.5	0.5	0.0
Beef, Touch of Taste*	1 Serving/15ml	11	73	7.5	9.5	0.5	0.0
Chicken, Benedicta*	1fl oz/30ml	23	75	4.0	8.0	3.0	5.6
Fish, Benedicta*	1fl oz/30ml	21	69	7.5	9.0	0.3	0.0
Swiss Vegetable, Powder, Marigold*	1 teaspoon/4g	8	202	18.4	17.7	6.3	0.7
Vegetable, Benedicta*	1fl oz/30ml	30	101	7.5	17.0	0.3	0.0
BOUNTY,							
Calapuno, Mars*	1 Pack/175g	919	525	6.3	54.3	31.4	0.0
Dark, Mars*	1 Funsize/29g	137	471	3.2	54.1	26.8	0.0
Milk, Mars*	1 Funsize/29g	137	471	3.7	56.4	25.6	0.0
BOURNVITA,							
Powder, Made Up With Semi-Skimmed Milk	1 Mug/227ml	132	58	3.5	7.8	1.6	0.0
Powder, Made Up With Whole Milk	1 Mug/227ml	173	76	3.4	7.6	3.8	0.0
BOVRIL,							
Beef Extract, Bovril*	1 Tsp/5g	9	181	39.7	3.9	0.6	0.0
Chicken Savoury Drink, Bovril*	1 Serving/12.5g	15	129	9.7	19.4	1.4	2.1
BOYSENBERRIES, Canned, In Syrup	1oz/28g	25	88	1.0	20.4	0.1	1.6
BRAN, Wheat	1 Tbsp/7g	14	206	14.1	26.8	5.5	36.4
BRANDY,							
37.5% Volume	1 Shot/25ml	52	207	0.0	0.0	0.0	0.0
40% Volume	1 Shot/25ml	56	222	0.0	0.0	0.0	0.0
Cherry	1 Shot/25ml	64	255	0.0	32.6	0.0	0.0
BRANDY SNAP, Baskets, Askeys*	1 Basket/20g	98	490	1.9	72.7	21.3	0.0
BRATWURST, Frozen, Lidl*	1 Sausage/80g	235	294	12.8	0.5	26.8	0.0
BRAZIL NUTS,							
Asda*	1 Serving/25g	172	688	16.0	2.9	68.0	4.3
Average	6 Whole/20g	136	682	14.1	3.1	68.2	4.3
Crazy Jacks*	1 Nut/3g	21	694	17.0	2.1	69.0	7.2
Kernels, Safeway*	1 Serving/28g	191	682	14.1	3.1	68.2	4.3
Whole, Sainsbury's*	2 Nuts/13g	90	691	16.3	3.1	68.2	4.3
BREAD, BAGEL,							
4 Everything, Finest, Tesco*	1 Bagel/100g	268	268	11.1	51.9	1.8	2.5
Bagel Factory	1 Serving/100g	260	260	10.0	52.0	0.0	2.0
Caramelised Onion & Poppyseed, Waitrose*	1 Bagel/86g	222	258	9.7	49.2	2.5	2.4
Cinamon & Raisin, Starbucks*	1 Bagel/83g	190	229	44.8	9.4	1.4	1.3
Cinnamon & Raisin, GFY, Asda*	1 Bagel/83.8g	223	266	10.0	52.0	2.0	2.7
Cinnamon & Raisin, Marks & Spencer*	1 Bagel/85g	223	262	9.6	52.5	1.8	2.2

INFO/WEIGHT	Measure per Measure KCAL	Nutrition Values per 100g / 100ml				
		KCAL	PROT	CARB	FAT	FIBRE
BREAD, BAGEL,						
Cinnamon & Raisin, New York Bagel Co*	1 Bagel/85g 240	282	10.5	56.0	1.8	2.2
Cinnamon & Raisin, Tesco*	1 Bagel/85g 207	243	9.3	47.5	1.7	2.3
Cinnamon & Raisin, Waitrose*	1 Bagel/86g 229	266	10.5	50.9	2.3	2.1
Fruit & Spice, Sainsbury's*	1 Bagel/85.1g 234	275	9.7	54.3	2.1	3.8
Multigrain, Sainsbury's*	1 Bagel/113g 293	259	10.0	49.6	3.1	2.0
Onion & Poppy Seed, Marks & Spencer*	1 Roll/85g 223	262	9.6	52.5	1.8	2.2
Onion & Poppy Seed, Tesco*	1 Bagel/85g 217	255	10.0	46.7	3.1	3.6
Onion, New York Bagel Co*	1 Bagel/85g 233	274	11.1	53.9	1.6	2.1
Onion, Tesco*	1 Bagel/85g 233	274	10.5	52.4	2.4	1.9
Original, New York Bagel Co*	1 Bagel/85g 230	271	11.2	53.2	1.5	2.2
Original, Organic, New York Bagel Co*	1 Bagel/85g 220	259	9.3	52.2	1.4	4.1
Plain, Good For You, Asda*	1 Bagel/84.2g 218	259	10.0	50.0	2.1	1.8
Plain, Marks & Spencer*	1 Bagel/85g 230	270	10.4	51.7	2.1	1.3
Plain, New York Bagel Co.*	1 Bagel/85g 216	254	10.6	49.2	1.7	3.6
Plain, Tesco*	1 Bagel/85g 214	252	9.9	48.6	2.0	1.8
Plain, Waitrose*	1 Bagel/85g 226	266	10.4	50.7	2.4	1.5
Poppy Seed, New York Bagel Co.*	1 Bagel/85g 233	274	11.4	50.8	2.8	3.2
Sesame Seed, GFY, Asda*	1 Bagel/83.8g 228	271	11.0	51.0	2.5	2.6
Sesame, New York Bagel Co*	1 Bagel/84g 228	272	11.4	52.7	1.8	2.2
Simply Plain, Marks & Spencer*	1 Bagel/85g 230	270	10.4	51.7	2.1	1.3
White, Asda*	1 Bagel/86g 227	264	10.0	49.0	3.1	0.0
BREAD, BAGUETTE,						
Budgens*	1 Baguette/125g 335	268	8.5	55.7	1.2	2.3
Chicken & Spicy Tomato, Snack, Sainsbury's*	1 Baguette/160g 344	215	14.1	31.2	3.7	2.2
Co-Op*	1 Baguette/125g 275	220	7.0	46.0	0.9	3.0
French, Tesco*	1 Serving/150g 360	240	7.8	49.5	1.2	3.4
Homebake, Half, Tesco*	1 Baguette/150g 353	235	7.8	49.1	0.8	1.2
Mediterranean Herb, Sainsbury's*	1 Serving/85g 288	339	8.5	40.8	15.7	2.3
Part Baked, Half, Tesco*	½ Baguette/150g 360	240	7.8	49.5	1.2	3.4
Part Baked, Happy Shopper*	½ Baguette/55g 142	258	8.2	53.9	1.0	2.2
Ready To Bake, Sainsbury's*	½ Baguette/62g 188	303	9.5	62.9	1.5	3.1
Ready To Bake, St Pierre*	1 Baguette/150g 336	224	7.6	46.2	1.0	1.6
Ready To Bake, Waitrose*	½ Baguette/65g 170	262	8.9	53.8	1.2	2.5
Soft Bake, Somerfield*	1 Serving/100g 284	284	10.3	57.3	1.5	1.9
Take & Bake, Budgens*	1 Baguette/110g 282	256	8.1	53.6	1.0	2.2
White, Ready To Bake, Asda*	1 Baguette/115g 322	280	10.0	56.0	1.8	2.6
White, Sainsbury's*	1 Serving/50g 132	263	9.3	53.1	1.5	2.7
With Garlic Butter, Half, Frozen, Oven Bake, Safeway*	1 Baguette/160g 568	355	6.7	39.8	19.8	2.5
BREAD, BALTIC RYE, Organic, The Village Bakery*	1oz/28g 68	243	8.0	50.3	1.4	2.9
BREAD, BAPS,						
Brown, Large, Asda*	1 Bap/58g 140	242	10.0	47.0	1.6	0.0
Brown, Malted Grain, Large, Tesco*	1 Bap/100g 238	238	8.5	44.0	3.1	1.9
Cheese Top, Sainsbury's*	1 Bap/75g 218	291	12.1	41.6	8.5	2.0
Cheese Topped, Marks & Spencer*	1 Bap/78.2g 215	275	11.6	34.1	11.1	1.8
Floured, Marks & Spencer*	1 Bap/60g 168	280	11.5	46.8	6.2	2.0
Multigrain, Tesco*	1 Serving/97.5g 239	244	8.7	45.1	3.2	1.9
White Sandwich, Kingsmill*	1 Bap/80g 209	261	10.1	46.2	4.0	2.2
White Soft, Somerfield*	1oz/28g 69	248	11.0	44.0	3.0	0.0
White, Giant, Sainsbury's*	1 Bap/103g 267	259	9.0	49.9	2.6	2.7
White, Giant, Waitrose*	1 Bap/104g 261	251	8.8	45.3	3.8	2.1
White, Large, Tesco*	1 Bap/100g 246	246	9.2	47.5	2.1	2.4
White, Medium, Morrisons*	1 Bap/62g 152	245	8.6	48.5	2.0	2.4
White, Sliced, Large, Asda*	1 Bap/58g 148	255	10.0	50.0	1.7	0.0

	Measure INFO/WEIGHT	per Measure KCAL	Nutrition Values per 100g / 100ml				
			KCAL	PROT	CARB	FAT	FIBRE
BREAD, BAPS,							
White, Soft, Floured, Marks & Spencer*	1 Bap/63g	176	280	11.5	46.8	6.2	2.0
White, Warburton's*	1 Bap/57g	144	252	9.8	43.4	4.3	2.7
Wholemeal, Diet Choice, Waitrose*	1 Bap/68g	171	252	9.6	41.4	5.3	5.6
Wholemeal, Giant, Sainsbury's*	1 Bap/110g	275	250	11.7	43.5	3.2	6.1
Wholemeal, Large, Tesco*	1 Bap/97g	228	235	10.5	39.1	4.1	7.6
Wholemeal, Sainsbury's*	1 Bap/60g	151	252	9.6	41.4	5.3	5.6
Wholemeal, Tesco*	1 Bap/46g	104	227	9.6	41.4	5.3	5.6
BREAD, BATCH,							
Seeded, Finest, Tesco*	1 Slice/65g	168	259	9.3	41.8	6.1	6.1
Seeded, Warburton's*	1 Slice/27g	76	280	11.3	39.6	8.5	3.2
White, Warburton's*	1 Slice/42g	98	233	9.8	43.6	2.1	2.7
BREAD, BEST OF BOTH, Hovis*	1 Slice/40g	88	219	9.0	40.8	2.3	4.5
BREAD, BLACK OLIVE, Finest, Tesco*	1 Serving/72g	184	255	9.7	39.7	6.4	2.9
BREAD, BLOOMER,							
Multiseed, Sliced, Marks & Spencer*	1 Slice/53.6g	151	280	10.5	43.6	7.2	3.1
Vienna, Marks & Spencer*	1oz/28g	79	281	9.6	55.8	2.1	2.7
White, Bake Off, Somerfield*	1oz/28g	69	246	9.0	47.0	3.0	0.0
White, Seeded, Bake Off, Somerfield*	1oz/28g	68	243	9.0	46.0	3.0	0.0
Wholemeal, Organic, Marks & Spencer*	1 Slice/120g	288	240	8.7	35.5	8.0	5.2
BREAD, BREADCAKES, Big Brown, Morrisons*	1 Breadcake/63g	154	245	9.0	44.6	3.4	4.3
BREAD, BRIOCHE,							
Loaf, Sainsbury's*	1/8 Loaf/50g	174	347	8.0	55.0	10.5	2.2
Continental Classics*	1 Roll/35g	122	349	8.2	58.3	9.3	0.0
Finest, Tesco*	1 Bun/52g	207	398	10.8	38.3	22.4	2.0
Marks & Spencer*	1 Brioche/50g	182	363	7.8	40.2	20.5	1.5
BREAD, BROWN,							
Average	1 Med Slice/34g	74	218	8.5	44.3	2.0	3.5
Crusty Golden, Hovis*	1 Slice/44g	102	231	8.7	43.0	2.7	3.3
Danish, Warburton's*	1 Slice/19g	38	200	8.6	37.7	1.6	9.6
Danish, Weight Watchers*	1 Slice/19g	38	200	8.6	37.7	1.6	9.6
Fibre Rich, Allinson*	1 Slice/24g	51	212	13.2	33.6	2.8	8.0
Good Health, Warburton's*	1 Slice/34.8g	79	226	10.3	39.6	2.9	7.2
Granary Malted, Waitrose*	1 Slice/40g	88	220	9.4	39.9	2.5	4.3
Harvest, Marks & Spencer*	1oz/28g	67	240	8.8	44.5	2.7	3.7
High Fibre, Ormo*	1 Slice/24g	57	239	9.2	42.9	2.6	7.5
Malted, Farmhouse Gold, Morrisons*	1 Slice/38g	96	253	10.3	49.9	1.4	3.1
Malted, Soft Granary With Sesame Seeds, Waitrose*	1 Slice/40g	98	246	9.7	42.1	4.3	6.7
Medium Sliced, Bettabuy, Morrisons*	1 Slice/31g	66	212	8.6	42.0	1.3	3.6
Medium Sliced, Tesco*	1 Serving/72g	157	218	8.0	41.6	2.2	4.5
New Look, Weight Watchers*	1 Slice/12.2g	28	235	14.1	39.9	2.6	5.1
Original Wheatgerm, Medium Sliced, Hovis*	1 Slice/33g	77	233	10.8	40.1	3.3	3.7
Premium Gold Malted, TTD, Sainsbury's*	1 Slice/43g	93	217	8.5	40.3	2.4	2.4
Sainsbury's*	1 Slice/34g	81	239	8.4	46.8	2.1	4.2
Sliced, Medium, Asda*	1 Slice/36g	80	223	8.0	44.0	1.7	4.6
Soda, Marks & Spencer*	1 Slice/40g	92	229	9.2	43.6	3.6	4.9
Thick, Country Baked, Lidl*	1 Slice/38g	82	217	8.1	42.6	1.6	4.5
Toasted	1 Med Slice/24g	65	272	10.4	56.5	2.1	4.5
Weight Watchers*	1 Slice/12g	25	209	11.9	36.5	1.8	6.3
BREAD, CIABATTA,							
Black Olive, Part Baked, Sainsbury's*	¼ Ciabatta/67g	172	257	8.8	46.8	3.8	2.4
Black Olive, Ready To Bake, Sainsbury's*	¼ Ciabatta/66g	170	257	8.8	46.8	3.8	2.4
Chicken Tomato & Basil, Boots*	1 Pack/207g	499	241	11.0	20.0	13.0	3.0
Finest, Tesco*	¼ Ciabatta/70g	185	264	9.3	42.5	6.3	2.3

B

	Measure	per Measure		Nutrition Values per 100g / 100ml			
	INFO/WEIGHT	KCAL	KCAL	PROT	CARB	FAT	FIBRE

BREAD, CIABATTA,

	Measure	KCAL	KCAL	PROT	CARB	FAT	FIBRE
Garlic, Asda*	¼ Loaf/50g	173	345	9.5	41.6	15.6	1.1
Garlic, BGTY, Sainsbury's*	½ Ciabatta/105g	306	291	8.7	36.2	12.4	2.7
Garlic, Finest, Tesco*	1 Serving/65g	200	307	7.7	41.3	12.3	1.8
Garlic, Healthy Living, Tesco*	¼ Bread/60g	149	249	8.2	46.8	3.2	2.5
Garlic, Safeway*	½ Ciabatta/105g	279	266	6.1	38.6	9.7	1.7
Green Olive, Tesco*	¼ Loaf/70g	151	215	7.4	36.3	4.4	1.9
Half, Marks & Spencer*	1 Loaf/135g	354	262	10.3	48.1	4.1	2.1
Half, Organic, Sainsbury's*	½ Roll/63g	152	241	9.1	48.7	1.0	2.3
Half, TTD, Sainsbury's*	½ Ciabatta/133g	346	260	8.9	47.7	3.7	2.2
Italian Garlic, Sainsbury's*	1 Serving/145g	454	313	10.0	41.6	11.8	2.9
Italian Style, Flutes, The Best, Safeway*	1 Flute/125g	319	255	8.8	47.2	3.5	2.2
Italian Style, Safeway*	¼ Loaf/75g	194	258	8.9	47.7	3.5	2.2
Marks & Spencer*	1 Ciabatta/130g	341	262	10.3	48.1	4.1	2.1
Organic, Marks & Spencer*	1oz/28g	59	209	7.8	42.5	0.9	1.9
Organic, Tesco*	1/3 Loaf/100g	240	240	7.6	44.7	3.4	2.1
Part Baked, Half, Sainsbury's*	½ Ciabatta/67g	174	260	8.9	47.7	3.7	2.2
Plain, Tesco*	1 Serving/100g	260	260	8.7	42.8	6.0	2.1
Ready To Bake, Marks & Spencer*	1 Serving/150g	393	262	10.3	48.1	4.1	2.1
Ready To Bake, Sainsbury's*	½ Ciabatta/66g	172	260	8.9	47.7	3.7	2.2
Spicy Topped Topped, Finest, Tesco*	1 Serving/73g	163	223	9.2	34.0	5.5	1.7
Sun Dried Tomato & Basil, Tesco*	¼ Loaf/75g	193	257	8.9	42.4	5.7	2.4
Sun Dried Tomato, Safeway*	1 Serving/127g	375	295	8.8	46.6	8.3	2.8
Tomato & Basil, Good For You, Asda*	1 Serving/55g	143	260	9.0	51.0	2.2	0.0
Tomato & Mozzarella, Iceland*	1 Ciabatta/150g	374	249	10.0	29.6	10.1	3.3
With Garlic & Herb Butter, Sainsbury's*	½ Loaf/105g	345	329	8.5	38.8	15.5	0.0
BREAD, COUNTRY GRAIN, COU, Marks & Spencer*	1 Slice/25g	58	233	11.0	42.8	2.0	5.6
BREAD, CRUSTY LOAF, Harvest Blend, Warburton's*	1 Slice/28.6g	64	220	11.3	37.4	2.8	4.3
BREAD, FARMHOUSE LOAF, Hovis*	1 Slice/44g	100	228	9.0	44.6	1.5	2.3

BREAD, FOCACCIA,

	Measure	KCAL	KCAL	PROT	CARB	FAT	FIBRE
Garlic & Herb, Italian Style, Morrisons*	1/6 Focaccia/76g	259	341	8.5	44.7	14.3	2.5
Garlic & Herb, Safeway*	1/6 Focaccia /50g	154	308	9.1	42.9	11.1	2.1
Garlic & Onion, Good for You, Asda*	¼ Focaccia/55g	150	272	12.0	47.0	4.0	0.0
Garlic Butter & Rosemary, Sainsbury's*	¼ Focaccia/75g	219	292	8.0	43.0	9.8	2.8
Mini, Sun Dried Tomato & Basil, Sainsbury's*	1oz/28g	90	321	8.0	41.8	13.6	0.0
Onion & Herb, Tesco*	½ Pack/190g	547	288	8.7	35.2	12.5	3.7
Safeway*	1/6 Slice/47g	131	279	9.5	46.9	5.9	3.4
Sun Dried Tomato & Cheese, Marks & Spencer*	½ Focaccia/111g	316	285	9.7	40.4	9.6	3.2
BREAD, FOUGASSE, Caramelised Onion & Cheese, Tesco*	1oz/28g	80	284	11.1	43.1	6.3	3.5

BREAD, FRENCH

	Measure	KCAL	KCAL	PROT	CARB	FAT	FIBRE
Average	2" Stick/40g	108	270	9.6	55.4	2.7	1.5
Part Baked For Home Baking, Budgens*	1 Stick/200g	526	263	8.4	54.8	1.2	2.3
Safeway*	1/5 Slice/41g	110	268	9.8	58.5	0.5	2.4

BREAD, FRUIT

	Measure	KCAL	KCAL	PROT	CARB	FAT	FIBRE
& Cinnamon Loaf, Finest, Tesco*	1 Slice/37g	134	363	6.4	54.6	13.2	1.5
Loaf, Apple & Cinnamon, Soreen*	1 Serving/10g	31	307	6.9	60.5	4.2	0.0
Loaf, Apple, Marks & Spencer*	1 Slice/39.2g	99	255	8.5	51.9	1.5	3.3
Loaf, Asda*	1 Slice/16g	45	280	8.0	54.0	3.5	2.1
Loaf, Banana, Soreen*	1 Slice/25g	78	313	6.8	60.9	4.7	0.0
Loaf, Co-Op*	1 Slice/36g	97	270	10.0	51.0	3.0	1.0
Loaf, Rich, Soreen*	1/10 Loaf/30g	93	310	7.4	60.7	4.1	0.0
Loaf, Sliced, Sainsbury's*	1 Slice/40g	104	260	8.9	47.9	3.6	2.4
Loaf, Sliced, Tesco*	1 Slice/27g	66	246	8.2	46.7	2.9	2.6
Loaf, With Orange, Warburton's*	1 Slice/33.3g	89	270	7.9	51.7	3.5	3.0

	Measure	per Measure	Nutrition Values per 100g / 100ml				
	INFO/WEIGHT	KCAL	KCAL	PROT	CARB	FAT	FIBRE

BREAD, FRUIT

	Measure	per Measure KCAL	KCAL	PROT	CARB	FAT	FIBRE
Raisin Swirl, Sun-Maid*	1 Slice/33.1g	95	287	8.3	50.4	5.8	2.6

BREAD, GARLIC

	Measure	per Measure KCAL	KCAL	PROT	CARB	FAT	FIBRE
25% Less Fat, Sainsbury's*	½ Baguette/85g	268	315	7.8	39.4	14.0	3.1
30% Less Fat, Morrisons*	1 Serving/80g	226	283	5.9	41.1	10.8	1.9
& Herb, Giant Feast, Sainsbury's*	1 Serving/50g	159	317	8.0	42.1	12.9	2.6
Asda*	½ Baguette/85g	302	355	7.6	39.4	18.6	2.0
Baguette, 50% Less Fat, Asda*	¼ Baguette/43g	126	294	9.2	45.8	8.2	1.3
Baguette, Asda*	¼ Baguette/42g	158	375	8.9	43.3	18.5	1.2
Baguette, BGTY, Sainsbury's*	1oz/28g	93	333	9.1	49.9	12.6	2.4
Baguette, Co-Op*	½ Baguette/80g	308	385	9.0	47.0	18.0	2.0
Baguette, Extra Strong, Sainsbury's*	½ Baguette/85g	278	327	8.4	40.0	14.8	3.4
Baguette, Frozen, Lidl*	1 Baguette/175g	555	317	7.6	44.7	12.0	0.0
Baguette, GFY, Asda *	¼ Baguette/42.5g	120	280	9.0	43.0	8.0	2.0
Baguette, Good Choice, Iceland*	1/3 Stick/54g	158	292	8.7	45.1	8.5	2.9
Baguette, Good Intentions, Somerfield*	½ Baguette/85g	209	246	7.0	37.8	7.4	1.6
Baguette, Healthy Eating, Tesco*	1 Serving/42g	111	264	8.0	41.1	7.5	2.6
Baguette, Iceland*	1 Serving/85g	302	355	7.5	38.2	19.1	1.8
Baguette, Italiano, Tesco*	1 Slice/19g	63	334	7.1	43.8	14.5	2.2
Baguette, Morrisons*	½ Baguette/95g	295	311	6.3	37.8	15.0	1.5
Baguette, Reduced Fat, Healthy Choice, Safeway*	½ Baguette/92g	306	333	7.3	45.4	13.6	2.1
Baguette, Sainsbury's*	1 Serving/50g	196	391	8.9	48.6	19.2	2.3
Baguette, Slices, Tesco*	1 Serving/35g	109	312	9.8	33.8	15.3	1.7
Baguette, Tesco*	1 Slice/19g	67	355	7.6	39.4	18.6	2.0
Baguette, Value, Asda*	½ Baguette/85g	252	297	9.0	47.0	8.0	1.6
Baguette, White, Homebake, Tesco*	3rd Baguette/55g	160	290	7.0	43.1	10.0	1.9
BGTY, Sainsbury's*	1 Serving/40g	126	315	7.8	39.4	14.0	3.1
Caramelised, TTD, Sainsbury's*	¼ Bread/75g	218	290	9.8	41.5	9.4	3.0
Finest, Tesco*	¼ Loaf/60g	187	311	7.7	40.3	13.2	1.8
Flatbread, BGTY, Sainsbury's*	¼ Bread/56g	177	316	9.6	46.6	10.1	2.7
Flatbread, Tesco*	1 Serving/82.5g	251	302	6.7	45.3	10.4	3.0
Good Choice, Iceland*	1 Slice/40g	156	389	7.7	43.9	22.8	0.0
Good For You, Asda*	1 Slice/31g	104	337	11.0	53.0	9.0	1.1
Homebake, Tesco*	1 Serving/60g	209	348	7.1	33.7	20.5	1.5
Italian Style Stone Baked, Morrisons*	½ Pack/115g	420	365	7.9	40.4	19.1	1.9
Marks & Spencer*	1 Slice/20g	76	380	7.5	39.5	21.6	1.0
Micro, McCain*	½ Bread/54g	202	374	7.8	45.1	18.0	0.0
Organic, Waitrose*	1 Baguette/170g	536	315	8.7	39.1	13.7	1.8
Pizza Bread, Co-Op*	1 Pizza/240g	756	315	8.0	41.0	13.0	2.0
Pizza, Domino's Pizza*	1 Slice/40g	115	295	12.0	41.4	9.0	2.3
Pizza Express*	1 Serving/100g	278	278	7.5	43.0	9.9	0.0
Pizza Hut*	1 Slice/24g	101	419	8.7	48.1	21.3	2.7
Reduced Fat, Waitrose*	1 Pack/170g	551	324	6.9	49.4	11.0	0.9
Safeway*	¼ Baguette/72g	242	336	8.2	45.9	13.3	2.7
Slices, BGTY, Sainsbury's*	1 Slice/27g	82	305	9.4	48.9	8.0	2.9
Slices, Farmfoods*	1oz/28g	106	379	8.8	37.9	21.4	3.3
Slices, Good For You, Asda*	1 Slice/31g	104	337	11.0	53.0	9.0	1.1
Slices, Healthy Living, Tesco*	1 Slice/52g	129	249	7.9	43.9	4.6	1.7
Slices, Morrisons*	1 Slice/30g	76	254	6.8	36.5	9.0	1.5
Slices, Safeway*	1 Slice/27g	105	388	8.8	37.5	22.5	1.8
Slices, Sainsbury's*	1 Slice/25g	108	433	8.5	39.2	26.9	2.3
Stonebake, Marks & Spencer*	1 Loaf/85g	242	285	8.1	41.7	9.4	1.1
To Share, Marks & Spencer*	¼ Loaf/82.1g	230	280	6.5	33.2	13.0	1.3
With Cheese, Asda*	1 Slice/34g	130	382	11.0	44.0	18.0	0.0

B

	Measure INFO/WEIGHT	per Measure KCAL	Nutrition Values per 100g / 100ml				
			KCAL	PROT	CARB	FAT	FIBRE
BREAD, GINGER,							
Organic, Sunnyvale*	1oz/28g	62	222	10.8	51.2	1.0	0.0
BREAD, GRANARY							
Average Granary	1 Slice/25g	59	235	9.3	46.3	2.7	4.3
COU, Marks & Spencer*	1 Slice/25g	62	246	11.7	45.1	2.1	5.7
Crusty, Farmhouse, Marks & Spencer*	1 Slice/50g	120	240	9.4	43.4	3.0	2.6
Hovis*	1 Slice/35g	79	225	9.1	42.7	2.0	3.3
Malted, Medium Brown, Asda*	1 Slice/35g	81	231	9.0	43.0	2.6	3.3
New, Hovis*	1 Slice/44g	101	229	9.0	42.2	2.6	3.3
Waitrose*	1 Slice/40g	88	220	9.4	39.9	2.5	4.3
BREAD, HI BRAN,							
Marks & Spencer*	1 Slice/26.2g	55	210	12.6	32.5	3.0	6.3
Medium Sliced, Allinson*	1 Slice/34g	72	212	13.2	33.6	2.8	8.0
BREAD, IRISH							
Barm Brack, Tesco*	1 Serving/75g	233	310	16.0	47.6	6.9	3.0
Brown Soda, Tesco*	1 Serving/50g	110	219	9.2	36.2	3.8	6.4
Brown, Ormo*	1 Serving/100g	229	229	9.2	43.6	3.6	4.9
Brown, Soda, Sainsbury's*	1 Serving/100g	208	208	8.8	36.4	3.0	5.3
Cottage Wheaten, Tesco*	1 Serving/40g	79	198	9.1	35.4	1.9	6.1
BREAD, ITALIAN STYLE							
Pesto, TTD Sainsbury's*	¼ Bread/99g	247	249	9.1	39.4	6.1	4.4
Red Pepper, Safeway*	1 Serving/80g	184	230	9.1	42.2	2.3	2.1
Cheese & Garlic, Morrisons*	½ Pack/135g	431	319	10.8	45.1	10.6	2.1
BREAD, LIGHT GRAIN, Eat Smart, Safeway*	1 Slice/26.5g	66	245	9.7	45.5	2.5	3.5
BREAD, MALT LOAF,							
Fruit, Sainsbury's*	1oz/28g	86	308	7.9	63.8	2.4	2.4
Organic, Tesco*	1 Slice/28g	82	292	7.2	61.2	2.0	2.3
Ready Spread Snack, Soreen*	2 Slices/64g	220	344	6.4	57.0	10.0	3.0
Sticky, Marks & Spencer*	3 Slices/47.5g	139	295	6.9	64.9	2.3	3.1
Tesco*	1 Slice/50g	146	291	8.6	58.0	2.7	4.8
Value, Tesco*	1 Slice/25g	72	289	8.9	60.2	1.4	3.3
BREAD, MALTED							
Brown, Granary, Medium Sliced, Hovis*	1 Slice/35g	79	225	9.1	42.7	2.0	3.3
Brown, Hovis*	1 Slice/36g	82	229	9.0	42.2	2.6	3.3
Brown, Kingsmill*	1 slice/44g	103	234	9.4	43.4	2.5	2.7
Brown, Morrisons*	1 Slice/38g	96	253	10.3	49.9	1.4	3.1
Brown, Slice, BGTY, Sainsbury's*	1 Slice/22g	53	239	12.1	41.4	2.8	5.8
Brown, TTD, Sainsbury's*	1 Slice/44g	103	234	8.8	42.9	3.0	3.1
Brown, Thick Sliced, Organic, Tesco*	1 Slice/44g	116	264	7.8	53.8	2.0	3.3
Danish, Nimble*	1 Slice/22g	49	222	8.3	43.7	1.6	5.3
Grain, Co-Op*	1 Slice/43g	99	230	8.4	46.0	2.0	3.0
Oat, Duchy Originals*	1 Serving/80g	195	244	8.8	43.6	3.8	3.7
Wheat Country, Kingsmill Gold*	1 Slice/41g	96	234	9.4	43.4	2.5	2.7
Wheat Loaf, Thick Sliced, Village Green, Aldi*	1 Slice/38g	96	253	10.3	49.9	1.4	3.1
Wheat, Eat Smart, Safeway*	1 Slice/26g	60	230	10.0	42.8	1.8	5.3
Wheat, Gold, Kingsmill*	1 Slice/45g	108	240	9.8	43.8	2.9	3.6
Wheat, The Best, Safeway*	1 Slice/44g	103	235	9.1	45.6	1.8	4.7
Crusty, Sainsbury's*	1 Slice/42.1g	109	259	8.6	48.6	3.3	4.4
Danish, Sliced, Warburton's*	1 Slice/19g	41	218	10.2	41.3	1.4	6.9
Danish, Weight Watchers*	1 Slice/19g	41	218	10.2	41.3	1.4	6.9
Floury Batch, Sainsbury's*	1 Roll/68g	190	280	8.7	51.6	4.3	4.2
Wheat Loaf, Crusty, Finest, Tesco*	1 Slice/50g	115	230	9.8	44.2	1.5	4.4
BREAD, MEDITERRANEAN							
Olive, Waitrose*	1 Slice/30g	82	273	7.4	40.1	9.2	4.9

B

	Measure INFO/WEIGHT	per Measure KCAL	Nutrition Values per 100g / 100ml				
			KCAL	PROT	CARB	FAT	FIBRE
BREAD, MEDITERRANEAN							
Style Seed, Safeway*	1 Slice/25g	65	259	11.4	37.2	7.2	9.1
BREAD, MULTIGRAIN,							
Bakers Choice, Marks & Spencer*	1 Slice/25g	61	242	13.4	33.7	6.0	6.4
Batch, Finest, Tesco*	1 Slice/50g	127	254	9.8	47.7	2.7	4.2
Gluten Free, Sainsbury's*	1 Slice/17g	39	229	5.1	40.8	5.0	5.6
Sliced Loaf, Gluten-Free, Dietary Specials*	2 Slices/66.4g	151	229	5.1	40.8	5.1	5.6
Soft Batch, Sainsbury's*	1 Slice/44g	106	242	11.3	34.5	6.5	5.6
TTD, Sainsbury's*	1 Slice/44g	106	242	10.2	35.9	6.4	5.3
Tesco*	1 Slice/31g	66	214	11.1	36.8	3.2	8.9
Thick Sliced, Tesco*	1 Slice/50g	113	225	8.4	42.2	2.5	3.9
BREAD, NAAN							
Average Naan	1 Naan/160g	538	336	8.9	50.1	12.5	1.9
Co-Op*	1oz/28g	60	216	7.7	36.9	4.2	1.3
Fresh, BGTY, Sainsbury's*	1 Serving/150g	368	245	9.4	44.9	3.1	2.2
Fresh, Sharwood's*	1oz/28g	70	251	7.3	48.0	3.3	2.0
Garlic & Coriander, Asda*	½ Naan/74g	260	352	7.0	45.0	16.0	2.3
Garlic & Coriander, Fresh, Sharwood's*	1oz/28g	71	252	7.7	47.8	3.3	2.2
Garlic & Coriander, Mini, Asda*	1 Naan/49.7g	165	330	7.0	44.0	14.0	1.2
Garlic & Coriander, Mini, Long Life, Sharwood's*	1oz/28g	71	255	7.4	45.3	4.9	2.3
Garlic & Coriander, Mini, Sainsbury's*	1 Naan/50g	148	295	8.6	44.2	9.3	3.7
Garlic & Coriander, Mini, Sharwood's*	1 Naan/59g	144	244	7.1	46.2	3.4	2.0
Garlic & Coriander, Mini, Tesco*	1 Naan/60g	178	296	7.6	47.0	8.6	2.5
Garlic & Coriander, Tesco*	1 Naan/150g	374	249	7.1	36.5	8.3	2.1
Indian Style, Lidl*	1 Naan/140g	332	237	8.7	44.2	2.5	0.0
Indian Style, Mini, Asda*	1 Mini Naan/50g	152	304	8.0	50.0	8.0	2.8
Keema Filled, Mini, Indian Takeaway, Safeway*	1 Naan/23g	58	253	10.1	38.3	6.6	2.1
King Prawn, Marks & Spencer*	1 Serving/185g	360	195	9.1	25.3	6.3	2.5
Long Life, Sharwood's*	1oz/28g	72	258	7.3	45.8	5.1	2.0
Marks & Spencer*	1 Bread/84g	260	310	12.0	43.8	9.8	2.1
Mini, Asda*	1 Serving/100g	304	304	8.0	50.0	8.0	2.8
Mini, Plain, Tesco*	1 Naan/60g	175	292	9.3	47.6	7.2	2.5
Mini, Sainsbury's*	1 Serving/50g	157	314	8.7	41.5	12.4	4.3
Northern Indian,, Sainsbury's*	1 Serving/125.3g	356	285	8.7	45.9	7.4	1.9
Onion & Mint, Marks & Spencer*	½ Naan/135g	351	260	8.9	35.8	8.7	2.5
Onion Bhaji, Sharwood's*	1 Pack/130g	378	291	7.3	48.4	7.6	2.2
Peshwari, Fresh, Sharwood's*	1oz/28g	67	240	6.8	41.9	5.0	2.5
Peshwari, Long Life, Sharwood's*	1oz/28g	71	252	6.2	42.0	6.6	2.6
Peshwari, Marks & Spencer*	1 Serving/127g	394	310	9.2	45.8	10.1	1.9
Peshwari, Tesco*	1 Naan/215.0g	544	253	6.8	38.8	7.8	3.0
Plain, Mini, Asda*	1 Nann/50g	144	288	7.0	47.0	8.0	1.5
Plain, Mini, Fresh, Sharwood's*	1oz/28g	70	251	7.3	48.0	3.3	2.0
Plain, Mini, Tesco*	1 Serving/60g	158	263	7.5	43.9	6.4	2.1
Plain, Nisa Heritage*	1 Naan/150g	401	267	9.0	44.2	6.2	1.9
Plain, Original, Mild, Patak's*	1 Serving/130g	399	307	9.5	48.0	8.6	0.0
Plain, Sainsbury's*	½ Naan/74.9g	209	279	7.3	46.7	7.0	2.7
Plain, Sharwood's*	1 Bread/120g	294	245	10.1	43.1	3.6	3.4
Plain, Tesco*	1 Naan/150g	429	286	7.8	47.6	7.2	2.5
Plain, Value, Tesco*	1 Naan/135g	363	269	8.1	42.9	7.2	1.6
Plain, Waitrose*	1 Naan/144.8g	473	326	7.2	49.9	10.8	2.4
Safeway*	1 Naan/120g	346	288	8.4	51.4	5.4	2.6
Tandoori, Large, The Bombay Brasserie, London*	1 Lge Naan/110g	270	245	10.1	43.1	3.6	3.4
Tandoori, Sharwood's*	1 Bread/130g	330	254	7.3	45.0	5.0	2.0
BREAD, OAT, Waitrose*	1oz/28g	71	253	8.5	44.9	4.4	3.6

B

Measure INFO/WEIGHT	per Measure KCAL	Nutrition Values per 100g / 100ml				
		KCAL	PROT	CARB	FAT	FIBRE

BREAD, OATMEAL,

	Measure	per Measure KCAL	KCAL	PROT	CARB	FAT	FIBRE
Batch, Tesco*	1 Slice/50g	135	269	9.3	50.1	3.5	4.0
Farmhouse, Soft, Marks & Spencer*	1 Slice/45g	110	245	11.1	39.5	4.4	5.2
Sliced Loaf, Tesco*	1 Slice/50g	111	222	7.4	40.5	3.4	2.8
BREAD, OLIVE, Waitrose*	1 Slice/28g	86	306	9.0	43.6	10.6	2.0
BREAD, PETIT PAIN,							
Harvester, Somerfield*	1 Serving/70g	188	269	10.6	52.2	2.0	3.2
Homebake Mini, Tesco*	1 Roll/50g	118	235	7.8	49.1	0.8	1.2
Homebake, Mini, Tesco*	1 Serving/50g	118	235	7.8	49.1	0.8	0.0
Organic, Tesco*	1 Roll/100g	235	235	7.8	49.1	0.8	1.2
Ready To Bake, Sainsbury's*	1 Petit Pain/44g	132	299	9.4	61.6	1.7	3.2
Waitrose*	1 Roll/69g	190	275	9.3	55.9	1.6	3.1
White, Soft Bake, Somerfield*	1 Roll/70g	174	248	9.2	49.9	1.3	1.8
BREAD, PITTA							
Pockets, Sainsbury's*	1 Serving/75g	188	250	8.5	52.0	1.0	3.5
Brown, Organic, Waitrose*	1 Pitta/61g	138	226	6.4	47.5	1.4	6.6
Cypriana Supreme*	1oz/28g	67	239	8.5	48.6	1.2	0.0
Garlic & Coriander, Asda*	1 Bread/57g	149	261	8.0	53.0	1.9	0.0
Garlic & Herb, Tesco*	1 Pitta/56g	138	246	8.4	50.3	1.2	2.1
Garlic, Co-Op*	1 Pitta/63g	161	255	9.0	53.0	1.0	2.0
Garlic, Morrisons*	1 Pitta/60g	149	249	9.7	51.1	1.8	0.0
Garlic, Sainsbury's*	1 Pitta/60g	153	255	9.5	52.0	1.0	2.5
Iceland*	1 Pitta/50g	126	251	8.6	50.0	1.8	2.3
Mexican, Santa Maria*	1 Pitta/66g	165	250	7.5	52.0	1.0	0.0
Mini, Marks & Spencer*	1 Pitta/13g	34	260	9.2	52.1	2.4	1.8
Mini, Sainsbury's*	1 Pitta/30g	75	249	10.3	49.3	1.2	3.5
Organic, Tesco*	1 Pitta/60g	124	206	8.3	40.2	1.4	5.7
Sesame, Sainsbury's*	1 Pitta/59g	156	264	9.8	50.8	2.4	3.1
Somerfield*	1 Pitta/56g	141	251	8.6	50.0	1.8	2.3
Tesco*	1oz/28g	69	247	8.4	50.7	1.2	2.6
Value, Tesco*	1oz/28g	64	227	6.0	48.8	0.9	2.0
White	1 Pitta/75g	199	265	9.2	57.9	1.2	2.2
White Picnic, Waitrose*	1 Pitta/30g	75	249	10.3	49.3	1.2	3.5
White, Asda*	1 Pitta/56g	141	252	9.0	50.0	1.8	2.3
White, Co-Op*	1 Pitta/63g	151	240	10.0	47.0	1.0	3.0
White, Greek Style, Asda*	1 Pitta/50g	127	253	8.0	51.0	1.9	0.0
White, Iceland*	1 Pitta/50g	126	251	8.6	50.0	1.8	2.3
White, Marks & Spencer*	1 Pitta/61g	156	255	8.9	51.6	2.4	0.0
White, Mini, Safeway*	1 Pitta/54g	119	220	8.0	49.4	1.2	1.9
White, Mini, Sainsbury's*	1 Pitta/31g	88	285	9.8	58.0	1.5	3.5
White, Safeway*	1 Pitta/54g	119	220	8.0	49.4	1.2	1.9
White, Sainsburys*	1 Pittta/59g	151	256	9.5	52.0	1.1	2.3
White, Somerfield*	1 Pitta/55.8g	141	251	8.6	50.0	1.8	2.3
White, Tesco*	1 Pitta/56g	147	262	10.1	51.2	1.9	2.6
White, Waitrose*	1 Pitta/60g	149	249	10.3	49.3	1.2	3.5
Wholemeal, Arnaouti*	1 Pitta/88.5g	199	226	11.5	43.0	1.7	7.2
Wholemeal, Asda*	1 Pitta/56g	128	229	11.0	41.0	2.3	0.0
Wholemeal, Healthy Eating, Co-Op*	1 Pitta/63g	135	215	12.0	37.0	2.0	9.0
Wholemeal, Marks & Spencer*	1 Pitta/60.9g	140	230	10.7	40.6	2.8	7.2
Wholemeal, Morrisons*	1 Pitta/60g	135	225	11.9	46.4	2.0	0.0
Wholemeal, Safeway*	1 Pitta/54g	125	232	9.7	44.2	1.9	6.5
Wholemeal, Sainsbury's*	1 Pitta/59g	146	247	12.4	46.0	1.5	5.3
Wholemeal, Somerfield*	1 Pitta/55.9g	127	227	10.6	41.0	2.3	6.2
Wholemeal, Tesco*	1 Pitta/60g	151	251	11.9	46.4	2.0	6.6

	Measure INFO/WEIGHT	per Measure KCAL	Nutrition Values per 100g / 100ml				
			KCAL	PROT	CARB	FAT	FIBRE
BREAD, PITTA							
Wholemeal, Tesco*	1 Pitta/62g	138	222	9.1	42.5	1.7	5.8
Wholemeal, Waitrose*	1 Pitta/60g	151	251	11.3	53.4	0.6	0.0
BREAD, POTATO & Rosemary, Tesco*	1oz/28g	67	241	8.2	42.0	4.5	2.2
BREAD, PUMPERNICKEL Rye, Kelderman*	1 Slice/50g	93	185	6.0	38.0	1.0	0.0
BREAD, PUMPKIN Seed, Raisin & Sunflower, Sainsbury's*	1 Slice/30g	77	255	11.6	45.9	2.8	3.4
BREAD, RAISIN							
& Pumpkin Seed, Organic, Tesco*	1 Slice/30g	76	253	9.7	40.6	5.8	3.8
Loaf With Cinnamon, Warburton's*	1 Slice/33g	91	276	7.5	52.9	3.8	4.2
BREAD, ROASTED ONION, Marks & Spencer*	1 Slice/50g	125	250	9.0	46.7	3.3	2.1
BREAD, ROLLS,							
American Style Deli, Tesco*	1 Roll/65g	162	249	7.8	46.8	3.4	1.6
Batched Sandwich, Warburton's*	1 Roll/60g	148	246	9.6	42.7	4.1	0.0
Best of Both, Hovis*	1 Roll/29g	68	235	9.8	39.5	4.2	4.2
Blackpool Milk, Warburton's*	1 Slice/18g	45	251	10.8	45.3	3.0	2.8
Brown, Crusty	1 Roll/50g	128	255	10.3	50.4	2.8	3.5
Brown, Large, Asda*	1 Roll/57g	138	242	10.0	47.0	1.6	0.0
Brown, Malted Grain, Somerfield*	1 Roll/60g	147	245	8.7	45.2	3.2	3.0
Brown, Malted Grain, Tesco*	1 Roll/58g	142	244	8.7	45.1	3.2	1.9
Brown, Morning, Farmfoods*	1 Roll/50g	135	269	12.0	47.0	3.7	4.2
Brown, Soft	1 Roll/50g	134	268	10.0	51.8	3.8	3.5
Brown, Soft, Marks & Spencer*	1 Roll/45.7g	106	230	8.7	44.0	2.2	5.2
Brown, Soft, Somerfield*	1oz/28g	68	243	9.0	42.0	3.0	0.0
Brown, Soft, Tesco*	1 Roll/50g	118	235	9.0	41.6	3.6	4.5
Cheese Topped, Village Green*	1 Roll/56g	159	284	13.1	41.2	7.4	4.8
Ciabatta, Best, Safeway*	1 Serving/100g	211	211	7.3	39.1	2.9	1.8
Ciabatta, Finest, Tesco*	1 Roll/45g	93	206	7.7	33.5	4.6	2.3
Ciabatta, Marks & Spencer*	1 Roll/80g	210	262	10.3	48.1	4.1	2.1
Ciabatta, Ready To Bake, Sainsbury's*	1 Roll/75g	198	264	9.1	48.9	3.6	2.3
Ciabatta, Ready to Bake, TTD, Sainsbury's*	1 Roll/72g	187	260	8.9	47.7	3.7	2.2
Ciabatta, Tesco*	1 Serving/75g	200	267	9.0	44.0	6.1	2.1
Crisp, Original, Organic, Kallo*	1 Roll/8.7g	35	390	11.0	74.0	5.6	3.0
Crusty, French, Marks & Spencer*	1 Roll/65g	159	245	8.1	50.5	1.2	3.3
Crusty, Part-Baked, Budgens*	1 Roll/50g	148	296	9.4	61.4	1.4	2.5
Finger, Morrisons*	1 Roll/46g	119	259	10.7	50.0	1.8	2.3
Finger, Sainsbury's*	1 Roll/40g	102	256	10.3	47.9	2.6	2.4
For Hamburgers	1 Roll/50g	132	264	9.1	48.8	5.0	1.5
Granary Malted Wheatgrain, Soft, Marks & Spencer*	1 Roll/80g	208	260	9.3	47.2	3.9	2.3
Granary, Bakers Premium, Tesco*	1 Roll/65g	158	243	9.9	47.8	1.3	2.3
Granary, Waitrose*	1 Roll/59g	160	271	10.0	47.2	6.4	3.8
Green Olive, Marks & Spencer*	1 Roll/75g	210	280	11.2	44.0	6.0	1.8
Hot Dog, Farmfoods*	1 Roll/53g	125	235	8.1	47.0	1.7	2.2
Hot Dog, Sliced, Asda*	1 Roll/84g	197	234	7.0	44.0	3.3	0.0
Hot Dog, Tesco*	1 Roll/85g	200	235	7.3	44.0	3.3	1.9
Lidl*	1 Roll/75g	209	279	11.0	51.0	3.0	2.3
Malted Grain Submarine, Marks & Spencer*	1 Serving/109.1g	300	275	8.9	53.6	4.3	3.0
Malted Grain, Soft, Weight Watchers*	1 Roll/42g	95	226	9.8	42.2	2.0	4.5
Malted Wheat & Poppy Seed, Safeway*	1 Roll/54g	140	260	10.6	48.7	2.8	3.4
Malted, Sainsbury's*	1 Roll/68g	190	280	8.7	51.6	4.3	4.2
Mini Submarine, Marks & Spencer*	1 Roll/23g	63	275	11.4	47.7	4.9	1.1
Morning Breakfast, Marks & Spencer*	1 Roll/55g	160	290	10.3	53.8	4.3	0.6
Morning, Tesco*	1 Roll/48g	117	243	10.4	44.8	2.5	4.7
Multigrain, Torpedo, Sainsbury's*	1 Roll/111.9g	328	293	10.5	47.7	6.7	6.3
Oatmeal, Soft, Marks & Spencer*	1 Roll/80g	224	280	12.3	43.4	6.4	2.7

B

BREAD, ROLLS,

	Measure INFO/WEIGHT	per Measure KCAL	Nutrition Values per 100g / 100ml				
			KCAL	PROT	CARB	FAT	FIBRE
Pain Raisin, Mini, Marks & Spencer*	1oz/28g	87	310	5.3	42.3	13.6	1.3
Panini, Marks & Spencer*	1 Roll/86g	211	245	8.3	39.3	6.2	1.6
Poppy Seeded Knot, Waitrose*	1 Roll/65g	179	275	9.3	55.9	1.6	3.1
Scottish, White, Tesco*	1 Roll/48g	117	243	10.4	44.8	2.5	4.7
Seeded, Sandwich, Warburton's*	1 Roll/77g	240	312	13.3	41.2	10.4	0.0
Snack, Mini, Tesco*	1 Roll/35g	95	271	19.0	43.0	6.0	4.0
Sun Dried Tomato, Homebake, Tesco*	1 Roll/50g	123	246	11.3	44.0	3.0	0.0
Sunflower Seed, Toasting, Good & Hot*	1 Roll/65g	163	250	8.5	41.0	5.0	8.0
White, BGTY, Sainsbury's*	1 Roll/50g	114	227	9.1	45.3	1.0	3.0
White, Basics, Somerfield*	1 Roll/44g	107	243	8.9	48.2	1.6	2.1
White, Cheese Topped, Asda*	1 Roll/46g	121	264	10.0	46.0	4.4	2.0
White, Cheese Topped, Sainsbury's*	1 Roll/75g	218	291	12.1	41.6	8.5	2.0
White, Co-Op*	1 Roll/55g	138	250	8.0	46.0	4.0	2.0
White, Crusty	1 Roll/50g	140	280	10.9	57.6	2.3	1.5
White, Deli Tesco*	1 Roll/65g	180	277	8.7	52.0	3.8	2.7
White, Finger, Co-Op*	1 Roll/46g	129	280	10.0	52.0	4.0	2.0
White, Finger, SmartPrice, Asda*	1 Roll/50g	121	242	9.0	48.0	1.6	2.1
White, Finger, Tesco*	1 Roll/50g	125	251	9.7	55.5	0.4	1.5
White, Finger, Waitrose*	1 Roll/49g	121	247	9.4	45.6	3.0	2.7
White, Floured, Warburton's*	1 Roll/50g	124	247	9.8	43.3	3.8	2.7
White, Floury Batch, Sainsbury's*	1 Roll/65g	167	257	8.7	46.6	4.0	3.1
White, Floury, Roberts*	1 Roll/63.0g	160	254	8.4	49.5	2.5	2.0
White, Hot Dog, Sainsbury's*	1 Roll/85g	235	277	7.3	48.8	5.8	2.4
White, Kingsmill*	1 Roll/60g	151	252	9.3	44.5	4.1	2.4
White, Low Price, Sainsbury's*	1 Roll/44g	107	243	8.9	48.2	1.6	2.1
White, Morning, Co-Op*	1 Roll/47g	134	285	12.0	53.0	3.0	2.0
White, Morning, Marks & Spencer*	1 Roll/50g	136	272	8.8	53.8	1.5	2.7
White, Old Fashioned, Waitrose*	1 Roll/57g	157	275	8.8	49.8	4.5	2.8
White, Organic, Sainsbury's*	1 Roll/65g	170	262	8.7	49.9	3.0	1.0
White, Ploughman's, Sainsbury's*	1 Roll/65g	185	285	8.6	54.1	3.8	2.3
White, Premium Soft, Rathbones*	1 Roll/65g	190	293	9.3	50.3	6.0	2.7
White, Savers, Safeway*	1 Roll/40g	113	283	10.4	54.6	1.8	20.0
White, Scottish, Morning, Safeway*	1 Roll/40g	113	283	10.4	56.4	1.8	1.6
White, Seeded, Sainsbury's*	1 Roll/80g	217	271	10.9	43.4	5.9	4.8
White, Seeded, Soft, Marks & Spencer*	1 Roll/72g	205	285	11.7	46.2	5.7	1.8
White, Smart Price, Asda*	1 Roll/44g	106	242	9.0	48.0	1.6	2.1
White, Snack, Sainsbury's*	1 Roll/67g	159	237	7.9	49.2	1.0	2.3
White, Soft	1 Roll/45g	121	268	9.2	51.6	4.2	1.5
White, Soft, Boulders, Hovis*	1 Roll/74g	206	279	11.0	51.5	3.0	2.3
White, Soft, COU, Marks & Spencer*	1 Roll/37g	94	255	10.7	47.1	2.7	1.5
White, Soft, Finger, Marks & Spencer*	1 Roll/64g	189	295	10.1	47.5	7.2	2.2
White, Soft, Marks & Spencer*	1 Roll/60g	150	250	10.3	45.2	3.1	2.7
White, Soft, Morrisons*	1 Roll/42g	100	238	9.1	46.4	1.9	2.4
White, Soft, Premium, Village Green, Aldi*	1 Roll/65g	168	259	8.3	47.5	4.0	1.9
White, Soft, Sandwich, Warburtons*	1 Roll/79g	209	264	11.0	45.0	4.4	0.0
White, Soft, Somerfield*	1 Roll/40g	104	260	10.0	48.0	3.0	0.0
White, Softgrain, Good For You, Asda*	1 Roll/54.0g	128	237	9.0	46.0	1.9	2.9
White, Split, Asda*	1 Roll/45g	113	251	10.0	45.0	3.4	2.8
White, Value, Tesco*	1 Roll/35g	81	231	8.0	45.7	1.8	2.3
White, Warburton's*	1 Roll/57g	141	248	9.7	42.8	4.2	0.0
Wholemeal	1 Roll 45g	108	241	9.0	48.3	2.9	5.9
Wholemeal With Cracked Wheat, Allinson*	1 Roll/58g	134	231	11.0	38.0	3.9	7.0
Wholemeal, Asda*	1 Roll/58g	131	225	11.0	39.0	2.8	6.0

INFO/WEIGHT	Measure per Measure KCAL	KCAL	Nutrition Values per 100g / 100ml PROT	CARB	FAT	FIBRE

BREAD, ROLLS,

	Measure INFO/WEIGHT	per Measure KCAL	KCAL	PROT	CARB	FAT	FIBRE
Wholemeal, Deli, With Cracked Wheat, Tesco*	1 Roll/65g	156	240	9.0	40.2	4.8	5.7
Wholemeal, Finger, Soft, Marks & Spencer*	1 Roll/60g	162	270	13.5	37.9	7.4	4.7
Wholemeal, Floury Batch, Sainsbury's*	1 Roll/68g	150	220	10.7	36.0	3.7	6.6
Wholemeal, Food Explorers, Waitrose*	1 Roll/32.0g	74	231	10.6	40.2	3.1	5.7
Wholemeal, Healthy Eating, Co-Op*	1 Roll/60g	141	235	13.0	37.0	4.0	8.0
Wholemeal, Healthy Eating, Tesco*	1 Roll/67g	135	202	8.9	37.4	1.9	7.0
Wholemeal, Kingsmill*	1 Roll/68g	167	245	10.7	41.5	4.0	5.1
Wholemeal, Milk, Warburton's*	1 Roll/22g	51	231	12.5	38.1	3.2	7.0
Wholemeal, Mini, Assorted, Waitrose*	1 Roll/35.6g	85	236	9.0	38.1	5.3	5.2
Wholemeal, Mini, Tesco*	1 Roll/34g	82	240	10.9	36.4	5.6	5.8
Wholemeal, Old Fashioned, Waitrose*	1 Roll/57g	135	236	11.1	37.2	4.8	6.6
Wholemeal, Organic, Sainsbury's*	1 Roll/66g	152	230	10.7	41.0	2.7	6.6
Wholemeal, Ploughman's, Sainsbury's*	1 Roll/65g	171	263	9.0	45.9	4.8	5.7
Wholemeal, Sandwich Warburton's*	1 Roll/58g	132	228	10.8	37.7	3.8	0.0
Wholemeal, Soft, Marks & Spencer*	1 Roll/55g	128	233	12.4	36.6	4.1	5.8
Wholemeal, Square, Hovis*	1 Roll/52g	118	227	11.1	36.3	4.2	6.1
Wholemeal, Sunflower & Honey, Sainsbury's*	1 Roll/85g	225	265	9.2	45.4	5.1	4.5
Wholemeal, Tasty, Kingsmill*	1 Roll/53g	125	236	10.7	39.2	4.0	7.4
Wholemeall With Jumbo Oat Fakes, Eat Smart, Safeway*	1 Roll/53g	125	235	10.6	41.8	2.8	6.2
Wholewhite, Kingsmill*	1 Roll/63g	158	251	9.5	43.7	4.2	3.5
Wholmeal, Deli, Tesco*	1 Roll/65g	156	240	9.0	40.2	4.8	5.7

BREAD, RYE

Average Rye	1 Slice/25g	55	219	8.3	45.8	1.7	4.4
With Sunflower Seeds, Organic, Sunnyvale*	1 Slice/25g	50	198	5.1	30.3	6.3	0.0
German Style, Kelderman*	1 Slice/62g	96	155	5.6	30.2	1.4	7.7
Organic, Waitrose*	1 Serving/100g	207	207	6.4	42.7	1.2	5.1
Swedish Style, Kelderman*	1 Slice/50g	93	185	7.2	31.5	3.2	4.3
BREAD, SCOTTISH Plain, Mothers Pride*	1oz/28g	64	227	8.7	44.6	1.5	3.0
BREAD, SFILATINO, Ready to Bake, TTD, Sainsbury's*	1 Sfilatino/125.9g	327	260	8.9	47.7	3.7	2.2

BREAD, SODA

Average Soda	1oz/28g	72	258	7.7	54.6	2.5	2.1
Farls, Marks & Spencer*	1 Farl/110g	267	243	9.6	50.1	2.7	2.3
Farls, Tesco*	1 Farl/142g	325	229	7.1	42.2	3.2	2.6

BREAD, SOFTGRAIN,

Farmhouse, Marks & Spencer*	1 Slice/25g	60	238	8.4	42.8	3.7	3.2
Medium Sliced, Good For You, Asda*	1 Slice/35g	79	226	7.0	46.0	1.5	3.7
Mighty White*	1 Slice/36g	81	224	7.2	45.5	1.5	3.7
Bread, Soya & Linseed, Burgen*	1 Slice/36g	89	246	14.7	29.5	7.7	5.6

BREAD, STROMBOLI,

Four Cheese & Sun Dried Tomato, Finest, Tesco*	1 Serving/67g	206	307	10.8	34.2	14.1	3.4
Sunblush Tomato Mozzarella & Basil, TTD, Sainsbury's*	1 Pack/300g	723	241	8.9	35.1	7.5	3.0

BREAD, SUBMARINE,

Malted Grain, Marks & Spencer*	1 Roll/109g	300	275	8.9	53.8	4.3	3.0
Sainsbury's*	1 Roll/117g	381	326	10.6	60.2	4.8	2.8

BREAD, SUNFLOWER

& Honey, Marks & Spencer*	1 Serving/67g	206	308	12.9	34.0	13.4	5.6
& Pumpin Seed, Batched, Organic, Tesco*	1 Slice/30g	73	243	11.0	33.1	7.4	5.2
BREAD, SUNNY, Hovis*	1 Slice/44g	110	250	8.2	41.5	5.7	2.0

BREAD, TOASTED,

Brown	1 Med Slice/30g	72	239	8.4	46.8	2.1	4.2
White	1 Med Slice/33g	79	238	7.5	48.5	1.6	1.8
Wholemeal	1 Med Slice/26g	58	224	8.6	42.3	2.2	5.8

B

	Measure INFO/WEIGHT	per Measure KCAL	Nutrition Values per 100g / 100ml				
			KCAL	PROT	CARB	FAT	FIBRE
BREAD, TOMATO							
& Garlic, Morrisons*	1 Serving/125g	271	217	5.9	31.4	7.6	2.5
Cheese & Olive, Sharing Bread, BGTY, Sainsbury's*	1 Serving/67g	168	250	9.8	43.4	4.1	2.5
BREAD, VEDA Malt, St Michael*	1 Serving/45g	99	219	7.1	45.3	1.1	2.2
BREAD, WALNUT, Waitrose*	1 Slice/33g	104	315	10.8	43.2	11.0	4.3
BREAD, WHEAT FREE, Organic, The Stamp Collection*	1 Slice/35g	66	188	6.5	39.5	0.4	0.4
BREAD, WHEATEN,							
Marks & Spencer*	1 Slice/33g	74	225	9.3	42.9	3.5	3.9
Sliced, Healthy, Irwin's*	2 Slices/80g	152	190	9.0	40.5	1.9	6.2
BREAD, WHEATGERM							
Brown, Original, Medium, Hovis*	1 Slice/33g	77	233	10.8	40.1	3.3	3.7
Thin Sliced, Hovis*	1 Slice/21g	47	222	10.1	38.5	3.0	4.6
BREAD, WHITE							
Average White	1 Slice/25g	59	235	8.4	49.3	1.9	1.5
Bakers Gold, Thick Sliced, Asda*	1 Slice/44g	103	233	8.0	46.0	1.9	2.2
COU, Marks & Spencer*	1 Slice/26g	60	231	10.6	41.9	2.3	4.6
Country Maid*	1 Slice/33.2g	76	229	8.5	44.1	2.1	3.0
Crusty, Gold, Kingsmill*	1 Slice/27g	70	258	9.4	48.5	2.9	2.7
Crusty, Hovis*	1 Slice/44g	103	233	8.8	44.3	2.2	2.1
Crusty, Sliced Loaf, Tesco*	1 Slice/50g	117	233	7.4	46.0	2.1	2.0
Crusty, Sliced, Finest, Tesco*	1 Slice/113g	255	226	9.5	44.3	1.2	2.7
Crusty, Sliced, Harvestime*	1 Slice/44g	98	222	6.6	45.6	1.5	1.9
Crusty, Sliced, Premium, Budgens*	1 Slice/50g	121	242	8.8	46.9	2.2	2.2
Danish, Medium Sliced, Morrisons*	1 Slice/17g	42	245	10.2	49.1	1.8	2.2
Danish, Soft & Light, Thick Cut, Asda*	1 Slice/26g	60	230	9.0	45.0	1.6	2.1
Danish, Tesco*	1 Slice/22g	56	254	9.4	49.7	1.9	2.8
Danish, Thick Sliced, Iceland*	1 Slice/22g	51	232	8.9	45.4	1.6	2.1
Danish, Thick Sliced, Tesco*	2 Slices/47g	105	223	7.4	45.3	1.3	2.6
Danish, Warburton's*	1 Slice/25g	61	243	10.7	46.9	1.4	2.7
Danish, Weight Watchers*	1 Slice/19g	42	222	8.7	43.9	1.3	2.8
Eat Smart, Safeway*	1 Slice/26g	60	230	8.8	45.0	1.8	2.3
Extra Thick Sliced, Kingsmill*	1 Slice/57g	132	232	8.8	43.8	2.4	2.8
Farmhouse Crusty, Marks & Spencer*	1 Slice/34g	85	250	8.8	48.0	2.6	2.3
Farmhouse Gold Premium, Morrisons*	1 Slice/38g	91	239	9.5	47.3	1.3	2.2
Farmhouse Soft, Warburton's*	1 Slice/26g	63	241	10.2	44.3	2.5	2.7
Farmhouse, Hovis	1 Slice/37g	84	228	9.0	44.6	1.5	2.3
Farmhouse, The Best, Safeway*	1 Slice/44.3g	104	237	8.4	47.5	1.5	3.1
Farmhouse, Waitrose*	1 Slice/40g	94	235	9.5	45.4	1.7	2.6
Fibre, Morrisons*	2 Slices/80g	192	240	8.0	48.4	1.7	0.3
Floury Batch, Sainsbury's*	1 Serving/62g	166	267	8.0	48.8	4.5	2.3
Fried in Blended Oil	1 Slice/28g	141	503	7.9	48.5	32.2	1.6
Gluten & Wheat Free, Free From, Sainsbury's*	1 Serving/70g	159	227	1.9	35.5	8.6	1.0
Gold Seeded, Kingsmill*	1 Slice/44g	108	245	9.7	38.8	5.7	3.5
Gold Toastie, Kingsmill*	1 Slice/44g	103	234	9.3	42.3	3.1	0.6
Good Health, Warburton's*	1 Slice/38g	84	220	9.4	41.6	1.8	4.1
Great, Hovis*	1 Slice/40g	90	226	8.8	44.4	1.5	2.2
Harvest Crust Premium, Ormo*	1 Slice/40g	92	229	9.4	47.4	1.5	2.7
Medium Sliced	1 Med Slice/39g	93	238	7.5	48.5	1.6	1.8
Medium Sliced, 7 Days Fresh, Kingsmill*	1 Slice/38.1g	88	231	8.1	44.3	2.4	2.8
Medium Sliced, Asda*	1 Slice/37g	84	226	7.0	46.0	1.5	2.8
Medium Sliced, BGTY, Sainsbury's*	1 Slice/20g	45	225	10.2	43.9	0.9	4.6
Medium Sliced, Brace's*	1 Slice/31.7g	73	227	9.6	43.4	1.7	2.2
Medium Sliced, Budgens*	1 Slice/35.8g	82	229	8.0	45.6	1.6	3.0
Medium Sliced, Co-Op*	1 Slice/36g	83	230	8.0	46.0	2.0	2.0

BREAD, WHITE

INFO/WEIGHT	Measure per Measure	KCAL	Nutrition Values per 100g / 100ml KCAL	PROT	CARB	FAT	FIBRE
Medium Sliced, Economy, Sainsbury's*	1 Slice/44g	104	236	7.6	48.6	1.3	1.8
Medium Sliced, Hovis*	1 Slice/35g	78	223	8.4	44.5	1.2	2.0
Medium Sliced, Keep Fresh, Safeway*	1 Slice/34g	76	224	7.3	44.3	1.9	2.7
Medium Sliced, Kingsmill*	1 Slice/38g	89	233	8.8	44.1	2.4	2.5
Medium Sliced, Long Life, Asda*	1 Slice/36g	82	228	8.0	45.0	1.8	2.7
Medium Sliced, Longer Life, Co-Op*	1 Slice/44g	99	225	8.0	45.0	2.0	2.0
Medium Sliced, Longerlife, Sainsbury's*	1 Slice/36g	87	243	8.3	47.6	2.2	1.7
Medium Sliced, Makes Sense, Somerfield*	1 Slice/36.3g	81	226	7.5	46.4	1.2	2.4
Medium Sliced, Marks & Spencer*	1 Slice/35g	81	230	7.4	45.9	1.7	2.4
Medium Sliced, Mother's Pride*	1 Slice/36g	82	229	8.0	45.6	1.6	3.0
Medium Sliced, New Look, Weight Watchers*	1 Slice/12.2g	30	247	12.5	45.2	1.9	3.2
Medium Sliced, Nimble*	1 Slice/20g	46	232	9.7	44.3	1.8	2.9
Medium Sliced, Sainsbury's*	1 Slice/36g	83	231	8.0	46.4	1.5	2.1
Medium Sliced, SmartPrice, Asda*	1 Slice/36g	81	226	7.0	46.0	1.5	2.8
Medium Sliced, Soft & Light, Danish, Safeway*	1 Slice/20.2g	47	233	8.7	45.1	2.0	2.2
Medium Sliced, Soft, Danish, Somerfield*	1 Slice/21g	48	229	8.6	44.8	1.4	2.4
Medium Sliced, Spinaca, Aldi*	1 Slice/25g	59	237	7.2	46.7	1.8	2.3
Medium Sliced, Superlife, Morrisons*	1 Slice/30g	79	263	9.6	47.4	3.9	2.5
Medium Sliced, Tesco*	1 Slice/73g	166	228	8.0	45.5	1.6	3.0
Medium Sliced, Top Grade, Kingsmill*	1 Slice/38g	88	232	8.8	43.8	2.4	2.8
Medium Sliced, Value, Tesco*	1 Slice/36g	81	225	7.9	46.1	1.0	2.1
Medium Sliced, Warburton's*	1 Slice/24g	57	237	10.2	44.9	1.8	2.7
Medium Sliced, Weight Watchers*	1 Slice/12g	27	226	10.3	42.6	1.6	3.6
Organic, Marks & Spencer*	1 Slice/36g	94	261	7.6	52.5	2.4	2.2
Organic, Sainsbury's*	1 Slice/35.9g	84	234	8.9	45.5	1.8	2.3
Premium Farmhouse, Lidl*	1 Slice/44g	99	225	7.4	45.4	1.5	2.5
Premium Gold, TTD, Sainsbury's*	1 Slice/44g	103	233	8.4	45.6	1.9	2.2
Premium, Marks & Spencer*	1 Slice/40.4g	94	235	8.5	45.8	1.9	2.7
Sandwich, Bakery, Sainsbury's*	1 Slice/50g	121	242	10.3	49.0	0.6	2.9
Soft Batch, Sliced, Sainsbury's*	1 Slice/44.0g	102	232	8.2	45.4	1.9	2.3
Soft Crusty, Marks & Spencer*	1 Slice/25g	64	256	9.3	49.0	2.5	2.4
Soft, Batch Loaf, Sliced, Tesco*	1 Slice/50g	117	233	7.5	46.1	2.1	2.1
Soft, Farmhouse, Marks & Spencer*	1 Slice/25g	60	239	9.8	42.6	3.3	2.5
Soft, Gold, Kingsmill*	1 Slice/47g	111	236	8.9	42.9	3.2	2.8
Soft, Medium Slice, Warburton's*	1 Slice/27g	88	326	12.2	61.5	3.3	4.1
Soft, Organic, Warburton's*	1 Slice/26.7g	62	228	9.7	44.6	3.0	2.6
Softgrain, Sliced, Tesco*	1 Med Slice/36g	81	224	7.2	45.5	1.5	3.7
Square Cut, Hovis*	1 Med Slice/40g	90	226	8.8	44.4	1.5	2.2
Stay Fresh, Tesco*	1 Slice/40g	100	249	8.6	48.3	2.4	1.5
Sunblest*	1 Med Slice/33g	77	232	7.4	46.4	1.9	2.1
Super Toastie, Warburton's*	1 Serving/57g	134	235	10.1	44.6	1.8	2.7
Thick Cut, Lidl*	1 Slice/35g	87	249	8.6	45.4	2.4	2.9
Thick Sliced, Aldi*	1 Slice/38g	90	237	7.2	46.7	1.8	2.3
Thick Sliced, Co-Op*	1 Slice/43g	99	230	8.0	46.0	2.0	2.0
Thick Sliced, Family Favourite*	1 Slice/37g	83	225	8.5	44.5	1.4	2.3
Thick Sliced, Fine Lady*	1 Slice/44.4g	112	254	7.8	53.1	1.2	2.3
Thick Sliced, Golden Sun*	1 Slice/44g	100	228	7.5	46.1	1.5	2.4
Thick Sliced, Healthy, Warburtons*	1 Slice/38g	84	222	10.3	41.2	1.8	4.1
Thick Sliced, Kingsmill*	1 Slice/42g	98	233	8.8	44.1	2.4	2.5
Thick Sliced, Long Life, Somerfield*	1 Slice/44g	100	227	7.5	44.9	1.9	2.4
Thick Sliced, Marks & Spencer*	1 Slice/42g	96	228	7.3	46.7	1.3	2.8
Thick Sliced, Organic, Tesco*	1 Slice/44g	110	249	7.4	51.3	1.6	2.1
Thick Sliced, Sainsbury's*	1 Slice/44g	100	228	7.1	46.4	1.5	2.8

B

BREAD, WHITE

INFO/WEIGHT	Measure	per Measure KCAL	KCAL	PROT	CARB	FAT	FIBRE
Thick Sliced, SmartPrice Asda*	1 Slice/47g	106	226	7.0	46.0	1.5	2.8
Thick Sliced, Square Cut, Asda*	1 Slice/43.9g	101	230	8.0	46.0	1.5	2.1
Thick Sliced, Tesco*	1 Slice/44g	100	228	7.1	46.4	1.5	2.8
Thick Sliced, Value, Tesco*	1 Slice/44g	109	248	8.4	49.3	1.9	1.5
Thick Sliced, Warbuton's*	1 Slice/28g	65	233	9.8	43.6	2.1	2.7
Thick Sliced, Woolworths*	1 Slice/38g	93	246	7.9	47.6	2.4	3.0
Thin Sliced, Sainsbury's*	1 Slice/29g	66	228	7.1	46.4	1.5	2.8
Toasted	1 Med Slice/33g	87	265	9.3	57.1	1.6	1.8
Toastie, Thick Cut, Hovis*	1 Slice/50g	113	226	8.8	44.4	1.5	2.2
Toastie, Thick Sliced, Warburton's*	1 Slice/44g	103	235	10.1	44.6	1.8	2.7
Whole, Extra Thick, Kingsmill*	1 Slice/57g	130	228	9.0	42.3	2.5	4.0
Whole, Kingsmill*	1 Slice/38g	87	230	9.0	42.9	2.5	3.4
Wholesome, Medium Sliced, Asda*	1 Slice/35.0g	78	223	7.0	43.0	2.6	5.0
With Wheatgerm, Best of Both, Hovis*	1 Slice/40g	89	223	8.8	42.3	2.0	3.8
BREAD, WHOLE & WHITE, Kingsmill*	1 Slice/38.2g	87	228	9.0	42.3	2.5	4.0
BREAD, WHOLE WHEAT, Nature's Own*	1 Slice/28g	66	236	14.3	39.3	3.6	10.7

BREAD, WHOLEMEAL

INFO/WEIGHT	Measure	per Measure KCAL	KCAL	PROT	CARB	FAT	FIBRE
Average Wholemeal	1 Slice/25g	54	215	9.2	41.6	2.5	5.8
BGTY, Sainsburys*	1 Slice/20g	41	207	12.6	36.8	1.0	7.3
Bake Off, Somerfield*	1oz/28g	62	222	11.0	40.0	2.0	0.0
Bakers Gold, Asda*	2 Slices/87g	196	225	12.0	37.0	3.2	6.0
Batch, Organic, Waitrose*	1 Slice/40g	88	219	10.0	38.8	2.6	7.2
Batch, Stoneground, Warburton's*	1 Slice/42g	91	217	9.8	39.3	2.3	7.2
COU, Marks & Spencer*	1 Slice/21g	45	213	13.6	33.7	2.6	7.0
Country Grain, Hovis*	1 Slice/44g	98	222	11.2	37.4	3.1	5.7
Crusty, Finest, Tesco*	1 Slice/50g	103	206	10.8	37.0	1.7	6.9
Danish, Better For You, Morrisons*	1 Slice/17g	39	228	11.2	47.9	1.8	6.2
Danish, Warburton's*	1 Slice/25g	57	229	13.3	38.5	2.4	7.2
Dove's Farm*	1 Slice/40g	83	208	8.5	40.5	2.5	6.4
Economy, Sainsbury's*	1 Slice/28g	61	217	10.3	38.4	2.5	6.5
Family Loaf, Safeway*	1 Slice/45g	96	213	9.5	37.4	2.8	6.0
Farmhouse Gold, Morrisons*	1 Slice/38g	78	204	9.2	38.3	1.6	6.0
Farmhouse Soft Golden, Marks & Spencer*	1 Slice/30g	65	215	11.0	35.1	3.1	7.4
Farmhouse, Hovis*	1 Slice/44g	91	206	10.2	36.6	2.1	5.3
Farmhouse, Organic, Marks & Spencer*	1oz/28g	63	224	11.2	42.7	4.2	7.4
Fresher For Longer, Sainsbury's*	1 Slice/44.1g	98	222	10.9	36.2	3.7	6.5
Gold, Kingsmill*	1 Slice/44g	95	217	10.9	36.8	2.9	7.0
Golden Wheat, Kingsmill*	1 Slice/44g	97	221	10.9	37.8	2.9	6.0
Good Health, Warburton's*	1 Slice/35.2g	82	233	10.9	41.0	2.7	7.2
Greggs*	1 Slice/36g	77	215	9.2	41.6	2.5	5.8
Heavenly, Hovis*	1 Slice/40.1g	87	217	11.4	38.0	2.2	6.5
Hovis*	1 Slice/35g	75	215	10.1	37.3	2.8	5.9
Iceland*	1 Slice/35.9g	78	217	10.3	38.4	2.5	6.5
Keep Fresh, Medium Sliced, Safeway*	1 Slice/37g	75	204	9.1	36.6	2.4	6.2
Kingsmill*	1 Slice/45g	99	221	10.9	37.8	2.9	6.0
Longer Life, Medium Sliced, Sainsbury's*	1 Slice/36g	73	203	8.6	37.6	2.1	5.1
Longer Life, Sainsbury's*	1 Med Slice/36g	85	237	10.7	41.0	3.4	6.2
Longer Life, Thick Slice, Sainsbury's*	1 Slice/45g	101	224	10.6	37.4	3.6	5.9
Marks & Spencer*	1 Slice/38g	80	210	9.6	33.5	4.2	7.2
Medium Cut, Allinson*	1 Slice/36g	78	216	9.5	39.2	2.4	6.5
Medium Cut, Small Sliced, Allinson*	1 Slice/23g	50	219	10.3	38.3	2.7	6.1
Medium Sliced, Asda*	1 Slice/37g	80	215	10.0	38.0	2.5	6.0
Medium Sliced, Co-Op*	1 Slice/36g	77	215	11.0	38.0	2.0	6.0

BREAD, WHOLEMEAL

	Measure INFO/WEIGHT	per Measure KCAL	Nutrition Values per 100g / 100ml				
			KCAL	PROT	CARB	FAT	FIBRE
Medium Sliced, Fresh For A Week, Asda*	1 Slice/35g	82	233	9.0	39.0	3.4	6.0
Medium Sliced, Fresher for Longer, Sainsbury's*	1 Slice/36g	80	222	10.9	36.2	3.7	6.5
Medium Sliced, Hovis*	1 Slice/36g	79	220	10.5	38.0	2.9	6.3
Medium Sliced, Kingsmill*	1 Slice/38g	87	228	10.1	39.2	3.4	5.2
Medium Sliced, Longerlife, Sainsbury's*	1 Slice/36g	73	203	8.6	37.6	2.1	5.1
Medium Sliced, Marks & Spencer*	1 Slice/37g	80	215	10.2	32.5	4.5	7.1
Medium Sliced, Morrisons*	1 Slice/32g	68	214	9.9	38.0	2.5	5.8
Medium Sliced, Organic, Asda*	1 Slice/43.3g	93	217	9.0	40.0	2.3	6.0
Medium Sliced, Organic, Tesco*	2 Slices/53g	111	209	9.2	37.2	2.8	6.0
Medium Sliced, Premium, Waitrose*	1 Med Slice/35g	83	237	10.7	41.0	3.4	6.2
Medium Sliced, Safeway*	1 Slice/36g	73	204	9.1	36.6	2.4	6.2
Medium Sliced, Sainsbury's*	1 Slice/36g	80	221	10.8	38.1	2.8	5.9
Medium Sliced, Stay Fresh, Somerfield*	1 Slice/36g	72	200	9.2	36.6	1.8	0.5
Medium Sliced, Stayfresh, Tesco*	1 Slice/36g	84	232	10.5	42.2	2.3	6.3
Medium Sliced, Tesco*	1 Slice/36g	81	226	9.2	41.6	2.5	5.8
Medium Sliced, Warburton's*	1 Slice/36g	84	234	10.3	40.1	3.6	7.2
Medium Sliced, Xtra Life, Waitrose*	1 Slice/36g	85	237	10.7	41.0	3.4	6.2
Multigrain, Country, Hovis*	1 Slice/36g	80	222	11.2	37.4	3.1	5.7
Multigrain, Premium Gold, TTD, Sainsbury's*	1 Slice/44g	106	242	10.2	35.9	6.4	5.3
Multigrain, Soft Batch, Sainsbury's*	1 Slice/44g	106	242	11.3	34.5	6.5	5.6
Nimble*	1 Slice/20g	43	216	11.2	36.9	2.7	6.9
Sandwich, Warburton's*	1 Slice/31g	72	232	10.7	40.2	3.1	7.2
Sliced, McCambridge*	1 Slice/38g	90	237	7.9	44.7	1.8	0.0
Sliced, Organic, Harvestime*	2 Slices/88g	190	216	9.0	38.8	2.7	5.6
Sliced, Organic, Warburton's*	1 Slice/27g	57	212	11.2	34.6	3.2	7.2
Sliced, Premium, Budgens*	1 Slice/45g	101	224	9.3	39.1	3.3	8.2
Small Sliced, Warburton's*	1 Slice/23.5g	57	238	10.6	41.7	3.0	7.2
Small, Allinson*	1 Slice/23g	49	213	10.1	37.3	2.6	7.5
Small, Kingsmill*	1 Slice/25g	56	224	10.7	38.0	3.2	5.8
Soft Crusty, Marks & Spencer*	1 Slice/25g	58	230	11.4	39.1	3.1	6.5
Soft, Medium Sliced, Morrisons*	1 Slice/32g	68	214	9.9	38.0	2.5	5.8
Square, Tasty, Kingsmill*	1 Slice/42g	96	228	10.1	39.2	3.4	5.2
Stoneground, Organic, Sainsbury's*	1 Slice/29g	63	217	7.9	39.9	2.9	5.8
Stoneground, Organic, Waitrose*	1 Slice/40g	95	237	10.7	41.0	3.4	6.2
Tasty, Kingsmill*	1 Slice/27g	59	220	10.7	37.0	3.2	6.9
Thick Cut, Allinson*	1 Slice/44g	94	213	10.1	37.3	2.6	7.5
Thick Sliced Loaf, Tesco*	1 Slice/45g	90	201	8.8	36.4	2.3	5.3
Thick Sliced, Asda*	1 Slice/45g	97	215	10.0	38.0	2.5	6.0
Thick Sliced, COU, Marks & Spencer*	1 Slice/26g	56	215	13.6	33.7	2.6	7.0
Thick Sliced, Healthy Living, Co-Op*	1 Slice/44g	95	215	11.0	38.0	2.0	7.0
Thick Sliced, Hovis*	1 Slice/44g	97	220	10.5	38.0	2.9	6.3
Thick Sliced, Kingsmill*	1 Slice/42g	96	228	10.1	39.2	3.4	5.2
Thick Sliced, Organic, Sainsbury's*	1 Slice/44g	92	210	10.0	40.1	1.0	6.7
Thick Sliced, Organic, Tesco*	1 Slice/44g	101	229	9.0	42.2	2.7	5.8
Thick Sliced, Organic, Warburton's*	1 Slice/26.5g	57	219	11.0	36.4	3.3	7.2
Thick Sliced, Sainsbury's*	1 Slice/45g	101	224	8.6	42.3	2.2	5.8
Thick Sliced, Stayfresh, Tesco, *	1 Slice/34g	69	204	10.2	34.5	2.9	6.0
Thick Sliced, Waitrose*	1 Slice/44g	111	252	10.9	36.0	7.2	5.8
Toastie, Warburton's*	1 Slice/44g	101	230	10.3	40.2	2.9	7.2
Unsliced, Organic, Dove's Farm*	1 Med Slice/35g	73	208	8.5	40.5	2.5	6.4
Value, Tesco*	1 Slice/36g	78	217	10.3	38.4	2.5	6.5
With Kibbled Malted Wheat, Kingsmill*	1 Slice/42g	96	228	10.1	39.2	3.4	5.2
With Oat Flakes & Seeds, Waitrose*	1 Slice/44.4g	111	252	10.9	36.0	7.2	5.8

	Measure INFO/WEIGHT	per Measure KCAL	Nutrition Values per 100g / 100ml				
			KCAL	PROT	CARB	FAT	FIBRE
BREAD, WHOLEMEAL							
With Pumpkin & Sunflower Seeds, Tesco*	1 Slice/25g	61	243	11.0	33.1	7.4	5.2
BREAD & BUTTER PUDDING,							
5% Fat, Marks & Spencer*	1 Pudding/237g	367	155	4.4	24.8	4.2	0.4
Asda*	1 Serving/125g	280	224	4.9	24.0	12.0	0.0
BGTY, Sainsbury's*	1 Serving/120g	161	134	5.6	23.0	2.2	0.8
COU, Marks & Spencer*	1 Pot/140g	189	135	5.5	24.6	1.7	0.6
Co-Op*	½ Pudding/170g	425	250	7.0	28.0	13.0	1.0
Finest, Tesco*	1 Serving/153g	379	248	4.9	24.6	14.4	0.9
Individual, Waitrose*	1 Pudding/116g	247	213	5.4	24.4	10.4	0.3
Marks & Spencer*	1 Serving/125g	359	287	5.3	24.1	19.4	0.8
Reduced Fat, Waitrose*	1 Serving/205g	299	146	7.4	23.3	2.6	2.0
Sainsbury's*	1 Pudding/230g	446	194	4.8	21.9	9.7	0.4
BREADCRUMBS,							
Golden, Sainsbury's*	1oz/28g	93	333	10.5	69.0	1.7	4.6
Homemade	1oz/28g	99	354	11.6	77.5	1.9	2.2
Manufactured	1oz/28g	99	354	10.1	78.5	2.1	0.0
Natural, Sainsbury's*	1oz/28g	100	358	10.8	74.3	2.0	3.4
BREADFRUIT,							
Boiled in Unsalted Water	1oz/28g	33	119	1.6	29.0	0.4	0.0
Canned, Drained	1oz/28g	18	66	0.6	16.4	0.2	1.7
Raw	1oz/28g	27	95	1.3	23.1	0.3	0.0
BREADSTICKS,							
Asda*	1 Serving/5g	21	412	12.0	73.0	8.0	2.9
Classic, Somerfield*	1 Breadstick/6g	24	396	10.0	82.5	2.9	1.0
Farleys*	1 Serving/12g	50	414	14.0	76.5	5.8	1.1
Grissini Italian, Sainsbury's*	1 Breadstick/5g	20	408	11.6	72.9	7.8	2.9
Grissini, Waitrose*	1 Breadstick/6.3g	24	397	12.0	72.5	6.2	3.1
Italian Cheese, Tesco*	4 Breadsticks/21g	84	399	14.2	67.5	8.0	3.4
Italian Original, Tesco*	1 Pack/125g	510	408	11.6	72.9	7.8	2.9
Onion, Marks & Spencer*	1 Serving/40g	166	415	12.6	59.6	14.1	4.8
Original Italian, Mini, Tesco*	1oz/28g	114	408	11.6	72.9	7.8	2.9
Original, Organic, Kallo*	1 Breadstick/6g	24	393	11.8	69.5	7.6	4.7
Pesto Flavour, Safeway*	1 Stick/6g	24	394	13.4	67.5	7.8	5.2
Plain, Asda*	1 Stick/5g	21	412	12.0	73.0	8.0	0.0
Safeway*	1 Breadstick/6.3g	24	395	12.9	72.7	9.3	4.3
Sesame Seed Grissini, Sainsbury's*	1 Breadstick/5g	21	419	12.7	65.5	11.8	3.2
BREAKFAST,							
All Day, With Heinz Baked Beans, Heinz*	1 Pack/403g	463	115	5.8	13.3	4.3	2.4
Big Breakfast, McDonald's*	1 Breakfast/256g	591	231	10.2	15.6	14.2	1.6
Farmhouse, Ready Meals, Waitrose*	½ Pack/250g	385	154	2.9	11.0	10.0	1.2
BREAKFAST, JUICE,							
Del Monte*	1 Glass/200ml	86	43	0.6	9.6	0.0	0.0
Tesco*	1 Glass/200ml	88	44	0.5	9.7	0.0	0.0
BREAKFAST CEREAL,							
Advantage, Weetabix*	1 Serving/30g	105	350	10.2	72.0	2.4	9.0
All Bran Flakes, Kellogg's*	1 Serving/40g	128	320	10.0	66.0	2.5	15.0
All Bran Splitz, Kellogg's*	1 Serving/40g	130	325	9.0	69.0	2.0	9.0
All Bran, Apricot Bites, Kellogg's*	1 Serving/45g	126	280	10.0	56.0	3.0	17.0
All Bran, Kellogg's	1 Serving/40g	108	270	13.0	45.0	4.0	29.0
Alpen, Caribbean Crunch, Weetabix*	1 Serving/40g	155	388	8.8	67.9	9.0	4.6
Alpen, Crunchy Bran, Weetabix*	1 Serving/40g	120	299	11.8	52.3	4.7	24.8
Alpen, No Added Sugar, Weetabix*	1 Serving/40g	143	357	12.1	61.3	7.1	9.0
Alpen, Nutty Crunch, Weetabix*	1 Serving/40g	159	398	10.7	63.6	11.2	6.5

BREAKFAST CEREAL,	Measure INFO/WEIGHT	per Measure KCAL	KCAL	PROT	CARB	FAT	FIBRE
Alpen, Original, Weetabix*	1 Serving/40g	146	365	10.0	66.0	6.8	7.7
Alpen, Strawberry, Weetabix*	1 Serving/40g	144	359	9.4	69.5	4.8	7.9
Alpen, Wheat Flakes, Weetabix*	1 Serving/40g	140	350	10.2	72.0	2.4	9.0
Apple & Cinnamon Flakes, Marks & Spencer*	1 Serving/30g	111	370	6.0	82.7	1.9	3.4
Apple & Cinnamon, Crisp, Sainsbury's*	1 Serving/50g	217	433	6.2	69.1	14.7	3.4
Apple, Blackberry & Raspberry Flakes, GFY, Asda*	1 Serving/40g	138	344	9.0	73.0	1.8	11.0
Apricot Bites, Kellogg's*	1 Serving/45g	126	280	12.0	51.0	3.5	21.0
Apricot Wheats, Adsa*	1 Serving/50g	165	330	7.8	71.0	1.5	8.0
Apricot Wheats, Whole Grain, Sainsbury's*	1 Serving/50g	165	330	7.8	71.4	1.5	8.0
Balance With Red Fruit, Sainsbury's*	1 Serving/40g	148	369	9.9	78.1	1.9	3.1
Banana, Papaya & Honey Oat, Crunchy, Waitrose*	1 Serving/40g	170	426	9.6	69.8	12.0	5.5
Berries, Cherries & Flakes, COU, Marks & Spencer*	1 Serving/40g	152	380	8.5	82.2	1.9	3.2
Blueberry & Cranberry, Pat Crunchy, Waitrose*	1 Serving/60g	262	437	8.0	67.0	15.2	7.4
Bran Flakes, Asda*	1 Serving/47g	157	333	11.0	65.0	3.2	14.0
Bran Flakes, Basics, Somerfield*	1 Serving/50g	154	308	12.3	58.9	2.6	19.3
Bran Flakes, Co-Op*	1 Serving/30g	99	330	11.0	65.0	3.0	15.0
Bran Flakes, Harvest Home, Nestle*	1 Serving/30g	99	331	10.2	67.1	2.4	14.1
Bran Flakes, Healthwise, Kellogg's*	1 Serving/40g	128	320	10.0	66.0	2.5	15.0
Bran Flakes, Honey & Nut, Safeway*	1 Serving/47g	168	358	9.6	70.0	4.4	11.0
Bran Flakes, Honey Nut, Asda*	1 Serving/50g	179	358	9.6	70.0	4.4	11.0
Bran Flakes, Honey Nut, Sainsbury's*	1 Serving/40g	143	358	9.6	70.0	4.4	11.0
Bran Flakes, Honey Nut, Tesco*	1 Serving/40g	143	358	9.6	70.0	4.4	11.0
Bran Flakes, Kellogg's*	1 Serving/30g	99	330	10.0	66.0	2.5	15.0
Bran Flakes, Morrisons*	1 Serving/25g	83	331	11.1	64.6	3.2	14.5
Bran Flakes, Oat With Apple & Raisin, Kellogg's*	1 Serving/40g	140	350	10.0	66.0	5.0	10.0
Bran Flakes, Organic, Tesco*	1 Serving/30g	99	330	10.2	67.0	2.4	14.1
Bran Flakes, Safeway*	1 Serving/40g	132	331	10.2	67.1	2.4	14.1
Bran Flakes, Tesco*	1 Serving/30g	99	331	10.2	67.1	2.4	14.1
Bran Flakes, Value, Tesco*	1 Serving/50g	160	320	11.4	63.2	2.4	17.1
Bran Flakes, Waitrose*	1 Serving/30g	100	333	10.1	67.7	2.4	12.7
Bran Flakes, Whole Grain, Sainsbury's*	1 Serving/30g	99	331	10.2	67.1	2.4	14.1
Cheerios, Honey Nut, Nestle*	1 Serving/40g	150	374	7.0	78.9	3.4	5.2
Cheerios, Nestle*	1 Serving/40g	148	369	7.9	75.9	3.8	6.2
Cheerios, Whole Grain, Nestle*	1 Serving/30g	110	366	8.1	74.6	3.9	6.5
Choco Corn Flakes, Asda*	1 Serving/50g	187	374	6.0	86.0	0.7	2.6
Choco Corn Flakes, Kellogg's*	1 Serving/30g	114	380	6.0	83.0	2.5	3.0
Choco Crackles, Morrisons*	1 Serving/30g	115	383	5.5	84.8	2.4	1.9
Choco Flakes, Tesco*	1 Serving/30g	112	374	5.6	86.3	0.7	2.6
Choco Hoops, Co-Op*	1 Serving/30g	116	385	7.0	80.0	4.0	5.0
Choco Snaps, Tesco*	1 Serving/30g	114	379	5.5	83.9	2.4	2.3
Chocolate Cereal, Tesco*	1 Serving/40g	169	423	8.0	66.3	14.0	6.0
Cinnamon & Apple, Sensations, Asda*	1 Serving/30g	112	373	10.0	72.0	5.0	7.0
Cinnamon Grahams, Nestle*	1 Serving/40g	166	416	4.6	75.1	10.9	4.2
Clusters, Nestle*	1 Serving/40g	153	382	10.0	70.2	6.8	8.5
Coco Pops Crunchers, Kellogg's*	1 Serving/30g	114	380	7.0	81.0	3.5	3.0
Coco Pops, Kellogg's*	1 Serving/30g	114	380	5.0	85.0	2.5	2.5
Corn Flakes, Asda*	1 Serving/30g	111	370	7.0	84.0	0.7	3.0
Corn Flakes, Banana Crunch, Kellogg's*	1 Serving/40g	159	398	6.0	80.0	7.0	2.5
Corn Flakes, Co-Op*	1 Serving/30g	113	375	8.0	84.0	1.0	1.0
Corn Flakes, Crunchy Nut, Kellogg's*	1 Serving/30g	117	390	7.0	82.0	3.5	3.0
Corn Flakes, Harvest Home, Nestle*	1 Serving/25g	92	367	7.3	82.7	0.8	3.6
Corn Flakes, Honey Nut With Cranberries, Sainsbury's*	1 Serving/40g	166	416	7.4	74.4	9.9	0.0
Corn Flakes, Honey Nut With Cranberries, Tesco*	1 Serving/50g	208	416	7.4	74.4	9.9	3.1

BREAKFAST CEREAL,	Measure INFO/WEIGHT	per Measure KCAL	Nutrition Values per 100g / 100ml				
			KCAL	PROT	CARB	FAT	FIBRE
Corn Flakes, Honey Nut, Co-Op*	1 Serving/40g	154	385	7.0	81.0	4.0	1.0
Corn Flakes, Honey Nut, Harvest Home, Nestle*	1 Serving/30g	118	392	7.4	81.1	4.2	2.5
Corn Flakes, Honey Nut, Morrisons*	1 Serving/30g	116	387	7.1	80.0	4.3	3.0
Corn Flakes, Honey Nut, Rumblers*	1 Pack/40g	207	518	17.3	91.3	8.8	3.0
Corn Flakes, Honey Nut, Sainsbury's*	1 Serving/30g	116	387	7.3	80.0	4.2	2.9
Corn Flakes, Honey Nut, Tesco*	1 Serving/30g	116	387	7.3	80.0	4.2	2.0
Corn Flakes, Kellogg's*	1 Serving/30g	111	370	8.0	82.0	0.8	3.0
Corn Flakes, Safeway*	1 Serving/25g	92	367	7.3	82.7	0.8	3.6
Corn Flakes, Sainsbury's*	1 Serving/25g	92	367	7.3	82.7	0.8	3.6
Corn Flakes, Tesco*	1 Serving/25g	92	367	7.3	82.7	0.8	3.6
Corn Pops, Kellogg's*	1 Serving/40g	152	380	6.0	87.0	1.0	2.0
Country Crisp Four Nut Combo, Jordans*	1 Serving/50g	240	480	8.9	54.2	25.3	5.9
Country Crisp Wild About Berries, Jordans*	1 Serving/50g	222	443	7.5	68.0	15.7	3.1
Country Crisp With Strawberries, Jordans*	1 Serving/40g	174	435	7.4	64.5	16.4	8.0
Country Crisp With Whole Raspberries, Jordans*	1 Serving/40g	174	435	7.4	64.5	16.4	8.0
Cranberry Wheats, Tesco*	1 Serving/40g	130	325	7.3	70.9	1.4	7.7
Cranberry, Cherry & Almond, Dorset Cereals*	1 Serving/25g	89	355	9.2	60.5	8.5	8.4
Crispy Rice & Wheat Flakes, Asda*	1 Serving/50g	185	370	11.0	78.0	1.5	3.2
Crunchy Bran Curls, Weetabix*	1 Serving/40g	120	299	11.8	52.3	4.7	24.8
Crunchy Cereal, Safeway*	1 Serving/45g	207	459	9.2	65.4	17.8	6.3
Crunchy Choco, Crisp & Square, Tesco*	1 Serving/50g	212	423	8.0	66.3	14.0	6.0
Crunchy Nut Clusters, Kellogg's*	1 Serving/40g	178	444	7.0	68.0	16.0	4.0
Crunchy Nut, Red, Kellogg's*	1 Serving/40g	164	410	7.0	73.0	10.0	3.0
Crunchy Oat With Raisins, Almonds & Honey, Tesco*	1 Serving/50g	213	425	9.1	62.8	15.3	4.7
Crunchy Oat, Golden Sun, Lidl*	1 Serving/50g	206	411	8.6	65.0	12.9	6.2
Crunchy Raisin & Coconut, Organic, Jordans*	1 Serving/40g	168	419	8.1	66.3	13.5	6.4
Fibre 1, Nestle*	1 Serving/40g	107	267	10.8	50.2	2.6	30.5
Fibre Bran, Safeway*	1 Serving/48.3g	124	259	13.3	43.4	3.6	31.0
Fitness & Fruits, Nestle*	1 Serving/40g	140	350	5.6	77.0	2.2	5.6
Flakes & Grains, Exotic Fruit, BGTY, Sainsbury's*	1 Serving/30g	113	377	6.8	76.4	4.9	5.9
Flakes & Orchard Fruits, BGTY, Sainsbury's*	1 Serving/40g	154	385	13.0	80.6	1.2	4.5
Force, Nestle*	1 Serving/40g	138	344	10.6	70.3	2.3	9.2
Frosted Flakes, Sainsbury's*	1 Serving/30g	112	374	4.9	87.8	0.4	2.4
Frosted Flakes, Tesco*	1 Serving/30g	112	374	4.9	87.8	0.4	2.4
Frosted Wheats, Kellogg's*	1 Serving/30g	102	340	10.0	72.0	2.0	9.0
Frosties, Caramel, Kellogg's*	1 Serving/30g	113	377	5.0	88.0	0.6	2.0
Frosties, Chocolate, Kellogg's*	1 Serving/40g	160	400	5.0	84.0	4.5	2.0
Frosties, Kellogg's*	1 Serving/30g	114	380	5.0	88.0	0.6	2.0
Fruit & Fibre, Flakes, Waitrose*	1 Serving/40g	140	350	8.2	65.7	6.0	10.1
Fruit & Fibre, Harvest Morn, Aldi*	1 Serving/40g	149	372	8.9	68.9	6.8	8.0
Fruit & Fibre, Morrisons*	1 Serving/30g	110	366	8.8	66.5	7.2	8.5
Fruit & Fibre, Organic, Sainsbury's*	1 Serving/40g	147	367	10.0	72.4	4.1	7.8
Fruit & Fibre, Safeway*	1 Serving/40g	143	358	9.0	66.4	6.4	9.0
Fruit & Fibre, Sainsbury's*	1 Serving/30g	108	361	8.1	68.5	6.1	8.9
Fruit & Fibre, Tesco*	1 Serving/30g	113	375	8.5	66.3	8.4	7.8
Fruit 'n' Fibre, Kellogg's*	1 Serving/50g	175	350	9.0	69.0	4.5	9.0
Fruit Nuts & Flakes, Marks & Spencer*	1 Serving/30g	117	391	9.1	69.6	8.5	3.5
Golden Grahams, Nestle*	1 Serving/40g	152	381	5.6	81.6	3.6	3.2
Golden Nuggets, Nestle*	1 Serving/40g	152	381	6.2	87.4	0.7	1.5
Golden Puffs, Sainsbury's*	1 Serving/28g	107	383	6.6	86.3	1.2	3.0
Grape Nuts, Kraft*	1 Serving/30g	104	345	10.5	72.5	1.9	8.6
Harvest Crunch, Nut, Quaker*	1 Serving/40g	184	459	8.0	62.5	19.5	6.0
Harvest Crunch, Real Red Berries, Quaker*	1 Serving/50g	224	447	7.0	66.0	17.0	4.5

BREAKFAST CEREAL,	INFO/WEIGHT	KCAL	KCAL	PROT	CARB	FAT	FIBRE
Harvest Crunch, Soft Juicy Raisins, Quaker*	1 Serving/50g	221	442	6.0	67.0	16.0	4.0
Hawaiian Crunch, Mornflake*	1 Serving/60g	247	411	8.1	66.8	12.4	6.8
High Fibre Bran, Asda*	1 Serving/50g	137	273	13.0	44.0	5.0	29.0
High Fibre Bran, Co-Op*	1 Serving/40g	108	270	13.0	44.0	5.0	29.0
High Fibre Bran, New, Tesco*	1 Serving/30g	73	242	14.0	38.4	3.5	31.0
High Fibre Bran, Sainsbury's*	1 Serving/40g	114	286	13.4	50.7	3.3	23.6
High Fibre Bran, Tesco*	1 Serving/40g	108	271	13.0	43.6	5.0	29.0
High Fibre Bran, Waitrose*	1 Serving/40g	112	281	14.4	47.2	3.8	26.0
Honey Loops, Kellogg's*	1 Serving/30g	111	370	8.0	77.0	3.0	7.0
Honey Nut & Flakes, Marks & Spencer*	1 Serving/40g	164	411	9.8	73.4	8.7	2.6
Honey Raisin & Almond, Crunchy, Waitrose*	1 Serving/40g	170	425	10.5	68.8	12.0	5.7
Hot Cereal, Flaxomeal*	1 Serving/40g	130	325	52.5	2.5	15.0	30.0
Hot Oats, Instant, Tesco*	1 Serving/30g	107	356	11.5	58.8	8.3	8.9
Hot Oats, Safeway*	1 Serving/20g	71	356	11.6	58.8	8.3	8.9
Hunny B's, Kellogg's*	1 Serving/28g	106	380	6.0	83.0	2.5	3.0
Just Right, Kellogg's*	1 Serving/40g	144	360	7.0	78.0	2.5	4.5
Malt Bites, Safeway*	1 Serving/40g	137	343	10.0	69.2	2.9	10.0
Malted Wheaties, Asda*	1 Serving/50g	171	342	10.0	69.0	2.9	10.0
Malties, Sainsbury's*	1 Serving/40g	137	343	10.0	69.2	2.9	10.0
Malty Flakes With Cranberry & Apple, BGTY, Sainsbury's*	1 Serving/40g	142	356	9.4	76.2	1.5	3.7
Malty Flakes With Peach & Raspberry, BGTY, Sainsbury's*	1 Serving/40g	146	364	10.8	76.4	1.7	3.3
Malty Flakes With Red Berries, Tesco*	1 Serving/30g	111	369	9.9	78.1	1.9	3.1
Malty Flakes, Tesco*	1 Serving/40g	148	371	11.0	78.4	1.5	4.3
Maple & Pecan, Crisp, Asda*	1 Serving/30g	135	451	8.0	62.0	19.0	6.0
Maple & Pecan, Crisp, Tesco*	1 Serving/60g	277	461	8.2	60.6	20.6	6.2
Maple & Pecan, Luxury Crunchy, Jordans*	1 Serving/50g	224	448	9.9	59.9	18.7	6.5
Maple & Pecan, Sainsbury's*	1 Serving/60g	318	530	13.3	69.7	22.0	5.3
Minibix, Banana, Weetabix*	1 Serving/40g	148	370	8.8	73.0	5.0	8.1
Minibix, Chocolate, Weetabix*	1 Serving/39g	149	383	8.4	73.3	6.2	6.7
Minibix, Fruit & Nut, Weetabix*	1 Serving/40g	141	353	8.8	71.2	3.8	8.1
Minibix, Honey, Weetabix*	1 Serving/40g	144	359	8.8	76.1	2.2	0.0
Minibix, Weetabix*	1 Serving/40g	134	335	8.8	71.2	3.8	8.1
Muesli, 12 Fruit & Nut, Sainsbury's*	1 Serving/50g	166	332	8.1	64.2	4.7	7.8
Muesli, BGTY, Sainsbury's*	1 Serving/64.8g	211	324	6.7	70.8	1.6	6.2
Muesli, COU, Marks & Spencer*	1 Serving/60g	201	335	7.6	70.2	2.5	8.1
Muesli, Creamy Tropical Fruit, Finest, Tesco*	1 Serving/80g	283	354	7.2	68.8	5.6	6.9
Muesli, Crunchy Bran, Nature's Harvest*	1 Serving/50g	176	352	8.8	62.9	9.9	6.4
Muesli, Crunchy, Organic, Sainsbury's*	1 Serving/40g	168	420	10.6	62.0	14.4	9.2
Muesli, De Luxe, No Added Salt or Sugar, Sainsbury's*	1 Serving/40g	161	403	11.9	57.6	13.9	8.4
Muesli, Eat Smart, Safeway*	1 Serving/40g	134	335	8.7	68.6	2.8	7.4
Muesli, Fruit & Bran, Unsweetened, Marks & Spencer*	1 Serving/40g	128	320	8.1	68.0	2.7	9.4
Muesli, Fruit & Fibre, COU, Marks & Spencer*	1 Serving/40g	130	325	7.5	74.5	2.8	7.5
Muesli, Fruit & Nut, Iceland*	1 Serving/30g	105	350	9.3	61.0	7.5	8.1
Muesli, Fruit & Nut, Jordans*	1 Serving/50g	189	378	7.3	60.6	11.8	6.7
Muesli, Fruit & Nut, Luxury, Co-Op*	1 Serving/40g	150	375	8.0	64.0	10.0	6.0
Muesli, Fruit & Nut, Luxury, Marks & Spencer*	1 Serving/50g	175	349	7.7	62.2	7.7	7.3
Muesli, Fruit & Nut, Luxury, Waitrose*	1 Serving/40g	145	363	9.0	60.3	9.5	6.5
Muesli, Fruit & Nut, Marks & Spencer*	1 Serving/40g	128	320	7.4	74.5	2.8	7.4
Muesli, Fruit & Nut, Organic, Marks & Spencer*	1 Serving/50g	167	333	8.2	61.6	6.0	7.6
Muesli, Fruit & Nut, Sainsbury's*	1 Serving/30g	121	402	10.4	51.3	17.2	9.2
Muesli, Fruit & Nut, Tesco*	1 Serving/65g	237	365	7.4	57.9	11.5	8.0
Muesli, Fruit Sensation, Marks & Spencer*	1 Serving/50g	158	315	6.0	66.0	3.0	7.4
Muesli, Fruit, 55%, Asda*	1 Serving/35g	111	318	6.0	67.0	2.9	7.0

B

	Measure INFO/WEIGHT	per Measure KCAL	Nutrition Values per 100g / 100ml				
			KCAL	PROT	CARB	FAT	FIBRE

BREAKFAST CEREAL,

	Measure INFO/WEIGHT	per Measure KCAL	KCAL	PROT	CARB	FAT	FIBRE
Muesli, Fruit, GFY, Asda*	1 Serving/50g	152	304	8.0	64.0	1.8	10.0
Muesli, Fruit, Healthy Eating, Tesco*	1 Serving/40g	129	322	7.0	66.6	4.2	6.9
Muesli, Fruit, Sainsbury's*	1 Serving/40g	132	330	8.1	64.3	4.5	9.6
Muesli, Fruit, Tesco*	1 Serving/50g	167	333	7.0	66.0	4.2	6.9
Muesli, Fruit, The Best, Safeway*	1 Serving/40g	138	346	5.3	71.3	4.3	5.0
Muesli, Gluten Free, Nature's Harvest, Holland & Barrett*	1 Serving/60g	234	390	14.1	54.1	13.0	3.3
Muesli, Golden Sun, Lidl*	1 Serving/40g	144	360	8.0	60.0	9.8	7.5
Muesli, Luxury Fruit, Perfectly Balanced, Waitrose*	1 Serving/50g	162	324	7.1	66.4	3.3	7.0
Muesli, Luxury Fruit, Safeway*	1 Serving/40g	139	347	7.1	74.3	1.0	2.2
Muesli, Luxury Fruit, Sainsbury's*	1 Serving/50g	162	324	7.1	66.4	3.3	7.0
Muesli, Luxury Fruit, Waitrose*	1 Serving/30g	101	337	7.7	66.3	4.5	6.9
Muesli, Luxury, Dorset Cereals*	1 Serving/28g	92	328	8.4	63.0	6.5	9.0
Muesli, Luxury, Jordans*	1 Serving/40g	154	384	9.6	58.4	12.5	8.2
Muesli, Luxury, Sainsbury's*	1 Serving/40g	144	359	8.5	57.1	10.7	7.7
Muesli, Natural, Jordans*	1 Serving/40g	141	352	10.4	62.4	6.7	8.9
Muesli, No Added Sugar or Salt, Organic, Jordans*	1 Serving/50g	191	381	9.9	62.3	10.2	9.3
Muesli, No Added Sugar, Waitrose*	1 Serving/40g	146	364	12.0	64.9	6.3	6.7
Muesli, Organic, Jordans*	1 Serving/40g	150	374	10.9	54.2	12.6	10.5
Muesli, Organic, Waitrose*	1 Serving/50g	179	358	10.8	59.1	8.7	7.8
Muesli, Organic, Whole Earth*	1 Serving/25g	87	347	10.5	61.0	6.4	8.0
Muesli, Original, Holland & Barrett*	1 Serving/30g	105	351	11.1	61.2	8.4	7.1
Muesli, Original, Sainsbury's*	1 Serving/60g	226	376	9.3	65.7	8.4	7.1
Muesli, Special, Jordans*	1 Serving/40g	143	358	8.4	60.8	9.0	8.1
Muesli, Swiss Style, Co-Op*	1 Serving/40g	148	370	11.0	67.0	6.0	6.0
Muesli, Swiss Style, No Added Salt Or Sugar, Sainsbury's*	1 Serving/40g	143	358	10.7	64.3	6.4	7.0
Muesli, Swiss Style, No Added Sugar or Salt, Asda*	1 Serving/50g	182	363	11.0	64.0	7.0	8.0
Muesli, Swiss Style, SmartPrice, Asda*	1 Serving/60g	222	370	9.0	70.0	6.0	10.0
Muesli, Swiss Style, Somerfield*	1 Serving/50g	180	359	11.0	64.0	6.5	8.0
Muesli, Swiss Style, Tesco*	1 Serving/40g	141	353	10.9	65.1	5.4	8.2
Muesli, Swiss Style, Waitrose*	1 Serving/40g	146	364	10.2	66.1	6.5	7.6
Muesli, Tropical Fruit, Holland & Barrett*	1 Bowl/60g	197	328	7.5	69.8	3.2	5.1
Muesli, Tropical, Tesco*	1 Serving/50g	173	346	7.8	68.2	4.7	9.1
Muesli, Unsweetened Wholewheat, Safeway*	1 Serving/50g	180	360	7.7	68.0	6.3	7.2
Muesli, Unsweetened, Marks & Spencer*	1 Serving/40g	129	322	8.1	68.0	2.7	9.4
Muesli, Value, Tesco*	1 Serving/50g	171	342	7.5	67.6	4.6	8.6
Muesli, Wholewheat, Co-Op*	1 Serving/40g	140	350	11.0	61.0	7.0	7.0
Muesli, Wholewheat, No Added Salt or Sugar, Sainsbury's	1 Serving/40g	140	351	8.2	58.9	9.2	8.1
Muesli, Wholewheat, No Added Sugar & Salt, Tesco*	1 Serving/40g	152	379	9.6	60.2	11.1	8.1
Muesli, Wholewheat, No Added Sugar, Tesco*	1 Serving/40g	154	386	9.5	59.1	12.4	7.4
Muesli, Wholewheat, Sainsbury's*	1 Serving/40g	136	339	8.5	60.6	6.9	7.6
Multi Fruit & Flake, COU, Marks & Spencer	1 Serving/39g	142	365	6.5	81.8	1.1	4.0
Multi Fruit & Flake, Perfectly Balanced, Waitrose*	1 Serving/40g	134	335	8.2	68.8	3.0	14.0
Multigrain Flakes With Apple, Eat Smart, Safeway*	1 Serving/45g	160	355	8.0	74.7	2.5	7.0
Multigrain, Start, Kellogg's*	1 Serving/40g	144	360	8.0	79.0	2.0	6.0
Natural Wheatgerm, Jordans*	1 Serving/40g	138	345	26.5	39.6	9.0	13.7
Natures Wholegrains, Jordans*	1 Serving/25g	98	390	9.4	61.7	11.7	7.7
Oat & Bran Flakes, Sainsbury's*	1 Serving/50g	172	344	12.6	60.0	5.9	15.0
Oat Bran, Crispies, Quaker*	1 Serving/40g	153	383	11.0	69.0	6.5	9.0
Oat Krunchies, Quaker*	1 Serving/30g	118	393	9.5	72.0	7.0	5.5
Oat With Tropical Fruits, Crunchy, Tesco*	1 Serving/35g	157	448	8.7	66.0	16.6	3.2
Oat, Crunchy, Sainsbury's*	1 Serving/50g	227	453	8.2	59.3	20.3	6.6
Oatbran Flakes, Nature's Path*	1 Serving/30g	124	414	8.7	83.0	4.7	6.7
Oatmeal, Instant, Quaker*	1 Serving/35g	126	360	13.6	57.0	8.7	9.7

BREAKFAST CEREAL,	Measure INFO/WEIGHT	per Measure KCAL	Nutrition Values per 100g / 100ml KCAL	PROT	CARB	FAT	FIBRE
Oatso Simple, Apple & Cinnamon, Quaker*	1 Satchet/38g	136	358	8.0	68.0	5.5	2.5
Oatso Simple, Baked Apple Flavour, Quaker*	1 Serving/38g	141	370	8.0	70.0	6.0	5.5
Oatso Simple, Berry Burst, Quaker*	1 Serving/38g	141	370	8.0	70.0	6.0	6.5
Oatso Simple, Country Honey, Quaker*	1 Serving/36g	134	373	8.5	69.0	6.5	6.0
Oatso Simple, Fruit Muesli, Quaker*	1 Sachet/39g	140	360	7.5	69.0	6.0	7.0
Oatso Simple, Golden Syrup Flavour, Quaker*	1 Serving/39g	142	364	7.5	70.0	5.5	5.0
Oatso Simple, Quaker*	1 Serving/27g	100	372	11.0	62.0	8.5	7.0
Orange, Banana, Etc, Flakes & Grains, BGTY, Sainsbury's*	1 Serving/35g	130	370	8.4	80.6	1.5	4.7
Perfect Balance, Weight Watchers*	1 Serving/30g	90	300	7.8	63.3	1.7	15.6
Porage Oats, Scot's, Quaker*	1 Serving/30g	110	368	11.0	62.0	8.0	7.0
Porridge Flakes, Organic, Barkat*	1 Serving/30g	109	362	8.5	74.1	3.0	0.0
Porridge Oats & Bran, Co-Op*	1 Serving/40g	141	353	12.5	60.0	7.0	12.0
Porridge Oats & Bran, Somerfield*	1 Serving/40g	154	385	12.0	68.0	7.0	0.0
Porridge Oats, Jordans*	1 Serving/40g	145	363	12.5	61.5	7.4	8.0
Porridge Oats, Organic, Evernat*	1 Serving/40g	167	418	13.0	69.0	9.6	7.4
Porridge Oats, Organic, Jordans*	1 Serving/45g	163	363	12.5	61.5	7.4	8.0
Porridge Oats, Organic, Tesco*	1 Serving/28g	100	357	13.5	57.8	8.0	9.0
Porridge Oats, Quick & Easy, Morrisons*	1 Serving/28g	103	367	11.8	62.0	8.0	7.0
Porridge Oats, Scott, Co-Op*	1 Serving/40g	146	364	11.8	62.0	7.6	7.2
Porridge Oats, Scottish, Asda*	1 Serving/50g	192	383	10.0	75.0	4.8	7.0
Porridge Oats, Scottish, Organic, Sainsbury's*	1 Serving/45g	172	383	10.0	74.4	5.0	7.9
Porridge Oats, Scottish, Safeway*	1 Serving/30g	109	364	11.8	62.0	7.6	7.2
Porridge Oats, Scottish, Tesco*	1 Serving/50g	182	364	11.8	62.0	7.6	7.2
Porridge Oats, SmartPrice, Asda*	1 Serving/50g	178	356	11.0	60.0	8.0	8.0
Porridge Oats, So-Easy, Scotts*	1 Serving/30g	109	364	11.0	60.0	8.5	9.0
Porridge Oats, Somerfield*	1 Serving/40g	154	385	12.0	68.0	7.0	0.0
Porridge Oats, Value, Tesco*	1 Serving/50g	192	384	11.8	68.0	7.2	7.2
Porridge Oats, Whole Rolled, Scottish, Sainsbury's*	1 Serving/50g	191	381	9.7	74.7	4.8	7.0
Porridge, COU, Marks & Spencer*	1 Pot/200g	180	90	3.9	13.3	2.2	0.9
Porridge, Instant, Quakers*	1 Serving/34g	125	368	12.8	66.7	7.6	5.0
Porridge, Quick, Marks & Spencer*	1 Serving/40g	159	398	15.5	55.1	12.8	5.9
Porridge, Weight Watchers*	1 Pack/220g	114	52	1.1	9.5	1.1	0.9
Precise, Sainsbury's*	1 Serving/40g	148	371	6.4	79.9	2.9	3.5
Puffed Rice, Kallo*	1 Serving/25g	95	380	8.0	80.0	3.0	9.0
Puffed Wheat, Quaker*	1 Serving/15g	49	328	15.3	62.4	1.3	5.6
Puffed Wheat, Tesco*	1 Serving/28g	104	373	13.9	72.2	3.2	5.7
Quaker Oats Crunch, Quaker*	1 Serving/40g	178	445	8.0	66.5	16.0	5.0
Quaker Oats, Quaker*	1 Serving/30g	110	368	11.0	62.0	8.0	7.0
Raisin & Almond, Crunchy, Jordans*	1 Serving/56g	230	411	8.4	66.0	12.5	5.0
Raisin Wheats, Kellogg's*	1 Serving/30g	96	320	9.0	69.0	2.0	9.0
Raisin Wheats, Sainsbury's*	1 Serving/50g	166	332	8.2	71.5	1.5	8.0
Raisin, Bran Flakes, Asda*	1 Serving/50g	166	331	7.0	69.0	3.0	10.0
Raisin, Honey & Almond Crunch, Asda*	1 Serving/60g	265	442	8.0	62.0	18.0	6.0
Ready Brek, Banana, Weetabix*	1 Serving/40g	146	365	8.9	68.0	6.4	6.7
Ready Brek, Chocolate, Weetabix*	1 Serving/40g	144	360	9.6	63.7	7.4	8.1
Ready Brek, Strawberry, Weetabix*	1 Serving/40g	146	365	8.7	68.6	6.2	6.8
Ready Brek, Weetabix*	1 Serving/40g	142	356	11.6	58.8	8.3	8.9
Red Berry & Almond Luxury Crunch, Jordans*	1 Serving/40g	176	441	8.2	60.5	18.5	6.6
Rice & Wheat Flake, Special Choice, Waitrose*	1 Serving/30g	111	370	11.4	77.7	1.5	3.2
Rice Krispies, Honey, Kellogg's*	1 Serving/30g	114	380	4.0	89.0	0.7	1.0
Rice Krispies, Kellogg's*	1 Serving/30g	111	370	6.0	85.0	1.0	1.5
Rice Pops, Blue Parrot Cafe, Sainsbury's*	1 Serving/30g	111	370	7.2	82.3	1.3	2.2
Rice Pops, Organic, Dove's Farm*	1 Serving/30g	107	357	6.8	86.1	0.8	2.0

B

B

	Measure INFO/WEIGHT	per Measure KCAL	KCAL	PROT	CARB	FAT	FIBRE
BREAKFAST CEREAL,							
Rice Pops, Sainsbury's*	1 Serving/30g	113	378	7.4	84.2	1.3	1.5
Rice Snaps, Asda*	1 Serving/28g	105	376	7.0	84.0	1.3	1.5
Rice Snaps, Harvest Home, Nestle*	1 Serving/25g	95	378	7.4	84.2	1.3	1.5
Rice Snaps, Healthy Eating, Tesco*	1 Pack/25g	93	370	7.2	82.3	1.3	2.2
Rice Snaps, Tesco*	1 Serving/30g	113	378	7.3	84.2	1.3	1.5
Ricicles, Kellogg's*	1 Serving/30g	114	380	4.0	89.0	0.7	1.0
Right Balance, Morrisons*	1 Serving/50g	181	362	6.9	78.6	2.2	5.3
Shredded Wheat, Bitesize, Nestle*	1 Serving/50g	168	335	11.5	67.7	2.2	11.6
Shredded Wheat, Fruitful, Nestle*	1 Serving/50g	177	353	8.4	66.9	5.8	10.3
Shredded Wheat, Honey Nut, Nestle*	1 Serving/40g	151	378	10.9	68.8	6.6	10.4
Shredded Wheat, Nestle*	1 Piece/22g	72	325	11.2	65.2	2.1	12.4
Shreddies, Coco, Nestle*	1 Serving/50g	177	353	8.0	76.1	1.9	9.2
Shreddies, Frosted, Kellogg's*	1 Serving/50g	162	323	0.7	78.5	1.8	4.7
Shreddies, Frosted, Nestle*	1 Serving/50g	178	356	7.3	78.5	1.4	8.3
Shreddies, Frosted, Variety Pack, Nestle*	1 Pack/45g	163	363	6.7	81.1	1.3	6.8
Shreddies, Malt Wheats, Tesco*	1 Serving/45g	151	335	8.3	70.7	2.1	9.7
Shreddies, Nestle*	1 Serving/45g	154	343	9.8	71.7	1.9	11.2
Smart Start, Kellogg's*	1 Serving/70g	252	360	6.0	86.0	1.0	4.0
Smoothies, Strawberry, Quaker*	1 Sachet/29g	117	402	6.5	67.0	12.0	5.5
Special K, Apricot & Peach, Kellogg's*	1 Serving/30g	111	369	15.0	75.0	1.0	3.0
Special K, Kellogg's*	1 Serving/30g	111	370	15.0	75.0	1.0	2.5
Special K, Red Berries, Kellogg's*	1 Serving/30g	111	370	14.0	74.0	1.0	3.0
Start Right, Asda*	1 Serving/40g	150	376	8.0	74.0	6.0	5.0
Strawberry & Almond Crunch, Marks & Spencer*	1 Serving/40g	186	465	8.0	66.0	18.6	4.9
Sugar Puffs, Quaker*	1 Serving/30g	116	387	6.5	86.5	1.0	3.0
Sultana Bran, Asda*	1 Serving/30g	98	327	9.0	66.0	3.0	11.0
Sultana Bran, Co-Op*	1 Serving/40g	130	325	9.0	66.0	3.0	11.0
Sultana Bran, Healthwise, Kellogg's*	1 Serving/40g	128	320	9.0	66.0	2.0	13.0
Sultana Bran, Healthy Eating,Tesco*	1 Serving/48g	156	326	8.1	69.0	1.9	9.8
Sultana Bran, Morrisons*	1 Serving/30g	98	325	8.8	65.8	3.0	11.4
Sultana Bran, Safeway*	1 Serving/50g	162	324	8.2	68.6	1.9	11.6
Sultana Bran, Sainsbury's*	1 Serving/30g	97	324	8.2	68.6	1.9	11.6
Sultana Bran, Somerfield*	1 Serving/30g	97	324	8.2	68.6	1.9	11.6
Super High Fibre, Dorset Cereals*	1 Serving/60g	214	357	8.0	60.1	9.4	8.4
Superfast Oats, Mornflake*	1 Serving/40g	144	359	11.0	60.4	8.1	8.5
Triple Chocolate Crisp, Sainsbury's*	1 Serving/40g	180	451	7.7	63.8	18.3	6.0
Tropical, Crunchy, Jordans*	1 Serving/40g	170	425	8.5	65.8	14.2	6.2
Tropicana, Weight Watchers*	1 Serving/50g	120	240	5.1	52.0	1.0	7.0
Weetabix*	2 Biscuits/37.5g	128	340	11.2	67.6	2.7	10.5
Weetabix, Organic, Weetabix*	2 Biscuits/35g	117	335	10.9	66.2	3.0	11.3
Weetos, Weetabix*	1 Serving/30g	115	384	6.2	78.4	5.0	5.6
Wheat Biscuits, Healthy Eating, Tesco*	2 Biscuits/55g	191	348	11.0	70.0	2.7	8.0
Wheat Biscuits, Nature's Own, Organic, Weetabix*	1 Biscuit/17g	58	339	10.3	69.2	2.4	10.4
Wheat Biscuits, Somerfield*	2 Biscuits/37.5g	129	339	11.2	67.6	2.7	10.5
Wheat Biscuits, Value, Tesco*	2 Biscuits/30g	103	342	13.7	69.5	1.0	7.5
Wheat Bisks, Asda*	1 Serving/29g	99	340	11.0	68.0	2.7	10.0
Wholewheat Biscuits, Sainsbury's*	1 Biscuit/36g	122	340	11.2	67.6	2.7	10.5
Yoghurt & Raspberry, Crisp, Sainsbury's*	1 Serving/45g	199	442	7.5	66.0	16.4	5.4
BREAKFAST COMPOTE,							
In Apple Juice, Tesco*	1 Can/300g	219	73	0.4	17.0	0.4	2.1
Sainsbury's*	1 Can/300g	327	109	1.7	24.4	0.5	3.1
BREAKFAST FRUITS, Grapefruit & Orange Del Monte*	1 Can/411g	193	47	1.0	10.2	0.1	1.0
BREAM, Sea, Raw	1oz/28g	27	96	17.5	0.0	2.9	0.0

Nutrition Values per 100g / 100ml

	Measure INFO/WEIGHT	per Measure KCAL	Nutrition Values per 100g / 100ml				
			KCAL	PROT	CARB	FAT	FIBRE
BRESAOLA,							
Della Valtellina, Sainsbury's*	1 Slice/14g	23	163	34.7	0.1	2.6	0.1
Marks & Spencer*	1oz/28g	56	200	34.6	0.0	6.8	0.0
BROCCOLI,							
Baby Courgette & Baby Leeks, Safeway*	1oz/28g	7	24	2.4	2.1	0.8	2.0
Carrot & Mange Tout, Marks & Spencer*	1oz/28g	10	35	2.9	5.6	0.2	2.1
Cauliflower & Baby Carrots, Safeway*	1 Serving/150g	38	25	2.0	3.0	0.6	2.3
Cauliflower & Carrots, Frozen, Great Value, Asda*	1 Serving/100g	25	25	2.2	2.6	0.6	5.0
Courgette & Peppers, COU, Marks & Spencer*	1 Pack/283g	156	55	1.7	2.7	4.1	1.7
Florets, Asda*	1 Serving/17g	4	24	3.1	1.1	0.8	2.3
Florets, Fresh, Frozen, Tesco*	1 Serving/250g	83	33	4.4	1.7	0.9	2.6
Florets, Freshly Frozen, Morrisons*	1 Pack/250g	60	24	3.1	1.1	0.8	0.0
Florets, Individually Frozen, Sainsbury's*	1 Serving/85g	26	31	3.3	2.3	0.9	3.6
Florets, Organic, Iceland*	1oz/28g	9	31	3.3	2.5	0.9	3.6
Florets, Sainsbury's*	½ Pack/150g	36	24	3.1	1.1	0.8	2.3
Florets, Tesco*	1oz/28g	7	24	3.1	1.1	0.8	2.3
Florets, Waitrose*	1 Serving/75g	25	33	4.4	1.8	0.9	3.0
Green, Boiled in Salted Water	1 Serving/90g	22	24	3.1	1.1	0.8	2.3
Green, Boiled in Unsalted Water	1 Serving/90g	22	24	3.1	1.1	0.8	2.3
Green, Raw, Fresh	1oz/28g	9	33	4.4	1.8	0.9	2.6
Mornay, Asda*	1 Pack/434g	434	100	4.5	7.0	6.0	0.3
Prepared Tender Stem, Marks & Spencer*	1oz/28g	11	38	4.1	4.9	0.2	0.2
Purple Sprouting, Boiled in Salted Water	1 Serving/90g	17	19	2.1	1.3	0.6	2.3
Purple Sprouting, Boiled in Unsalted Water	1 Serving/90g	17	19	2.1	1.3	0.6	2.3
Purple Sprouting, Raw	1oz/28g	10	35	3.9	2.6	1.1	3.5
BROCCOLI & CAULIFLOWER, Floret Mix, Frozen, Tesco*	1 Serving/150g	50	33	4.0	2.3	0.9	2.2
BROCCOLI CHEESE, Morrisons*	1 Pack/350g	406	116	6.2	6.6	7.1	0.8
BRUSSELS SPROUTS,							
& Sweet Chestnuts, Asda*	1 Serving/100g	73	73	3.1	11.0	1.7	4.2
Boiled in Salted Water	1 Med Serving/90g	32	35	2.9	3.5	1.3	3.1
Boiled in Unsalted Water	1 Med Serving/90g	32	35	2.9	3.5	1.3	3.1
Button, Frozen, Sainsbury's*	1 Serving/100g	37	37	3.5	2.7	1.3	4.3
Canned, Drained	1oz/28g	8	28	2.6	2.4	1.0	2.6
Frozen, Basics, Somerfield*	1 Serving/90g	39	43	4.0	4.0	1.0	0.0
Iceland*	1 Serving/100g	35	35	3.5	2.5	1.3	4.3
Peeled, Sainsbury's*	1 Pack/250g	93	37	2.9	3.5	1.3	1.3
Prepared, Marks & Spencer*	1oz/28g	7	26	4.0	2.7	0.0	4.2
Raw	1oz/28g	12	42	3.5	4.1	1.4	4.1
Trimmed, Fresh, Asda*	1 Pack/300g	111	37	2.9	3.5	1.3	3.1
BUBBLE & SQUEAK,							
Aunt Bessie's*	1 Serving/100g	145	145	2.7	17.5	7.1	1.3
Fried in Vegetable Oil	1oz/28g	35	124	1.4	9.8	9.1	1.5
Safeway*	1 Serving/200g	160	80	1.8	10.7	3.3	1.4
Tesco*	1 Pack/325g	325	100	1.3	13.5	4.5	1.3
Waitrose*	½ Pack/225g	216	96	1.6	13.4	4.0	1.8
BUCKWHEAT, Average	1oz/28g	102	364	8.1	84.9	1.5	2.1
BULGAR WHEAT,							
Cracked, Organic, Evernat*	1oz/28g	31	110	3.6	23.7	0.1	3.2
Tesco*	1 Serving/50g	180	359	9.7	76.3	1.7	9.1
Average	1oz/28g	99	353	9.7	76.3	1.7	0.0
BUNS,							
American, Safeway*	1 Bun/60.1g	152	253	8.9	44.5	4.4	3.7
Bath, Marks & Spencer*	1 Bun/71g	217	305	8.3	49.8	8.0	1.9
Bath, Tesco*	1 Bun/80g	262	328	8.0	48.9	11.1	5.8

BUNS,	Measure INFO/WEIGHT	per Measure KCAL	Nutrition Values per 100g / 100ml				
			KCAL	PROT	CARB	FAT	FIBRE
Belgian, Co-Op*	1 Bun/118g	413	350	5.0	54.0	13.0	2.0
Belgian, Dairy Cream, Somerfield*	1 Serving/120.8g	401	331	5.2	52.6	11.1	2.0
Belgian, Tesco*	1 Bun/125g	451	361	4.4	56.7	12.9	2.7
Burger, Sainsbury's*	1 Bun/56g	162	289	7.8	49.4	6.7	2.4
Burger, Sliced, Tesco*	1 Bun/60g	168	280	7.9	47.3	6.6	2.1
Burger, Sliced, Waitrose*	1 Bun/61g	158	264	10.0	47.2	3.9	1.8
Burger, With Sesame Seeds, Co-Op*	1 Bun/55g	143	260	9.0	44.0	5.0	2.0
Chelsea	1 Bun/78g	285	366	7.8	56.1	13.8	1.7
Chelsea, Sainsbury's*	1 Bun/85g	239	281	6.9	51.6	5.2	2.9
Chelsea, Tesco*	1 Bun/85g	269	316	7.9	53.9	7.6	2.3
Currant	1 Bun/60g	178	296	7.6	52.7	7.5	0.0
Currant, Healthy Eating, Tesco*	1 Bun/62g	157	253	6.6	50.8	2.6	3.2
Currant, Healthy Living, Tesco*	1 Bun/63g	155	246	6.6	51.8	1.4	2.4
Currant, Safeway*	1 Bun/65.0g	178	274	7.0	50.0	5.1	2.8
Currant, Sainsbury's	1 Bun/72g	197	274	7.0	50.0	5.1	2.8
Currant, Somerfield*	1 Bun/52.7g	150	283	8.0	50.8	5.3	2.4
Custard Choux, Marks & Spencer*	1 Bun/85g	234	275	4.2	15.0	22.0	0.3
Dairy Cream, Somerfield*	1 Bun/98g	304	310	6.0	46.9	10.9	0.0
Fruit, Waitrose*	1 Bun/54g	171	316	7.8	55.7	6.9	1.6
Hot Cross	1 Bun/50g	155	310	7.4	58.5	6.8	1.7
Hot Cross, Apple & Cinnamon, Marks & Spencer*	1 Bun/71g	170	240	8.1	46.9	2.1	3.7
Hot Cross, BGTY, Sainsbury's*	1 Bun/70g	176	252	9.3	48.7	1.6	2.0
Hot Cross, Budgens*	1 Bun/64g	201	314	7.9	54.2	7.3	2.9
Hot Cross, Chocolate & Raisin, Mini, Tesco*	1 Bun/40g	127	318	8.1	47.0	10.9	2.8
Hot Cross, Chocolate, Mini, Sainsbury's*	1 Bun/39g	127	325	7.7	48.1	11.3	2.5
Hot Cross, Co-Op*	1 Bun/60g	165	275	8.0	47.0	6.0	3.0
Hot Cross, Extra Spicy, Marks & Spencer*	1 Bun/76g	175	230	8.6	44.1	1.9	4.2
Hot Cross, Finest, Tesco*	1 Bun/75g	203	270	6.9	49.0	5.2	2.6
Hot Cross, Golden Wholemeal, 3% Fat, Marks & Spencer*	1 Bun/67g	144	215	8.9	39.6	2.2	6.7
Hot Cross, Golden Wholemeal, Sainsbury's*	1 Bun/65g	180	277	9.9	45.4	6.2	4.3
Hot Cross, Healthy Eating, Tesco*	1 Bun/60g	155	258	8.6	50.3	2.5	2.6
Hot Cross, Healthy Living, Tesco*	1 Bun/62g	155	250	6.7	51.4	1.9	2.3
Hot Cross, Less Than 3% Fat, Marks & Spencer*	1 Bun/70g	175	250	8.1	49.8	1.8	2.2
Hot Cross, Luxury, Cafe, Marks & Spencer*	1 Bun/78g	199	255	8.6	46.2	4.0	2.1
Hot Cross, Luxury, Marks & Spencer*	1 Bun/79g	201	255	8.6	46.2	4.0	2.1
Hot Cross, Mini, Marks & Spencer*	1 Bun/36g	90	250	8.1	49.8	1.8	2.2
Hot Cross, Mini, Tesco*	1 Bun/36g	99	274	7.9	48.1	5.5	2.7
Hot Cross, Morning Fresh, Safeway*	1 Bun/64g	170	265	6.0	50.9	4.1	1.7
Hot Cross, Morrisons*	1 Bun/60g	163	272	8.5	47.4	5.4	3.3
Hot Cross, Perfectly Balanced, Waitrose*	1 Bun/68g	166	244	7.6	48.7	2.1	3.2
Hot Cross, Reduced Fat, Good For You, Asda*	1 Bun/67g	179	267	7.0	53.0	3.0	2.1
Hot Cross, Reduced Fat, Waitrose*	1 Bun/67g	171	255	8.1	54.3	2.1	3.3
Hot Cross, Safeway*	1 Bun/65g	174	268	7.9	46.9	5.4	2.2
Hot Cross, Sainsbury's*	1 Bun/70g	205	293	7.6	53.2	5.5	2.1
Hot Cross, So Good, Somerfield*	1 Bun/72g	184	256	7.4	46.3	4.6	2.3
Hot Cross, Tesco*	1 Bun/55g	144	262	7.4	46.8	5.0	2.8
Hot Cross, White, Low Fat, Safeway*	1 Bun/65g	161	248	8.7	47.4	2.6	3.0
Hot Cross, Wholemeal, Organic, Tesco*	1 Bun/55g	140	254	7.6	44.8	4.9	4.5
Hot Cross, Wholemeal, Tesco*	1 Bun/62g	166	268	9.9	43.6	6.0	4.7
Hot Cross, Wholemeal, Waitrose*	1 Bun/64g	177	276	8.8	45.2	6.7	4.9
Iced & Spiced Soft, Marks & Spencer*	1 Bun/42g	118	280	7.9	55.0	2.9	1.9
Iced Finger, Tesco*	1 Finger/69g	241	349	6.4	58.3	10.0	1.7
Iced Fruit, Marks & Spencer*	1 Bun/95g	285	300	8.5	57.9	4.3	1.3

	Measure INFO/WEIGHT	per Measure KCAL	Nutrition Values per 100g / 100ml				
			KCAL	PROT	CARB	FAT	FIBRE
BUNS,							
Iced Lemon, Tesco*	1 Bun/48g	156	325	5.2	56.5	8.7	1.9
Iced, Marks & Spencer*	1 Bun/42g	138	328	8.3	53.7	8.9	2.0
Iced, Tesco*	1 Bun/35g	113	323	7.0	58.9	6.6	2.1
Spiced, Perfectly Balanced, Waitrose*	1 Bun/65g	177	272	8.0	52.3	3.4	2.9
Swiss, Tesco*	1 Bun/100g	334	334	4.0	52.8	11.9	1.4
Vanilla, Soft Iced, Marks & Spencer*	1 Bun/41g	131	320	8.2	55.5	7.6	1.8
White, Stay Fresh, Tesco*	1 Bun/56g	152	271	7.5	45.5	6.6	0.0
BURGERS,							
Aberdeen Angus Beef, Mega, Bird's Eye*	1 Burger/101g	279	276	16.3	2.4	22.4	0.1
American Style, Asda*	1 Burger/41.7g	157	374	25.0	10.0	26.0	1.1
American Style, Tesco*	1 Burger/125g	250	200	13.0	20.4	7.3	3.9
BGTY, Sainsbury's*	1 Burger/110g	177	161	20.8	7.1	5.5	1.1
Bacon & Cheese, McDonald's*	1 Burger/141g	358	254	14.1	23.9	11.3	1.9
Bacon Double Cheeseburger, Bunless, Burger King*	1 Burger/138g	607	440	30.0	4.0	31.0	0.0
Bean, Quarter Pounders, Mexican Style, Tesco*	1 Burger/101g	215	213	4.3	25.0	10.6	2.8
Beef With Onion, Bird's Eye*	1 Burger/41g	114	278	15.3	3.5	22.5	0.2
Beef With Onion, Sainsbury's*	1 Burger/42g	102	243	20.7	6.9	14.8	1.0
Beef, 100% Beef, Somerfield*	1 Burger/113.5g	329	289	17.0	1.0	24.0	0.0
Beef, 100% With Seasoning, No Onion, Bird's Eye*	1 Burger/41g	134	326	16.1	0.2	29.0	0.0
Beef, 100%, Bird's Eye*	1 Burger/41g	120	292	17.3	0.0	24.8	0.0
Beef, 100%, Sainsbury's*	1 Burger/44g	133	302	21.4	0.9	23.6	0.9
Beef, Aberdeen Angus, Marks & Spencer*	1 Burger/142g	298	210	18.3	4.1	13.3	0.1
Beef, Aberdeen Angus, Waitrose*	1 Burger/114g	269	236	18.2	0.3	18.0	0.0
Beef, Asda*	1 Burger/114g	259	227	22.2	5.7	12.8	0.6
Beef, Barbecue, Tesco*	1 Burger/113.5g	259	227	16.4	1.3	17.4	1.2
Beef, Farmfoods*	1 Burger/50g	128	255	14.4	5.4	19.6	0.1
Beef, Flame Grilled, Dalepak*	1 Burger/44g	131	304	15.3	2.1	26.0	0.4
Beef, Frozen, Safeway*	1 Burger/44g	123	279	21.3	1.3	20.2	0.0
Beef, Giant Chargrilled, Farmfoods*	1 Burger/170g	352	207	17.3	5.6	12.8	1.2
Beef, Herbs, Finest, Tesco*	1 Burger/170g	284	167	16.9	3.6	9.4	0.3
Beef, In a Bun, Healthy Eating, Tesco*	1 Pack/189g	282	149	13.6	20.7	1.3	2.1
Beef, Mega, Bird's Eye*	1 Burger/109g	300	275	14.3	2.7	23.0	0.3
Beef, Morrisons*	1 Burger/56.7g	170	298	12.3	5.5	25.2	0.6
Beef, Organic, Marks & Spencer*	1 Burger/110g	239	217	18.2	0.0	16.0	0.2
Beef, Organic, Tesco*	1 Burger/56.8g	148	260	15.5	4.2	20.1	0.5
Beef, Quarter Pounders, 100% Prime, Asda*	1 Burger/86g	254	299	26.0	1.6	21.0	0.0
Beef, Quarter Pounders, Aberdeen Angus, M&S*	1 Burger/113g	254	225	19.8	1.6	15.5	0.0
Beef, Quarter Pounders, Bird's Eye*	1 Burger/139g	386	278	15.3	3.5	22.5	0.2
Beef, Quarter Pounders, Farmfoods*	1 Burger/113g	289	256	14.4	5.4	19.6	0.1
Beef, Quarter Pounders, Flame Grilled, Tesco*	1 Burger/88g	246	280	13.1	4.8	23.2	0.8
Beef, Quarter Pounders, Grilled, Bird's Eye*	1 Burger/113.5g	231	203	14.1	2.7	15.0	0.3
Beef, Quarter Pounders, Reduced Fat, Tesco*	1 Burger/95g	171	180	14.0	1.8	13.0	0.8
Beef, Quarter Pounders, Safeway*	1 Burger/100g	227	227	22.2	5.7	12.8	0.6
Beef, Quarter Pounders, Somerfield*	1 Burger/113.9g	319	280	14.7	5.6	22.1	1.2
Beef, Quarter Pounders, Steak Country, Lidl*	1 Burger/68g	188	276	16.3	2.4	22.2	0.1
Beef, Quarter Pounders, Tesco*	1 Burger/113g	292	258	17.8	0.7	20.4	1.3
Beef, Quarterpounders, Flame Grilled, Rustlers*	1 Burger/190g	557	293	14.9	24.3	15.1	0.0
Beef, Sainsbury's*	1 Burger/57g	150	267	29.6	1.3	15.9	1.5
Beef, Spicy Jalapeno, Finest, Tesco*	1 Burger/170g	277	163	17.2	2.4	9.4	0.4
Beef, Tesco*	1 Burger/47g	110	234	22.3	8.7	12.1	1.1
Big Mac, McDonald's*	1 Big Mac/215g	492	229	12.4	20.5	10.7	2.5
Big Tasty, McDonald's*	1 Pack/348g	804	231	11.7	14.6	14.5	1.6
Chargrilled Style, Vegetarian, Safeway*	1 Burger/57g	95	167	18.8	3.7	8.5	4.0

B

BURGERS,

INFO/WEIGHT	Measure per Measure KCAL	Nutrition Values per 100g / 100ml				
		KCAL	PROT	CARB	FAT	FIBRE
Cheeseburger, Bacon Double, Burger King*	1 Pack/191g 510	267	19.0	16.0	14.0	1.0
Cheeseburger, Burger King*	1 Burger/141g 379	269	15.6	30.0	13.4	1.4
Cheeseburger, Double, McDonalds*	1 Burger/171g 438	256	15.5	19.4	11.7	1.8
Cheeseburger, McDonald's*	1 Burger/122g 300	246	13.0	27.2	9.5	2.1
Cheeseburger, Wth Relish, American Style, Tesco*	1 Burger/61.4g 131	215	14.2	17.5	9.8	4.2
Chicken Fillet, Kentucky Fried Chicken*	1 Burger/213g 469	220	15.0	19.0	9.2	1.6
Chicken Flamer, Burger King*	1 Sandwich/162g 308	190	12.6	18.6	7.3	1.9
Chicken Sandwich, Burger King*	1 Sandwich/224g 659	294	11.2	23.6	17.4	1.3
Chicken Whopper, Lite, Burger King*	1 Whopper/159g 339	213	15.3	18.4	8.7	0.0
Chicken, Bird's Eye*	1 Burger/57g 147	258	13.6	16.8	15.2	0.4
Chicken, Breaded, Asda*	1 Burger/54.8g 145	263	14.0	18.0	15.0	0.0
Chicken, Crispy Crumb, Farmfoods*	1 Burger/242g 707	292	10.5	20.2	18.8	1.1
Chicken, Crunch Crumb, Tesco*	1 Burger/57g 161	282	12.3	15.6	18.9	0.0
Chicken, Quarter Pounders, Bird's Eye*	1 Burger/117g 280	239	13.5	15.2	13.8	0.6
Chicken, Sainsbury's*	1 Serving/46g 115	247	15.6	12.2	15.1	1.3
Chicken, Southern Fried, Sainsbury's*	1 Burger/52g 154	297	12.6	17.2	19.8	1.3
Chicken, Spar*	1 Burger/67g 163	244	16.1	20.8	11.2	1.5
Chicken, With Sesame Seed Bun, Breaded, Tesco*	1 Burger/205g 588	287	10.2	26.2	15.7	2.9
Chicken, Without Mayo, Nando's*	1 Burger/100g 399	399	32.3	45.2	9.5	0.0
Chilli Flavour Brown Rice & Tofu, Cauldron Foods*	1 Burger/75g 185	246	16.2	13.5	14.1	4.3
Chilli, Quarter Pounders, Asda*	1 Burger/87.7g 222	252	25.0	2.0	16.0	0.0
Chilli, Quarter Pounders, Farmfoods*	1 Burger/115g 285	248	13.5	2.9	20.3	0.9
Chilli, Quarter Pounders, Iceland*	1 Burger/84g 265	316	18.6	6.5	23.9	0.4
Classic, 3oz, Big Al's*	1 Burger/100g 169	169	15.0	0.0	12.2	0.0
Double Whopper With Cheese, Burger King*	1 Pack/378g 934	247	14.0	13.0	16.0	1.0
Double Whopper, Burger King*	1 Sandwich/353g 918	260	13.5	15.0	16.1	1.1
Economy, SmartPrice, Asda*	1 Burger/48.5g 141	293	14.0	12.0	21.0	1.1
Filet-O-Fish, McDonald's*	1 Pack/161g 388	241	10.0	25.0	11.0	0.7
Fillet Towermeal, Kentucky Fried Chicken*	1 Pack/283g 656	232	13.0	19.8	11.2	1.5
Hamburger, Burger King*	1 Burger/128g 339	265	14.8	23.4	12.5	1.5
Hamburger, McDonald's*	1 Burger/108g 254	235	12.2	30.6	7.1	2.3
Juicy Mushroom & Sweet Onion, Cauldron Foods*	1 Burger/87.5g 99	113	6.4	9.9	5.3	2.7
Lamb, Quarter Pounders, Bird's Eye*	1 Burger/112g 232	207	13.9	3.8	15.1	0.3
Lamb, Quarter Pounders, Farmfoods*	1oz/28g 76	272	12.3	6.6	21.8	1.0
Less Than 7% Fat, Sainsbury's*	1 Burger/102g 164	161	20.8	7.1	5.5	1.1
Low Fat, Iceland*	1 Serving/85g 148	174	27.8	5.0	4.8	1.1
McChicken Grill With BBQ Sauce, McDonald's*	1 Pack/215g 309	144	12.1	18.1	2.6	2.2
McChicken Premiere, McDonald's*	1 Burger/244g 547	224	11.0	15.9	11.5	1.3
McChicken Sandwich, McDonald's*	1 Pack/167g 376	225	9.9	23.1	10.3	2.2
Meat Free, Asda*	1 Burger/60g 138	230	24.0	11.0	10.0	0.3
Meat Free, Sainsbury's*	1 Burger/57g 92	161	19.6	3.9	7.4	4.8
Mushroom & Red Onion, Tesco*	1 Burger/87.1g 135	155	5.4	21.3	5.4	1.6
Mushroom, Cauldron Foods*	1 Burger/87.5g 135	153	7.1	15.1	7.1	2.7
Mushroom, Tesco*	1 Burger/87g 144	166	2.8	20.4	8.1	3.1
Pork, Quarter Pounders, Bird's Eye*	1 Burger/122g 292	239	13.9	3.2	19.0	0.2
Prime Beef, Asda*	1 Burger/45g 123	274	22.0	6.0	18.0	0.6
Quarter Pounder With Cheese & Buns, Sainsbury's*	1 Burger/198g 471	238	15.6	19.1	11.5	1.4
Quarter Pounder With Cheese, McDonald's*	1 Burger/206g 515	250	15.1	18.2	13.0	1.8
Quarter Pounders, 95% Fat Free, Good Choice, Iceland*	1 Burger/86g 150	174	27.8	5.0	4.8	1.1
Quarter Pounders, Big Country*	1 Burger/90g 271	301	22.1	1.8	23.1	0.0
Quarter Pounders, Chargrilled, BGTY, Sainsbury's*	1 Burger/114g 184	161	20.8	7.1	5.5	1.1
Quarter Pounders, Deluxe, McDonald's*	1 Burger/253g 521	206	11.4	16.1	10.6	1.7
Quarter Pounders, Healthy Living, Tesco*	1 Burger/114g 188	165	18.7	3.6	8.4	0.6

BURGERS,

	Measure INFO/WEIGHT	per Measure KCAL	KCAL	PROT	CARB	FAT	FIBRE
			Nutrition Values per 100g / 100ml				
Quarter Pounders, Iceland*	1 Burger/83g	253	305	20.4	5.1	22.6	0.6
Quarter Pounders, Marks & Spencer*	1oz/28g	69	247	18.5	3.2	17.9	0.6
Quarter Pounders, McDonald's*	1 Burger/178g	424	238	14.5	20.9	10.7	2.1
Quarter Pounders, TTD, Sainsbury's*	1 Burger/100g	182	182	22.6	5.5	7.7	1.5
Quorn*	1 Burger/50g	56	112	12.4	5.3	4.6	3.6
Quorn*, New Improved	2 Burgers/100g	137	137	17.8	8.8	3.4	3.7
Quorn*, Original	1 Burger/50g	55	109	12.0	6.9	3.7	4.9
Quorn*, Premium	1 Burger/81g	96	118	11.4	7.1	4.9	3.5
Quorn*, Southern Style	1 Burger/63g	113	180	10.7	12.3	9.8	3.1
Salmon, Quarter Pounders, Morrisons*	1 Burger/109.8g	235	214	21.4	5.5	11.8	1.7
Savoury Tofu, Cauldron Foods*	1 Burger/75g	162	216	14.8	13.2	11.5	3.5
Spicy Bean, Burger King*	1 Burger/239g	504	211	7.9	26.2	8.3	3.9
Spicy Bean, Dalepak*	1 Burger/118g	242	205	4.6	22.8	10.6	3.0
Spicy Bean, Quarter Pounders, Asda*	1 Serving/108g	257	238	4.5	28.0	12.0	3.0
Spicy Bean, Sainsbury's*	1 Burger/110g	262	240	5.0	27.1	12.4	2.0
Spicy Black Bean, Cauldron Foods*	1 Burger/88g	158	180	10.8	13.4	9.2	5.1
Spicy Vegetable Bean, BGTY, Sainsbury's*	1 Burger/76g	119	156	5.6	24.3	3.2	3.3
Spicy Vegetable, Asda*	1 Burger/56g	108	193	3.4	20.0	11.0	0.0
Steak Premiere, McDonald's*	1 Burger/229g	453	198	14.9	19.4	6.2	1.6
Tuna, Bird's Eye*	1 Burger/50g	125	250	15.0	16.2	14.0	0.8
Tuna, Quarter Pounders, Sainsbury's*	1 Serving/100g	179	179	24.0	10.0	4.8	0.4
Tuna, Sainsbury's*	1 Serving/105g	194	185	20.8	3.4	9.8	1.2
Turkey Cheese, Somerfield*	1oz/28g	79	281	14.0	16.0	18.0	0.0
Turkey Cheeseburgers, Tesco*	1 Burger/105g	252	240	15.4	12.8	14.1	1.3
Turkey, Crispy Crumb, Bernard Matthews*	1 Burger/71g	222	313	11.3	19.3	19.8	0.9
Value, Farmfoods*	1 Burger/49g	138	282	11.4	9.6	22.1	0.9
Vegeburger Mix, Realeat*	1 Serving/62.5g	233	370	30.0	40.0	10.0	6.0
Vegeburger, Herb & Vegetable, Realeat*	1 Burger/125g	433	346	32.0	32.0	10.0	0.0
Vegeburger, Linda McCartney*	1 Burger/59g	79	134	22.6	2.9	3.6	1.6
Vegeburger, Retail, Grilled	1oz/28g	55	196	16.6	8.0	11.1	4.2
Vegetable & Cheese, Tesco*	1 Burger/85g	167	197	7.7	19.5	9.8	1.4
Vegetable With Tofu, Organic, Evernat*	1oz/28g	52	186	7.9	16.9	8.3	0.0
Vegetable, Captains, Bird's Eye*	1 Burger/48g	96	200	4.7	25.5	8.8	2.0
Vegetable, Deluxe, McDonald's*	1 Burger/210g	422	201	4.6	25.8	8.9	2.8
Vegetable, Organic, Tesco*	1 Burger/90g	108	120	2.6	17.6	4.3	2.1
Vegetable, Quarter Pounders, Bird's Eye*	1 Burger/100g	166	166	4.3	19.8	8.0	1.6
Vegetable, Quarter Pounders, Dalepak*	1 Burger/114g	251	220	4.4	20.8	13.2	2.7
Vegetarian, Bean, Mexican Quarter Pounders, Tesco*	1 Burger/101g	215	213	4.3	25.0	10.6	2.8
Vegetarian, Cheeseburger, Chicken Style, Safeway*	1 Burger/100g	234	234	16.6	11.4	13.5	3.0
Vegetarian, Flame Grilled, Linda McCartney*	1 Burger/60g	80	134	22.6	2.9	3.6	1.6
Vegetarian, Mushroom & Red Onion, Tesco*	1 Burger/78g	105	135	4.7	18.6	4.6	1.4
Vegetarian, Quarterpounders, Chargrilled, Tesco*	1 Burger/113.5g	187	164	16.0	7.0	8.0	2.5
Vegetarian, Spicy Bean, Linda McCartney*	1 Burger/85g	190	223	4.3	26.2	11.2	2.9
Vegetarian, Tesco*	1 Burger/56g	92	164	16.0	7.0	8.0	2.5
Veggie, Burger King*	1 Burger/223g	433	194	6.6	24.9	7.6	3.4
Whopper Junior With Cheese, Burger King*	1 Burger/167g	421	252	12.0	18.0	14.0	1.0
Whopper With Cheese, Burger King*	1 Pack/299g	724	242	11.0	16.0	15.0	1.0
Whopper With Mayo, Burger King*	1 Whopper/278g	678	244	10.4	19.0	14.0	1.4
Whopper, Burger King*	1 Whopper/274g	641	234	11.0	17.0	14.0	1.0
Zinger Fillet, Kentucky Fried Chicken*	1 Serving/185g	445	241	13.9	22.4	10.6	1.4
Zinger Tower, Kentucky Fried Chicken*	1 Serving/256g	620	242	12.4	20.2	12.5	1.3
Zinger, Meal, Kentucky Fried Chicken*	1 Meal/305g	735	241	22.4	10.6	14.0	1.4
BURRITO, Dinner Kit, Old El Paso*	1 Serving/100g	294	294	8.0	55.0	4.8	0.0

	Measure	per Measure	Nutrition Values per 100g / 100ml				
	INFO/WEIGHT	KCAL	KCAL	PROT	CARB	FAT	FIBRE
BUTTER,							
Alpine Unsalted, TTD, Sainsbury's*	1 Serving/10g	75	748	0.7	0.6	82.5	0.0
Brandy, With Cognac, Sainsbury's*	1/8 Pot/25g	137	549	0.2	44.1	37.6	0.0
Butter Me Up, Tesco*	1 Serving/15g	95	631	1.0	1.5	69.0	0.0
Creamery, Asda*	1 Serving/10g	73	734	0.5	0.7	81.0	0.0
Creamery, Co-Op*	Thin Spread/7g	52	737	0.5	0.0	81.7	0.0
Dairy, Marks & Spencer*	Thin Spread/7g	29	415	0.9	78.1	11.0	0.0
Don't Flutter With Butter, Safeway*	Thin Spread/7g	45	636	0.4	1.0	70.0	0.0
English, Unsalted, Country Life*	Thin Spread/7g	52	746	0.5	0.0	82.7	0.0
Fresh	Thin Spread/7g	52	737	0.5	0.0	81.7	0.0
Fresh, Spreadable, Kerrygold*	Thin Spread/7g	50	720	0.4	0.0	80.0	0.0
Garlic, Somerfield*	1oz/28g	192	686	1.0	2.0	75.0	0.0
Golden Churn, St Ivel*	Thin Spread/7g	44	628	0.8	1.0	69.0	0.0
Half Fat, Anchor*	Thin Spread/7g	25	363	0.1	0.8	40.0	0.8
Half Fat, Healthy Choice, Asda*	Thin Spread/7g	26	370	2.0	0.5	40.0	0.0
Half Fat, Marks & Spencer*	Thin Spread/7g	26	370	1.8	2.0	39.5	0.5
Half Fat, Tesco*	Thin Spread/7g	25	361	2.1	0.4	39.0	0.6
I Can't Believe It's Not Butter*	Thin Spread/7g	44	625	0.4	0.7	69.0	0.0
Light, Good For You, Asda*	1 Serving/10g	37	368	2.0	0.0	40.0	0.0
Lighter Spreadable, Reduced Fat, Lurpak*	Thin Spread/7g	38	540	0.5	0.5	60.0	0.0
Low Fat, Connacht Gold*	1 Serving/15g	58	384	7.0	0.0	40.0	0.0
Low Fat, Marks & Spencer*	Thin Spread/7g	26	374	3.5	0.0	40.0	0.0
Salted, Marks & Spencer*	1oz/28g	205	733	0.5	0.5	81.0	0.0
Salted, Organic, Marks & Spencer*	1oz/28g	202	720	0.1	0.1	81.0	0.0
Slightly Salted, Organic, Sainsbury's*	1 Serving/10g	72	724	0.5	0.6	80.0	0.0
Spreadable, Anchor*	Thin Spread/7g	52	741	0.4	0.6	81.9	0.0
Spreadable, Country Life*	Thin Spread/7g	51	728	0.3	0.5	80.5	0.0
Spreadable, Fresh	Thin Spread/7g	52	745	0.5	0.0	82.5	0.0
Spreadable, Lurpak*	Thin Spread/7g	51	724	0.5	0.5	80.0	0.0
Sunflower, Asda*	1 Serving/25g	160	638	0.9	1.2	70.0	0.0
Utterly Butterly*	1 Tbsp/10g	63	630	1.0	1.5	69.0	0.0
Utterly Butterly* Scandinavian Style	1 Serving/25g	152	606	0.3	0.5	67.0	0.0
Value, Tesco*	Thin Spread/7g	51	732	0.5	0.7	81.0	0.0
With Crushed Garlic, Lurpak*	1 Serving/10g	70	700	1.0	4.0	75.0	0.0
You'd Butter Believe It, Low Fat, Dairy, Asda*	1 Serving/10g	63	627	0.5	1.0	69.0	0.0
BUTTERMILK,							
Average	1oz/28g	10	37	3.4	5.0	0.5	0.0
Low Fat, Yoplait*	1 Pot/284ml	133	47	5.2	6.0	0.2	0.0
BUTTONS,							
Cadbury's*	1 Treat Pack/14g	74	525	7.8	56.8	29.4	0.0
White, Cadbury's*	1 Bag/32g	171	535	8.8	56.5	30.3	0.0

	Measure	per Measure	Nutrition Values per 100g / 100ml				
	INFO/WEIGHT	KCAL	KCAL	PROT	CARB	FAT	FIBRE

CABBAGE,

Boiled in Salted Water, Average	1 Serving/90g	14	16	1.0	2.2	0.4	1.8
Boiled in Unsalted Water, Average	1 Serving/90g	14	16	1.0	2.2	0.4	1.8
Braised Red, Safeway*	½ Pack/150g	159	106	0.8	17.6	3.6	2.2
Chinese, Raw	1oz/28g	3	12	1.0	1.4	0.2	1.2
Cut, Fresh, Frozen, Tesco*	1oz/28g	6	22	1.3	3.2	0.5	0.3
Green, Frozen, Asda*	1 Serving/60g	13	22	1.3	3.1	0.5	2.9
Green, Tesco*	1 Serving/100g	16	16	1.0	2.2	0.4	1.8
Greens, Hand Trimmed, Marks & Spencer*	1oz/28g	6	22	2.8	2.8	0.0	3.4
Greens, Marks & Spencer*	1 Serving/75g	26	35	3.0	3.1	1.0	3.4
Mash, Eat Smart, Safeway*	½ Pack/225g	146	65	2.0	9.2	1.8	1.7
Medley, Marks & Spencer*	1 Serving/300g	270	90	1.7	2.7	8.2	1.5
Raw, Average	1oz/28g	7	26	1.7	4.1	0.4	2.4
Red & Cranberry Slaw, Tesco*	½ Pack/125g	75	60	0.7	11.3	1.3	0.0
Red, Boiled in Salted Water	1 Serving/90g	14	15	0.8	2.3	0.3	2.0
Red, Pickled, Asda*	1oz/28g	8	30	0.9	4.5	0.1	1.2
Red, Raw	1oz/28g	6	21	1.1	3.7	0.3	2.5
Red, Raw, Tesco*	1 Serving/100g	27	27	1.2	5.0	0.2	2.1
Red, in Sweet Vinegar, Heinz*	1 Serving/100g	23	23	0.9	4.7	0.2	1.9
Savoy, Boiled in Salted Water	1 Serving/90g	15	17	1.1	2.2	0.5	2.0
Savoy, Raw	1 Serving/90g	24	27	2.1	3.9	0.5	3.1
White, Boiled in Salted Water	1 Serving/90g	13	14	1.0	2.2	0.2	1.5
White, Raw	1oz/28g	8	27	1.4	5.0	0.2	2.1
White, Raw, Tesco*	1 Serving/100g	27	27	1.4	5.0	0.2	2.1
CADBURY'S BYTE, McDonald's*	1 Byte/14g	67	478	6.5	64.7	20.7	1.7

CAKE,

Action Man, Birthday, Memory Lane Cakes*	1/12 Portion/83g	322	388	3.0	57.0	16.4	0.8
Alabama Chocolate Fudge, Farmfoods*	1/6 Cake/61g	201	329	4.7	55.7	9.7	2.7
Almond Flavour Slices, Good For You, Asda*	1 Slice/25g	67	268	4.0	56.0	3.1	0.7
Almond Flavoured Rounds, Country Garden Cakes*	1 Cake/45.4g	181	403	4.3	62.4	14.7	2.3
Almond Slices, Lyons*	1 Slice/26.8g	115	426	7.1	41.3	25.8	1.6
Almond Slices, Mr Kipling*	1 Slice/35g	141	403	6.8	58.6	13.4	0.0
Angel Layer, Tesco*	1 Serving/25g	101	403	4.5	57.4	17.3	0.9
Angel Slices, Mr Kipling*	1 Slice/38g	138	362	2.6	49.8	16.9	0.4
Angel, Co-Op*	1/8 Cake/35g	131	375	4.0	52.0	17.0	0.7
Angel, Sainsbury's*	1/8 Cake/41g	171	417	4.1	55.7	19.8	0.8
Apple Bakes, Go Ahead, McVitie's*	1 Cake/35g	129	368	2.8	74.7	8.3	1.2
Apple Crumble, Co-Op*	1/8 Cake/52g	151	290	4.0	41.0	12.0	2.0
Apple Crumble, Eat Smart, Safeway*	1 Serving/28g	85	305	5.2	64.5	2.4	1.2
Apple Sponge, Marks & Spencer*	1 Portion/63g	178	283	3.8	32.0	16.4	0.7
Apple, Home Style, Marks & Spencer*	1 Cake/54g	189	350	5.3	49.4	14.7	1.5
Apple, Pret A Manger*	1 Av Pack/120g	432	360	5.3	38.8	21.9	2.1
Apricot & Almond, Bakers Delight*	1oz/28g	106	379	5.5	53.2	16.0	1.8
Apricot & Apple, Trimlyne*	1 Cake/50g	134	267	4.3	58.4	2.7	1.9
Assorted Cup, Sainsbury's*	1 Cake/38g	130	341	2.2	69.3	6.1	0.4
Bakewell Slices, Mr Kipling*	1 Slice/35g	153	436	3.7	59.5	20.4	0.0
Banana & Date Loaf, Starbucks*	1 Slice/105g	292	278	5.9	57.1	2.9	2.7
Banana Loaf, Organic, Respect*	1 Slice/40g	151	377	3.5	48.7	19.5	0.9
Banana Loaf, Waitrose*	1 Slice/70g	236	337	5.0	55.2	10.7	1.7
Banana, Date & Walnut Slices, BGTY, Sainsbury's*	1 Slice/28g	78	280	5.3	56.1	4.9	2.2
Battenberg, Lyons*	1 Serving/26g	112	431	6.9	70.3	13.7	1.3
Battenburg, Mini, Mr Kipling*	1 Serving/35g	119	339	3.1	65.6	7.0	0.7
Best Chocolate Orange Explosion, Safeway*	1 Serving/59g	248	421	4.1	48.8	23.3	0.9
Birthday Present, Tesco*	1 Serving/79g	347	439	3.5	66.6	17.6	0.4

CAKE,

	Measure INFO/WEIGHT	per Measure KCAL	Nutrition Values per 100g / 100ml				
			KCAL	PROT	CARB	FAT	FIBRE
Birthday, Marks & Spencer*	1 Serving/60g	240	400	2.3	70.9	11.9	0.8
Birthday, McDonald's*	1 Portion/158g	406	257	1.6	39.6	9.5	0.3
Bounty Bar, McVitie's*	1 Cake/36g	166	461	5.1	55.2	24.5	0.0
Brownie, Pret A Manger*	1 Av Pack/50g	328	656	7.2	81.0	33.8	1.0
Butterfly, Mr Kipling*	1 Cake/29g	114	392	4.4	43.4	22.2	0.6
Buttons, Cadbury's*	1 Cake/25g	110	440	7.2	50.0	22.8	0.0
Cappuccino, Finest, Tesco*	1oz/28g	105	374	2.8	40.4	22.3	0.2
Caramel Bar, Cadbury's*	1 Bar/6g	25	411	6.4	57.0	16.8	0.0
Caramel Slice, Marks & Spencer*	1 Slice/64g	304	475	4.9	60.4	25.2	2.6
Caramel, Milk Chocolate, Holly Lane*	1 Cake/25g	110	441	6.9	57.6	20.3	1.1
Carrot & Apple, Safeway*	1 Serving/50g	158	315	3.2	50.4	11.2	0.8
Carrot & Mango Slices, Eat Smart, Safeway*	1 Slice/31g	95	305	3.4	65.3	2.9	2.3
Carrot & Orange Slices, Good For You, Asda*	1 Slice/24g	70	291	3.3	62.0	3.3	1.0
Carrot & Orange Slices, Healthy Eating, Tesco*	1 Slice/29g	75	257	3.0	56.4	2.7	1.9
Carrot & Orange, Finest, Tesco*	1 Serving/50g	171	342	4.1	49.1	14.3	1.0
Carrot & Orange, Waitrose*	1/6 Cake/47g	165	350	5.3	46.8	15.7	1.8
Carrot & Walnut, Marks & Spencer*	1/6 Cake/82g	279	340	5.8	34.8	19.5	1.5
Carrot Loaf, Starbucks*	1 Slice/100g	352	352	4.7	38.4	19.9	2.3
Carrot Slices, BGTY, Sainsbury's*	1 Slice/27g	81	313	3.4	68.7	2.7	2.4
Carrot Slices, Weight Watchers*	1oz/28g	81	290	3.0	56.7	2.7	1.9
Carrot Wedge, Tesco*	1 Pack/175g	576	329	4.6	41.7	16.0	1.5
Carrot, Entenmann's*	1 Serving/40g	156	391	4.1	47.4	20.5	1.5
Carrot, Farmfoods*	1/8 Cake/59g	187	317	3.7	35.4	17.8	1.6
Carrot, Marks & Spencer*	1oz/28g	98	350	6.1	34.5	21.0	1.5
Carrot, Traditional, Farringford Foods*	1oz/28g	115	412	4.4	44.8	25.2	0.0
Carrot, Ultimate, Entenmann's*	1/8 Cake/63.8g	235	367	4.7	51.4	15.8	0.3
Cherry Bakewell, Gluten Free, Bakers Delight*	1 Cake/50g	211	422	2.9	66.1	16.3	0.4
Cherry Bakewell, Marks & Spencer*	1 Cake/44g	185	420	4.5	61.7	17.7	1.0
Cherry Bakewell, Mini, Sainsbury's*	1 Tart/27.3g	100	370	3.4	62.2	12.0	0.4
Cherry Bakewell, Mr Kipling*	1 Cake/45g	186	414	3.9	59.3	17.9	1.2
Cherry Bakewell, Safeway*	1 Bakewell/47.0g	203	432	3.5	58.7	20.3	3.9
Cherry Bakewell, Sara Lee*	1/5 Slice/69.9g	228	326	4.1	51.9	11.3	1.4
Cherry Bakewell, SmartPrice, Asda*	1 Cake/38g	157	413	2.7	60.0	18.0	2.6
Cherry Bakewell, Somerfield*	1 Cake/50g	216	431	3.5	58.7	20.3	3.9
Cherry Bakewell, Tesco*	1 Tart/50g	208	416	3.6	65.8	15.4	1.8
Cherry Bakewell, Weight Watchers*	1 Cake/43g	156	363	3.7	65.1	11.6	3.3
Cherry Genoa, Marks & Spencer*	1oz/28g	99	355	4.5	59.3	10.9	1.6
Cherry, Co-Op*	1/8 Cake/47g	195	415	5.0	49.0	22.0	0.5
Cherry, Marks & Spencer*	1 Serving/75g	285	380	5.0	60.6	12.7	0.8
Chewy Fruity Corn Flake, Doves Farm*	1 Bar/40g	155	388	5.8	64.5	14.0	4.5
Chewy Rice Pop & Chocolate, Doves Farm*	1 Bar/35g	156	447	3.9	69.9	20.2	2.3
Choc Chip Bar, Go Ahead, McVitie's*	1 Bar/28g	100	356	6.4	56.9	12.1	1.0
Choc Chip Mini Bar, Go Ahead, McVitie's	1 Bar/27g	93	343	5.7	55.3	12.1	0.9
Chocolate	1oz/28g	128	456	7.4	50.4	26.4	0.0
Chocolate & Orange Bar, Go Ahead, McVitie's*	1 Cake Bar/33g	109	330	4.3	64.9	6.0	1.0
Chocolate & Orange Rolls, Marks & Spencer*	1 Roll/60g	228	380	3.6	27.0	28.4	1.3
Chocolate & Orange Slices, Good For You, Asda*	1 Slice/30g	84	281	3.0	61.0	2.8	0.7
Chocolate Birthday, Asda*	1/10 Cake/61.1g	281	460	6.0	46.0	28.0	0.9
Chocolate Birthday, Marks & Spencer*	1 Serving/68g	279	410	4.5	43.7	24.1	1.3
Chocolate Birthday, Tesco*	1 Serving/58g	276	475	6.3	50.3	27.6	0.9
Chocolate Box, Asda*	1 Serving/60g	263	439	5.0	53.0	23.0	0.7
Chocolate Brownie, Fudge, Entenmann's*	1/8 Cake/55g	168	306	4.0	62.7	4.4	1.5
Chocolate Brownie, Fudgy, Marks & Spencer*	1 Brownie/87g	400	460	4.8	56.9	25.2	3.0

CAKE,

INFO/WEIGHT	Measure per Measure	KCAL	Nutrition Values per 100g / 100ml KCAL	PROT	CARB	FAT	FIBRE
Chocolate Brownie, Slices, Marks & Spencer*	1 Brownie/36g	158	440	5.3	51.1	24.1	1.3
Chocolate Brownie, Topped With M&M's Minis, McVitie's*	1 Cake/92.5g	424	456	4.6	59.4	22.2	0.0
Chocolate Brownie, Waitrose*	1 Brownie/45g	192	426	6.3	55.6	19.8	2.7
Chocolate Chip Bar, Mr Kipling*	1 Bar/33g	148	448	6.1	45.2	27.0	0.0
Chocolate Chip Bar, Sainsbury's*	1 Cake Bar/25g	108	430	6.1	51.2	22.3	0.6
Chocolate Chip Brownie, McDonald's*	1 Brownie/19g	68	360	4.9	58.8	12.7	1.9
Chocolate Chip, Co-Op*	1/6 Cake/62.5g	273	440	5.0	44.0	27.0	0.5
Chocolate Cup, 5% Fat, Sainsbury's*	1 Cake/38g	133	349	2.5	74.8	4.4	1.7
Chocolate Cup, BGTY, Sainsbury's*	1 Cake/38g	121	318	2.5	66.5	4.6	0.8
Chocolate Cup, Fabulous Bakin' boys*	1 Cake/40g	164	410	3.0	44.0	24.0	1.0
Chocolate Cup, Lyons*	1 Cake/39g	125	321	2.4	67.5	4.6	0.8
Chocolate Dream Bar, Go Ahead, McVitie's*	1 Bar/36g	141	391	4.6	63.2	13.4	0.9
Chocolate Flavour Slice, Eat Smart, Safeway*	1 Slice/28g	95	340	5.3	73.6	2.4	4.0
Chocolate Flavour Slices, Good For You, Asda*	2 Slices/55g	141	257	4.3	54.0	2.6	1.4
Chocolate Flavour Slices, Healthy Eating, Tesco*	1 Slice/25g	79	314	4.7	65.5	2.4	3.7
Chocolate Fudge & Vanilla Cream, Marks & Spencer*	1/6 Cake/69g	306	450	5.2	49.8	26.0	1.3
Chocolate Fudge Slice, Waitrose*	1 Slice/60g	230	383	4.7	54.6	16.2	1.5
Chocolate Fudge, Entenmann's*	1 Serving/48g	173	361	4.4	51.8	15.1	0.9
Chocolate Fudge, Marks & Spencer*	1oz/28g	109	390	3.7	50.8	20.6	1.4
Chocolate Fudge, Pizza Express*	1 Cake/100g	395	395	4.0	57.2	17.0	0.0
Chocolate Fudge, Somerfield*	1oz/28g	114	406	5.0	48.0	22.0	0.0
Chocolate Heaven, Extra Special, Asda*	1/6 Cake/65.7g	256	388	4.0	48.0	20.0	1.0
Chocolate Indulgence, Finest, Tesco*	1 Slice/52g	203	390	3.8	47.8	20.4	0.4
Chocolate Loaf, Somerfield*	1oz/28g	111	396	6.0	44.0	22.0	0.0
Chocolate Log, Iceland*	1 Cake/31g	157	505	5.3	48.0	32.4	1.2
Chocolate Orange Slices, BGTY, Sainsbury's*	1 Slice/30g	90	301	3.9	62.8	4.8	1.3
Chocolate Orange Slices, BGTY, Sainsbury's*	1 Cake/30g	83	275	3.9	54.8	4.5	1.5
Chocolate Party, Tesco*	1 Slice/62g	244	394	4.6	46.3	21.2	0.9
Chocolate Slice, Go Ahead, McVitie's*	1 Slice/32g	94	293	4.5	49.4	8.2	1.9
Chocolate Slices, Mr Kipling*	1oz/28g	108	386	4.8	50.4	18.3	0.0
Chocolate Sponge Roll, Marks & Spencer*	¼ Cake/66g	251	380	3.9	50.5	18.4	1.8
Chocolate Sponge, Less Than 5% Fat, Asda*	1 Sponge/110g	198	180	4.4	32.0	3.8	1.1
Chocolate Swiss Roll, Mini, Tesco*	1 Roll/22g	87	396	4.6	61.0	14.8	0.0
Chocolate Truffle, Extra Special, Asda*	1 Serving/103g	402	390	5.0	34.0	26.0	1.8
Chocolate Victoria Sponge, Co-Op*	1 Slice/61g	201	330	5.0	42.0	16.0	1.0
Chocolate With Butter Icing	1oz/28g	135	481	5.7	50.9	29.7	0.0
Chocolate, Double Dream, Nestle*	1 Serving/150g	638	425	5.0	44.7	25.1	0.9
Chocolate, Home Bake, McVitie's*	1oz/28g	99	355	5.7	54.4	14.1	1.4
Chocolate, Low Fat, Safeway*	1 Slice/73.4g	176	241	5.8	45.0	4.8	1.3
Chocolate, Morrisons*	1 Serving/31.5g	157	505	5.3	48.0	32.4	1.2
Chocolate, Sainsbury's*	1 Serving/30g	119	395	4.1	52.6	18.5	1.3
Chocolate, Sara Lee*	¼ Cake/88g	339	385	4.1	54.3	16.8	0.0
Chocolate, Thorntons*	1 Serving/87g	408	469	5.2	47.1	28.8	0.6
Chocolate, Viennese, Marks & Spencer*	1oz/28g	105	375	4.4	54.1	13.6	1.6
Choux Buns, Fresh Cream, Tesco*	1 Bun/95g	340	358	4.9	28.5	24.9	0.9
Choux Buns, Marks & Spencer*	1oz/28g	89	317	5.4	25.6	22.2	0.3
Christmas, Conoisseur, Marks & Spencer*	1 Slice/60g	216	360	4.1	64.7	9.2	3.3
Christmas, Iced, Slices, Tesco*	1 Slice/45g	168	369	2.9	67.6	9.6	1.2
Christmas, Rich Fruit, All Iced, Sainsbury's*	1/16 Cake/85g	307	361	4.0	66.4	8.9	1.5
Christmas, Rich Fruit, Free From, Tesco*	1 Serving/100g	301	301	2.9	56.0	7.3	0.9
Christmas, TTD, Sainsbury's*	1/16 Cake/85g	315	371	3.7	67.1	8.9	1.3
Classic Lemon Drizzle, Marks & Spencer*	1/6 Cake/67.5g	255	375	4.7	55.0	15.3	0.6
Coconut	1 Slice/70g	304	434	6.7	51.2	23.8	2.5

CAKE,

INFO/WEIGHT	Measure	per Measure KCAL	KCAL	PROT	CARB	FAT	FIBRE
Coconut Delight, Burton's*	1 Cake/25.1g	104	415	4.1	65.0	15.4	1.6
Coconut Macaroons, Sainsbury's*	1 Macaroon/33g	144	436	4.8	65.1	17.3	1.6
Coconut Snowball, Bobby's*	1 Cake/18.3g	78	436	2.2	57.3	22.1	0.0
Coconut Sponge, Mini Classics, Mr Kipling*	1 Cake/38g	155	409	3.7	47.0	22.9	0.9
Coffee & Walnut Slices, Healthy Eating,Tesco*	1 Slice/23g	69	301	4.4	65.7	2.3	2.8
Coffee & Walnut, Mrs Beeton's*	1 Slice/54g	219	405	3.7	41.4	25.0	0.3
Coffee & Walnut, Somerfield*	1oz/28g	123	440	5.0	46.0	26.0	0.0
Coffee Sponge Roll, Marks & Spencer*	1 Serving/40g	150	375	3.5	51.1	17.3	0.6
Coffee, Entenmann's*	1 Portion/41g	159	388	4.0	54.7	17.3	0.6
Coffee, Iced, Marks & Spencer*	1 Slice/33g	135	410	4.4	54.5	19.6	1.6
Country Slices, Good Intentions, Somerfield*	1 Cake/22g	70	318	5.5	70.0	1.8	1.8
Country Slices, Mr Kipling*	1oz/28g	104	371	4.8	53.7	15.2	0.0
Cream Oysters, Marks & Spencer*	1 Oyster/72g	227	315	3.6	27.5	21.2	3.0
Cream Slices, Marks & Spencer*	1 Slice/80g	310	387	2.3	45.7	22.9	0.6
Crispy Fruit Slices, Apple & Sultana, Go Ahead, McVitie's*	1 Slice/14g	54	386	6.0	72.7	7.9	3.3
Crispy Fruit Slices, Forest Fruit, Go Ahead, McVitie's*	1 Biscuit/14g	56	400	5.5	73.0	8.8	3.7
Crispy Fruit Slices, Orange & Sultana, GA, McVitie's*	1 Biscuit/15g	60	400	5.1	75.7	8.1	3.0
Crunchie Cake Bar, Cadbury's*	1 Cake Bar/32g	147	460	5.9	58.3	22.6	0.0
Custard Slices, Tesco*	1 Slice/108g	320	296	2.4	37.5	15.2	0.5
Date & Walnut Loaf, Sainsbury's*	1/10 Slice/40g	148	371	6.7	40.1	20.4	1.0
Date & Walnut, Bakers Delight*	1oz/28g	88	315	5.2	55.5	8.0	1.2
Double Chocolate Ganache, Marks & Spencer*	1/12 Cake/61g	281	460	5.9	46.1	27.6	2.5
Double Chocolate Wedge, Tesco*	1 Piece/100g	416	416	5.0	53.4	20.3	0.9
Dundee, Co-Op*	1/8 Cake/71g	238	335	5.0	53.0	11.0	2.0
Dundee, Somerfield*	1/10 Cake/75g	254	339	5.0	57.0	11.0	0.0
Easter Lemon Bakewells, Morrisons*	1 Cake/45g	186	413	3.1	64.8	15.7	1.8
Eccles	1 Cake/45g	214	475	3.9	59.3	26.4	1.6
Eccles, Weight Watchers*	1 Cake/48g	190	396	4.4	57.5	16.5	2.0
Fairy, Co-Op*	1oz/28g	105	375	4.0	43.0	21.0	0.8
Fairy, Holly Lane*	1 Cake/25.7g	120	460	3.7	52.5	26.1	3.5
Fairy, Iced, Somerfield*	1 Cake/15.1g	59	392	4.9	62.9	13.4	1.4
Fairy, Mini, Tesco*	1 Cake/13g	55	424	6.1	54.6	20.1	1.3
Fairy, Smartprice, Asda*	1 Cake/15g	66	438	6.0	54.0	22.0	1.0
Fairy, Value,Tesco*	1 Cake/16g	70	436	6.1	53.7	21.9	1.0
Farmhouse Fruit, Bakers Delight*	1oz/28g	107	381	5.2	55.5	15.3	2.1
Farmhouse Slice, Weight Watchers*	1 Slice/23g	73	317	5.5	64.9	4.0	1.3
Flake Cake Bar, Cadbury's*	1 Cake/22g	97	442	6.5	51.8	23.3	0.5
Flake, Cadbury's*	1 Cake/26g	114	439	6.0	54.1	22.1	0.7
Fondant Fancies, Sainsbury's*	1 Cake/27g	95	353	2.4	65.7	9.0	0.4
French Fancies, Mr Kipling*	1 Cake/28g	100	356	2.3	65.1	9.6	0.0
Fresh Cream Bramley Apple Sponge, Tesco*	1/6 Slice/43g	130	303	3.6	35.4	16.3	1.0
Fruit & Nut Crisp Bar, Go Ahead, McVitie's*	1 Bar/22g	95	430	5.3	71.3	13.7	1.7
Fruit Cake With Marzipan & Icing, Asda*	1/12 Slice/76g	280	369	3.9	68.0	9.0	0.0
Fruit Slice, Value, Tesco*	1 Slice/22.6g	85	372	4.0	48.7	17.7	1.3
Fruit, Fully Iced, Luxury Rich, Co-Op*	1oz/28g	99	355	3.0	64.0	9.0	4.0
Fruit, Healthy Selection, Somerfield*	1oz/28g	73	260	5.0	55.0	2.0	0.0
Fruit, Plain, Retail	1 Slice/90g	319	354	5.1	57.9	12.9	0.0
Fruit, Rich, Connoisseur, Somerfield*	1oz/28g	91	326	4.0	54.0	10.0	0.0
Fruit, Rich, Iced	1 Slice/70g	249	356	4.1	62.7	11.4	1.7
Fruit, Rich, Retail	1 Slice/70g	225	322	4.9	50.7	12.5	1.7
Fruit, Rich, Somerfield*	1oz/28g	97	348	4.0	57.0	12.0	0.0
Fudge, Pret A Manger*	1 Av Pack/140g	537	384	4.1	46.1	20.3	1.3
Fudgy Chocolate Slices, COU, Marks & Spencer*	1 Slice/36g	95	265	4.6	66.4	2.2	2.1

CAKE,

INFO/WEIGHT	KCAL	KCAL	PROT	CARB	FAT	FIBRE
Galaxy Cake Bar, McVitie's*	1oz/28g	138	494	5.1	57.5	27.0	0.3
Genoa, Home Bake, McVitie's*	1oz/28g	107	383	4.7	55.9	15.6	1.4
Genoa, Tesco*	1 Serving/50g	162	324	4.0	58.6	8.2	3.2
Ginger Drizzle, Iced, Co-Op*	1/6 Cake/64.5g	226	350	3.0	58.0	12.0	1.0
Ginger, Jamaica Bar, McVitie's*	1 Mini Cake/33g	128	388	3.5	60.2	14.7	1.2
Ginger, Marks & Spencer*	1/6 Cake/41g	156	380	6.3	62.3	11.5	1.7
Golden Syrup Bar, McVitie's*	1 Mini Cake/33g	127	385	3.6	60.2	14.4	1.2
Happy Birthday, Sainsbury's*	1 Slice/50g	207	414	2.8	64.5	16.1	0.6
Heavenly Chocolate Brownie, Safeway*	1 Pack/300g	900	300	6.2	38.5	13.4	0.8
Iced Madeira, Sainsbury's*	1/8 Cake/47g	182	388	3.6	61.6	14.1	0.7
Jaffa Cake Bar, McVitie's	1 Bar/31g	126	408	3.9	59.0	17.4	0.0
Jaffa Cakes, Asda*	1 Serving/11g	42	378	4.2	70.0	9.0	1.4
Jaffa Cakes, Co-Op*	1 Cake/12g	45	375	4.0	70.0	9.0	2.0
Jaffa Cakes, Continental, Bahlsen*	1oz/28g	117	419	4.0	55.9	25.5	0.0
Jaffa Cakes, Dark Chocolate, Marks & Spencer*	1 Cake/11g	43	395	4.0	62.4	14.1	3.1
Jaffa Cakes, Lunch Box, McVitie's*	1 Cake/6.6g	28	395	4.2	74.3	9.0	1.4
Jaffa Cakes, McVitie's*	1 Biscuit/12g	46	384	4.4	73.3	8.1	1.3
Jaffa Cakes, Mini Roll XL, McVitie's*	1 Cake/44g	169	384	3.5	66.9	11.4	0.0
Jaffa Cakes, Mini, Asda*	1 Cake/5g	21	412	3.9	63.0	16.0	1.9
Jaffa Cakes, Mini, Co-Op*	1 Biscuit/5g	19	385	4.0	65.0	12.0	3.0
Jaffa Cakes, Mini, Marks & Spencer*	1oz/28g	113	405	3.9	62.8	15.8	1.9
Jaffa Cakes, Mini, McVitie's*	1 Cake/5.9g	26	441	5.1	83.1	10.2	1.7
Jaffa Cakes, Mini, Morrisons*	1 Cake/5g	20	405	3.9	62.8	15.8	1.9
Jaffa Cakes, Morrisons*	1 Cake/13g	50	384	4.4	73.2	8.1	0.0
Jaffa Cakes, Plain Chocolate, Sainsbury's*	1 Cake/13g	46	384	4.4	73.3	8.1	1.3
Jaffa Cakes, Roll Bites, Mini, McVitie's*	1 Cake/15.9g	62	389	3.7	66.7	12.0	1.4
Jaffa Cakes, Tesco*	1 Cake/12g	45	378	4.2	70.4	8.8	1.4
Jaffa Cakes, Value, Tesco*	1 Cake/11g	42	386	4.2	72.7	8.7	0.6
Jamaica Ginger With Lemon Filling, McVitie's*	1 Cake/32.9g	143	434	4.0	48.3	25.0	0.8
Jammy Strawberry Rolls, Mini, Cadbury's*	1 Roll/29g	119	411	4.9	59.8	16.5	0.5
Lemon Bakewell, Mr Kipling*	1 Cake/48.0g	199	415	3.9	59.8	17.9	0.9
Lemon Buttercream & Lemon Curd, The Cake Shop*	1 Cake/28g	124	444	3.5	43.4	27.8	0.6
Lemon Drizzle Slices, Good For You, Asda*	1 Slice/25g	69	274	3.6	56.0	4.0	0.7
Lemon Drizzle, Marks & Spencer*	1/6 Cake/63g	230	365	4.2	55.8	13.9	1.4
Lemon Iced Madeira, Co-Op*	1 Cake/290g	1131	390	4.0	53.0	18.0	0.6
Lemon Slices, BGTY, Sainsbury's*	1 Slice/26.0g	84	323	3.7	74.0	1.4	1.3
Lemon Slices, Healthy Eating, Tesco*	1 Slice/26g	86	329	3.4	69.1	2.6	3.0
Lemon Slices, Mr Kipling*	1oz/28g	117	417	4.1	58.2	16.3	0.0
Lemon Slices, Sponge, Mr Kipling*	1 Slice/30g	119	397	4.1	58.5	16.2	0.0
Lemon Smoothie Bake, Go Ahead, McVitie's*	1 Bar/35g	130	372	3.0	75.1	8.1	1.0
Lemon Sponge Slices, Zesty, Marks & Spencer*	1 Slice/27g	107	395	3.7	54.4	18.0	0.7
Lemon Tartlette, Go Ahead, McVitie's*	1 Cake/45g	161	357	3.7	67.9	9.5	1.1
Lemon, Entenmann's*	1 Serving/55.6g	214	383	3.7	56.9	15.7	1.1
Lemon, Half Moon, Bobby's*	1/6 Cake/60g	244	406	4.1	55.7	18.4	0.0
Lemon, Home Bake, McVitie's*	1oz/28g	108	384	4.6	53.9	18.2	1.0
Lemon, Low Fat, Weight Watchers*	1 Cake/26g	79	304	3.7	68.8	1.6	3.5
Leo the Lion, Birthday, Asda*	1 Slice/80.8g	326	402	2.6	62.0	16.0	0.5
Madeira	1 Slice/40g	157	393	5.4	58.4	16.9	0.9
Madeira, Tesco*	1 Serving/50g	197	394	5.5	57.9	15.6	1.2
Manor House, Mr Kipling*	1 Serving/69.2g	277	402	5.1	49.1	20.5	1.4
Marble, Home Bake, McVitie's*	1oz/28g	115	411	3.7	56.9	18.8	0.9
Milk Chocolate Bar, Cadbury's*	1 Bar/35g	140	401	6.8	48.8	19.8	0.8
Milky Way Cake Bar, McVitie's*	1 Bar/26g	138	530	5.3	53.8	32.6	0.2

CAKE,

INFO/WEIGHT	Measure	per Measure KCAL	Nutrition Values per 100g / 100ml				
			KCAL	PROT	CARB	FAT	FIBRE
Mini Rolls, Cadbury's*	1 Roll/26g	113	434	5.5	55.6	20.6	0.6
Mini Rolls, Chocolate & Vanilla, Somerfield*	1oz/28g	112	399	5.0	62.0	15.0	0.0
Mini Rolls, Chocolate, Tesco*	1 Roll/31g	137	442	6.0	56.3	21.4	0.8
Mini Rolls, Chocolate, Weight Watchers*	1 Cake/23g	85	371	5.3	61.9	15.0	2.0
Mini Rolls, Easter Selection, Cadbury's*	1oz/28g	122	434	5.5	55.6	20.6	0.0
Nut Munch, Pret A Manger*	1 Av Pack/100g	493	493	8.0	38.5	34.6	7.9
Orange Marmalade Loaf, Aldi*	1 Slice/33.0g	88	267	4.5	57.4	2.2	1.8
Pecan Pie, Pret A Manger*	1 Av Pack/70g	333	476	6.1	44.4	30.3	0.7
Piece of Cake, Birthday, Marks & Spencer*	1 Serving/85g	395	465	4.3	39.7	28.7	0.9
Raisin, Dernys*	1 Cake/45g	175	388	5.0	54.0	17.0	0.0
Raspberry & Vanilla Swiss Roll, Morrisons*	1 Serving/28g	98	350	4.2	61.8	9.5	0.0
Raspberry Jam & Buttercream Sandwich, Somerfield*	1oz/28g	102	364	4.0	61.0	12.0	0.0
Raspberry Smoothie Bake, Go Ahead, McVitie's*	1 Bar/35g	131	373	3.1	74.9	8.2	1.4
Raspberry Swiss Roll, Lyons*	1 Swiss Roll/175g	485	277	5.2	60.6	1.4	0.0
Raspberry Swiss Roll, Somerfield*	1 Swiss Roll/80g	245	306	5.0	66.0	3.0	0.0
Rich Choc' Roll, Cadbury's*	1/6 Portion/39g	149	381	4.8	50.2	15.6	1.0
Rock	1 Sm Cake/40g	158	396	5.4	60.5	16.4	1.5
Rollers, Culi d'Or*	1 Roll/20.8g	69	330	5.8	50.0	12.0	0.0
Seriously Chocolatey Celebration, Sainsbury's*	1/8 Cake/77g	336	437	6.3	45.0	25.7	0.3
Shrek Birthday, Tesco*	1/16 Cake/72g	248	344	3.3	64.0	12.2	0.5
Snowball, Chocolate, Tunnock's*	1 Snowball/25g	97	388	3.9	47.0	21.8	0.0
Snowballs, Sainsbury's*	1 Snowball/18g	80	445	2.5	55.6	23.0	3.6
Sponge	1 Slice/53g	243	459	6.4	52.4	26.3	0.9
Sponge With Butter Icing	1 Slice/65g	319	490	4.5	52.4	30.6	0.6
Sponge, Fatless	1 Slice/53g	156	294	10.1	53.0	6.1	0.9
Sponge, Iced, Marks & Spencer*	1 Serving/100g	400	400	3.4	58.4	17.0	1.3
Sponge, Jam Filled	1 Slice/65g	196	302	4.2	64.2	4.9	1.8
Spooky, Birthday, Memory Lane*	1 Slice/75g	295	393	3.5	50.8	19.5	0.7
Stem Ginger, 96% Fat Free, Trimlyne*	¼ Cake/62.5g	170	273	4.4	58.1	3.6	1.2
Sticky Toffee Slices, Eat Smart, Safeway*	1 Cake/85g	259	305	3.6	65.8	2.7	1.3
Stollen Slices, Somerfield*	1oz/28g	115	411	7.0	54.0	19.0	0.0
Stollen, Christmas Range, Tesco*	1oz/28g	99	355	5.0	52.9	13.7	1.8
Stollen, Marks & Spencer*	2 Lge Slices/175g	656	375	7.3	46.3	17.0	2.4
Strawberry Swiss Roll, Luxury, Somerfield*	1oz/28g	84	301	4.0	62.0	4.0	0.0
Sultana & Cherry Slice, Co-Op*	1oz/28g	87	310	3.0	48.0	12.0	2.0
Sultana & Cherry, Tesco*	1 Cake/37g	124	334	4.7	54.4	10.8	2.5
Sultana, Apple & Cranberry, 99% Fat Free, Trimlyne*,	1/6 Cake/66.6g	130	195	4.6	45.5	0.9	3.3
Summer Fruit Cream, GFY, Asda*	1 Serving/74.0g	165	223	3.6	41.0	4.9	2.5
Summer Strawberry Bakes, Go Ahead, McVitie's*	1 Bar/35g	128	367	2.7	75.1	8.0	1.0
Swiss Roll	1oz/28g	77	276	7.2	55.5	4.4	0.8
Swiss Roll, Chocolate Flavour, Value, Tesco*	1 Slice/20g	79	394	5.5	49.2	19.5	1.4
Swiss Roll, Chocolate, Individual	1 Roll/26g	88	337	4.3	58.1	11.3	0.0
Swiss Roll, Chocolate, Jumbo, Safeway*	1/12 Roll/35g	129	369	4.1	47.1	18.2	0.9
Swiss Roll, Chocolate, Somerfield*	¼ Roll/43.5g	167	384	6.0	55.0	16.0	0.0
Syrup & Ginger, Tesco*	1 Serving/32g	134	420	4.5	51.4	21.8	0.7
The Ultimate Carrot Passion, Entenmann's*	1 Slice/52g	206	403	4.6	42.4	24.3	1.0
Toffee & Pecan Loaf, Safeway*	1/6 Cake/62g	225	363	3.6	35.5	22.9	0.5
Toffee & Pecan Slices, Marks & Spencer*	1 Slice/36g	160	445	4.7	54.0	23.7	1.3
Toffee Flavour Slices, Low Fat, Weight Watchers*	1 Slice/27g	80	297	4.2	63.9	2.6	3.2
Toffee Fudge, Entenmann's*	1 Serving/65g	274	421	3.4	53.0	21.7	0.5
Toffee Temptation, Tesco*	1 Slice/67g	228	340	2.9	39.1	19.1	0.3
Triple Chocolate, TTD, Sainsbury's*	1/8 Cake/52g	210	412	4.7	42.6	24.7	0.5
Turkish Delight, Fry's*	1 Cake/26g	96	371	4.5	62.4	10.8	0.5

	Measure INFO/WEIGHT	per Measure KCAL	Nutrition Values per 100g / 100ml KCAL	PROT	CARB	FAT	FIBRE
CAKE,							
Victoria Ring, Asda*	1 Serving/50g	153	305	6.0	59.0	5.0	1.3
Victoria Sandwich, Co-Op*	1oz/28g	101	360	4.0	48.0	17.0	1.0
Victoria Sponge Sandwich, Somerfield*	1oz/28g	112	400	4.0	53.0	19.0	0.0
Victoria Sponge, Fresh Cream, Tesco*	1 Slice/46.7g	157	334	3.9	40.8	17.3	0.7
Victoria Sponge, Lemon, Co-Op*	1 Slice/42g	151	360	4.0	44.0	19.0	0.7
Victoria Sponge, Mini, Bobby's*	1 Cake/35g	164	469	4.0	51.3	27.5	0.2
Victoria Sponge, Mini, Mr Kipling*	1 Cake/37g	142	383	3.8	48.7	19.2	0.6
Viennese Whirl, Mr Kipling*	1 Whirl/28g	139	497	4.1	51.5	30.5	1.2
Viennese Whirl, Somerfield*	1oz/28g	133	475	4.0	56.0	26.0	0.0
Viennese Whirl, Tesco*	1 Cake/39g	181	465	4.0	53.2	26.2	1.2
Walnut & Coffee, Co-Op*	¼ Cake/65g	254	390	5.0	47.0	20.0	0.7
Walnut Layer, Somerfield*	¼ Cake/77.5g	295	381	6.0	45.0	20.0	0.0
Welsh	1oz/28g	121	431	5.6	61.8	19.6	1.5
Wild Blueberry & Apple, Bakers Delight*	1oz/28g	99	354	4.6	48.8	15.6	1.5
Winnie The Pooh Birthday, Nestle*	1 Serving/100g	361	361	2.4	63.3	10.9	0.5
Yoghurt & Berry Loaf, Low Fat, Starbucks*	1 Cake/94g	254	270	5.3	50.8	5.1	1.7
Yorkshire Parkin, Bakers Delight*	1oz/28g	111	395	5.1	60.3	14.8	1.5
Yum Yums, Tesco*	1 Cake/61g	232	380	6.1	51.6	16.6	1.7
CAKE MIX,							
Free From, Sainsbury's*	1 Serving/50g	173	346	1.3	84.4	0.3	2.2
CALAMARI,							
Battered With Tartar Sauce Dip, Tesco*	1 Pack/210g	573	273	8.9	15.4	19.5	0.6
Battered, Marks & Spencer*	1 Pack/160g	424	265	14.3	15.8	16.1	0.7
Battered, Young's*	1 Serving/150g	266	177	7.8	13.0	10.4	1.5
Marks & Spencer*	1oz/28g	65	231	13.9	11.5	14.4	0.5
Rings In Batter, Waitrose*	½ Pack/85g	227	267	13.9	14.2	17.2	0.6
CAMPINO,							
Oranges & Cream, Bendicks*	1oz/28g	116	416	0.1	85.8	8.1	0.0
Strawberries & Cream, Bendicks*	1oz/28g	117	418	0.1	86.2	8.1	0.0
CANAPES,							
Caponata, Puff Pastry, Occasions, Sainsbury's*	1 Square/12g	30	249	4.1	22.9	15.7	2.1
Red Onion & Goats Cheese, Puff Pastry, Sainsbury's*	1 Square/12g	36	296	6.3	25.7	18.7	1.5
Spinach & Ricotta, Puff Pastry, Sainsbury's*	1 Square/12g	35	290	10.1	19.3	19.1	1.5
CANNELLONI,							
Beef, BGTY, Sainsbury's*	1 Pack/300g	249	83	5.5	10.1	2.3	1.7
Beef, Geat Value, Asda*	1 Pack/400g	384	96	6.0	12.0	2.7	1.6
Beef, Italiano, Tesco*	1 Serving/340g	442	130	5.3	12.4	6.6	0.7
Findus*	1 Pack/342g	445	130	5.6	11.1	6.7	1.0
Five Cheese & Spinach, Finest, Tesco*	½ Pack/300g	468	156	7.0	9.6	9.9	1.7
Iceland*	1 Pack/400g	584	146	7.2	13.0	7.2	0.6
Italian Chicken & Pesto, Sainsbury's*	1 Pack/450g	675	150	6.1	14.4	7.5	1.1
Mediterranean Vegetable, Waitrose*	1 Serving/170g	330	194	9.7	18.7	9.0	1.9
Parmesan & Basil, Marks & Spencer*	1 Pack/360g	504	140	5.9	11.4	7.9	0.8
Pork, Marks & Spencer*	1 Pack/400g	460	115	6.2	8.7	6.2	1.1
Ricotta & Spinach, COU, Marks & Spencer*	1 Pack/360g	288	80	5.8	9.7	1.9	1.5
Ricotta & Spinach, Co-Op*	1 Pack/340g	357	105	5.0	10.0	5.0	3.0
Ricotta & Spinach, Waitrose*	½ Pack/170g	323	190	10.2	21.9	6.9	1.2
Roasted Vegetable, Morrisons*	1 Pack/350g	312	89	3.9	12.5	2.5	2.3
Smoked Salmon & Spinach, Sainsbury's*	1 Pack/450g	599	133	5.7	13.5	6.2	0.4
Spinach & Ricotta, BGTY, Sainsbury's*	1 Serving/300g	297	99	4.9	15.9	1.7	1.0
Spinach & Ricotta, Eat Smart, Safeway*	1 Pack/350g	333	95	6.2	12.0	2.2	1.3
Spinach & Ricotta, GFY, Asda*	1 Pack/303g	418	138	6.0	21.0	3.3	0.5
Spinach & Ricotta, Healthy Choice, Asda*	1 Pack/400g	448	112	4.0	15.0	4.0	0.5

C

	Measure INFO/WEIGHT	per Measure KCAL	Nutrition Values per 100g / 100ml				
			KCAL	PROT	CARB	FAT	FIBRE
CANNELLONI,							
Spinach & Ricotta, Healthy Eating, Tesco*	1 Pack/340g	326	96	4.5	13.7	2.6	1.3
Spinach & Ricotta, Healthy Living, Tesco*	1 Pack/340g	316	93	4.3	12.7	2.8	1.6
Spinach & Ricotta, Italiano, Tesco*	1 Pack/425g	510	120	4.7	12.4	5.7	0.9
Spinach & Ricotta, Ross*	1 Pack/300g	300	100	4.3	13.7	3.1	0.5
Spinach & Ricotta, Safeway*	1 Pack/401g	565	141	6.5	14.4	6.4	0.4
Spinach & Ricotta, Sainsbury's*	1 Pack/288g	372	129	5.1	10.5	7.4	1.2
Spinach & Ricotta, Somerfield*	1 Pack/300g	393	131	5.0	13.0	7.0	0.0
Spinach & Ricotta, Tesco*	1 Pack/340g	490	144	4.5	6.4	11.2	0.5
Spinach & Wild Mushroom, Linda McCartney*	1 Pack/340g	381	112	4.9	14.1	4.0	1.7
Vegetarian, Tesco*	1 Pack/400g	552	138	5.3	9.8	8.6	1.5
CAPPELLETTI,							
Chicken & Ham, Fresh, Safeway*	½ Pack/177g	320	181	9.7	27.7	3.5	1.8
Fresh, Sainsbury's*	1 Serving/125g	294	235	12.9	33.5	5.5	2.7
CAPRI SUN, Orange, The Coca Cola Co*	1 Pouch/200ml	90	45	0.0	11.0	0.0	0.0
CARAMAC, Nestle*	1 Bar/30g	163	563	5.8	54.4	35.8	0.0
CARAMEL,							
Cadbury's*	1 Bar/50g	240	480	4.3	61.3	24.3	0.0
Egg, Cadbury's*	1 Egg/39g	191	490	4.3	58.9	26.1	0.0
Mighty, Asda*	1 Serving/40g	186	464	5.0	66.0	20.0	1.5
CARO, Instant Beverage, No Caffeine, Nestle Uk Ltd*	1 Pot/50g	133	265	5.5	60.0	0.3	0.0
CAROB POWDER, Average	1 Tsp/2g	3	159	4.9	37.0	0.1	0.0
CARROT & SWEDE,							
Crush, Marks & Spencer*	1 Serving/150g	83	55	0.7	2.8	4.5	3.1
Julienne, Frozen, Great Value, Asda*	1 Serving/100g	20	20	0.5	3.7	0.3	1.8
Mash, BGTY, Sainsbury's*	1 Serving/225g	200	89	1.3	16.0	2.2	1.2
Mash, Eat Smart, Safeway*	1 Serving/225g	146	65	1.6	11.8	1.2	1.3
Mash, Fresh, Tesco*	1oz/28g	22	80	1.2	11.1	3.4	1.4
Mix, Freshly Prepared, Asda*	½ Pack/250g	48	19	0.5	3.6	0.3	1.6
CARROT JUICE,							
Organic, Evernat*	1 Glass/200ml	44	22	0.6	4.8	0.0	0.3
P & J*	1 Glass/250ml	60	24	0.5	5.7	0.0	0.0
CARROTS,							
& Peas, Sainsbury's*	1 Serving/200g	100	50	3.3	8.3	0.5	3.8
Baby, Extra Sweet, Organic, Iceland*	1oz/28g	6	22	0.4	4.7	0.3	2.3
Baby, Flavoursome, Tesco*	1 Serving/100g	31	31	0.7	6.0	0.5	2.4
Baby, Frozen, Sainsbury's*	1 Serving/60g	14	23	0.4	4.7	0.3	2.3
Baby, Frozen, Somerfield*	1 Serving/75g	21	28	1.0	6.0	0.0	0.0
Baby, In Sugared Salt Water, Tesco*	1 Serving/100g	20	20	0.5	3.9	0.3	1.9
Baby, In Water, Salt Added, Sainsbury's*	½ Can/86g	19	22	0.5	4.2	0.3	1.9
Baby, Peeled, Ready to Cook, Sainsbury's*	1 Serving/100g	35	35	0.6	7.5	0.3	3.0
Baby, Safeway*	1 Serving/75g	23	31	0.7	5.9	0.5	0.0
Baby, Tesco*	1 Serving/75g	17	22	0.4	4.5	0.3	2.3
Baby, With Fine Beans, Tesco*	1 Pack/200g	58	29	1.3	4.7	0.5	2.3
Batons, Fresh 'N' Ready, Sainsbury's*	1 Serving/100g	26	26	0.6	4.9	0.4	2.5
Batons, Marks & Spencer*	1oz/28g	9	33	0.7	8.3	0.0	2.9
Batons, Tesco*	1 Serving/100g	37	37	0.6	7.9	0.3	2.4
Broccoli & Cauliflower Florets, Marks & Spencer*	1oz/28g	8	30	1.8	6.1	0.0	2.8
Canned, Drained, Sainsbury's*	1oz/28g	6	22	0.5	4.2	0.3	1.9
Canned, Re-Heated, Drained	1oz/28g	6	20	0.5	4.2	0.3	1.9
Cauliflower & Broccoli Florets, Safeway*	1 Serving/125g	44	35	2.6	4.6	0.7	2.3
Cauliflower & Broccoli, Tesco*	1oz/28g	10	35	2.5	4.9	0.6	2.3
Crunchies, Blue Parrot Cafe, Sainsbury's*	1 Pack/80g	28	35	0.6	7.5	0.3	3.0
Crunchies, Shapers, Boots*	1 Pack/80g	28	35	0.6	7.5	0.3	3.0

	Measure	per Measure	Nutrition Values per 100g / 100ml				
	INFO/WEIGHT	KCAL	KCAL	PROT	CARB	FAT	FIBRE
CARROTS,							
Fresh, Sainsbury's*	1 Carrot/70g	17	24	0.6	4.9	0.4	2.8
Frozen, Co-Op*	1oz/28g	7	25	0.6	5.0	0.4	2.0
Frozen, Iceland*	1 Serving/100g	22	22	0.4	4.7	0.3	2.3
Grated, Asda*	1oz/28g	9	31	0.7	6.0	0.5	2.4
Julienne, Farmfoods*	1oz/28g	10	37	0.6	7.9	0.3	2.4
Mini, Tesco*	1 Pack/270g	111	41	1.0	8.4	0.4	2.9
Peeled, Mini, Sainsbury's*	1 Pack/270g	95	35	0.6	7.5	0.3	3.0
Raw, Asda*	1 Serving/50g	12	23	0.6	4.9	0.4	2.3
Raw, Organic, Tesco*	1 Serving/100g	37	37	0.6	7.9	0.3	2.4
Sliced, Asda*	1oz/28g	6	20	0.7	4.4	0.0	1.9
Sliced, Basics, Frozen, Somerfield*	1oz/28g	10	37	1.0	8.0	0.0	0.0
Sliced, Freshly Frozen, Iceland*	1 Serving/100g	22	22	0.4	4.7	0.3	2.3
Sliced, Frozen, Sainsburys*	1 Serving/60g	13	22	0.4	4.4	0.3	2.3
Sliced, Frozen, Tesco*	1oz/28g	8	30	0.7	5.7	0.5	2.4
Sliced, In Brine, Asda*	1oz/28g	6	20	0.7	4.4	0.0	1.9
Sliced, In Water, Somerfield*	1oz/28g	6	20	1.0	4.0	0.0	0.0
Sliced, In Water, Tinned, Tesco*	1 Serving/180g	36	20	0.5	3.9	0.3	1.9
Sliced, No Added Salt, Sainsbury's*	1 Serving/150g	33	22	0.5	4.2	0.3	1.9
Sliced, Tesco*	1 Serving/175g	72	41	1.0	8.4	0.4	2.9
Sliced, Tinned, SmartPrice, Asda*	1 Can/180g	36	20	0.7	4.4	0.0	1.9
Sliced, Value, Tesco*	½ Can/90g	18	20	0.5	3.9	0.3	1.9
Whole, In Salted Water, Asda*	¼ Can/75g	15	20	0.7	4.4	0.0	1.9
Whole, Tesco*	1oz/28g	6	20	0.5	3.9	0.3	1.9
Whole, in Water, Salt Added, Sainsbury's*	1 Serving/180g	40	22	0.5	4.2	0.3	1.9
Young, Boiled in Salted Water	1oz/28g	6	22	0.6	4.4	0.4	2.3
Young, Boiled in Unsalted Water	1oz/28g	6	22	0.6	4.4	0.4	2.3
Young, Raw, Fresh	1oz/28g	8	30	0.7	6.0	0.5	2.4
Corn & Mange Tout, Baby, Safeway*	1 Pack/200g	48	24	2.1	3.2	0.3	0.0
CASHEW NUTS,							
Honey Roasted, Waitrose*	½ Pack/50g	298	595	17.8	35.0	42.6	3.2
Organic, Crazy Jack*	1 Pack/100g	573	573	7.7	18.2	48.2	3.2
Plain	10 Whole/10g	57	573	17.7	18.1	48.2	3.2
Roasted & Salted	10 Whole/10g	61	611	20.5	18.8	50.9	3.2
Roasted & Salted, Co-Op*	1 Serving/20g	124	620	20.0	21.0	51.0	4.0
Roasted Salted, Waitrose*	1 Serving/100g	615	615	16.1	19.5	52.5	3.2
Roasted Salted, Whole, Tesco*	1 Serving/25g	133	531	20.1	36.9	33.7	3.8
Roasted Unsalted, Sainsbury's*	1/3 Pack/50g	298	595	18.3	18.7	49.7	3.3
Roasted, Salted, KP*	1 Pack/50g	310	619	19.8	20.5	50.9	4.0
Salted, Morrisons*	1 Serving/50g	294	588	16.7	17.0	50.4	0.0
Whole, Holland & Barrett*	1 Pack/100g	573	573	17.7	18.2	48.2	3.2
Whole, Tesco*	1oz/28g	173	619	19.8	20.5	50.9	4.0
CASHEWS &							
Peanuts, Honey Roasted, Planters*	1 Serving/50g	290	579	21.6	26.6	42.9	4.2
Peanuts, Honey Roasted, Tesco*	1 Bag/25g	145	579	21.6	26.6	42.9	4.2
CASSAVA,							
Baked	1oz/28g	43	155	0.7	40.1	0.2	1.7
Boiled in Unsalted Water	1oz/28g	36	130	0.5	33.5	0.2	1.4
Chips	1oz/28g	99	353	1.8	91.4	0.4	4.0
Gari	1oz/28g	100	358	1.3	92.9	0.5	0.0
Raw	1oz/28g	40	142	0.6	36.8	0.2	1.6
Steamed	1oz/28g	40	142	0.6	36.8	0.2	1.6
CASSEROLE,							
Bean & Lentil, Morrisons*	1 Can/410g	287	70	4.1	12.5	0.4	0.0

C

C

CASEROLE,

Measure INFO/WEIGHT	per Measure KCAL	KCAL	PROT	CARB	FAT	FIBRE

CASSEROLE,

	Measure INFO/WEIGHT	per Measure KCAL	KCAL	PROT	CARB	FAT	FIBRE
Beef & Ale, Finest, Tesco*	½ Pack/300g	222	74	12.2	3.9	1.1	0.4
Beef & Dumplings, Marks & Spencer*	1 Pack/454g	522	115	10.5	7.7	4.7	1.0
Beef & Dumplings, Safeway*	1 Pack/390g	215	55	1.6	7.5	1.9	1.2
Beef & Red Wine, BGTY, Sainsbury's*	1 Pack/300g	192	64	8.0	6.7	0.6	0.9
Beef Bourguignon, Finest, Tesco*	1 Serving/300g	258	86	10.8	1.9	3.9	0.8
Beef With Dumplings, COU, Marks & Spencer*	½ Pack/226g	215	95	9.0	9.1	2.4	0.6
Beef, Marks & Spencer*	1 Serving/200g	240	120	8.1	9.2	5.7	1.0
Beef, Ready Meals, Marks & Spencer*	1 Meal/454g	622	137	11.1	9.9	6.4	0.7
Beef, Traditional British, TTD, Sainsbury's*	1 Serving/100g	136	136	22.5	0.1	5.1	0.1
Chicken & Asparagus in White Wine, Tesco*	½ Pack/300g	444	148	11.5	7.7	7.9	0.8
Chicken & Dumplings, Healthy Eating, Tesco*	1 Pack/450g	441	98	7.4	11.1	2.7	0.6
Chicken & Dumplings, Healthy Living, Tesco*	1 Pack/450g	441	98	7.4	11.1	2.7	0.6
Chicken & Herb Dumplings, BGTY, Sainsbury's*	1 Pack/450g	446	99	6.1	9.5	4.1	0.6
Chicken & Tomato, Asda*	¼ Pack/273g	569	208	16.0	2.2	15.0	0.5
Chicken & Vegetable, Apetito*	1 Pack/330g	286	87	6.3	9.4	3.0	1.6
Chicken & White Wine, BGTY, Sainsbury's*	1 Serving/300g	216	72	7.2	5.9	2.2	1.3
Chicken Filled Yorkshire Pudding, Farmfoods*	1 Pack/280g	347	124	6.5	19.3	2.3	1.3
Chicken Mediterranean, Tesco*	1 Pack/400g	260	65	6.7	4.5	2.3	0.9
Chicken With Dumplings, Marks & Spencer*	½ Pack/227g	261	115	9.7	9.0	4.4	0.9
Chicken With Herb Dumplings, COU, Marks & Spencer*	½ Pack/227.8g	205	90	10.6	7.2	1.9	0.6
Chicken, GFY, Asda*	1 Pack/400g	280	70	5.0	8.0	2.0	1.5
Chicken, Green Isle*	1 Pack/400g	300	75	5.7	9.2	1.7	1.0
Chicken, Leek & Mushroom, Tesco*	1 Pack/350g	382	109	4.5	8.6	6.3	1.0
Chicken, Marks & Spencer*	1 Pack/200g	230	115	7.4	10.9	4.4	0.9
Chicken, Perfectly Balanced, Waitrose*	1 Pack/400g	392	98	6.6	9.8	3.6	1.2
Chunky Vegetables, Marks & Spencer*	1 Bag/450g	90	20	0.7	3.4	0.3	1.4
Country Vegetable, Sainsbury's*	1 Can/400g	300	75	2.2	11.0	2.5	1.1
Cowboy, Iceland*	1 Pack/400g	500	125	5.8	10.9	6.5	1.7
Lamb & Rosemary, BGTY, Sainsbury's*	1 Serving/300g	192	64	7.1	6.8	0.9	0.6
Lamb & Rosemary, Marks & Spencer*	1 Pack/454g	409	90	9.7	5.5	3.3	1.0
Lamb, BGTY, Sainsbury's*	1 Serving/200g	242	121	20.7	0.1	4.3	0.1
Lamb, Braised, British Classics, Tesco*	1 Pack/350g	333	95	7.5	4.6	5.2	1.2
Lamb, Marks & Spencer*	1 Pack/200g	260	130	6.2	10.6	6.8	1.2
Lentil & Vegetable, Granose*	1 Pack/400g	220	55	2.8	7.9	1.4	0.0
Minced Lamb With Mint Dumplings, Sainsbury's*	1 Pack/450g	558	124	5.4	10.4	6.8	1.1
Normandy Style Pork, Finest, Tesco*	1 Pack/450g	405	90	7.6	4.1	4.8	2.3
Pork With Apple & Cider, Safeway*	1 Pack/450g	729	162	8.3	13.4	8.4	1.1
Prime Steak, Sainsbury's*	1oz/28g	34	122	22.6	0.1	3.5	0.1
Quorn*, Dumplings	1oz/28g	36	127	4.5	14.2	5.8	1.7
Rabbit	1oz/28g	29	102	11.6	2.6	5.1	0.4
Roasted Vegetable With Herb Dumplings, COU, M&S*	½ Pack/227g	204	90	1.7	13.1	2.7	2.2
Sausage & Potato, Marks & Spencer*	1 Serving/200g	190	95	3.3	7.5	5.9	0.9
Steak & Ale, Sainsbury's*	1 Pack/300g	288	96	10.6	5.6	3.5	0.4
Steak & Mushroom With Mustard Mash, Finest, Tesco*	1 Pack/550g	523	95	5.9	9.0	3.9	1.1
Vegetable & Chicken, Long Life, Sainsbury's*	1 Pack/300g	186	62	4.6	7.4	1.5	0.8
Vegetable With Dumplings, Asda*	1 Pack/350g	343	98	2.7	12.0	4.3	2.1
Vegetable With Herb Dumplings, COU, Marks & Spencer*	1 Pack/450g	270	60	1.6	10.1	1.2	1.0
Vegetable With Potato Crush, Safeway*	1 Pack/450g	293	65	1.3	7.7	3.1	2.0
Vegetable, Tesco*	1 Serving/220g	66	30	0.8	6.1	0.3	1.5

CASSEROLE MIX,

	Measure INFO/WEIGHT	per Measure KCAL	KCAL	PROT	CARB	FAT	FIBRE
Beef, Authentic, Schwartz*	1 Pack/43g	111	257	7.4	54.5	1.0	0.4
Beef, Colman's*	1 Pack/40g	119	297	5.2	67.0	0.6	0.0
Beef, Schwartz*	½ Pack/21g	58	276	9.9	53.9	2.3	0.0

	Measure INFO/WEIGHT	per Measure KCAL	Nutrition Values per 100g / 100ml KCAL	PROT	CARB	FAT	FIBRE
CASEROLE MIX,							
Chicken Chasseur, Asda*	1 Pack/80g	273	341	9.0	74.0	1.0	1.4
Chicken, Colman's*	1 Pack/40g	109	272	5.3	60.0	0.7	0.0
Chicken, Schwartz*	½ Pack/18g	55	304	10.6	62.8	1.2	0.0
Liver & Bacon, Colman's*	1 Pack/40g	116	289	9.3	59.0	1.2	0.0
Pork, Colman's*	1 Serving/40g	117	293	5.3	65.5	1.1	3.4
Sausage, Asda*	¼ Pack/25g	80	321	6.0	65.0	4.1	5.0
Sausage, Colman's*	1 Serving/40g	122	304	8.1	65.7	1.0	5.4
CAULIFLOWER,							
& Broccoli Florets, Asda*	1 Serving/100g	26	26	2.7	2.1	0.7	2.4
& Broccoli Florets, Marks & Spencer*	½ Pack/125g	31	25	3.0	1.6	0.8	2.0
& Broccoli Florets, Morrisons*	1 Serving/60g	16	26	2.7	2.3	0.7	0.0
& Broccoli Florets, Sainsbury's*	1 Serving/180g	47	26	3.0	1.6	0.8	2.0
& Broccoli Florets, Tesco*	1oz/28g	9	33	4.0	2.3	0.9	2.2
Boiled in Salted Water	1oz/28g	8	28	2.9	2.1	0.9	1.6
Boiled in Unsalted Water	1oz/28g	8	28	2.9	2.1	0.9	1.6
Florets, Fresh, Frozen, Tesco*	1 Serving/75g	22	29	3.1	2.4	0.8	2.3
Florets, Frozen, Boiled, Iceland*	1 Serving/100g	20	20	2.0	2.0	0.5	1.2
Florets, Frozen, Safeway*	1 Serving/100g	21	21	2.0	2.0	0.5	1.2
Florets, Frozen, Sainsbury's*	1 Serving/100g	20	20	2.0	1.9	0.5	1.2
Florets, In Cheese Sauce, Tesco*	1 Pack/500g	345	69	5.9	4.8	2.9	1.9
Florets, Morrisons*	1oz/28g	10	34	3.6	3.0	0.9	0.0
Florets, Waitrose*	1 Serving/75g	26	35	3.6	3.0	0.9	2.5
Florets, in a Cheese Sauce, Healthy Living, Tesco*	½ Pack/250g	160	64	6.5	3.8	2.6	1.0
Frozen, Asda*	1 Serving/115g	38	33	3.6	2.8	0.9	1.8
Organic, Waitrose*	1oz/28g	10	35	3.6	3.0	0.9	1.8
Peas & Carrots, Bird's Eye*	1oz/28g	9	32	2.2	4.8	0.4	2.6
Raw, Asda*	1 Serving/50g	14	28	2.9	2.1	0.9	1.6
Raw, Fresh	1oz/28g	10	34	3.6	3.0	0.9	1.8
CAULIFLOWER CHEESE,							
Asda*	1 Pack/454g	431	95	4.8	3.1	7.0	0.7
BGTY, Sainsbury's*	1 Pack/403g	238	59	5.4	6.5	1.3	1.0
Better For You, Morrisons*	1 Pack/300g	231	77	4.5	5.4	4.1	1.2
Bird's Eye*	1 Pack/329g	354	108	4.8	7.7	6.4	0.8
COU, Marks & Spencer*	1 Pack/300g	195	65	5.3	5.7	2.2	1.3
Eat Smart, Safeway*	1 Pack/300g	165	55	4.5	4.0	2.1	1.0
Great Value, Asda*	1 Pack/396g	352	89	3.9	4.9	6.0	0.8
Healthy Eating, Tesco*	1 Pack/500g	345	69	5.9	4.8	2.9	1.9
Healthy Living , Tesco*	1 Pack/400g	212	53	3.1	4.1	2.7	1.5
Healthy Living, Co-Op*	1 Pack/300g	155	52	5.3	4.7	1.3	1.3
Improved Recipe, Marks & Spencer*	½ Pack/225g	214	95	6.4	5.2	5.6	2.4
Lattice Bake, Asda*	1 Serving/132g	355	269	6.0	23.0	17.0	1.1
Marks & Spencer*	1 Pack/300g	360	120	6.7	5.6	7.9	1.8
Morrisons*	1 Pack/350g	361	103	5.9	5.1	6.9	0.6
Ready Meal, Tesco*	1 Pack/300g	264	88	4.2	5.2	5.6	1.2
Ross*	1 Pack/300g	300	100	4.9	5.5	6.6	0.1
Safeway*	½ Pack/185g	205	111	5.7	3.7	8.1	1.5
Sainsbury's*	1 Pack/300g	357	119	6.4	7.8	6.9	0.9
TTD, Sainsbury's*	½ Pack/150g	252	168	6.9	8.0	12.0	0.9
Vegetable Recipes, Less Than 5% Fat, Ross*	1 Pack/300g	213	71	3.1	5.6	4.0	1.1
Vegetarian, Safeway*	1 Serving/150g	138	92	4.7	5.2	5.8	1.4
With Half Fat Cheese, Healthy Eating, Tesco*	½ Pack/250g	160	64	6.5	3.8	2.6	1.0
With Roasted Potatoes, Marks & Spencer*	1 Pack/200g	290	145	5.4	9.6	9.6	1.2
CAVATELLI, Egg, Asda*	1 Serving/100g	203	203	9.0	34.0	3.4	3.0

C

	Measure INFO/WEIGHT	per Measure KCAL	Nutrition Values per 100g / 100ml				
			KCAL	PROT	CARB	FAT	FIBRE
CAVIAR,							
Lumpfish, John West*	1oz/28g	26	92	13.0	1.0	4.0	0.0
CAVIARE, Bottled in Brine, Drained	1oz/28g	26	92	10.9	0.0	5.4	0.0
CELERIAC,							
Boiled in Salted Water	1oz/28g	4	15	0.9	1.9	0.5	3.2
Raw	1oz/28g	5	18	1.2	2.3	0.4	3.7
CELERY,							
Boiled in Salted Water	1 Med Serving/50g	4	8	0.5	0.8	0.3	1.2
Hearts, Tesco*	½ Can/133g	12	9	0.9	1.1	0.1	2.3
Raw	1 Med Stalk/40g	3	7	0.5	0.9	0.2	1.1
CELLANTANI, Buitoni*	1 Serving/195g	706	362	12.2	74.4	1.7	0.0
CHAMPAGNE, Average	1 Glass/120ml	89	76	0.3	1.4	0.0	0.0
CHANNA MASALA,							
Indian, Sainsbury's*	1 Serving/149g	165	111	4.2	12.4	4.9	3.3
Marks & Spencer*	1 Pack/200g	320	160	5.6	11.2	10.5	8.2
Safeway*	1 Pack/400g	540	135	5.3	16.2	5.4	2.5
CHAPATIS,							
Brown Wheat Flour, Waitrose*	1 Chapatis/42g	128	305	8.6	49.4	8.0	4.6
Gujarati Style, Safeway*	1 Chapatis/40g	111	277	8.1	50.0	4.9	2.8
Indian Style, Asda*	1 Chapatis/43g	121	282	7.0	50.0	6.0	0.0
Made With Fat	1 Chapatis/60g	197	328	8.1	48.3	12.8	0.0
Made Without Fat	1 Chapatis/55g	111	202	7.3	43.7	1.0	0.0
Morrisons*	1 Chapatis/40g	105	269	8.6	49.8	6.9	0.0
Patak's*	1 Chapatis/42g	121	287	7.5	53.1	6.4	3.2
Spicy, Safeway*	1 Chapatis/41g	115	280	8.9	47.6	6.6	4.5
Wholemeal, Patak's*	1 Chapatis/42g	130	310	11.2	44.9	9.5	9.0
CHARD,							
Swiss, Boiled in Unsalted Water	1oz/28g	6	20	1.9	3.2	0.1	0.0
Swiss, Raw	1oz/28g	5	19	1.8	2.9	0.2	0.0
CHEDDAR MASH, Waitrose*	1 Pack/450g	464	103	3.8	13.4	3.8	1.3
CHEDDARS,							
Cheese & Ham, Mini, McVitie's*	1 Bag/30g	160	534	11.0	55.5	29.8	2.0
Mini, McVitie's*	1 Bag/30g	161	535	11.0	54.4	30.3	2.0
Tangy Salsa, Mini, McVitie's*	1 Bag/50g	266	532	11.0	54.7	29.9	2.1
CHEESE,							
15% Fat, Sainsbury's*	1 Serving/100g	261	261	31.5	0.1	15.0	0.0
Ail & Fines Herbes, Boursin*	1oz/28g	116	414	7.0	2.0	42.0	0.0
Alternative To, Tesco*	1 Serving/60g	238	396	22.5	0.1	34.0	0.0
Appenzellar, Sainsbury's*	1 Serving/25g	97	386	25.4	0.0	31.6	0.0
Applewood, Somerfield*	1oz/28g	119	426	28.0	0.0	35.0	0.0
Asiago, Marks & Spencer*	1oz/28g	105	375	33.0	0.1	27.0	0.0
Aufschnitt in Scheiben Gouda, Edam, Tilsiter, Du Darfst*	1 Slice/19g	51	269	29.0	0.0	17.0	0.0
Austrian Smoked Flavour, Sainsbury's*	½ Pack/50g	143	286	17.4	0.0	24.0	0.0
Babybel With Cheddar, Mini, Fromageries Bel*	1 Cheese/25g	94	374	25.0	1.0	30.0	0.0
Babybel, Fromageries Bel*	1 Cheese/20g	62	308	23.0	0.0	24.0	0.0
Babybel, Light, Mini, Fromageries Bel*	1 Mini Cheese/20g	43	214	26.5	0.0	12.0	0.0
Bavarian Smoked, Processed, Somefield*	1oz/28g	85	302	29.0	0.0	21.0	0.0
Bleu d' Auvergne, Sainsbury's*	1 Serving/25g	84	335	22.0	2.0	26.5	0.0
Blue, Philadelphia, Kraft*	1 Serving/28g	76	270	6.8	3.4	25.5	0.2
Bresse Bleu, Marks & Spencer*	1oz/28g	99	355	19.0	0.3	31.0	0.0
Brie	1oz/28g	89	319	19.3	0.0	26.9	0.0
Brie, 50% Less Fat, Sainsbury's*	1 Serving/30g	62	207	25.6	0.1	11.6	0.0
Brie, Continental, Healthy Eating, Tesco*	1 Serving/50g	85	170	20.0	0.0	10.0	0.0
Brie, Cornish, Organic, Waitrose*	1oz/28g	74	265	16.8	0.1	22.0	0.0

	Measure INFO/WEIGHT	per Measure KCAL	Nutrition Values per 100g / 100ml KCAL	PROT	CARB	FAT	FIBRE
CHEESE,							
Brie, French Creamy, Budgens*	1oz/28g	102	364	19.0	0.1	32.0	0.0
Brie, French, Mild, Sainsbury's*	1 Serving/10g	36	360	19.0	0.1	31.5	0.0
Brie, French, Organic, Tesco*	1 Serving/25g	69	277	22.0	0.0	21.0	0.0
Brie, French, Sainsbury's*	1 Serving/30g	85	284	17.0	0.1	24.0	0.0
Brie, Half Fat, Marks & Spencer*	1 Serving/100g	207	207	23.5	1.3	12.0	0.0
Brie, Organic, Marks & Spencer*	1oz/28g	87	310	19.0	0.1	26.0	0.0
Brie, Somerset, Tesco*	1 Serving/40g	122	306	22.0	0.5	24.0	0.0
Brie, Tesco*	1 Serving/100g	309	309	21.5	1.3	24.2	0.0
Buffalo Mozzarella, Marks & Spencer*	1oz/28g	80	284	18.0	0.1	23.5	0.0
Caerphilly	1oz/28g	105	375	23.2	0.1	31.3	0.0
Caerphilly, Sainsbury's*	1 Serving/50g	187	373	22.8	0.1	31.3	0.0
Cambozola Blue Brie, Somerfield*	1oz/28g	122	434	14.0	1.0	42.0	0.0
Camembert	1oz/28g	83	297	20.9	0.0	23.7	0.0
Camembert, French, Sainsbury's*	1 Serving/30g	84	279	20.0	0.2	22.0	0.0
Camembert, French, Tesco*	1 Serving/50g	136	272	20.5	0.2	21.0	0.0
Camembert, Half, Fat, Coeur De Lion*	1 Serving/125g	261	209	23.5	0.5	12.5	0.0
Camembert, In Crispy Crumb, Kitchen Range Foods*	1oz/28g	98	349	13.3	14.5	26.5	0.0
Cantal, French, Sainsbury's*	1 Serving/30g	106	353	23.0	0.1	29.0	0.0
Chaumes, Marks & Spencer*	1oz/28g	85	305	20.2	1.0	26.0	0.0
Cheddar, 3% Fat, Marks & Spencer*	1oz/28g	48	172	36.2	0.1	2.8	0.0
Cheddar, Average	1oz/28g	115	412	25.5	0.1	34.4	0.0
Cheddar, Campbeltown Mature, Safeway*	1 Serving/50g	205	410	25.0	0.1	34.4	0.0
Cheddar, Canadian, Somerfield*	1oz/28g	114	406	25.0	0.0	34.0	0.0
Cheddar, Canadian, Waitrose*	1 Serving/25g	103	410	25.0	0.1	34.4	0.0
Cheddar, Cathedral City, Dairy Crest Ltd*	1oz/28g	115	410	25.0	0.1	34.4	0.0
Cheddar, Davidstow Extra Mature, Sainsbury's*	1 Serving/100g	410	410	25.0	0.1	34.4	0.0
Cheddar, Davidstow Mature, Marks & Spencer*	1 Slice/10g	41	410	25.0	0.1	34.4	0.0
Cheddar, English Mature, Co-Op*	1 Serving/30g	123	410	25.0	0.1	34.4	0.0
Cheddar, English Mature, Somerfield*	1 Serving/30g	123	410	25.0	0.1	34.4	0.0
Cheddar, English Mature, Tesco*	1oz/28g	115	410	25.0	0.1	34.4	0.0
Cheddar, English Medium, Sainsbury's*	1 Serving/40g	164	410	25.0	0.1	34.4	0.0
Cheddar, English Mild, Tesco*	1 Serving/35g	144	410	25.0	0.1	34.4	0.0
Cheddar, English, Extra Mature, Asda*	1oz/28g	114	406	25.0	0.1	34.0	0.0
Cheddar, Extra Mature, Canadian, Tesco*	1 Serving/30g	123	410	25.0	0.1	34.4	0.0
Cheddar, Extra Mature, Horlicks Farms*	1oz/28g	115	412	25.5	0.1	34.4	0.0
Cheddar, Extra Mature, Safeway*	1 Serving/60g	246	410	25.0	0.1	34.4	0.0
Cheddar, Extra Mature, Vintage, Marks & Spencer*	1oz/28g	115	410	25.0	0.1	34.4	0.0
Cheddar, Full Flavour, Value, Tesco*	1 Serving/30g	123	410	25.0	0.1	34.4	0.0
Cheddar, Grated, Medium, Tesco*	1 Serving/60g	248	413	24.4	1.4	34.4	0.0
Cheddar, Grated, Mild, Safeway*	1 Serving/50g	205	410	25.0	0.1	34.4	0.0
Cheddar, Half Fat, Tesco*	1oz/28g	73	259	30.9	0.1	15.0	0.0
Cheddar, Irish Mature, Tesco*	1 Serving/100g	410	410	25.0	0.1	34.4	0.0
Cheddar, Mature English, Sainsbury's*	1 Slice/20g	82	410	25.0	0.1	34.4	0.0
Cheddar, Mature Grated, Tesco*	1 Serving/50g	207	413	24.4	1.4	34.4	0.0
Cheddar, Mature Reduced Fat, Marks & Spencer*	1oz/28g	91	325	29.4	0.1	23.0	0.0
Cheddar, Mature Style, Half Fat, Marks & Spencer*	1oz/28g	78	277	31.0	0.1	17.0	0.0
Cheddar, Mature West Country Farmhouse, Sainsbury's*	1 Serving/28g	115	410	25.0	0.1	34.4	0.0
Cheddar, Mature White, Iceland*	1 Serving/100g	410	410	25.0	0.1	34.4	0.0
Cheddar, Mature White, Morrisons*	1 Serving/28g	115	410	25.0	0.1	34.4	0.0
Cheddar, Mature White, Westacre, Aldi*	1oz/28g	115	410	25.0	0.1	34.4	0.0
Cheddar, Mature, 16% Fat, BGTY, Sainsbury's*	1 Serving/100g	260	260	29.3	0.1	15.8	0.0
Cheddar, Mature, GFY, Asda*	1 Serving/28g	73	259	31.0	0.0	15.0	0.0
Cheddar, Mature, Half Fat, Iceland*	1oz/28g	73	260	29.3	0.1	15.8	0.0

C

CHEESE,

	Measure INFO/WEIGHT	per Measure KCAL	Nutrition Values per 100g / 100ml				
			KCAL	PROT	CARB	FAT	FIBRE
Cheddar, Mature, Half Fat, Safeway*	1 Serving/25g	66	264	30.0	0.1	16.0	0.0
Cheddar, Mature, Half Fat, Tesco*	1 Serving/25g	65	259	30.9	0.1	15.0	0.0
Cheddar, Mature, Half Fat, Waitrose*	1 Serving/40g	105	262	29.1	0.1	16.0	0.0
Cheddar, Mature, Sainsbury's*	1 Serving/50g	205	410	25.0	0.1	34.4	0.0
Cheddar, Mature, Tesco*	1 Serving/25g	103	410	25.0	0.1	34.4	0.0
Cheddar, Medium, Asda*	1 Serving/28g	114	406	25.0	0.1	34.0	0.0
Cheddar, Medium, Half Fat, Marks & Spencer*	1oz/28g	92	327	30.0	0.1	23.0	0.0
Cheddar, Medium, Organic, Somerfield*	1oz/28g	114	406	25.0	0.0	34.0	0.0
Cheddar, Medium, Organic, Waitrose*	1 Serving/25g	103	410	25.0	0.1	34.4	0.0
Cheddar, Mild, Asda*	1 Serving/50g	203	406	25.0	0.1	34.0	0.0
Cheddar, Mild, Netto*	1 Serving/90g	369	410	25.0	0.1	34.4	0.0
Cheddar, Mild, Organic, Somerfield*	1oz/28g	114	406	25.0	0.0	34.0	0.0
Cheddar, Mild, Sainsbury's*	1 Serving/50g	205	410	25.0	0.1	34.4	0.0
Cheddar, Oak Smoked, Marks & Spencer*	1oz/28g	115	410	25.0	0.1	34.4	0.0
Cheddar, Reduced Fat	1 Sm Serving/20g	52	261	31.5	0.0	15.0	0.0
Cheddar, Scottish Extra Mature, Sainsbury's*	1 Serving/100g	410	410	25.0	0.1	34.4	0.0
Cheddar, Scottish Medium, Marks & Spencer*	1oz/28g	115	410	25.0	0.1	34.4	0.0
Cheddar, Slow Matured, Anchor*	1oz/28g	120	429	24.0	0.0	37.0	0.0
Cheddar, Smoked, Marks & Spencer*	1oz/28g	115	412	25.5	0.1	34.4	0.0
Cheddar, Tesco*	1oz/28g	115	410	25.0	0.1	34.4	0.0
Cheddar, Vegetarian	1oz/28g	119	425	25.8	0.0	35.7	0.0
Cheddar, Vintage Davidstow, Safeway*	1oz/28g	115	410	25.0	0.1	34.4	0.0
Cheddar, Vintage Truckle, Marks & Spencer*	1oz/28g	115	410	25.0	0.1	34.4	0.0
Cheddar, Welsh Extra Mature, Tesco*	1 Serving/25g	103	410	25.0	0.1	34.4	0.0
Cheddar, West Country Farmhouse, Mature, Tesco*	1 Serving/25g	103	410	25.0	0.1	34.4	0.0
Cheddar, West Country Farmhouse, Mature, Waitrose*	1 Serving/28g	115	410	25.0	0.1	34.4	0.0
Cheddar, West Country, TTD, Sainsbury's*	1 Serving/28g	115	410	25.0	0.1	34.4	0.0
Cheddar, White, Medium, Co-Op*	1 Serving/28g	115	410	25.0	0.1	34.0	0.0
Cheddar, White, Mild, Grated, Kerrygold*	¼ Pack/63g	260	413	24.4	1.4	34.4	0.0
Cheddar, Wickedly Extra Mature, Marks & Spencer*	1oz/28g	115	410	25.0	0.1	34.4	0.0
Cheddar, With Caramelised Onion, Sainsbury's*	1 Serving/28g	109	391	22.8	5.1	31.0	0.0
Cheddar, With Caramelised Onion, Tesco*	1 Serving/50g	183	366	21.4	7.1	28.0	0.4
Cheddar, With Onion & Chives, Davidson*	1 Serving/25g	100	400	24.3	0.6	33.3	0.0
Cheestrings, Golden Vale*	1 Stick/21g	69	328	28.0	0.0	24.0	0.0
Cheshire	1oz/28g	106	379	24.0	0.1	31.4	0.0
Chevre Du Berry, Marks & Spencer*	1oz/28g	55	195	11.8	3.1	15.0	0.0
Chevre Pave d'Affinois, Finest, Tesco*	1 Pack/150g	404	269	18.5	0.0	21.7	0.0
Coloured, Low Fat, Weight Watchers*	1oz/28g	51	182	34.2	0.1	5.0	0.0
Cotswold, Full Fat With Herbs, Somerfield*	1oz/28g	113	405	25.0	0.0	34.0	0.0
Cottage, Arla*	1 Serving/25g	23	90	12.0	2.0	4.0	0.0
Cottage, BGTY, Sainsbury's*	1oz/28g	25	91	12.1	8.4	0.9	0.2
Cottage, Bettabuy, Morrisons*	1 Tub/200g	210	105	11.0	5.0	5.0	0.0
Cottage, Better For You, Morrisons*	1 Pot/125g	110	88	13.0	6.9	0.9	0.0
Cottage, Danone*	1 Serving/100g	89	89	11.2	2.3	3.9	0.0
Cottage, Healthy Choice, Asda*	1oz/28g	25	88	13.0	4.0	2.0	0.0
Cottage, Iceland*	1 Serving/100g	77	77	11.8	3.4	1.8	0.3
Cottage, Jocca, Kraft*	1 Serving/50g	55	109	9.3	5.0	5.5	0.0
Cottage, Less Than 5% Fat, Sainsbury's*	½ Pot/125g	131	105	12.3	4.4	4.2	0.0
Cottage, Lidl*	1 Pot/200g	204	102	13.2	2.0	4.6	0.0
Cottage, Low Fat, Longley Farm*	1oz/28g	32	114	11.5	3.4	6.0	0.0
Cottage, Low Fat, Loseley*	1 Pot/125g	148	118	13.3	2.0	6.0	0.0
Cottage, Low Fat, Westacre, Aldi*	1 Pot/100g	85	85	14.6	3.6	1.3	0.1
Cottage, Natural	1oz/28g	29	105	12.0	4.0	4.0	0.0

CHEESE,	Measure INFO/WEIGHT	per Measure KCAL	Nutrition Values per 100g / 100ml				
			KCAL	PROT	CARB	FAT	FIBRE
Cottage, Natural, 95% Fat Free, Marks & Spencer*	1oz/28g	28	99	11.6	3.5	4.0	0.0
Cottage, Natural, Asda*	¼ Pot/113g	118	104	12.0	4.0	4.2	0.0
Cottage, Natural, BGTY, Sainsbury's*	1oz/28g	25	88	13.0	6.9	0.9	0.0
Cottage, Natural, Deliciously Creamy, Marks & Spencer	1 Serving/50g	48	95	12.5	4.1	2.9	0.0
Cottage, Natural, Diet Choice, Waitrose*	1oz/28g	27	98	11.4	3.6	4.2	0.0
Cottage, Natural, Eat Smart, Safeway*	1 Pot/115g	93	81	11.8	3.4	1.8	0.3
Cottage, Natural, GFY, Asda*	1 Serving/113g	97	86	12.0	4.3	2.0	0.0
Cottage, Natural, Good Intentions, Somerfield*	1 Pot/125g	110	88	13.0	6.9	0.9	0.0
Cottage, Natural, Healthy Choice, Safeway*	1oz/28g	24	87	12.7	4.0	2.0	0.0
Cottage, Natural, Healthy Eating, Tesco*	1 Pot/125g	98	78	11.9	3.6	1.8	0.0
Cottage, Natural, Healthy Living, Co-Op*	1 Pot/250g	188	75	10.0	4.0	2.0	0.0
Cottage, Natural, Kwik Save*	1 Serving/25g	21	85	13.8	4.4	1.4	0.0
Cottage, Natural, Less Than 5% Fat, Sainsbury's*	½ Pot/131g	138	105	12.3	4.4	4.2	0.0
Cottage, Natural, Morrisons*	1 Serving/100g	88	88	13.0	6.9	0.9	0.0
Cottage, Natural, Organic, Loseley*	1 Pot/250g	265	106	13.7	1.5	5.0	0.0
Cottage, Natural, Organic, Sainsbury's*	1 Pot/201g	185	92	12.8	6.3	1.8	0.0
Cottage, Natural, Organic, Tesco*	½ Pot/100g	78	78	11.9	3.6	1.8	0.0
Cottage, Natural, Perfectly Balanced, Watirose*	1 Serving/250g	198	79	11.9	3.8	1.8	0.0
Cottage, Natural, Simply, KwikSave*	1 Pot/200g	158	79	11.7	5.5	1.1	0.0
Cottage, Natural, Smartprice, Asda	½ Pot/100g	86	86	12.0	4.3	2.0	0.0
Cottage, Natural, Somerfield*	1 Serving/100g	105	105	12.3	4.4	4.2	0.0
Cottage, Natural, Tesco*	1 Serving/50g	49	97	11.2	3.5	4.2	0.0
Cottage, Natural, Waitrose*	½ Pot/125g	113	90	10.0	3.1	4.2	0.0
Cottage, Plain	1oz/28g	27	98	13.8	2.1	3.9	0.0
Cottage, Plain, Reduced Fat	1oz/28g	22	78	13.3	3.3	1.4	0.0
Cottage, Slimline*	1 Serving/70g	43	62	12.0	3.0	0.2	0.0
Cottage, Very Low Fat, Nisa Heritage*	1 Tub/227g	193	85	13.8	4.4	1.4	0.0
Cottage, Virtually Fat Free, Eden Vale*	1oz/28g	22	80	12.9	6.5	0.3	0.0
Cottage, Virtually Fat Free, Longley Farm*	½ Pot/125g	84	67	13.4	3.0	0.1	0.0
Cottage, Virtually Fat Free, Sainsbury's*	1oz/28g	22	80	12.9	6.5	0.3	0.0
Cottage, With Apricot, Mango & Peach, Low Fat, Safeway*	1 Pot/125g	113	90	10.2	7.9	1.7	0.2
Cottage, With Black Pepper, Healthy Eating, Tesco*	1 Pot/125g	101	81	12.1	4.0	1.8	0.0
Cottage, With Chargrilled Vegetables, BGTY, Sainsbury's*	1oz/28g	25	88	12.1	7.8	0.9	0.6
Cottage, With Chives, Good Intentions, Somerfield*	1 Pot/125g	101	81	10.8	3.2	2.8	0.0
Cottage, With Chives, Low Fat, Westacre, Aldi*	1 Pot/100g	81	81	13.7	3.5	1.4	1.2
Cottage, With Chives, Marks & Spencer*	1oz/28g	28	100	11.9	3.5	3.9	0.0
Cottage, With Chives, Somerfield*	1oz/28g	29	105	12.0	5.0	4.0	0.0
Cottage, With Coronation Chicken, BGTY, Sainsbury's*	1oz/28g	25	91	11.3	8.7	1.2	0.1
Cottage, With Crunchy Vegetables, HE, Tesco*	1 Pot/125g	91	73	9.9	5.0	1.5	0.2
Cottage, With Crunchy Vegetables, PB, Waitrose*	½ Pot/125g	81	65	10.0	2.6	1.8	1.0
Cottage, With Cucumber & Mint, BGTY, Sainsbury's*	½ Pot/125g	103	82	12.0	6.6	0.9	0.0
Cottage, With Cucumber & Mint, COU, Marks & Spencer*	1 Pot/113g	85	75	11.6	3.1	1.5	0.2
Cottage, With Cucumber & Mint, Good for You, Asda*	1 Pot/227g	177	78	11.0	4.1	1.9	0.1
Cottage, With Cucumber & Mint, Healthy Eating, Tesco*	½ Pot/125g	91	73	10.7	3.8	1.7	0.1
Cottage, With Lime & Coriander, Low Fat, Safeway*	½ Pot/126g	113	90	12.2	5.2	2.0	0.0
Cottage, With Mango & Peach, Healthy Eating, Tesco*	1 Pot/250g	188	75	10.4	4.8	1.6	0.1
Cottage, With Mango & Pineapple, BGTY, Sainsbury's*	½ Pot/125g	113	90	10.7	10.4	0.7	0.2
Cottage, With Mango & Pineapple, Morrisons*	1 Pot/125g	113	90	10.7	10.4	0.7	0.0
Cottage, With Mango, COU, Marks & Spencer*	1 Serving/100g	100	100	10.3	11.0	1.1	0.5
Cottage, With Oak Smoked Cheddar, Longley Farm*	½ Pot/125g	160	128	11.1	4.7	6.7	0.0
Cottage, With Onion & Chive, BGTY, Sainsbury's*	1 Serving/50g	42	83	12.4	6.4	0.9	0.1
Cottage, With Onion & Chive, GFY, Asda*	1 Serving/50g	43	85	12.0	4.4	1.9	0.1
Cottage, With Onion & Chive, Good Choice, Iceland*	1 Serving/100g	74	74	11.1	3.8	1.6	0.3
Cottage, With Onion & Chive, Healthy Choice, Asda*	1oz/28g	23	82	12.0	4.0	2.0	0.1

C

CHEESE,	Measure INFO/WEIGHT	per Measure KCAL	Nutrition Values per 100g / 100ml				
			KCAL	PROT	CARB	FAT	FIBRE
Cottage, With Onion & Chive, Healthy Choice, Safeway*	1 Pot/125g	105	84	12.0	4.2	1.9	0.1
Cottage, With Onion & Chive, Healthy Eating, Tesco*	1oz/28g	22	77	11.0	4.5	1.7	0.2
Cottage, With Onion & Chive, Iceland*	½ Pot/100g	81	81	8.5	8.9	1.3	0.3
Cottage, With Onion & Chive, PB, Waitrose*	1 Serving/20g	14	70	10.0	3.4	1.8	0.0
Cottage, With Onion & Chive, Tesco*	1 Serving/250g	235	94	10.9	3.7	4.0	0.0
Cottage, With Onion & Chives, Low Fat, Sainsbury's*	1oz/28g	28	99	11.6	4.4	4.0	0.1
Cottage, With Onion & Chives, Marks & Spencer*	1 Serving/100g	90	90	11.9	4.3	2.8	0.1
Cottage, With Onion & Chives, Nisa Heritage*	1 Pot/227g	168	74	11.1	3.8	1.6	0.3
Cottage, With Onions & Chives, Better For You, Morrisons*	1oz/28g	22	78	12.4	6.4	0.3	0.1
Cottage, With Peach & Mango, COU, Marks & Spencer*	1 Pot/113g	96	85	9.1	9.7	1.0	0.4
Cottage, With Pineapple, Asda*	1oz/28g	31	109	10.0	8.0	3.9	0.0
Cottage, With Pineapple, BGTY, Sainsbury's*	1oz/28g	24	84	10.5	8.9	0.7	0.1
Cottage, With Pineapple, Balanced Lifestyle, Aldi*	1 Serving/200g	140	70	11.0	4.4	0.9	1.5
Cottage, With Pineapple, GFY, Asda*	1 Serving/200g	184	92	10.0	9.0	1.6	0.2
Cottage, With Pineapple, Good Intentions, Somerfield*	1 Pot/125g	105	84	10.5	8.9	0.7	0.1
Cottage, With Pineapple, Healthy Choice, Safeway*	1oz/28g	25	89	10.8	6.9	1.8	0.0
Cottage, With Pineapple, Healthy Eating, Tesco*	1oz/28g	21	75	10.1	5.3	1.5	0.1
Cottage, With Pineapple, Healthy Living, Tesco*	½ Pot/125g	119	95	10.0	9.0	2.0	0.2
Cottage, With Pineapple, Iceland*	½ Pot/100g	81	81	8.5	8.9	1.3	0.3
Cottage, With Pineapple, Less Than 3% Fat, M&S*	1 Serving/200g	190	95	9.4	9.3	2.2	0.2
Cottage, With Pineapple, Low Fat, Waitrose*	1 Serving/40g	34	84	10.4	6.7	1.7	0.2
Cottage, With Pineapple, Morrisons*	1 Serving/100g	84	84	10.5	8.9	0.7	0.0
Cottage, With Pineapple, Sainsbury's*	½ Pot/125g	121	97	9.9	6.8	3.4	2.1
Cottage, With Pineapple, Shape*	1oz/28g	20	73	9.8	8.0	0.2	0.1
Cottage, With Pineapple, Somerfield*	1oz/28g	27	97	10.0	7.0	3.0	0.0
Cottage, With Pineapple, Tesco*	1 Serving/150g	158	105	9.1	9.8	3.3	0.1
Cottage, With Poached Salmon & Cucumber, PB, Waitrose*	1 Pot/200g	156	78	10.0	2.3	3.2	1.0
Cottage, With Poached Salmon & Dill, GFY, Asda*	1/3 Pot/75g	65	86	12.0	2.3	2.7	0.6
Cottage, With Prawn & Cucumber, Safeway*	1 Serving/200g	184	92	12.0	4.7	2.5	0.1
Cottage, With Prawn Cocktail, BGTY, Sainsbury's*	1oz/28g	25	91	12.3	8.3	0.9	0.1
Cottage, With Prawn, GFY, Asda*	1oz/28g	25	91	13.0	6.0	1.5	0.0
Cottage, With Prawns, Marks & Spencer*	1 Serving/100g	95	95	13.4	4.3	2.6	0.0
Cottage, With Red Onion & Chive, COU, M&S*	1 Pot/113g	90	80	11.5	3.6	1.7	0.2
Cottage, With Roasted Tomatoes & Black Pepper, M&S*	½ Pot/100g	95	95	11.7	5.5	2.5	0.0
Cottage, With Roasted Vegetables, Low Fat, Safeway*	1 Pot/125g	96	77	10.5	4.3	1.7	1.8
Cottage, With Salmon & Dill, Healthy Eating, Tesco*	1oz/28g	25	89	12.0	4.7	2.5	0.5
Cottage, With Smoked Cheese & Onion, GFY, Asda*	½ Pot/114g	100	88	13.0	4.4	1.8	0.1
Cottage, With Smoked Salmon & Dill, BGTY, Sainsbury's*	1oz/28g	25	89	13.8	6.4	0.9	0.1
Cottage, With Sweet Chilli Chicken, Marks & Spencer*	1 Serving/200g	190	95	13.8	4.7	2.1	0.5
Cottage, With Tomato & Cracked Black Pepper, Asda*	½ Pot/113g	86	76	10.0	3.1	2.1	1.3
Cottage, With Tuna & Pesto, Asda*	1 Serving/170g	184	108	10.0	3.5	6.0	0.7
Cottage, With Tuna & Sweetcorn, BGTY, Sainsbury's*	1oz/28g	25	91	12.1	8.4	0.9	0.2
Cottage, With Tuna & Sweetcorn, Healthy Choice, Asda*	1oz/28g	25	91	12.0	6.0	1.9	0.1
Cottage, With Tuna & Sweetcorn, Healthy Living, Tesco*	1 Serving/150g	113	75	10.6	4.9	1.5	0.1
Cottage, With Tuna, Cucumber & Mint, Low Fat, Safeway*	½ Pot/100g	87	87	12.0	3.7	2.5	0.1
Cream	1 Portion/30g	132	439	3.1	0.0	47.4	0.0
Cream, 95% Fat Free, Marks & Spencer*	1oz/28g	31	111	13.0	4.2	4.5	0.0
Cream, Extra Light, Tesco*	1oz/28g	36	128	15.0	3.5	6.0	0.0
Cream, Garlic & Herbs, Light, Boursin*	1 Portion/20g	28	140	12.0	2.5	9.0	0.0
Cream, Light, Benecol*	1 Serving/34g	58	170	7.8	3.3	14.0	0.7
Cream, Low Fat, BGTY, Sainsbury's*	1oz/28g	31	111	11.0	4.3	5.5	0.4
Cream, With Onion & Chives, Morrisons*	1 Serving/20g	38	190	11.0	3.0	15.0	0.0
Cream, With Red Peppers & Onion, GFY, Asda*	1 Serving/32.3g	42	130	13.0	6.0	6.0	0.0

CHEESE,	Measure INFO/WEIGHT	per Measure KCAL	Nutrition Values per 100g / 100ml				
			KCAL	PROT	CARB	FAT	FIBRE
Creamy Chaumes, Marks & Spencer*	1oz/28g	80	287	17.6	1.0	23.6	0.0
Danish Blue	1oz/28g	97	347	20.1	0.0	29.6	0.0
Demi Pont L'eveque, Finest, Tesco*	1 Serving/46g	138	301	21.1	0.4	23.0	0.0
Dolcelatte, Marks & Spencer*	1oz/28g	89	317	19.2	0.1	26.0	0.0
Dolcelatte, Tesco*	1oz/28g	108	385	17.3	0.2	35.0	1.1
Double Gloucester	1oz/28g	113	405	24.6	0.1	34.0	0.0
Double Gloucester, Organic, Marks & Spencer*	1oz/28g	113	404	24.4	0.1	34.0	0.0
Double Gloucester, Soft & Chives, Marks & Spencer*	1oz/28g	100	358	20.0	9.2	26.8	0.0
Dubliner, Kerrygold*	1oz/28g	110	392	26.0	0.1	32.0	0.0
Dutch Edam, 50% Less Fat, BGTY, Sainsbury's*	1 Serving/30g	69	231	31.9	0.1	11.4	0.0
Dutch Edam, Safeway*	1 Serving/10g	33	326	25.6	0.0	24.7	0.0
Edam	1oz/28g	93	333	26.0	0.0	25.4	0.0
Edam Hard, Medium Fat, Healthy Eating, Tesco*	1 Serving/100g	229	229	32.6	0.1	10.9	0.0
Edam Type, Reduced Fat	1oz/28g	64	229	32.6	0.0	10.9	0.0
Edam, Dutch Mature, Tesco*	1 Serving/80g	265	331	25.5	0.0	25.4	0.0
Edam, Slices, Asda*	1 Serving/100g	316	316	25.0	0.0	24.0	0.0
Emmental	1oz/28g	107	382	28.7	0.0	29.7	0.0
Emmental, President*	1 Serving/10g	36	355	28.0	0.0	27.0	0.0
Farmhouse Mature, Healthy Eating, Tesco*	1 Serving/50g	131	261	31.5	0.0	15.0	0.0
Farmhouse, 16% Fat, Sainsbury's*	1oz/28g	73	260	29.3	0.1	15.8	0.0
Feta	1oz/28g	70	250	15.6	1.5	20.2	0.0
Feta, Cow's Milk, Asda*	1 Serving/100g	239	239	17.0	0.0	19.0	0.0
Feta, French, Sainsbury's*	1 Serving/100g	283	283	15.1	1.2	24.2	0.0
Feta, Greek, Co-Op*	1 Serving/30g	78	260	16.0	2.0	21.0	0.0
Feta, Marks & Spencer*	1 Serving/20g	62	310	15.0	2.0	26.8	0.0
Feta, Safeway*	1 Serving/20g	61	303	17.0	2.1	25.0	0.0
Feta, Tesco*	1 Serving/70g	212	303	17.0	2.5	25.0	0.0
Fingers, Eat Smart, Safeway*	1 Finger/50g	86	172	36.2	0.1	2.8	0.0
Full Flavour, Economy, Sainsbury's*	1oz/28g	115	410	25.0	0.1	34.4	0.0
Garlic & Herb, Light, Philadelphia, Kraft*	1 Serving/30g	54	180	7.2	3.4	15.5	0.2
Garlic & Herb, Soft & Creamy, Extra Light, Asda*	¼ Pack/50g	65	130	13.0	6.0	6.0	0.0
Garlic & Herb, Soft, Lite, Somerfield*	½ Pot/100g	191	191	9.0	4.9	15.0	0.0
Garlic & Herb, Soft, Marks & Spencer*	1oz/28g	58	206	8.5	2.7	18.0	0.0
Garlic & Herb, Soft, Medium Fat, Safeway*	1 Serving/10g	20	195	9.3	4.9	15.0	0.0
Garlic & Parsley Roule, Light, BGTY, Sainsbury's*	1 Pack/100g	176	176	17.6	1.6	11.0	0.0
Garlic Roule With Herbs, Somerfield*	1oz/28g	92	329	10.0	3.0	31.0	0.0
Goats Camembert, Marks & Spencer*	1oz/28g	85	304	20.0	2.0	24.0	0.0
Goats Milk, Soft	1oz/28g	55	198	13.1	1.0	15.8	0.0
Goats With Roasted Vegetables, Somerfield*	1oz/28g	55	196	8.0	26.0	7.0	0.0
Goats, Crumbled, Tesco*	1 Serving/20g	56	282	14.8	4.3	22.8	0.0
Goats, Disc, Marks & Spencer*	1 Pack/100g	296	296	15.4	2.9	24.3	0.0
Goats, French Chevre Blanc, Safeway*	1 Serving/10g	31	314	21.0	0.0	25.6	0.0
Goats, French Chevre Blanc, Sainsbury's*	1 Serving/50g	163	326	23.0	0.0	26.0	0.0
Goats, French, Fresh, Finest, Tesco*	1 Serving/40g	66	166	11.5	2.8	12.1	0.0
Goats, French, Mild, Sainsbury's*	1 Serving/30g	48	160	11.0	3.2	11.5	0.0
Goats, Organic, Marks & Spencer*	1oz/28g	77	275	14.9	2.5	22.8	0.1
Goats, Sainsbury's*	1oz/28g	79	283	15.0	4.0	23.0	0.0
Goats, St Helen's Farm*	1oz/28g	105	374	24.8	0.5	30.2	0.0
Gorgonzola, Creamy, Marks & Spencer*	1oz/28g	92	330	19.0	0.1	26.0	0.0
Gorgonzola, Somerfield*	1oz/28g	95	338	21.0	0.0	28.0	0.0
Gouda	1oz/28g	105	375	24.0	0.0	31.0	0.0
Gouda, Slices, Waitrose*	1 Slice/25g	94	376	24.0	0.0	32.0	0.0
Grana Padano, Italian Cheese, Waitrose*	1 Serving/14g	54	388	33.0	0.0	28.4	0.0

C

CHEESE,

INFO/WEIGHT	Measure per Measure KCAL	KCAL	PROT	CARB	FAT	FIBRE
Grated, BGTY, Sainsbury's*	1 Serving/50g	132	264	31.0	0.6	15.0	0.0
Grated, Good For You, Asda*	1 Serving/10g	22	220	31.0	1.5	10.0	0.0
Grated, Healthy Living, Tesco*	1 Pack/75g	201	268	34.2	1.4	14.0	0.0
Great for Pizza, Grated, Tesco*	1 Serving/100g	326	326	25.0	2.5	24.0	0.0
Gruyere	1oz/28g	115	409	27.2	0.0	33.3	0.0
Half Fat, BGTY, Sainsbury's*	1 Serving/30g	80	268	34.5	1.4	14.0	0.0
Half Fat, GFY, Asda*	1 Serving/20g	52	259	31.0	0.0	15.0	0.0
Hard Coloured, Medium Fat, Tesco*	1 Serving/100g	259	259	30.9	0.1	15.0	0.0
Havarti, Danish, Sainsbury's*	1 Serving/100g	426	426	20.0	1.0	38.0	0.0
Herbs & Garlic, Creamery Light, Soft, Sainsbury's*	1 Serving/30g	54	180	7.2	3.4	15.5	0.3
Italian Dolcelatte, Asda*	1 Serving/50g	198	395	17.0	0.8	36.0	0.0
Italian Ricotta, Marks & Spencer*	1oz/28g	42	149	10.5	2.0	11.0	0.0
Italian, Dried, Grated, Asda*	1 Serving/28g	135	482	44.0	0.0	34.0	0.0
Italian, Grated, Sainsbury's*	1 Serving/30g	146	485	44.1	0.3	34.2	0.0
Italian, Hard, Finely Grated, Safeway*	1 Serving/10g	48	476	44.0	3.0	32.0	0.0
Jarlsberg, Marks & Spencer*	1oz/28g	98	351	27.0	0.1	27.0	0.0
Lancashire	1oz/28g	104	373	23.3	0.1	31.0	0.0
Leerdammer* Wedge	1 Wedge/250g	933	373	28.3	0.0	28.6	0.0
Leicester	1oz/28g	112	401	24.3	0.1	33.7	0.0
Light, Boursin*	1oz/28g	43	153	12.5	4.5	9.5	0.0
Light, Snack, Philadelphia, Kraft*	1 Pack/50g	123	246	8.4	23.0	13.2	1.6
Lite, Anchor*	1 Slice/21g	50	240	20.9	6.6	15.0	0.0
Low Fat, Healthy Living, Tesco*	1 Serving/15g	29	193	36.1	6.0	2.7	0.0
Mascarpone, Marks & Spencer*	1oz/28g	133	474	5.2	4.1	46.6	0.0
Mascarpone, Sainsbury's*	1 Serving/100g	404	404	5.5	4.8	40.3	0.0
Mature, 95% Fat Free, Weight Watchers*	1 Serving/50g	91	182	34.2	0.1	5.0	0.0
Mature, BGTY, Sainsbury's*	1oz/28g	73	260	29.3	0.1	15.8	0.0
Mature, Extra, Reduced Fat, Tesco*	1 Serving/70g	207	295	26.4	0.1	21.0	0.0
Mature, Grated, Half Fat, Morrisons*	1 Serving/25g	65	259	30.9	1.4	15.0	0.0
Mature, Half Fat, Safeway*	1 Piece/25g	66	264	30.0	0.1	16.0	0.0
Mature, Healthy Eating, Tesco*	1oz/28g	73	259	30.9	0.1	15.0	0.0
Mature, Living, Shape*	1oz/28g	87	309	30.0	0.1	21.0	0.0
Mature, Low Fat, Weight Watchers*	1 Serving/40g	75	188	36.1	5.8	2.3	0.0
Mature, Medium, Fat Hard, Tesco*	1 Serving/100g	261	261	31.5	0.0	15.0	0.0
Medium Fat, BGTY, Sainsbury's*	1 Serving/30g	80	268	31.0	0.1	15.9	0.0
Mild Coloured, Healthy Eating, Tesco*	1 Serving/30g	78	259	30.9	0.1	15.0	0.0
Mild, BGTY, Sainsbury's*	1 Serving/35g	91	261	31.5	0.1	15.0	0.0
Mild, Half Fat, Morrisons*	1 Serving/25g	66	264	31.0	0.0	15.0	0.0
Mild, Low Fat, Weight Watchers*	1/5 Pack/40g	73	182	34.2	0.1	5.0	0.0
Mild, Value, Tesco*	1 Serving/25g	103	410	25.0	0.1	34.4	0.0
Mozzarella, Italian, Castelli*	1 Pack/125g	308	246	20.0	1.0	18.0	0.0
Mozzarella	1oz/28g	81	289	25.1	0.0	21.0	0.0
Mozzarella, Breaded, Asda*	1 Serving/24.5g	66	274	17.0	11.0	18.0	0.7
Mozzarella, For Pizza, Tesco*	¼ Pack/50g	151	301	25.5	1.4	21.5	0.0
Mozzarella, Good For You, Asda*	1 Serving/125g	229	183	21.0	0.0	11.0	0.0
Mozzarella, Grated Italian, Sainsbury's*	1 Serving/25g	74	294	24.5	0.6	21.5	0.1
Mozzarella, Grated, Asda*	1 Serving/20g	62	308	25.0	2.5	22.0	0.0
Mozzarella, Grated, Soft, Full Fat, Tesco*	1 Serving/28g	84	301	25.5	1.4	21.5	0.0
Mozzarella, Grated, Somerfield*	1 Serving/50g	155	310	25.3	0.9	22.8	0.0
Mozzarella, Half Fat, Healthy Eating, Tesco*	1 Serving/125g	231	185	20.0	0.7	10.0	0.0
Mozzarella, Italian, Asda*	1 Serving/45g	132	293	20.0	1.5	23.0	0.0
Mozzarella, Italian, Light, Safeway*	1 Pot/100g	152	152	18.5	1.5	8.0	0.0
Mozzarella, Italian, Tesco*	1 Serving/50g	134	268	18.0	2.0	20.0	0.0

	Measure	per Measure	Nutrition Values per 100g / 100ml				
	INFO/WEIGHT	KCAL	KCAL	PROT	CARB	FAT	FIBRE
CHEESE,							
Mozzarella, Light, BGTY, Sainsbury's*	1oz/28g	48	172	19.0	1.5	10.0	0.0
Mozzarella, Light, Galbani*	1 Serving/50g	95	190	21.2	1.2	11.0	0.0
Mozzarella, Light, Santa Lucia, Galbani*	1 Pack/125g	216	173	20.0	0.8	10.0	0.0
Mozzarella, Marks & Spencer*	1 Pack/125g	300	240	18.0	1.5	18.0	0.0
Mozzarella, Sainsbury's*	1 Serving/75g	194	258	18.0	1.5	21.6	0.2
Mozzarella, Santa Lucia, Galbani*	1 Pack/125g	323	258	18.0	1.5	20.0	0.0
Norvegia, Sliced Light, Tine*	1 Slice/10g	27	272	32.0	0.0	16.0	0.0
Onion & Chive, Low Fat, Soft, BGTY, Sainsbury's*	1 Serving/30g	35	115	13.5	4.0	5.0	1.0
Parmesan	1oz/28g	127	452	39.4	0.0	32.7	0.0
Parmesan Shavings, Asda*	1 Serving/25g	97	388	33.0	0.0	28.4	0.0
Parmesan, Continental Fresh, Grated, Tesco*	1 Tbsp/6g	25	415	34.0	0.1	31.0	0.0
Parmesan, Freshly Grated, Parmigiano Reggiano*	1 Serving/10g	39	388	33.0	0.1	28.4	0.1
Parmesan, Grated, Marks & Spencer*	1 Serving/10g	39	390	33.0	0.1	28.4	0.0
Parmesan, Grated, Sainsbury's*	1 Serving/30g	146	485	44.1	0.3	34.2	0.0
Parmesan, Kraft*	2 Tsp/5g	20	400	40.0	0.0	30.0	0.0
Parmesan, Organic, Marks & Spencer*	1oz/28g	110	392	33.0	0.1	28.4	0.0
Patros Feta, Somerfield*	1oz/28g	75	267	19.0	1.0	21.0	0.0
Pizza, Grated, Safeway*	1 Serving/50g	163	325	25.0	0.6	24.8	0.0
Poivre, Boursin*	1oz/28g	116	414	7.0	2.0	42.0	0.0
Port Salut, Marks & Spencer*	1oz/28g	90	322	21.0	1.0	26.0	0.0
Processed, Plain	1oz/28g	92	330	20.8	0.9	27.0	0.0
Processed, Smoked	1oz/28g	85	303	20.5	0.2	24.5	0.0
Quark, Asda*	1 Serving/20g	12	61	11.0	3.9	0.2	0.0
Quark, Sainsbury's*	1 Serving/16g	11	67	12.3	4.1	0.2	0.1
Quark, Virtuallty Fat Free, Orchard Dairy*	1 Serving/100g	70	70	12.3	4.1	0.2	0.0
Red Leicester, Asda*	1 Serving/15g	60	402	24.0	0.1	34.0	0.0
Red Leicester, BGTY, Sainsbury's*	1 Serving/50g	130	259	31.0	0.1	15.0	0.0
Red Leicester, Economy, Sainsbury's*	1oz/28g	112	399	23.8	0.1	33.7	0.0
Red Leicester, Half Fat, Asda*	¼ Pack/75g	194	259	31.0	0.0	15.0	0.0
Red Leicester, Half Fat, Morrisons*	1oz/28g	74	264	31.0	0.0	15.0	0.0
Red Leicester, Healthy Eating, Tesco*	1oz/28g	73	262	29.1	0.1	16.1	0.0
Red Leicester, Marks & Spencer*	1oz/28g	112	399	23.0	0.1	33.7	0.0
Red Leicester, Medium, Half Fat, Waitrose*	1oz/28g	73	261	29.1	0.1	16.0	0.0
Red Leicester, Organic, Marks & Spencer*	1oz/28g	112	399	23.8	0.1	33.7	0.0
Red Leicester, Tesco*	1oz/28g	112	399	23.8	0.1	33.7	0.0
Ricotta	1oz/28g	40	144	9.4	2.0	11.0	0.0
Ricotta, Italian, Tesco*	1 Serving/50g	63	125	10.5	2.8	8.0	0.0
Ricotta, Sainsbury's*	1 Serving/100g	146	146	8.0	3.8	11.0	0.0
Roquefort	1oz/28g	105	375	19.7	0.0	32.9	0.0
Roule, French, Sainsbury's*	1 Serving/30g	96	321	8.5	3.0	30.5	0.0
Sage Derby	1oz/28g	113	402	24.2	0.1	33.9	0.0
Shaved Pamesan, Fresh, Marks & Spencer*	1 Serving/10g	39	392	33.0	0.1	28.4	0.0
Shredded Monterey Jack, Kraft*	¼ Cup/28g	101	360	22.0	3.6	28.8	0.0
Shropshire, Blue, Sainsbury's*	1 Serving/100g	373	373	20.1	0.1	32.5	0.0
Shropshire, Blue, Somerfield*	1oz/28g	115	409	22.0	0.0	36.0	0.0
Soft & Creamy With Onions & Garlic, GFY, Asda*	1 Serving/25g	32	126	13.0	5.0	6.0	0.0
Soft & Creamy With Pineapple, Asda*	1 Serving/32.1g	62	193	8.0	11.0	13.0	0.0
Soft & Creamy, Extra Light, Asda*	1 Serving/20g	26	128	15.0	3.5	6.0	0.0
Soft & Creamy, Light, Asda*	1 Serving/65g	127	195	12.0	3.0	15.0	0.0
Soft Cream, Lite, Somerfield*	1 Serving/20g	39	195	12.0	3.0	15.0	0.0
Soft, Creamy, Light, Sainsbury's*	1 Serving/30g	56	187	7.8	4.1	15.5	0.3
Soft, Creamy, TTD, Sainsbury's*	1 Serving/20g	52	261	6.5	2.5	25.0	0.0
Soft, Creamy, With Onion & Chives, BGTY, Sainsbury's*	1 Serving/20g	23	115	13.5	4.0	5.0	1.0

INFO/WEIGHT	Measure	per Measure KCAL	Nutrition Values per 100g / 100ml				
			KCAL	PROT	CARB	FAT	FIBRE
CHEESE,							
Soft, Creamy, With Shallots & Chives, BGTY, Sainsbury's*	1 Serving/20g	47	235	5.8	2.2	22.5	0.0
Soft, Extra Light, Co-Op*	1oz/28g	36	128	15.0	3.5	6.0	0.0
Soft, Extra Light, Healthy Choice, Safeway*	1/8 Pack/25g	32	126	15.0	3.0	6.0	0.0
Soft, Extra Light, Low Fat, BGTY, Sainsbury's*	1oz/28g	31	111	11.0	4.3	5.5	0.4
Soft, Extra Light, Morrisons*	1 Serving/20g	26	130	15.0	3.5	6.0	0.0
Soft, Extra Light, Philadelphia, Kraft*	1 Serving/30g	30	101	11.0	3.0	5.0	0.6
Soft, Extra Light, Tesco*	1oz/28g	36	128	15.0	3.5	6.0	0.0
Soft, Full Fat	1oz/28g	88	313	8.6	0.0	31.0	0.0
Soft, Full Fat, Sainsbury's*	1 Serving/50g	156	312	8.0	2.5	30.0	0.0
Soft, Full Fat, Tesco*	1 Serving/25g	78	312	8.0	2.5	30.0	0.0
Soft, Less Than 5% Fat, Marks & Spencer*	1oz/28g	31	111	13.0	4.2	4.5	0.3
Soft, Light, Co-Op*	1 Serving/50g	98	195	12.0	3.0	15.0	0.0
Soft, Light, Tesco*	1oz/28g	55	195	12.0	3.0	15.0	0.0
Soft, Light, Waitrose*	1 Serving/30g	37	122	14.1	3.0	6.0	0.0
Soft, Low Fat, Asda*	1oz/28g	27	96	6.8	5.7	5.1	0.1
Soft, Low Fat, Waitrose*	1oz/28g	36	128	15.0	3.5	6.0	0.0
Soft, Medium Fat	1oz/28g	50	179	9.2	3.1	14.5	0.0
Soft, Natural, Extra Lite, Good Intentions, Somerfield*	1 Serving/20g	26	128	15.0	3.5	6.0	0.0
Soft, Onion & Chive, Extra Light, BFY, Morrisons*	1 Tsp/10g	12	121	12.9	5.0	5.5	0.0
Soft, Reduced Fat, Marks & Spencer*	1oz/28g	53	190	8.0	3.0	16.0	0.0
Soft, Smooth & Cream Light, Morrisons*	1/8 Pack/25g	50	200	12.0	3.0	15.0	0.0
Soft, With Chives, Light, Philadelphia, Kraft*	1 Serving/15g	28	185	7.5	3.4	15.5	0.3
Soft, With Cracked Pepper, Marks & Spencer*	1 Serving/40g	44	110	13.0	4.2	4.5	0.3
Soft, With Garlic & Herb, Extra Light, HE, Tesco*	1 Serving/50g	63	126	13.5	5.6	5.5	0.0
Soft, With Onion & Chives, Extra Light, Tesco*	1 Serving/30g	36	121	12.9	5.0	5.5	0.0
Somerset Camenbert, Safeway*	½ Pack/110g	341	310	22.0	0.5	24.0	0.0
Somerset Goats, Waitrose*	1oz/28g	95	340	20.6	0.0	28.6	0.0
Soya	1oz/28g	89	319	18.3	0.0	27.3	0.0
Stilton, Blue	1oz/28g	115	411	22.7	0.1	35.5	0.0
Stilton, Blue, Budgens*	1oz/28g	115	410	22.7	0.0	35.5	0.0
Stilton, English Blue, Asda*	1 Serving/50g	208	416	23.0	0.1	36.0	0.0
Stilton, Mature, Marks & Spencer*	1oz/28g	115	411	22.7	0.1	35.5	0.0
Stilton, Mature, Safeway*	1 Serving/200g	818	409	22.3	0.1	35.5	0.0
Stilton, White	1oz/28g	101	362	19.9	0.1	31.3	0.0
Taleggio, Tesco*	1 Serving/25g	74	297	18.0	0.0	25.0	0.0
Vinney, Blue, BGTY, Sainsbury's*	1oz/28g	90	320	30.4	0.1	22.0	0.0
Welsh Goats, Sainsbury's*	1 Serving/30g	85	283	15.0	4.0	23.0	0.0
Wensleydale	1oz/28g	106	377	23.3	0.1	31.5	0.0
Wensleydale With Cranberries, Co-Op*	1 Serving/25g	91	365	18.0	12.0	27.0	3.0
Wensleydale With Cranberries, Sainsbury's*	1 Serving/50g	180	359	20.7	6.4	27.8	0.0
Wensleydale, Handmade, Finest, Tesco*	1 Serving/50g	188	375	22.8	0.1	31.5	0.0
Wensleydale, Organic, Sainsbury's*	1 Serving/28g	105	375	22.8	0.1	31.5	0.0
Wexford Mature, Sainsbury's*	1 Serving/83g	340	410	25.0	0.1	34.4	0.0
White Stilton & Apricot, Marks & Spencer*	1oz/28g	94	337	13.8	18.5	23.1	0.0
White Stilton & Cranberry, Marks & Spencer*	1oz/28g	101	362	18.2	15.5	25.3	0.0
White Stilton With Apricot, Somerfield*	1oz/28g	103	369	16.0	8.0	30.0	0.0
White Stilton With Cranberries, Tesco*	1 Serving/50g	184	368	15.8	9.5	29.7	0.7
White, Grated, 14% Fat, Somerfield*	1oz/28g	71	253	30.0	1.0	14.0	0.0
White, Mature, Good Choice, Iceland*	1 Serving/100g	266	266	30.5	0.1	15.9	0.0
White, Mild, Arla*	1 Serving/20g	42	209	22.0	1.0	13.0	0.0
CHEESE PUFFS,							
Farmfoods*	1 Bag/18g	96	532	7.0	54.3	31.9	1.0
Sainsbury's*	1 Pack/100g	530	530	9.1	51.4	32.0	1.9

	Measure INFO/WEIGHT	per Measure KCAL	Nutrition Values per 100g / 100ml KCAL	PROT	CARB	FAT	FIBRE
CHEESE PUFFS,							
Shapers, Boots*	1 Bag/16g	84	523	6.4	59.0	29.0	1.6
SmartPrice, Asda*	1 Bag/18g	92	512	7.0	58.0	28.0	1.3
Value, Tesco*	1 Bag/18g	90	498	7.7	54.1	27.9	1.7
CHEESE SINGLES,							
50% Less Fat, Asda*	1 Slice/20g	38	190	19.0	6.0	10.0	0.0
50% Less Fat, BGTY, Sainsbury's*	1 Slice/20g	38	190	18.0	7.0	10.0	0.0
American, 2% Milk, Kraft*	1 Slice/19g	45	237	21.0	5.3	15.8	0.0
Half Fat, Co-Op*	1 Slice/20g	47	235	25.0	7.0	12.0	0.0
Healthy Eating, Tesco*	1 Slice/20g	39	194	21.7	4.2	10.0	0.0
Light, Kraft*	1 Slice/20g	41	205	20.0	6.0	11.0	0.0
Light, Safeway*	1 Slice/20g	38	192	21.2	4.2	10.0	0.0
CHEESE SLICES							
40% Less Fat, Iceland*	1 Slice/20.1g	41	204	18.0	6.0	12.0	0.0
97% Fat Free, Kraft*	1 Slice/20g	31	155	23.3	9.9	2.3	0.0
Bavarian Smoked, Asda*	1 Slice/18g	50	277	17.0	0.4	23.0	0.0
Better For You, Morrisons*	1 Slice/20g	39	196	21.0	5.4	10.0	0.0
Cheddar, Mature, Marks & Spencer*	1 Slice/30g	124	412	25.5	0.1	34.4	0.0
Cheddar, Mild, Marks & Spencer*	1 Slice/30g	124	412	25.5	0.1	34.4	0.0
Cheddar, Mild, Tesco*	1 Slice/30g	123	410	25.0	0.1	34.4	0.0
Cheddar, Reduced Fat, Weight Watchers*	1 Slice/21g	50	239	21.9	5.0	14.7	0.0
Cheese Food, Asda*	1 Slice/20g	58	289	18.0	7.0	21.0	0.0
Cheese Food, Sainsbury's*	1 Slice/20g	52	260	14.5	5.4	20.0	0.0
Dairylea, Kraft*	1 Slice/25g	76	305	13.0	8.0	24.5	0.0
Farmfoods*	1 Slice/17g	49	286	18.0	4.0	22.0	0.0
Half Fat, Asda*	1 Slice/20g	39	194	20.6	5.4	10.0	0.0
Half Fat, Co-Op*	1 Slice/20g	47	235	25.0	7.0	12.0	0.0
Half Fat, Marks & Spencer*	1 Slice/30g	83	277	31.0	0.1	17.0	0.0
Jarlsberg*	1 Slice/15g	54	360	27.0	0.0	27.0	0.0
Kraft*	1 Slice/20g	56	280	13.5	6.6	21.5	0.0
Leerdammer*	1 Slice/28g	101	360	27.1	0.0	27.7	0.0
Light, Aldi*	1 Slice/19.9g	41	206	20.1	8.1	10.4	0.9
Light, Dairylea, Kraft*	1 Slice/25g	55	220	18.5	7.0	12.5	0.0
Light, Laughing Cow*	1 Slice/20g	41	203	21.0	6.0	10.5	0.0
Light, Thick, Dairylea, Kraft*	1 Slice/25g	51	205	17.3	8.6	10.5	0.0
Lightlife, Leerdammer*	1 Slice/20g	55	273	30.6	0.0	16.4	0.0
Low Fat, Healthy Living, Tesco*	1 Slice/27g	52	193	36.1	6.0	2.7	0.0
Mature Cheddar, Tesco*	1 Slice/30g	123	410	25.0	0.1	34.4	0.0
Mature, Asda*	1 Slice/20g	52	259	31.0	0.1	15.0	0.0
Mature, BGTY, Sainsbury's*	1 Slice/24g	63	261	31.5	0.1	15.0	0.0
Mature, Medium Fat, Healthy Eating, Tesco*	1 Slice/30g	78	259	30.9	0.0	15.0	0.0
Reduced Fat, GFY, Asda*	1 Slice/19.9g	38	191	21.0	4.2	10.0	0.0
Safeway*	1 Slice/20.1g	56	279	15.2	7.2	21.0	0.0
Singles, Half Fat, Tesco*	1 Serving/20g	39	194	21.7	4.2	10.0	0.0
Singles, Lite, Somerfield*	1 Slice/20g	42	212	20.0	6.0	12.0	0.0
Smartprice, Asda*	1 Slice/16.6g	48	283	14.0	5.0	23.0	0.0
Somerfield*	1 oz/28g	84	300	19.0	2.0	24.0	0.0
Swiss, Leerdammer*	1 Slice/25g	90	360	27.1	0.0	27.7	0.0
Tesco*	1 Slice/20g	55	275	14.2	7.2	21.0	0.0
CHEESE SPREAD							
60% Less Fat, Asda*	1 Serving/30g	52	174	16.0	7.3	9.0	0.0
Asda*	1 Serving/33g	92	280	9.0	7.0	24.0	0.0
BGTY, Sainsbury's*	1 Serving/25g	28	111	11.0	4.3	5.5	0.4
Cheese & Garlic, Primula*	1 Serving/20g	49	247	15.7	4.3	18.6	0.0

	Measure INFO/WEIGHT	per Measure KCAL	Nutrition Values per 100g / 100ml				
			KCAL	PROT	CARB	FAT	FIBRE
CHEESE SPREAD							
Cheese & Salmon With Dill, Primula*	3 Inches/10g	26	261	17.6	3.8	19.5	0.0
Cheez Whiz, Original, Light, 41% Less Fat, Kraft*	2 Tbsp/30g	63	210	15.7	11.7	11.3	0.0
Chunky Triangles, BGTY, Sainsbury's*	1 Triangle/25g	43	171	14.8	10.0	8.0	0.0
Chunky, Triangles, Kerrygold*	2 Triangles/47g	119	254	9.1	9.5	20.0	0.0
Cream, Extra Light, Philadelphia, Kraft*	1oz/28g	28	101	11.0	3.0	5.0	0.6
Cream, Light, Sainsbury's*	1 Serving/50g	94	187	7.8	4.1	15.5	0.3
Creamery, Light, Sainsbury's*	1 Serving/25g	46	185	9.0	3.5	15.0	0.0
Dairylea Light, Half Fat, Kraft*	1 Serving/25g	40	161	12.0	8.2	8.7	0.0
Dairylea, Kraft*	1oz/28g	71	255	7.6	8.0	21.5	0.0
Flavoured	1oz/28g	72	258	14.2	4.4	20.5	0.0
Garlic & Herbs, Light, Benecol*	1 Serving/20g	35	174	7.8	4.2	14.0	0.7
Garlic & Herbs, Light, Philadelphia, Kraft*	1oz/28g	50	180	7.2	3.4	15.5	0.2
Happy Shopper*	1 Serving/30g	64	213	11.0	8.5	15.0	0.0
Healthy Eating, Tesco*	¼ Pot/25g	47	187	20.0	6.5	9.0	0.0
Kerrygold*	1oz/28g	60	213	11.0	8.5	15.0	0.0
Light, Laughing Cow*	1 Triangle/18g	25	141	13.5	6.5	7.0	0.0
Light, Philadelphia, Kraft*	1oz/28g	53	190	7.6	3.4	16.0	0.3
Light, Primula*	1oz/28g	48	171	16.0	6.6	9.0	0.0
Light, Triangles, Dairylea, Kraft*	1oz/28g	52	185	14.5	7.6	11.0	0.0
Light, Tub, Dairylea, Kraft*	1oz/28g	52	186	14.0	7.3	11.0	0.0
Low Fat, Weight Watchers*	1 Serving/50g	56	112	18.1	3.4	2.9	1.2
Mediterranean Soft & Creamy, Extra Light, Asda*	1 Serving/32g	42	130	13.0	6.0	6.0	0.0
Mini Tubs, Extra Light, Philadelphia, Kraft*	1 Mini Tub/35g	39	111	11.0	4.8	5.2	0.0
Mini Tubs, Light, Philadelphia, Kraft*	1 Serving/35g	39	111	10.9	4.9	5.1	0.0
Original, Primula*	1oz/28g	72	257	16.0	1.0	21.0	0.0
Philadelphia, Kraft*	1oz/28g	78	280	6.0	2.5	27.5	0.1
Portions, Good for You, Asda*	1 Triangle/22.4g	35	161	14.0	6.0	9.0	0.0
Soft Cream, Full Fat, Philadelphia, Kraft*	1 Serving/25g	63	250	5.9	3.2	24.0	0.2
Soft, Low Fat, Marks & Spencer*	1 Pack/100g	111	111	13.0	4.2	4.5	0.3
The Laughing Cow*	1 Portion/17.5g	46	269	10.0	6.5	22.5	0.0
Tomato & Basil, Light, Philadelphia, Kraft*	1 Tbsp/20g	38	190	7.6	4.3	16.0	0.5
Triangles, Chunky, Dairylea, Kraft*	1 Triangle/14g	32	225	9.9	7.3	17.5	0.0
With Chives, Light, Philadelphia, Kraft*	1oz/28g	52	185	7.5	3.4	15.5	0.3
With Chives, Primula*	1oz/28g	71	253	15.0	1.0	21.0	0.0
With Ham, Light, Philadelphia, Kraft*	1oz/28g	52	184	7.9	4.3	15.0	0.2
With Ham, Primula*	1oz/28g	71	253	15.0	1.0	21.0	0.0
With Shrimp, Primula*	1 Tbsp/15g	38	253	15.0	1.0	21.0	0.0
With Sun Dried Tomato & Basil, Weight Watchers*	1 Serving/50g	53	106	15.9	4.1	2.9	1.2
CHEESE STRAWS							
Cheddar, Marks & Spencer*	1 Straw/11g	59	535	14.9	40.1	34.9	2.4
Selection, Sainsbury's*	1 Straw/7g	41	558	16.6	34.5	39.3	2.8
CHEESE STRIPS, Dairylea, Kraft*	1 Pack/21g	72	345	23.5	0.4	27.0	0.0
CHEESE TRIANGLES,							
BGTY, Sainsbury's*	1 Pack/20g	71	354	5.6	78.2	2.1	2.3
Big Portions, Laughing Cow*	1 Triangle/18g	48	269	10.0	6.5	22.5	0.0
Chunky, Better For You, Morrisons*	1 Triangle/28.3g	50	180	14.5	9.2	9.5	0.0
Chunky, Light, Dairylea, Kraft*	1 Triangle/23g	37	161	13.5	6.9	8.7	0.0
Half Fat, Safeway*	1oz/28g	52	184	16.0	8.5	9.5	0.0
Healthy Eating, Tesco*	1oz/28g	52	187	16.8	6.4	10.5	0.0
Kids, Tesco*	1 Triangle/14.1g	36	254	12.0	6.5	20.0	0.0
Light, Dairylea, Kraft*	1 Triangle/23g	43	185	14.5	7.6	11.0	0.0
Light, Laughing Cow*	1 Triangle/17.5g	25	143	13.0	7.0	7.0	0.0

CHEESECAKE,	Measure INFO/WEIGHT	per Measure KCAL	KCAL	PROT	CARB	FAT	FIBRE
			Nutrition Values per 100g / 100ml				
American Red White & Blueberry, Sainsbury's*	1/6th/83g	264	318	3.8	35.1	18.5	0.4
Blackcurrant Devonshire, McVitie's*	1/6 Cake/67g	190	288	3.8	29.7	17.1	1.7
Blackcurrant Swirl, Heinz*	1/5 Portion/87g	241	277	4.1	30.3	15.4	3.6
Blackcurrant, Marks & Spencer*	1oz/28g	82	293	3.3	29.4	17.9	0.9
Blackcurrant, Sainsbury's*	1oz/28g	75	267	3.2	29.5	15.1	1.1
Blackcurrant, Tesco*	1 Cake/100g	252	252	3.9	32.2	12.0	0.7
Blackcurrant, Value, Tesco*	1 Serving/70g	174	248	2.8	31.4	12.3	1.0
Blueberry & Lemon Flavour Wedges, Sainsbury's*	1 Serving/80g	262	327	5.1	29.2	21.1	1.2
Caramel Swirl, Cadbury's*	1 Slice/91g	373	410	6.0	40.1	25.8	0.0
Cherry, BGTY, Sainsbury's*	1 Serving/91g	181	199	4.6	35.5	4.3	0.5
Cherry, Low Fat, Tesco*	1 Serving/91g	185	203	3.4	38.0	4.1	0.9
Chocolate & Hazlenut, Gold, Sara Lee*	1 Slice/65g	205	316	5.9	28.7	19.7	1.1
Chocolate & Vanilla, Reduced Fat, Marks & Spencer*	1 Portion/114g	319	280	7.0	37.9	12.0	1.5
Chocolate Brownie, Tesco*	1 Serving/101g	400	396	4.8	31.8	27.7	0.8
Chocolate Chip, Marks & Spencer*	1oz/28g	109	391	5.1	39.7	23.6	0.2
Chocolate Swirl, Deeply Delicious, Heinz*	1/5 Slice/81.5g	221	271	4.6	37.4	11.5	4.7
Chocolate, American Style, Asda*	1 Cake/390g	1486	381	5.0	43.0	21.0	6.0
Chocolate, Baked, Ultimate, Entenmann's*	1 Cake/100g	331	331	5.7	34.2	19.0	2.8
Chocolate, Family, Safeway*	1/6 Cake/100g	385	385	7.2	35.0	23.8	1.6
Chocolate, Marks & Spencer*	1oz/28g	106	380	6.5	40.3	21.5	0.4
Chocolate, Pure Indulgence, Thorntons*	1 Serving/75g	308	410	5.6	44.3	23.4	0.6
Chocolate, Weight Watchers*	1 Cake/95g	143	151	7.5	20.7	4.0	0.7
Citrus, Good Choice, Iceland*	1 Cake Mini/111g	198	178	3.5	31.6	4.2	0.4
Devonshire Strawberry, McVitie's*	1/6 Portion/66g	192	291	4.4	31.8	16.2	3.6
Domino's Pizza*	1 Serving/132g	396	300	5.0	28.5	18.6	0.0
Double Chocolate Wedge, Sainsbury's*	1 Portion/75g	327	436	5.7	29.0	33.0	1.7
Homestyle Chocolate, Marks & Spencer*	1oz/28g	105	376	6.0	38.0	22.2	0.7
Irish Cream, McVitie's*	¼ Slice/190g	616	324	4.4	33.0	19.4	0.4
Lemon Creamy & Light, Marks & Spencer*	1/6 Cake/67.5g	238	350	3.5	32.3	20.4	0.4
Lemon Meringue, Tesco*	1 Wedge/94g	353	375	3.8	30.1	26.6	0.3
Lemon, BGTY, Sainsbury's*	1/6 Cake/71g	142	200	4.4	37.0	3.8	0.5
Lemon, Marks & Spencer*	1oz/28g	92	330	5.7	38.7	17.1	0.2
Lemon, Pret A Manger*	1 Pot/150g	382	255	1.8	14.6	20.9	0.2
Mandarin, Co-Op*	1 Slice/99g	297	300	4.0	32.0	17.0	0.3
Mandarin, Good For You, Asda*	1 Serving/97g	194	200	4.0	36.0	4.4	0.8
Mandarin, Healthy Choice, Safeway*	1 Serving/92g	189	205	3.8	37.1	4.6	0.4
Mandarin, Low Fat, Tesco*	1 Serving/70g	145	207	3.3	37.0	4.7	1.4
Pizza Express*	1 Slice/100g	347	347	5.9	24.8	24.8	0.0
Praline, Asda*	1/8 Cake/62g	226	364	7.0	30.0	24.0	3.2
Raspberry Brulee, Marks & Spencer*	1 Serving/100g	255	255	5.7	29.7	12.9	2.1
Raspberry Rapture, Tesco*	1 Serving/109.5g	332	302	3.8	25.4	20.6	0.6
Raspberry Ripple, Marks & Spencer*	1oz/28g	84	300	5.9	32.8	15.6	0.3
Raspberry Swirl, Heinz*	1 Serving/100g	266	266	3.9	30.1	14.5	2.8
Raspberry, Marks & Spencer*	1 Slice/105g	331	315	5.0	32.2	20.5	1.0
Raspberry, Perfectly Balanced, Waitrose*	1 Serving/106g	212	200	4.0	36.2	3.5	1.7
Rhubarb Crumble, Sainsbury's*	1 Serving/114g	268	235	3.1	34.8	9.3	2.4
Sticky Toffee, Iceland*	1 Serving/116g	331	285	3.8	33.9	14.9	0.1
Sticky Toffee, Tesco*	1 Slice/66g	248	375	4.0	35.3	24.2	0.5
Strawberry Shortcake, Sara Lee*	1/6 Slice/68.2g	229	337	4.9	27.6	23.0	0.5
Strawberry, 95% Fat Free, Marks & Spencer*	1 Slice/98g	187	191	5.1	33.8	4.0	0.3
Strawberry, Baked New York, Sara Lee*	1 Serving/100g	248	248	4.7	34.9	9.9	0.7
Strawberry, Co-Op*	1 Cake/100g	225	225	4.0	27.0	11.0	1.0
Strawberry, Deep Dish, Iceland*	¼ Cake/120g	292	243	4.2	32.3	10.8	2.0

	Measure INFO/WEIGHT	per Measure KCAL	Nutrition Values per 100g / 100ml				
			KCAL	PROT	CARB	FAT	FIBRE
CHEESECAKE,							
Strawberry, Fresh, Marks & Spencer*	¼ Cake/125g	300	240	2.8	23.1	15.4	1.1
Strawberry, Heinz*	1 Pack/245g	588	240	3.4	28.1	12.7	2.4
Strawberry, Iceland*	1 Cake/101g	226	224	3.5	31.0	9.5	0.1
Strawberry, Individual, Weight Watchers*	1 Cake/103g	199	193	5.5	33.9	3.2	1.8
Strawberry, Sainsbury's*	1 Serving/90g	221	246	3.5	24.4	14.9	4.6
Strawberry, SmartPrice, Asda*	1 Cake/90g	239	265	5.0	32.0	13.0	1.1
Strawberry, Tesco*	1 Serving/100g	254	254	3.9	32.5	12.0	0.0
Summerfruit, Good For You, Asda*	¼ Cake/130g	259	199	2.8	36.0	4.7	2.0
The Ultimate New York Baked, Entenmann's*	1 Cake/100g	347	347	4.2	35.7	21.3	0.9
Toffee & Banana, Marks & Spencer*	1oz/28g	88	315	5.0	35.7	16.7	0.2
Toffee & Pecan, Wedge, Sainsbury's*	1 Serving/75g	296	395	5.4	28.1	29.0	3.1
Toffee, Asda*	1 Cake/87g	295	339	4.3	31.0	22.0	3.5
Toffee, Co-Op*	1oz/28g	74	265	5.0	35.0	11.0	1.0
Toffee, Marks & Spencer*	1 Serving/105g	357	340	5.2	37.2	21.5	0.9
Toffee, Morrisons*	1 Serving/100g	341	341	5.5	40.4	17.4	0.0
Toffee, Tesco*	1 Serving/100g	265	265	4.3	33.1	12.9	0.8
Triple Chocolate, Waitrose*	1/6 Cake/76g	262	349	5.4	38.3	19.3	1.2
Ultimate Vanilla New York Baked, Entenmann's*	1 Cake/100g	327	327	4.1	34.2	19.3	1.7
Vanilla, Tesco*	1 Serving/115g	417	363	5.7	29.4	24.7	0.6
CHEETOS, Cheese, Walkers*	1 Bag/24g	120	500	6.5	61.0	26.0	1.3
CHERRIES,							
Fresh, Raw, Weighed With Stones	1oz/28g	11	39	0.7	9.5	0.1	0.7
Fresh, Raw, Weighed Without Stones	1oz/28g	13	48	0.9	11.5	0.1	0.9
Glace	1oz/28g	70	251	0.4	66.4	0.0	0.9
In Kirsch, Marks & Spencer*	1oz/28g	35	125	0.4	28.3	0.3	0.4
Stewed With Sugar	1oz/28g	23	82	0.7	21.0	0.1	0.7
Stewed Without Sugar	1oz/28g	12	42	0.8	10.1	0.1	0.8
CHERRYADE, Sugar Free, Tesco*	1 Glass/250ml	3	1	0.0	0.0	0.0	0.0
CHESTNUTS, Average	1 Nut/10g	17	170	2.0	36.6	2.7	4.1
CHEWING GUM,							
Airwaves, Wrigleys*	1 Piece/1g	2	150	0.0	62.0	0.0	0.0
Doublemint, Wrigleys*	1 Piece/3g	9	306	0.0	73.0	0.0	0.0
Extra Peppermint Maltitol, Wrigleys*	1 Piece/1g	2	165	0.0	63.0	0.0	0.0
Orbit, Spearmint, Wrigleys*	1 Piece/3g	6	190	0.0	62.0	0.0	0.0
Spearmint, Wrigleys*	1 Piece/3g	9	295	0.0	73.0	0.0	0.0
CHICK PEAS,							
Asda*	1 Serving/90g	103	114	7.0	15.0	2.9	4.4
Canned, Asda*	1 Can/179g	197	110	7.0	14.0	2.9	4.1
Canned, Re-Heated, Drained	1oz/28g	32	115	7.2	16.1	2.9	4.1
Dhal, Sainsbury's*	½ Can/200g	432	216	10.8	22.7	9.1	7.1
Dried, Tesco*	1 Serving/100g	315	315	21.4	45.2	5.4	10.7
Gigante Verde*	1 Serving/100g	92	92	6.1	14.1	1.2	0.0
In Salted Water, Safeway*	1 Serving/100g	119	119	7.2	16.1	2.9	4.1
In Salted Water, Sainsbury's*	1 Can/130g	144	111	7.2	14.1	2.9	4.1
In Salted Water, Tesco*	1 Can/240g	266	111	7.2	14.1	2.9	4.1
In Water, Salt Added, Drained, Sainsbury's*	1oz/28g	33	119	7.2	16.1	2.9	4.3
Morrisons*	1 Can/130g	155	119	7.2	16.1	2.9	0.0
Organic, Dried, Evernat*	1oz/28g	88	315	21.4	45.2	5.4	10.7
Organic, Waitrose*	1oz/28g	33	119	7.5	20.0	1.0	3.5
Sainsbury's*	1oz/28g	33	119	7.2	16.1	2.9	4.1
Split, Dried, Boiled in Unsalted Water	1 Tbsp/28g	32	114	7.7	17.4	2.0	0.0
Split, Dried, Raw	1 Tbsp/28g	91	325	22.7	49.6	5.4	0.0
Tesco*	1oz/28g	31	111	7.2	14.1	2.9	4.1

	Measure INFO/WEIGHT	per Measure KCAL	Nutrition Values per 100g / 100ml				
			KCAL	PROT	CARB	FAT	FIBRE
CHICK PEAS,							
Tinned, Organic, Tesco*	½ Can /120g	137	114	7.2	14.7	2.9	4.1
Whole, Dried, Boiled in Unsalted Water	1 Tbsp/28g	34	121	8.4	18.2	2.1	4.3
Whole, Dried, Raw	1oz/28g	90	320	21.3	49.6	5.4	10.7
Zeta, Zeta*	1 Can /250g	265	106	7.5	16.4	1.2	8.3
CHICKEN, BREAST,							
Boneless, Free Range, Sainsbury's*	1 Breast/160g	234	146	25.7	0.1	4.7	0.1
Boneless, Grade A, Frozen, Sainsbury's*	1 Serving/100g	164	164	27.2	0.1	6.1	0.1
Boneless, Roast, Marks & Spencer*	1oz/28g	48	170	25.7	0.7	4.5	0.0
Boneless, Sainsbury's*	1 Serving/150g	221	147	21.9	0.1	6.5	0.5
Char Grill, Bernard Matthews*	¼ Pack/50g	100	200	23.2	1.3	11.3	0.0
Cooked, 85% Meat, Somerfield*	1oz/28g	29	103	21.0	2.0	1.0	0.0
Cooked, Safeway*	1 Breast/100g	155	155	27.7	0.0	4.9	0.0
Cooked, Sliced, Iceland*	1 Serving/100g	110	110	25.0	0.1	1.1	0.0
Cooked, Sliced, Organic, Marks & Spencer*	1 Slice/13g	18	135	28.3	0.0	2.4	0.0
Cured, Marks & Spencer*	1 Serving/50g	41	82	18.4	0.0	1.0	0.0
Diced, BGTY, Sainsbury's*	1 Pack/375g	386	103	24.0	0.3	1.1	0.1
Diced, Less Than 5% Fat, Asda*	1 Serving/225g	362	161	30.0	0.0	4.6	0.0
Double, Boneless, Tesco*	1 Serving/150g	222	148	18.8	5.7	5.6	0.3
Eastern Spices, Bird's Eye*	1 Portion/175g	308	176	13.5	3.8	11.9	1.5
Fajita, Sliced, Sainsbury's*	½ Pack/70g	91	130	24.0	4.1	2.0	0.0
Fillets, Asda*	1 Breast/142g	210	148	32.0	0.0	2.2	0.0
Fillets, BBQ, Sliced, Safeway*	1 Serving/80g	120	150	28.1	3.2	2.2	0.6
Fillets, BGTY, Sainsbury's*	1 Fillet/100g	134	134	29.3	0.1	1.9	0.2
Fillets, Breaded, BGTY, Sainsbury's*	1 Fillet/113g	247	219	19.8	24.3	4.7	1.9
Fillets, Breaded, Farmfoods*	1oz/28g	57	204	0.0	16.0	13.8	9.4
Fillets, Breaded, Tesco*	1 Portion/95g	213	224	13.0	16.9	11.6	0.4
Fillets, British, Diced, Healthy Eating, Tesco*	1 Pack/400g	424	106	24.0	0.0	1.1	0.0
Fillets, Chinese Style, Simple Solutions, Tesco*	1 Serving/192g	278	145	19.9	2.5	6.2	0.0
Fillets, Co-Op*	1 Breast/117g	123	105	23.0	0.0	2.0	0.0
Fillets, Crunchy Coated, Mini, Marks & Spencer*	1 Serving/150g	345	230	15.8	18.1	10.5	2.0
Fillets, Extra Hot, American, Asda*	1 Fillet/154.2g	313	203	15.0	11.0	11.0	2.9
Fillets, Frozen, Marks & Spencer*	1 Fillet/125g	150	120	24.1	0.0	2.5	0.0
Fillets, Frozen, Tesco*	1 Serving/115g	133	116	21.8	0.0	3.2	0.0
Fillets, Healthy Choice, Safeway*	1oz/28g	50	180	19.7	18.0	3.7	1.4
Fillets, Healthy Eating, Tesco*	1 Fillet/155g	180	116	21.8	0.0	3.2	0.0
Fillets, Iceland*	1 Fillet/130g	192	148	32.0	0.0	2.2	0.0
Fillets, In Crispy Breadcrumbs, Safeway*	1 Fillet/112.5g	244	216	20.8	11.0	9.9	1.2
Fillets, Korma Sliced, Safeway*	1 Serving/100g	131	131	28.7	0.8	2.8	0.7
Fillets, Korma Style, Ready to Eat, Tesco*	½ Pack/100g	132	132	26.1	0.8	2.7	0.4
Fillets, Less Than 2% Fat, Asda*	1 Breast/150g	159	106	24.0	0.0	1.1	0.0
Fillets, Mini, British, Free Range, Tesco*	1 Pack/300g	297	99	23.9	0.0	0.4	0.0
Fillets, Mini, Tesco*	1 Serving/150g	174	116	21.8	0.0	3.2	0.0
Fillets, Organic, Marks & Spencer*	1 Fillet/180g	189	105	24.0	0.0	1.1	0.0
Fillets, Organic, Waitrose*	1 Serving/150g	149	99	23.9	0.0	0.4	0.0
Fillets, Prime, Sainsbury's*	1 Serving/230g	244	106	24.0	0.1	1.1	0.1
Fillets, Sainsbury's*	1 Fillet/130g	215	165	36.5	0.1	2.2	0.1
Fillets, Skinless & Boneless, Marks & Spencer*	1 Fillet/130g	130	100	22.7	0.4	0.9	0.3
Fillets, Skinless, Fresh, Value, Tesco*	1 Breast/170g	197	116	21.8	0.0	3.2	0.0
Fillets, Skinless, Healthy Eating, Tesco*	1 Serving/140g	146	104	23.6	0.0	1.1	0.0
Fillets, Skinless, Sainsbury's*	1 Pack/520g	551	106	24.0	0.0	1.1	0.0
Fillets, Skinless, Waitrose*	1 Pack/190g	236	124	27.6	0.6	1.6	0.6
Fillets, Skinned & Boned, Sainsbury's*	1 Breast/140g	148	106	24.0	0.1	1.1	0.1
Fillets, SmartPrice, Asda*	1 Serving/175g	186	106	24.0	0.0	1.1	0.0

C

CHICKEN, BREAST,

INFO/WEIGHT	Measure	per Measure KCAL	KCAL	PROT	CARB	FAT	FIBRE
Fillets, Somerfield*	1 Serving/262g	388	148	32.0	0.0	2.2	0.0
Fillets, Stir Fry, Mini, Tesco*	1 Serving/200g	204	102	21.8	0.0	1.6	0.0
Fillets, in Breadcrumbs, Marks & Spencer*	1 Fillet/125g	250	200	17.0	13.5	8.6	0.5
Fresh, Good Intentions, Somerfield*	1 Serving/262g	388	148	32.0	0.0	2.2	0.0
Garlic & Herb Flavour, Co-Op*	1 Serving/170g	281	165	19.0	2.0	9.0	0.3
Golden Roasted, Bernard Matthews*	1oz/28g	31	110	23.4	0.6	1.5	0.0
Hot & Spicy, Simple Solutions, Tesco*	1 Serving/192g	278	145	19.5	0.9	7.0	0.9
In BBQ Sauce, Weight Watchers*	1 Pack/339g	336	99	5.8	11.0	3.5	0.9
In Low Fat White Sauce, Safeway*	1 Serving/200g	190	95	11.5	2.1	4.5	0.2
Joint With Pork, Stuffing & Chipolatas, Tesco*	½ Pack/340g	524	154	16.7	3.4	8.2	0.5
Kentucky Fried Chicken*	1 Breast/161g	370	230	24.8	6.8	11.8	0.0
Marks & Spencer*	1/3 Serving/166g	266	160	19.6	5.4	6.9	0.0
Meat Only, Minced	1oz/28g	31	110	23.1	0.0	1.2	0.0
Original Recipe, Kentucky Fried Chicken*	1 Breast/161g	596	370	40.0	11.0	19.0	0.0
Part Boned, Tesco*	1 Pack/200g	340	170	25.9	0.5	7.2	0.0
Pieces, Co-Op*	1 Serving/100g	125	125	27.0	1.0	2.0	0.0
Premium, Bernard Matthews*	1 Slice/20g	24	122	19.3	3.0	3.6	0.0
Roast, Low Fat, Safeway*	1oz/28g	29	105	20.3	3.2	1.2	1.0
Roast, Marks & Spencer*	½ Pack/250g	388	155	15.4	10.6	5.6	0.7
Roast, Part-Boned, Co-Op*	1 Pack/200g	290	145	26.0	0.7	4.0	0.0
Roast, Portion, Sainsbury's*	1oz/28g	55	196	22.6	0.1	11.7	0.1
Roast, Premium, Sainsbury's*	1oz/28g	31	110	24.8	0.9	0.9	0.3
Roast, Sliced, Tesco*	1 Slice/120g	146	122	26.0	0.8	1.6	0.0
Roast, Traditional, Tesco*	1 Breast/200g	342	171	26.5	1.7	6.5	0.0
Sage & Onion, Slices, Sainsbury's*	1 Pack/140g	158	113	23.1	1.0	1.8	0.5
Seasoned, Marks & Spencer*	1oz/28g	35	126	20.5	2.6	3.8	0.0
Skinless & Boneless, Iceland*	1 Serving/150g	222	148	32.0	0.0	2.2	0.0
Skinless, Boneless, Ready To Eat, Asda*	1oz/28g	31	111	24.3	0.7	1.3	0.0
Sliced, Good For You, Asda*	1 Pack/140g	172	123	27.0	0.0	1.7	0.0
Slices, Cooked, Sainsbury's*	1 Slice/5g	5	105	20.9	2.2	1.4	0.2
Smoked, Premium, Bernard Matthews*	1 Slice/20g	21	107	17.2	1.6	3.5	0.0
Smoked, Premium, Sainsbury's*	1 Slice/20g	23	114	24.8	0.5	1.7	0.4
Steaks in Breadcrumbs, Asda*	1 Steak/100g	282	282	21.0	18.0	14.0	0.6
Strips, Stir Fry, Asda*	1 Pack/250g	383	153	31.1	0.6	3.0	0.0
Strips, Tesco*	1 Serving/280g	288	103	23.1	0.1	1.1	0.6
Supreme, Sainsbury's*	1 Serving/187g	421	225	20.6	0.3	15.8	0.6
Tandoori, Pieces, Sainsbury's*	1 Serving/100g	140	140	28.6	0.9	2.8	0.9
Tandoori, Simple Solutions, Tesco*	1 Serving/180g	221	123	16.0	3.7	4.7	1.1
Tikka Pieces, Sainsbury's*	½ Pack/113.5g	169	148	27.8	2.1	3.1	1.1
Wafer Thin, Bernard Matthew*	1 Serving/100g	111	111	18.0	3.1	3.0	0.0
With Sticky Honey & Chilli Sauce, Asda*	1 Serving/175g	247	141	20.0	8.0	3.2	0.0
In Barbeque Sauce, COU, Marks & Spencer*	1 Pack/350g	420	120	8.5	20.6	1.9	0.6
Chilli & Ginger, COU, Marks & Spencer*	1 Breast/120g	156	130	19.5	8.6	2.0	1.7
Honey & Mustard, Bird's Eye*	1 Portion/97g	175	180	19.6	4.2	9.4	0.1
In Tikka Masala Sauce, GFY, Asda*	1 Pack/380g	426	112	13.0	6.0	4.0	0.7
Breasts, In Wild Mushroom Sauce, Healthy Living, Tesco*	1 Serving/212g	191	90	15.1	2.1	2.4	1.5
Breasts, Plum Tomatoes, Basil, Bird's Eye*	1 Portion/172.4g	200	116	13.3	5.0	4.7	0.6
With Garlic Mushrooms, Simple Solution, Tesco*	1 Serving/200g	304	152	16.1	2.0	8.8	0.5
With Mushroom & Garlic Butter, Sainsbury's*	1 Serving/195g	384	197	21.6	5.0	10.0	0.1
With Thai Green Curry, Finest, Tesco*	1 Serving/200g	292	146	16.5	2.0	8.0	0.7
With Tomato & Basil Sauce, Healthy Living, Tesco*	1 Serving/225g	221	98	14.6	4.4	2.5	0.9
With a Sea Salt & Black Pepper Crust, Asda*	1 Serving/153.7g	186	121	19.0	5.0	2.8	0.0
In Sweet & Sour Sauce, Good Choice, Iceland*	1 Pack/340g	350	103	15.3	8.8	0.7	0.8

	Measure INFO/WEIGHT	per Measure KCAL	Nutrition Values per 100g / 100ml KCAL	PROT	CARB	FAT	FIBRE
CHICKEN, BREAST,							
In White Wine & Tarragon Sauce, Finest, Tesco*	½ Pack/200g	326	163	16.8	1.3	10.1	0.0
In Barbecue Sauce, COU, Marks & Spencer*	1 Pack/350g	420	120	8.5	17.1	1.7	0.6
CHICKEN, DICED,							
Frozen, Tesco*	1oz/28g	36	128	21.4	0.0	4.7	0.0
Tesco*	1oz/28g	36	128	21.4	0.0	4.7	0.0
CHICKEN, DIPPERS, Bird's Eye*	5 Dippers/93.3g	209	225	12.7	12.0	14.0	0.6
CHICKEN, DRUMSTICKS							
Roast, Sainsbury's*	1 Piece/100g	162	162	21.6	0.2	7.2	0.5
BBQ, Frozen, Tesco*	1 Serving/200g	306	153	18.8	1.6	7.9	1.0
CHICKEN, FILLETS,							
Burger King*	1 Serving/72g	101	140	27.9	0.4	3.1	0.0
Diced, Sainsbury's*	1 Serving/150g	248	165	36.5	0.0	2.2	0.0
Fresh, Mini, Sainsbury's*	½ Pack/225g	371	165	36.5	0.1	2.3	0.1
Honey & Maple, Roast, Mini, Waitrose*	½ Pack/100g	131	131	23.0	8.6	0.5	1.5
Iceland*	1 Pack/200g	146	73	13.5	2.2	1.1	0.1
In Peppers, Sainsbury's*	1 Pack/360g	378	105	13.7	4.2	3.7	1.1
Lime & Coriander, Mini, Waitrose*	1 Serving/100g	126	126	25.4	3.1	1.3	1.4
Meal, American, Asda*	1 Pack/345g	838	243	9.0	27.0	11.0	2.3
Mini, BGTY, Sainsbury's*	1 Serving/100g	129	129	29.7	0.1	1.1	0.1
Mini, Battered, Sainsbury's*	1 Fillet/29.8g	57	191	19.0	9.7	8.5	0.6
Mini, Eat Smart, Safeway*	½ Pack/100g	150	150	35.3	0.8	0.7	0.6
Parmesan & Sun Dried Tomato, Mini, Sainsbury's*	1 Pack/200g	278	139	22.1	6.0	2.9	0.5
Sweet Chilli, Roast, Mini, Waitrose*	1 Pack/200g	216	108	23.0	3.8	0.2	0.9
Thai Style, Mini, Sainsbury's*	1 Serving/100g	125	125	20.9	6.8	1.6	0.8
CHICKEN, LEG,							
Asda*	1 Serving/160g	379	237	21.0	0.0	17.0	0.0
Hot & Spicy, Tesco*	1 Serving/330g	482	146	11.3	0.4	11.1	0.5
Portion, Free Range, Organic, Sainsbury's*	1 Serving/100g	186	186	27.2	0.0	8.4	0.0
Portion, Ready To Roast, Sainsbury's	1 Leg/200g	428	214	21.6	0.1	14.1	0.1
Portion, Roast, Somerfield*	1oz/28g	57	203	23.0	0.0	12.0	0.0
Roasted, Marks & Spencer*	1oz/28g	64	230	22.7	0.3	15.3	0.0
CHICKEN, LIGHT MEAT,							
Raw	1oz/28g	30	106	24.0	0.0	1.1	0.0
Roasted	1oz/28g	43	153	30.2	0.0	3.6	0.0
CHICKEN, MEAT,							
& Skin Portions, Deep Fried	1oz/28g	73	259	26.9	0.0	16.8	0.0
& Skin, Raw	1oz/28g	64	230	17.6	0.0	17.7	0.0
& Skin, Roasted	1oz/28g	60	216	22.6	0.0	14.0	0.0
Average, Raw	1oz/28g	30	108	22.3	0.0	2.1	0.0
Average, Roasted	1oz/28g	50	177	27.3	0.0	7.5	0.0
CHICKEN, MINCE,							
BGTY, Sainsbury's*	1 Serving/250g	375	150	21.4	0.1	7.1	0.1
Sainsbury's*	1 Serving/125g	201	161	18.1	0.1	9.8	0.5
CHICKEN, STEAKS,							
Hot & Spicy, Iceland*	1 Steak/95g	273	287	18.2	11.1	18.9	1.0
Safeway*	1 Steak/130.2g	306	235	15.1	11.0	14.5	1.4
Southern Fried, Safeway*	1 Serving/140g	332	237	17.4	7.8	15.1	1.3
CHICKEN, THIGH,							
Chinese, Forest Farms*	1oz/28g	68	242	20.2	1.4	17.3	9.0
Fillets, Fresh, Asda*	1 Serving/100g	195	195	24.0	0.0	11.0	0.0
Fillets, Large, Sainsbury's*	1 Thigh/125g	270	216	28.0	0.1	11.6	0.1
Fillets, Skinless, Tesco*	2 Thighs/180g	227	126	19.1	0.0	5.5	0.0
Frozen, Sainsbury's*	1 Thigh/130g	319	245	16.4	0.0	20.0	0.0

	Measure	per Measure	Nutrition Values per 100g / 100ml				
	INFO/WEIGHT	KCAL	KCAL	PROT	CARB	FAT	FIBRE
CHICKEN, THIGH,							
Meat & Skin, Casseroled	1oz/28g	65	233	21.5	0.0	16.3	0.0
Meat Only, Diced, Casseroled	1oz/28g	50	180	25.6	0.0	8.6	0.0
Roast, Asda*	1 Pack/500g	1305	261	22.2	0.0	19.1	0.0
Roast, Marks & Spencer*	1oz/28g	76	270	24.8	0.8	18.7	0.0
Roast, Sainsbury's*	1 Serving/100g	182	182	26.5	0.6	8.2	0.1
CHICKEN, WHOLE,							
Garlic Basted, Asda*	1oz/28g	60	214	20.0	0.0	14.9	0.2
Roast, Asda*	1oz/28g	56	199	20.9	1.4	12.2	0.0
Rotisserie, Marks & Spencer*	1oz/28g	62	220	23.7	0.4	14.0	0.4
CHICKEN, WING,							
Quarter, Meat & Skin, Casseroled	1oz/28g	59	210	24.4	0.0	12.5	0.0
Quarter, Meat & Skin, Raw	1oz/28g	54	193	20.3	0.0	12.4	0.0
Quarter, Meat & Skin, Roasted	1oz/28g	63	226	24.8	0.0	14.1	0.0
Quarter, Meat Only, Casseroled	1oz/28g	46	164	26.9	0.0	6.3	0.0
CHICKEN &,							
Apricot Rice, COU, Marks & Spencer*	1 Pack/400g	360	90	9.4	10.6	0.9	0.7
Asparagus Pasta, Easy Steam, Healthy Living, Tesco*	1 Pack/400g	312	78	8.7	8.4	1.1	1.0
Asparagus in a Champagne Sauce, Finest, Tesco*	1 Pack/500g	615	123	8.8	7.0	6.7	0.9
Asparagus, BGTY, Sainsbury's*	1 Pack/450g	504	112	8.5	17.4	1.0	0.8
Asparagus, Long Grain & Wild Rice, BGTY, Sainsbury's*	1 Pack/451g	555	123	9.2	17.1	2.0	0.8
Bacon Parcels, Finest, Tesco*	1 Pack/232.5g	380	163	16.1	3.7	9.3	0.5
Bacon Parcels, Sainsbury's*	½ Pack/170g	406	239	21.9	0.1	16.8	0.0
Black Bean Noodles, Sainsbury's*	1 Serving/130g	155	119	4.3	23.9	0.7	0.8
Black Bean Sauce & Egg Fried Rice, BGTY, Sainsbury's*	1 Pack/450g	527	117	7.2	14.7	3.3	0.5
Black Bean With Chinese Rice, COU, Marks & Spencer*	1 Pack/400g	320	80	7.4	7.6	2.4	1.1
Black Bean With Egg Fried Rice, New, BGTY, Sainsbury's*	1 Pack/450g	446	99	6.4	16.6	0.8	0.6
Black Bean With Noodles, Tesco*	1 Pack/475g	470	99	7.6	13.6	1.6	0.2
Black Bean With Rice, Healthy Living, Tesco*	1 Pack/450g	464	103	7.6	15.2	1.3	1.1
Black Bean With Vegetable Rice, COU, Marks & Spencer*	1 Pack/400g	340	85	6.6	10.7	1.9	0.9
Black Bean, Chinese Takeaway, Tesco*	1 Serving/200g	190	95	8.3	8.0	3.3	0.5
Broccoli With Rigatoni Pasta, BGTY, Sainsbury's*	1 Pack/450g	590	131	10.5	15.2	3.1	0.7
Broccoli, White Wine Sauce & Potato, HE, Tesco*	1 Pack/400g	312	78	6.0	10.2	1.5	1.0
Cashew Nut With Egg Fried Rice, Somerfield*	1 Pack/340g	435	128	7.0	13.0	5.0	0.0
Cashew Nuts & Veg Rice, COU, Marks & Spencer*	1 Pack/400g	320	80	6.9	8.6	2.0	1.0
Cashew Nuts With Egg Fried Rice, Healthy Living, Tesco*	1 Pack/450g	441	98	8.9	12.7	1.3	1.3
Cashew Nuts With Egg Rice, Good For You, Asda*	1 Pack/396g	384	97	6.0	16.0	1.0	6.0
Cashew Nuts, Asda*	1 Pack/400g	528	132	8.2	4.2	9.1	0.8
Cashew Nuts, Cantonese, Sainsbury's*	1 Pack/350g	350	100	9.4	3.8	5.2	1.8
Cashew Nuts, Chinese, Sainsbury's*	1 Pack/350g	312	89	7.8	5.7	4.0	1.2
Cashew Nuts, Chinese, Tesco*	1 Pack/350g	378	108	9.5	4.9	5.6	0.6
Cashew Nuts, Marks & Spencer*	1 Pack/300g	300	100	10.3	5.0	4.0	1.2
Cashew Nuts, Ready Meals, Waitrose*	1 Pack/400g	416	104	11.3	8.2	2.9	1.0
Chargrilled Vegetable Roll, Healthy Living, Tesco*	1 Pack/221.1g	336	152	10.1	21.8	2.7	2.3
Coconut, Lime & Ginger Rice, PB, Waitrose*	1 Pack/400g	432	108	7.2	15.1	2.7	0.9
Cous Cous, Healthy Eating, Tesco*	1 Pack/351g	263	75	10.3	7.3	0.5	1.4
Gravy, COU, Marks & Spencer*	1 Pack/300g	216	72	7.2	7.8	1.3	1.6
King Prawn Special Fried Rice, Finest, Tesco*	1 Pack/450g	734	163	7.7	17.0	7.1	0.7
Mushroom With Vegetable Rice, BGTY, Sainsbury's*	1 Pack/400g	376	94	6.4	13.0	1.8	0.9
Mushroom in Oyster Sauce, Tesco*	1 Pack/350g	252	72	8.0	6.3	1.6	0.7
Mushroom in White Wine Sauce, GFY, Asda*	1 Pack/400g	272	68	6.0	7.0	1.8	1.2
Mushroom, Chinese, Iceland*	1 Pack/400g	276	69	8.2	3.8	2.3	0.4
Mushroom, Chinese, Sainsbury's*	½ Pack/175g	116	66	7.6	4.4	2.0	0.9
Mushroom, Chinese, Tesco*	1 Pack/460g	474	103	5.7	13.8	2.8	1.0

C

	Measure INFO/WEIGHT	per Measure KCAL	Nutrition Values per 100g / 100ml				
			KCAL	PROT	CARB	FAT	FIBRE
CHICKEN &,							
Mushroom, With Vegetable Rice, BGTY, Sainsbury's*	1 Pack/400g	376	94	6.4	13.0	1.8	0.9
Noodles, Chinese Style, Healthy Eating, Tesco*	1 Pack/370g	422	114	8.5	15.9	1.7	1.5
Peppers In A Black Bean Sauce, Marks & Spencer*	1 Pack/320g	256	80	9.4	7.3	1.5	1.2
Pineapple Pasta, Shapers, Boots*	1 Pack/221g	210	95	5.4	15.0	1.5	0.9
Pineapple With Egg Fried Rice, Tesco*	1 Pack/450g	450	100	7.6	12.1	2.4	1.2
Pineapple With Rice, Healthy Living, Tesco*	1 Pack/450g	401	89	6.6	12.0	1.6	1.0
Pineapple With Vegetable Rice, Marks & Spencer*	1 Pack/400g	400	100	7.2	13.0	1.9	1.6
Pineapple, Chilled, Tesco*	1 Pack/350g	364	104	9.6	11.1	2.4	5.5
Prawn Yaki Udan Noodles, Marks & Spencer*	1 Pack/395g	435	110	8.1	11.9	3.6	0.8
Red Pepper Dressing, Simple Solutions, Tesco*	1 Serving/140g	228	163	19.2	0.1	9.5	0.5
Red Wine Penne, Italiana, Weight Watchers*	1 Pack/395g	249	63	3.7	10.1	0.7	0.6
Red Wine Sauce With Potato Gratin, HE, Tesco*	1 Pack/450g	410	91	7.7	8.9	2.7	2.2
Roast Med Vegetables in Red Pepper Sauce, Sainsbury's*	½ Pack/300g	228	76	10.1	4.7	1.9	0.7
Spinach Pasta, Waitrose*	1 Pack/350g	483	138	7.0	14.0	6.0	0.8
Tomato & Basil, COU, Marks & Spencer*	½ Pack/200g	180	90	14.3	3.4	2.3	0.8
Tomato Saag With Pilau Rice, BGTY, Sainsbury's*	1 Pack/400g	404	101	7.3	15.6	1.0	1.0
Vegetable Savoury Rice, Safeway*	½ Pack/185g	231	125	2.9	25.9	1.1	0.8
White Wine With Rice, Healthy Eating, Tesco*	1 Pack/450g	450	100	7.1	14.8	1.4	1.0
CHICKEN A L' ORANGE, Lean Cuisine*	1 Pack/334g	384	115	5.6	18.0	2.1	0.4
CHICKEN AL FORNO, Arrabbiata, Sainsbury's*	1 Pack/900g	1026	114	6.5	16.4	2.5	1.4
CHICKEN ARRABBIATA,							
Bistro, Waitrose*	½ Pack/175g	156	89	12.9	2.5	3.0	0.5
Perfectly Balanced, Waitrose*	1 Serving/240g	211	88	12.4	4.0	2.4	0.6
Good for You, Asda*	1 Pack/340g	228	67	4.7	9.0	1.3	0.0
CHICKEN - BBQ,							
Chunky, Ready To Eat, Tesco*	½ Pack/85g	118	139	29.0	3.2	1.1	0.3
Thigh, Asda*	1oz/28g	60	216	22.6	0.0	14.0	0.0
Wings, Flavoured, Farmfoods*	1oz/28g	69	247	21.1	8.0	14.5	1.0
Wings, McCain*	1 Serving/135g	298	221	22.3	6.6	11.7	0.0
CHICKEN - BALLS,							
Chinese, Marks & Spencer*	1 Ball/16g	45	280	10.8	29.2	13.6	2.1
Crispy, Marks & Spencer*	1 Ball/16g	35	220	13.3	23.7	8.1	0.5
Lemon, Asda*	1 Ball/15g	42	279	14.0	19.0	17.0	1.6
CHICKEN - BARBECUE,							
Breast in a Sauce, COU, Marks & Spencer*	1 Pack/420g	504	120	8.5	17.1	1.7	0.6
Breast, Steaks, Spicy, Marks & Spencer*	1 Serving/100g	135	135	17.7	2.0	6.3	0.9
Fillets, Mini, Marks & Spencer*	1oz/28g	36	130	25.3	5.9	0.6	0.8
Southern Style, Good For You, Asda*	1 Serving/165g	213	129	19.0	5.0	3.7	1.0
CHICKEN - BATTERED,							
Breast, Steaks, Iceland*	1 Breasteak/95g	224	236	15.4	14.2	13.1	0.9
Crispy, Asda*	1 Piece/95g	225	237	14.0	16.0	13.0	0.0
CHICKEN - BREADED,							
Breast, Fillets, Marinated in Lemon & Pepper, Sainsbury's*	1 Fillet/89g	114	128	25.7	2.5	1.6	1.2
Breast, Steaks, Iceland*	1 Breasteak/84g	206	245	18.9	12.9	13.1	1.4
Fillet, Asda*	1 Piece/98g	196	200	21.0	11.0	8.0	0.0
CHICKEN BREADED,							
Fillet, Lemon & Pepper, BGTY, Sainsbury's*	1 Serving/112g	202	180	18.2	18.9	3.5	1.3
Portions, Crunchy, Asda*	1 Piece/92g	199	216	14.0	13.0	12.0	0.0
Steaks, Tesco*	1 Steak/95g	213	224	13.0	16.9	11.6	0.4
CHICKEN BUTTER,							
Sainsbury's*	1 Pack/400g	592	148	12.1	4.4	9.1	1.2
Waitrose*	1 Serving/100g	114	114	13.6	3.2	5.2	1.8

C

INFO/WEIGHT	per Measure KCAL	Nutrition Values per 100g / 100ml				
Measure		KCAL	PROT	CARB	FAT	FIBRE

CHICKEN - CAJUN,

	Measure INFO/WEIGHT	per Measure KCAL	KCAL	PROT	CARB	FAT	FIBRE
& Pasta, Safeway*	1 Pack/455g	501	110	8.6	10.5	3.4	2.1
& Potato Hash, Healthy Eating, Tesco*	1 Pack/450g	428	95	6.6	11.7	2.4	0.9
Asda*	1 Serving/150g	327	218	22.0	7.0	11.0	0.4
Breast, Fillet, Good Choice, Iceland*	1 Fillet/80.3g	106	132	26.1	3.5	1.5	0.0
Breast, Fillets, Marinated, Sainsbury's*	1 Fillet/93g	113	122	24.7	2.6	1.4	0.5
Breast, Pieces, Sainsbury's*	1 Serving/100g	142	142	22.0	6.3	3.2	0.9
Fettuccine, Marks & Spencer*	1 Pack/500g	600	120	8.7	11.4	4.4	0.9
Healthy Eating, Tesco*	1 Pack/365g	412	113	7.9	17.3	1.3	0.7
Somerfield*	1 Pack/149g	282	189	6.2	24.4	7.5	1.1
CHICKEN CALIFORNIAN, Creamy Lime, Wedges, Safeway*	1 Pack/400g	460	115	8.8	9.2	4.5	2.5
CHICKEN CALYPSO, Turmeric Rice, BGTY, Sainsbury's*	1 Pack/450g	495	110	6.7	16.3	2.1	1.0
CHICKEN CARBONARE, SC, Marks & Spencer*	1 Pack/400g	560	140	10.4	9.8	6.9	1.2
CHICKEN CARIBBEAN, With Rice & Peas, BGTY, Sainsbury's*	1 Pack/400g	412	103	7.3	14.8	1.6	1.5

CHICKEN - CHARGRILLED,

	Measure INFO/WEIGHT	per Measure KCAL	KCAL	PROT	CARB	FAT	FIBRE
& Lime & Coriander, Asda*	1 Serving/190g	352	185	24.0	2.0	9.0	1.1
& Vegetable Medley, Healthy Eating, Tesco*	1 Pack/450g	270	60	6.5	5.8	1.2	0.9
Asda*	1 Slice/25g	27	109	23.9	0.5	1.3	0.0
Breast, Cured, Marks & Spencer*	1 Slice/19g	19	100	20.9	0.3	1.7	0.0
Breast, In Mushroom & Madeira Sauce, COU, M&S*	½ Pack/180g	162	90	16.9	1.1	2.0	0.7
Breast, In Mango Ginger Marinade, GFY, Asda*	½ Pack/190g	234	123	17.0	11.0	1.2	0.5
Breast, Lemon & Herb, Bernard Matthews*	1 Serving/100g	154	154	23.7	4.7	4.5	0.0
Breast, Thai Style Marinade, GFY, Asda*	½ Pack/178g	178	100	17.0	1.3	3.0	0.5
Breast, Mushroom & Bacon Smoked Garlic Sauce, M&S*	½ Pack/190g	266	140	14.4	1.9	8.5	0.4
Breasts, Bird's Eye*	1 Piece/93.8g	196	208	22.2	2.5	12.1	0.1
Fillets, Good For You, Asda*	1 Fillet/64g	90	140	30.0	0.4	2.0	1.1
Fillets, Sainsbury's*	1 Serving/119g	214	180	22.1	1.4	9.5	0.7
Fillets, Sliced, Marks & Spencer*	1 Serving/140g	182	130	29.8	0.6	1.0	0.5
Herb & Red Pepper Sauce, COU, Marks & Spencer*	1oz/28g	25	90	15.9	1.2	2.1	0.4
In BBQ Sauce, GFY, Breast, Asda*	1 Serving/166g	214	129	19.0	5.0	3.7	1.0
In Tomato & Basil Sauce, Marks & Spencer*	1 Serving/235g	223	95	12.9	2.1	3.8	1.3
In a Coriander & Lime Marinade, Asda*	½ Pack/163.4g	285	175	23.0	0.5	9.0	0.0
Lemon, COU, Marks & Spencer*	½ Pack/175g	158	90	16.1	5.5	0.6	0.9
Pasta Salsa, Healthy Eating, Tesco*	1 Pack/450g	396	88	7.3	11.7	1.3	1.0
Spicy, Breast, With Rice, Asda*	1 Pack/400g	372	93	6.0	16.0	0.6	1.0
With Caramelised Peppers, Marks & Spencer*	½ Pack/237g	225	95	12.9	2.1	3.8	1.3
With Lime & Coriander Marinade, Asda*	1 Portion/163.4g	285	175	23.0	0.5	9.0	0.0
With Mushrooms & Garlic Dressing, Good For You, Asda*	½ Pack/280g	330	118	20.0	2.9	2.9	0.5
With Olive Oil, Coriander & Lemon, Sainsbury's*	1 Serving/122g	310	254	22.7	2.2	17.1	0.7
With Red Peppers, Spinach, Goats Cheese, COU, M&S*	1 Pack/320g	304	95	18.2	1.3	1.8	0.0
With Tomato, Tesco*	1 Pot/300g	381	127	6.0	14.6	4.9	1.0

CHICKEN - CHARGRILLS,

	Measure INFO/WEIGHT	per Measure KCAL	KCAL	PROT	CARB	FAT	FIBRE
Garlic, Bird's Eye*	1 Piece/76g	169	222	19.2	1.2	15.6	0.0
Original, Birds Eye*	1 Serving/79g	179	227	18.5	1.1	16.5	0.0

CHICKEN CHASSEUR,

	Measure INFO/WEIGHT	per Measure KCAL	KCAL	PROT	CARB	FAT	FIBRE
& Colcannon, Healthy Living, Tesco*	1 Pack/400g	348	87	9.7	6.7	2.4	0.6
BGTY, Sainsbury's*	1 Pack/320g	243	76	6.8	9.5	1.1	1.0
Finest, Tesco*	1 Serving/200g	266	133	12.6	1.6	8.4	0.4

CHICKEN - CHILLI,

	Measure INFO/WEIGHT	per Measure KCAL	KCAL	PROT	CARB	FAT	FIBRE
& Lemongrass, With Egg Noodles, BGTY, Sainsbury's*	1 Pack/450g	500	111	10.0	10.2	3.4	1.2
Chunks, Breast, Safeway*	1 Serving/100g	142	142	22.2	6.3	3.2	0.0
Grande, Stagg*	1oz/28g	27	95	10.0	10.4	0.4	2.0
Sweet, Findus*	1 Pack/350g	420	120	6.0	15.0	3.5	1.5
With Lime, Breast, Simple Solutions, Tesco*	1 Pack/400g	564	141	22.5	0.8	5.3	1.4

	Measure INFO/WEIGHT	per Measure KCAL	Nutrition Values per 100g / 100ml				
			KCAL	PROT	CARB	FAT	FIBRE
CHICKEN - CHINESE,							
Marks & Spencer*	1 Serving/140g	182	130	22.8	8.5	0.3	0.8
Oriental Express*	1 Pack/350g	326	93	5.7	15.9	0.7	2.2
Sliced, Breast, Fillets, Marks & Spencer*	1 Pack/140g	182	130	22.8	8.5	0.3	0.8
Style, & Noodles, Healthy Eating, Tesco*	1 Pack/370g	278	75	6.9	9.4	1.1	0.7
Style, Breast, Fillets, Asda*	1oz/28g	41	148	31.2	1.1	2.1	0.7
Style, GFY, Asda*	1 Serving/200g	220	110	18.0	3.5	2.7	0.5
Style, Mini, Breast, Fillets, Tesco*	½ Pack/100g	121	121	24.9	2.9	1.1	0.2
Style, Mini, Fillets, Marks & Spencer*	1 Pack/190g	228	120	22.0	7.5	0.7	1.2
Wings, Sainsbury's*	1 Wing/33.9g	87	257	24.1	5.0	15.6	0.6
CHICKEN - CIDER,							
COU, Marks & Spencer*	1 Pack/400g	300	75	7.2	6.7	2.3	0.8
With Colcannon, Perfectly Balanced, Waitrose*	1 Pack/401.1g	353	88	6.2	8.9	3.1	1.1
CHICKEN - CORONATION,							
COU, Marks & Spencer*	1oz/28g	34	120	16.3	8.6	2.2	0.7
Marks & Spencer*	1 Serving/200g	420	210	12.6	10.6	13.2	1.3
CHICKEN DRUMSTICKS,							
American Style, Frozen, Sainsbury's*	1 Drumstick/84g	195	232	21.9	7.3	12.8	0.8
BBQ, Asda*	1oz/28g	53	189	25.0	2.0	9.0	0.3
BBQ, Safeway*	1 Serving/48g	84	176	23.8	3.4	7.9	0.0
BBQ, Sainsbury's*	1 Drumstick/100g	195	195	22.4	6.5	8.7	0.1
Chinese Style, Asda*	1oz/28g	52	184	24.2	1.9	8.8	0.6
Chinese, Sainsbury's*	1 Drumstick/100g	171	171	20.9	5.2	7.4	0.8
Extra Crispy, Kentucky Fried Chicken*	1 Drumstick/67g	195	291	22.3	10.4	17.9	1.4
Hot & Spicy, Asda*	1oz/28g	49	176	25.0	1.0	8.0	0.4
Jumbo Size, Marks & Spencer*	1oz/28g	53	190	26.0	0.6	9.5	0.0
Roast, Asda*	1oz/28g	50	180	24.9	1.0	8.5	0.0
Roast, Safeway*	1 Serving/85g	150	176	24.9	0.3	8.3	0.0
Roasted, Tesco*	1 Drumstick/70g	125	179	26.1	0.3	8.1	0.0
Sainsbury's*	1 Drumstick/100g	183	183	25.3	0.1	9.1	0.1
Tesco*	1 Serving/100g	230	230	17.6	0.0	17.7	0.0
With Skin, Asda*	1 Drumstick/125g	231	185	26.0	0.0	9.0	0.0
Without Skin, Tesco*	1 Drumstick/121g	152	126	19.0	0.0	5.5	0.0
CHICKEN - DUNKERS, Domino's Pizza*	1oz/28g	62	220	23.5	1.5	13.3	0.5
CHICKEN ESCALOPE,							
Bernard Matthews*	1 Escalope/143g	390	273	9.5	18.3	18.0	0.0
Marinated in Sun Dried Tomatoes, Olive Oil & Basil, M&S*	1 Portion/145g	232	160	18.9	1.1	8.6	0.4
Breast, Pesto Chargrilled, Marks & Spencer*	1 Serving/100g	135	135	19.6	0.7	6.2	0.6
Breast, Quick Cook, Healthy Living, Tesco*	1 Serving/100g	106	106	23.7	0.0	1.2	0.0
Breast, Tesco*	1 Serving/100g	103	103	23.0	0.6	1.0	0.8
Breast, Smoked Ham, Cheddar Cheese & Mushrooms, M&S*	1 Portion/155g	202	130	19.5	0.5	5.6	0.6
Crispy Crumb, Sainsbury's*	1 Escalope/121g	381	315	15.8	21.0	18.6	1.7
Good For You, Asda*	1 Escalope/128g	330	258	15.0	18.0	14.0	0.4
Tomato & Basil, Safeway*	1 Escalope/150g	242	161	21.2	2.2	7.5	1.2
Topped With Cheese, Ham & Mushrooms, Asda*	½ Pack/149g	259	174	25.0	0.6	8.0	0.0
CHICKEN FILLETS,							
Baked, Breast, Farmfoods*	1 Serving/100g	79	79	17.4	0.2	1.0	0.8
Chilli & Ginger, Marks & Spencer*	1 Serving/120g	156	130	19.5	8.6	2.0	1.7
Coronation, BGTY, Sainsbury's*	1 Fillet/100g	136	136	27.1	2.4	2.6	1.0
Crumbed, Breast, Sainsbury's*	1 Fillet/107g	230	215	16.4	15.6	9.7	1.1
Hickory Barbecue & Chilli, BGTY, Sainsbury's*	1 Fillet/100g	133	133	26.9	3.6	1.2	0.9
Honey & Mustard, Mini, Marks & Spencer*	1 Serving/105g	142	135	24.9	3.9	2.0	1.3
Hot & Spicy, Breast, Sainsbury's*	1 Fillet/108g	211	195	18.5	14.6	7.0	1.2
Hot & Spicy, Iceland*	1 Serving/92g	171	186	18.2	10.9	7.8	0.9

C

CHICKEN FILLETS,	Measure INFO/WEIGHT	per Measure KCAL	KCAL	PROT	CARB	FAT	FIBRE
Lime & Coriander, Mini, Breast, Tesco*	½ Pack/100g	122	122	25.0	2.5	1.3	0.2
Lime & Coriander, Mini, Marks & Spencer*	1 Fillet/42g	44	105	22.4	2.1	1.2	0.3
Mini, Marks & Spencer*	1oz/28g	35	125	26.6	0.0	2.1	0.0
Red Pepper, Mini, BGTY, Sainsbury's*	1 Serving/100g	126	126	26.5	3.7	0.6	0.7
Roast, Boneless, Breast, Sainsbury's*	1 Breast/120g	221	184	25.1	0.2	9.2	0.1
Roast, Breast, Morrisons*	1 Fillet/120g	221	184	25.1	0.2	9.2	0.1
Roast, Sliced, Skinless, Breast, Marks & Spencer*	1 Serving/240g	312	130	29.8	0.6	1.0	0.5
Skinless, Cooked, Breast, Marks & Spencer*	1 Serving/100g	130	130	29.8	0.6	1.0	0.5
Skinless, Cooked, Breast, Waitrose*	1 Breast/85g	201	236	52.4	1.2	3.0	1.2
Sun Dried Tomato & Parmesan, BGTY, Sainsbury's*	½ Pack/100g	138	138	22.1	6.0	2.9	0.5
Sweet Chilli & Lime, Mini, Marks & Spencer*	1 Serving/210g	284	135	24.5	5.6	1.8	1.1
Tandoori, Mini, Eat Smart, Safeway*	1 Serving/50g	65	130	26.2	1.4	2.0	0.5
Tandoori, Mini, Marks & Spencer*	1 Serving/100g	125	125	23.2	3.7	2.1	0.2
Tomato & Basil, Mini, Breast, Tesco*	1 Pack/200g	262	131	25.2	2.1	2.4	0.2
Tomato & Basil, Mini, Marks & Spencer*	1oz/28g	32	115	21.7	2.9	1.8	0.5
With Gravy & Carrot Swede Mash, COU, M&S*	1 Pack/360g	288	80	8.6	7.2	1.6	1.5
With Mushroom Sauce Herby Rice, Marks & Spencer*	1 Pack/380g	475	125	7.7	12.0	5.1	1.3
CHICKEN FINGERS,							
Safeway*	1 Finger/23g	60	259	14.0	20.8	13.1	1.7
Tesco*	1 Serving/75g	181	241	13.4	16.7	13.4	0.6
CHICKEN - FORRESTIERE, GFY, Asda*	1 Pack/442g	402	91	15.0	2.5	2.3	0.3
CHICKEN - FRIED, Spicy, Sainsbury's*	1 Serving/150g	414	276	28.8	2.9	16.6	2.1
CHICKEN - FU YUNG, Chinese Takeaway, Tesco*	1 Pack/350g	315	90	5.6	14.5	1.0	0.8
CHICKEN - GARLIC, Crunchy, Bird's Eye*	1 Piece/99g	259	262	14.4	16.9	15.2	0.9
CHICKEN GOUJONS,							
Asda*	1 Serving/100g	148	148	32.0	0.0	2.2	0.0
Bernard Matthews*	1 Goujon/32g	87	271	13.8	16.8	16.5	0.0
Breast, Fresh, Asda*	1oz/28g	30	106	24.0	0.0	1.1	0.0
Caesar, Marks & Spencer*	½ Pack/128g	250	195	18.6	9.2	9.2	2.0
Cracked Black Pepper, American, Asda*	1 Serving/150g	333	222	16.0	8.0	14.0	2.5
Garlic & Herb, Breaded, American, Asda*	½ Pack/150g	377	251	17.0	12.0	15.0	2.1
Hot & Spicy, Sainsbury's*	½ Pack/125g	253	202	20.0	13.1	7.7	1.2
Sainsbury's*	1 Goujon/25g	69	276	12.9	14.7	18.9	1.2
Southern Fried, Somerfield*	1 Goujon/21g	55	261	18.6	11.2	15.8	1.0
CHICKEN - GRIDDLERS, BBQ, Mini, Bird's Eye*	½ Pack/50g	109	217	15.8	6.7	14.1	0.2
CHICKEN - HAWAIIAN, With Rice, Bird's Eye*	1 Pack/350g	406	116	5.5	20.2	1.5	0.6
CHICKEN - HERB, Steam Cuisine, Marks & Spencer*	1 Pack/400g	280	70	8.2	6.0	1.6	0.9
CHICKEN - HONEY,							
& Mustard, BGTY, Sainsbury's*	1 Pack/451g	528	117	8.6	15.5	2.3	0.6
& Mustard, Bird's Eye*	1 Piece/87g	185	213	18.2	3.0	14.2	0.0
& Mustard, Good For You, Asda*	1 Pack/402g	478	119	7.0	17.0	2.5	0.1
& Mustard, Shapers, Boots*	1 Pack/241g	304	126	7.0	19.0	2.4	1.7
Cantonese, Sesame, Sainsbury's*	1/3 Pack/135g	116	86	9.8	5.5	2.7	0.8
CHICKEN - HONEY ROAST,							
Asda*	1 Slice/25g	30	118	24.0	1.1	1.9	0.1
Thin Sliced, Asda*	1 Slice/13g	15	116	19.1	3.2	3.0	0.1
CHICKEN IN,							
Asparagus Sauce & New Potatoes, Sainsbury's*	1 Pack/495g	545	110	7.4	9.5	4.7	0.9
BBQ Sauce, GFY, Asda*	1 Pack/380g	414	109	13.0	13.0	0.5	1.3
BBQ Sauce, Weight Watchers*	1 Pack/339g	332	98	5.8	10.8	3.5	0.9
Barbecue Sauce, COU, Marks & Spencer*	1 Pack/352g	370	105	8.6	13.8	1.6	1.2
Barbeque Sauce, Healthy Eating, Tesco*	1 Breast/170g	177	104	18.3	4.5	1.4	0.9
Basil & Chilli Sauce Jasmine Rice, BGTY, Sainsbury's*	1 Pack/400g	404	101	6.3	15.6	1.5	0.4

CHICKEN IN,

	Measure INFO/WEIGHT	per Measure KCAL	KCAL	PROT	CARB	FAT	FIBRE
Black Bean & Rice, Healthy Eating, Tesco*	1 Pack/450g	387	86	7.4	12.4	0.7	1.6
Black Bean Sauce & Rice, Morrisons*	1 Pack/400g	408	102	3.9	16.4	2.3	1.2
Black Bean Sauce With Egg Fried Rice, Somerfield*	1 Pack/340g	384	113	7.0	13.0	4.0	0.0
Black Bean Sauce With Noodles, Pro Cuisine*	1 Pack/600g	366	61	5.6	8.5	0.6	0.0
Black Bean Sauce With Rice, Asda*	1 Pack/400g	500	125	7.0	20.0	1.9	0.6
Black Bean Sauce With Rice, BGTY, Sainsbury's*	1 Pack/450g	446	99	6.4	16.6	0.8	0.6
Black Bean Sauce With Rice, Iceland*	1 Pack/400g	388	97	5.1	15.8	1.5	0.8
Black Bean Sauce, BGTY, Sainsbury's*	1 Can/400g	308	77	9.3	7.9	0.9	0.7
Black Bean Sauce, Budgens*	1 Pack/350g	333	95	9.9	4.9	4.0	0.9
Black Bean Sauce, Chinese Takeaway, Iceland*	1 Pack/400g	348	87	9.3	5.3	3.2	0.7
Black Bean Sauce, Marks & Spencer*	1 Pack/350g	298	85	8.7	8.0	2.0	1.1
Black Bean Sauce, Safeway*	1 Pack/350g	284	81	9.4	7.9	1.3	1.0
Black Bean Sauce, Somerfield*	½ Pack/175g	133	76	10.7	6.1	1.0	1.9
Black Bean Sauce, Tesco*	1 Pack/450g	387	86	7.4	12.4	0.7	1.6
Black Bean Sauce, Waitrose*	1 Pack/300g	243	81	10.9	6.6	1.2	0.8
Broccoli & Mushroom With Rice, Healthy Eating, Tesco*	1 Pack/400g	440	110	7.5	17.1	1.2	0.7
Broccoli & Mushroom, Good Choice, Iceland*	1 Pack/400g	436	109	7.5	17.1	1.2	0.7
Chilli & Lemon Grass With Rice, Sainsbury's*	1 Pack/450g	527	117	6.2	17.4	2.5	0.7
Creamy Mushroom Sauce, Weight Watchers*	1 Pack/330g	264	80	6.8	7.5	2.5	0.5
Creamy Mustard Sauce, GFY, Asda*	1 Pack/400g	468	117	6.0	18.0	2.3	0.4
Creamy Thai Sauce, Somerfield*	1 Pack/440g	748	170	22.0	2.0	8.0	0.0
Creamy Tikka Style Sauce, Tesco*	1 Breast/190g	215	113	15.1	0.7	5.5	0.8
Creamy White Wine Sauce, Sainsbury's*	1 Pack/324g	285	88	8.9	4.7	3.7	1.0
Garlic & Herbs, Breast, Sainsbury's*	1 Serving/200g	316	158	28.3	5.4	2.6	0.1
Ginger & Chilli With Veg Noodles, COU, Marks & Spencer*	1 Pack/400g	300	75	6.4	10.7	0.6	1.1
Gravy, Chunky, Marks & Spencer*	1 Can/489g	465	95	13.6	1.4	3.9	0.8
Honey & Mustard Sauce With Wild Rice, HL, Tesco*	1 Pack/400g	508	127	7.2	20.3	1.9	1.0
Hot Ginger Sauce With Jasmine Rice, BGTY, Sainsbury's*	1 Pack/400g	400	100	6.6	15.4	1.4	0.5
Hot Ginger Sauce With Thai Sticky Rice, Sainsbury's*	1 Pack/450g	603	134	6.8	16.3	4.6	0.5
Italian Style Tomato & Herb Sauce, Tesco*	1 Serving/180g	144	80	15.8	1.6	1.2	0.6
Leek & Bacon Sauce, Chilled, Co-Op*	1 Pack/400g	460	115	15.0	2.0	5.0	0.2
Lemon Flavour Sauce, Breast Fillets, Safeway*	1 Fillet/92g	200	217	17.0	16.0	9.4	1.4
Lemon Sauce With Rice, Sainsbury's*	1 Pack/450g	513	114	8.1	17.0	1.5	0.7
Lemon Sauce, Breast, Healthy Eating, Tesco*	1 Pack/385g	385	100	15.9	4.7	1.9	0.5
Mediterranean Sauce, Iceland*	1 Pack/500g	640	128	7.4	21.8	1.2	0.5
Mexican Salsa, Tesco*	1 Pack/320g	368	115	19.5	3.1	2.7	0.6
Mild & Fruity Curry, Breasts, Healthy Eating, Tesco*	2 Breasts/345g	321	93	15.8	4.1	1.5	0.5
Mushroom & Ham Sauce With Rice, BGTY, Sainsbury's*	1 Pack/450g	581	129	9.7	18.9	1.6	0.3
Mushroom & Wine Sauce, Roast Potatoes, ES, Safeway*	1 Pack/400g	380	95	7.7	12.1	1.4	1.5
Mushroom Sauce With Mash, Healthy Living, Tesco*	1 Pack/400g	384	96	9.9	8.0	2.7	0.6
Pesto Style Dressing, Asda*	1 Serving/150g	210	140	18.7	1.3	6.7	0.0
Pesto Style Dressing, Simple Solutions, Tesco*	1 Serving/142g	268	189	20.1	2.5	11.0	1.6
Red Pepper Sauce, Eat Smart, Safeway*	1 Serving/175g	166	95	18.4	2.3	1.3	1.4
Red Pepper Sauce, Tesco*	1 Serving/140g	228	163	19.2	0.1	9.5	0.5
Red Wine & Bacon Sauce, Breast, Somerfield*	1 Breast/150g	131	87	14.0	3.0	2.0	0.0
Red Wine & Mushrooms, Asda*	½ Pack/190g	174	92	17.0	1.8	1.9	0.5
Red Wine & Potato Grattin, Healthy Eating, Tesco*	1 Pack/450g	410	91	7.7	8.9	2.7	2.2
Red Wine With Cabbage & Spring Onion Mash, M&S*	1 Pack/440g	265	60	10.1	2.4	1.4	3.6
Red Wine With Mash, Eat Smart, Safeway*	1 Pack/400g	300	75	9.1	6.1	1.3	1.4
Red Wine, Mushrooms, Bacon & Onions, M&S*	½ Pack/215g	247	115	15.7	2.4	4.6	0.4
Satay Sauce, Safeway*	1 Serving/250g	363	145	10.5	7.1	8.0	1.4
Shiraz Wine Sauce, Finest, Tesco*	1 Pack/600g	420	70	10.9	2.9	1.6	1.3
Spicy Tomato Sauce & Basil Mash, PB, Waitrose*	1 Pack/400g	376	94	6.3	10.0	3.2	0.8

	Measure	per Measure	Nutrition Values per 100g / 100ml				
	INFO/WEIGHT	KCAL	KCAL	PROT	CARB	FAT	FIBRE
CHICKEN IN,							
Sweet & Sour Sauce, GFY, Asda*	1 Pack/400g	424	106	6.0	19.0	0.7	1.2
Sweet & Sour With Noodles, Feeling Great, Findus*	1 Pack/350g	385	110	5.0	17.0	2.5	1.5
Tomato & Basil Sauce With Rice, Eat Smart, Safeway*	1 Pack/400g	360	90	8.9	10.2	1.1	1.0
Tomato & Basil Sauce, Breast Fillets, HC, Asda*	1 Pack/400g	484	121	22.0	1.2	3.2	2.0
Tomato & Basil Sauce, Breast, Good For You, Asda*	1 Pack/392g	447	114	12.0	9.0	3.4	1.5
Tomato & Basil Sauce, Good Choice, Iceland*	½ Pack/170g	153	90	13.3	3.3	2.6	0.6
White Sauce, BGTY, Sainsbury's*	1 Can/200g	250	125	14.5	2.5	6.3	1.0
White Sauce, Healthy Eating, Tesco*	1 Serving/100g	94	94	12.0	4.8	3.0	0.0
White Wine & Asparagus Panzerotti, Asda*	½ Pack/150g	239	159	8.0	28.0	1.7	0.0
White Wine & Mushroom Sauce, Marks & Spencer*	1 Serving/200g	260	130	15.6	1.6	6.8	1.0
White Wine Sauce, Simple Solutions, Tesco*	½ Pack/200g	198	99	19.3	0.9	2.0	0.5
Zesty Orange Sauce, Asda*	1 Serving/200g	340	170	16.0	13.0	6.0	0.4
CHICKEN - INDIAN, Style, Fillets, Sainsbury's*	1 Pack/200g	233	112	13.7	4.4	4.4	1.2
CHICKEN - ITALIAN,							
Good Choice, Iceland*	1 Pack/400g	400	100	5.0	19.0	0.4	0.5
Iceland*	1 Pack/250g	208	83	13.6	4.8	1.0	0.5
Style, BGTY, Sainsbury's*	1 Pack/400g	364	91	6.0	14.5	1.1	0.9
Style, Dinner, Asda*	1 Pack/400g	244	61	6.0	7.0	1.0	1.1
Style, Meal, Asda*	1 Pack/408g	241	59	6.0	7.0	0.8	0.8
Style, Sainsbury's*	½ Pack/190g	222	117	16.3	3.9	4.0	0.1
CHICKEN - KUNG PO,							
Sainsbury's*	½ Pack/175g	131	75	9.2	4.0	2.5	1.0
Waitrose*	1 Pack/350g	319	91	8.2	12.1	1.1	1.2
With Egg Fried Rice, Asda*	1 Pack/450g	689	153	6.0	21.0	5.0	1.0
CHICKEN - LAKSA, COU, Marks & Spencer*	1 Pack/450g	360	80	7.5	7.0	2.2	1.1
CHICKEN - LEMON,							
& Ginger With Apricot Rice, COU, Marks & Spencer*	1 Pack/400g	320	80	7.9	9.7	0.9	2.0
& Pepper, Marks & Spencer*	1 Serving/100g	125	125	24.1	5.2	0.7	0.0
Battered, Sainsbury's*	1 Pack/350g	462	132	8.9	16.0	3.6	0.5
Breast, Fillets, BGTY, Sainsbury's*	1 Fillet/112.5g	195	173	18.4	19.9	2.1	1.9
COU, Marks & Spencer*	1 Pack/150g	150	100	17.9	5.6	0.9	0.8
Cantonese Style, With Egg Fried Rice, Farmfoods*	1 Pack/324g	486	150	4.9	21.8	4.8	0.1
Cantonese, Sainsbury's*	½ Pack/140g	217	156	11.0	13.9	6.3	0.6
Cream, With Rice, Perfectly Balanced, Waitrose*	1 Pack/400g	592	148	7.6	21.7	3.4	0.3
Crispy, Take It Away, Marks & Spencer*	1 Carton/227g	329	145	9.4	19.2	3.4	0.7
Pepper, Bird's Eye*	1 Piece/113g	273	242	15.4	17.5	12.3	0.6
Steam Cuisine, COU, Marks & Spencer*	1 Pack/400g	420	105	9.8	11.8	2.2	2.0
Tesco*	½ Pack/175g	214	122	11.0	10.1	4.2	0.6
With Rice, Healthy Living, Tesco*	1 Pack/450g	477	106	5.9	14.4	2.7	0.9
With Vegetable Rice, BGTY, Sainsbury's*	1 Pack/400g	428	107	6.5	16.8	1.6	0.8
CHICKEN MCNUGGETS, McDonald's*	6 Pieces/109g	254	233	17.1	10.6	13.6	1.9
CHICKEN - MEXICAN,							
Spicy, Bird's Eye*	1 Piece/103g	254	247	14.6	16.5	13.6	0.6
Style With Rice, Better For You, Morrisons*	1 Pack/400g	360	90	5.1	14.1	1.3	0.8
Style, BGTY, Sainsbury's*	1 Serving/260g	255	98	6.9	12.1	2.5	2.2
Style, Good For You, Asda*	½ Pack/200g	256	128	17.0	3.7	5.0	0.3
CHICKEN - MUSTARD,							
New Potatoes, Leeks, Spinach & Leaves, SC, M&S*	1 Pack/400g	400	100	10.2	8.2	3.4	1.3
With Gratin Potatoes, Healthy Living, Tesco*	1 Pack/450g	464	103	9.0	10.7	2.7	2.5
CHICKEN NUGGETS,							
Battered, Somerfield*	1oz/28g	69	248	14.0	16.0	14.0	0.0
Breaded, Crunchy, Asda*	1 Nugget/14g	35	253	16.0	18.0	13.0	1.9
Breaded, Iceland*	1 Nugget/13g	35	270	19.4	15.8	14.3	1.1

	Measure INFO/WEIGHT	per Measure KCAL	Nutrition Values per 100g / 100ml				
			KCAL	PROT	CARB	FAT	FIBRE
CHICKEN NUGGETS,							
Breaded, SmartPrice, Asda*	1 Nugget/16g	51	320	15.0	29.0	16.0	1.2
Breaded, Waitrose*	1 Nugget/14.2g	31	219	12.2	17.0	11.4	3.4
Breast, Maitre Choice, Lidl*	1 Serving/100g	184	184	16.4	12.9	7.4	0.0
Crispy, Premium, Sun Valley*	5 Nuggets/108g	295	273	13.0	17.0	17.0	0.0
Crunchy Crumb, Tesco*	1 Serving/100g	257	257	13.1	18.6	14.5	0.7
Iceland*	1 Nugget/15g	44	290	14.5	18.9	17.4	2.3
In Crispy Breadcrumbs, Sainsbury's*	4 Nuggets/54g	137	253	12.9	18.1	14.3	1.2
Organic, Tesco*	1 Nugget/20g	52	258	13.5	22.3	12.7	1.1
Southern Fried, Bird's Eye*	1 Nugget/17g	42	248	12.9	17.8	14.0	1.2
Tesco*	1oz/28g	68	243	13.3	16.2	13.9	0.7
CHICKEN - PAPRIKA,							
& Savoury Rice, BGTY, Sainsbury's*	1 Pack/401g	441	110	6.8	19.2	0.7	0.4
COU, Marks & Spencer*	1 Pack/400g	380	95	9.0	11.7	1.6	2.0
With Savoury Vegetables & Rice, BGTY, Sainsbury's*	1 Pack/451g	555	123	7.2	17.8	2.6	0.8
CHICKEN - PEPPER, Fry, Sainsburys*	1 Pack/400g	508	127	15.0	2.9	6.2	1.6
CHICKEN PICCATA, Healthy Eating, Tesco*	1 Pack/405g	518	128	15.7	7.7	3.8	0.5
CHICKEN PIRI PIRI,							
Marks & Spencer*	1 Pack/300g	420	140	10.0	7.3	7.7	1.3
Safeway*	1 Pack/350g	508	145	11.2	9.4	6.6	1.1
Sainsbury's*	½ Pack/200g	248	124	14.0	4.8	5.4	0.5
Tesco*	1 Serving/290g	307	106	15.8	1.4	4.1	0.5
CHICKEN - POLENTA Paupiettes, PB, Waitrose*	½ Pack/225g	254	113	19.1	5.0	1.8	0.8
CHICKEN - RENDANG, Sainsbury's*	1 Pack/350g	690	197	9.6	5.1	15.3	1.7
CHICKEN - ROAST,							
Dinner, Bird's Eye*	1 Pack/368g	364	99	8.9	8.9	3.1	1.3
Drumsticks, With Brown Sugar, Sainsbury's*	1 Drumstick/78g	144	185	22.9	2.0	9.5	1.1
Healthy Living, Tesco*	1 Slice/25g	30	118	23.0	2.2	1.9	0.2
In Sugar Marinade, Marks & Spencer*	1 Portion/200g	370	185	26.4	0.4	8.6	0.1
In a Pot, Sainsbury's*	1 Pack/450g	477	106	9.6	10.3	2.9	0.7
Leg Quarter, Waitrose*	1 Quarter/120g	230	192	20.3	0.7	12.1	0.5
Meal, Marks & Spencer*	1 Pack/250g	375	150	14.6	5.3	7.7	0.1
Tesco*	1 Slice/20g	27	133	24.0	2.8	2.8	0.3
CHICKEN ROLL,							
Asda*	1 Slice/10g	17	174	15.0	3.8	11.0	0.0
Breast, Sainsbury's	1 Slice/10g	15	153	18.4	1.9	8.0	0.7
Broccoli & Mushroom, Sainsbury's*	½ Roll/175g	441	252	8.7	24.3	13.3	1.0
SmartPrice, Asda*	1 Slice/14g	24	174	15.0	3.8	11.0	0.0
With Pork, Sage & Onion Stuffing, Value, Tesco*	1 Roll/125g	166	133	9.4	7.8	7.1	0.5
CHICKEN - SALSA,							
Mango, Breast, Sainsbury's*	1 Breast/178g	271	152	26.2	6.4	2.4	0.1
Roast, Chunks, Breast, Waitrose*	1oz/28g	36	127	25.9	3.6	1.0	1.1
CHICKEN SELECT, McDonald's*	2 Selects/82.1g	184	224	13.7	14.8	11.7	1.3
CHICKEN SLICES,							
Breast, Bernard Matthews*	1 Slice/20g	24	122	19.3	3.0	3.6	0.0
Cooked, Sainsbury's*	1 Slice/19g	20	106	21.4	2.1	1.3	0.3
Roast, Mattessons*	1 Slice/25g	33	131	24.8	2.2	3.4	0.5
Roast, Premium, Somerfield*	1 Slice/20g	23	114	25.0	1.0	1.0	0.0
CHICKEN - SOUTHERN FRIED,							
Bird's Eye*	1 Steak/98g	272	278	14.6	13.4	18.4	0.9
Drumsticks, Tesco*	1oz/28g	57	202	17.6	8.8	10.7	0.5
Fillets, Asda*	1 Fillet/86g	175	203	21.0	14.0	7.0	0.5
Fillets, Fresh, Sainsbury's*	1 Fillet/104g	220	212	18.2	12.4	9.9	1.0
Fillets, Frozen, Morrisons*	1 Piece/100g	181	181	15.1	9.7	9.1	2.3

	Measure INFO/WEIGHT	per Measure KCAL	Nutrition Values per 100g / 100ml				
			KCAL	PROT	CARB	FAT	FIBRE
CHICKEN - SOUTHERN FRIED,							
Fillets, Mini, Breast, Tesco*	1 Piece/43.7g	87	199	16.5	13.0	9.0	2.3
Portions, Asda*	1 Portion/95g	210	221	14.0	12.0	13.0	0.0
Steaks, Tesco*	1 Steak/137g	293	214	15.4	11.1	12.0	0.9
Strips, Tesco*	1 Pack/300g	699	233	18.7	18.3	9.4	1.4
Thigh, Tesco*	1oz/28g	68	242	14.7	10.1	15.9	0.5
Wing, Tesco*	1 Serving/100g	238	238	15.0	11.7	14.6	0.5
CHICKEN - SPANISH, Style, Asda*	½ Pack/275.2g	322	117	14.0	4.1	4.9	0.7
CHICKEN - STEAKS, Hot & Spicy, Tesco*	1 Steak/95g	200	211	13.5	11.4	12.4	0.8
CHICKEN - STRIPPERS, Domino's Pizza*	1oz/28g	61	219	23.3	13.4	8.0	1.0
CHICKEN - STRIPS, Crispy, Kentucky Fried Chicken*	1 Strip/50g	134	268	18.6	14.5	15.1	1.5
CHICKEN - STUFFED, Breast, With Mushrooms, HE, Tesco*	1 Serving/175g	152	87	16.3	1.5	1.8	0.2
CHICKEN - SUPREME,							
BGTY, Sainsbury's*	1 Pack/350g	417	119	9.4	17.2	1.4	0.5
With Rice, Asda*	1 Pack/450g	549	122	6.0	18.0	2.9	0.5
With Rice, Bird's Eye*	1 Pack/375g	499	133	6.7	19.1	3.3	0.5
With Rice, Healthy Eating, Tesco*	1 Pack/400g	384	96	4.9	15.6	1.6	1.5
With Rice, Weight Watchers*	1 Pack/300g	255	85	5.6	11.9	1.6	0.5
CHICKEN - SZECHUAN,							
Chilli & Peppercorn, Sainsbury's*	1 Pack/400g	352	88	9.9	3.2	4.0	0.5
With Noodles, Sainsbury's*	1 Pack/450g	423	94	6.0	10.4	3.1	0.9
CHICKEN - THAI,							
Bird's Eye*	1 Portion/86g	189	220	18.1	3.1	15.0	0.1
Chiang Mai, & Noodles, BGTY, Sainsbury's*	1 Pack/448g	484	108	6.9	11.0	4.0	1.7
Coconut, & Noodles, Marks & Spencer*	1 Pack/400g	320	80	7.2	8.1	1.8	0.7
Green, Fillets, Mini, Sainsbury's*	½ Pack/100g	130	130	27.9	0.9	1.6	0.8
Red, Fillets, Mini, BGTY, Sainsbury's*,	1 Serving/100g	125	125	20.9	6.8	1.6	0.8
Red, Fillets, Mini, Marks & Spencer*	1 Serving/210g	273	130	22.5	4.1	2.5	0.4
Style, Red, Fillets, Mini, Breast, Tesco*	½ Pack/100g	135	135	26.8	2.8	1.8	0.5
Style, Steam Cuisine, Marks & Spencer*	1 Pack/400g	440	110	8.8	10.4	3.8	1.7
Style, With Noodles, Tesco*	1 Pack/400g	332	83	7.5	9.5	1.7	1.0
CHICKEN TIKKA,							
& Cous Cous, Boots*	1 Pack/160g	307	192	6.2	17.0	11.0	1.3
& Lemon Rice, Deli Meal, Marks & Spencer*	1 Pack/360g	342	95	9.8	10.2	2.0	0.7
& Rice Salad, COU, Marks & Spencer*	1 Pack/390g	351	90	5.9	14.6	0.7	0.6
& Salad Pitta Pocket, Rainbow Service Station*	1 Serving/110g	248	225	1.0	1.9	23.8	0.0
BGTY, Sainsbury's	1 Serving/188g	265	141	10.5	21.2	1.6	0.0
Bird's Eye*	1 Serving/98g	195	199	22.1	3.5	10.7	0.1
Breast Chunks, Safeway*	1 Pack/200g	356	178	32.2	4.1	3.7	0.0
Breast Fillets, Mini, Asda*	1oz/28g	34	123	26.0	1.5	1.7	1.0
Breast Fillets, Sliced, Marks & Spencer*	1 Pack/140g	154	110	21.9	3.2	1.7	0.8
Breast Pieces, Sainsbury's*	1 Serving/150g	233	155	26.1	3.2	4.1	0.5
Breast, Ready Cooked, Frozen, Fullers Foods, Aldi*	1 Serving/100g	127	127	24.0	2.4	2.4	2.0
Chunky, Tesco*	1 Pack/170g	221	130	27.4	0.5	2.1	0.3
Fillets, Mini, Eat Smart, Safeway*	1 Serving/100g	120	120	27.9	1.2	0.3	0.8
Fillets, Mini, Marks & Spencer*	1 Serving/100g	125	125	24.2	1.1	2.6	1.3
Fillets, Roast, Asda*	1oz/28g	36	127	26.0	2.3	1.5	0.3
Pieces, Ready Cooked, Iceland*	1 Serving/100g	135	135	26.8	1.6	2.5	0.0
Portions, Asda*	1oz/28g	47	169	17.2	0.5	11.0	1.0
Sliced, Asda*	1 Serving/140g	274	196	40.0	2.3	3.0	0.0
With Basmati Rice, GFY, Asda*	1 Pack/400g	592	148	9.0	24.0	1.8	1.6
CHICKEN VINDALOO,							
Asda*	1 Pack/411g	649	158	7.0	19.0	6.0	0.0
Sainsbury's*	1 Pack/400g	460	115	14.6	4.8	4.2	0.6

	Measure	per Measure	Nutrition Values per 100g / 100ml				
	INFO/WEIGHT	KCAL	KCAL	PROT	CARB	FAT	FIBRE
CHICKEN VINDALOO,							
Waitrose*	1 Pack/340g	398	117	10.6	6.4	5.4	1.6
CHICKEN - WAFER THIN,							
American Fried, Bernard Matthews*	1oz/28g	31	111	18.0	3.1	3.0	0.0
Marks & Spencer*	1oz/28g	28	100	18.8	1.5	2.1	0.0
Roast, Asda*	1oz/28g	31	110	21.0	3.6	1.3	0.0
Roast, Safeway*	1 Serving/25g	28	112	20.6	2.4	2.2	0.0
Roast, Sainsbury's*	1oz/28g	34	121	18.3	3.7	3.6	1.6
Roast, Tesco*	1oz/28g	36	129	19.3	3.6	4.1	0.0
Sage & Onion, Breast, Bernard Matthews*	1 Serving/25g	30	120	19.8	3.5	3.0	0.0
Sainsbury's*	1 Pack/100g	114	114	20.4	1.9	2.7	0.1
CHICKEN - WINGS,							
Chinese Style, Asda*	1oz/28g	70	250	28.0	3.0	14.0	0.5
Chinese Style, Marks & Spencer*	1 Serving/100g	260	260	20.5	7.3	17.0	0.6
Hot & Spicy, Asda*	1 Pack/450g	1076	239	21.0	4.9	15.0	1.3
Hot & Spicy, Tesco*	½ Pack/325g	725	223	22.7	5.4	12.3	0.4
Microwave, Tesco*	1oz/28g	72	256	22.7	7.8	14.9	0.4
Take Away, Pizza Hut*	1 Pack/178g	466	262	22.5	1.7	18.4	1.3
With Sour Cream & Chive Dip, Pizza Hut*	1 Pack/178g	680	382	22.8	1.9	31.5	1.3
CHICKEN WITH,							
Apricots & Almonds, Healthy Eating, Tesco*	1 Pack/500g	465	93	11.8	7.3	1.9	0.5
Broccoli & Pesto Pasta, BGTY, Sainsbury's*	1 Pack/299g	296	99	10.3	12.3	0.9	2.5
Cheese & Bacon, Tesco*	1 Pack/475g	546	115	8.1	9.6	4.9	0.4
Chunky Tomato Sauce, COU, Marks & Spencer*	1 Pack/400g	360	90	7.9	9.3	2.3	0.9
Citrus Ginger, Pepper, Apricot & Coconut Rice, Sainsbury's*	1 Pack/450g	846	188	10.6	18.8	7.8	0.4
Coriander & Lime, Asda*	1 Serving/105g	122	116	24.0	2.9	0.9	0.2
Cranberry & Orange Stuffing, Sainsbury's*	1 Serving/100g	201	201	23.0	4.1	10.3	0.8
Cranberry Stuffing, Breast, Finest, Tesco*	½ Pack/200g	252	126	16.2	9.9	2.4	0.9
Creamy Mushroom Sauce & Mash, Healthy Living Tesco*	1 Pack/400g	384	96	10.0	8.0	2.7	0.6
Garlic & Herbs, Asda*	1 Slice/25g	29	114	23.9	1.1	1.5	0.0
Garlic & Mushrooms, Somerfield*	½ Pack/190g	287	151	17.3	0.9	8.7	0.8
Grapes & Asparagus, Sainsbury's*	½ Pack/200g	240	120	13.3	1.8	6.6	1.0
Green Peppers, Black Bean Sauce & Rice, Farmfoods*	1 Meal/324g	408	126	5.5	17.1	3.9	0.4
Hoi Sin Sauce, Ooodles Of Noodles, Oriental Express*	1 Pack/425g	400	94	5.3	13.2	2.2	1.7
Leek & Bacon Sauce, Good Intentions, Somerfield*	1 Pack/400g	284	71	5.4	7.2	2.3	2.9
Leek, Cheese & Smoked Bacon, Breast, M&S*	1 Breast/200g	290	145	18.4	0.6	7.8	0.3
Mango Salsa & Potato Wedges, BGTY, Sainsbury's*	1 Pack/400g	336	84	7.0	10.4	1.6	1.5
Mushroom & Madeira Ragout, TTD, Sainsbury's*	½ Pack/225g	218	97	13.6	3.7	3.1	0.1
Mushroom In Madeira Sauce, Healthy Eating, Tesco*	½ Pack/200g	182	91	15.0	5.4	1.0	0.4
Mushrooms in Oyster Sauce, Tesco*	1 Pack/350g	189	54	8.0	3.5	0.9	0.8
Pancakes & Plum Sauce, COU Marks & Spencer*	1 Pack/245g	257	105	7.9	12.7	2.3	0.3
Pancetta & Mozzarella, Finest, Tesco*	1 Serving/150g	297	198	11.6	11.5	11.8	0.9
Pasta & Spicy Arrabbiata Sauce, COU, Marks & Spencer*	1 Pack/360g	252	70	5.2	8.7	1.4	1.3
Pork, Parsnip Herb Stuffing, Sainsbury's*	1 Serving/100g	181	181	22.9	2.1	9.0	0.7
Potato Wedges, BBQ, Eat Smart, Safeway*	1 Pack/350g	368	105	9.6	14.0	0.9	1.8
Prosciutio, Dolcelatte & 3 Cheese Sauce, Asda*	½ Pack/195g	355	182	30.0	1.9	6.0	1.2
Rice 'n' Peas, Sainsbury's*	1 Pack/300g	489	163	12.5	14.4	6.1	2.1
Rice, Fiesta, Weight Watchers*	1 Pack/330g	307	93	6.1	12.8	2.0	0.4
Spicy Vegetable Rice, Tandoori, Safeway*	1 Pack/345g	345	100	9.7	11.1	1.7	2.0
Spinach & Pasta, Marks & Spencer*	1oz/28g	64	228	9.4	14.0	15.0	1.3
Spinach, Honey Mustard, American Style, Asda*	1 Serving/240g	394	164	14.0	4.4	10.0	0.3
Stuffing & Roast Potatoes, Tesco*	1 Pack/440g	480	109	10.1	11.5	2.5	1.0
Stuffing, Breast, TTD, Sainsbury's*	1oz/28g	50	180	21.5	5.2	8.1	0.9
Sun Dried Tomato & Basil Butter, Sainsbury's*	1 Breast/185g	363	196	25.0	2.5	9.5	0.2

C

	Measure INFO/WEIGHT	per Measure KCAL	Nutrition Values per 100g / 100ml				
			KCAL	PROT	CARB	FAT	FIBRE
CHICKEN WITH,							
Sun Dried Tomato & Basil Sauce, Bistro, Waitrose*	½ Pack/175g	254	145	14.2	3.7	8.1	0.3
Tagine, Cous Cous, BGTY, Sainsbury's*	1 Pack/450g	626	139	10.1	15.9	3.9	1.5
Tagine, Cous Cous, Perfectly Balanced, Waitrose*	1 Pack/400g	516	129	8.2	16.2	3.5	1.0
Tomato & Basil & Roasted Potatoes, BGTY, Sainsbury's*	1 Pack/450g	369	82	9.0	7.9	1.6	1.2
Tomato & Basil, Healthy Eating, Tesco*	1 Serving/225g	189	84	11.2	6.1	1.7	1.2
Tomato & White Wine Sauce, Bird's Eye*	1 Pack/382.4g	325	85	9.4	9.7	0.9	0.8
CHILLI,							
& Lemongrass Prawns With Noodles, BGTY, Sainsbury's*	1 Pack/400g	328	82	5.0	13.8	0.7	1.3
& Potato Wedges, Good Choice, Iceland*	1 Pack/400g	368	92	5.5	9.8	3.4	1.2
& Potato Wedges, Sainsbury's*	1 Pack/370g	393	106	7.2	10.1	4.1	2.2
& Rice, Frozen, Sainsbury's*	1 Pack/400g	436	109	4.8	18.4	1.9	0.6
& Rice, Good for You, Asda*	1 Pack/400g	352	88	5.0	16.0	0.4	1.8
Beef & Chilli Sauce, Chinese Takeaway, Farmfoods*	1oz/28g	66	234	6.7	20.0	13.0	0.3
Beef & Potato Wedge Superbowl, Good for you, Asda*	1 Pack/450g	477	106	6.0	14.0	2.9	1.5
Beef Jacket, Marks & Spencer*	1 Pack/360g	288	80	5.9	9.6	2.0	0.9
Beef, Asda*	½ Pack/200g	190	95	7.0	8.0	3.9	1.2
Beef, Crispy, Sainsbury's*	1 Pack/400g	628	157	12.8	4.9	9.6	1.2
Beef, With Rice, Sainsbury's*	1 Serving/300g	360	120	5.6	20.6	1.7	1.1
Bowl, American Style, Sainsbury's*	½ Pack/300g	255	85	8.8	4.6	3.5	2.0
Bowl, Safeway*	1 Pack/300g	327	109	8.8	8.3	4.5	2.7
Chicken With Fettucine, Marks & Spencer*	1 Pack/350g	368	105	7.9	13.9	2.1	1.1
Con Carne & Rice, Co-Op*	1 Pack/300g	195	65	4.0	8.0	2.0	1.0
Con Carne & Rice, Healthy Eating, Tesco*	1 Pack/450g	446	99	9.1	10.9	2.1	1.6
Con Carne & Rice, Healthy Living, Tesco*	1 Pack/450.5g	473	105	5.5	14.8	2.6	1.2
Con Carne & Rice, Somerfield*	1 Pack/500g	490	98	5.0	18.0	1.0	0.0
Con Carne With Rice, BGTY, Sainsbury's*	1 Pack/400g	432	108	6.2	16.9	1.7	1.0
Con Carne With Rice, COU, Marks & Spencer*	1oz/28g	25	90	6.3	14.0	1.1	1.4
Con Carne With Rice, Eat Smart, Safeway*	1 Pack/400g	340	85	5.3	12.2	1.3	1.4
Con Carne With Rice, Healthy Choice, Asda*	1 Pack/400g	412	103	6.0	15.0	2.1	0.9
Con Carne With Rice, Organic, Sainsbury's*	1 Pack/400g	472	118	5.0	18.5	2.7	1.8
Con Carne With Rice, Perfectly Balanced, Waitrose*	1 Pack/400g	508	127	5.6	19.9	2.8	0.9
Con Carne, 99% Fat Free, Stagg*	1oz/28g	28	99	7.2	14.2	0.4	2.2
Con Carne, Asda*	1 Can/392g	376	96	7.0	9.0	3.5	0.0
Con Carne, Baked Bean, Heinz*	1 Can/390g	324	83	7.0	10.3	1.5	2.8
Con Carne, Bird's Eye*	1 Pack/300g	324	108	3.9	17.8	2.3	1.6
Con Carne, Classic, Stagg*	1 Can/410g	521	127	8.8	8.6	6.4	2.3
Con Carne, Co-Op*	1 Serving/200g	240	120	7.0	15.0	3.3	0.0
Con Carne, Dynamite Hot, Stagg*	1 Serving/250g	310	124	7.6	9.6	6.2	2.5
Con Carne, Frozen, Co-Op*	1 Pack/340g	306	90	6.0	15.0	1.0	1.0
Con Carne, Homepride*	1 Can/390g	234	60	2.5	11.2	0.6	0.0
Con Carne, Marks & Spencer*	1 Pack/285g	285	100	8.7	7.4	3.7	2.0
Con Carne, Morrisons*	1 Tin/197g	227	115	8.1	11.5	4.1	1.7
Con Carne, New Lower Fat, BGTY, Sainsbury's*	1 Pack/400g	400	100	5.5	18.4	0.5	1.0
Con Carne, Silverado Beef, Stagg*	1 Can/410g	406	99	7.8	10.9	2.7	1.5
Con Carne, Tesco*	1 Can/392g	463	118	8.0	10.5	4.9	2.4
Crispy Beef, Ready Meals, Marks & Spencer*	1oz/28g	74	265	8.9	33.1	10.5	0.7
Crispy Beef, Tesco*	1 Pack/250g	455	182	11.4	19.8	6.3	1.2
Extra Hot, Marks & Spencer*	1oz/28g	28	100	8.7	9.1	3.1	1.8
Meat Free, Sainsbury's*	1 Pack/400g	308	77	4.0	4.1	5.0	5.2
Medium, Uncle Ben's*	1 Jar/500g	305	61	1.8	11.1	0.8	0.0
Mexican Chilli With Potato Wedges, Weight Watchers*	1 Pack/300g	252	84	5.1	10.3	2.5	1.7
Mexican Style, Aldi*	½ Can/196g	231	118	8.7	9.2	5.2	2.1
Mixed Vegetable, Tesco*	1 Pack/400g	352	88	3.9	11.0	2.9	3.2

C

	Measure INFO/WEIGHT	per Measure KCAL	Nutrition Values per 100g / 100ml				
			KCAL	PROT	CARB	FAT	FIBRE
CHILLI,							
Non Carne, Linda McCartney*	1 Pack/340g	252	74	5.8	9.2	2.3	1.7
Quorn*	1oz/28g	23	81	4.7	6.9	4.2	2.5
Spicy Bean & Vegetable, Safeway*	1 Pack/311g	196	63	3.3	9.6	1.3	2.5
Uncle Ben's*	1oz/28g	17	59	1.8	11.1	0.8	0.0
Vegetable	1oz/28g	16	57	3.0	10.8	0.6	2.6
Vegetable & Rice, BGTY, Sainsbury's*	1 Pack/450g	401	89	3.4	17.8	0.5	2.4
Vegetable, & Rice, Healthy Eating,Tesco*	1 Pack/450g	392	87	2.8	16.1	1.2	1.5
Vegetable, & Rice, Safeway*	1 Pack/500g	530	106	3.4	21.2	0.8	1.7
Vegetable, 99% Fat Free, Stagg*	1oz/28g	16	58	3.1	9.3	0.5	3.1
Vegetable, Chesswood*	½ Can/200g	138	69	3.3	13.3	0.3	2.1
Vegetable, Retail	1oz/28g	20	70	4.0	9.4	2.1	0.0
Vegetable, Waitrose*	1 Can/392g	227	58	2.9	6.6	2.2	0.0
Vegetarian, Quorn, Tesco*	1 Pack/400g	340	85	4.4	15.0	0.8	2.1
Wedge Bowl, COU, Marks & Spencer*	1 Pack/400g	380	95	7.2	11.3	2.3	1.8
Weight Watchers*	1 Pack/320g	269	84	5.1	10.4	2.5	1.7
CHILLI POWDER, Average	1 Tsp/4g	16	405	12.3	54.7	16.8	34.2
CHILLIES,							
Green, Tesco*	1oz/28g	4	16	0.8	2.6	0.3	1.6
Jalapeno, Discovery*	1 Serving/100g	32	32	0.8	3.4	0.7	0.3
Mixed, Tesco*	1oz/28g	8	27	1.8	4.2	0.3	1.6
Red, Raw, Tesco*	1 Serving/28g	8	27	1.8	4.2	0.3	0.0
Very Lazy, EPC*	1 serving/10g	11	114	4.2	15.3	4.0	0.5
CHINESE HOUSE SPECIAL, Healthy Living, Tesco*	1 Pack/450g	369	82	6.5	10.5	1.6	1.1
CHINESE LEAVES, Tesco*	1 Serving/100g	18	18	3.5	0.3	0.3	2.6
CHINESE MEAL,							
For One, Safeway*	1 Serving/584g	993	170	5.5	25.8	4.7	1.3
For Two, Tesco*	1 Pack/500g	480	96	4.4	16.0	1.6	1.1
For One, Good For You, Asda*	1 Pack/570g	946	166	7.0	28.0	2.9	0.0
CHINESE TAKEAWAY, Ready Meals, Marks & Spencer*	1oz/28g	38	135	7.5	17.0	4.2	1.1
CHIPLETS, Salt & Vinegar, Marks & Spencer*	1 Bag/35g	170	485	6.4	59.5	25.5	2.4
CHIPS,							
11mm Fresh, Deep Fried, McCain*	1oz/28g	66	235	3.2	31.8	10.6	0.0
14mm Fresh, Deep Fried, McCain*	1oz/28g	59	209	2.7	34.2	6.8	0.0
14mm Friers Choice, Deep Fried, McCain*	1oz/28g	56	199	3.5	29.3	8.0	0.0
3 Way Cook, Somerfield*	1 Serving/96g	145	151	2.5	24.0	5.0	1.6
9/16" Straight Cut Caterpack, Deep Fried, McCain*	1oz/28g	63	225	3.1	32.1	9.4	0.0
American Style Oven, Co-Op*	1 Serving/150g	255	170	2.0	26.0	6.0	3.0
American Style Oven, Safeway*	1 Serving/125g	288	230	4.1	38.2	6.8	3.0
American Style Oven, Sainsbury's*	1 Serving/165g	314	190	5.4	23.6	8.3	1.3
American Style Southern Fried, Iceland*	1 Serving/100g	251	251	4.0	34.0	11.0	3.0
American Style,Thin Oven, Tesco*	1 Serving/125g	210	168	2.7	24.6	6.5	2.1
Beefeater, Deep Fried, McCain*	1oz/28g	71	253	3.3	37.7	9.9	0.0
Beefeater, Oven Baked, McCain*	1oz/28g	55	195	4.0	32.2	5.6	0.0
Chunky Oven, Harry Ramsden's*	1 Serving/150g	185	123	2.8	19.9	3.6	1.6
Chunky, Baked, Organic, Marks & Spencer*	1 Serving/100g	150	150	1.7	27.1	3.7	2.2
Chunky, COU, Marks & Spencer*	1 Serving/150g	135	90	1.6	17.6	1.7	1.5
Chunky, Eat Smart, Safeway*	1 Serving/158g	150	95	1.6	18.3	1.6	1.4
Crinkle Cut Oven, 5% Fat, McCain*	1 Serving/100g	163	163	2.9	30.2	5.4	2.9
Crinkle Cut Oven, Asda*	1 Serving/100g	244	244	3.8	37.0	9.0	3.0
Crinkle Cut Oven, Ultimate Seasoned, McCain*	1 Serving/85g	190	223	3.5	34.0	8.2	3.5
Crinkle Cut, Frozen, Fried in Corn Oil	1oz/28g	81	290	3.6	33.4	16.7	2.2
Crinkle Cut, Oven Baked, McCain*	1oz/28g	51	182	3.3	29.7	5.6	0.0
Family Fries Oven, Tesco*	1 Serving/125g	164	131	2.0	22.4	3.7	1.8

CHIPS,	Measure INFO/WEIGHT	per Measure KCAL	Nutrition Values per 100g / 100ml				
			KCAL	PROT	CARB	FAT	FIBRE
Fine Cut, Frozen, Fried in Blended Oil	1oz/28g	102	364	4.5	41.2	21.3	2.4
Fine Cut, Frozen, Fried in Corn Oil	1oz/28g	102	364	4.5	41.2	21.3	2.7
French Fries, Retail	1oz/28g	78	280	3.3	34.0	15.5	2.1
Homefries, Crinkle Cut, Oven Baked, McCain*	1 Serving/225g	448	199	3.2	34.8	6.9	0.0
Homefries, Jacket Oven, McCain*	1 Serving/100g	220	220	3.9	37.9	7.4	0.0
Homemade, Fried in Blended Oil	1oz/28g	53	189	3.9	30.1	6.7	2.2
Homemade, Fried in Corn Oil	1oz/28g	53	189	3.9	30.1	6.7	2.2
Homemade, Fried in Dripping	1oz/28g	53	189	3.9	30.1	6.7	2.2
Homestyle Oven, Sainsbury's*	1 Serving/125g	206	165	2.4	29.2	4.3	2.1
Just Bake, Low Fat, Marks & Spencer*	1oz/28g	37	133	2.0	24.7	3.7	1.7
Low Fat, Good Choice, Iceland*	1oz/28g	41	147	2.0	25.3	2.6	1.8
Micro, Asda*	1 Serving/112g	221	197	3.5	30.0	7.0	4.0
Micro, McCain*	1oz/28g	54	194	3.3	27.3	7.9	0.0
Oven Baked, Crinke Cut, New, McCain*	1oz/28g	55	198	3.5	33.4	5.6	0.0
Oven Baked, McCain*	1oz/28g	48	173	2.8	29.3	4.9	0.0
Oven Baked, Straight Cut, New, McCain*	1oz/28g	51	182	3.6	31.4	4.7	0.0
Oven, BGTY, Sainsbury's*	1oz/28g	42	151	2.7	27.1	3.5	2.1
Oven, Champion, Aldi*	1oz/28g	44	158	2.5	27.0	4.5	0.0
Oven, Chunky, Ross*	1 Serving/100g	177	177	3.1	26.6	6.5	3.9
Oven, Cooked, Value, Tesco*	1 Serving/125g	308	246	4.5	39.5	7.8	2.9
Oven, Crinkle Cut, Safeway*	1 Serving/130g	234	180	3.3	29.5	5.4	2.4
Oven, Crinkle Cut, Sainsbury's*	1 Serving/165g	297	180	3.3	29.5	5.5	2.4
Oven, Crinkle Cut, Tesco*	1oz/28g	40	142	2.1	23.3	4.5	2.0
Oven, Curly, Safeway*	1 Serving/125g	376	301	3.8	34.0	16.6	4.1
Oven, Frozen, Baked	1oz/28g	45	162	3.2	29.8	4.2	2.0
Oven, Frozen, McCain*	1oz/28g	39	138	2.5	26.2	4.0	1.9
Oven, Good Choice, Iceland*	1 Serving/150g	171	114	2.5	20.3	2.5	1.9
Oven, Healthy Choice, Safeway*	1 Serving/150g	227	151	2.8	27.1	3.5	2.1
Oven, Morrisons*	1 Serving/100g	134	134	2.4	22.2	3.9	0.0
Oven, New, BGTY, Sainsbury's*	1 Serving/165g	185	112	2.4	19.2	2.8	1.9
Oven, Organic, Waitrose*	1 Serving/165g	233	141	1.5	25.1	3.8	1.6
Oven, Reduced Fat, Waitrose*	1oz/28g	37	133	2.3	24.3	3.0	1.6
Oven, Safeway*	1oz/28g	42	151	2.8	27.1	3.5	2.1
Oven, Steak Cut, Asda*	1 Serving/100g	153	153	2.0	27.0	4.1	2.5
Oven, Steak Cut, Sainsbury's*	1 Serving/165g	266	161	2.6	27.1	4.7	2.8
Oven, Steakhouse, Tesco*	1 Serving/125g	165	132	2.7	22.7	3.4	1.7
Oven, Straight Cut, 4% Fat, Healthy Eating, Tesco*,	1oz/28g	35	124	2.3	21.8	3.1	1.9
Oven, Straight Cut, 5% Fat, Sainsbury's*	1 Serving/165g	281	170	3.4	28.0	4.9	2.5
Oven, Straight Cut, Better For You, Morrisons*	1 Serving/165g	249	151	2.8	27.1	3.5	2.1
Oven, Straight Cut, Budgens*	1 Portion/180g	205	114	2.3	21.9	1.9	2.7
Oven, Straight Cut, Good For You, Asda*	1oz/28g	42	150	2.6	27.0	3.5	2.4
Oven, Straight Cut, Great Value Asda*	1 Serving/100g	199	199	3.5	35.0	5.0	3.0
Oven, Straight Cut, Healthy Eating, Tesco*	1oz/28g	35	124	2.3	21.8	3.1	1.9
Oven, Straight Cut, Iceland*	1 Serving/100g	197	197	3.6	31.6	6.2	2.3
Oven, Straight Cut, Reduced Fat, Tesco*	1 Serving/100g	127	127	2.3	22.7	3.0	2.1
Oven, Straight Cut, Safeway*	1 Serving/125g	226	181	3.6	30.0	5.2	2.5
Oven, Straight Cut, Tesco*	1oz/28g	46	166	2.6	27.8	4.9	1.7
Oven, Stringfellows, McCain*	1oz/28g	72	256	4.1	37.0	10.2	0.0
Oven, Thick Cut, Frozen, Baked	1oz/28g	44	157	3.2	27.9	4.4	1.8
Steak Cut, 3 Way Cook, Somerfield*	1 Serving/200g	294	147	2.4	23.0	5.0	1.5
Steak Cut, Oven, Tesco*	1 Serving/165.2g	233	141	2.0	24.4	3.9	2.0
Steak, Cut Frying, Safeway*	1 Serving/125g	289	231	3.3	27.1	12.1	2.2
Straight Cut, Frozen, Fried in Blended Oil	1oz/28g	76	273	4.1	36.0	13.5	2.4

	Measure INFO/WEIGHT	per Measure KCAL	Nutrition Values per 100g / 100ml				
			KCAL	PROT	CARB	FAT	FIBRE
CHIPS,							
Straight Cut, Frozen, Fried in Corn Oil	1oz/28g	76	273	4.1	36.0	13.5	2.4
Straight Cut, Low Fat, Good Choice, Iceland*	1 Serving/150g	171	114	2.5	20.3	2.5	0.3
Straight Cut, Microwave Baked, McCain*	1oz/28g	70	251	3.5	35.0	10.7	0.0
Thick Cut, Caterpack, Deep Fried, McCain*	1oz/28g	60	215	3.1	28.8	9.7	0.0
Thick Cut, Frozen, Fried in Corn Oil	1oz/28g	66	234	3.6	34.0	10.2	2.4
Three Way Cook, Co-Op*	1 Serving/100g	140	140	2.0	19.0	6.0	3.0
Vending 3/8" Straight Cut, Deep Fried, McCain*	1oz/28g	62	220	3.3	29.6	9.8	0.0
Waffle, Bird's Eye*	1 Serving/75g	156	208	2.5	24.3	11.2	2.6
CHIPSTICKS,							
Ready Salted, Smiths, Walkers*	1 Bag/22g	105	476	6.8	59.5	23.5	0.0
Salt & Vinegar, Smiths, Walkers*	1 Bag/22g	105	476	6.8	59.5	23.5	0.0
CHIVES, Fresh	1oz/28g	6	23	2.8	1.7	0.6	1.9
CHOC ICES,							
Chocolate, Real Milk, Sainsbury's*	1 Ice/48.4g	150	312	3.5	30.3	19.7	0.8
Chunky, Wall's*	1 Ice/81g	162	200	2.6	18.9	13.1	0.0
Dark, Sainsbury's*	1 Ice/43.2g	135	315	3.8	25.5	22.0	0.4
Dark, Somerfield*	1 Ice/62ml	186	300	3.0	25.0	21.0	0.0
Dark, Tesco*	1 Ice/43.4g	136	316	3.0	27.4	21.4	0.7
Light, Sainsburys*	1 Ice/43g	135	313	3.2	27.0	21.4	0.3
Light, Tesco*	1 Ice/43g	138	322	3.4	27.1	22.1	0.5
Milk Chocolate, Marks & Spencer*	1oz/28g	86	306	4.1	28.7	19.4	0.5
Mini Mix, Magnum Style, Eis Stern, Lidl*	1 Ice/38.6g	130	334	4.2	29.0	23.0	0.0
Morrisons*	1 Ice/31g	86	279	3.0	24.7	19.3	0.4
Neapolitan Chocolate, Co-Op*	1 Ice/62g	120	194	2.0	16.9	13.2	0.4
Neopolitan, Safeway*	1 Ice/41.4g	119	290	2.6	25.4	19.5	0.3
Real Milk, Sainsbury's*	1 Ice/71ml	133	187	2.0	20.0	11.0	0.1
Real Plain, Sainsbury's*	1 Ice/48.4g	149	310	2.9	29.5	20.0	2.2
Real White, Tesco*	1 Ice/54g	185	343	4.2	27.4	24.1	0.1
Rum & Rasin, Safeway*	1 Ice/45g	136	303	3.3	28.9	19.3	1.1
Safeway*	1 Ice/70g	217	310	2.8	25.9	21.6	0.9
SmartPrice, Asda*	1 Ice/31g	81	262	2.8	20.0	19.0	0.0
Value, Tesco*	1 Ice/31g	87	281	2.6	24.8	19.0	0.6
Vanilla, Co-Op*	1 Ice/70g	130	186	3.6	3.6	17.1	0.0
CHOCOLATE,							
A Darker Shade of Milk, Green & Black's*	1 Serving/20g	108	542	9.5	54.0	32.0	0.0
All Gold Plain, Terry's*	1oz/28g	134	477	3.8	60.9	24.0	1.1
Animal Bar, Nestle*	1 Bar/19g	97	513	5.8	63.6	26.1	0.0
Assortment, Diabetic, Thorntons*	1oz/28g	108	385	4.3	57.0	24.0	2.5
Assortment, Occasions, Tesco*	1 Serving/150g	705	470	4.6	65.8	20.9	0.5
Belgian Assortment, Waitrose*	1oz/28g	127	453	6.3	45.5	27.3	3.8
Belgian Dark, Extra Special, Asda*	2 Squares/20g	102	508	11.0	26.0	40.0	16.0
Belgian Milk, TTD, Sainsbury's*	2 Squares/20g	108	540	9.8	50.9	33.0	2.3
Belgian Plain With Ginger, TTD, Sainsbury's*	2 Squares/20g	114	571	7.2	31.2	46.4	10.9
Belgian Plain, Organic, Waitrose*	1 Bar/100g	505	505	9.6	32.0	37.6	5.6
Belgian Seashells, Woolworths*	1 Box/63g	347	550	5.5	52.9	31.1	0.0
Belgian White With Coffee, TTD, Sainsbury's*	2 Squares/20g	110	548	6.5	56.9	32.7	0.0
Belgian White With Lemon, TTD, Sainsbury's*	2 Squares/20g	109	546	5.7	61.2	30.9	0.1
Belgian, Finest, Tesco*	1 Chocolate/12g	62	520	5.9	55.6	28.4	5.2
Black Magic, Nestle*	1oz/28g	128	456	4.4	62.6	20.8	1.6
Bournville, Cadbury's*	1 Bar/50g	248	495	4.6	59.6	26.7	0.0
Bournville, Extra Dark, Cadbury's*	1 Square/10g	56	560	8.5	30.8	44.8	0.0
Brandy Liqueurs, Asda*	1 Chocolate/8.3g	33	409	4.0	60.0	17.0	0.8
Brazil Nut Assortment, Marks & Spencer*	1oz/28g	163	581	9.6	37.5	45.3	1.5

C

INFO/WEIGHT	KCAL	KCAL	PROT	CARB	FAT	FIBRE
	Measure per Measure		Nutrition Values per 100g / 100ml			

CHOCOLATE,

	Measure INFO/WEIGHT	per Measure KCAL	KCAL	PROT	CARB	FAT	FIBRE
Bubble Bar, Marks & Spencer*	1 Bar/25g	136	542	9.5	51.8	33.1	2.2
Cafe au Lait, Thorntons*	1 Chocolate/16g	77	481	5.3	58.1	25.0	0.6
Cappuccino Bar, Thorntons*	1 Bar/38g	201	529	5.2	49.7	34.7	0.5
Cappuccino Mountain Bar, Marks & Spencer*	1oz/28g	149	533	8.4	52.0	32.5	2.6
Chocolat Noir, Lindt*	1/6 Bar/17g	87	510	6.0	50.0	32.0	0.0
Chocolate Orange Bar, Milk, Terry's*	1 Bar/85g	459	540	7.5	55.6	32.0	0.3
Chomp, Cadbury's*	1 Treatsize/12g	56	465	3.5	67.9	19.8	0.0
Chunky Hazelnut Bar, Marks & Spencer*	1 Bar/52g	293	563	8.8	48.1	37.3	1.7
Classic Chocolate Bar, Cadbury's*	1 Bar/26g	134	514	6.5	62.3	26.5	0.8
Coconut, White, Excellence, Lindt*	1 Square/10g	61	610	6.0	48.0	44.0	0.0
Continental, Cappuccino, Thorntons*	1 Bar/38.0g	201	529	5.2	49.7	34.7	0.1
Creamy Vanilla White, Green & Black's*	1 Serving/20g	115	577	7.5	52.5	37.5	0.0
Credit Card, Solid Milk, Marks & Spencer*	1 Bar/20g	108	540	8.1	54.1	32.4	1.3
Crispy, Sainsbury's*	4 Squares/19g	99	521	9.1	56.9	28.5	2.1
Dairy Milk, Bubbly, Cadbury's*	1 Bar/35.2g	184	525	7.6	56.4	29.7	0.0
Dairy Milk, Cadbury's*	1 Treatsize/15g	80	530	7.8	57.1	29.9	0.0
Dairy Milk, Caramel Centre, Cadbury's*	1 Square/10g	50	495	5.7	61.1	25.3	0.0
Dairy Milk, Crispies, Cadbury's*	1 Serving/100g	510	510	7.6	58.6	27.4	0.0
Dairy Milk, Mint Chips, Cadbury's*	1 Serving/50g	253	505	6.5	61.2	26.1	0.0
Dairy Milk, Snack Size, Cadbury's*	1 Bar/30g	159	530	7.8	57.1	29.9	0.0
Dairy Milk, Turkish, Cadbury's*	1 Serving/100g	455	455	5.3	63.0	20.0	0.0
Dairy Milk, With Shortcake Biscuit, Cadbury's*	1 Square/6g	31	520	7.5	59.0	28.0	0.0
Dark, Bar, Thorntons*	1 Sm Bar/48g	245	511	9.3	31.6	38.8	15.9
Dark, Belgian, Luxury Continental, Sainsbury's*	1 Bar/100g	490	490	11.1	24.2	38.7	7.4
Dark, Co-Op*	1 Bar/50g	253	505	4.0	57.0	29.0	6.0
Dark, Orange With Slivered Almonds, Excellence, Lindt*	1 Square/10g	50	500	6.0	46.0	30.0	0.0
Dark, Organic, Green & Black's*	1 Bar/20g	114	571	10.0	51.0	37.0	0.0
Dark, TTD, Sainsbury's*	1 Square/10g	57	569	7.2	31.2	46.3	10.9
Dark, With 70% Cocoa Solids, Organic, Green & Black's*	1 Serving/20g	115	576	7.5	45.5	40.5	0.0
Dark, With Cherries, Green & Black's*	1 Serving/75g	390	520	7.0	57.3	32.8	0.0
Dark, With Hazelnuts & Currants, Green & Black's*	1 Serving/60g	323	539	8.4	51.6	36.4	0.0
Dark, With a Soft Mint Centre, Green & Black's*	4 Squares/30g	136	452	4.8	56.0	23.2	0.0
Divine, Milk, Co-Op*	1 Bar/45g	243	540	7.0	57.0	32.0	2.0
Excellence, 85% Cocoa Solids, Lindt*	1 Square/8.3g	44	530	11.0	32.0	46.0	0.0
Extremely Chocolatey Mini Bites, Marks & Spencer*	1 Cake/17g	76	445	5.5	51.4	24.6	2.0
Ferrero Rocher, Ferrero*	1 Sweet/12.5g	74	593	7.0	49.0	41.0	0.0
Freddo, Dairy Milk, Cadbury's*	1 Frog/20g	106	530	7.8	57.1	29.9	0.0
Fruit & Nut Assortment, Marks & Spencer*	1oz/28g	148	527	7.6	49.8	34.3	1.3
Fruit & Nut, Cadbury's*	1 Bar/49g	240	490	8.0	55.7	26.3	0.0
Fruit & Nut, Dark, Tesco*	4 Squares/25g	124	494	5.8	54.8	27.9	6.5
Fudge, Keto Bar*	1 Serving/65g	250	385	36.9	36.9	10.8	32.3
Ginger, Dark, Thorntons*	1 Bar/100g	509	509	5.8	44.3	35.1	8.8
Ginger, Terry's*	1oz/28g	111	395	2.6	68.0	12.4	3.4
Jazz Orange Bar, Thorntons*	1 Bar/56g	304	543	6.8	55.7	32.3	1.2
Kinder Bueno, Ferrero*	1 Twin Bar/43g	245	570	8.5	47.6	38.5	0.0
Kinder Maxi, Ferrero*	1 Bar/21g	116	550	10.0	51.0	34.0	0.0
Kinder Surprise, Ferrero*	1 Egg/20g	110	550	10.0	51.0	34.0	0.4
Kinder, Ferrero*	1 Bar/12.5g	69	550	10.0	51.0	34.0	0.0
Kinder, Riegel, Ferrero*	1 Bar/21g	117	558	10.0	53.0	34.0	0.0
Lemon Mousse, Bar, Thorntons*	1oz/28g	141	503	4.1	55.3	29.3	0.0
Limes, Pascall*	1 Sweet/8g	27	333	0.3	77.2	2.5	0.0
Luxury Dark Continental, Tesco*	1 Bar/100g	571	571	11.3	46.5	37.8	0.1
Maya Gold, Green & Black's*	1 Bar/20g	110	552	6.0	56.5	33.5	0.0

	Measure INFO/WEIGHT	per Measure KCAL	Nutrition Values per 100g / 100ml				
			KCAL	PROT	CARB	FAT	FIBRE
Milk	1oz/28g	146	520	7.7	56.9	30.7	0.8
Milk & White Belgian, Shells, Waitrose*	1 Serving/15g	77	511	5.0	53.1	31.0	2.8
Milk Caramel, Green & Black's*	1 Serving/20g	92	461	5.9	57.5	22.9	0.0
Milk Chocolate Excellence, Lindt*	1 Bar/100g	570	570	6.6	48.9	39.6	0.0
Milk, Co-Op*	1 Sm Bar/50g	265	530	9.0	55.0	31.0	2.0
Milk, Extra Fine Swiss, Marks & Spencer*	1oz/28g	155	553	8.9	50.4	35.3	2.4
Milk, Extra au Lait, Milch Extra, Lindt*	½ Bar/50g	268	535	6.5	57.0	31.0	0.0
Milk, Organic, Green & Black's*	1oz/28g	147	524	9.5	54.0	32.0	0.0
Milk, Sainsbury's*	4 Squares/25g	133	533	9.2	54.6	30.8	2.2
Milk, SmartPrice, Asda*	1 Square/6g	32	536	8.0	54.0	32.0	2.4
Milk, Tesco*	1 Serving/25g	133	533	9.5	54.7	30.7	2.2
Milk, Thorntons*	1 Sm Bar/50g	269	538	7.5	54.8	32.0	1.0
Milk, With Whole Almonds, Green & Black's*	1 Serving/20g	114	572	11.5	41.5	40.0	0.0
Mini Bites, Chunky, Moments, Fox's*	1 Roll/20g	90	450	5.7	52.4	24.6	2.2
Mini Eggs, Milk, Cadbury's*	1 Egg/3g	15	495	5.6	67.7	22.2	0.0
Mint Crisp, Cadbury's*	1oz/28g	141	505	6.4	70.3	22.2	0.0
Mint Crisp, Sainsbury's*	4 Squares/19g	95	501	5.0	63.7	25.0	3.6
Mint Crisps, Marks & Spencer*	1 Mint/8g	40	494	5.4	54.8	29.6	3.1
Mint Thins, Plain, Safeway*	1 Thin/10g	48	480	2.3	67.5	22.3	0.7
Neapolitans, Terry's*	1oz/28g	146	522	6.0	57.3	29.7	4.1
Nuts About Caramel, Cadbury's*	1 Bar/55g	272	495	5.8	56.6	27.4	0.0
Old Jamaica, Cadbury's*	1oz/28g	129	460	5.8	56.9	23.3	0.0
Orange Mini Bites, Marks & Spencer*	1 Bite/22g	95	430	5.5	54.6	21.6	1.8
Orange Tree, Lidl*	1 Bar/28g	150	537	9.6	53.0	31.8	2.1
Pain Au Chocolat, Asda*	1 Serving/23g	106	462	8.0	49.0	26.0	0.0
Pain Au Chocolat, Waitrose*	1 Serving/90g	380	422	8.1	34.9	27.8	1.1
Peppermint Patty, Hershey*	3 Patties/41g	160	390	2.4	80.5	7.3	0.0
Plain	1oz/28g	143	510	5.0	63.5	28.0	2.5
Plain, 72%, Finest, Tesco*	1 Square/10g	60	603	7.7	44.0	44.0	3.7
Plain, Cocoa Solids, Finest, Tesco*	1 Square/10g	58	581	7.7	38.5	44.0	5.8
Plain, Organic, Tesco*	1 oz/28g	145	519	6.4	44.7	34.9	9.6
Plain, With Hazelnuts, Tesco*	4 Squares/25g	135	539	6.1	48.3	35.7	6.5
Refrigerator Squares, Marks & Spencer*	1 Square/24g	180	750	5.0	113.8	30.4	3.3
Rich Dark Fruit & Nut Plain, Sainsbury's*	4 Squares/25g	117	489	5.2	53.9	27.9	5.7
Rich Dark Plain, Co-Op*	1 Bar/200g	1010	505	4.0	57.0	29.0	6.0
Rich Dark Plain, Sainsbury's*	1oz/28g	144	514	3.7	65.0	29.5	0.9
Rocher, Thorntons*	1 Chocolate/15g	76	507	6.8	45.3	33.3	2.0
Swiss Dark Extra Fine, Marks & Spencer*	1 Bar/150g	773	515	6.4	46.7	34.5	9.7
Swiss Milk Chocolate & Hazelnut Bar, Marks & Spencer*	1oz/28g	156	556	6.4	51.9	36.0	3.3
Swiss Milk, Marks & Spencer*	1oz/28g	150	535	5.1	60.9	30.1	1.9
Swiss Mountain Bar, Marks & Spencer*	1 Bar/100g	555	555	6.5	55.2	35.3	0.2
Swiss Plain With Ginger, Waitrose*	4 Squares/17g	88	519	5.3	58.3	29.4	2.0
Swiss White, Bar, Marks & Spencer*	1oz/28g	152	543	8.0	58.3	30.9	0.0
Taz Chocolate Bar, Cadbury's*	1 Bar/25g	121	485	4.8	62.0	24.0	0.0
Teddy, Milk, Thorntons*	1 Teddy/250g	1358	543	7.6	52.6	33.5	1.0
Triple Crunch, Marks & Spencer*	1 Serving/60g	280	467	6.8	66.3	19.4	3.4
White	1oz/28g	148	529	8.0	58.3	30.9	0.0
White, Crispy, Fair Trade, Co-Op*	½ Bar/50g	278	555	9.0	51.0	35.0	0.1
White, Nestle*	4 Pieces/40g	220	550	7.5	55.0	32.5	0.0
White, Organic, Green & Black's*	1 Bag/30g	173	577	7.5	52.5	37.5	0.0
White, Organic, Waitrose*	1oz/28g	160	572	6.1	53.9	36.8	0.0
White, Thorntons*	1 Bar/50g	273	546	6.7	59.4	31.4	0.0
White, With Honey & Almond Nougat, Toblerone*	1 Serving/25g	133	530	6.2	60.5	29.0	0.2

C

CHOCOLATE,	Measure INFO/WEIGHT	per Measure KCAL	KCAL	PROT	CARB	FAT	FIBRE
Whole Nut, Cadbury's*	1 Bar/49g	270	550	9.3	48.8	35.2	0.0
Whole Nut, Plain, Belgian, Waitrose*	4 Squares/25g	135	540	6.3	45.4	38.0	7.8
Wholenut, SmartPrice, Asda*	½ Bar/16.4g	90	562	8.0	47.0	38.0	3.3
Wildlife Bar, Cadbury's*	1 Bar/21g	109	520	7.8	56.8	29.3	0.0
With Almonds, Dark, Organic, Evernat*	1oz/28g	169	604	16.3	37.4	43.2	0.0
With Orange & Spices, Green & Black's*	1 Serving/20g	110	552	6.0	56.5	33.5	0.0
CHOCOLATE CREAM, Fry's*	1 Serving/50g	215	430	2.6	68.6	15.4	0.0
CHOCOLATE DRINK, Instant Break, Milk, Cadbury's*	4 Tsp/28g	119	425	10.9	64.2	14.0	0.0
CHOCOLATE DROPS,							
Plain, Sainsbury's*	1 Serving/125g	638	510	5.3	60.1	27.6	4.0
White, For Cooking & Decorating, Sainsbury's*	1oz/28g	152	544	6.5	60.3	30.8	0.0
CHOCOLATE ECLAIRS,							
Asda*	1 Eclair/50g	192	383	6.0	20.0	31.0	0.5
Ashbury, The Sweet Partnership/Childline*	1 Sweet/12g	59	490	4.1	63.1	22.4	0.0
Cadbury's*	1 Sweet/8g	39	485	4.6	75.0	18.8	0.0
Dairy Cream, Co-Op*	1 Eclair/29g	122	420	6.0	23.0	34.0	0.6
Dairy Cream, Safeway*	1 Eclair/27g	101	373	4.1	32.1	26.2	0.4
Fresh Cream, Co-Op*	1 Eclair/8g	38	470	3.0	71.0	19.0	0.1
Fresh Cream, Jumbo, Co-Op*	1 Eclair/94g	357	380	4.0	27.0	28.0	2.0
Fresh Cream, Marks & Spencer*	1 Eclair/62g	234	378	4.1	18.8	32.3	0.2
Fresh Cream, Mini, Tesco*	1 Cake/28g	111	397	4.8	33.6	27.0	0.4
Fresh Cream, Safeway*	1 Eclair/59g	210	356	4.1	24.8	26.7	0.4
Fresh Cream, Sainsbury's*	1 Eclair/29g	104	360	4.2	32.7	23.6	0.1
Fresh, Cream, Tesco*	1 Eclair/66g	244	370	4.0	31.2	25.5	0.4
Marks & Spencer*	1 Sweet/7g	34	482	1.9	73.9	20.1	0.0
Mini, Iceland*	1 Eclair/13g	55	426	4.9	21.5	35.6	0.4
Weight Watchers*	1 Eclair/31g	71	230	4.0	22.9	12.8	11.4
CHOCOLATE FOOTBALL, Thorntons*	1 Football/200g	1088	544	7.6	52.9	33.5	1.0
CHOCOLATE ORANGE,							
Milk Bar, Terrys*	1 Bar/40g	212	531	7.2	57.5	30.2	0.0
Milk, Mini Segments, Terry's*	1 Segment/8g	42	527	7.7	57.9	29.4	2.1
Milk, Terry's*	1 Orange/175g	928	530	7.5	57.3	30.0	2.1
Plain, Terry's*	1 Orange/175g	889	508	3.8	56.8	29.4	6.2
White, Terry's*	1 Segment/11.4g	59	535	6.3	60.9	29.4	0.0
CHOCOLATE PEANUTS,							
Assorted, Thorntons*	1 Bag/140g	785	561	13.8	34.8	40.8	3.6
Co-Op*	1oz/28g	153	545	15.0	34.0	39.0	4.0
Milk, Tesco*	1 Bag/227g	1221	538	17.5	31.8	37.9	4.4
CHOCOLATE RAISINS,							
Assorted, Thorntons*	1 Bag/140g	601	429	4.2	58.8	19.7	2.9
Bonds Sweetstars*	1 Serving/28g	109	391	4.7	57.0	16.0	0.0
Co-Op*	¼ Pack/50g	205	410	4.0	64.0	15.0	1.0
Marks & Spencer*	1oz/28g	116	414	4.5	66.5	14.6	1.2
Milk, Asda*	1 Serving/28g	127	452	6.0	62.0	20.0	1.2
Milk, Sainsbury's*	1oz/28g	117	418	4.7	62.7	16.5	1.4
CHOCOLATE SPREAD,							
Average	1 Tsp/12g	68	569	4.1	57.1	37.6	0.0
Cadbury's*	1 Tsp/12g	69	575	4.5	55.0	38.0	0.0
Hazelnut, Nutella, Ferrero*	1oz/28g	149	533	6.5	57.0	31.0	0.0
Milk, Belgian, Sainsbury's*	1 Serving/10g	56	559	11.9	47.2	35.8	1.4
Milk, SmartPrice, Asda*	1 Tbsp/16g	92	573	4.0	56.0	37.0	2.0
Nutella, Ferrero*	1 Tsp/12g	64	533	6.5	57.0	31.0	0.0
Snickers, Mars*	1 Serving/7g	38	548	8.7	43.3	37.8	0.0

C

	Measure INFO/WEIGHT	per Measure KCAL	Nutrition Values per 100g / 100ml				
			KCAL	PROT	CARB	FAT	FIBRE
CHOCOLATE SPREAD,							
Value, Tesco*	1 Serving/20g	116	581	3.0	54.5	39.0	1.5
With Nuts	1 Tsp/12g	66	549	6.2	60.5	33.0	0.8
CHOCOLATES,							
All Gold Milk, Terry's*	1oz/28g	137	490	5.6	61.5	24.5	0.6
Almond Mocca Mousse, Thorntons*	1 Chocolate/14g	76	543	8.5	40.7	37.9	2.9
Alpini, Thorntons*	1 Chocolate/13g	70	538	7.0	54.6	32.3	2.3
Bittermint, Bendicks*	1 Mint/18.2g	74	411	4.4	63.0	17.6	0.0
Buttons, Milk, Marks & Spencer*	1 Pack/75g	375	500	8.6	59.8	25.3	1.9
Buttons, Milk, Somerfield*	1 Pack/75g	390	520	8.0	58.0	28.0	0.0
Buttons, White, Co-Op*	1 Pack/70g	382	545	7.0	61.0	31.0	0.0
Cappuccino, Thorntons*	1 Chocolate/13g	70	538	5.9	48.5	36.2	0.8
Champagne, Thorntons*	1 Chocolate/16g	76	475	6.9	43.1	29.4	2.5
Chocolate Mousse, Thorntons*	1 Chocolate/13g	67	515	7.5	40.0	36.2	3.1
Coffee Creme, Dark, Thorntons*	1 Chocolate/13g	52	400	3.0	71.5	10.8	0.8
Coffee Creme, Milk, Thorntons*	1 Chocolate/13g	52	400	2.8	74.6	10.0	0.8
Country Caramel, Milk, Thorntons*	1 Chocolate/9g	45	500	4.6	62.2	26.7	0.0
Dairy Box, Milk, Nestle*	1 Sm Box/227g	1085	478	5.7	60.8	23.5	0.8
Dark, Elegant, Elizabeth Shaw*	1 Chocolate/8g	38	469	2.9	62.5	23.1	0.0
Liquers, Cognac Truffle, Thorntons*	1 Chocolate/14g	65	464	7.3	40.0	27.1	2.9
Milk Tray, Cadbury's*	1oz/28g	139	495	5.2	60.5	26.0	0.0
Mingles, Bendicks*	1 Chocolate/5g	26	528	6.5	55.0	32.9	0.0
Mint Crisp, Bendicks*	1 Mint/7.7g	40	494	5.2	55.0	29.9	0.0
Mint Crisp, Dark, Elizabeth Shaw*	1 Chocolate/6g	27	458	1.9	68.0	20.7	0.0
Mint Crisp, Milk, Elizabeth Shaw*	1 Chocolate/6g	30	493	4.0	70.9	21.4	0.0
Mint Crisp, Thorntons*	1 Chocolate/7g	34	486	7.7	40.0	31.4	4.3
Praline, Coffee, Thorntons*	1 Chocolate/7g	37	529	7.0	47.1	34.3	2.9
Praline, Roast Hazelnut, Thorntons*	1 Chocolate/13g	70	538	6.0	51.5	33.8	3.1
Praline, Hazelnut, Thorntons*	1 Chocolate/5g	27	540	7.0	48.0	36.0	4.0
Praline, Marzipan, Thorntons*	1 Chocolate/14g	63	450	5.9	58.6	21.4	2.1
Strawberry Parfait, Milk, Thorntons*	1 Chocolate/14g	67	479	3.6	65.7	22.9	0.7
Swiss Milk Discs, Marks & Spencer*	1 Disc/5g	28	553	8.9	50.4	35.3	2.4
Truffle, Lemon, White, Thorntons*	1 Chocolate/14g	63	450	4.6	64.3	25.0	0.7
Truffle, Seville, Thorntons*	1 Chocolate/14g	76	543	7.1	53.6	33.6	1.4
Truffle, Swiss, Somerfield*	1 Pack/125g	640	512	4.0	52.0	32.0	0.0
Truffle, Amaretto, Thorntons*	1 Chocolate/14g	66	471	5.5	55.0	25.7	2.9
Truffle, Brandy, Thorntons*	1 Chocolate/14g	68	486	6.1	52.1	27.1	0.7
Truffle, Caramel, Thorntons*	1 Chocolate/14g	67	479	4.2	57.9	25.7	2.1
Truffle, Champagne, Petit, Thorntons*	1 Chocolate/6g	31	517	7.5	48.3	31.7	3.3
Truffle, Champagne, Premier, Thorntons*	1 Chocolate/17g	88	518	6.9	45.3	32.9	2.4
Truffle, Cherry, Thorntons*	1 Chocolate/14g	58	414	4.2	50.7	21.4	1.4
Truffle, Continental Champagne, Thorntons*	1 Chocolate/16g	78	488	6.1	51.3	28.0	0.6
Truffle, Grand Marnier, Thorntons*	1 Chocolate/15g	77	513	7.2	40.7	34.0	4.0
Truffle, Irish Milk Chocolate Cream, Elizabeth Shaw*	1 Chocolate/12g	57	477	3.9	63.4	22.8	0.0
Truffle, Rum, Thorntons*	1 Chocolate/13g	63	485	4.8	58.5	24.6	4.8
Truffle, Thorntons*	1 Chocolate/7g	33	471	6.0	48.6	27.1	1.4
Truffle, Vanilla, Thorntons*	1 Chocolate/13g	64	492	4.8	57.7	26.9	1.5
Truffle, Viennese, Dark, Thorntons*	1 Chocolate/10g	53	530	5.9	47.0	36.0	3.0
Truffle, Viennese, Milk, Thorntons*	1 Chocolate/10g	56	560	4.9	54.0	36.0	0.0
Truffles, Rum	1oz/28g	146	521	6.1	49.7	33.7	1.9
CHOCOLATINE,							
All Butter, Sainsbury's*	1 Serving/58.1g	241	415	7.9	42.5	23.7	3.3
Sainsbury's*	1 Serving/58g	263	454	8.5	42.3	27.9	2.1
With Plain Chocolate, Tesco*	1 Serving/58g	264	455	8.5	42.3	27.9	2.1

	Measure INFO/WEIGHT	per Measure KCAL	Nutrition Values per 100g / 100ml				
			KCAL	PROT	CARB	FAT	FIBRE
CHOW MEIN,							
Beef, Sainsbury's*	1 Pack/450g	500	111	6.6	15.5	2.5	0.8
Cantonese Chicken, Sainsbury's*	1 Pack/450g	455	101	6.5	11.5	3.2	1.7
Cantonese Vegetable Stir Fry, Sainsbury's*	¼ Pack/100g	85	85	2.2	10.6	3.8	1.2
Chicken Stir Fry, Oriental Express*	1 Pack/350g	347	99	5.8	14.9	1.8	2.9
Chicken With Vegetable Spring Roll, Oriental Express*	1 Pack/300g	213	71	5.5	12.4	0.6	1.9
Chicken, Ainsley Harriott*	1 Serving/250g	447	179	14.0	21.2	4.7	2.0
Chicken, Asda*	1 Pack/460g	488	106	5.0	13.0	3.8	2.1
Chicken, BGTY, Sainsbury's*	1 Pack/450g	410	91	6.9	11.5	1.9	1.2
Chicken, COU, Marks & Spencer*	1 Pack/200g	180	90	9.3	8.1	2.3	1.1
Chicken, Chinese Takeaway, Sainsbury's*	1 Pack/316g	338	107	9.1	11.6	2.7	0.7
Chicken, Co-Op*	1 Pack/300g	270	90	8.0	9.0	3.0	0.9
Chicken, Great Value, Asda*	1 Pack/400g	408	102	5.0	14.0	2.9	0.8
Chicken, Healthy Eating, Tesco*	1 Pack/450g	392	87	8.2	10.8	1.2	0.4
Chicken, Healthy Living, Tesco*	1 Pack/450g	392	87	8.2	10.8	1.2	0.4
Chicken, New BGTY, Sainsbury's*	1 Pack/450g	374	83	6.0	11.4	1.4	1.1
Chicken, New Improved Recipe, Sainsbury's*	1 Pack/449g	395	88	5.7	11.7	2.0	1.2
Chicken, Oriental Express*	1 Pack/300g	210	70	4.4	13.1	0.6	1.9
Chicken, Tesco*	1 Pack/350g	322	92	5.1	14.5	1.5	0.8
Chinese Style, Safeway*	1 Serving/150g	167	111	4.0	13.0	4.4	1.1
Pork, Perfectly Balanced, Waitrose*	½ Pack/310g	332	107	7.6	17.2	0.9	1.6
Special Chinese, Farmfoods*	1 Pack/400g	276	69	4.3	6.7	2.8	0.8
Special, COU, Marks & Spencer*	1 Pack/400g	320	80	7.4	9.9	1.0	1.0
Special, Good For You, Asda*	1 Pack/400g	360	90	7.0	14.0	0.7	1.2
Special, Marks & Spencer*	1 Pack/340g	289	85	6.6	8.2	2.7	1.2
Special, Ready Meals, Marks & Spencer*	1oz/28g	38	135	7.4	18.2	3.7	1.1
Stir Fry, Asda*	1 Pack/350g	270	77	2.1	6.0	5.0	0.0
Stir Fry, Somerfield*	1 Pack/300g	474	158	6.0	32.0	1.0	0.0
Stir Fry, Tesco*	1 Pack/500g	335	67	2.5	10.8	1.5	1.0
Vegetable & Cashew Nut, Eat Smart, Safeway*	1 Pack/380g	323	85	7.0	11.4	1.2	1.1
Vegetable, Asda*	1oz/28g	25	90	2.9	15.5	1.8	1.2
Vegetable, Healthy Eating, Tesco*	1 Pack/350g	221	63	6.8	7.9	0.5	1.3
Vegetables & Noodles in Sauce, Safeway*	1 Serving/200g	110	55	3.7	9.5	0.2	1.3
With Vegetable Spring Roll, Oriental Express*	1 Roll/120g	196	163	5.3	28.5	3.2	3.0
CHRISTMAS PUDDING,							
Average	1oz/28g	81	291	4.6	49.5	9.7	1.3
Less Than 5% Fat, Good For You, Asda*	½ Pudding/100g	279	279	2.6	58.0	4.1	1.6
Luxury, Safeway*	1/8 Pudding/114g	316	277	3.1	47.9	8.1	1.3
Nut Free & Alcohol Free, Healthy Eating, Tesco*	1 Serving/100g	258	258	2.8	55.6	2.7	4.3
Rich Fruit, Laced With Brandy, Tesco*	1 Serving/100g	305	305	3.7	50.8	9.7	1.3
Rich Fruit, Tesco*	1 Serving/114g	331	290	2.4	55.0	5.9	0.0
Sticky Toffee, Tesco*	¼ Pudding/114g	372	326	2.5	64.5	6.4	0.8
Tesco*	1 Serving/113g	305	270	2.4	55.0	5.9	1.5
Toffee Sauce Coated, Morrisons*	1 Pudding/100g	324	324	2.5	64.5	6.4	0.0
Traditional Style, Asda*	1 Pudding/100g	296	296	2.6	58.0	6.0	1.6
Vintage, Marks & Spencer*	1/8 Pudding/113g	335	295	2.6	59.8	5.6	1.4
With Cider, Value, Tesco*	1 Serving/100g	312	312	2.7	59.6	7.0	3.3
CHUTNEY,							
Albert's Victorian, Baxters*	1 Serving/25g	38	150	35.0	6.0	0.1	0.0
Apricot & Ginger, Safeway*	1 Tsp/15g	24	162	1.4	38.0	0.2	2.0
Apricot, Sharwood's*	1 Tsp/16g	21	131	0.6	32.0	0.1	2.3
Bengal Hot, Sharwood's*	1oz/28g	56	200	0.5	48.7	0.3	1.1
Bengal Spice Mango, Sharwood's*	1 Tsp/5g	12	236	0.5	58.0	0.2	1.2
Caramalised Onion, Sainsbury's*	1 Serving/25g	28	111	1.1	23.5	1.4	1.1

	Measure INFO/WEIGHT	per Measure KCAL	Nutrition Values per 100g / 100ml KCAL	PROT	CARB	FAT	FIBRE
CHUTNEY,							
Cranberry & Caramelised Red Onion, Baxters*	1 Serving/20g	31	154	0.3	38.0	0.1	0.3
Flame Roasted Tomato & Pepper, TTD, Sainsbury's*	1 Serving/5g	9	189	1.0	45.3	0.4	1.1
Fruit, Spiced, Baxters*	1 Tsp/16g	23	143	6.0	34.8	0.1	0.0
Fruit, Traditional, Marks & Spencer*	1oz/28g	43	155	0.9	37.2	0.3	1.7
Hot Mango, TTD, Sainsbury's*	1 Tbs/15g	36	240	0.7	54.7	2.0	2.0
Lime & Chilli, Geeta's*	1 Serving/25g	69	277	2.0	64.0	1.4	1.9
Major Grey Mango, Patak's*	1oz/28g	71	255	0.4	66.0	0.2	0.7
Mango & Apple, Sharwood's*	1oz/28g	65	233	0.4	57.6	0.1	1.1
Mango & Ginger, Baxters*	1 Jar/320g	598	187	5.0	45.7	0.2	0.9
Mango & Lime, Sharwood's*	1oz/28g	58	206	0.4	50.5	0.3	0.8
Mango, Budgens*	1oz/28g	66	235	0.3	58.2	0.1	0.0
Mango, Green Label, Sharwood's*	1 Serving/10g	23	234	0.3	57.8	0.2	0.9
Mango, Hot, Patak's*	1oz/28g	72	258	0.4	67.1	0.2	0.7
Mango, Premium, Geetas*	1 Serving/50g	131	262	0.8	63.0	0.3	0.9
Mango, Somerfield*	1oz/28g	40	143	1.0	35.0	0.0	0.0
Mango, Sweet	1 Heaped Tsp/16g	30	189	0.7	48.3	0.1	0.0
Mixed Fruit	1 Heaped Tsp/16g	25	155	0.6	39.7	0.0	0.0
Peach Fruit, Sharwoods*	1oz/28g	48	172	0.4	42.3	0.1	0.9
Ploughman's Plum, EPC*	1 Tsp/10g	16	160	1.3	38.1	0.2	1.6
Spicy Fruit, Safeway*	1 Tsp/16g	16	109	0.5	25.5	0.1	0.1
Spicy Mango, Marks & Spencer*	1oz/28g	52	185	0.1	46.1	0.3	1.8
Sweet Mango, Marks & Spencer*	1oz/28g	67	240	0.3	58.8	0.2	1.5
Sweet Mango, Patak's*	1oz/28g	73	259	0.3	67.4	0.1	0.7
Tomato	1 Heaped Tsp/16g	20	128	1.2	31.0	0.2	1.3
Tomato & Red Pepper, Baxters*	1 Jar/312g	512	164	2.0	38.0	0.4	1.5
Tomato, TTD, Sainsbury's*	1 Tbsp/15g	29	193	2.0	44.7	1.3	2.7
Tomato, Waitrose*	1 Pot/100g	195	195	1.3	46.8	0.3	1.5
CIDER,							
Dry	1 Pint/568ml	204	36	0.0	2.6	0.0	0.0
Low Alcohol	1 Pint/568ml	97	17	0.0	3.6	0.0	0.0
Medium Sweet, Somerfield*	1 Pint/568ml	233	41	0.0	5.0	0.0	0.0
Sweet	1 Pint/568ml	239	42	0.0	4.3	0.0	0.0
Value, Tesco*	1 Pint/568ml	153	27	0.0	0.8	0.0	0.0
CINNAMON, Powder	1 Tsp/3g	8	261	3.9	55.5	3.2	0.0
CLAMS,							
Baby, In Brine, John West*	1/3 Can/47g	38	81	16.0	3.0	0.6	0.0
Canned in Brine, Drained	1oz/28g	22	77	16.0	1.9	0.6	0.0
CLEMENTINE JUICE, Morrisons*	1 Serving/100ml	48	48	0.5	10.9	0.1	0.1
CLEMENTINES,							
Weighed With Peel & Pips	1oz/28g	8	28	0.7	6.5	0.1	0.9
Weighed Without Peel	1 Med/60g	22	37	0.9	8.7	0.1	1.2
COCKLES,							
Boiled	1 Cockle/4g	2	53	12.0	0.0	0.6	0.0
Bottled in Vinegar, Drained	1oz/28g	17	60	13.3	0.0	0.7	0.0
COCOA BUTTER, Average	1oz/28g	251	896	0.0	0.0	99.5	0.0
COCOA POWDER,							
Cadbury's*	1 Tbsp/16g	52	322	23.1	10.5	20.8	0.0
Made Up With Semi-Skimmed Milk	1 Mug/227ml	129	57	3.5	7.0	1.9	0.2
Made Up With Skimmed Milk	1 Mug/227ml	100	44	3.5	7.0	0.5	0.0
Made Up With Whole Milk	1 Mug/227ml	173	76	3.4	6.8	4.2	0.2
COCONUT,							
Cream	1oz/28g	98	350	4.0	5.9	34.7	0.0
Creamed, Block	1oz/28g	187	669	6.0	7.0	68.8	0.0

C

	Measure INFO/WEIGHT	per Measure KCAL	Nutrition Values per 100g / 100ml				
			KCAL	PROT	CARB	FAT	FIBRE
COCONUT,							
Creamed, Sharwood's*	1oz/28g	185	662	6.0	6.4	68.0	14.0
Desiccated	1oz/28g	169	604	5.6	6.4	62.0	13.7
Fresh	1oz/28g	98	351	3.2	3.7	36.0	7.3
Ice	1oz/28g	104	371	1.7	66.7	12.7	2.6
Milk, Amoy*	1oz/28g	39	140	1.9	1.1	17.0	0.0
Milk, BGTY, Sainsbury's*	¼ Can/100ml	96	96	1.0	3.6	8.6	0.0
Milk, Blue Dragon*	1 Can/400ml	640	160	2.2	2.2	15.7	0.0
Milk, Light, Reduced Fat, Blue Dragon*	1 Can/400ml	408	102	0.9	2.4	9.8	0.0
Milk, Low Fat, Blue Dragon*	1 Can/400ml	272	68	0.7	1.0	6.7	0.0
Milk, Sococo*	1 Serving/50ml	125	250	0.0	0.0	25.0	20.0
COD,							
& Chips, Oven Baked, Safeway*	1 Pack/250g	523	209	8.4	25.0	8.4	3.5
& Parsley Sauce, Frozen, Marks & Spencer*	1 Pack/184g	156	85	11.1	1.9	3.9	1.0
& Salmon, Steam Cuisine, COU, Marks & Spencer*	1 Pack/400g	340	85	6.8	8.9	1.8	1.2
Baked	1oz/28g	27	96	21.4	0.0	1.2	0.0
Battered, Chip Shop Style, Aldi*	1 Serving/150g	293	195	13.3	7.7	12.3	1.4
Battered, Chip Shop, Youngs*	1 Portion/113g	237	210	11.5	14.3	12.1	0.6
Breaded, In Oven Crisp Crumb, Morrisons*	1 Serving/100g	201	201	12.4	17.5	9.0	1.0
Breaded, Portions, GFY, Asda*	1 Portion/125g	169	135	14.0	15.0	2.1	1.0
Breaded, Portions, Value, Tesco*	1 Portion/127.5g	257	201	12.4	17.5	9.0	1.0
Cakes, Big Time, Bird's Eye*	1 Cake/114g	185	162	7.6	16.7	7.2	1.0
Captains Coins, Bird's Eye*	1 Coin/20g	34	168	10.1	13.3	8.3	0.9
Dried, Salted, Boiled	1oz/28g	39	138	32.5	0.0	0.9	0.0
Fillets, Battered, Iceland*	1 Fillet/115g	292	254	13.9	20.9	12.8	1.7
Fillets, Battered, Tesco*	1 Fillet/150g	266	177	11.6	16.2	7.3	1.1
Fillets, Breaded, Chunky, Prime, Tesco*	1 Fillet/135g	246	182	12.9	12.4	9.0	1.7
Fillets, Breaded, Chunky, Reduced Fat, Tesco*	1 Fillet/135g	201	149	14.1	10.4	5.7	2.0
Fillets, Breaded, Extra Chunky, Marks & Spencer*	1 Fillet/217.5g	316	145	15.2	7.3	6.3	0.9
Fillets, Breaded, GFY, Asda*	1 Fillet/123g	185	150	14.0	17.0	2.9	1.5
Fillets, Breaded, Marks & Spencer*	1 Fillet/128g	256	200	11.2	14.3	11.3	1.1
Fillets, Breaded, Tesco*	1 Fillet/110g	220	200	12.2	17.6	9.0	1.1
Fillets, Breaded, Waitrose*	1 Fillet/150g	282	188	13.4	17.0	7.4	1.5
Fillets, Chargrilled, Sainsbury's*	1 Fillet/112g	184	164	15.4	0.8	11.0	0.0
Fillets, Chip Shop, Youngs*	1 Fillet/135g	315	233	11.0	15.1	14.6	0.6
Fillets, Chunky In Breadcrumbs, Better for You, Morrisons*	1 Fillet/124g	166	134	12.3	16.2	2.1	1.4
Fillets, Chunky In Breadcrumbs, Sainsbury's*	1 Fillet/145g	219	151	15.7	9.4	5.6	2.1
Fillets, Chunky, Asda*	1 Fillet/198g	176	89	21.0	0.0	0.5	0.0
Fillets, Chunky, BGTY, Sainsbury's*	1 Fillet/139g	228	165	16.1	12.9	5.4	1.3
Fillets, Chunky, In Breadcrumbs, Sainsbury's*	1 Fillet/125g	264	211	14.9	16.3	9.6	1.2
Fillets, Chunky, Tesco*	1 Fillet/170g	255	150	14.1	11.6	5.2	1.1
Fillets, Chunky, in Breadcrumbs, New, BGTY, Sainsbury's*	1 Fillet/119.2g	180	151	15.8	15.3	2.9	1.4
Fillets, Extra Large, Harry Ramsdens*	1 Fillet/190g	433	228	10.3	18.7	12.8	0.8
Fillets, Fresh Icelandic Prime, Waitrose*	1 Fillet/140g	112	80	18.3	0.0	0.7	0.0
Fillets, Fresh, Asda*	1 Serving/100g	95	95	21.0	0.0	1.2	0.0
Fillets, Frozen, Sainsbury's*	1 Fillet/110g	99	90	20.8	0.1	0.8	0.1
Fillets, In A Crunchy Ovencrisp Crumb, Tesco*	1 Fillet/127g	202	159	12.8	12.9	6.2	1.0
Fillets, In Breadcrumbs, Safeway*	1 Fillet/135g	234	173	17.5	11.8	6.3	1.2
Fillets, In Crisp Crumb, Prime Cut Skinless, Waitrose*	1 Fillet/160g	269	168	14.2	11.7	7.1	0.5
Fillets, In Crispy Batter, Boned, Asda*	1 Fillet/157g	360	229	13.0	15.0	13.0	1.1
Fillets, In Crispy Breadcrumbs, Asda*	1 Fillet/142g	291	205	16.0	15.0	9.0	1.1
Fillets, In Crispy Breadcrumbs, Healthy Eating, Tesco*	1 Portion/120g	166	138	15.1	13.4	2.7	1.9
Fillets, In Crispy Crumb, Good Choice, Iceland*	1 Serving/127g	267	210	16.2	17.5	8.4	0.9
Fillets, In Crunchy Breadcrumbs, Sainsbury's*	1 Fillet/125g	273	218	13.6	17.1	10.6	1.3

COD,

	Measure INFO/WEIGHT	per Measure KCAL	KCAL	PROT	CARB	FAT	FIBRE
Fillets, In Light Breadcrumbs, Premium, Bird's Eye*	1 Fillet/113g	202	179	12.7	15.0	7.6	0.6
Fillets, In Light Crispy Batter, Premium, Bird's Eye*	1 Fillet/112.5g	246	218	14.2	16.0	10.7	0.6
Fillets, In Ovencrisp Breadcrumbs, Tesco*	1 Fillet/120g	236	197	13.7	15.3	9.0	1.2
Fillets, In a Light & Crispy Breadcrumbs, Youngs*	1 Serving/135g	267	198	11.0	18.5	8.9	1.1
Fillets, In a Sweet Red Pepper Sauce, GFY, Asda*	½ Pack/170g	143	84	15.0	2.3	1.6	0.1
Fillets, Mediterranean Style, GFY, Asda*	1 Serving/200g	138	69	9.0	2.5	2.5	0.9
Fillets, Mornay, Sainsbury's*	1 Serving/153g	236	154	15.2	2.2	9.4	0.9
Fillets, Morrisons*	1 Fillet/100g	76	76	17.4	0.0	0.7	0.1
Fillets, Prime Fresh Icelandic, Waitrose*	1 Fillet/130g	104	80	18.3	0.0	0.7	0.0
Fillets, Safeway*	1 Serving/200g	190	95	20.8	0.0	1.3	0.0
Fillets, Sainsbury's*	1 Fillet/208g	196	94	20.9	0.0	1.1	0.0
Fillets, Skinless, Iceland*	1 Fillet/100g	95	95	20.8	0.0	1.3	0.0
Fillets, Smoked, Sainsbury's*	1 Serving/150g	152	101	21.6	0.0	1.6	0.0
Fillets, Somerfield*	1oz/28g	22	79	18.0	0.0	1.0	0.0
Fillets, Tesco*	1 Fillet/100g	80	80	18.3	0.0	0.7	0.0
Fillets, With A Mediterranean Pepper Sauce, Waitrose*	1 Pack/370g	241	65	12.2	1.1	1.3	0.9
Fillets, in Breadcrumbs, Bird's Eye*	1 Serving/112g	190	170	12.8	14.2	6.9	0.5
Fillets, in Chip Shop Batter, Marks & Spencer*	1 Serving/135g	285	211	12.5	11.3	12.6	1.0
Fillets, in Ovencrisp Batter, Tesco*	1 Portion/142g	240	169	12.1	16.3	6.1	0.3
Fillets, in Parsley Sauce, BGTY, Sainsbury's*	1 Pack/351g	316	90	11.6	1.3	4.3	0.7
Fish & Chips, Waitrose*	1 Pack/283g	849	300	14.4	33.7	12.0	4.8
Fritters, Cafe Culture, Marks & Spencer*	½ Pack/68.6g	121	175	8.5	10.8	11.1	1.2
In Breadcrumbs, COU, Marks & Spencer*	1 Serving/136g	170	125	13.2	13.7	1.6	1.3
In Breadcrumbs, Somerfield*	1 Av Fillet/135g	277	205	9.9	17.5	10.6	1.3
In Bubble Batter, Youngs*	1 Fish/135g	315	233	11.0	15.1	14.6	0.6
In Butter Sauce, Ross*	1 Serving/150g	126	84	9.1	3.2	3.9	0.1
In Butter Sauce, Sainsbury's*	1 Serving/170g	184	108	10.5	3.1	5.9	0.3
In Cheese Sauce, BGTY, Sainsbury's*	1 Serving/170g	145	85	12.8	3.1	2.4	0.0
In Mushroom Sauce, BGTY, Sainsbury's*	1 Serving/170g	112	66	9.9	2.8	1.7	0.1
In Oceancrisp Breadcrumbs, Tesco*	1 Fillet/125g	214	171	12.1	11.5	8.5	3.9
In Parsley Sauce, BGTY, Sainsbury's*	1 Pack/170g	143	84	11.4	2.4	3.2	0.3
In Parsley Sauce, COU, Marks & Spencer*	1 Pack/185g	130	70	10.6	1.4	2.5	0.6
In Parsley Sauce, Eat Smart, Safeway*	1 Serving/200g	150	75	11.5	2.4	1.9	0.9
In Parsley Sauce, Marks & Spencer*	1oz/28g	30	107	11.5	3.9	5.1	0.5
Loins, 5 Minute Fish, Tesco*	1 Serving/145g	110	76	16.8	0.3	0.8	0.6
Loins, Sainsbury's*	1 Serving/125g	104	83	18.6	0.1	0.9	0.0
Loins, Smoked, Sainsbury's*	1 Serving/125g	126	101	21.6	0.1	1.6	0.1
Loins, Tesco*	1 Loin/150g	120	80	18.3	0.0	0.7	0.0
Mediterranean, COU, Marks & Spencer*	1 Pack/400g	320	80	6.5	11.2	0.7	2.3
Mornay, Sainsbury's*	1 Serving/180g	277	154	15.2	2.2	9.4	0.9
Natural Fillets, Farmfoods*	1oz/28g	19	68	15.9	0.0	0.6	0.0
Pieces, Tesco*	1 Serving/100g	85	85	18.1	0.0	1.1	0.0
Poached	1oz/28g	26	94	20.9	0.0	1.1	0.0
Portions, Asda*	1 Cod Steak/92g	78	85	21.0	0.0	0.1	0.0
Portions, Breaded, Somerfield*	1 Portion/100g	206	206	13.0	13.0	12.0	0.0
Portions, In Butter Sauce, Asda*	1 Serving/151g	134	89	10.0	3.5	3.9	0.1
Portions, In Parsley Sauce, Sainsbury's*	1 Pack/170g	143	84	11.4	2.4	3.2	0.3
Portions, Low Fat, Tesco*	1 Portion/92g	63	68	15.6	0.0	0.6	0.0
Portions, Peche Ocean*	1 Serving/200g	154	77	18.0	0.0	0.5	0.0
Portions, Safeway*	1 Serving/100g	72	72	16.7	0.0	0.6	0.0
Portions, in Breadcrumbs, Marks & Spencer*	1oz/28g	57	203	10.7	15.4	11.0	0.8
Portions, in Crispy Breadcrumbs, Youngs*	1 Serving/141g	289	205	12.0	17.0	10.0	0.9
Portions, in Parsley Sauce, Asda*	1 Serving/150g	116	77	11.0	3.8	2.0	0.1

	Measure	per Measure	Nutrition Values per 100g / 100ml				
	INFO/WEIGHT	KCAL	KCAL	PROT	CARB	FAT	FIBRE
COD,							
Raw	1oz/28g	22	80	18.3	0.0	0.7	0.0
Smoked, Poached	1oz/28g	28	101	21.6	0.0	1.6	0.0
Smoked, Raw	1oz/28g	22	79	18.3	0.0	0.6	0.0
Steak, in Crunch Crumb, Bird's Eye*	1 Steak/107g	235	220	14.1	17.5	10.4	0.8
Steaks, Battered, Sainsbury's*	1 Steak/95.5g	188	198	11.3	14.2	10.7	0.7
Steaks, Haches With Vegetables, Peche Ocean*	1 Serving/200g	184	92	12.0	2.1	3.9	0.0
Steaks, In Parsley Sauce, Frozen, Bird's Eye*	1 Pack/172.2g	155	90	10.5	5.6	2.8	0.1
Steaks, Skinless & Boneless, Sainsbury's*	1 Steak/72g	62	86	21.4	0.0	0.1	0.1
Steaks, in Batter, Morrisons*	1 Serving/100g	220	220	11.2	14.7	13.0	0.6
Steaks, in Breadcrumbs, Morrisons*	1 Serving/150g	327	218	11.3	19.4	10.6	0.7
Steaks, in Butter Sauce, Bird's Eye*	1 Pack/170g	165	97	10.0	3.9	4.6	0.1
Steaks, in Cheese Sauce, Bird's Eye*	1 Pack/182g	175	96	10.9	5.2	3.5	0.1
Steaks, in Crispy Batter, Bird's Eye*	1 Steak/124g	241	194	10.4	11.0	12.0	1.1
Steaks, in Parsley Sauce, Bird's Eye*	1 Pack/176g	150	85	10.4	5.0	2.6	0.1
Steaks, in Parsley Sauce, Iceland*	1 Serving/151.2g	130	86	9.1	2.1	4.6	0.7
Steaks, in Parsley Sauce, Sainsbury's*	1 Serving/150g	126	84	11.4	2.4	3.2	0.3
Steamed	1oz/28g	23	83	18.6	0.0	0.9	0.0
Sweet Chilli, COU, Marks & Spencer*	1 Pack/400g	360	90	7.7	13.1	0.5	1.6
With Mediterranean Butter, Sainsbury's*	1 Pack/170.4g	196	115	17.0	0.1	5.2	0.1
With Roasted Vegetables, Marks & Spencer*	1 Serving/280g	238	85	8.0	4.9	3.8	1.7
With Salsa & Rosemary Potatoes, BGTY, Sainsbury's*	1 Pack/450g	356	79	4.7	13.1	0.9	1.6
With Sunblush Tomato Sauce, GFY, Asda*	½ Pack/177.3g	117	66	13.0	0.1	1.5	1.0
With a Thai Crust, Perfectly Balanced, Waitrose*	1 Pack/280g	249	89	15.1	1.6	2.5	0.6
in Batter, Chunky, Marks & Spencer*	1oz/28g	48	172	13.8	10.6	8.6	0.8
in Batter, Fried in Blended Oil	1oz/28g	69	247	16.1	11.7	15.4	0.5
in Breadcrumbs, Chunky, Marks & Spencer*	1oz/28g	46	166	13.6	9.9	8.0	1.3
COFFEE,							
Black	1 Mug/270ml	5	2	0.2	0.3	0.0	0.0
Cafe Vanilla, Nescafe*	1 Sachet/18.5g	82	432	9.7	73.0	11.4	0.0
Caffe Mocha, Starbucks*	1 Tall/200ml	278	139	4.9	15.0	7.9	0.7
Cappuccino, Cafe Mocha, Dry, Maxwell House*	1 Serving/23g	100	434	4.3	78.2	10.8	0.0
Cappuccino, Cafe Specials, Dry, Marks & Spencer*	1 Serving/14g	55	395	14.0	59.0	11.5	0.7
Cappuccino, Chocolate, Tall, Pret A Manger*	1 Serving/355ml	106	30	1.7	2.1	1.6	0.0
Cappuccino, Dry, Maxwell House*	1 Mug/15g	53	350	12.0	64.0	9.6	0.4
Cappuccino, For Filter Systems, Kenco*	1 Sachet/6g	23	375	19.0	44.0	13.5	0.0
Cappuccino, Instant, Kenco*	1 Sachet/20g	80	401	13.5	55.7	13.8	0.0
Cappuccino, Instant, Made Up, Maxwell House*	1 Serving/280g	123	44	0.6	5.8	1.9	0.0
Cappuccino, Instant, Unsweetened, Douwe Egberts*	1 Serving/12g	48	400	11.0	53.0	16.0	0.0
Cappuccino, Low Sugar, Tesco*	1 Serving/13g	55	425	18.4	43.3	19.8	0.4
Cappuccino, Marks & Spencer*	1 Serving/164g	66	40	1.5	4.4	1.6	0.1
Cappuccino, Nescafe*	1 Sachet/13g	52	398	11.5	66.6	9.5	0.0
Cappuccino, Sainsbury's*	1 Serving/12g	49	411	14.9	52.9	15.5	0.4
Cappuccino, Swiss Chocolate, Nescafe*	1 Sachet/20g	81	404	10.5	63.5	11.5	2.9
Cappuccino, Unsweetened Taste, Maxwell House*	1 Serving/15g	65	434	17.4	47.6	19.3	0.0
Cappuccino, Unsweetened, Dry, Nescafe*	1 Sachet/12g	51	427	14.9	54.7	16.6	0.0
Caramel Macchiato, Starbucks*	1 Grande/100ml	250	250	9.0	36.0	9.0	0.0
Frappe Iced, Nestle*	1 Serving/25g	96	384	15.0	72.0	4.0	0.5
Frappuccino, Blended Coffee, Starbucks*	1 Serving/454ml	260	57	1.1	11.5	0.8	0.0
Frappuccino, Caramel, Coffee Based, Starbucks*	1 Grande/473ml	279	59	1.0	11.6	0.7	0.0
Frappuccino, Mango Citrus Tea, Starbucks*	1 Tall/220ml	180	82	0.5	18.2	0.0	0.0
Frappuccino, Starbucks*	1 Drink/281ml	190	68	2.1	13.9	1.1	0.0
Frappuccino, Strawberries & Cream, Starbucks*	1 Grande/473ml	581	123	3.2	19.5	3.6	0.0
Ice Mocha Drink, Nescafe, Nestle*	1 Bottle/280ml	160	57	1.1	10.5	1.2	0.0

	Measure INFO/WEIGHT	per Measure KCAL	Nutrition Values per 100g / 100ml				
			KCAL	PROT	CARB	FAT	FIBRE
COFFEE,							
Infusion, Average With Semi-Skimmed Milk	1 Cup/220ml	14	7	0.6	0.7	0.2	0.0
Infusion, Average With Single Cream	1 Cup/220ml	31	14	0.4	0.3	1.2	0.0
Infusion, Average With Whole Milk	1 Cup/220ml	15	7	0.5	0.5	0.4	0.0
Infusion, Average, Made With Skimmed Milk	1 Cup/220ml	13	6	0.6	0.7	0.0	0.0
Instant, Made With Water & Semi-Skimmed Milk	1 Serving/350ml	25	7	0.4	0.5	0.4	0.0
Latte, 'A' Mocha, Cafe Met*	1 Bottle/290ml	174	60	3.2	9.0	1.4	0.0
Latte, Cafe, Marks & Spencer*	1 Serving/190g	143	75	4.3	8.3	2.8	0.0
Latte, Nescafe*	1 Sachet/21g	98	469	14.5	52.4	22.5	0.0
Latte, Pret A Manger*	1 Serving/336g	194	58	3.1	3.9	3.3	2.1
Latte, Skimmed Milk, Starbucks*	1 Serving/260ml	88	34	3.4	5.0	0.1	0.0
Latte, Whole Milk, Starbucks*	1 Tall/355.2ml	180	51	2.8	3.9	2.8	0.0
Moch'a'Latte, CafeMet*	1 Bottle/290ml	174	60	3.2	9.0	1.4	0.0
Regular, Ground or Instant	1 Cup (6fl oz)/177g	6	4	0.2	0.7	0.0	0.0
UHT Creamer, McDonald's*	1 Cup/14ml	17	123	4.2	4.2	10.0	0.0
COFFEE BEANS, Solid Dark Chocolate, Marks & Spencer*	1 Serving/10g	53	532	4.7	42.4	37.6	11.6
COFFEE MATE,							
Lite, Nestle*	2 Tsps/5g	20	398	2.5	83.9	6.9	0.0
Nestle*	2 Tsp/7g	36	520	1.2	60.5	30.3	0.0
COFFEE WHITENER,							
Half Fat, Co-Op*	1 Tsp/5g	22	430	0.9	78.0	13.0	0.0
Light, Healthy Eating, Tesco*	1 Tsp/6g	27	449	3.5	71.0	16.8	0.0
Tesco*	1 Tsp/3g	16	533	1.2	61.3	31.4	0.0
COGNAC, 40% Volume	1 Shot/25ml	56	222	0.0	0.0	0.0	0.0
COINTREAU, Liqueur Specialite De France	1 Serving/37g	80	215	0.0	0.0	0.0	0.0
COLA,							
Average	1 Can/330ml	135	41	0.0	10.9	0.0	0.0
Burger King*	1 Med/400g	172	43	0.0	10.6	0.0	0.0
Cherry Coke, The Coca Cola Co*	1fl oz/30ml	13	42	0.0	10.0	0.0	0.0
Coca Cola, McDonald's*	1 Med/400ml	172	43	0.0	10.5	0.0	0.0
Coke, The Coca Cola Co*	1 Can/330ml	139	42	0.0	10.9	0.0	0.0
Diet, Classic, Sainsbury's*	1 Can/330ml	1	0	0.0	0.0	0.0	0.0
Diet Coke, Caffeine Free, The Coca Cola Co*	1 Can/330ml	1	0	0.0	0.1	0.0	0.0
Diet Coke, The Coca Cola Co*	1 Can/330ml	1	0	0.0	0.0	0.0	0.0
Diet, Just, Asda*	1 Bottle/250ml	1	0	0.0	0.0	0.0	0.0
Diet, Marks & Spencer*	1 Can/330ml	3	1	0.0	0.3	0.0	0.0
Diet, Pepsi*	1 Can/330ml	1	0	0.0	0.0	0.0	0.0
Diet, Virgin*	1 Glass/250ml	1	0	0.1	0.1	0.1	0.0
Pepsi Max*	1fl oz/30ml	0	1	0.1	0.1	0.0	0.0
Pepsi-Cola, Pepsi*	1 Can/330ml	145	44	0.0	11.1	0.0	0.0
With Lemon, Diet Coke, Coca Cola*	1 Can/330ml	5	1	0.0	0.0	0.0	0.0
With Vanilla, Diet Coke, The Coca Cola Co*	1 Glass/200ml	1	0	0.0	0.1	0.0	0.0
COLA BOTTLES, Fizzy, Marks & Spencer*	1 Pack/200g	650	325	6.4	75.0	0.0	0.0
COLCANNON,							
Co-Op*	1 Pack/500g	325	65	2.0	10.0	2.0	2.0
Healthy Eating, Tesco*	1 Pack/330g	244	74	2.1	12.2	1.9	1.0
Tesco*	1 Serving/250g	245	98	2.3	11.7	4.7	1.7
Waitrose*	½ Pack/150g	138	92	1.7	12.8	3.8	1.4
COLESLAW,							
3 Cheese, Tesco*	½ Pot/125g	230	184	4.0	4.8	16.5	1.2
3% Fat, Marks & Spencer*	1oz/28g	47	167	1.3	9.0	14.0	1.4
50% Less Fat, Asda*	1oz/28g	17	61	2.1	6.8	2.8	0.9
99% Fat Free, Kraft*	1 Serving/40ml	50	126	1.0	28.9	1.0	0.0
Aldi*	1 Serving/100g	206	206	0.8	8.6	18.7	0.0

COLESLAW,

INFO/WEIGHT	Measure	per Measure KCAL	Nutrition Values per 100g / 100ml KCAL	PROT	CARB	FAT	FIBRE
Apple, Marks & Spencer*	1oz/28g	53	190	1.4	9.2	16.6	1.4
BGTY, Sainsbury's*	1oz/28g	19	69	0.9	6.6	4.3	1.9
Better For You, Morrisons*	1oz/28g	17	62	1.5	6.7	3.5	0.0
Betterbuy, Morrisons*	1 Serving/20g	23	113	0.8	9.2	8.1	0.0
Bryn Wharf Food Co*	1 Serving/90g	109	121	1.4	5.7	10.4	1.8
Budgens*	1 Serving/50g	103	206	1.2	9.5	18.1	2.0
Cheese, Co-Op*	1 Serving/125g	344	275	6.0	6.0	25.0	1.0
Cheese, Marks & Spencer*	1 Serving/30g	98	325	4.2	2.0	33.5	1.7
Cheese, Somerfield*	1oz/28g	48	171	3.0	7.0	14.0	0.0
Chunky, Asda*	1oz/28g	54	194	1.0	7.1	18.0	1.6
Classic, Marks & Spencer*	1 Pot/190g	124	65	1.9	8.8	2.3	1.3
Co-Op*	1 Serving/50g	65	130	1.0	7.0	11.0	2.0
Creamy, Asda*	1oz/28g	55	195	1.0	7.8	17.7	1.0
Creamy, Healthy Eating, Tesco*	1 Serving/30g	29	95	2.4	6.8	6.4	1.4
Creamy, Kwik Save*	1 Serving/10g	27	274	1.1	5.1	27.7	1.3
Creamy, Sainsbury's*	1oz/28g	69	245	1.3	4.6	24.6	1.6
Creamy, Tesco*	1oz/28g	52	186	1.1	7.6	16.8	1.5
Deli-Style, Marks & Spencer*	½ Pack/150g	285	190	1.6	3.9	18.5	1.3
Eat Smart, Safeway*	¼ Pack/50g	30	60	1.8	7.2	2.6	1.9
Finest, Tesco*	1 Serving/50g	107	214	1.2	6.1	20.5	1.6
Fruity, Asda*	½ Pot/125g	101	81	1.3	8.0	4.9	1.7
Garlic & Herb, Asda*	1oz/28g	60	216	1.1	7.2	20.3	1.5
Good For You, Asda*	1 Serving/50g	48	96	1.4	9.0	6.0	1.6
Good Intentions, Somerfield*	1 Serving/50g	36	72	1.6	7.6	3.9	1.5
Half Fat, Safeway*	1 Serving/70g	60	86	1.5	7.4	5.7	1.6
Healthy Choice, Safeway*	1 Pot/250g	215	86	1.5	7.4	5.7	1.6
Healthy Eating, Tesco*	1 Serving/100g	85	85	1.3	7.0	5.8	1.6
Healthy Living, Tesco*	1 Serving/60g	51	85	1.3	7.0	5.8	1.6
Heinz*	1oz/28g	38	135	1.6	9.4	10.2	1.2
Iceland*	1 Serving/110g	112	102	0.7	7.8	7.5	1.6
Kentucky Fried Chicken*	1 Portion/142g	231	163	1.4	18.3	9.5	2.1
Kwik Save*	1 Serving/50g	51	101	0.8	7.7	7.5	2.1
Less Than 3% Fat, Marks & Spencer*	1oz/28g	18	65	1.9	8.8	2.3	1.3
Light, Morrisons*	1oz/28g	33	118	1.1	8.3	7.8	0.0
Low Fat Mayonnaise, Tesco*	1oz/28g	18	64	1.4	4.7	4.4	1.4
Luxury, Asda*	1 Serving/50g	109	217	0.9	6.0	21.0	0.0
Luxury, Lidl*	1 Serving/50g	102	203	0.9	5.9	19.4	0.0
Luxury, Marks & Spencer*	1oz/28g	43	152	1.0	6.0	13.8	1.0
Marks & Spencer*	1oz/28g	50	180	1.7	6.1	16.5	1.1
Organic, Marks & Spencer*	1oz/28g	41	145	1.1	7.3	12.4	1.0
Perfectly Balanced, Waitrose*	1 Serving/84g	46	55	1.8	6.8	2.3	1.5
Prawn, Asda*	1oz/28g	54	192	2.4	6.6	17.3	1.4
Premium, Safeway*	1 Serving/125g	334	267	1.9	3.8	27.2	2.3
Reduced Calorie, Budgens*	½ Pot/125g	124	99	1.0	8.3	6.9	2.3
Reduced Calorie, Iceland*	1 Serving/50g	51	102	0.7	7.8	7.5	1.6
Reduced Calorie, Waitrose*	1 Serving/125g	74	59	2.3	5.5	3.1	1.7
Reduced Fat, Asda*	1 Pot/250g	218	87	1.5	6.0	6.3	1.6
Reduced Fat, Co-Op*	1 Serving/50g	45	90	0.9	6.0	7.0	2.0
Reduced Fat, Sainsbury's*	1/3 Pot/87g	89	102	1.2	7.3	8.0	1.7
Reduced Fat, Traditional, Marks & Spencer*	1oz/28g	57	205	1.1	5.4	20.0	2.8
Safeway*	1 Serving/75g	128	170	0.7	6.7	15.6	0.0
Sainsbury's*	1/3 Pot/75g	108	144	1.3	6.8	12.5	1.7
Salad, Reduced Fat, Sainsbury's*	1 Serving/250g	255	102	1.2	7.3	8.0	1.7

	Measure INFO/WEIGHT	per Measure KCAL	Nutrition Values per 100g / 100ml				
			KCAL	PROT	CARB	FAT	FIBRE
COLESLAW,							
SmartPrice, Asda*	1oz/28g	30	107	0.8	8.0	8.0	2.0
Supreme, Waitrose*	1oz/28g	53	190	1.8	4.9	18.1	1.7
TTD, Sainsbury's*	1oz/28g	74	263	1.6	6.1	25.8	1.5
Tesco*	1 Serving/50g	79	158	2.2	5.2	14.3	1.6
The Best, Safeway*	1 Serving/10g	30	296	1.0	7.2	29.2	0.8
Three Cheese, Asda*	1oz/28g	54	192	5.0	7.4	16.4	1.2
Traditional, Marks & Spencer*	1oz/28g	84	301	1.2	3.9	31.2	1.7
Value, Tesco*	1oz/28g	32	115	1.2	6.8	9.2	1.6
With 60% Less Fat, Good For You, Asda*	1 Serving/41g	36	88	1.5	7.0	6.0	1.7
With Mayonnaise, Retail	1oz/28g	72	258	1.2	4.2	26.4	1.4
With Reduced Calorie Dressing, Retail	1oz/28g	19	67	0.9	6.1	4.5	1.4
COLESLAW MIX,							
Shredded, Waitrose*	1 Serving/100g	29	29	1.1	5.6	0.2	2.2
Tesco*	1 Pack/400g	124	31	1.1	6.2	0.2	2.1
COLEY,							
Portions, Frozen, Sainsbury's*	1 Portion/92g	72	78	17.0	0.0	0.5	0.0
Portions, Tesco*	1 Serving/92g	68	74	16.4	0.0	0.9	0.0
Raw	1oz/28g	23	82	18.3	0.0	1.0	0.0
Steak, Skinless & Boneless, Sainsbury's*	1 Portion/72g	66	92	21.8	0.0	0.5	0.0
Steamed	1oz/28g	29	105	23.3	0.0	1.3	0.0
CONCHIGLIE,							
Asda*	1 Serving/50g	173	346	12.0	71.0	1.5	3.0
Dried, Napolina*	1oz/28g	99	352	11.5	73.0	1.5	2.2
Dried, Sainsbury's*	1 Serving/90g	321	357	12.3	73.1	1.7	2.5
Egg, Fresh, Waitrose*	1 Serving/125g	334	267	11.6	50.0	2.3	3.9
Safeway*	1 Serving/50g	174	348	13.2	70.1	1.7	2.9
Shells, Asda*	1 Serving/50g	173	346	12.0	71.0	1.5	3.0
Shells, Tesco*	1 Serving/100g	345	345	13.2	68.5	2.0	2.9
Whole Wheat, Asda*	1oz/28g	90	323	14.0	60.0	3.0	10.0
Wholewheat, Organic, Sainsbury's*	1 Serving/100g	316	316	12.7	61.9	2.0	10.0
CONSERVE,							
Apricot, 50% Fruit, Marks & Spencer*	1 Tbsp/15g	35	235	0.4	57.3	0.2	1.3
Apricot, Continental Soft Set, Sainsbury's*	1 Tbsp/15g	38	255	0.5	62.3	0.4	0.4
Apricot, Sainsbury's*	1 Tbsp/15g	36	241	0.5	58.4	0.1	2.8
Blackcurrant, Marks & Spencer*	1 Tbsp/15g	35	235	0.7	57.1	0.1	1.4
Blueberry, Marks & Spencer*	1 Tsp/7.5g	16	206	0.3	51.1	0.1	1.3
Raspberry, Continental Extra Jam, Waitrose*	1 Tbsp/15g	33	222	0.4	54.7	0.2	0.7
Raspberry, Extra Jam, Morrisons*	1 Serving/20g	51	254	0.6	63.0	1.1	0.0
Raspberry, Extra Jam, Organic, Sainsbury's*	1 Tbsp/15g	37	247	0.7	60.5	0.2	2.5
Raspberry, Finest, Tesco*	1 Tbsp/15g	42	277	0.6	67.7	0.1	1.0
Raspberry, Sainsbury's*	1 Tbsp/15g	37	244	0.7	59.2	0.1	2.2
Red Cherry, Finest, Tesco*	1 Tbsp/15g	42	277	0.6	67.6	0.1	0.8
Rhubarb & Ginger, Marks & Spencer*	1 Tbsp/15g	29	194	0.3	47.9	0.1	1.0
Strawberry, Continental, Asda*	1 Tbsp/15g	36	242	0.4	60.0	0.0	0.0
Strawberry, Continental, Extra Jam, Co-Op*	1 Tbsp/18g	50	275	0.3	68.0	0.0	0.9
Strawberry, Marks & Spencer*	1 Tbsp/15g	35	236	0.4	57.6	0.2	0.8
Strawberry, Set, Traditional, Sainsbury's*	1 Tbsp/15g	37	245	0.5	59.6	0.1	1.6
Strawberry, Soft, Set, Continental, Sainsbury's*	1 Tbsp/15g	38	251	0.5	61.1	0.5	0.4
Strawberry, Soft-Set Fruit, Premium, Co-Op*	1 Tbsp/20g	48	240	0.4	60.0	0.0	0.0
Strawberry, Tiptree*	1 Tbsp/15g	40	268	0.0	67.0	0.0	0.0
CONSOMME, Average	1oz/28g	3	12	2.9	0.1	0.0	0.0
COOKIES,							
All Butter Chocolate Chunk, Marks & Spencer*	1 Cookie/26g	130	500	5.2	62.4	25.2	2.6

C

COOKIES,

INFO/WEIGHT	Measure KCAL	per Measure	KCAL	PROT	CARB	FAT	FIBRE
All Butter Fruity Flapjack, Marks & Spencer*	1 Cookie/24.1g	100	415	4.6	53.4	20.2	4.2
All Butter Sultana, Marks & Spencer*	1 Cookie/16g	73	455	5.2	66.0	19.0	2.7
Apple & Raisin, Go Ahead, McVitie's*	1 Cookie/15g	66	443	5.3	76.8	12.7	3.4
Apple Crumble, Marks & Spencer*	1 Cookie/26g	90	345	4.6	76.8	2.0	2.9
Apricot, COU, Marks & Spencer*	1 Cookie/26g	88	340	5.4	75.0	2.4	2.0
Big Milk Chocolate Chunk, Cookie Coach Co*	1 Cookie/35g	174	497	6.2	61.4	25.1	0.0
Brazil Nut, Prewett's*	1 Cookie/50g	122	244	2.6	25.2	14.8	1.0
Butter & Sultana, Sainsbury's*	1 Cookie/13g	61	473	4.5	68.4	20.1	1.6
Cherry Bakewell, COU, Marks & Spencer*	1 Cookie/27g	95	350	5.8	72.3	2.6	2.3
Choc Chip, Asda*	1 Cookie/11g	56	506	5.0	63.0	26.0	1.8
Choc Chip, Maryland*	1 Cookie/11g	56	511	6.2	68.0	23.9	0.0
Choc Chip, McVitie's*	1 Cookie/10g	45	453	5.2	75.5	14.5	1.7
Choc Chunk & Hazelnut, Co-Op*	1 Cookie/17g	89	525	6.0	56.0	31.0	3.0
Choc Chunk, Fabulous Bakin Boys*	1 Cookie/60g	270	450	5.0	59.0	21.0	3.0
Chocolate & Ginger, The Best, Safeway*	1 Cookie/135g	709	525	5.5	62.0	28.0	2.6
Chocolate & Nut, Organic, Evernat*	1 Cookie/69g	337	489	7.2	64.1	22.6	0.0
Chocolate & Roasted Hazelnut, TTD, Sainsbury's*	1 Cookie/17g	89	521	6.4	56.3	30.3	2.2
Chocolate Chip & Hazelnut, Asda*	1 Cookie/12g	62	516	6.0	60.0	28.0	0.0
Chocolate Chip & Peanut, Trufree*	1 Cookie/11g	55	496	4.0	66.0	24.0	2.0
Chocolate Chip, BGTY, Sainsbury's*	1 Cookie/16.8g	73	428	4.5	75.6	11.9	2.5
Chocolate Chip, Chips Ahoy*	1 Cookie/11g	55	500	6.0	65.0	25.0	3.0
Chocolate Chip, Co-Op*	1 Cookie/11g	55	500	5.0	65.0	24.0	1.0
Chocolate Chip, Doves Farm*	1 Cookie/17g	82	485	4.1	58.7	25.9	2.7
Chocolate Chip, GFY, Asda*	1 Cookie/10.4g	46	463	5.0	68.0	19.0	3.5
Chocolate Chip, Handbaked, Border*	1 Cookie/15g	72	480	5.9	67.4	22.6	0.0
Chocolate Chip, Marks & Spencer*	1 Cookie/12g	61	506	6.0	62.1	25.9	1.2
Chocolate Chip, Mini, McVitie's*	1 Pack/50g	260	520	5.7	66.7	25.6	1.9
Chocolate Chip, Mini, Tesco*	1 Bag/30g	148	493	5.4	64.6	23.7	1.7
Chocolate Chip, Organic, Sainsbury's*	1 Cookie/16.8g	90	530	5.0	61.8	29.2	0.3
Chocolate Chip, Organic, Tesco*	1 Cookie/17g	88	520	0.0	63.3	27.4	2.8
Chocolate Chip, Sainsbury's*	1 Cookie/11g	56	508	6.2	67.0	23.9	1.3
Chocolate Chip, SmartPrice, Asda*	1 Cookie/10g	52	508	5.0	68.0	24.0	0.0
Chocolate Chunk & Hazelnut, Tesco*	1 Cookie/22g	118	538	6.2	60.2	30.3	1.9
Chocolate Chunk & Hazelnut, So Good, Somerfield*	1 Cookie/22.3g	117	530	6.3	55.7	31.3	2.4
Chocolate Chunk, Cadbury's*	1 Cookie/22g	119	540	6.5	58.0	31.2	0.0
Chocolate Chunk, Double Chocolate, Asda*	1 Cookie/26g	137	526	6.0	58.0	30.0	1.9
Chocolate Orange, Half Coated, Finest, Tesco*	1 Cookie/22g	107	488	4.9	59.6	25.5	1.2
Chocolate, Belgian, Extra Special, Asda*	1 Cookie/25.8g	139	535	6.0	58.0	31.0	2.0
Chocolate, Half Coated Triple, Finest, Tesco*	1 Cookie/25g	129	517	5.8	58.8	28.7	2.2
Chocolate, Soft, American Style, Budgens*	1 Cookie/50g	216	431	5.1	60.8	18.6	2.2
Coconut & Raspberry, Gluten Free, Sainsbury's*	1 Cookie/20g	102	511	5.9	56.0	29.3	6.7
Coconut, Gluten-Free, Sainsbury's*	1 Cookie/20g	103	516	5.6	54.4	30.7	4.1
Cranberry & Orange, Go Ahead, McVitie's*	1 Cookie/17g	77	452	5.3	78.0	13.2	2.4
Cranberry & Orange, Weight Watchers*	2 Cookies/23g	103	448	4.3	72.2	15.7	3.0
Dark Treacle, Weight Watchers*	2 Cookies/23g	97	423	5.2	66.7	15.1	1.7
Double Choc Chip, Mini, Marks & Spencer*	1 Cookie/22g	108	490	5.3	63.6	23.7	1.8
Double Choc Chunk, Luxury, Cadbury's*	1oz/28g	146	521	5.7	59.0	29.0	0.0
Double Choc, Maryland*	1 Cookie/10g	46	510	5.2	64.4	25.7	0.0
Double Chocolate Chip, Organic, Waitrose*	1 Cookie/18g	96	535	5.1	58.6	31.0	1.9
Double Chocolate Chip, Somerfield*	1 Cookie/11g	56	513	5.2	64.9	25.8	1.3
Fruit, Giant, Cookie Coach Co*	1 Cookie/60g	280	466	4.9	62.0	22.0	0.0
Fudge Brownie American Cream, Sainsbury's*	1 Cookie/12g	60	499	4.8	67.9	23.2	2.2
Ginger & Lemon, Weight Watchers*	2 Cookies/23g	104	452	4.3	73.9	15.7	2.2

	Measure INFO/WEIGHT	per Measure KCAL	Nutrition Values per 100g / 100ml				
			KCAL	PROT	CARB	FAT	FIBRE
COOKIES,							
Ginger Crunch, Hand Baked, Border*	1 Cookie/11.5g	52	470	4.7	71.4	20.4	0.0
Ginger, Low Fat, Marks & Spencer*	1 Cookie/23g	82	358	5.1	74.9	4.3	2.4
Ginger, Safeway*	1 Cookie/22g	106	480	4.7	66.5	22.7	2.4
Glace Cherry, Border*	1 Cookie/15.0g	74	493	5.4	64.3	25.6	0.0
Lemon Zest, Organic, Doves Farm*	1 Cookie/16.8g	74	435	3.0	57.0	21.5	1.9
Oat & Cranberry, BGTY, Sainsbury's*	1 Cookie/28g	126	449	6.8	65.0	18.0	5.1
Oat & Raisin, Safeway*	1 Cookie/12g	50	414	7.5	77.5	8.8	0.0
Oatflake & Honey, Organic, Sainsbury's*	1 Cookie/17g	82	480	6.3	66.0	21.2	2.6
Oatflake & Raisin, Waitrose*	1 Cookie/17g	80	469	5.8	61.7	22.1	4.7
Oreo, Nabisco*	3 Cookies/34g	160	470	6.0	71.0	21.0	3.0
Peanut, Hellema*	1 Cookie/16g	81	509	11.8	47.3	30.3	0.7
Pecan & Maple, Mini, Bronte*	1 Pack/100g	509	509	5.4	60.3	27.3	1.6
Praline Nougatine, Belle France*	1 Cookie/16.6g	86	506	8.0	63.0	25.0	0.0
Raisin & Cinnamon, Low Fat, Marks & Spencer*	1 Cookie/22g	78	355	6.2	73.0	4.1	3.2
Real Chocolate Chip, Weight Watchers*	2 Cookies/23g	98	427	5.3	66.1	15.7	1.6
Shortbread Rings, Handbaked, Border*	1 Cookie/16.5g	88	520	6.2	61.2	29.5	0.0
Shortbread, Organic, Evernat*	1oz/28g	149	532	5.9	56.7	31.3	0.0
Smarties, Asda*	1 Cookie/100g	175	175	2.3	28.0	6.0	0.6
Spiced Apple, COU, Marks & Spencer*	1 Cookie/25g	83	330	5.0	72.8	2.5	2.1
Spiced Apple, Marks & Spencer*	1 Cookie/25g	90	360	5.2	75.6	2.8	2.0
Stem Ginger, BGTY, Sainsbury's*	1 Cookie/17g	78	458	5.3	68.2	18.2	2.2
Stem Ginger, Half Coated, Finest, Tesco*	1 Cookie/25g	127	508	4.4	62.4	26.8	3.6
Stem Ginger, Less Than 5% Fat, Marks & Spencer*	1 Cookie/22g	79	360	6.2	73.9	4.3	3.0
Stem Ginger, Reduced Fat, Waitrose*	1 Cookie/16.7g	76	448	4.5	71.0	16.2	1.6
Stem Ginger, TTD, Sainsbury's*	1 Cookie/17g	84	496	4.5	63.4	24.9	1.7
Stem Ginger, Tesco*	1 Cookie/20g	98	489	4.2	64.0	24.0	2.0
Sultana & Cinnamon, Weight Watchers*	2 Cookies/23g	92	398	5.0	67.1	12.1	1.8
Sultana, All Butter, Reduced Fat, Marks & Spencer*	1 Cookie/16.7g	71	420	4.9	68.6	14.2	2.6
Tennessee American Style, Stiftung & Co, Lidl*	1 Cookie/19g	96	504	6.0	66.0	24.0	0.0
White Chocolate & Raspberry, McVitie's*	1 Cookie/17g	88	518	4.8	65.1	26.5	1.8
White Chocolate, Asda*	1 Cookie/54g	256	474	5.0	64.0	22.0	2.1
COQ AU VIN,							
Finest, Tesco*	1 Serving/273g	251	92	14.3	0.7	3.6	1.8
Healthy Living, Tesco*	½ Pack/200g	172	86	15.2	2.1	1.9	0.4
Marks & Spencer*	1 Serving/295g	398	135	14.2	1.5	7.7	1.0
Perfectly Balanced, Waitrose*	1 Pack/500g	445	89	12.6	2.7	3.1	0.6
Sainsbury's*	1 Pack/400g	484	121	16.8	3.5	4.4	0.2
COQUILLE, St Jacques, Marks & Spencer*	1 Serving/150g	165	110	5.0	8.8	6.1	1.1
CORDIAL,							
Blackcurrant, Diluted, Jucee, Princes*	1fl oz/30ml	3	11	0.0	1.6	0.0	0.0
Elderflower, Undiluted, Waitrose*	1 Cordial/20ml	22	110	0.0	27.5	0.0	0.0
Lime With Aromatic Bitters & Ginger, Sainsbury's*	1 Serving/40ml	12	29	0.0	6.9	0.3	0.3
CORIANDER,							
Leaves, Dried	1oz/28g	78	279	21.8	41.7	4.8	0.0
Leaves, Fresh	1oz/28g	6	20	2.4	1.8	0.6	0.0
CORN,							
Baby, & Asparagus Tips, Tesco*	1 Pack/150g	38	25	2.6	2.5	0.5	1.9
Baby, & Mange Tout, Tesco*	1 Serving/100g	27	27	2.9	3.3	0.3	2.1
Baby, & Sugar Snap Peas, Safeway*	½ Pack/100g	27	27	2.9	3.3	0.2	0.0
Baby, Fine Beans & Baby Carrots, Tesco*	1 Pack/250g	68	27	1.7	4.0	0.5	2.2
Baby, Organic, Tesco*	½ Pack/63g	15	24	2.5	2.7	0.4	2.0
Baby, Safeway*	1oz/28g	6	23	2.9	1.9	0.4	0.0
Baby, Sweet	1 Serving/100g	24	24	2.5	2.7	0.4	2.0

	Measure INFO/WEIGHT	per Measure KCAL	Nutrition Values per 100g / 100ml				
			KCAL	PROT	CARB	FAT	FIBRE
CORN,							
Cobs, Baby, Asda*	¼ Can/51g	9	17	0.8	3.4	0.0	0.4
Cobs, Baby, Boiled, Unsalted, Budgens*	1 Serving/150g	36	24	2.5	2.6	0.4	2.0
Cobs, Baby, Green Giant*	1 Serving/62g	16	26	2.9	2.4	0.5	1.9
Cobs, Baby, Sainsbury's*	1 Serving/68g	16	24	2.5	2.5	0.4	2.0
Creamed, Green Giant*	1 Can/418g	238	57	1.2	11.9	0.5	3.0
On The Cob, Kentucky Fried Chicken*	1 Cob/162g	150	93	3.0	21.6	0.9	1.2
On The Cob, Mini, Fresh Frozen, Tesco*	1 Cob/112g	77	69	2.5	11.6	1.4	1.3
On The Cob, Mini, Sainsbury's*	1oz/28g	20	72	2.6	12.2	1.4	1.4
On The Cob, Mini, Tesco*	1 Serving/75g	40	53	1.9	9.1	1.0	0.9
On The Cob, Prepared, Marks & Spencer*	1 Cob/175g	95	54	2.0	9.9	1.0	0.9
On The Cob, Supersweet, Marks & Spencer*	1 Serving/160g	88	55	2.0	9.9	1.0	0.9
On The Cob, Supersweet, Tesco*	1 Cob/250g	143	57	2.0	9.9	1.0	0.9
On The Cob, Whole, Boiled in Salted Water	1oz/28g	18	66	2.5	11.6	1.4	1.3
On The Cob, Whole, Boiled in Unsalted Water	1oz/28g	18	66	2.5	11.6	1.4	1.3
On The Cob, Whole, Raw	1oz/28g	15	54	2.0	9.9	1.0	0.9
Whole Kernel, Del Monte*	½ Can/125g	60	48	1.6	8.8	0.8	2.4
CORN SNACKS, Paprika Flavour, Shapers, Boots*	1 Pack/13g	64	494	8.7	54.0	27.0	2.2
CORNED BEEF,							
100%, Hydale, Aldi*	1 Serving/100g	217	217	26.9	0.0	14.0	0.0
Asda*	1 Slice/31g	68	218	26.4	0.2	12.4	0.0
BGTY, Saisnbury's*	1 Serving/100g	184	184	26.8	1.2	8.0	0.1
Fray Bentos*	1 Serving/115g	251	218	25.4	0.8	12.6	0.0
John West*	1oz/28g	62	221	25.0	1.0	13.0	0.0
Lean, Marks & Spencer*	1oz/28g	59	210	26.0	1.5	11.0	0.0
Lean, Princes*	½ Can/100g	194	194	25.0	1.0	10.0	0.0
Lean, Traditional, Marks & Spencer*	1 Slice/44g	86	195	29.3	0.9	8.0	0.0
Premium, Sainsbury's*	1oz/28g	58	208	26.8	1.2	10.7	0.1
Premium, Sliced, Sainsbury's*	1 Slice/42g	90	214	27.3	0.5	11.4	0.1
Princes*	1 Can/200g	446	223	24.8	0.5	13.5	0.0
Sliced, Somerfield*	1 Slice/27.9g	64	229	26.7	0.5	13.4	0.0
Slices, Economy, Sainsbury's*	1 Slice/37g	87	236	26.5	1.0	14.0	0.1
Slices, Value, Tesco*	1 Slice/31g	62	201	26.2	0.1	10.6	0.0
SmartPrice, Asda*	1oz/28g	64	228	25.0	0.4	14.0	0.0
Tesco*	1 Serving/175g	352	201	26.0	0.5	10.6	0.0
Thin Sliced, Asda*	1oz/28g	60	213	26.0	0.2	12.0	0.0
Value, Tesco*	1oz/28g	63	225	24.8	1.0	13.5	0.0
CORNFLOUR,							
Average	1oz/28g	99	354	0.6	92.0	0.7	0.1
Bestfoods*	1oz/28g	96	343	0.6	83.6	0.7	0.1
COURGETTE,							
& Sweetcorn, Fresh 'n' Ready, Sainsbury's*	1oz/28g	12	42	2.3	6.7	0.9	1.3
Baby, Tesco*	1 Serving/100g	18	18	1.8	1.8	0.4	0.9
Boiled in Unsalted Water	1oz/28g	5	19	2.0	2.0	0.4	1.2
Fried in Blended Oil	1oz/28g	18	63	2.6	2.6	4.8	1.2
Fried in Butter	1oz/28g	18	63	2.6	2.6	4.8	1.2
Raw	1 Sm/60g	11	18	1.8	1.8	0.4	0.9
COUS COUS,							
& Chargrilled Vegetables, Marks & Spencer*	1 Serving/200g	200	100	3.9	17.3	1.5	1.6
& Wok Oriental, Findus*	½ Pack/300g	510	170	4.5	19.0	8.5	0.0
Average	1oz/28g	64	227	5.7	51.3	1.0	0.0
Chargrilled Red & Yellow Pepper, Tesco*	1 Pack/200g	212	106	4.6	17.8	1.8	0.5
Chargrilled Vegetables & Olive Oil, Delphi*	½ Pot/75g	105	140	3.8	22.5	3.9	1.9
Citrus Kick, Ainsley Harriott*	½ Pack/134.3g	184	137	4.3	28.5	0.6	2.4

COUS COUS,

	Measure INFO/WEIGHT	per Measure KCAL	KCAL	PROT	CARB	FAT	FIBRE
Cooked, Sainsbury's*	1 Serving/75g	177	236	8.0	38.8	5.4	2.8
Coriander & Lemon, Good For You, Asda*	½ Pack/145g	189	130	4.2	27.0	0.6	1.8
Coriander & Lemon, Sainsbury's*	½ Pack/165g	200	121	4.8	23.5	0.7	0.8
Garlic & Coriander, Waitrose*	1 Serving/70g	235	336	11.7	64.2	3.6	6.2
Indian Style, Sainsbury's*	½ Pack/143g	204	143	4.5	25.1	2.7	1.0
Lemon & Coriander, Tesco*	1 Serving/137g	207	151	4.0	28.3	2.4	2.0
Made Up, Asda*	1oz/28g	43	155	4.2	21.4	5.8	2.4
Mediterranean Style, Tesco*	1 Pack/110g	369	335	11.9	65.1	3.0	5.6
Mediterranean Tomato, GFY, Asda*	½ Pack/141g	192	136	5.0	27.0	0.9	1.7
Moroccan Style, Sainsbury's*	½ Pack/150g	195	130	5.0	21.5	2.7	1.0
Moroccan Sultana & Pine Nuts, Sammy's*	1 Serving/50g	172	343	12.0	72.0	3.0	6.0
Mushroom, Morrisons*	1 Serving/100g	164	164	5.7	28.7	3.0	1.7
Mushrooms, Onion, Garlic & Herbs, Tesco*	½ Pack/50g	167	333	11.3	66.2	2.6	4.9
Plain, Dry Weight, Tesco*	1oz/28g	102	363	15.1	73.1	1.1	0.8
Plain, Organic, Crazy Jack*	1 Serving/50g	178	355	13.5	72.5	1.9	0.0
Red Pepper & Chilli, Waitrose*	1 Pack/200g	344	172	4.5	23.0	6.9	1.3
Roast Garlic & Olive Oil, Sammy's*	1 Serving/49.9g	170	339	12.0	71.5	3.0	0.0
Roasted Vegetable, Finest, Tesco*	1 Serving/175g	263	150	4.0	17.4	7.1	1.3
Roasted Vegetables, Waitrose*	1 Serving/200g	324	162	5.2	22.4	5.7	0.0
Salad Bar, BGTY, Sainsbury's*	1 Md Bowl/28g	29	103	3.7	18.5	1.6	0.0
Spice Sensation, Ainsley Harriott*	½ Pack/50g	62	123	4.3	24.5	0.9	3.4
Spicy Moroccan Chicken & Veg, COU, Marks & Spencer*	1 Pack/400g	380	95	9.1	10.3	1.7	1.9
Spicy Vegetable, GFY, Asda*	½ Pack/141g	183	130	5.0	25.0	1.1	2.0
Spicy Vegetable, Morrisons*	1 Serving/50g	85	170	5.1	26.2	5.0	2.9
Spicy, Healthy Eating, Tesco*	1 Pot/250g	325	130	3.6	25.1	1.7	0.6
Sun Dried Tomato, Somerfield*	1 Jar/110g	176	160	3.0	25.0	5.0	0.0
Tomato & Onion, Waitrose*	½ Pack/55g	188	342	12.6	64.9	3.6	5.1
Tomato & Vegetable, Snack Pack, Sammy's*	1 Serving/70g	228	326	12.0	67.9	3.5	6.3
Tomato tango, Ainsley Harriott*	½ Pack/132.8g	166	125	4.6	25.3	0.6	3.3
Wild Mushroom & Garlic, Sainsbury's*	1 Serving/166g	239	144	4.2	22.9	4.0	0.6
With Lemon & Garlic, Waitrose*	½ Pack/55g	188	341	11.8	65.5	3.3	4.5
Zesty Lemon & Coriander, Sammy's*	1 Serving/50g	171	342	13.0	74.0	2.8	6.0

CRAB,

	Measure INFO/WEIGHT	per Measure KCAL	KCAL	PROT	CARB	FAT	FIBRE
Boiled	1oz/28g	36	128	19.5	0.0	5.5	0.0
8Cakes, Goan, Marks & Spencer*	1 Pack/190g	228	120	8.0	12.9	4.0	1.8
Cakes, Iceland*	1 Serving/18g	52	288	7.2	25.6	18.0	1.3
Cakes, Tesco*	1 Serving/130g	281	216	11.0	15.4	12.3	1.1
Canned In Brine, Sainsbury's*	½ Can/60g	46	77	18.1	0.1	0.5	0.1
Canned in Brine, Drained	1 Sm Can/85g	65	77	18.1	0.0	0.5	0.0
Claws, Asda*	1oz/28g	25	89	11.0	9.0	1.0	0.2
Cocktail, Waitrose*	1 Serving/100g	217	217	10.8	3.8	17.6	0.4
Dressed Layered, Marks & Spencer*	½ Pack/100g	150	150	15.0	1.7	9.2	0.6
Dressed, In Shell, Asda*	1 Crab/142g	64	45	6.8	0.0	1.9	0.0
Dressed, John West*	1 Can/43g	61	143	18.0	2.0	7.0	0.0
Meat White, Raw*	1 Serving/50g	50	100	20.8	2.8	0.6	0.0
Meat, Orkney, Marks & Spencer*	1 Pack/100g	100	100	20.8	2.8	0.6	0.0
Meat, White, In Brine, Drained, Marks & Spencer*	1 Serving/61g	45	74	15.0	2.7	0.4	0.5
Meat, White, In Brine, Glenryck*	1 Can/122g	96	79	16.7	2.0	0.5	0.0
Meat, White, In Brine, John West*	½ Can/60g	43	72	17.0	0.7	0.1	0.0
Orkney, Dressed in Shell, Marks & Spencer*	½ Pack/62.5g	107	170	17.5	8.6	7.6	0.1
Sticks, Average	1oz/28g	19	68	10.0	6.6	0.4	0.0
Sticks, Sainsbury's*	1 Stick/16g	18	113	7.0	21.0	0.1	0.1
Sticks, Sealord*	1 Serving/16g	15	94	10.0	11.9	0.6	0.0

	Measure INFO/WEIGHT	per Measure KCAL	Nutrition Values per 100g / 100ml				
			KCAL	PROT	CARB	FAT	FIBRE
CRACKERBREAD,							
Golden Wheat, Ryvita*	1 Slice/6g	19	317	8.3	65.0	3.3	3.3
High Fibre, Ryvita*	1oz/28g	89	318	12.6	60.5	2.8	16.8
Wheat, Original, Ryvita*	1oz/28g	107	383	9.8	79.3	3.0	2.6
Wholemeal, Ryvita*	1 Slice/5.6g	19	319	10.8	71.5	4.2	6.5
CRACKERS,							
99% Fat Free, Rakusen's*	1 Cracker/5g	18	366	10.9	88.9	0.9	0.0
99% Fat Free, Snax, Rakusen's*	1 Cracker/1.7g	8	385	9.4	84.5	1.0	0.0
Bath Oliver, Jacob's*	1 Cracker/12g	52	432	9.6	67.6	13.7	2.6
Biscuits For Cheese, TTD, Sainsbury's*	1 Cracker/8g	39	493	8.6	61.0	23.8	3.1
Black Olive, Marks & Spencer*	1 Cracker/4.1g	19	485	8.3	59.4	23.5	4.3
Blazing BBQ, JacoBites, Jacob's*	1 Pack/9g	41	461	5.2	55.8	24.2	1.7
Bran, Jacob's*	1 Cracker/7g	32	454	9.7	62.8	18.2	3.2
Cheddars, McVitie's*	1 Cracker/4g	22	543	10.0	55.1	31.3	2.6
Cheese Biscuit Thins, Safeway*	1 Cracker/4g	22	545	11.9	52.6	31.9	2.5
Cheese Melts, Carr's*	1 Cracker/4g	19	468	9.4	58.0	22.1	3.0
Cheese Thins, Asda*	1 Cracker/4g	21	532	12.0	49.0	32.0	0.0
Cheese Thins, Co-Op*	1 Cracker/4g	21	530	12.0	49.0	32.0	3.0
Chinese, Pop Pan*	2 Crackers/15g	80	533	13.3	53.3	33.3	0.0
Chives, Jacob's*	1 Cracker/6.1g	27	457	9.5	67.5	16.5	2.7
Choice Grain, Jacob's*	1 Cracker/7g	30	435	9.2	65.4	15.2	4.7
Corn Thins, 97% Fat Free, Real Foods*	1 Cracker/6g	19	378	10.2	81.7	3.0	8.6
Cornish Wafer, Jacob's*	1 Cracker/9g	48	528	8.0	54.4	31.2	2.4
Cream	1 Cracker/7g	31	440	9.5	68.3	16.3	2.2
Cream With Flaked Salt, TTD, Sainsbury's*	1 Cracker/7.4g	35	500	8.5	64.8	22.9	2.7
Cream, Asda*	1 Cracker/8g	35	443	10.0	67.0	15.0	0.0
Cream, BGTY, Sainsbury's*	1 Cracker/8g	32	400	10.9	71.7	7.7	3.1
Cream, Better For You, Morrisons*	1 Cracker/8g	32	406	10.9	74.4	7.2	2.8
Cream, Biscuits For Cheese, Tesco*	1 Cracker/8g	35	438	10.2	66.7	14.5	2.8
Cream, Half Fat, Safeway*	1 Cracker/8g	32	406	74.4	2.4	7.2	2.9
Cream, Jacob's*	1 Cracker/8g	35	438	10.2	66.9	14.4	2.9
Cream, Lower Fat, Tesco*	1 Cracker/5g	20	393	11.0	72.4	6.6	3.1
Cream, Roasted Onion, Jacob's*	1 Cracker/8g	35	441	10.2	66.8	14.8	2.9
Cream, Sainsbury's*	1 Cracker/8.3g	34	422	9.5	66.7	15.2	2.8
Cream, Sun Dried Tomato Flavour, Jacob's*	1 Cracker/8g	35	434	10.2	66.7	14.0	3.0
Cream, Tesco*	1 Cracker/5g	22	444	8.4	70.0	14.5	3.1
Harvest Grain, Sainsbury's*	1 Cracker/6g	27	458	8.5	64.5	18.4	4.1
Herb & Onion, 99% Fat Free, Rakusen's*	1 Cracker/4g	14	361	10.0	78.0	1.0	0.0
Herb & Onion, Trufree*	1 Cracker/6g	25	418	2.5	75.0	12.0	10.0
Herb & Spice, Jacob's*	1 Cracker/6g	27	457	9.5	67.5	16.5	2.7
Herbs & Spice Selection, Jacob's*	1 Cracker/6g	27	451	9.5	68.0	15.7	2.7
Hovis, Jacob's*	1 Cracker/6g	27	447	10.2	60.0	18.5	4.4
Krackawheat, McVitie's*	1 Cracker/7g	36	515	9.1	62.4	25.4	4.8
Light & Crispy, Sainsbury's*	1 Cracker/11g	42	384	11.3	61.0	10.5	13.0
Lightly Salted, Italian, Jacob's*	1 Cracker/6g	26	429	10.3	67.6	13.0	2.9
Matzo, Rakusen's*	1 Cracker/4g	15	370	8.8	80.2	1.5	4.0
Mediterranean, Jacob's*	1 Cracker/6g	27	450	9.7	66.5	16.1	2.7
Melts, Carr's*	1 Cracker/4g	18	451	10.2	57.0	20.2	5.0
Multigrain, Tesco*	1 Cracker/6g	27	458	8.5	64.5	18.4	4.1
Olive Oil & Oregano, Italian, Jacob's*	1 Cracker/6g	26	437	10.3	66.3	14.5	4.0
Oriental Style, Safeway*	1 Serving/25g	88	350	1.5	82.2	1.2	6.2
Oriental, Asda*	1 Serving/30g	146	485	1.0	62.0	26.0	3.5
Passionately Pizza, JacoBites, Jacob's*	1 Pack/150g	708	472	5.7	55.3	25.4	1.7
Pesto, Jacob's*	1 Cracker/6g	27	450	9.7	66.5	16.1	2.7

C

	Measure INFO/WEIGHT	per Measure KCAL	Nutrition Values per 100g / 100ml				
			KCAL	PROT	CARB	FAT	FIBRE
CRACKERS,							
Ritz, Original, Jacob's*	1 Cracker/3g	15	509	6.9	55.6	28.8	2.0
Rye, Organic, Doves Farm*	1 Cracker/7.1g	28	393	7.0	58.4	14.6	8.7
Salt & Black Pepper, Jacob's*	1 Cracker/6g	27	457	9.5	67.5	16.5	2.7
Sesame & Poppy, Tesco*	1 Cracker/3g	15	506	9.4	53.7	28.2	3.4
Spicy Indonesian Vegetable, Waitrose*	1 Pack/60g	295	492	1.2	60.6	27.2	2.2
Spicy Vegetable, Tesco*	1 Serving/60g	340	566	2.6	52.4	38.4	1.2
Tangy Malaysian Chutney, Oriental, Sensations, Walkers*	1 Serving/35g	170	485	0.9	62.0	26.0	3.5
Tempting Tandoori, JacoBites, Jacob's*	1 Pack/150g	711	474	5.7	55.5	25.5	1.7
Tuc, Jacob's*	1 Cracker/4.5g	23	512	7.8	57.7	27.8	2.1
Tuc, McVitie's*	1 Cracker/4g	21	530	7.8	62.2	27.8	2.1
Wheaten, Marks & Spencer*	1oz/28g	129	460	11.0	54.0	22.0	5.0
Wholemeal, Tesco*	1 Cracker/7g	29	414	9.4	60.6	14.9	10.4
Wholmeal, Organic, Nairn's*	1 Cracker/14g	58	413	9.0	61.4	14.6	8.7
CRANBERRIES,							
Dried, Sainsbury's*	1 Pack/75g	253	337	0.1	81.1	1.4	5.1
Fresh, Raw	1oz/28g	4	15	0.4	3.4	0.1	3.0
CRANBERRY &							
Apple Juice Drink, Ocean Spray*	1 Glass/200ml	92	46	0.0	11.1	0.0	0.0
& Blackberry Juice, Ocean Spray*	1 Glass/250ml	120	48	0.1	11.3	0.1	0.2
& Blackcurrant Juice Drink, Ocean Spray*	1 Bottle/500ml	265	53	0.2	12.7	0.0	0.0
& Lime Juice Drink, Ocean Spray*	1 Glass/250ml	140	56	0.1	13.2	0.0	0.0
& Orange Juice Drink, Healthy Eating, Tesco*	1 Glass/200ml	10	5	0.0	0.8	0.0	0.0
& Passion Fruit Juice Drink, Ocean Spray*	1 Glass/250ml	135	54	0.1	12.8	0.0	0.0
& Raspberry Juice, Low Sugar, Sainsbury's*	1 Glass/250ml	10	4	0.1	0.7	0.1	0.1
& Raspberry Juice, Ocean Spray*	1 Glass/200ml	104	52	0.0	12.7	0.0	0.0
& Raspberry Juice Drink, Asda*	1 Glass/250ml	135	54	0.2	13.0	0.0	0.0
CRANBERRY CLASSIC Light, Ocean Spray*	1 Glass/200ml	48	24	0.0	5.6	0.0	0.0
CRANBERRY GRAPE & Apple Juice, Ocean Spray*	1 Glass/200ml	108	54	0.1	12.9	0.0	0.0
CRANBERRY JUICE,							
Low Sugar, Sainsbury's*	1 Glass/200ml	10	5	0.1	0.9	0.1	0.1
Marks & Spencer*	1 Glass/200ml	120	60	0.0	14.5	0.0	0.0
No Added Sugar, Asda*	1 Glass/200ml	12	6	0.1	0.8	0.0	0.0
Sainsbury's*	1 Bottle/250ml	133	53	0.2	12.8	0.1	0.4
Solevita, Lidl*	1 Glass/250ml	123	49	0.0	11.7	0.0	0.0
CRANBERRY JUICE DRINK,							
Classic, Ocean Spray*	1 Glass/200ml	98	49	0.0	11.7	0.0	0.0
Del Rivo, Aldi*	1 Glass/100ml	40	40	0.0	9.6	0.0	0.0
Light, Classic, Ocean Spray*	1 Glass/200ml	48	24	0.0	6.0	0.0	0.0
Morrisons*	1 Glass/200ml	92	46	0.0	11.6	0.0	0.0
No Added Sugar, Tesco*	1 Glass/200ml	8	4	0.0	0.7	0.0	0.0
Tesco*	1 Glass/200ml	100	50	0.0	12.0	0.0	0.0
Tropical, Ocean Spray*	1 Glass/200ml	96	48	0.1	11.5	0.0	0.0
CRAYFISH, Raw	1oz/28g	19	67	14.9	0.0	0.8	0.0
CREAM,							
Aerosol, Elmlea*	1oz/28g	71	253	1.5	6.3	24.8	0.0
Aerosol, Marks & Spencer*	1fl oz/30ml	110	365	2.0	6.1	37.0	0.0
Clotted, Fresh, Waitrose*	1 Serving/28g	157	560	1.5	2.5	60.5	0.0
Dairy, UHT Sweetened, Reduced Fat, Tesco*	1 Tbsp/15g	36	240	2.5	11.2	20.6	0.0
Double, Asda*	1 Tbsp/13g	58	449	1.7	2.6	48.0	0.0
Double, Elmlea*	1 Serving/25ml	87	349	2.4	3.9	36.0	0.3
Double, Fresh, Marks & Spencer*	1 Tbsp/15ml	67	445	1.7	2.6	47.5	0.0
Double, Fresh, Sainsbury's*	1 Tbsp/15ml	67	445	1.7	2.6	47.5	0.0
Double, Pasturised, Somerfield*	1 Serving/30g	134	445	1.7	2.6	47.5	0.0

C

	Measure INFO/WEIGHT	per Measure KCAL	Nutrition Values per 100g / 100ml				
			KCAL	PROT	CARB	FAT	FIBRE
CREAM,							
Double, Tesco*	1 Tbsp/15ml	68	450	1.7	2.7	48.0	0.0
Extra Thick Double, Tesco*	1 Tbsp/15ml	68	450	1.7	2.7	48.0	0.0
Extra Thick, Canned, Sterilised, Nestle*	1 Tbsp/50g	117	233	2.6	3.6	23.1	0.0
Extra Thick, Reduced Fat, Waitrose*	1 Serving/30ml	73	242	2.5	3.9	24.1	0.0
For Coffee, UHT, Kerrygold*	1 Tbsp/15ml	29	190	2.7	3.9	18.3	0.0
Fresh Double, Waitrose*	1 Tbsp/15ml	67	445	1.7	2.6	47.5	0.0
Fresh Pasteurised Soured, Co-Op*	1 Tbsp/15ml	28	188	2.6	3.9	18.0	0.0
Fresh Single, Extra Thick, Marks & Spencer*	1 Tbsp/15ml	34	227	2.8	3.3	22.5	0.0
Fresh, Clotted	1 Tbsp/15ml	88	586	1.6	2.3	63.5	0.0
Fresh, Double	1 Tbsp/15ml	67	449	1.7	2.7	48.0	0.0
Fresh, Single	1 Tbsp/15ml	30	198	2.6	4.1	19.1	0.0
Fresh, Soured	1 Tbsp/15ml	31	205	2.9	3.8	19.9	0.0
Fresh, Whipping	1 Tbsp/15ml	56	373	2.0	3.1	39.3	0.0
Half Fat, Thick, Marks & Spencer*	1 Tbsp/15ml	36	241	2.9	3.4	24.0	0.0
Light Double, Elmlea*	1 Tbsp/15ml	37	248	2.8	4.1	24.5	0.3
Light Single, Elmlea*	1 Tbsp/15ml	19	124	3.1	6.4	9.5	0.3
Light Whipping, Elmlea*	1 Tbsp/15ml	30	197	3.1	4.6	18.5	0.2
Light, Real Dairy Aerosol, Anchor*	1 Serving/55ml	25	45	0.6	1.8	3.9	0.0
Pasteurised Double, Morrisons*	1 Serving/50g	225	449	1.7	2.6	48.0	0.0
Pasteurised Single, Fresh, Tesco*	1 Sm Pot/142ml	283	199	2.6	4.1	19.1	0.0
Portion, UHT, Kerrygold*	1 Portion/14g	27	196	2.6	4.0	19.0	0.0
Single, British, Asda*	1 Serving/37.5ml	71	188	2.6	3.9	18.0	0.0
Single, Elmlea*	1 Tbsp/15ml	22	148	3.1	4.6	13.0	0.2
Single, Extra Thick, Waitrose*	1 Serving/50ml	94	188	2.6	3.9	18.0	0.0
Single, Fresh, Sainsbury's*	1 Tbsp/15ml	28	188	2.6	3.9	18.0	0.0
Single, Reduced Fat, Waitrose*	1 Serving/20ml	28	140	3.1	4.2	12.3	0.0
Soured, Fresh, Sainsbury's*	1 Tbsp/15ml	28	188	2.6	3.9	18.0	0.0
Soured, Tesco*	1Tbsp/15ml	28	188	2.6	3.9	18.0	0.0
Squirty, Anchor*	1 Squirt/20ml	16	79	0.5	1.4	8.0	0.0
Sterilised, Nestle*	1 Tbsp/15ml	35	233	2.6	3.6	23.1	0.0
Swirls Light, Half Fat, Anchor*	1 Serving/30ml	14	45	0.6	1.8	3.9	0.0
UHT, Canned Spray	1 Tbsp/15g	46	309	1.9	3.5	32.0	0.0
UHT, Single	1 Tbsp/15g	29	196	2.6	4.0	19.0	0.0
Whipping, Elmlea*	1 Tbsp/15ml	43	285	2.4	3.5	29.0	0.2
Whipping, Tesco*	1 Tbsp/15ml	56	374	1.9	3.1	39.3	0.0
CREAM SODA, Traditional Style, Tesco*	1 Can/330ml	139	42	0.0	10.4	0.0	0.0
CREMA CATALANA, Cafe Culture, Marks & Spencer*	1 Pot/110g	385	350	3.5	12.2	31.7	0.4
CREME BRULEE,							
Marks & Spencer*	1 Pot/100g	360	360	3.3	13.0	32.6	0.0
Nestle*	1 Serving/100g	305	305	4.0	14.6	25.6	0.0
Somerfield*	1 Pot/100g	316	316	4.0	15.0	27.0	0.0
CREME CARAMEL,							
Average	1oz/28g	31	109	3.0	20.6	2.2	0.0
Carmelle, Green's*	1 Pack/70g	82	117	3.0	17.0	4.0	0.0
La Laitiere*	1 Pot/100g	135	135	5.0	20.0	4.0	0.0
Marks & Spencer*	1oz/28g	48	172	4.5	18.9	8.7	0.0
Organic, Evernat*	1oz/28g	37	132	4.2	20.1	3.9	0.0
Sainsbury's*	1 Pot/100g	102	102	2.5	21.1	0.9	0.0
SmartPrice, Asda*	1 Pot/100g	102	102	2.5	21.0	0.9	0.0
Somerfield*	1 Pot/100g	114	114	3.0	24.0	1.0	0.0
Tesco*	1 Pot/100g	113	113	2.4	20.0	2.6	0.0
CREME COMPOSE, Strothmann*	1 Pot/150g	209	139	3.5	22.2	4.0	0.0
CREME EGG, Cadbury's	1 Egg/39g	174	445	4.0	70.8	15.9	0.0

	Measure INFO/WEIGHT	per Measure KCAL	Nutrition Values per 100g / 100ml				
			KCAL	PROT	CARB	FAT	FIBRE
CREME FRAICHE,							
BGTY, Sainsbury's*	1oz/28g	46	164	3.5	5.0	15.0	0.0
Better For You, Morrisons*	1 Serving/100ml	165	165	3.0	4.5	15.0	0.0
Epaisse, Langley Farm*	1 Pot/295g	870	295	3.0	2.6	30.0	0.0
Half Fat, Asda*	1 Serving/50g	87	173	4.9	4.6	15.0	0.0
Half Fat, Marks & Spencer*	1fl oz/30ml	60	200	4.3	3.5	18.7	0.0
Half Fat, Morrisons*	1 Serving/25g	42	169	3.0	4.4	15.2	0.0
Half Fat, Organic, Yeo Valley*	1 Pack/200g	356	178	2.1	3.1	17.6	0.0
Half Fat, Safeway*	1 Serving/200ml	330	165	2.7	5.8	14.5	0.0
Half Fat, Somerfield*	1fl oz/30ml	51	171	4.0	6.0	15.0	0.0
Half Fat, Spelga*	1 Serving/50g	103	205	3.5	5.5	19.0	0.0
Half Fat, Waitrose*	1fl oz/30ml	50	165	2.7	5.8	14.6	0.0
Healthy Choice, Safeway*	1fl oz/30ml	50	165	2.7	5.8	14.6	0.0
Healthy Eating, Tesco*	1fl oz/30ml	51	170	3.5	5.0	15.0	0.0
Light, Tine*	1 Carton/110g	223	203	2.6	3.2	20.0	0.0
Low Fat, Marks & Spencer*	1oz/28g	58	207	4.6	4.3	19.0	0.0
Somerfield*	1oz/28g	106	377	2.0	2.0	40.0	0.0
d'Isigny, Tesco*	1 Tbs/35g	133	380	2.3	2.8	40.0	0.0
CREPES,							
Lobster, Finest, Tesco*	1 Serving/160g	250	156	10.7	14.0	6.4	1.2
Mushroom, Marks & Spencer*	1 Pack/186g	195	105	5.7	17.1	2.4	2.5
CREVETTES, Asda*	1oz/28g	11	41	8.6	0.0	0.7	0.0
CRISPBAKES,							
Cheese & Chive, Sainsbury's*	1 Serving/108g	273	253	7.1	24.5	14.8	1.7
Cheese & Onion, Marks & Spencer*	1 Piece/114g	285	250	6.4	19.4	16.2	1.7
Cheese & Onion, Tesco*	1 Piece/109g	275	252	7.9	19.6	15.8	2.1
Chicken & Broccoli, Marks & Spencer*	1 Piece/114g	225	197	6.1	16.5	11.9	1.9
Dutch, Asda*	1 Toast/10g	39	394	14.0	77.0	3.3	3.9
Dutch, Safeway*	1 Bake/10g	39	394	14.0	77.0	3.3	3.9
Dutch, Tesco*	1 Slice/8g	30	371	17.0	72.0	1.7	4.0
Mushroom & Garlic, Ovenbaked, Iceland*	1 Piece/140g	241	172	4.3	23.7	6.7	2.9
Spinach, Feta & Soft Cheese, Mini, Safeway*	1 Pack/191.5g	449	235	6.6	20.8	13.4	2.5
Tuna & Sweetcorn, Lakeland*	1 Serving/170g	391	230	11.3	20.1	11.6	0.0
Vegetable, Marks & Spencer*	1 Piece/114.3g	160	140	2.8	14.9	7.7	1.8
Vegetable, Sainsbury's*	1 Serving/114g	246	216	2.0	26.2	11.4	2.0
CRISPBREAD,							
Corn, Orgran*	1 Crispbread/5g	18	360	7.5	83.0	1.8	3.0
Currant Crunch, Ryvita*	1oz/28g	94	334	8.7	69.9	2.5	12.8
Dark Rye, Ryvita*	1 Serving/9g	27	303	9.9	62.0	1.7	18.5
Emmental Cheese & Pumpkin Seed, Dr Karg*	1 Crispbread/25g	82	327	14.6	39.0	14.3	8.0
Harvest Wheat, Finn Crisp*	1 Serving/50g	195	390	10.0	72.0	6.7	5.8
Hi-Fibre Rye, Organic, Finn Crisp*	1 Piece/12.9g	40	310	9.8	63.0	1.8	16.0
Light, Marks & Spencer*	1 Crispbread/4g	14	360	11.4	71.8	5.0	5.2
Light, Ryvita*	1 Slice/5g	19	383	9.8	79.3	3.0	2.6
Multigrain, Ryvita*	1 Slice/11g	37	335	11.5	58.5	6.1	16.2
Organic, Trimlyne*	1 Crispbake/10g	38	380	16.0	73.0	2.3	6.0
Original, Rye, Trimlyne*	1 Crispbread/11g	36	325	10.3	65.4	2.5	12.8
Original, Ryvita*	1 Crispbread/9g	27	305	9.4	63.3	1.6	17.4
Pagen*	1 Crispbread/3g	11	370	12.0	65.0	7.0	9.5
Rye, Harvest Slims, Finn Crisp*	3 Slices/18g	58	320	11.0	63.0	2.3	16.0
Rye, Original, Ryvita*	1 Crispbread/9g	28	315	8.5	67.2	1.4	16.5
Sesame, Ryvita*	1oz/28g	95	339	10.5	58.5	7.0	16.0
Wasa*	1 Crispbread/11g	35	315	9.0	67.0	1.4	14.0
Wheat, Cracottes*	1 Slice/6.9g	26	367	9.8	75.2	3.0	3.2

	Measure INFO/WEIGHT	per Measure KCAL	Nutrition Values per 100g / 100ml				
			KCAL	PROT	CARB	FAT	FIBRE
CRISPBREAD,							
Wholegrain, Classic, Organic, Dr Karg*	1 Crispbread/25g	89	355	13.4	38.2	16.5	10.2
Wholemeal Rye, Kallo*	1 Crispbread/10g	31	314	9.7	65.0	1.7	15.4
Wholemeal, Light, Allinson*	1 Slice/5g	17	349	11.7	69.7	2.6	11.0
Wholemeal, Organic, Allinson*	1 Crispbread/5g	17	336	14.2	66.0	1.7	12.2
With Currants, Oats & Honey, Ryvita*	1 Crisp/14.8g	50	333	8.0	69.5	2.5	12.0
With Sesame, Spar*	1 Crispbread/15g	62	410	12.0	66.0	11.0	5.0
CRISPIES, Dairy Milk, Cadbury's*	1 Bar/49g	250	510	7.6	58.6	27.4	0.0
CRISPS,							
Apple, Thyme & Sage, Marks & Spencer*	1 Bag/55g	253	460	5.5	55.3	24.3	6.1
BBQ Chilli & Mesquite, Pan-Fried, TTD, Sainsbury's*	1 Sm Pack/50g	239	478	8.0	51.3	26.7	5.4
Bacon Bites, Eat Smart, Safeway*	1 Bag/12g	41	340	10.8	70.3	1.6	3.5
Bacon Crispies, Sainsbury's*	1 Bag/25g	117	468	19.9	45.8	22.8	4.8
Bacon Flavour Rashers, BGTY, Sainsbury's*	1 Pack/10g	34	340	10.8	70.3	1.6	3.5
Bacon Rashers, Blazin, Tesco*	1 Bag/25g	119	477	15.4	44.7	26.3	4.4
Bacon Rashers, COU, Marks & Spencer*	1 Bag/20g	72	360	9.4	77.5	2.9	3.5
Bacon Rashers, Marks & Spencer*	1 Bag/40g	192	480	8.1	59.9	22.9	2.2
Bacon Rice Bites, Asda*	1 Bag/30g	136	452	7.0	70.0	16.0	0.4
Bacon, Shapers, Boots*	1 Bag/23g	99	431	8.0	66.0	15.0	3.0
Bagels, Sour Cream & Chive, Shapers, Boots*	1 Bag/25g	94	377	9.7	78.0	2.9	1.9
Baked Beans, Walkers*	1 Bag/35g	184	525	6.5	50.0	33.0	4.0
Baked Potato, COU, Marks & Spencer*	1 Bag/25g	88	350	8.5	76.4	2.3	5.7
Barbecue, Handcooked, Tesco*	1 Bag/40g	187	468	6.6	53.8	25.1	5.2
Barbecue, Walkers*	1 Bag/35g	186	530	6.5	50.0	33.0	4.1
Beef & Onion, Asda*	1 Bag/25g	135	539	7.0	49.0	35.0	4.5
Beef & Onion, Potato, Marks & Spencer*	1 Bag/24.5g	133	530	6.6	48.2	34.5	5.0
Beef & Onion, Safeway*	1 Bag/25g	125	501	5.2	55.7	31.5	0.0
Beef & Onion, Walkers*	1 Bag/35g	186	530	6.5	50.0	33.0	4.1
Beefy, Smiths, Walkers*	1 Bag/25g	133	531	4.3	45.2	37.0	0.0
Butter & Chive, COU, Marks & Spencer*	1 Bag/26g	95	365	7.7	77.3	1.9	4.6
Caramalised Onion & Mature Cheddar Cheese, M&S*	1 Bag/40.4g	208	520	6.6	50.1	33.0	5.0
Chargrilled Chicken Crinkles, Shapers, Boots*	1 Bag/20g	96	482	6.6	60.0	24.0	4.0
Chargrilled Steak, Max, Walkers*	1 Bag/55g	289	525	6.5	50.0	33.0	4.0
Cheddar & Chive, Pret A Manger*	1 Bag/40g	187	468	7.0	53.8	24.8	6.0
Cheddar & Onion, Thick & Crunchy, McCoys*	1 Bag/49g	250	511	6.6	52.4	30.6	4.7
Cheese & Branston Pickle Flavour, Walkers*	1 Bag/34.5g	176	510	7.0	49.0	32.0	4.5
Cheese & Chive Flavour, Good For You, Asda*	1 Bag/25g	119	476	6.0	59.0	24.0	6.0
Cheese & Chives, Walkers*	1 Bag/35g	186	530	6.5	50.0	33.0	4.1
Cheese & Onion, Asda*	1 Bag/25g	133	530	6.0	50.0	34.0	4.5
Cheese & Onion, BGTY, Sainsbury's*	1 Bag/25g	120	479	7.0	57.0	24.8	5.7
Cheese & Onion, Big Eat, Walkers*	1 Bag/55g	289	525	6.5	50.0	33.0	4.0
Cheese & Onion, Flavour Crinkles, Shapers, Boots*	1 Bag/20g	96	482	6.6	60.0	24.0	4.0
Cheese & Onion, GFY, Asda*	1 Pack/26g	122	471	7.00	59.0	23.0	6.0
Cheese & Onion, Golden Wonder*	1 Bag/25g	131	524	6.1	49.2	33.6	2.0
Cheese & Onion, KP*	1 Bag/25g	134	534	6.6	48.7	34.8	4.8
Cheese & Onion, Lites, Walkers*	1 Bag/28g	130	465	7.5	61.0	21.0	4.0
Cheese & Onion, Lower Fat, Asda*	1 Bag/25g	120	481	6.0	58.0	25.0	4.8
Cheese & Onion, Marks & Spencer*	1 Bag/25g	134	535	5.5	48.8	35.5	5.0
Cheese & Onion, Max, Walkers*	1 Bag/55g	289	525	6.5	50.0	33.0	4.0
Cheese & Onion, McCoys*	1 Bag/35g	177	506	6.4	53.8	29.5	4.0
Cheese & Onion, Morrisons*	1 Bag/30g	152	508	7.1	50.5	30.8	4.6
Cheese & Onion, Organic, Tesco*	1 Bag/25g	129	514	5.2	49.9	32.6	7.0
Cheese & Onion, Potato Triangles, Waitrose*	1 Bag/20g	89	447	8.8	48.3	23.0	11.0
Cheese & Onion, Safeway*	1 Bag/25g	143	570	5.8	52.5	37.5	0.0

CRISPS,	INFO/WEIGHT	KCAL	KCAL	PROT	CARB	FAT	FIBRE
Cheese & Onion, Sainsbury's*	1 Bag/25g	132	527	4.6	48.8	34.8	3.9
Cheese & Onion, Select, Tesco*	1 Bag/25g	134	535	6.6	48.5	34.9	4.8
Cheese & Onion, Smiths, Walkers*	1 Bag/25g	133	531	4.3	45.2	37.0	0.0
Cheese & Onion, SnackRite*	1 Pack/25g	132	527	5.3	51.3	33.4	0.0
Cheese & Onion, Sprinter, Aldi*	1 Bag/25g	137	549	5.4	49.4	36.6	0.0
Cheese & Onion, Square, Smiths, Walkers*	1 Bag/25g	113	452	6.9	62.5	19.4	0.0
Cheese & Onion, Square, Walkers*	1 Bag/25g	106	425	6.5	59.0	18.0	4.4
Cheese & Onion, Tayto*	1 Bag/25g	137	546	5.8	53.7	34.2	0.0
Cheese & Onion, Value, Tesco*	1 Bag/20g	108	541	6.0	48.3	36.0	4.8
Cheese & Onion, Walkers*	1 Bag/35g	194	553	6.5	50.0	33.0	4.1
Cheese Curls, Asda*	1 Bag/14g	71	507	4.3	50.0	32.1	2.9
Cheese Curls, Shapers Boots*	1 Bag/13.9g	74	525	4.5	57.0	31.0	2.7
Cheese Curls, Sprinters, Aldi*	1 Bag/14g	68	483	4.1	56.4	26.8	0.0
Cheese Flavour Puffs, Morrisons*	1 Bag/25g	136	542	6.7	50.2	34.9	1.1
Cheese Tasters, Marks & Spencer*	1 Sm Bag/30g	156	520	8.5	51.0	31.0	3.2
Cheese XL, Golden Wonder*	1 Bag/30g	155	516	6.2	50.6	32.1	4.2
Cheesy Curls, Bobby's*	1 Bag/40g	225	563	7.6	50.1	36.9	0.0
Cheesy Puffs, Co-Op*	1 Bag/60g	321	535	3.0	54.0	34.0	2.0
Chicken & Thyme Flavour, Oven Roasted, Walkers*	1 Bag/40g	194	485	6.5	54.0	27.0	4.5
Chicken Flavour, Healthy Eating, Tesco*	1 Bag/12g	43	357	5.1	81.0	1.4	3.4
Chicken Tikka Masala, Great British Takeaways, Walkers*	1 Bag/25g	131	525	6.5	50.0	33.0	4.0
Chicken, Firecracker, McCoys*	1 Bag/35g	177	506	6.2	54.0	29.5	1.0
Chill, Coriander & Lime, Marks & Spencer*	1 Bag/40g	194	485	6.4	53.6	27.1	5.0
Chinese Spare Rib, Walkers*	1 Bag/25g	131	525	6.5	50.0	33.0	4.0
Chip Shop Curry, Max, Walkers*	1 Bag/55g	289	525	6.5	50.0	33.0	4.0
Cool Cheese Curly, Tesco*	1 Bag/14g	71	510	4.5	51.0	32.0	2.6
Cool Sour Cream & Chive Jacket, Half Fat, M&S*	1 Bag/40g	172	430	5.8	61.0	17.0	7.7
Coronation Chicken, Walkers*	1 Bag/25g	131	525	6.5	50.0	33.0	4.0
Cream Cheese & Cracked Peppercorn, Finest, Tesco*	1 Bag/150g	726	484	7.6	52.1	27.2	5.0
Creme Fraiche & Black Pepper, Crinkle, M&S*	1 Bag/24.7g	121	485	6.5	61.0	24.0	3.5
Crinkle Cut, Lower Fat, No Added Salt, Waitrose*	1 Bag/40g	193	483	6.5	58.0	25.0	3.9
Crispy Bacon Bites, Shapers, Boots*	1 Bag/21g	97	464	13.0	58.0	20.0	1.8
Double Cheddar & Chives, Deli Style, Brannigans*	1oz/28g	148	529	7.6	49.5	33.4	3.8
Flame Grilled Steak, Thick & Crunchy, McCoys*	1 Bag/50g	254	508	6.4	52.9	30.1	4.7
Four Cheese & Red Onion Sensations, Walkers*	1 Bag/40g	194	485	6.5	54.0	27.0	4.5
Garlic & Herbs Creme Fraiche, Kettle Chips*	1 Bag/50g	249	497	6.0	54.7	28.3	4.2
Golden Lights, Golden Wonder*	1 Bag/21g	91	435	5.4	64.5	17.2	0.0
Handcooked, Marks & Spencer*	1 Bag/40g	198	495	5.4	56.9	27.2	4.5
Honey Roast Ham, Marks & Spencer*	1 Bag/24.5g	133	530	6.6	49.0	34.1	4.6
Honey Roasted Ham, Sensations, Walkers*	1 Bag/40g	196	490	6.5	55.0	27.0	4.0
Hot & Spicy Salami, Tesco*	1 Bag/50g	216	431	26.2	0.7	35.9	0.0
Lamb & Mint, Sensations, Walkers*	1 Bag/35g	170	485	6.5	54.0	27.0	4.5
Lightly Salted Crinkle Cut Potato, Lower Fat, Waitrose*	1 Bag/40g	193	483	6.5	58.0	25.0	3.9
Lightly Salted, COU, Marks & Spencer*	1 Bag/26g	91	350	8.5	76.4	2.3	5.7
Lightly Salted, Golden Lights, Golden Wonder*	1 Bag/21g	92	440	5.1	64.3	18.0	4.3
Lightly Salted, Kettle Chips*	1 Bag/50g	124	247	6.4	51.5	3.0	6.0
Lightly Salted, Pret A Manger*	1 Bag/40g	198	495	5.8	58.0	28.5	4.3
Lightly Salted, Traditional Pan Fried, TTD, Sainsbury's*	1 Bag/50g	236	472	6.2	53.6	25.8	5.1
Lightly Sea Salted, Jonathan Crisp*	1 Bag/35g	176	503	6.5	52.0	29.0	5.4
Marmite Flavour, Walkers*	1 Bag/34.5g	176	510	6.5	49.0	32.0	4.0
Mediterranean Baked Potato, COU, Marks & Spencer*	1 Bag/26g	91	350	7.6	73.8	2.6	6.6
Merry Crispmas Turkey With Paxo Sage & Onion, Walkers*	1 Bag/34.5g	184	525	6.5	50.0	33.0	4.0
Mixed Pepper Flavour Burst, Marks & Spencer*	1 Bag/55g	286	520	6.0	50.1	33.5	4.0

CRISPS,

	Measure INFO/WEIGHT	per Measure KCAL	Nutrition Values per 100g / 100ml				
			KCAL	PROT	CARB	FAT	FIBRE
New York Cheddar, Kettle Chips*	1 Bag/50g	242	483	6.7	53.9	26.7	4.5
Nicely Spicy, Shots, Walkers*	1 Bag/18g	87	485	5.5	60.0	25.0	1.5
Oven Roasted Chicken & Thyme Sensations, Walkers*	1 Bag/40g	194	485	6.5	54.0	27.0	4.5
Paprika, Handcooked, Shapers, Boots*	1 Bag/20g	99	493	7.2	62.0	24.0	5.0
Paprika, Max, Walkers*	1 Bag/29g	152	525	6.5	50.0	33.0	4.0
Paprika, Mini Hoops, Shapers, Boots*	1 Bag/13.0g	64	494	8.7	54.0	27.0	2.2
Pastrami & Cheese, Crinkle, Marks & Spencer*	1 Bag/24.7g	121	485	6.5	61.0	24.0	3.5
Peking Spare Rib & Five Spice, Sensations, Walkers*	1 Bag/24g	116	485	1.3	62.0	26.0	3.5
Pickled Onion, Golden Wonder*	1 Bag/25g	131	524	5.6	49.0	34.0	2.0
Pickled Onion, Monster Bites, Sainsbury's*	1 Bag/20g	107	535	5.2	53.5	33.3	1.0
Pickled Onion, Pret A Manger*	1 Bag/40g	177	443	7.5	52.0	22.8	7.3
Pickled Onion, Walkers*	1 Bag/35g	186	530	6.5	50.0	33.0	4.1
Potato	1oz/28g	148	530	5.7	53.3	34.2	5.3
Potato, Low Fat	1oz/28g	128	458	6.6	63.5	21.5	5.9
Prawn Cocktail Flavour, Morrisons*	1 Bag/25g	132	528	8.0	48.8	32.8	5.2
Prawn Cocktail, Asda*	1 Bag/25g	134	535	6.0	49.0	35.0	4.3
Prawn Cocktail, BGTY, Sainsbury's*	1 Bag/25g	118	473	6.3	58.6	23.7	5.7
Prawn Cocktail, Golden Wonder*	1 Bag/25g	130	521	5.8	49.0	33.5	2.0
Prawn Cocktail, KP*	1 Bag/25g	133	531	5.9	48.4	34.9	4.7
Prawn Cocktail, Lites, Shapers, Boots*	1 Bag/21g	92	438	5.1	64.0	18.0	4.1
Prawn Cocktail, Sainsbury's*	1 Bag/25g	130	521	4.3	47.5	34.9	3.9
Prawn Cocktail, Seabrook*	1 Bag/31.8g	182	569	5.3	54.4	36.8	3.9
Prawn Cocktail, Select, Tesco*	1 Bag/25g	134	535	6.2	49.1	34.9	4.3
Prawn Cocktail, Smiths, Walkers*	1 Bag/25g	133	531	4.3	45.2	37.0	0.0
Prawn Cocktail, Walkers*	1 Bag/35g	186	530	6.5	50.0	33.0	4.1
Prawn Crackers, Tesco's*	1 Bag/60g	316	527	3.2	62.8	29.2	0.8
Punching Paprika, Max, Walkers*	1 Bag/55g	256	465	7.5	61.0	21.0	4.0
Ready Salted Crinkle, Reduced Fat, Marks & Spencer*	1 Bag/40g	190	475	6.5	58.0	24.0	6.5
Ready Salted, BGTY, Sainsbury's*	1 Bag/25g	122	486	6.8	55.7	26.2	6.6
Ready Salted, Betterbuy, Morrisons*	1 Bag/22g	118	538	6.5	49.3	35.0	4.2
Ready Salted, GFY, Asda*	1 Bag/25g	118	471	6.0	60.0	23.0	6.0
Ready Salted, Golden Lights, Golden Wonder*	1 Bag/21g	92	440	5.1	64.3	18.0	0.0
Ready Salted, Golden Wonder*	1 Bag/25g	135	539	5.5	49.9	35.3	2.0
Ready Salted, KP*	1 Bag/24g	131	545	5.6	47.9	36.8	4.9
Ready Salted, Lidl*	1 Bag/25g	139	554	4.9	50.3	37.0	0.0
Ready Salted, Lites, Walkers*	1 Bag/28g	132	470	7.5	60.0	22.0	4.0
Ready Salted, Lower Fat, Asda*	1 Bag/25g	120	481	6.0	58.0	25.0	4.8
Ready Salted, Lower Fat, Sainsbury's*	1 Bag/25g	111	444	7.0	55.0	21.8	5.1
Ready Salted, Made With Sunflower Oil, Walkers*	1 Bag/24g	113	470	7.5	60.0	22.0	5.0
Ready Salted, Marks & Spencer*	1 Bag/25g	136	545	5.6	47.8	36.6	4.9
Ready Salted, Organic, Tesco*	1 Bag/25g	130	520	4.3	49.0	34.1	7.3
Ready Salted, Potato Chips, Tesco*	1 Bag/25g	132	526	5.6	51.7	33.0	3.8
Ready Salted, Potato Squares, Sainsbury's*	1 Bag/50g	192	384	6.5	53.8	15.9	7.8
Ready Salted, Safeway*	1 Bag/25g	143	570	5.8	52.5	37.5	0.0
Ready Salted, Sainsbury's*	1 Bag/25g	135	538	4.3	47.4	36.8	4.1
Ready Salted, Select, Tesco*	1 Bag/25g	136	544	6.2	47.9	36.6	4.5
Ready Salted, SmartPrice, Asda*	1 Bag/20g	111	553	5.0	50.0	37.0	3.0
Ready Salted, Smiths, Walkers*	1 Bag/25g	133	531	4.3	45.2	37.0	0.0
Ready Salted, Square, Smiths, Walkers*	1 Bag/25g	113	452	6.9	62.5	19.4	0.0
Ready Salted, Squares, Marks & Spencer*	1 Bag/35g	151	430	6.8	63.5	18.1	3.9
Ready Salted, Thick & Crunchy, McCoys*	1 Bag/49g	253	517	6.0	52.3	31.5	4.9
Ready Salted, Value, Tesco*	1 Bag/21g	115	548	6.0	50.0	36.0	0.0
Ready Salted, Walkers*	1 Bag/35g	186	530	6.5	55.0	34.0	4.1

CRISPS,	Measure INFO/WEIGHT	per Measure KCAL	Nutrition Values per 100g / 100ml				
			KCAL	PROT	CARB	FAT	FIBRE
Red Leicester & Spring Onion, Marks & Spencer*	1 Bag/40g	194	485	6.2	58.7	27.2	4.9
Roast Beef & Mustard, Thick Cut, Brannigans*	1 Bag/40g	203	507	7.6	51.7	30.0	3.7
Roast Beef, KP*	1 Bag/25g	134	534	6.6	47.5	35.3	4.7
Roast Chicken & Sage Flavour, Marks & Spencer*	1 Bag/25g	135	540	5.9	50.6	34.6	4.6
Roast Chicken Flavour, BGTY, Sainsbury's*	1 Bag/25g	118	473	6.2	58.9	23.6	5.7
Roast Chicken Flavour, Budgens*	1 Bag/25g	129	516	7.3	47.6	33.0	3.6
Roast Chicken, Golden Wonder*	1 Bag/25g	131	522	6.2	48.6	33.6	2.0
Roast Chicken, Highlander*	1 Bag/25g	139	554	5.3	46.0	38.9	5.1
Roast Chicken, Select, Tesco*	1 Bag/25g	134	536	6.6	48.6	35.0	4.4
Roast Chicken, Smiths, Walkers*	1 Bag/25g	133	531	4.3	45.2	37.0	0.0
Roast Chicken, Walkers*	1 Bag/35g	184	525	6.5	50.0	33.0	4.0
Salsa With Mesquite, Kettle Chips*	1 Bag/50g	229	458	6.1	54.0	24.3	5.7
Salt & Balsamic Vinegar, Marks & Spencer*	1 Bag/40g	192	480	6.2	52.5	27.6	5.3
Salt & Black Pepper, Handcooked, Marks & Spencer*	1 Bag/40g	180	450	5.7	55.0	22.9	5.2
Salt & Malt Vinegar Flavour, Sainsbury's*	1 Bag/25g	135	538	4.9	50.3	35.2	2.3
Salt & Malt Vinegar, Thick & Crunchy, McCoys*	1 Bag/50g	253	506	6.5	52.6	30.0	4.7
Salt & Shake, Walkers*	1 Bag/24g	127	530	6.5	49.0	34.0	4.5
Salt & Vinegar Flavour Crinkles, Reduced Fat, Boots*	1 Bag/35g	165	471	7.1	59.0	23.0	3.0
Salt & Vinegar Flavour, Asda*	1 Bag/25g	133	530	6.0	50.0	34.0	4.5
Salt & Vinegar Flavour, Half Fat, Marks & Spencer*	1 Bag/40g	168	420	5.8	61.0	17.0	7.7
Salt & Vinegar Flavour, Sprinters*	1 Bag/25g	133	532	4.8	49.1	35.2	0.0
Salt & Vinegar, BGTY, Sainsbury's*	1 Bag/25g	121	482	6.5	57.3	25.2	5.2
Salt & Vinegar, Big Eat, Walkers*	1 Bag/55.0g	289	525	6.5	50.0	33.0	4.0
Salt & Vinegar, Crinkle Cut, Seabrook*	1 Bag/31.8g	182	569	5.4	54.4	36.7	3.9
Salt & Vinegar, Everyday, Co-Op*	1 Bag/17g	77	455	6.0	62.0	20.0	2.0
Salt & Vinegar, Fish Shapes, Food Explorers, Waitrose*	1 Bag/20g	86	430	2.4	69.1	16.0	1.3
Salt & Vinegar, Golden Lights, Golden Wonder*	1 Bag/21g	91	435	4.9	64.1	17.8	4.3
Salt & Vinegar, Golden Wonder*	1 Bag/25g	131	522	5.4	48.5	34.0	2.0
Salt & Vinegar, Good For You, Asda*	1 Bag/25.7g	121	467	6.0	59.0	23.0	10.0
Salt & Vinegar, Healthy Eating, Tesco*	1 Bag/17g	61	357	3.2	82.4	1.6	3.0
Salt & Vinegar, KP*	1 Bag/25g	133	532	5.5	48.7	35.0	4.7
Salt & Vinegar, Lites, Walkers*	1 Bag/28g	130	465	7.5	61.0	21.0	4.0
Salt & Vinegar, Lower Fat, Asda*	1 Bag/25g	120	481	5.0	58.0	25.0	4.8
Salt & Vinegar, Marks & Spencer*	1 Bag/25g	131	525	5.4	48.8	34.5	4.6
Salt & Vinegar, Max, Walkers*	1 Bag/55g	289	525	6.5	50.0	33.0	4.0
Salt & Vinegar, Morrisons*	1 Bag/25g	124	497	7.2	48.7	30.4	4.5
Salt & Vinegar, Potato Twirls, Co-Op*	1 Bag/40g	170	425	5.0	57.5	20.0	5.0
Salt & Vinegar, Pret A Manger*	1 Bag/40g	186	465	6.8	55.0	25.3	6.0
Salt & Vinegar, Red Mill*	1 Bag/40g	174	436	3.9	65.8	17.5	2.4
Salt & Vinegar, Reduced Fat, Marks & Spencer*	1 Bag/40g	190	475	7.0	58.0	24.0	6.5
Salt & Vinegar, Sainsbury's*	1 Bag/25g	131	522	4.1	46.9	35.3	3.9
Salt & Vinegar, Select, Tesco*	1 Bag/25g	132	529	5.9	47.8	34.9	4.3
Salt & Vinegar, Simply, Kwik Save*	1 Bag/20g	106	531	5.1	47.5	35.6	4.2
Salt & Vinegar, Smiths, Walkers*	1 Bag/25g	133	531	4.3	45.2	37.0	0.0
Salt & Vinegar, Square, Smiths, Walkers*	1 Bag/25g	113	452	6.9	62.5	19.4	0.0
Salt & Vinegar, Square, Walkers*	1 Bag/25g	105	420	6.0	58.0	18.0	4.5
Salt & Vinegar, Value, Tesco*	1 Bag/20g	109	547	5.7	47.7	37.0	4.8
Salt & Vinegar, Walkers*	1 Bag/35g	186	530	6.5	50.0	33.0	4.1
Salt'n'Shake, Smiths, Walkers*	1 Bag/25g	136	543	4.1	44.2	38.9	0.0
Salted Tubes, Shapers, Boots*	1 Bag/15g	67	448	5.1	62.0	20.0	3.6
Screaming Salt & Vinegar, Max, Walkers*	1 Bag/55g	256	465	7.5	61.0	21.0	4.0
Sea Salt & Balsamic Vinegar, Kettle Chips*	1 Bag/50g	234	468	5.6	60.9	24.4	4.4
Sea Salt & Black Pepper, Good For You, Asda*	1 Bag/100g	476	476	6.0	59.0	24.0	6.0

	Measure INFO/WEIGHT	per Measure KCAL	KCAL	PROT	CARB	FAT	FIBRE
CRISPS,							
Sea Salt & Black Pepper, Pret A Manger*	1 Bag/40g	180	450	5.8	55.0	23.0	5.3
Sea Salt & Black Pepper, Shapers, Boots*	1 Bag/19.9g	96	482	6.6	60.0	24.0	4.0
Sea Salt & Cracked Black Pepper, Sensations, Walkers*	1 Bag/40g	194	485	6.5	54.0	27.0	4.5
Sea Salt & Malt Vinegar, Sensations, Walkers*	1 Bag/40g	194	485	6.5	54.0	27.0	4.5
Sea Salt & Vinegar, Mini Bagels, Shapers, Boots*	1 Bag/25g	95	378	11.0	77.0	2.9	3.1
Sea Salt With Crushed Black Peppercorns, Kettle Chips*	1 Bag/50g	225	449	5.7	55.0	22.9	5.2
Sea Salt, Original, Crinkle Cut, Seabrook*	1 Bag/31.8g	182	569	5.4	54.4	36.7	3.9
Sizzling Beef, Spice, McCoys*	1 Bag/35g	175	501	6.4	51.7	29.8	4.0
Smoked Ham & Pickle, Thick Cut, Brannigans*	1 Bag/40g	203	507	7.0	52.8	29.8	3.8
Smokey Bacon, Budgens*	1 Bag/25g	130	519	6.2	49.3	33.0	4.8
Smokey Bacon, Select, Tesco*	1 Bag/25g	134	536	6.4	49.0	34.9	4.3
Smokey Bacon, Smiths, Walkers*	1 Bag/25g	133	531	4.3	45.2	37.0	0.0
Smokey Bacon, Walkers*	1 Bag/34g	179	525	6.5	50.0	33.0	4.0
Smoky Bacon, Asda*	1 Bag/25g	133	530	6.0	50.0	34.0	4.5
Smoky Bacon, BGTY, Sainsbury's*	1 Bag/25g	118	472	6.5	58.5	23.6	5.7
Smoky Bacon, Golden Wonder*	1 Bag/25g	131	523	5.9	49.1	33.7	2.0
Smoky Bacon, Sainsbury's*	1 Bag/25g	132	529	5.7	49.5	34.2	4.4
Smoky Bacon, Walkers*	1 Bag/35g	186	530	6.5	50.0	33.0	4.1
Sour Cream & Chive Crinkles, Shapers, Boots*	1 Bag/20g	96	482	6.6	60.0	24.0	4.0
Sour Cream & Chive, Reduced Fat, Marks & Spencer*	1 Bag/40g	192	480	6.5	60.0	24.0	6.5
Sour Cream & Chives, Jordans*	1 Bag/30g	125	417	7.3	69.9	12.0	2.7
Sour Cream & Onion, Lights, Golden Wonder*	1 Bag/21g	91	435	5.4	64.5	17.2	5.9
Spare Rib Flavour, Chinese, Walkers*	1 Bag/34.5g	184	525	6.5	50.0	33.0	4.0
Spiced Chilli, McCoys*	1 Bag/50g	250	500	6.1	54.2	28.8	4.2
Spring Onion Flavour, Marks & Spencer*	1 Bag/40g	210	525	5.9	48.7	34.3	5.1
Spring Onion, Seabrook*	1 Bag/32g	182	569	5.4	54.4	36.7	3.9
Strawberry Raisin Snack, Fruitwonders, Golden Wonder*	1 Bag/29.5g	115	383	3.8	62.9	12.9	0.0
Sweet & Sour, Great British Takeaways, Walkers*	1 Bag/25g	131	525	6.5	50.0	33.0	4.0
T Bone Steak, Roysters*	1 Bag/31g	160	516	5.7	52.6	31.4	3.6
Tangy Tomato & Red Pepper Salsa, Sensations, Walkers*	1 Bag/35g	168	480	6.5	53.0	27.0	4.5
Thai Curry Flavour Curls, Marks & Spencer*	1 Bag/25g	90	360	1.3	82.5	2.5	3.1
Thai Green Curry, TTD, Sainsbury's*	1 Bag/50g	235	470	6.1	55.6	24.8	5.2
Thai Sweet Chilli, Sensations, Walkers*	1 Bag/35g	170	485	6.5	54.0	27.0	4.5
Tomato & Herb, Shapers, Boots*	1 Bag/20g	94	468	3.7	66.0	21.0	3.9
Tomato Ketchup, Potato Hoops, Waitrose*	1 Bag/20g	83	416	4.8	65.2	15.1	4.5
Tomato Ketchup, Walkers*	1 Bag/35g	186	530	6.5	50.0	33.0	4.1
Tomato Sauce, Golden Wonder*	1 Bag/25g	130	521	5.7	49.2	33.5	2.0
Tomato, Olive Oil & Basil, TTD, Sainsbury's*	1 Bag/50g	235	469	7.5	51.4	26.0	5.4
Traditional, Hand Cooked, Finest, Tesco*	1 Bag/150g	708	472	6.4	52.9	26.1	5.1
Vegetable Chips, Pret A Manger*	1 Bag/25g	126	504	5.6	37.2	36.8	10.0
Vegetable, Pan Fried, Sainsbury's*	¼ Bag/25g	102	407	4.6	36.5	27.0	6.4
Wild Chilli, Thick & Crunchy, McCoys*	1 Bag/50g	255	510	6.0	53.2	30.3	4.8
Worcester Sauce, Walkers*	1 Bag/25g	133	530	6.5	50.0	33.0	4.1
Worscester Sauce Flavour, Hunky Dorys*	1 Bag/45g	211	469	6.3	49.3	28.7	0.0
CRISPY PANCAKE,							
Beef Bolognese, Findus*	1 Pancake/65g	104	160	6.6	25.0	4.3	1.2
Chicken & Bacon, Findus*	1 Pancake/62g	90	145	6.1	23.6	2.8	0.9
Chicken, Bacon & Sweetcorn, Findus*	1 Pancake/63g	101	160	5.8	24.8	4.1	1.1
Minced Beef & Onion, Green Isle*	1 Pancake/60g	140	234	6.0	31.2	9.5	2.7
Three Cheeses, Findus*	1 Pancake/62g	115	185	7.2	24.4	6.5	0.9
CROISSANT,							
All Butter, BGTY, Sainsbury's*	1 Croissant/44g	176	401	9.8	44.2	20.5	2.2
All Butter, Budgens*	1 Croissant/45g	185	412	7.9	39.7	24.6	3.3

CROISSANT,

	Measure INFO/WEIGHT	per Measure KCAL	KCAL	PROT	CARB	FAT	FIBRE
All Butter, Finest, Tesco*	1 Croissant/77g	328	426	8.6	44.9	23.6	1.9
All Butter, Marks & Spencer*	1 Croissant/53g	227	420	7.2	44.4	25.0	1.6
All Butter, Mini, Sainsbury's*	1 Croissant/35g	156	446	9.3	38.2	28.4	2.0
All Butter, Mini, Tesco*	1 Croissant/35g	151	430	9.3	45.2	23.5	2.0
All Butter, Reduced Fat, Marks & Spencer*	1 Croissant/54g	181	335	6.8	38.4	16.9	1.5
All Butter, Reduced Fat, Tesco*	1 Croissant/52g	164	315	7.5	47.4	10.6	1.8
All Butter, Sainsbury's*	1 Croissant/44g	196	446	9.3	38.2	28.4	2.0
All Butter, TTD, Sainsbury's*	1 Croissant/75g	362	483	8.3	40.2	32.1	2.9
All Butter, Tesco*	1 Croissant/77g	297	386	6.5	40.4	22.1	1.9
Asda*	1 Croissant/47g	186	405	9.0	45.0	21.0	0.0
Au Beurre, St Pierre*	1 Croissant/45g	180	401	7.0	48.2	20.0	1.6
Butter, Asda*	1 Croissant/46g	191	416	8.0	42.0	24.0	1.9
Butter, GFY, Asda*	1 Croissant/43g	151	352	6.0	46.0	16.0	2.0
Butter, Mini, Waitrose*	1 Croissant/35g	156	446	9.3	38.2	28.4	2.0
Butter, Starbucks*	1 Croissant/82g	289	352	5.9	34.9	21.1	0.0
Chocolate, Pret A Manger*	1 Croissant/70g	322	460	9.3	35.6	31.3	0.0
Flaky Pastry With A Plain Chocolate Filling, Tesco*	1 Croissant/78g	318	408	6.5	41.0	24.3	2.0
Low Fat, Marks & Spencer*	1 Croissant/45g	180	400	8.2	46.0	20.2	1.8
Reduced Fat Butter, Tesco*	1 Croissant/52g	165	318	6.6	45.0	12.4	2.1
Reduced Fat, Sainsbury's*	1 Croissant/44g	173	393	9.8	49.2	17.5	2.2
Smoked Ham & Cheese, Marks & Spencer*	1 Croissant/105g	341	325	13.4	22.2	21.6	3.9

CROQUETTE,

Morrisons*	1 Serving/150g	231	154	3.3	23.1	5.4	1.1
Parsnip, Finest, Tesco*	1 Croquette/37g	77	207	5.9	26.2	8.7	1.3
Potato, Asda*	1 Pack/127g	224	176	2.3	26.0	7.0	1.8
Potato, Bird's Eye*	1 Croquette/29g	44	152	2.6	22.6	5.7	1.2
Potato, Fried in Blended Oil	1oz/28g	60	214	3.7	21.6	13.1	1.3
Potato, Frozen, Tesco*	1 Croquette/30g	58	193	3.7	23.0	9.7	1.0
Potato, Iceland*	1 Serving/100g	198	198	3.3	30.0	7.2	3.0
Potato, Marks & Spencer*	1 Serving/125g	206	165	2.4	19.3	8.8	2.2
Potato, Sainsbury's*	1 Croquette/28g	50	180	3.9	23.0	8.0	1.0
Potato, Tesco*	1 Croquette/30g	43	142	3.0	19.2	5.9	1.5
Potato, Waitrose*	1 Croquette/29g	47	157	3.0	17.9	8.1	1.5
Vegetable, Sainsbury's*	1 Serving/175g	392	224	5.8	23.3	11.9	2.2

CROUTONS,

Cracked Pepper & Sea Salt, Safeway*	1 Serving/10g	45	454	12.8	56.5	19.6	3.9
Fresh, Marks & Spencer*	1 Serving/10g	53	530	11.4	50.0	32.8	3.2
Herb & Garlic, Rochelle*	¼ Pack/18g	106	587	6.9	49.8	40.0	2.1
Herb, Sainsbury's*	1 Serving/15g	64	429	13.4	68.2	11.4	2.8
Italian Salad, Sainsbury's*	1 Pack/40g	204	510	8.5	62.7	25.0	2.5
Rochelle*	1 Bag/70g	400	572	7.0	49.0	40.0	0.0
CRUDITE PLATTER, Sainsbury*	1 Pack/275g	96	35	1.4	6.6	0.3	1.6

CRUMBLE,

Apple & Blackberry, Asda*	1 Serving/175g	427	244	2.7	38.0	9.0	1.2
Apple & Blackberry, Marks & Spencer*	1 Serving/135g	398	295	3.5	44.9	11.2	1.6
Apple & Blackberry, Sainsbury's*	1 Serving/110g	232	211	3.0	37.1	5.6	2.1
Apple & Blackberry, Tesco*	1 Crumble/335g	667	199	2.6	40.1	3.1	1.9
Apple & Custard, Asda*	1 Serving/125g	250	200	2.3	32.0	7.0	0.0
Apple & Toffee, Weight Watchers*	1 Pot/98g	206	210	2.1	37.6	5.7	1.6
Apple With Custard, Individual, Sainsbury's*	1 Pudding/120g	286	238	2.0	31.4	11.6	2.4
Apple, Farmfoods*	½ Pack/185g	411	222	2.9	39.3	5.9	2.3
Apple, Frozen, Iceland*	1 Portion/97g	240	247	2.1	36.9	10.1	1.8
Apple, Somerfield*	1 Serving/195g	454	233	2.5	36.8	8.4	1.1

	Measure INFO/WEIGHT	per Measure KCAL	Nutrition Values per 100g / 100ml				
			KCAL	PROT	CARB	FAT	FIBRE
CRUMBLE,							
Apple, Tesco*	1 Serving/150g	342	228	2.0	33.6	9.5	1.2
Apple, With Sultanas, Weight Watchers*	1 Dessert/110g	196	178	1.4	34.2	3.9	1.3
Bramley Apple, Marks & Spencer*	1 Serving/149g	387	260	4.4	40.3	9.2	1.1
Bramley Apple, Sainsbury's*	1 Serving/100g	248	248	2.0	35.4	10.9	2.3
Fish & Prawn, Youngs*	1 Pie/375g	476	127	5.8	9.7	7.2	1.3
Fruit	1oz/28g	55	198	2.0	34.0	6.9	1.7
Fruit, Wholemeal	1oz/28g	54	193	2.6	31.7	7.1	2.7
Gooseberry, Marks & Spencer*	1 Serving/133g	379	285	3.5	43.3	10.7	1.7
Ocean, Good Choice, Iceland*	1 Pack/340g	377	111	7.2	14.4	2.7	1.1
Ocean, Low Fat, Ross*	1 Crumble/300g	219	73	5.1	11.4	0.8	0.4
Rhubarb, Co-Op*	¼ Crumble/110g	0	245	2.0	42.0	7.0	1.0
Rhubarb, Farmfoods*	1oz/28g	54	192	2.0	35.0	4.9	2.3
Rhubarb, Marks & Spencer*	1 Serving/133g	366	275	3.4	42.6	9.9	1.4
Rhubarb, Sainsbury's*	1 Serving/50g	112	224	3.1	40.4	5.6	1.8
Rhubarb, Somerfield*	¼ Crumble/130g	281	216	3.0	38.0	6.0	0.0
Rhubarb, Tesco*	1/6 Crumble/116g	228	195	2.8	27.3	8.3	1.7
Salmon, Youngs*	1 Pie/339g	380	112	4.6	13.0	4.6	0.7
Topping, Sainsbury's*	1 Serving/47g	188	401	5.9	50.3	19.6	5.3
CRUMBLE MIX, Luxury, Tesco*	1 Pack/225g	992	441	5.7	67.9	16.3	3.2
CRUMBLE TOPPING, Morrisons*	1 Serving/40g	179	448	5.4	69.5	16.5	2.8
CRUMPETS,							
Asda*	1 Crumpet/45g	94	208	6.0	44.0	0.9	0.0
Co-Op*	1 Crumpet/55g	102	185	8.0	36.0	1.0	2.0
Finger, Safeway*	1 Crumpet/30g	55	182	6.9	36.7	0.1	1.8
Finger, Sainsbury's*	1 Crumpet/30g	55	182	7.0	36.6	0.8	1.8
Iceland*	1 Crumpet/46.6g	97	206	6.1	43.8	0.7	1.8
KwikSave*	1 Crumpet/41.1g	79	192	5.9	39.9	1.0	2.5
Less Than 1% Fat, Warburton's*	1 Crumpet/45.6g	71	155	5.6	31.7	0.7	0.0
Less Than 2% Fat, Marks & Spencer*	1 Crumpet/61g	116	190	8.0	36.9	1.3	2.1
Morning Fresh*	1 Crumpet/20g	36	180	7.3	34.8	1.3	5.2
Morrisons*	1 Crumpet/41g	78	191	6.1	38.6	1.4	0.0
Mother's Pride*	1 Crumpet/48g	90	187	5.6	38.9	1.0	1.7
Perfectly Balanced, Waitrose*	1 Crumpet/55g	94	171	6.1	36.1	0.3	4.4
Premium, Safeway*	1 Crumpet/60g	111	185	7.5	36.3	1.1	2.4
Premium, Sainsbury's*	1 Crumpet/50g	96	191	6.1	38.6	1.4	1.7
Safeway*	1 Crumpet/44g	80	182	7.0	36.6	0.8	1.8
Sainsbury's*	1 Crumpet/44g	91	207	5.6	44.0	0.9	0.5
SmartPrice, Asda*	1 Crumpet/42g	84	199	6.0	42.0	0.8	1.7
Soldier, Mother's Pride*	1 Crumpet/30g	58	193	7.8	37.1	1.6	1.6
Tesco*	1 Crumpet/46g	92	201	6.0	42.6	0.7	1.8
Toasted	1 Crumpet/40g	80	199	6.7	43.4	1.0	2.0
Toaster, Organic, Waitrose*	1 Crumpet/55g	95	172	7.3	34.4	0.6	4.6
Value, Tesco*	1 Crumpet/50g	102	204	6.0	43.0	0.9	1.8
Warburton's*	1 Crumpet/50g	89	178	7.1	35.8	0.7	0.0
CRUNCHIE,							
Cadbury's	1 Std Bar/41g	193	470	4.4	72.1	18.1	0.0
Nuggets, Cadbury's*	1 Bag/125g	569	455	3.8	73.1	16.4	0.0
CRUNCHY STICKS,							
Salt & Vinegar, Sainsburys*	1 Bag/25g	119	474	5.9	58.0	24.3	2.4
Salt & Vinegar, Shapers, Boots*	1 Bag/23g	99	430	7.8	66.0	15.0	3.1
CRUSH,							
Morello Cherry, Finest, Tesco*	1 Bottle/250ml	115	46	0.0	11.2	0.0	0.0
Orange & Raspberry, Freshly Squeezed, Finest, Tesco*	1fl oz/30ml	17	56	0.5	12.6	0.1	0.2

INFO/WEIGHT	Measure per Measure KCAL	Nutrition Values per 100g / 100ml KCAL PROT CARB FAT FIBRE

	Measure	per Measure	Nutrition Values per 100g / 100ml				
INFO/WEIGHT		KCAL	KCAL	PROT	CARB	FAT	FIBRE
CRUSH,							
Orange & Raspberry, Safeway*	1 Serving/100ml	57	57	0.5	13.6	0.1	0.2
Orange, Cool, Diet, Sainsbury*	1 Can/330ml	10	3	0.1	0.6	0.1	0.1
CUCUMBER,							
Portion, Tesco*	1 Serving/14g	1	10	0.7	1.5	0.1	0.6
Raw, Fresh	1oz/28g	3	10	0.7	1.5	0.1	0.6
CUCUMBER & MINT Raita, Patak's*	1oz/28g	33	117	3.9	12.9	5.5	0.1
CURACAO, Average	1 Shot/25ml	78	311	0.0	28.3	0.0	0.0
CURLY KALE,							
Boiled in Salted Water	1oz/28g	7	24	2.4	1.0	1.1	2.8
Raw	1oz/28g	9	33	3.4	1.4	1.6	3.1
CURLY WURLY,							
Cadbury's*	1 Bar/28g	126	450	4.8	69.9	16.7	0.0
Squirlies, Cadbury's*	1 Squirl/3g	14	450	3.9	69.0	17.8	0.0
CURRANTS, Average	1oz/28g	75	267	2.3	67.8	0.4	1.9
CURRY,							
& Rice, Ross*	1 Pack/328.2g	279	85	3.4	14.7	1.3	0.5
Aubergine	1oz/28g	33	118	1.4	6.2	10.1	1.5
Beef & Rice, Iceland*	1 Pack/400g	492	123	8.7	16.0	2.6	0.6
Beef With Rice, Asda*	1 Pack/406g	547	135	6.0	19.0	3.9	1.2
Beef With Rice, Bird's Eye*	1 Pack/388g	524	135	6.9	20.8	2.8	0.8
Beef With Rice, Healthy Choice, Asda*	1 Pack/400g	476	119	6.0	18.0	2.6	0.9
Beef With Rice, Tesco*	1 Pack/400g	456	114	4.5	16.7	3.3	0.6
Beef With Rice, Weight Watchers*	1 Pack/328g	249	76	4.2	12.5	1.0	0.3
Beef, Marks & Spencer*	1oz/28g	34	120	12.2	3.9	6.1	1.0
Beef, SmartPrice, Asda*	1 Serving/392g	223	57	4.0	9.0	0.5	1.0
Bhuna Chicken, Tesco*	1 Serving/300g	396	132	11.4	4.5	7.6	0.5
Blackeye Bean, Gujerati	1oz/28g	36	127	7.2	16.1	4.4	2.8
Bombay Potato	1oz/28g	33	117	2.0	13.7	6.8	1.2
Butter Chicken, Fresh, Tesco*	1 Pack/350g	487	139	11.8	7.1	7.0	1.8
Cabbage	1oz/28g	23	82	1.9	8.1	5.0	2.1
Caribbean Style Chicken With Rice & Beans, ES, Safeway*	1 Pack/380g	342	90	6.2	12.5	1.3	1.8
Cauliflower & Potato	1oz/28g	17	59	3.4	6.6	2.4	1.8
Chick Pea, Whole	1oz/28g	50	179	9.6	21.3	7.5	4.5
Chick Pea, Whole & Tomato, Punjabi With Vegetable	1oz/28g	31	112	5.6	12.4	4.9	2.9
Chick Pea, Whole, Basic	1oz/28g	30	108	6.0	14.2	3.6	3.3
Chicken & Rice, Asda*	1 Pack/300g	351	117	4.7	15.0	4.2	0.3
Chicken & Rice, Fresh, Co-Op*	1 Pack/300g	270	90	3.0	13.0	3.0	1.0
Chicken & Rice, Iceland*	1 Pack/399g	455	114	7.5	13.6	3.3	0.9
Chicken & Rice, International Cuisine*	1 Pack/300g	264	88	3.1	12.6	2.8	1.0
Chicken Malaysian With Rice, Bernard Matthews*	1 Pack/400g	512	128	6.1	17.0	3.9	0.0
Chicken With Naan Bread, Iceland*	1 Portion/260g	484	186	10.1	22.3	6.3	1.4
Chicken With Rice, Asda*	1 Pack/400g	440	110	5.0	17.0	2.4	1.0
Chicken With Rice, Bird's Eye*	1 Pack/380g	475	125	5.8	20.5	2.2	0.8
Chicken With Rice, Dunnes Stores*	1 Pack/375g	400	107	4.2	20.2	1.7	0.8
Chicken With Rice, Healthy Choice, Asda*	1 Pack/400g	492	123	6.0	18.0	3.0	1.0
Chicken With Rice, Morrisons*	1 Pack/300g	345	115	5.5	18.7	2.0	0.4
Chicken With Rice, Sainsbury's*	1 Pack/400g	500	125	5.4	17.5	3.7	0.8
Chicken With Rice, Tesco*	1 Pack/300g	300	100	5.7	14.4	2.2	0.4
Chicken With Rice, Weight Watchers*	1 Pack/300g	273	91	4.7	14.3	1.7	0.5
Chicken With Vegetables, Value, Tesco*	1 Serving/196g	123	63	3.1	7.2	2.4	0.7
Chicken, & Potato Wedges, Healthy Eating, Tesco*	1 Pack/450g	428	95	7.6	10.3	2.7	1.1
Chicken, Asda*	1 Can/200g	210	105	10.0	5.0	5.0	0.0
Chicken, Canned, Sainsbury's*	1 Serving/100g	136	136	11.1	9.1	6.1	1.0

C

CURRY,

INFO/WEIGHT	per Measure KCAL	KCAL	PROT	CARB	FAT	FIBRE
Chicken, Extra Strong, Marks & Spencer*	1oz/28g	28	100	13.8	2.5	3.9	1.4
Chicken, Fruity With Rice, Healthy Living, Tesco*	1 Pack/450g	495	110	6.5	18.2	1.2	1.2
Chicken, Green Thai, Jasmine Rice, PB, Waitrose*	1 Pack/400g	512	128	6.5	19.0	3.2	0.5
Chicken, Hot, Can, Tesco*	1 Can/418g	514	123	9.7	6.9	6.3	0.9
Chicken, Hot, Canned, Asda*	1 Can/398g	462	116	10.0	5.5	6.0	0.0
Chicken, Medium Hot, Marks & Spencer*	1 Serving/200g	310	155	7.8	14.3	7.1	0.8
Chicken, Mild, Bilash, Aldi*	½ Can/200g	180	90	9.5	4.5	3.8	0.7
Chicken, Mild, Iceland*	½ Can/200g	234	117	10.6	8.5	4.5	0.7
Chicken, Mild, Marks & Spencer*	1oz/28g	28	100	13.8	2.5	3.9	1.4
Chicken, Mild, Sainsbury's*	1 Can/400g	472	118	10.5	3.5	6.9	1.3
Chicken, Newgate*	1 Serving/196g	220	112	8.0	6.6	6.0	0.0
Chicken, Red Thai, Jasmine Rice, PB, Waitrose*	1 Pack/400g	496	124	6.2	18.5	2.9	0.4
Chicken, Reduced Fat, Asda*	1 Pack/400g	476	119	6.0	18.0	2.6	0.9
Chicken, SmartPrice, Asda*	1 Can/392g	282	72	4.0	11.0	1.3	1.0
Chicken, Value, Tesco*	1 Pack/300g	399	133	5.5	15.9	5.2	1.7
Chicken, Yellow Thai Style, Healthy Living, Tesco*	1 Pack/450g	504	112	9.3	12.6	2.7	0.5
Chinese Chicken With Vegetable Rice, Marks & Spencer*	1 Pack/400g	320	80	7.1	8.4	2.0	1.3
Chinese Chicken, Morrisons*	1 Pack/340g	347	102	10.3	5.0	4.6	0.8
Chinese Chicken, Oriental Express*	1 Pack/340g	286	84	4.8	16.2	0.6	0.8
Courgette & Potato	1oz/28g	24	86	1.9	8.7	5.2	1.2
Dudhi, Kofta	1oz/28g	32	113	2.6	9.4	7.4	2.8
Fish & Vegetable, Bangladeshi	1oz/28g	33	117	9.1	1.4	8.4	0.5
Fish, Bangladeshi	1oz/28g	35	124	12.2	1.5	7.9	0.3
Gobi Aloo Sag, Retail	1oz/28g	27	95	2.2	7.1	6.9	1.4
Green Bean	1oz/28g	37	131	1.7	3.6	12.7	1.6
Green Thai & Rice, Good For You, Asda*	1 Pack/400g	460	115	5.0	19.0	2.1	0.5
Green Thai Chicken, Safeway*	1 Pack/350g	490	140	12.5	3.5	8.0	1.4
Green Thai Chicken, Sainsbury's*	1 Serving/200g	306	153	13.6	3.0	9.6	1.6
Green Thai Style Chicken & Sticky Rice, Asda*	1 Pack/450g	585	130	7.0	20.0	2.4	0.1
Hot Chicken With Rice, Asda*	1 Pack/400g	440	110	5.0	18.0	2.0	1.1
King Prawn, Goan, Eat Smart, Safeway*	1 Pack/400g	340	85	3.7	12.7	1.7	2.1
Lamb With Rice, Bird's Eye*	1 Pack/382g	520	136	5.6	20.8	3.4	0.9
Lamb, Extra Strong, Marks & Spencer*	1oz/28g	35	125	11.5	4.6	6.9	0.9
Malai Prawn, Sainsbury's*	1 Serving/171g	299	175	7.7	1.4	15.4	1.1
Mango Chicken, Thai, Sainsbury's*	½ Pack/200g	288	144	11.2	4.8	8.9	1.9
Potato & Pea	1oz/28g	26	92	2.9	13.0	3.8	2.4
Prawn & Mushroom	1oz/28g	47	168	7.3	2.5	14.4	1.0
Prawn & Rice, Iceland*	1 Pack/400g	432	108	4.5	15.4	3.2	1.0
Prawn Malai, With Jeera Rice, PB, Waitrose*	1 Pack/450g	590	131	6.3	18.2	3.7	1.3
Prawn With Rice, Asda*	1 Pack/400g	420	105	3.5	17.0	2.6	1.1
Red Kidney Bean, Punjabi	1oz/28g	30	106	4.7	10.1	5.6	3.8
Red Thai Chicken With Jasmine Rice, ES, Safeway*	1 Pack/380g	380	100	6.9	13.1	1.7	1.3
Red Thai Chicken With Jasmine Rice, PB, Waitrose*	1 Pack/400g	496	124	6.2	18.5	2.9	0.4
Red Thai Chicken, New Recipe, Waitrose*	1 Pack/350g	389	111	8.9	5.0	6.2	0.9
Red Thai Fish, Waitrose*	1 Pack/500g	275	55	5.2	3.7	2.2	1.0
Red Thai Style Chicken, Healthy Eating, Tesco*	1 Pack/420g	462	110	6.0	17.7	1.7	0.2
Red Thai, Oriental, Tesco*	1 Pack/350g	469	134	11.0	3.6	8.4	1.1
Red Thai, Quorn*	1 Pack/400g	464	116	4.6	15.5	3.9	4.0
Red Thai, Safeway*	1 Pack/324g	369	114	10.0	4.8	6.1	1.6
Thai Chicken With Rice, Oriental Express*	1 Pack/340g	303	89	4.1	15.3	1.3	1.2
Thai Chicken, COU, Marks & Spencer*	1 Pack/400g	320	80	7.2	8.8	1.9	1.0
Thai Chicken, Tom Yum, Sainsbury's*	1 Pot/400g	416	104	11.1	3.5	5.1	1.9
Thai Green Chicken, Jasmine Rice, BGTY, Sainsbury's*	1 Pack/400g	424	106	6.8	15.8	1.7	0.9

	Measure INFO/WEIGHT	per Measure KCAL	Nutrition Values per 100g / 100ml				
			KCAL	PROT	CARB	FAT	FIBRE
CURRY,							
Thai Green Chicken, BGTY, Sainsbury's*	1 Pack/400g	376	94	9.3	6.1	3.6	0.4
Thai Green Chicken, Bird's Eye*	1 Pack/450g	536	119	4.7	15.2	4.4	0.3
Thai Green Chicken, Marks & Spencer*	½ Pack/107g	171	160	12.3	1.8	11.6	0.6
Thai Green With Sticky Rice, Healthy Living, Tesco*	1 Pack/450g	518	115	7.7	14.9	2.7	0.6
Thai Peanut Chicken, Sainsbury's*	½ Pack/200g	314	157	12.8	4.9	9.6	1.2
Thai Red Chicken With Fragrant Rice, Somerfield	1 Pack/340g	503	148	8.0	18.0	5.0	0.0
Thai Red Chicken With Jasmine Rice, BGTY, Sainsbury's*	1 Pack/400g	428	107	6.9	16.0	1.7	0.2
Thai Red Chicken, Thai Jasmine Rice, BGTY, Sainsbury's*	1 Pack/450g	545	121	6.2	14.9	4.1	1.1
Thai Red Chicken, 97% Fat Free, Birds Eye*	1 Pack/366g	425	116	5.7	19.0	1.9	0.5
Thai Red Chicken, Asda*	1 Pack/360g	461	128	9.1	5.5	7.7	1.0
Thai Red Chicken, COU, Marks & Spencer*	1 Pack/400g	420	105	7.1	13.4	2.3	1.4
Thai Red Chicken, Sainsbury's*	1 Serving/200g	300	150	14.3	5.5	7.9	1.0
Thai Red, Sizzle & Stir, Chicken Tonight*	1 Jar/485g	873	180	1.5	4.5	17.3	1.7
Thai Yellow Vegetable, Sainsburys*	½ Pack/200g	256	128	1.7	7.1	10.3	1.5
Vegetable & Pilau Rice, BGTY, Sainsbury's*	1 Pack/450g	396	88	2.5	17.4	0.9	1.4
Vegetable With Pilau Rice, BGTY, Sainsbury's*	1 Pack/450g	441	98	2.4	16.9	2.3	0.5
Vegetable With Pilau Rice, Linda McCartney*	1 Pack/339g	224	66	1.6	13.5	0.6	0.5
Vegetable With Rice, Asda*	1 Pack/392.7g	432	110	2.6	18.0	3.1	1.4
Vegetable With Rice, Co-Op*	1 Pack/340g	289	85	2.0	17.0	1.0	0.7
Vegetable With Rice, Tesco*	1 Pack/400g	440	110	2.1	18.7	3.0	1.0
Vegetable With Yoghurt	1oz/28g	17	62	2.6	4.6	4.1	1.4
Vegetable, Budgens*	1 Pack/350g	249	71	1.8	6.9	4.0	2.2
Vegetable, Frozen, Mixed Vegetables	1oz/28g	25	88	2.5	6.9	6.1	0.0
Vegetable, Health Eating, Tesco*	1 Pack/350g	280	80	4.5	13.6	0.8	1.3
Vegetable, Indian Meal For One, Tesco*	1 Serving/200g	220	110	1.9	10.5	6.7	1.4
Vegetable, Marks & Spencer*	1 Pack/250g	300	120	2.1	7.1	9.5	2.5
Vegetable, Medium Spicy, Tesco*	1 Pack/350g	385	110	1.9	10.5	6.7	1.4
Vegetable, Medium, Tesco*	1 Pack/350g	326	93	2.3	7.1	6.2	1.9
Vegetable, Mild, Tesco*	1 Can/425g	315	74	2.1	10.7	2.5	1.7
Vegetable, Pakistani	1oz/28g	17	60	2.2	8.7	2.6	2.2
Vegetable, Ready Meals, Marks & Spencer*	1 Pack/300g	495	165	2.4	7.2	14.2	2.1
Vegetable, Retail With Rice	1oz/28g	29	102	3.3	16.4	3.0	0.0
Vegetable, Safeway*	1 Pack/275g	239	87	2.4	7.3	5.4	2.8
Vegetable, SmartPrice, Asda*	½ Can/203g	132	65	2.0	13.0	0.5	1.7
Vegetable, Takeaway	1oz/28g	29	105	2.5	7.6	7.4	0.0
Vegetable, Tesco*	½ Can/200g	278	139	3.4	10.5	9.3	3.2
Vegetable, Tinned, Asda*	½ Can/200g	206	103	2.2	10.0	6.0	2.5
Vegetable, Tinned, Tesco*	1 Can/400g	312	78	2.4	10.5	2.9	1.7
Vegetable, Waitrose*	1 Pack/352g	285	81	3.5	4.9	5.3	2.1
Vegetable, Way to Five, Sainsbury's*	½ Pack/344g	227	66	2.5	11.6	1.1	1.4
Vegetable, With Rice, Bird's Eye*	1 Pack/413.6g	455	110	2.3	19.6	2.3	1.1
Yellow Vegetable Thai, Sainsbury's*	1 Pack/400g	624	156	2.2	9.4	12.2	1.1
Yellow Vegetable, Tesco*	1 Pack/355.6g	324	91	1.9	9.9	4.9	1.4
CURRY LEAVES, Fresh	1oz/28g	27	97	7.9	13.3	1.3	0.0
CURRY PASTE,							
Balti, Patak's*	1 Tbsp/15g	59	393	5.0	20.3	31.8	3.1
Balti, Sharwood's*	¼ Pack/72.5g	328	453	5.0	19.2	39.6	3.1
Balti, Tomato & Coriander, Patak's*	1 Serving/30g	117	391	4.1	17.2	34.0	2.2
Garam Masala, Cinnamon & Ginger, Hot, Patak's*	1 Tbsp/25g	101	403	3.2	17.9	35.4	0.6
Hot, Marks & Spencer*	1oz/28g	69	245	4.2	13.4	19.2	3.3
Hot, Sharwood's*	1oz/28g	123	439	5.1	18.6	38.3	2.6
Korma, Patak's*	1 Tbsp/10g	54	535	4.2	13.0	51.8	2.6
Madras, Patak's*	½ Jar/50g	293	586	4.3	21.6	53.6	5.2

C

	Measure INFO/WEIGHT	per Measure KCAL	Nutrition Values per 100g / 100ml				
			KCAL	PROT	CARB	FAT	FIBRE
CURRY PASTE,							
Medium, Marks & Spencer*	1oz/28g	64	230	2.5	10.7	19.5	4.9
Medium, Sharwood's*	1oz/28g	122	434	4.5	16.8	38.8	2.7
Mild, Original, Patak's*	1oz/28g	155	552	4.9	14.3	52.8	6.2
Mild, Sharwood's*	1oz/28g	78	279	3.6	17.7	21.5	3.4
Rogan Josh, Patak's*	1 Serving/30g	119	397	4.1	12.7	36.7	5.9
Tandoori, Sharwood's*	1oz/28g	64	228	5.9	15.5	15.8	1.9
Thai Green, Mild, Sainsbury's*	1 Tbsp/15g	23	156	2.2	14.5	9.9	2.7
Thai Red, Sainsbury's*	1oz/28g	43	154	2.0	8.0	12.0	3.0
Tikka Masala, Patak's*	1oz/28g	101	361	3.4	16.2	31.4	3.2
Tikka Masala, Sharwood's*	1oz/28g	53	191	3.2	9.9	15.4	2.6
Vindaloo, Patak's*	1 Tbsp/15g	84	557	4.8	16.0	52.6	6.1
CURRY POWDER,							
Average	1 Tsp/2g	7	325	12.7	41.8	13.8	0.0
Medium, Schwartz*	1 Tsp Heaped/4g	14	348	12.0	50.0	11.0	15.0
Medium, Sharwood's*	1 Pack/113g	336	297	12.2	52.9	13.4	18.5
Mild, Sharwood's*	1 Tsp/2g	6	300	12.7	54.1	12.3	16.4
Mixed Flavours	1 Tsp/2g	6	316	13.0	34.7	13.9	0.0
CUSTARD,							
Canned	1oz/28g	27	95	2.6	15.4	3.0	0.1
Chocolate, COU, Marks & Spencer*	1 Pot/140g	147	105	3.1	18.6	2.2	1.0
Confectioners'	1oz/28g	48	170	6.4	24.4	5.9	0.2
Dairy Free, Sainsbury's*	1 Serving/250g	210	84	3.0	14.2	1.7	0.2
Devon, Ambrosia*	1oz/28g	29	103	2.7	16.4	3.0	0.1
Devon, Chocolate Flavour, Ambrosia*	¼ Pack/125g	141	113	3.0	18.8	2.9	0.5
Devon, Low Fat, Ambrosia*	1/3 Pot/141g	102	72	2.9	12.7	1.1	0.1
Economy, Sainsbury's*	½ Can/198g	150	76	3.0	14.4	0.7	0.0
Egg	1oz/28g	33	118	5.7	11.0	6.0	0.0
Fresh, Co-Op*	1 Serving/125g	150	120	5.0	14.0	5.0	0.5
Fresh, Healthy Eating, Tesco*	1 Serving/100g	103	103	2.3	17.3	2.7	0.2
Fresh, Sainsbury's*	1 Serving/125g	158	126	2.6	15.4	6.0	0.1
Fresh, Thick & Creamy, BGTY, Sainsbury's*	1oz/28g	33	119	3.2	14.1	5.5	0.0
Good For You, Asda*	1 Serving/150g	137	91	2.9	17.0	1.3	0.1
Half Fat, Safeway*	1 Serving/100ml	105	105	2.3	17.3	2.7	0.7
Instant, Dry Weight, Bird's*	1oz/28g	119	425	4.5	76.0	11.5	0.0
Instant, Dry Weight, Low Fat, Bird's*	1oz/28g	113	405	4.3	78.5	8.2	0.0
Instant, Dry Weight, No Added Sugar, Tesco*	1 Serving/18g	73	406	5.3	77.0	8.5	0.0
Instant, Sainsbury's*	1 Serving/141g	109	77	0.8	14.0	2.0	0.0
Low Fat, Bird's Eye*	1 Serving/125g	105	84	2.9	15.0	1.3	0.0
Low Fat, Ready To Serve, Bird's*	1oz/28g	24	87	2.8	15.5	1.4	0.0
Low Fat, Ready To Serve, Budgens*	1oz/28g	21	74	2.9	14.0	0.7	0.0
Low Fat, Somerfield*	1 Pot/425g	391	92	3.0	17.0	1.0	0.0
Low Sugar Instant, Co-Op*	1 Pack/74g	56	75	1.1	13.4	1.9	0.1
Made Up With Semi-Skimmed Milk	1oz/28g	26	94	3.8	16.8	1.9	0.0
Made Up With Skimmed Milk	1oz/28g	22	79	3.8	16.8	0.1	0.0
Made Up With Whole Milk	1oz/28g	33	117	3.7	16.6	4.5	0.0
Mix, Instant, Co-Op*	1 Pack/76g	340	448	4.5	68.5	17.3	0.0
Mix, Instant, Made Up, Co-Op*	½ Pack/140ml	118	84	0.7	13.9	2.9	0.0
Original, Ready To Serve, Bird's*	1oz/28g	29	102	2.8	15.5	3.0	0.0
Pot, Forest Fruits Flavour, Hot 'n' Fruity, Bird's*	1 Pot/174g	171	98	0.9	18.5	2.4	0.1
Pot, Strawberry Flavour, Hot 'n' Fruity, Bird's*	1oz/28g	28	99	1.0	18.5	2.4	0.1
Powder	1oz/28g	99	354	0.6	92.0	0.7	0.1
Powder, Original Flavour, Bird's*	1oz/28g	99	355	0.4	87.0	0.5	0.0
Ready To Eat, Low Fat, Tesco*	1 Pot/150g	132	88	2.9	16.2	1.3	0.2

	Measure INFO/WEIGHT	per Measure KCAL	Nutrition Values per 100g / 100ml				
			KCAL	PROT	CARB	FAT	FIBRE
CUSTARD,							
Ready To Serve Low Fat, Co-Op*	1 Can/425g	319	75	3.0	14.0	0.7	0.0
Ready To Serve, BGTY, Sainsbury's*	1/3 Pot/166g	163	98	2.6	15.6	2.8	0.1
Ready To Serve, Co-Op*	1 Can/425g	425	100	3.0	16.0	3.0	0.0
Ready To Serve, Healthy Eating, Tesco*	1oz/28g	22	77	2.9	13.0	1.5	0.0
Ready To Serve, Low Fat, Asda*	¼ Pack/142g	109	77	2.9	13.0	1.5	0.0
Ready To Serve, Somerfield*	1oz/28g	29	103	3.0	17.0	3.0	0.0
Ready To Serve, Sweet Valley, Aldi*	½ Carton/200g	196	98	2.9	15.0	2.9	1.0
Ready to Eat, Good For You, Asda*	1 Serving/150g	137	91	2.9	17.0	1.3	0.1
Sauce, Fresh, Somerfield*	¼ Pack/100g	119	119	3.0	15.0	5.0	0.0
Smooth & Creamy, Fresh, Tesco*	1 Serving/100g	123	123	2.5	15.0	5.9	0.3
Strawberry Style, Shapers, Boots*	1 Pot/148g	83	56	4.0	8.2	0.8	0.1
Summer, Ambrosia*	1 Pack/500g	490	98	2.7	15.0	3.0	0.0
Thick & Creamy, Fresh, Marks & Spencer*	¼ Carton/125g	286	229	2.7	16.2	17.0	0.0
Vanilla With Apple Crunch, Ambrosia*	1 Pack/193g	276	143	3.4	22.4	4.5	0.8
Vanilla, COU, Marks & Spencer*	1 Pot/140g	147	105	4.3	16.6	2.5	0.6
CUTLETS, NUT,							
Goodlife*	1 Serving/88g	248	282	10.2	27.4	14.6	3.0
Grilled, Cauldron Foods*	1 Cutlet/87g	250	287	10.2	26.8	15.4	4.6
Retail, Fried in Vegetable Oil	1oz/28g	81	289	4.8	18.7	22.3	1.7
Retail, Grilled	1oz/28g	59	212	5.1	19.9	13.0	1.8
CUTLETS, VEGETABLE, Nut, Tesco*	1 Serving/88g	271	308	7.7	22.0	21.0	3.5
CUTTLEFISH, Raw	1oz/28g	20	71	16.1	0.0	0.7	0.0

C

	Measure INFO/WEIGHT	per Measuring KCAL	Nutrition Values per 100g / 100ml				
			KCAL	PROT	CARB	FAT	FIBRE
DAB,							
Raw	1oz/28g	21	74	15.7	0.0	1.2	0.0
DAIRYLEA							
Dunkers, Jumbo Munch, Dairylea, Kraft*	1 Serving/50g	150	300	7.2	26.5	18.5	1.2
Dunkers, Smokey Bacon, Dairylea, Kraft*	1 Pack/45g	135	300	7.3	24.0	19.5	0.0
Lunchables, Cheese & Pizza Crackers, Dairylea, Kraft*	1oz/28g	105	375	10.5	24.5	27.0	1.4
Lunchables, Chicken, Fun Pack, Dairylea, Kraft*	1 Pack/311g	454	146	5.5	15.0	6.2	0.2
Lunchables, Double Cheese, Dairylea, Kraft*	1 Pack/110g	413	375	18.0	17.0	26.0	0.3
Lunchables, Ham & Cheese Pizza, Dairylea, Kraft*	1 Pack/97g	247	255	11.5	26.0	11.0	1.6
Lunchables, Harvest Ham, Dairylea, Kraft*	1 Pack/110g	314	285	16.5	16.5	17.0	0.3
Lunchables, Tasty Chicken, Dairylea, Kraft*	1 Pack/110g	314	285	17.0	17.5	16.5	0.3
DAMSONS,							
Raw, Weighed With Stones	1oz/28g	10	34	0.5	8.6	0.0	1.6
Raw, Weighed Without Stones	1oz/28g	11	38	0.5	9.6	0.0	1.8
DANDELION & BURDOCK, Drink, Ben Shaws Original*	1 Can/440ml	128	29	0.0	7.0	0.0	0.0
DANISH PASTRY,							
Apple & Sultana, Tesco*	1 Pastry/72g	293	407	5.4	45.0	22.8	1.4
Custard Danish Bar, Sara Lee*	¼ Bar/100g	228	228	6.6	36.1	6.4	0.8
Danish Apple Bar, Sara Lee*	1/6 Bar/70g	160	229	4.3	42.1	5.7	1.7
Danish Twist, Apple & Cinnamon, Entenmann's*	1 Serving/52g	150	288	5.6	62.0	1.9	1.5
Danish Twist, Toasted Pecan, Entenmann's*	1 Slice/48g	171	351	7.0	47.2	15.6	1.4
Pecan, Marks & Spencer*	1 Serving/67g	287	428	6.2	45.0	26.0	1.3
DATES,							
Dried	1oz/28g	76	270	3.3	68.0	0.2	4.0
Dried, Stone-Out, Tesco*	4 Dates/23g	70	305	2.1	71.8	1.0	8.2
Dried, Weighed With Stones	1 Date/20g	45	227	2.8	57.1	0.2	3.4
Fresh, Raw	1oz/28g	35	124	1.5	31.3	0.1	1.8
Medjool	1oz/28g	76	273	2.3	65.5	0.2	2.2
Organic, Waitrose*	1oz/28g	81	290	3.3	67.7	0.7	4.0
Pitted, Asda*	1 Pack/50g	127	254	3.0	60.0	0.2	3.0
Raw, Weighed With Stones	1 Date/30g	32	107	1.3	26.9	0.1	1.5
DELIGHT,							
Butterscotch Flavour, No Added Sugar, Tesco*	½ Pack/25g	109	434	4.8	66.5	16.5	0.0
Chocolate Flavour, Dry, Tesco*	1 Pack/49g	204	417	6.3	63.0	15.5	0.5
Ravishing Raspberry, Made Up, Asda*	1/3 Pack/100g	112	112	3.2	16.0	3.9	0.0
Strawberry Flavour, No Added Sugar, Dry, Tesco*	½ Pack/25g	110	440	4.8	67.0	17.0	0.0
Strawberry, Shapers, Boots*	1 Pot/121g	96	79	4.5	13.0	1.0	0.1
DESSERT,							
Apple Rice, Classic Desserts, Marks & Spencer*	1 Pot/200g	210	105	2.5	20.0	1.7	0.3
Baked Lemon, COU, Marks & Spencer*	1 Serving/100g	140	140	6.8	22.0	2.5	0.8
Banana Flavour Custard, Ambrosia*	1 Pack/135g	136	101	2.6	16.2	2.9	0.1
Banoffee Layered, Sainsbury's**	1 Pot/115g	270	235	2.2	27.8	12.8	1.0
Banoffee, Frozen, Healthy Living, Tesco*	1 Serving/60g	92	153	2.5	29.9	2.6	0.6
Banoffee, Shape*	1 Pot/120g	175	146	3.3	28.0	2.3	0.5
Banoffee, Weight Watchers*	1 Pot/80g	154	192	4.5	35.3	3.7	0.8
Black Cherry & Chocolate, COU, Marks & Spencer*	1 Pack/115g	132	115	3.6	22.6	1.4	1.2
Black Forest, Tesco*	1 Pot/100g	287	287	3.5	35.8	14.4	2.4
Blackcurrant, Yoghurt & Sorbet, Mini, Eat Smart, Safeway*	1 Pot/75g	90	120	2.2	25.8	0.7	1.8
Blueberry Muffin, Tesco*	1 Pot/91g	265	291	2.0	24.5	20.6	3.0
Bounty, Mars*	1 Pot/110g	253	230	5.3	23.2	13.6	0.0
Bread & Butter, Eat Smart, Safeway*	1 Pudding/117g	140	120	5.1	20.4	1.8	0.8
Butterscotch Flavour Whip, Co-Op*	1 Pack/64g	241	377	0.6	93.4	0.1	0.1
Buttons, Cadbury's*	1 Pot/100g	295	295	6.4	34.9	14.7	0.0
Cafe Latte, COU, Marks & Spencer*	1 Pot/120g	162	135	5.0	24.0	2.2	0.9

DESSERT,	Measure INFO/WEIGHT	per Measure KCAL	Nutrition Values per 100g / 100ml				
			KCAL	PROT	CARB	FAT	FIBRE
Cafe Latte, Iced, BGTY, Sainsbury's*	1 Serving/75g	104	139	2.9	23.7	3.6	3.3
Cafe Mocha, COU, Marks & Spencer*	1 Dessert/115g	155	135	5.5	21.8	2.7	1.0
Cappuccino, BGTY, Sainsbury's*	1 Pot/119g	224	188	3.3	25.2	8.1	0.8
Cappuccino, Italian, Co-Op*	1 Pack/90g	257	285	5.0	39.0	12.0	0.1
Caramel, Marks & Spencer*	1oz/28g	41	147	3.9	22.3	4.1	0.0
Cherry & Chocolate, Eat Smart, Safeway*	1 Serving/100g	150	150	3.2	27.5	2.7	0.1
Cherry & Vanilla, BGTY, Sainsbury's*	1 Pot/115g	225	196	1.6	32.6	6.6	1.0
Chocolait, Luxury, Aldi*	1 Pot/200g	270	135	3.3	18.1	5.5	0.0
Chocolate & Cherry, COU, Marks & Spencer*	1 Pot/130g	156	120	2.6	24.5	1.6	0.9
Chocolate & Coconut, COU, Marks & Spencer*	1 Pot/125g	169	135	3.6	25.6	2.2	0.7
Chocolate & Honeycomb Iced, Weight Watchers*	1 Pot/58g	92	159	3.1	26.3	4.3	0.8
Chocolate & Mallow Iced, GFY, Asda*	1 Pot/150ml	140	93	2.0	18.7	1.2	2.3
Chocolate & Marshmallow Swirls, Iced, BGTY, Sainsbury's	¼ Pot/75g	130	173	3.9	33.8	2.5	2.8
Chocolate & Vanilla Caramel, Dairy, Yoplait Petits Filous*	1 Pot/60g	101	169	4.8	23.6	6.2	0.0
Chocolate & Vanilla, Heavenly Swirls, HL, Tesco*	1 Pot/73g	104	143	3.0	26.9	2.6	0.7
Chocolate & White Chocolate, BGTY, Sainsbury's*	1 Pot/67.1g	104	155	2.7	30.9	2.3	4.3
Chocolate Brownie, Asda*	1/6 Brownie/63g	171	271	5.0	38.0	11.0	4.4
Chocolate Brownie, Marks & Spencer*	¼ Pack/143.5g	612	425	4.7	39.6	27.5	1.0
Chocolate Chip Sponge & Custard, COU M&S*	1 Pot/125g	181	145	4.3	26.9	2.0	1.3
Chocolate Creme, Somerfield*	1 Pot/125g	180	144	4.0	22.0	4.0	0.0
Chocolate Dream, Delicious Dessert Co-Op*	1 Pot/110g	184	167	4.1	22.0	7.0	0.0
Chocolate Fudge Brownie, Tesco*	1 Pot/125g	374	299	4.6	40.2	13.3	1.3
Chocolate Hazelnut, Charolait, Aldi*	1 Serving/200g	270	135	3.3	18.1	5.5	0.0
Chocolate Mint Crisp, Iced, Marks & Spencer*	¼ Pot/85.2g	115	135	5.4	21.9	2.9	1.0
Chocolate Muffin, COU, Marks & Spencer*	1 Serving/110g	149	135	4.6	26.5	1.9	0.9
Chocolate Orange, Eat Smart, Safeway*	1 Pot/90g	153	170	4.5	32.5	1.9	0.5
Chocolate Profiterole, Sainsbury's*	1/6 Pot/95.0g	192	202	5.4	25.1	8.9	0.8
Chocolate Profiterole, Tesco*	1 Serving/76g	281	370	4.3	27.9	26.7	0.4
Chocolate Toffee, Weight Watchers*	1 Pot/90.1g	164	182	4.9	35.0	3.5	1.8
Chocolate With Cream, Campina*	1 Serving/100g	134	134	2.5	18.9	5.4	0.0
Chocolate, COU Marks & Spencers*	1 Serving/120g	168	140	5.6	26.4	2.1	1.1
Chocolate, Campina*	1 Pot/125g	186	149	3.2	18.5	6.9	0.0
Chocolate, Frozen, Healthy Eating, Tesco*	1 Serving/52g	68	131	3.5	23.7	2.5	0.9
Chocolate, Iced, Non-Dairy, Swedish Glace*	1 Serving/100g	200	200	3.0	24.0	10.0	1.0
Chocolate, Value, Tesco*	1 Pot/115g	112	97	2.8	15.7	2.6	0.0
Creme Brulee, Dairy, Waitrose*	1 Serving/100g	324	324	4.3	13.9	27.9	0.5
Creme Caramel, Sainsbury's*	1 Pot/100g	102	102	2.5	21.1	0.9	0.0
Crunchie, Milk Chocolate, Cadbury's*	1 Pot/100g	285	285	5.8	37.8	12.5	0.0
Dairy Vanilla Iced, Sainsbury's*	1 Serving/65g	77	119	3.0	19.9	3.0	3.7
Double Chocolate Brownie, Weight Watchers*	1 Serving/82g	151	184	4.5	33.3	3.6	2.2
Double Chocolate Fudge, Marks & Spencer*	1 Pot/119g	387	325	3.0	30.6	21.4	1.6
Double Chocolate, Eat Smart, Safeway*	1 Pot/90g	144	160	3.9	31.0	2.2	2.0
Dreaming of, Cherry Rice, Marks & Spencer*	1 Pot/200g	220	110	2.4	19.7	2.2	0.1
Dreamy Vanilla, BGTY, Sainsbury's*	1 Serving/58g	146	252	3.5	27.6	14.2	5.3
Flake, Milk Chocolate, Cadbury's*	1 Pot/100g	290	290	6.3	34.7	14.1	0.0
Fruit & Nut, Cadbury's*	1 Pot/100g	285	285	6.4	36.3	12.5	0.0
Galaxy, Mars*	1 Pot/75g	166	221	4.9	22.7	12.3	0.0
Gulabjam Indian, Waitrose*	1 Pot/180g	476	266	4.8	42.9	8.6	0.6
Irish Cream Caffe Latte, Marks & Spencer*	1 Pot/118.5g	161	135	5.0	24.0	2.2	0.9
Jaffa Cake, COU, Marks & Spencer*	1 Serving/120g	138	115	2.4	20.1	2.6	1.0
Lemon & Sultana Sponge, COU, Marks & Spencer*	1 Pot/130g	169	130	2.8	26.5	1.2	0.5
Lemon Meringue, Weight Watchers*	1 Pot/170g	321	189	2.4	43.1	0.5	0.6
Lemoncello, Italian, Co-Op*	1 Pot/90g	266	295	3.0	34.0	16.0	0.1

D

DESSERT,

	Measure INFO/WEIGHT	per Measuring KCAL	Nutrition Values per 100g / 100ml KCAL	PROT	CARB	FAT	FIBRE
Lemoncillo, Tesco*	1 Pot/100g	273	273	4.2	41.8	9.9	0.8
Mandarin, 95% Fat Free, Marks & Spencer*	1oz/28g	35	125	1.0	19.6	4.5	0.2
Mars, Mars*	1 Pot/110g	215	195	6.0	28.2	6.7	0.7
Natural Rice, Shape*	1 Pot/175g	149	85	3.5	15.4	1.0	0.1
Neapolitan, Frozen, GFY, Asda*	1 Scoop/100g	64	64	1.2	10.0	2.1	0.1
Peach & Raspberry, COU, Marks & Spencer*	1 Pot/90g	135	150	2.6	30.5	1.6	1.0
Peach, Iced, So-Lo, Iceland*	1 Lolly/92ml	98	107	2.3	23.5	0.0	2.2
Pineapple & Passionfruit, Marks & Spencer*	1 Pot/100g	130	130	0.8	21.7	3.8	0.3
Profiterole, Marks & Spencer*	1 Pot/61g	209	342	5.5	29.1	22.1	0.5
Pure Bliss, Aldi*	1 Pot/125.4g	158	126	2.5	20.3	3.9	0.2
Raspberry & Chardonnay, COU, Marks & Spencer*	1 Serving/135g	155	115	1.6	25.5	0.5	2.7
Raspberry Flavour Whip, Co-Op*	1 Whip/64g	241	377	1.2	92.5	0.2	0.1
Raspberry Swirl, Iced, Weight Watchers*	1 Scoop/60g	74	124	1.7	23.4	2.5	0.3
Raspberry With Light Lemon Sponge, Weight Watchers*	1 Dessert/85.2g	155	182	3.9	32.0	4.3	1.8
Red Devil, Simpsons, St Ivel*	1oz/28g	38	134	2.8	24.3	2.8	0.4
Rice, Lite, Muller*	1 Pot/150g	116	77	3.5	13.6	0.9	0.0
Rolo, Nestle*	1 Pot/78g	191	245	3.1	30.3	12.2	0.3
Strawberries & Cream, Better for You, Morrisons*	1 Serving/200g	244	122	2.2	26.0	1.1	0.1
Strawberry & Rhubarb, COU, Marks & Spencer*	1 Pot/110g	105	95	1.5	20.1	0.7	0.9
Strawberry Flavour, SmartPrice, Asda*	1 Pot/115g	113	98	2.4	17.0	2.3	0.0
Strawberry Flavour, With Cream, Somerfield*	1 Pot/100g	119	119	2.0	16.0	5.0	0.0
Strawberry, SmartPrice, Asda*	1 Pot/100g	120	120	2.3	16.0	5.0	0.0
Strawberry, Value, Tesco*	1 Pot/115g	113	98	2.4	16.9	2.3	0.0
Summer Fruits, COU, Marks & Spencer*	1 Serving/105g	110	105	2.1	21.6	1.1	1.2
Summer Fruits, Yoghurt, Iced, BGTY, Sainsbury's*	¼ Pot/85g	105	124	3.3	25.6	0.9	0.5
Summerberry, Healthy Living, Tesco*	1 Pot/102g	133	130	2.8	24.5	2.3	1.5
Supreme, No Added Sugar, Sainsbury's*	¼ Pack/91g	98	108	3.5	13.6	4.4	0.0
Tantalising Toffee Flavour, Iced, Weight Watchers*	1 Serving/57g	93	163	2.7	26.2	4.8	0.2
Tantalising Toffee, COU, Marks & Spencer*	¼ Pot/85g	145	170	3.1	32.8	2.9	0.5
Toffee & Vanilla, Weight Watchers*	1 Pot/67g	107	159	3.1	34.8	0.8	3.9
Toffee Apple, Eat Smart, Safeway*	1 Pot/100g	145	145	2.4	29.1	1.7	2.6
Toffee Banana Crunch, Farmfoods*	1/6 Dessert/82g	219	267	2.6	38.5	11.4	0.7
Toffee Chocolate, Weight Watchers*	1 Pot/100g	164	164	4.4	31.5	3.2	1.6
Toffee Flavour & Toffee Sauce, Iced, Weight Watchers*	1 Pot/57g	93	163	2.7	26.2	4.8	0.2
Toffee Flavour Custard, Ambrosia*	1 Pack/135g	139	103	2.7	16.4	2.9	0.1
Toffee Flavour Fudge Swirl, Iced, Weight Watchers*	1 Pot/57g	82	143	2.5	22.6	4.4	0.4
Toffee Flavour, Low Fat, So-Lo, Iceland*	1 Serving/100g	65	65	2.1	10.1	1.8	0.3
Toffee Flavoured Dairy, Iced, BGTY, Sainsbury's*	1 Serving/70g	103	147	2.7	24.0	4.5	0.2
Toffee Iced, 3% Fat, Marks & Spencer*	1oz/28g	51	183	3.1	37.2	2.4	0.5
Toffee Muffin, COU, Marks & Spencer*	1 Serving/100g	180	180	3.7	35.8	2.2	0.3
Toffee With Biscuit Pieces, Iced, Weight Watchers*	1 Pot/100ml	93	93	1.5	14.9	2.7	0.1
Triple Chocolate Layered, BGTY, Sainsbury's*	1 Pot/105g	147	140	4.2	24.4	2.8	0.5
Triple Chocolate Truffle, Entenmann's*	1 Serving/100g	304	304	4.5	28.4	19.1	2.2
Vanilla & Chocolate Iced, Healthy Living, Tesco*	1 Pot/73g	104	143	3.0	26.9	2.6	0.7
Vanilla & Raspberry Swirl, Weight Watchers*	1 Serving/100ml	81	81	1.5	13.3	2.2	0.2
Vanilla & Strawberry Compote, Iced, Weight Watchers*	1 Pot/57g	81	142	2.5	23.4	3.9	0.2
Vanilla & Toffee, Heavenly Swirls, Healthy Living. Tesco*	1 Pot/73g	106	145	2.5	28.1	2.5	0.5
Vanilla Flavour, Iced, Healthy Eating, Tesco*	1 Serving/50g	67	134	3.9	24.1	2.4	4.6
Vanilla Sponge & Custard, Raspberry Conserve, COU, M&S*	1 Serving/140g	189	135	2.4	28.3	1.2	1.7
Vanilla Supreme, Sainsbury's*	1 Pot/95g	116	122	3.0	18.0	4.0	0.0
Vanilla With Strawberries Swirl, Weight Watchers*	1 Pot/57g	81	142	2.5	23.4	3.9	0.2
Vanilla, Frozen, BGTY, Sainsbury's*	1 Serving/75g	89	119	3.0	19.9	3.0	3.7
Vanilla, Frozen, GFY, Asda*	1 Serving/52g	72	139	2.7	22.0	4.5	0.0

	Measure INFO/WEIGHT	per Measure KCAL	Nutrition Values per 100g / 100ml				
			KCAL	PROT	CARB	FAT	FIBRE
DESSERT,							
Vanilla, Iced, 3% Fat, Marks & Spencer*	1oz/28g	40	143	3.5	25.9	2.8	0.7
Vanilla, Iced, Non-Dairy, Swedish Glace*	1 Serving/100g	200	200	2.5	25.0	10.0	1.0
Vanilla, Luxury, Charolait, Aldi*	1 Serving/200g	248	124	3.0	16.6	5.1	0.0
Vanilla, Too Good To Be True, Frozen, Wall's*	1 Serving/50ml	35	70	2.0	14.9	0.4	0.1
DESSERT MIX,							
Instant Powder, Made Up With Skimmed Milk	1oz/28g	27	97	3.1	14.9	3.2	0.2
Instant Powder, Made Up With Whole Milk	1oz/28g	35	125	3.1	14.8	6.3	0.2
DHAL,							
Blackeye Bean, Patak's*	1oz/28g	29	102	3.6	12.4	4.6	1.8
Black Gram	1oz/28g	21	74	4.2	7.0	3.4	1.7
Chick Pea	1oz/28g	42	149	7.4	17.7	6.1	3.8
Chick Pea, Canned, Asda*	½ Can/194g	198	102	4.3	14.0	3.2	2.9
Lentil, Patak's*	1 Can/283g	156	55	2.8	9.3	1.0	1.0
Lentil, Red Masoor & Tomato With Butter	1oz/28g	26	94	4.0	9.7	4.9	0.9
Lentil, Red Masoor & Vegetable	1oz/28g	31	110	5.8	14.7	3.8	1.8
Lentil, Red Masoor With Vegetable Oil	1oz/28g	48	172	7.6	19.2	7.9	1.8
Lentil, Red Masoor, Punjabi	1oz/28g	39	139	7.2	19.2	4.6	2.0
Lentil, Red Masoorl & Mung Bean	1oz/28g	32	114	4.8	9.9	6.7	1.6
Lentil, Red, Way To Five, Sainsbury's*	½ Pack/94g	87	93	5.5	14.4	1.5	1.4
Lentil, Safeway*	1 Serving/200g	182	91	2.4	10.5	4.4	0.9
Lentil, Tesco*	1 Serving/200g	248	124	5.1	10.6	6.6	2.5
Mung Bean, Bengali	1oz/28g	20	73	4.2	7.4	3.3	1.7
Mung Beans, Dried, Boiled in Unsalted Water	1oz/28g	26	92	7.8	15.3	0.4	0.0
Mung Beans, Dried, Raw	1oz/28g	81	291	26.8	46.3	1.1	0.0
Toor, Cooked Dish	1oz/28g	31	109	4.6	13.3	4.6	0.0
DHANSAK,							
Chicken With Bagara Rice, Waitrose*	1 Pack/450g	549	122	8.2	18.2	1.8	1.2
Chicken, Ready Meals, Marks & Spencer*	1oz/28g	50	180	12.4	6.6	11.5	1.6
Vegetable, Sainsbury's*	1 Pack/400g	416	104	2.6	7.2	7.2	1.3
DIAMOND WHITE, Cider	1fl oz/30ml	11	36	0.0	2.6	0.0	0.0
DILL,							
Dried	1 Tsp/1g	3	253	19.9	42.2	4.4	13.6
Fresh	1oz/28g	7	25	3.7	0.9	0.8	2.5
DIME,							
Mini, Terry's*	1 Bag/100g	550	550	4.2	61.0	32.0	0.7
Single, Terry's*	1oz/28g	154	550	3.9	61.6	32.1	0.6
Terry's*	1oz/28g	154	550	4.6	68.5	33.8	0.6
DIP,							
Applewood Cheddar & Onion, Fresh, BGTY, Sainsbury's*	½ Pot/85g	85	100	7.3	7.3	4.6	0.5
Aubergine, Fresh, Waitrose*	1 Serving/85g	159	187	2.5	10.5	15.0	1.7
Aubergine, Taverna*	1 Serving/50g	139	277	4.7	11.4	23.6	0.0
Blue Cheese, Fresh, Sainsbury's*	1/5 Pot/34g	115	337	3.6	3.1	34.5	0.1
Cajun Red Pepper, Sainsbury's*	1 Serving/50g	25	50	1.4	7.0	1.8	1.4
Caramelised Onion & Garlic, Waitrose*	½ Pot/85g	389	458	1.7	5.8	47.6	0.5
Celery, Marks & Spencer*	1 pot/130g	163	125	1.8	4.4	11.0	1.2
Cheddar & Onion, Marks & Spencer*	1oz/28g	88	315	5.1	7.5	29.5	0.5
Cheese & Bacon With Breadsticks, Weight Watchers*	1 Pack/50g	98	196	16.0	24.0	4.2	1.4
Cheese & Chive, 50% Less Fat, Asda*	1 Pot/125g	261	209	4.5	9.0	17.2	0.0
Cheese & Chive, 50% Less Fat, Morrisons*	1 Serving/50g	86	172	8.8	5.2	12.7	0.2
Cheese & Chive, Classic, Tesco*	1 Serving/32g	164	511	3.3	3.1	54.0	0.1
Cheese & Chive, Fresh, Safeway*	1 Pot/170g	877	516	4.1	3.0	54.2	0.0
Cheese & Chive, Fresh, Sainsbury's*	1oz/28g	109	390	3.9	2.7	40.4	0.0
Cheese & Chive, Healthy Choice, Safeway*	1 Pack/100g	137	137	10.2	6.0	8.0	1.3

D

DIP,

INFO/WEIGHT	Measure per Measuring KCAL	Nutrition Values per 100g / 100ml KCAL	PROT	CARB	FAT	FIBRE
Cheese & Chive, Healthy Eating, Tesco*	1 Tsp/10g	23	228	5.7	6.4	19.9	0.0
Cheese & Chive, Healthy Selection, Somerfield*	1oz/28g	67	239	6.0	5.0	22.0	0.0
Cheese & Chive, Marks & Spencer*	1oz/28g	120	430	4.5	3.9	44.1	0.5
Cheese & Spring Onion, Weight Watchers*	1 Serving/50g	98	196	16.0	24.0	4.2	1.4
Chilli Cheese, Max, Walkers*	1 Jar/300g	390	130	3.3	9.4	9.1	0.3
Chilli, Marks & Spencer*	1 Pot/35g	103	295	0.4	73.2	0.2	0.4
Chunky Tomato Salsa, Tesco*	1 Pot/170g	68	40	1.1	5.9	1.3	1.1
Creamy Roasted Tomato & Herb, COU, M&S*	1 Serving/40g	30	75	7.7	7.2	1.7	0.9
Cucumber & Mint, Eat Smart, Safeway*	½ Pot/85g	55	65	7.3	4.9	1.3	0.8
Cucumber & Mint, Fresh, Sainsbury's*	1oz/28g	34	123	4.5	3.7	10.0	0.0
Doritos Hot Salsa, Walkers*	1 Jar/326g	130	40	0.9	8.5	0.2	2.2
Doritos Mild Salsa, Walkers*	1oz/28g	11	40	0.9	8.5	0.2	2.2
Feta Cheese, Fresh, Tesco*	1oz/28g	81	288	6.8	7.9	25.5	0.7
Garlic & Herb, Marks & Spencer*	1oz/28g	88	315	2.4	7.1	30.6	0.5
Garlic & Herb, Reduced Fat, Marks & Spencer*	1 Serving/10g	10	95	6.0	8.1	4.0	0.5
Garlic & Herb, Tesco*	¼ Pack/42.5g	260	604	0.9	3.2	65.4	0.3
Garlic& Herb, Domino's*	1 Pot/28g	194	693	1.4	2.5	75.4	0.4
Garlic, Olive Oil & Butter, Pizza Express*	½ Pot/17g	106	621	1.5	2.8	67.4	0.5
Mature Cheddar Cheese & Chive, Fresh, Waitrose*	½ Pot/85g	393	462	5.8	2.4	47.7	1.7
Mexican Bean, Doritos*	1 Tbsp/20g	18	89	2.7	12.1	3.3	2.4
Mustard & Honey, Fresh, Sainsbury's*	1oz/28g	100	356	2.2	5.1	36.3	0.0
Nacho Cheese, Marks & Spencer*	1oz/28g	76	270	9.8	3.8	23.7	0.4
Nacho Cheese, Sainsbury's*	1 Serving/50g	244	487	4.8	3.9	50.2	0.0
Onion & Garlic, 50% Less Fat, Asda*	1oz/28g	59	209	4.5	9.0	17.2	0.0
Onion & Garlic, Fresh, BGTY, Sainsbury's*	1oz/28g	56	201	4.4	4.8	18.2	0.8
Onion & Garlic, GFY, Asda*	1/5 Pot/34g	56	166	2.1	8.0	14.0	0.2
Onion & Garlic, Healthy Eating, Tesco*	1 Pot/170g	345	203	3.3	7.9	17.6	0.1
Onion & Garlic, Healthy Selection, Somerfield*	1oz/28g	62	222	3.0	5.0	21.0	0.0
Peanut, Satay Selection, Occasions, Sainsbury's*	1 Serving/2g	4	186	7.1	13.8	11.4	1.1
Pecorino, Basil & Pine Nut, Fresh, Waitrose*	½ Pot/85g	338	398	5.1	5.1	39.7	0.0
Philadelphia & Breadsticks, Light, Kraft*	1 Portion/50g	119	238	8.5	24.5	12.0	1.1
Philadelphia Light With Italian Breadsticks, Kraft*	1 Pack/50g	123	245	8.4	23.0	13.0	1.5
Red Pepper, Sainsbury's*	1 Pot/100g	103	103	2.3	14.6	4.0	0.0
Roast Onion, Garlic & Rocket, Reduced Fat, Waitrose*	1 Serving/25g	51	202	2.7	5.4	18.8	1.5
Salsa, Chunky, Fresh, Sainsbury's*	1 Serving/100g	51	51	1.1	7.8	1.7	1.2
Salsa, Kettle*	1 Serving/25g	10	39	1.7	8.0	0.0	0.0
Smoked Salmon & Dill, Fresh, Waitrose*	½ Pot/85g	373	439	5.1	4.1	44.7	0.1
Smoked Salmon & Dill, Reduced Fat, Waitrose*	½ Pot/85g	184	217	3.9	6.1	19.7	1.1
Sour Cream & Chive, Asda*	1/5 Pot/33g	116	350	2.4	4.0	36.0	0.1
Sour Cream & Chive, BGTY, Sainsbury's	1oz/28g	46	165	4.9	3.4	14.6	0.7
Sour Cream & Chive, Doritos*	1 Tbsp/20g	64	322	2.5	3.1	33.3	0.1
Sour Cream & Chive, Fresh, Tesco*	½ Pot/75g	305	407	2.1	4.1	42.4	0.0
Sour Cream & Chive, Primula*	1oz/28g	97	346	5.0	1.8	35.3	0.0
Sour Cream & Chive, Reduced Fat, Asda*	1oz/28g	55	197	2.3	7.1	17.9	0.1
Sour Cream & Chive, Sainsbury's*	1 Serving/50g	157	314	2.2	2.5	32.8	0.0
Sour Cream, Co-Op*	1oz/28g	137	490	2.0	3.0	52.0	0.0
Soured Cream & Chive, 95% Fat Free, Marks & Spencer*	1oz/28g	25	90	6.5	9.6	2.8	0.5
Soured Cream & Chive, BGTY, Sainsbury's*	1 Serving/170g	131	77	6.0	6.6	2.9	0.3
Soured Cream & Chive, Classic, Tesco*	1 Serving/25g	67	267	2.6	3.6	26.9	0.1
Soured Cream & Chive, Marks & Spencer*	1oz/28g	83	295	2.5	7.2	28.5	0.6
Soured Cream & Chive, Morrisons*	1 Serving/100g	317	317	2.6	3.3	32.6	0.0
Soured Cream & Chive, Reduced Fat, Tesco*	1 Serving/85g	159	187	3.6	6.1	16.5	0.4
Spicy Moroccan, BGTY, Sainsbury's*	½ Pot/84.8g	56	66	2.1	10.0	2.0	1.7

	Measure INFO/WEIGHT	per Measure KCAL	Nutrition Values per 100g / 100ml				
			KCAL	PROT	CARB	FAT	FIBRE
DIP,							
Sun Dried Tomato, Somerfield*	1oz/28g	155	552	1.0	5.0	59.0	0.0
Sweet & Sour, Marks & Spencer*	1oz/28g	36	130	0.7	31.4	0.1	0.5
Tangy Barbecue, Marks & Spencer*	1oz/28g	28	100	1.1	22.2	0.6	0.6
Thousand Island, Marks & Spencer*	1oz/28g	69	245	2.1	9.4	22.2	0.7
Tikka, Classic, Fresh, Healthy Choice, Safeway*	1oz/28g	38	137	10.2	6.0	8.0	1.3
Tomato Ketchip, Asda*	1 Pack/25g	18	71	1.6	16.0	0.1	1.0
Tortilla Chips, Cool Flavour, Big, Morrisons*	½ Pack/100g	453	453	6.4	57.4	22.0	8.1
Tzatzaki, Somerfield*	1oz/28g	37	131	6.0	3.0	11.0	0.0
Yoghurt & Cucumber Mint, Tesco*	1oz/28g	34	121	7.0	7.2	7.1	0.6
DIP POT, Barbeque Sauce, Burger King*	1 Serving/25g	31	125	0.6	28.7	0.3	0.4
DIPPERS,							
Chicken, Battered, Safeway*	5 Pieces/90g	219	243	13.4	16.4	13.8	1.2
Chicken, Chinese, Tesco*	½ Pack/150g	255	170	17.3	8.4	7.5	0.9
Chicken, Crispy, Bird's Eye*	1 Dipper/17g	48	280	12.5	12.9	19.8	0.2
Chicken, Crispy, Farmfoods*	1 Dipper/17g	42	247	14.2	16.4	13.9	0.4
Chicken, Tikka, Tesco*	1oz/28g	54	193	21.5	5.0	9.7	1.0
DISCOS,							
Pickled Onion, KP*	1 Bag/31g	155	500	3.7	58.6	27.8	2.9
Salt & Vinegar, KP*	1 Bag/31g	153	493	3.8	57.2	27.6	2.8
DOLLY MIXTURES, Marks & Spencer*	1 Pack/125g	479	383	1.5	90.7	1.5	0.0
DOPIAZA,							
Chicken, Safeway*	1 Pack/326g	450	138	10.4	5.3	8.4	1.4
Chicken, Tesco*	1 Pack/350g	448	128	10.8	5.3	7.1	0.6
Chicken, With Pilau Rice, Tesco*	1 Pack/400g	424	106	5.7	12.3	3.8	1.5
Mushroom, Retail	1oz/28g	19	69	1.3	3.7	5.7	1.1
Mushroom, Waitrose*	½ Pack/150g	81	54	2.2	4.3	3.1	2.3
DORITOS,							
Cheesy 3D's, Walkers*	1 Pack/20g	89	445	7.0	68.0	16.0	3.0
Cool Original, Walkers*	1 Bag/40g	204	510	7.5	62.0	26.0	3.5
Cool Spice 3Ds, Walkers*	1 Bag/24g	108	450	8.0	64.0	18.0	4.4
Dippas Dipping Chips, Doritos*	1 Bag/35g	172	490	7.5	63.0	23.0	3.5
Hint Of Chilli Dippas, Walkers*	1 Bag/35g	173	495	7.0	61.0	25.0	3.5
Hint of Lime, Walkers*	1 Bag/35g	170	485	7.5	58.0	25.0	7.5
Mexican Hot, Walkers*	1 Bag/40g	202	505	8.0	57.0	27.0	3.5
Roast Onion & Garlic Dippas, Walkers*	1 Tsp/25g	83	333	3.2	8.7	31.7	0.9
Tangy Cheese Flavour Corn Chips, Doritos*	1 Bag/35g	179	510	8.0	58.0	27.0	3.0
Tangy Cheese, Walkers*	1 Bag/40g	210	525	7.0	63.0	27.0	3.5
DOUBLE DECKER, Cadbury's*	1 Bar/51g	237	465	5.2	64.9	20.7	0.0
DOUGH BALLS,							
Cheese & Garlic, Occasions, Sainsbury's*	1 Ball/12g	41	341	10.3	33.4	18.5	2.1
Garlic & Herb, Occasions, Sainsbury's*	1 Ball/12g	41	343	8.4	38.7	17.2	2.2
Pizza Express*	8 Balls/50g	200	400	14.3	85.0	3.2	0.0
Sainsbury's*	1 Ball/12g	41	343	8.4	38.7	17.2	2.2
With Garlic & Herb Butter, Aldi*	1 Ball/12.3g	44	365	7.7	46.7	18.2	1.8
DOUGHNUTS,							
Chocolate Donut, McDonald's*	1 Donut/79g	329	417	4.9	45.9	23.8	2.4
Chocolate Donut, Mini, McDonald's*	1 Donut/17g	64	375	6.8	46.9	17.8	1.6
Chocolate, Somerfield*	1 Doughnut/57g	203	356	7.8	43.8	16.6	1.7
Cinnamon Donut, McDonald's*	1 Donut/72g	302	419	5.1	43.1	25.1	3.8
Cream & Jam, Tesco*	1 Doughnut/90g	324	360	4.1	39.7	20.5	1.3
Custard, Tesco*	1 Doughnut/91g	266	292	4.1	33.4	15.8	1.0
Custard-Filled	1 Doughnut/75g	269	358	6.2	43.3	19.0	0.0
Dairy Cream Finger, Safeway*	1 Doughnut/98g	342	349	5.5	36.4	20.1	1.8

D

	INFO/WEIGHT	KCAL	KCAL	PROT	CARB	FAT	FIBRE
DOUGHNUTS,							
Dairy Cream, Marks & Spencer*	1oz/28g	87	310	4.9	40.8	14.1	1.3
Finger, Co-Op*	1 Doughnut/82g	299	365	4.0	45.0	18.0	2.0
Jam	1 Doughnut/75g	252	336	5.7	48.8	14.5	0.0
Jam, American Style, Budgens*	1 Doughnut/46g	127	275	7.1	46.5	6.7	0.0
Jam, Marks & Spencer*	1 Doughnut/49g	141	287	5.0	57.6	4.0	1.3
Jam, Somerfield*	1 Doughnut/70g	213	304	6.8	47.9	9.5	1.6
Ring	1 Doughnut/60g	238	397	6.1	47.2	21.7	0.0
Ring, Co-Op*	1 Doughnut/106g	392	370	4.0	44.0	20.0	1.0
Ring, Iced	1 Doughnut/70g	268	383	4.8	55.1	17.5	0.0
Ring, Waitrose*	1 Doughnut/107g	396	370	4.2	43.5	19.9	0.7
Sugared Donut, McDonald's*	1 Donut/72g	303	421	5.0	42.6	25.6	3.7
Toffee, Tesco*	1 Doughnut/75g	235	313	8.0	44.2	11.6	1.6
DOVER SOLE, Raw	1oz/28g	25	89	18.1	0.0	1.8	0.0
DR PEPPER*, Soda, Diet	1fl oz/30ml	0	1	0.0	0.1	0.0	0.0
DRAMBUIE, 39% Volume	1 Shot/25ml	68	272	0.0	0.0	0.0	0.0
DREAM,							
Cadbury's*	1 Bar/45g	250	555	4.5	59.7	33.3	0.0
Double Fudge, Cadbury's*	1oz/28g	139	495	6.3	61.4	25.2	0.0
White Chocolate, Cadbury's*	1 Piece/8g	44	555	4.5	59.7	33.3	0.0
DREAM TOPPING,							
Dry, Bird's*	1oz/28g	193	690	6.7	32.5	58.5	0.5
Made Up, Skimmed Milk, Birds*	1oz/28g	21	75	2.0	4.8	5.3	0.0
DRESSING,							
Balsamic Vinegar & Oregano, Waitrose*	1 Serving/25g	101	404	0.6	8.2	41.0	0.4
Balsamic Vinegar & Red Pepper, PB, Waitrose*	1 Tbsp/15ml	22	148	0.6	28.5	3.5	1.1
Balsamic Vinegar & Smoked Garlic, Safeway*	1 Tbsp/15ml	19	125	0.1	28.3	0.9	0.5
Balsamic Vinegar, Asda*	1 Pack/44ml	121	275	0.9	7.0	27.0	0.0
Balsamic With Garlic & Herbs, Finest, Tesco*	1 Serving/10ml	13	133	0.3	3.4	13.1	0.1
Balsamic With Olive Oil, Pizza Express*	1 Serving/10g	42	421	0.3	10.3	41.2	0.0
Balsamic, Extra Virgin Olive Oil, TTD, Sainsbury's*	1 Tsp/5ml	19	376	0.5	12.8	36.0	0.4
Balsamic, Marks & Spencer*	1 Tbsp/15g	74	490	0.3	9.7	48.0	0.5
Balsamic, New, Sainsbury's*	1 Tbsp/15g	58	389	0.6	18.3	34.8	0.8
Balsamic, Sainsbury's*	1 Tbsp/15ml	47	316	0.4	13.8	28.8	0.4
Blue Cheese, BGTY, Sainsbury's*	1 Tbsp/15ml	16	108	2.9	3.6	6.0	0.7
Blue Cheese, Fresh, Sainsbury's*	1 Dtsp/10ml	42	423	2.3	0.5	45.7	0.1
Blue Cheese, Healthy Eating, Tesco*	1 Tsp/5g	4	82	4.4	9.0	3.1	0.1
Blue Cheese, Hellmann's*	1 Tbsp/15g	69	459	0.7	6.3	47.2	1.1
Blue Cheese, Low Fat, Weight Watchers*	1oz/28g	17	59	1.5	5.8	3.4	0.0
Blue Cheese, Salad, Waitrose*	1 Serving/50g	265	530	2.1	17.3	50.3	4.1
Caesar Salad, Finest, Tesco*	1 Serving/25ml	119	477	1.9	2.8	50.9	0.2
Caesar Salad, Marks & Spencer*	1 Serving/10ml	52	515	1.8	2.2	55.2	0.5
Caesar Salad, Safeway*	1 Serving/25g	122	488	3.7	13.7	48.5	0.1
Caesar Style, Good For You, Asda*	1 Sachet/44ml	34	77	5.0	9.0	2.3	0.0
Caesar Style, Kraft*	1 Tbsp/15ml	15	102	2.1	15.0	3.5	0.1
Caesar Style, Low Fat, Weight Watchers*	1 Tsp/6g	4	60	1.6	5.8	3.4	0.0
Caesar, 95% Fat Free, Tesco*	1 Tsp/6g	5	88	4.1	8.9	3.7	0.3
Caesar, BGTY, Sainsbury's*	1 Serving/25ml	27	108	1.3	8.3	7.8	0.9
Caesar, Chilled, Reduced Fat, Tesco*	1 Tsp/5ml	13	252	6.5	3.1	23.7	0.1
Caesar, Finest, Tesco*	1 Tbsp/15ml	72	477	1.9	2.8	50.9	0.2
Caesar, Fresh, Asda*	1 Dtsp/10ml	45	445	2.5	0.7	48.0	0.0
Caesar, Fresh, Marks & Spencer*	1 Tsp/6g	32	525	2.0	1.8	56.4	0.2
Caesar, Fresh, Sainsbury's*	1 Tsp/6g	29	479	3.0	1.1	51.4	0.2
Caesar, Gourmet, Fresh, Waitrose*	1 Tbsp/15ml	72	479	4.5	0.9	50.8	0.5

D

DRESSING,

INFO/WEIGHT	per Measure KCAL	KCAL	PROT	CARB	FAT	FIBRE
Caesar, Healthy Eating, Tesco*	1 Tbsp/15ml	11	74	3.0	8.4	2.8	0.2
Caesar, Hellmann's*	1 Tsp/6g	30	499	2.5	4.5	51.7	0.3
Caesar, Low Fat, Cardini's*	1 Tsp/6g	7	120	1.0	27.0	1.0	1.0
Caesar, Marks & Spencer*	1 Tsp/6g	31	523	2.0	1.8	56.4	0.2
Caesar, Original, Cardini's*	1 Serving/10g	56	560	2.0	2.0	60.0	0.0
Citrus Salad, BGTY, Sainsbury's*	1 Tbsp/15ml	14	90	0.3	14.4	3.1	0.3
Classic Caesar, Sainsbury's*	1 Tsp/5ml	22	442	2.7	4.6	45.9	0.5
Classic French, Fresh, Marks & Spencer*	1 Serving/10ml	52	515	0.6	8.2	53.1	0.2
Classic Italian, Fat Free, Kraft*	1fl oz/30ml	10	32	0.1	6.8	0.0	0.6
Cream Cheese & Chive, Creamy Ranch, Kraft*	1 Serving/15ml	31	205	1.2	11.0	17.0	0.0
Creamy Caesar, Waistline, Crosse & Blackwell*	1 Dtsp/11g	15	135	1.5	11.1	9.2	0.3
Creamy Ranch, 95% Fat Free, Kraft*	1 Tsp/6ml	7	111	1.4	14.5	5.0	0.3
Creamy Roasted Garlic, Good For You, Asda*	1 Tbsp/15g	11	70	0.8	8.0	3.9	0.6
Creamy, Waistline, 93% Fat Free, Crosse & Blackwell*	1 Tsp/6g	7	120	1.0	14.4	6.4	0.2
Creme Fraiche, Salad, Kraft*	2 Tbsp/30ml	23	78	0.8	12.5	2.5	0.0
Extra Virgin Olive Oil & Balsamic Vinegar, Fresh, Safeway*	1 Serving/20ml	86	432	0.5	6.8	44.7	0.0
Extra Virgin Olive Oil & Lemon, Fresh, Organic, Waitrose*	1 Serving/100ml	427	427	0.7	10.2	42.6	0.6
Fire Roasted Garlic & Thyme, Tesco*	1 Serving/10ml	45	447	0.9	4.7	47.2	0.0
For Tuna, Coronation Style, Weight Watchers*	1 Can/80g	122	152	10.2	6.5	9.5	0.6
French Classic, Marks & Spencer*	1 Tbsp/15ml	77	516	0.6	8.2	53.1	0.2
French Dressing, Fresh, Co-Op*	1 Tbsp/15ml	70	467	0.0	0.0	46.7	0.0
French Salad, Marks & Spencer*	1 Serving/25ml	156	625	0.5	3.8	67.3	0.1
French Style Calorie-Wise Salad, Kraft*	1 Tbsp/15ml	24	160	0.0	18.7	10.7	0.0
French Style, Eat Smart, Safeway*	1 Serving/15ml	22	145	0.7	28.9	2.5	0.7
French Style, Oil Free, Healthy Eating, Tesco*	1 Tbsp/15g	5	30	0.3	6.0	0.2	1.4
French, BGTY, Sainsbury's*	1 Tbsp/15ml	12	79	1.1	8.8	4.4	0.5
French, COU, Marks & Spencer*	1/3 Bottle/105g	74	70	0.7	11.5	2.6	0.7
French, Chilled, Tesco*	1 Tbsp/15ml	63	421	1.1	15.1	39.6	0.0
French, Fresh, Healthy Eating, Tesco*	1 Tbsp/15ml	8	56	1.1	6.7	2.8	0.0
French, Fresh, Morrisons*	1 Tbsp/15ml	75	499	1.5	13.6	48.7	0.0
French, Fresh, Organic, Sainsbury's*	1 Tbsp/15ml	45	301	0.4	5.5	31.0	0.4
French, Fresh, Safeway*	1 Tbsp/15ml	77	510	1.5	13.8	49.9	0.0
French, Fresh, Sainsbury's*	1 Tbsp/15ml	64	429	0.6	6.6	44.6	0.6
French, Fresh, Somerfield*	1 Tbsp/15ml	74	490	1.0	7.0	51.0	0.0
French, Good For You, Asda*	1 Tbsp/15g	8	50	0.7	7.0	2.1	0.1
French, Healthy Eating, Tesco*	1 Tbsp/15ml	3	23	0.8	3.1	0.8	0.0
French, Less Than 3% Fat, Marks & Spencer*	1 Tbsp/15ml	10	68	0.7	11.5	2.6	0.7
French, Low Fat, Hellmann's*	1 Tbsp/15g	9	62	0.1	10.8	1.6	0.5
French, Luxury, Hellmann's*	1 Tbsp/15g	45	297	0.4	14.9	25.9	0.3
French, Oil Free, Perfectly Balanced, Waitrose*	1 Serving/15ml	11	72	2.2	12.2	1.6	1.1
French, Organic, Marks & Spencer*	1 Tbsp/15g	98	655	0.2	7.5	69.4	0.3
French, Organic, Sainsbury's*	1 Tbsp/15ml	11	71	0.2	8.3	4.1	0.5
French, Organic, Tesco*	1 Tsp/5ml	23	451	0.6	11.0	44.9	0.2
French, Reduced Fat, Marks & Spencer*	1 Tbsp/15g	11	70	0.7	11.5	2.8	0.7
French, Sainsbury's*	1 Tbsp/15ml	33	219	0.6	9.8	19.1	0.5
Garlic & Herb, Perfectly Balanced, Waitrose*	1 Serving/50ml	68	135	0.6	29.9	1.4	0.8
Garlic & Herb, Reduced Calorie, Hellmann's*	1 Tbsp/15ml	35	232	0.6	12.8	19.3	0.4
Green Olive, Marks & Spencer*	1oz/28g	40	144	1.5	2.2	14.4	1.3
Green Thai, Coconut & Lemon Grass, Loyd Grossman*	1oz/28g	49	174	0.2	19.3	10.6	0.5
Healthy Choice, Safeway*	1 Tbsp/15ml	4	29	0.2	6.3	0.3	0.0
Herb 'n' Garlic, Kraft*	1 Tbsp/15ml	17	116	1.3	15.5	5.1	0.2
Herb, Eat Smart, Safeway*	1 Tbsp/15ml	9	60	0.5	9.5	2.0	0.5
Honey & Mustard, Burger King*	1 Sachet/40g	32	80	1.5	14.5	2.0	0.8

DRESSING,

INFO/WEIGHT	Measure per Measuring KCAL	KCAL	PROT	CARB	FAT	FIBRE
Honey & Mustard, Finest, Tesco*	1 Serving/25ml	72	288	1.7	19.6	22.5	0.7
Honey & Mustard, Fresh, Marks & Spencer*	1 Serving/10ml	43	430	1.7	9.7	42.4	0.5
Honey & Mustard, Fresh, Safeway*	1 Serving/80ml	309	386	1.3	13.4	36.3	0.0
Honey & Mustard, Good For You, Asda*	1 Tbsp/15g	13	89	1.5	13.0	3.4	0.8
Honey & Mustard, Healthy Eating, Tesco*	1 Tbsp/15g	12	79	1.5	12.1	2.7	0.9
Honey & Mustard, Kraft*	1 Serving/30ml	39	131	1.3	19.0	5.0	1.2
Honey & Mustard, Low Fat, Marks & Spencer*	1 Serving/28g	31	110	1.5	20.0	2.5	0.8
Honey & Mustard, Marks & Spencer*	1 Tbsp/15ml	64	427	1.7	9.7	42.4	0.6
Honey & Mustard, More Than A Dressing, EPC*	1 Tsp/7g	6	91	0.5	21.6	0.3	0.0
Honey & Mustard, Sainsbury's*	1 Serving/10ml	37	366	1.0	15.4	33.0	0.1
Honey, Orange & Mustard, BGTY, Sainsbury's*	1 Tbsp/15ml	16	105	1.8	18.6	2.5	1.8
Hot Lime & Coconut, BGTY, Sainsbury's*	1 Tbsp/15ml	8	51	0.7	5.7	2.9	1.2
Italian Balsamic, Loyd Grossman*	1 Serving/10g	36	357	0.9	13.1	33.5	0.1
Italian Salad, Hellmann's*	1 Serving/50g	103	206	0.7	12.8	16.7	0.0
Italian Style, Green Pesto & Black Olives, Finest, Tesco*	1 Serving/30ml	84	279	1.3	1.9	29.3	0.5
Italian, Reduced Calorie, Hellmann's*	1 Serving/25ml	65	269	0.5	19.5	20.8	0.3
Italian, Waistline, 99% Fat Free, Crosse & Blackwell*	1 Tsp/6g	2	39	0.7	7.0	0.9	0.3
Lemon & Black Pepper, Good Intentions, Somerfield*	1 Tbsp/15ml	36	241	2.6	10.5	21.0	0.4
Lemon & Cracked Black Pepper, Good For You, Asda*	1 Tbsp/15g	9	57	0.2	14.0	0.0	0.3
Lemon & Tarragon, Healthy Eating, Tesco*	1 Serving/10ml	11	113	1.1	21.6	2.4	0.0
Lemon, Feta & Oregano, Marks & Spencer*	1 Tbsp/15ml	24	160	1.3	8.2	13.4	0.6
Lime & Coriander, EPC*	1 Serving/50g	29	57	0.3	13.3	0.3	0.0
Lime & Corriander, Sainsbury's*	1 Tbsp/15ml	61	409	0.4	10.0	40.8	0.5
Lime Sublime Creamy, Ainsley Harriott*	1 Serving/28g	95	338	0.0	10.0	32.5	0.0
Mayonnaise Style, 90% Fat Free, Weight Watchers*	1 Tsp/11g	14	125	1.7	8.9	9.2	0.0
Mild Mustard, Low Fat, Weight Watchers*	1 Tbsp/10g	6	63	2.0	5.7	3.6	0.0
Miracle Whip, Kraft*	1 Tbsp/15ml	60	400	0.3	11.0	39.0	0.1
Mustard & Dill, Perfectly Balanced, Waitrose*	1 Tbsp/15ml	24	159	1.1	31.5	3.2	1.1
Oil & Lemon	1 Tbsp/15g	97	647	0.3	2.8	70.6	0.0
Oil Free Lime & Coriander, Waitrose*	1 Tsp/5ml	3	65	1.5	11.9	1.3	0.4
Oil Free, French, Waitrose*	1 Tsp/5ml	4	76	1.5	13.1	2.0	0.6
Oil Free, Safeway*	1 Serving/30ml	23	75	1.6	14.0	1.4	0.0
Olive Oil & Balsamic Vinegar, Sainsbury's*	1 Serving/25ml	104	415	0.9	9.4	41.8	0.2
Olive Oil, Pizza Express*	2 Tsp/5g	29	573	1.4	3.4	63.0	0.0
Orange & Honey, Luxury, Hellmann's*	1 Serving/15ml	17	110	0.8	17.5	3.5	0.8
Parmesan & Peppercorn, Loyd Grossman*	1oz/28g	98	349	2.1	5.9	35.2	0.5
Passion Fruit & Mango, Healthy Eating, Tesco*	1 Tbsp/15ml	25	169	0.6	36.7	2.2	0.4
Porcini Mushroom, TTD, Sainsbury's*	1 Tbsp/15g	46	308	1.3	3.3	32.1	5.4
Provencal Roasted Vegetable, Healthy Eating, Tesco*	1 Serving/10ml	8	75	1.0	12.1	2.5	0.4
Raspberry Balsamic Vinegar, EPC*	1 Serving/50g	34	67	0.4	15.7	0.1	0.6
Red Pepper, Marks & Spencer*	1 Tbsp/15ml	58	385	0.6	7.6	39.2	0.5
Roasted Garlic, More Than A Dressing, EPC*	1 Serving/100ml	55	55	0.6	12.4	0.3	0.0
Roasted Red Pepper, TTD, Sainsbury's*	1 Tbsp/15ml	52	347	1.3	10.0	34.0	1.3
Salad Cream Style, Weight Watchers*	1 Tbsp/10g	12	115	1.5	16.2	4.4	0.0
Salad, BGTY, Sainsbury's*	1 Tbsp/15g	21	140	0.8	10.8	9.9	0.3
Salad, Healthy Eating, Tesco*	1 Tbsp/15g	22	144	0.8	12.9	9.9	0.3
Salad, Italian, Light, Calorie-Wise, Kraft*	1 Tbsp/15ml	6	40	0.0	5.3	2.7	0.0
Salad, Italian, Newman's Own*	1 Tbsp/10g	55	545	0.2	1.0	59.8	0.0
Salad, Light, Heinz*	1 Serving/9.8g	24	244	1.8	13.5	19.9	0.0
Salad, Low Fat, Weight Watchers*	1 Tbsp/10g	11	106	1.5	15.4	4.3	0.0
Salad, Luxury Caesar, Hellmann's*	1 Serving/10ml	50	498	2.5	4.4	51.7	0.3
Salad, Pizza Express*	1 Serving/5g	29	573	1.4	3.4	63.0	0.0
Salad, Raspberry Balsamic, GFY, Asda*	1 Tbsp/15ml	6	40	0.7	9.3	0.7	1.3

	Measure INFO/WEIGHT	per Measure KCAL	Nutrition Values per 100g / 100ml				
			KCAL	PROT	CARB	FAT	FIBRE
DRESSING,							
Salad, Sun Dried Tomato & Chilli, Loyd Grossman*	1 Tsp/5g	18	361	0.9	5.3	37.3	0.9
Salad, Thousand Island, 95% Fat Free, Asda	1 Tsp/6g	6	99	1.6	12.6	4.7	0.5
Salad, Thousand Island, Hellmann's*	1oz/28g	97	347	0.9	15.2	31.0	1.0
Salad, Thousand Island, Reduced Calorie, Hellmann's*	1oz/28g	73	259	1.0	19.0	19.4	0.9
Salad, Vinaigrette Style, 95% Fat Free, Asda*	1 Tbsp/15ml	6	42	0.1	10.6	0.0	0.3
Seafood, Marks & Spencer*	1 Tsp/7g	39	555	0.9	4.9	59.3	0.9
Smoked Garlic & Parmesan, Sainsbury's*	1 Serving/20ml	83	415	3.0	4.0	41.1	0.3
Sun Dried Tomato, Safeway*	1 Serving/40ml	126	314	1.1	13.8	28.3	0.0
Sun Dried Tomato, Sainsbury's	1 Serving/15ml	27	179	1.5	10.9	14.4	0.6
Sweet Chilli, COU, Marks & Spencer*	1 Tbsp/15ml	9	60	0.5	14.5	0.5	0.4
Sweetfire Pepper, Healthy Eating, Tesco*	1 Serving/10ml	7	67	0.6	15.7	0.3	0.1
Texas Ranch, Frank Cooper*	1 Pot/28g	128	457	1.9	9.4	45.8	0.2
Thousand Island	1 Tsp/6g	19	323	1.1	12.5	30.2	0.4
Thousand Island, BGTY, Sainsbury's*	1 Serving/50g	53	105	1.2	21.6	1.1	2.9
Thousand Island, COU, Marks & Spencer*	1 Serving/30g	26	85	1.4	14.2	2.6	1.1
Thousand Island, Fat Free, Kraft*	1floz/30ml	27	90	0.5	20.5	0.2	2.8
Thousand Island, Frank Cooper*	1 Pot/28g	122	437	1.2	7.2	44.8	0.3
Thousand Island, Healthy Eating, Tesco*	1 Serving/25ml	47	189	2.9	10.0	15.1	0.0
Thousand Island, Original, Kraft*	1oz/28g	102	365	0.9	19.0	31.5	0.4
Thousand Island, Reduced Calorie	1 Tsp/6g	12	195	0.7	14.7	15.2	0.0
Thousand Island, Tesco*	1 Serving/30ml	130	433	1.0	12.3	42.2	0.0
Tomato & Basil, Fresh, Somerfield*	1 Tbsp/15ml	52	348	2.0	7.0	35.0	0.0
Tomato & Basil, Healthy Eating, Tesco*	1 Serving/10ml	7	73	0.5	12.9	2.0	0.5
Tomato & Herb, Less Than 1% Fat, Asda*	1 Tbsp/15g	6	43	0.7	8.0	0.9	0.4
Tomato & Olive, Eat Smart, Safeway*	1 Tbsp/15ml	15	100	0.7	22.8	0.7	1.8
Tomato & Red Pepper, BGTY, Sainsbury's*	1 Serving/50ml	42	83	1.1	10.0	4.3	0.6
Tuna Mayonnaise & Sweetcorn Style, Weight Watchers*	1 Can/80g	114	142	11.5	6.2	8.0	0.1
Tuna, Tomato & Herb, Weight Watchers*	1 Can/80g	79	99	11.6	5.1	3.6	0.5
Waistline, Reduced Fat, Crosse & Blackwell*	1oz/28g	29	105	0.8	11.6	6.0	0.3
Wholegrain Dijon Mustard & Honey, Loyd Grossman*	1oz/28g	93	331	1.2	9.9	31.8	1.3
Yoghurt & Mint, Good For You, Asda*	1 Tbsp/15ml	9	60	3.9	8.0	1.4	0.0
Yoghurt & Mint, Healthy Eating, Tesco*	1 Tbsp/15g	20	135	1.5	26.2	2.7	0.0
Yoghurt & Mint, Perfectly Balanced, Waitrose*	1 Serving/100ml	130	130	4.6	22.1	2.6	0.7
Yoghurt Mint Cucumber, Marks & Spencer*	1 Tsp/5ml	6	115	1.0	8.7	8.0	0.0
DRIED FRUIT,							
Exotic Mix, Sundora*	1 Sm Pack/50g	138	276	2.3	60.6	2.7	3.8
Exotic, Ready To Eat, Sainsbury's*	1/3 Pack/85g	241	284	0.2	70.6	0.1	2.4
Luxury Mixed, Co-Op*	1 Serving/40g	114	285	2.0	68.0	0.6	4.0
Mixed	1 Tbsp/25g	67	268	2.3	68.1	0.4	2.2
Mixed, Ready Washed, Asda*	1 Serving/100g	284	284	2.1	68.0	0.4	1.7
Mixed, Tesco*	1 Tbsp/25g	71	284	2.3	67.9	0.4	2.2
DRIFTER, Nestle*	1 Finger/31g	144	479	4.1	66.7	21.7	0.9
DRINKING CHOCOLATE,							
Asda*, Dry Weight	1 Serving/30g	111	370	6.0	73.0	6.0	0.0
BGTY, Sainsbury's*, Made-Up	1 Serving/178g	114	64	3.9	11.4	0.2	0.7
Cadbury's*, Dry Weight	1 Serving/18g	66	367	6.4	72.4	5.8	0.0
Granules, Impress*, Dry Weight	1oz/28g	102	365	5.6	77.0	3.7	6.0
Powder, Made Up With Skimmed Milk	1 Mug/227ml	134	59	3.5	10.8	0.6	0.0
Powder, Made Up With Whole Milk	1 Mug/227ml	204	90	3.4	10.6	4.1	0.0
Waitrose*, Dry Weight	3 Tsp/12g	48	403	7.2	79.9	6.1	2.9
DRIPPING, Beef	1oz/28g	249	891	0.0	0.0	99.0	0.0
DUCK,							
A L' Orange, Roast, Marks & Spencer*	½ Pack/270g	554	205	12.5	4.1	15.6	0.6

DIP,

	Measure per Measuring		Nutrition Values per 100g / 100ml				
	INFO/WEIGHT	KCAL	KCAL	PROT	CARB	FAT	FIBRE
Aromatic With Plum Sauce, Tesco*	½ Pack/250g	350	140	9.3	15.2	4.6	0.3
Aromatic With a Plum Sauce, Finest, Tesco*	1 Serving/250g	400	160	16.1	11.3	5.6	4.6
Breast, Fillet, Skinless, Gressingham, TTD, Sainsbury's	1 Serving/160g	192	120	25.4	0.1	2.0	0.4
Breast, Fillets, Sliced, Marks & Spencer*	1 Pack/100g	150	150	25.3	3.6	3.7	0.0
Crispy Aromatic, Asda*	1/3 Pack/165.7g	470	283	19.0	18.0	15.0	0.8
Crispy Aromatic, Ready Meals, Marks & Spencer*	1 Pack/275g	591	215	12.6	10.3	13.6	1.2
Crispy Aromatic, Somerfield*	1 Serving/265g	782	295	18.1	14.0	18.5	0.7
Crispy Aromatic, Tesco*	1 Serving/61g	131	214	14.6	12.3	11.8	0.9
Crispy in a Plum Sauce, Marks & Spencer*	1 Pack/325g	569	175	10.7	11.2	9.6	0.9
Fillet With Orange Sauce, Waitrose*	½ Pack/250g	418	167	12.0	7.1	9.9	3.9
Fillets, Free Range With Red Wine Sauce, Waitrose*	½ Pack/250g	378	151	16.4	4.1	7.7	2.2
Gressingham Fillets & Orange Sauce, TTD Sainsbury's*	½ Pack/250g	633	253	24.9	0.1	17.0	1.0
Gressingham, Sweet Plum & Red Chilli Sauce, Sainsbury's*	½ Pack/225g	540	240	14.4	13.8	13.8	0.9
In Orange Sauce, Iceland*	1 Serving/200g	336	168	11.3	7.4	10.4	1.2
In Oriental Sauce, Iceland*	1 Pack/201.1g	352	175	12.0	6.3	11.3	1.5
Leg, Crispy, Sainsbury's*	1 Pack/230g	598	260	15.4	28.3	9.5	0.0
Leg, Sainsbury's*	1 Leg/76.1g	237	312	21.3	0.0	25.2	0.1
Legs, Meat & Skin, Finest, Tesco*	1 Serving/150g	431	287	15.0	0.1	25.2	1.0
Peking, Crispy, Sainsbury's*	½ Pack/300g	1236	412	19.5	0.6	36.9	0.0
Raw, Meat Only	1oz/28g	38	137	19.7	0.0	6.5	0.0
Raw, Meat, Fat & Skin	1oz/28g	109	388	13.1	0.0	37.3	0.0
Roasted, & Plum Sauce, Sainsbury's*	½ Pack/150g	272	181	12.0	13.5	8.8	0.7
Roasted, Meat Only	1oz/28g	55	195	25.3	0.0	10.4	0.0
Roasted, Meat, Fat & Skin	1oz/28g	118	423	20.0	0.0	38.1	0.0
Shanghai Roast With Noodles, Sainsbury's*	1 Pack/450g	581	129	5.6	18.0	3.8	1.2
Traditional Norfolk Breast Fillets, Sainsbury's*	1 Fillet/170g	442	260	22.3	0.0	19.0	0.1
DUETTO, Pasta, Green & White, Pasta Reale*	1oz/28g	79	281	10.9	49.4	6.0	3.6

DUMPLINGS,

Average	1oz/28g	58	208	2.8	24.5	11.7	0.9
Homestyle, Aunt Bessie's*	1 Dumpling/49g	187	382	8.5	39.5	21.1	2.1
Prawn Sui Mai With Soy Sauce, Marks & Spencer*	1 Pack/130g	143	110	13.7	6.7	3.4	0.6
Prawn, Cantonese, Crispy, Sainsbury's*	1 Dumpling/11g	27	241	9.3	20.9	13.4	1.1

	Measure INFO/WEIGHT	per Measure KCAL	Nutrition Values per 100g / 100ml				
			KCAL	PROT	CARB	FAT	FIBRE
EASTER EGG,							
Buttons, Cadbury's*	1 Pack/105g	557	530	7.8	56.9	30.0	0.0
Easter Egg, Kit Kat, Chunky, Nestle*	1 Pack/245g	1279	522	6.0	60.0	28.7	0.8
Easter Egg, Mars*	1 Serving/62.6g	283	449	4.2	69.0	17.4	0.0
EEL,							
Jellied	1oz/28g	27	98	8.4	0.0	7.1	0.0
Raw	1oz/28g	47	168	16.6	0.0	11.3	0.0
EGGS,							
Boiled	1 Size One/67g	98	147	12.5	0.0	10.8	0.0
Dried	1oz/28g	159	568	48.4	0.0	41.6	0.0
Duck, Boiled & Salted	1 Egg/75g	149	198	14.6	0.0	15.5	0.0
Duck, Whole, Raw	1 Egg/75g	122	163	14.3	0.0	11.8	0.0
Fried	1 Med/60g	107	179	13.6	0.0	13.9	0.0
Poached	1 Med/50g	74	147	12.5	0.0	10.8	0.0
Quail, Whole, Raw	1oz/28g	42	151	12.9	0.0	11.1	0.0
Scrambled With Milk	2 Med Eggs/120g	296	247	10.7	0.6	22.6	0.0
Turkey, Whole, Raw	1oz/28g	46	165	13.7	0.0	12.2	0.0
White, Dried	1oz/28g	83	295	73.8	0.0	0.0	0.0
Whites, Raw	1oz/28g	10	36	9.0	0.0	0.0	0.0
Whole, Raw	1 Size Three/57g	84	147	12.5	0.0	10.8	0.0
Yolks, Raw	1oz/28g	95	339	16.1	0.0	30.5	0.0
ELDERBERRIES, Average	1oz/28g	10	35	0.7	7.4	0.5	0.0
ELDERFLOWER CORDIAL, Bottle Green*	1 Glass/200ml	46	23	0.0	5.6	0.0	0.0
ELICHE, Pasta, Buitoni*	1 Serving/80g	282	352	11.2	72.6	1.9	0.0
ENCHILADAS,							
Chicken, Iceland*	1 Pack/400g	536	134	9.7	13.3	4.7	0.9
Chicken, In A Spicy Salsa & Bean Sauce, Asda*	½ Pack/211.9g	373	176	10.0	16.0	8.0	0.0
Chicken, Marks & Spencer*	1 Serving/225g	405	180	9.2	11.5	10.6	2.2
Chicken, Perfectly Balanced, Waitrose*	1 Pack/450g	482	107	6.9	12.7	3.2	1.1
Chicken, Safeway*	1 Serving/230g	384	167	7.9	22.9	4.9	1.0
Quorn*	1 Pack/400g	384	96	5.3	11.7	3.1	1.9
Quorn, Marlow Foods*	1 Pack/401g	405	101	5.3	11.7	3.7	1.9
Vegetable, Good for You, Asda*	1 Pack/350g	399	114	4.4	14.0	4.5	1.3
Vegetable, Morrisons*	1 Pack/400g	468	117	4.5	14.4	4.6	1.8
ENDIVE, Raw	1oz/28g	4	13	1.8	1.0	0.2	2.0
ENERGY DRINK, Red Rooster, Cott Beverages Ltd*	1 Can/250ml	113	45	0.6	10.3	0.0	0.0
EXOTIC FRUIT, Marks & Spencer*	1 Pack/425g	213	50	0.7	11.8	0.3	0.0
EXOTIC FRUIT JUICE, Pure, Del Monte*	1 Glass/200ml	96	48	0.3	11.3	0.0	0.0

E

	Measure INFO/WEIGHT	per Measure KCAL	Nutrition Values per 100g / 100ml				
			KCAL	PROT	CARB	FAT	FIBRE
FAGGOTS,							
In Rich Gravy, Iceland*	1 Faggot/81g	116	143	6.5	15.9	6.4	1.1
Mushy Peas & Mash, Sainsbury's*	1 Pack/450g	576	128	6.0	16.3	4.3	1.6
Pork, Mr Brains*	1 Serving/189g	242	128	5.3	11.9	6.6	0.6
FAGOTTINI, Mushroom, Sainsbury's*	½ Pack/155g	339	219	10.2	27.7	7.5	2.7
FAJITA,							
Beef, Good For You, Asda*	½ Pack/208g	354	170	11.0	21.0	4.7	1.6
Chicken With Salsa & Sour Cream Dips, Safeway*	1 Pack/242g	390	161	9.8	16.7	6.1	1.9
Chicken, American Style, Tesco*	1 Pack/275g	388	141	9.5	14.2	5.1	1.0
Chicken, BGTY, Sainsbury's*	1 Pack/299g	389	130	11.0	18.3	1.4	1.6
Chicken, Boots*	1 Pack/223g	448	201	9.1	25.0	7.2	3.9
Chicken, COU, Marks & Spencer*	1 Pack/230g	288	125	10.0	16.5	2.3	1.5
Chicken, COU, Salt Balanced, Marks & Spencer*	1 Pack/230g	253	110	9.5	13.2	2.3	1.7
Chicken, Co-Op*	1 Serving/230g	391	170	11.0	15.0	7.0	3.0
Chicken, Eat Smart, Safeway*	1 Serving/248g	290	117	10.6	14.8	1.7	1.6
Chicken, Good For You, Asda*	1 Serving/225g	297	132	10.0	17.0	2.7	1.1
Chicken, Healthy Eating, Tesco*	½ Pack/225g	248	110	9.2	15.3	1.3	0.5
Chicken, Marks & Spencer*	1 Pack/230g	345	150	8.6	17.7	5.3	1.0
Chicken, Sainsbury's*	½ Pack/250g	360	144	11.5	13.8	4.8	1.2
Chicken, Shapers, Boots*	1 Pack/192g	307	160	9.3	24.0	3.0	1.7
Chicken, Somerfield*	4 Fajitas/440g	528	120	7.8	13.2	4.1	2.8
Chicken, Tesco*	1 Serving/275g	388	141	9.5	14.2	5.1	1.0
Chicken, Weight Watchers*	1 Pack/175g	271	155	8.6	24.1	2.7	1.2
Gammon Steaks, Tesco*	1 Serving/250g	368	147	17.5	5.3	6.2	0.0
Ready Meals, Quorn*	1oz/28g	41	148	6.9	22.1	3.5	2.7
Steak, Marks & Spencer*	1oz/28g	53	190	8.9	17.2	9.1	0.6
Tuna, Eat Smart, Safeway*	1 Pack/263g	302	115	9.7	15.0	1.8	1.4
Tuna, Sainsbury's*	1 Pack/450g	752	167	11.4	18.2	5.4	1.6
Vegetable, Somerfield*	1 Pack/500g	640	128	3.0	17.0	5.0	0.0
Vegetable, Tesco*	1 Wrap/112g	133	119	4.2	14.3	5.0	1.1
FALAFEL,							
Cauldron Foods*	1 Falafel/25g	37	149	7.6	15.3	6.4	7.1
Fried in Vegetable Oil	1oz/28g	50	179	6.4	15.6	11.2	3.4
Marks & Spencer*	1 Serving/165g	388	235	8.3	19.2	13.7	8.4
Mini, Marks & Spencer*	1 Falafel/13g	40	310	7.9	28.1	18.4	2.6
Mini, Sainsbury's*	1 Serving/168g	499	297	8.0	26.8	17.6	3.2
Organic, Cauldron Foods*	1 Falafel/25g	55	220	8.0	23.3	10.5	7.6
Vegetarian, Organic, Waitrose*	1 Felafel/25g	55	220	8.0	23.3	10.5	7.6
FANTA,							
Lemon, The Coca Cola Co*	1 Can/330ml	165	50	0.0	12.0	0.0	0.0
Light, The Coca-Cola Co*	1 Glass/250ml	5	2	0.0	0.5	0.0	0.0
Orange, McDonald's*	1 Reguar/251g	108	43	0.0	10.4	0.0	0.0
Orange, The Coca-Cola Co*	1 Can/330ml	142	43	0.0	10.4	0.0	0.0
FARFALLE,							
Asda*	1 Serving/100g	366	366	12.0	75.0	2.0	3.0
Bows, Morrisons*	1 Serving/75g	266	354	12.0	72.0	2.0	3.0
Bows, Tesco*	1 Serving/100g	354	354	11.0	73.1	1.9	2.7
Dried, Napolina*	1oz/28g	99	352	11.5	73.0	1.5	2.2
Sainsbury's*	1 Serving/100g	357	357	12.3	73.1	1.7	2.5
Salmon & Broccoli, Eat Smart, Safeway*	1 Pack/380g	361	95	6.4	11.6	2.4	1.1
FARFALLINE, Bows, Mini, Tesco*	1oz/28g	93	333	13.2	65.6	2.0	2.9
FARMHOUSE MIX, Vegetables, Frozen, Asda*	1 Serving/100g	25	25	2.5	2.2	0.8	0.0
FENNEL,							
Florence, Boiled in Salted Water	1oz/28g	3	11	0.9	1.5	0.2	2.3

	Measure INFO/WEIGHT	per Measure KCAL	KCAL	PROT	CARB	FAT	FIBRE
FENNEL,							
Florence, Raw	1oz/28g	3	12	0.9	1.8	0.2	2.4
FENUGREEK LEAVES, Raw	1oz/28g	10	35	4.6	4.8	0.2	0.0
FETTUCCINE,							
Buitoni*	1oz/28g	101	362	12.2	74.4	1.7	0.0
Cajun Chicken, COU, Marks & Spencer*	1 Pack/350g	368	105	7.9	13.9	2.1	1.1
Tricolour, Asda*	1 Serving/100g	162	162	7.0	28.0	2.4	3.9
FIBRE JUICE, Tropicana*	1 Serving/200ml	130	65	0.4	15.8	0.0	3.4
FIG ROLLS,							
Asda*	1 Biscuit/19g	71	372	4.8	68.0	9.0	0.0
Go Ahead, McVitie's*	1 Roll/15g	55	365	4.2	76.8	4.6	2.9
Jacob's*	1 Biscuit/17g	61	357	3.5	67.7	8.0	3.9
Sainsbury's*	1 Biscuit/18g	70	377	4.8	68.3	9.4	2.6
Vitalinea, Jacob's*	1 Biscuit/18g	61	339	3.7	68.2	5.8	3.8
FIGS,							
Dried	1 Fig/20g	45	227	3.6	52.9	1.6	7.5
Dried, Marks & Spencer*	1oz/28g	71	253	3.4	63.6	0.0	4.6
Dried, Organic, Waitrose*	1oz/28g	67	240	3.6	52.9	1.6	7.5
Dried, Ready to Eat, Sainsbury's*	1 Fruit/14g	31	220	3.3	48.4	1.5	6.9
Fresh, Tesco*	4 Figs/200g	92	46	1.3	9.5	0.3	1.5
Raw	1 Fig/35g	15	43	1.3	9.5	0.3	1.5
Sun Dried, Garland, Ready to Eat, Tesco*	1 Serving/50g	115	230	4.2	52.9	0.2	18.5
Whitworth*	1oz/28g	62	220	3.3	48.4	1.5	6.9
FILET-O-FISH, McDonald's*	1 Pack/161g	388	241	10.0	25.0	11.0	0.7
FIORELLI, Egg, Marks & Spencer*	1 Serving/100g	355	355	13.9	68.5	2.8	3.0
FISH,							
Battered, Portion, Ross*	1 Fish/100g	203	203	10.4	16.1	10.8	0.8
Breaded, Asda*	1 Serving/150g	351	234	15.0	12.0	14.0	0.5
Chip Shop Portion, Youngs*	1 Portion/135g	315	233	11.0	15.1	14.6	0.6
Fillets, Natural White, Tesco*	1 Fillet/100g	72	72	16.6	0.0	0.6	0.0
Fillets, Steaks, Crunch Crumb, Bird's Eye*	1 Steak/110g	264	240	15.0	18.0	12.0	0.9
Fillets, White, Breaded, Tesco*	1 Piece/95g	205	216	10.0	20.9	10.3	1.1
In Light Batter, Iceland*	1 Fillet/120g	230	192	13.6	11.6	10.1	0.7
Nuggets, Battered, Farmfoods*	1oz/28g	60	214	10.9	16.0	11.8	0.7
Parcel With Mushroom, Carrots & Broccoli, Bird's Eye*	1 Pack/250g	235	94	7.9	3.1	5.6	0.8
Salted, Chinese, Steamed	1oz/28g	43	155	33.9	0.0	2.2	0.0
Steaks, Chip Shop, Youngs*	1 Portion/100g	198	198	11.0	14.9	10.4	0.9
Steaks, In Butter Sauce, Ross*	1 Serving/150g	126	84	9.1	3.2	3.9	0.1
Steaks, in Parsley Sauce, Ross*	1 Serving/150g	123	82	9.1	3.1	3.7	0.1
White, Tesco*	1 Med Fillet/100g	78	78	16.6	0.0	0.6	0.0
in Batter, Youngs*	1 Serving/100g	315	315	14.9	20.4	19.7	0.8
in Crispy Batter, Bird's Eye*	1 Steak/120g	230	192	13.6	11.6	10.1	0.7
FISH & CHIPS,							
Budgens*	1 Pack/284g	625	220	8.0	24.5	10.0	2.3
Co-Op*	1 Pack/250g	388	155	6.0	18.0	6.0	2.0
Ross*	1 Serving/250g	415	166	6.2	18.1	7.6	1.6
Safeway*	1 Pack/249g	518	208	8.0	25.0	8.4	3.5
Somerfield*	1 Serving/283g	495	175	8.0	22.0	6.0	0.0
FISH BAKE,							
Cheese & Leek, Healthy Living, Tesco*	1 Pack/400g	340	85	11.0	5.8	2.0	0.8
Cheese Pastry, Bird's Eye*	1 Piece/171g	390	228	9.3	17.2	13.6	1.9
Haddock & Prawn, COU, Marks & Spencer*	1 Bake/340g	289	85	7.3	7.3	2.8	0.4
Italiano, Bird's Eye*	½ Pack/205g	180	88	11.5	3.6	3.1	0.3
Vegetable Tuscany, Bird's Eye*	½ Pack/201g	195	97	11.8	2.2	4.6	0.6

F

	Measure INFO/WEIGHT	per Measure KCAL	Nutrition Values per 100g / 100ml				
			KCAL	PROT	CARB	FAT	FIBRE
FISH BALLS,							
Gefilte, Marks & Spencer*	1 Pack/200g	280	140	14.1	11.9	3.9	1.0
Steamed	1oz/28g	21	74	11.8	5.5	0.5	0.0
FISH CAKES,							
Bubbly Batter, Youngs*	1 Fish Cake/44g	109	247	7.1	20.5	15.1	1.4
Captain's Coins, Mini, Bird's Eye*	1 Fish Cake/20g	34	168	10.1	13.3	8.3	0.9
Cod & Pancetta, Cafe Culture, Marks & Spencer*	1 Fish Cake/85g	166	195	9.2	7.2	15.5	2.0
Cod & Parsley, Waitrose*	1 Fish Cake/85g	157	185	10.7	13.1	10.0	2.0
Cod, Asda*	1 Fish Cake/72g	163	227	7.0	25.0	11.0	2.3
Cod, Homemade	1 Fish Cake/50g	121	241	9.3	14.4	16.6	0.7
Cod, In Crunch Crumb, Bird's Eye*	1 Fish Cake/52g	85	163	8.8	16.2	7.0	0.7
Cod, Macfisheries*	1 Fish Cake/85g	163	192	7.6	22.1	8.2	1.1
Cod, Marks & Spencer*	1 Fish Cake/85g	162	190	8.4	15.7	10.1	1.6
Cod, Sainsbury's*	1 Fish Cake/90g	176	195	9.5	17.5	9.0	0.8
Cod, Tesco*	1 Fish Cake/49g	94	192	8.6	18.8	9.1	0.8
Crab, Marks & Spencer*	1oz/28g	63	225	8.0	18.0	13.2	1.4
Fried in Blended Oil	1 Fish Cake/50g	109	218	8.6	16.8	13.4	0.0
Frozen	1oz/28g	37	132	8.6	16.7	3.9	0.0
Great Value, Iceland*	1 Fish Cake/42g	74	175	9.1	20.3	6.4	1.6
Grilled	1 Fish Cake/50g	77	154	9.9	19.7	4.5	0.0
Haddock, Asda*	1 Fish Cake/88g	181	206	8.0	21.0	10.0	1.5
Haddock, Marks & Spencer*	1 Pack/170g	289	170	8.6	13.7	9.2	1.3
Haddock, Sainsbury's*	1 Fish Cake/90g	173	192	11.7	18.1	8.1	0.7
Haddock, Smoked, Frozen, Waitrose*	1 Fish Cake/85g	157	185	11.0	12.4	10.1	2.1
Haddock, Smoked, Tesco*	1 Fish Cake/90g	171	190	8.6	22.5	7.3	1.1
Halibut Cod Loin, Finest, Tesco*	1 Serving/115g	213	185	8.8	21.3	7.2	1.4
Makes Sense, Somerfield*	1 Fish Cake/42g	70	166	8.2	18.7	6.5	1.5
Marks & Spencer*	1 Fish Cake/80g	180	225	8.0	18.0	13.3	0.0
Prawn, Sainsbury's*	1 Fish Cake/90g	154	171	10.3	15.6	7.5	0.7
Prawn, Tesco*	1 Fish Cake/90g	209	232	8.2	29.2	9.1	1.8
Ross*	1 Fish Cake/52g	102	196	9.6	18.6	9.2	0.8
Salmon & Broccoli, Morrisons*	1 Fish Cake/60g	126	210	9.8	17.2	11.9	1.3
Salmon & Broccoli, With Bubble & Squeak, Safeway*	1 Pack/389g	513	132	3.9	15.0	6.3	1.0
Salmon & Dill, Waitrose*	1 Fish Cake/85g	179	211	9.1	17.6	11.6	2.2
Salmon & Tarragon, Waitrose*	1 Fish Cake/85g	179	211	11.9	14.3	11.8	2.2
Salmon, Asda*	1 Fish Cake/86g	215	250	8.0	23.0	14.0	1.4
Salmon, Bird's Eye*	1 Fish Cake/50g	84	168	9.5	12.2	9.0	1.4
Salmon, Homemade	1 Fish Cake/50g	137	273	10.4	14.4	19.7	0.7
Salmon, Marks & Spencer*	1 Fish Cake/86g	181	210	9.1	15.1	12.7	1.7
Salmon, Morrisons*	1 Fish Cake/90g	241	268	10.1	27.6	13.1	1.5
Salmon, Sainsbury's*	1 Fish Cake/90g	167	186	13.2	17.4	7.1	1.2
Salmon, Tesco*	1 Fish Cake/50g	110	219	10.1	13.7	13.7	0.9
Salmon, With Parsley Sauce, Finest, Tesco*	½ Pack/170g	350	206	8.6	11.7	13.9	1.0
SmarPrice, Asda*	1 Fish Cake/41g	77	188	7.0	22.0	8.0	0.9
Smoked Haddock, Sainsbury's*	1 Fish Cake/63g	127	201	11.0	17.8	9.5	2.1
Thai Crab & Prawn, Tesco*	1 Fish Cake/115g	269	234	8.8	17.4	14.4	1.2
Thai Style, Sainsbury's*	1 Fish Cake/49g	69	141	12.0	13.8	4.2	1.7
Thai, Tesco*	4 Cakes/88g	148	166	17.4	12.8	5.0	1.1
Tuna & Red Pepper, Waitrose*	1 Fish Cake/85g	175	206	9.5	15.4	11.8	1.6
Tuna, Asda*	1 Fish Cake/87g	171	196	9.0	22.0	8.0	1.3
Tuna, Marks & Spencer*	1 Fish Cake/85g	170	200	10.0	14.9	11.0	1.6
Tuna, Tesco*	1 Fish Cake/90g	182	202	9.2	25.0	7.3	1.3
Value, Tesco*	1 Fish Cake/40g	73	183	7.1	21.2	7.8	1.2

F

	Measure INFO/WEIGHT	per Measure KCAL	Nutrition Values per 100g / 100ml				
			KCAL	PROT	CARB	FAT	FIBRE
FISH FINGERS,							
100% Cod Fillet, Bird's Eye*	1 Finger/30g	56	186	13.0	15.6	7.9	0.7
Chip Shop, Youngs*	1 Finger/30g	75	251	9.3	16.6	16.4	1.2
Cod Fillet, Asda*	1 Finger/31g	66	214	13.0	18.0	10.0	0.0
Cod Fillet, Bird's Eye*	1 Finger/30g	53	177	12.7	14.1	7.7	1.0
Cod Fillet, Chunky, Marks & Spencer*	1 Finger/40g	70	175	12.0	17.3	6.0	1.0
Cod Fillet, Waitrose*	1 Finger/30g	55	183	11.9	16.9	7.5	0.7
Cod, Fried in Blended Oil	1 Finger/28g	67	238	13.2	15.5	14.1	0.6
Cod, Frozen	1 Finger/28g	48	170	11.6	14.2	7.8	0.6
Cod, Grilled	1 Finger/28g	56	200	14.3	16.6	8.9	0.7
Cod, Tesco*	1 Finger/30g	56	188	12.3	16.8	7.9	1.6
Economy, Sainsbury's*	1 Finger/26g	51	198	12.6	17.7	8.5	1.3
Farmfoods*	1 Finger/27g	49	183	12.2	15.6	8.0	1.2
Free From, Sainsbury's*	1 Finger/30g	56	188	11.4	18.0	7.8	0.7
Haddock Fillet, Asda*	1 Finger/30g	62	205	14.0	17.0	9.0	0.0
Haddock Fillet, Bird's Eye*	1 Finger/29g	48	167	12.4	13.2	7.2	0.9
Hoki Fillet, Bird's Eye*	1 Finger/30g	58	193	12.6	15.6	8.9	0.7
Iceland*	1 Finger/23g	44	192	11.5	17.3	8.5	1.3
In Crispy Batter, Bird's Eye*	1 Finger/29g	63	218	10.4	15.8	12.6	0.4
In Crispy Batter, Jumbo, Morrisons*	1 Finger/71g	146	205	11.3	12.2	12.5	0.6
McDonald's*	3 Fingers/74g	164	221	13.5	20.2	9.6	3.1
Minced White Fish, Bird's Eye*	1 Finger/25g	47	187	12.7	16.7	7.7	0.7
Ross*	1 Finger/26g	48	186	12.1	17.6	7.5	0.8
Sainsbury's*	1 Finger/27g	52	194	13.4	16.0	8.5	0.7
SmartPrice, Asda*	1 Finger/25g	46	184	12.0	16.0	8.0	1.1
Value, Tesco*	1 Finger/25g	46	182	11.0	16.8	7.9	1.6
FISH MIX, For Smoked Haddock, Schwartz*	1 Pack/35g	154	440	13.8	46.9	21.9	0.0
FIVE FRUITS, Fruit Burst, Del Monte*	1 Carton/250ml	133	53	0.2	12.4	0.0	0.0
FIVE SPICE POWDER, Sharwood's*	1oz/28g	48	172	12.2	11.6	8.6	23.4
FLAKE, Cadbury's*	1 Std Bar/34g	180	530	8.1	55.7	30.7	0.0
FLAN,							
Cauliflower Cheese, Safeway*	1 Sm Flan/150g	420	280	7.3	25.0	16.5	2.0
Cauliflower, Cheese & Broccoli, Hot, Sainsbury's*	¼ Flan/100g	303	303	6.4	24.7	19.8	1.2
Cheese & Onion, Marks & Spencer*	1oz/28g	81	290	6.1	25.1	18.7	1.4
Cheese & Potato, Hot, Tesco*	¼ Flan/100g	282	282	6.0	20.0	19.7	2.3
Chicken & Smoked Bacon, Hot, Sainsbury's*	¼ Flan/100g	293	293	10.2	21.5	18.5	1.2
Mediterranean Vegetable, Co-Op*	¼ Flan/87.5g	189	215	4.0	22.0	12.0	3.0
Pastry, With Fruit	1oz/28g	33	118	1.4	19.3	4.4	0.7
Sponge With Fruit	1oz/28g	31	112	2.8	23.3	1.5	0.6
FLAN CASE,							
Golden Bake, Sainsbury's*	1 Case/113g	373	330	5.5	65.6	5.1	1.2
Sponge	1oz/28g	83	295	9.8	53.6	6.1	0.8
FLAPJACK,							
90% Fat Free, Cookie Coach Company*	1 Flapjack/75g	287	383	7.0	66.2	9.9	0.0
All Butter, Sainsbury's*	1 Flapjack/35g	156	446	5.7	54.5	22.8	2.7
Apple & Raisin, Lite, Crazy Jack*	1 Flapjack70g	227	324	9.8	72.0	2.1	0.0
Apple & Raspberry, Fox's*	1 Flapjack/26g	105	403	4.8	52.5	19.4	3.7
Apple & Sultana, Mr Kipling*	1 Flapjack/27g	124	460	4.6	59.6	22.5	0.0
Apricot & Raisin, Waitrose*	1 Flapjack/38g	143	376	4.7	64.3	11.1	5.8
Apricot, COU, Marks & Spencer*	1oz/28g	96	342	5.4	77.1	2.1	2.0
Apricot, Food To Go, Marks & Spencer*	1 Bar/86g	348	405	4.7	64.4	16.2	4.3
Average	1oz/28g	136	484	4.5	60.4	26.6	2.7
Cappuccino, Black Friars*	1 Flapjack/110g	481	437	5.0	61.0	25.0	0.0
Cherry & Sultana, 90% Fat Free, Cookie Coach Company*	1 Flapjack/75g	276	368	6.0	69.4	9.0	0.0

F

	Measure INFO/WEIGHT	per Measure KCAL	Nutrition Values per 100g / 100ml				
			KCAL	PROT	CARB	FAT	FIBRE
FLAPJACK,							
Cherry & Sultana, Cookie Coach Company*	1 Pack/90g	373	414	6.2	58.2	17.3	0.0
Cherry & Sultana, Marks & Spencer*	1oz/28g	111	395	5.4	63.7	13.0	5.1
Chewy Nutty, Coffee Republic	1 Flapjack/33g	145	440	7.1	50.9	23.2	2.0
Chocolate & Hazelnut, Marks & Spencer*	1 Flapjack/71g	330	465	7.3	55.6	25.5	3.8
Chocolate Chip, Boots*	1 Flapjack/75g	313	417	5.6	65.0	15.0	3.5
Chocolate Chip, Happy Shopper*	1 Flapjack/35g	163	467	5.7	58.7	23.3	0.0
Chocolate Chunk, Boots*	1 Slice/75g	351	468	5.7	55.0	25.0	3.0
Chocolate Dipped, Marks & Spencer*	1 Flapjack/96g	442	460	6.1	61.3	22.4	3.0
Chocolate, McVitie's*	1 Flapjack/85g	422	496	6.6	56.6	27.1	3.2
Co-Op*	1 Flapjack/37.6g	177	465	5.0	54.0	25.0	4.0
Crazy Raizin, The Fabulous Bakin' Boys*	1 Pack/90g	378	420	6.0	60.0	17.0	4.0
Fingers, Good for You, Asda*	1 Finger/37g	130	350	5.0	60.0	10.0	3.5
Fruit & Nut, Organic, Evernat*	1oz/28g	136	484	4.5	60.4	26.6	0.0
Fruit With Raisins, Boots*	1 Pack/75g	329	439	5.4	57.0	21.0	3.5
Fruit, Good for You, Asda*	1 Flapjack/45g	173	384	6.0	72.0	8.0	3.4
Fruit, Mr Kipling*	1 Flapjack/24g	103	430	4.8	51.4	22.9	0.0
Fruit, Somerfield*	1 Flapjack/45g	182	405	6.3	57.9	16.5	5.0
Fruity, Waitrose*	1 Serving/50g	199	398	6.1	62.9	13.5	3.9
Fudge, Black Friars*	1 Slice/110g	528	480	5.0	60.0	24.0	0.0
Golden Oaty Fingers, Tesco*	1 Finger/25g	113	450	5.7	59.6	21.1	3.4
Marks & Spencer*	1 Flapjack/53g	228	430	6.0	59.1	19.0	3.5
Mini Bites, Mark & Spencer*	1 Bite/14g	70	500	6.4	62.8	25.0	2.6
Mixed Fruit, Organic, Evernat*	1oz/28g	136	484	4.5	60.4	26.6	0.0
Organic, Wholebake*	1 Bar/90g	388	431	6.0	59.4	20.8	0.0
Safeway*	1 Flapjack/60g	255	425	5.9	55.1	20.1	2.7
Snickers, McVitie's*	1 Flapjack/65g	320	492	9.5	47.6	29.3	0.0
Sultana, Tesco*	1 Flapjack/50g	173	346	5.0	36.2	20.1	3.7
Syrup, McVitie's*	1 Flapjack/85g	417	490	6.5	56.0	26.7	3.4
Tropical Mix, Reduced Fat, The Fabulous Bakin' Boys*	1 Flapjack/90g	347	385	6.0	63.0	12.0	3.0
Weight Watchers*	1 Slice/30g	109	364	6.5	71.0	6.0	3.9
With Sultanas, Tesco*	1 Flapjack/49g	217	442	5.3	57.9	21.0	3.7
Yoghurt Flavour, Blackfriars*	1 Bar/110g	521	474	7.0	58.0	24.0	0.0
FLATBREAD,							
BBQ Style Chicken, Shapers, Boots*	1 Serving/108g	187	173	10.0	23.0	4.6	2.8
Cajun Style Chicken, GFY, Asda*	1 Wrap/176.3g	231	131	9.0	21.0	1.2	0.9
Cheese & Garlic, Sainsbury's*	¼ Bread/100g	340	340	9.3	39.3	16.2	2.2
Cheese & Onion Swedish Style, Shapers, Boots*	1 Flatbread/127g	265	209	10.0	24.0	8.1	1.3
Chicken & Black Bean Sauce, Shapers, Boots*	1 Pack/204g	249	122	8.7	20.0	0.8	1.7
Chicken Caesar, Shapers, Boots*	1 Serving/160g	254	159	13.0	22.0	2.1	2.0
Chicken Fajita, Shapers, Boots*	1 Serving/200g	276	138	9.0	20.0	2.4	2.6
Chicken Salsa, McDonald's*	1 Serving/100g	480	480	27.3	57.6	15.5	0.0
Chicken Tikka, BGTY, Sainsbury's*	1 Flatbread/188g	241	128	10.3	18.5	1.4	2.1
Chicken Tikka, Shapers, Boots*	1 Flatbread/164g	282	172	11.0	24.0	3.6	1.4
Chinese Chicken, COU, Marks & Spencer*	1 Flatbread/156g	281	180	13.9	24.3	2.8	2.2
Chinese Chicken, Shapers, Boots*	1 Pack/159.3g	273	172	11.0	29.0	1.3	1.8
Feta Cheese, Shapers, Boots*	1 Pack/165.6g	256	154	6.7	23.0	3.9	1.4
Garlic & Rosemary, Accompaniments, Sainsbury's*	¼ Flatbread/60g	184	306	8.7	40.3	12.2	2.7
Greek Style Salad, Waitrose*	1 Pack/171.8g	280	163	7.4	22.3	4.9	3.3
Greek Style, GFY, Asda*	1 Flatbread/165g	256	155	7.0	22.0	4.3	2.1
Greek, McDonald's*	1 Flatbread/100g	433	433	21.2	47.3	20.7	3.8
Italian Chicken, Shapers, Boots*	1 Pack/168.4g	265	158	10.0	22.0	3.3	1.3
Japapeno & Sweet Pepper, Sainsbury's*	1 Serving/100g	263	263	10.9	40.9	6.2	2.6
Mediterranean Chicken, Ginsters*	1 Pack/167.8g	302	180	10.6	25.5	4.0	0.0

F

INFO/WEIGHT	Measure per Measure KCAL	Nutrition Values per 100g / 100ml KCAL	PROT	CARB	FAT	FIBRE

FLATBREAD,

	Measure INFO/WEIGHT	per Measure KCAL	KCAL	PROT	CARB	FAT	FIBRE
Mediterranean Tuna, Ginsters*	1 Pack/166.9g	297	178	10.3	25.6	3.8	0.0
Mexican Style Chicken, Safeway*	1 Pack/150g	248	165	11.6	24.7	2.1	1.9
Peking Duck, Less Than 3% Fat, Shapers, Boots*	1 Pack/155.7g	246	158	7.2	27.0	2.4	1.9
Prawn Korma, Shapers, Boots*	1 Pack/169.0g	267	158	8.8	22.0	3.9	1.3
Rancher's Chicken, COU, Marks & Spencer*	1 Pack/174g	270	155	10.9	23.0	2.0	1.5
Ranchers Chicken, Shapers, Boots*	1 Pack/194.2g	303	156	12.0	22.0	2.2	1.5
Salsa Chicken, Shapers, Boots*	1 Pack/190.7g	329	172	11.0	22.0	4.4	1.6
Spicy Chicken & Salsa, Healthy Living, Tesco	1 Flatbread/183g	251	137	10.1	21.1	1.4	1.2
Spicy Mexican, Shapers, Boots*	1 Pack/190g	296	156	7.0	23.0	4.0	3.7
Sticky BBQ Style Chicken, Shapers, Boots*	1 Pack/158.4g	273	173	10.0	23.0	4.6	2.8
Tomata & Chilli, Sainsbury's*	¼ Bread/65g	155	238	11.9	36.9	4.7	2.8
Tomato & Chilli, BGTY, Sainsbury's*	¼ Flatbread/100g	155	155	7.7	24.0	3.1	1.8
Vegetable & Salsa, Healthy Living, Tesco*	1 Flatbread/193g	262	136	7.9	22.2	1.8	1.2
FLIPPER DIPPER, Penguin, McVitie's*	1 Pack/50.1g	267	533	8.2	60.7	28.7	1.5

FLOUR,

	Measure INFO/WEIGHT	per Measure KCAL	KCAL	PROT	CARB	FAT	FIBRE
Bread, Wholemeal, Strong, Organic, Doves Farm*	1 Serving/100g	319	319	12.0	62.8	2.2	9.0
Brown, Chapati,	1 Tbsp/20g	67	333	11.5	73.7	1.2	0.0
Brown, Wheat	1oz/28g	90	323	12.6	68.5	1.8	6.4
Chick Pea	1oz/28g	88	313	19.7	49.6	5.4	10.7
Corn, Tesco*	1 Serving/90g	316	351	0.4	87.0	0.1	0.1
Millet	1oz/28g	99	354	5.8	75.4	1.7	0.0
Plain, Economy, Sainsbury's*	1 Serving/100g	344	344	9.7	73.4	1.4	3.0
Plain, Organic, Marks & Spencer*	1oz/28g	95	340	10.9	70.4	1.9	3.7
Potato	1oz/28g	92	328	9.1	75.6	0.9	5.7
Rice	1oz/28g	102	366	6.4	80.1	0.8	2.0
Rye, Whole	1oz/28g	94	335	8.2	75.9	2.0	11.7
Self Raising, Bettabuy, Morrisons*	1 Serving/100g	337	337	9.8	71.4	1.3	3.0
Self Raising, Sainsbury's*	1 Serving/100g	335	335	8.9	72.0	1.3	3.3
Self-Raising, Organic, Marks & Spencer*	1oz/28g	92	330	10.3	68.1	1.6	5.3
Soya, Full Fat	1oz/28g	125	447	36.8	23.5	23.5	11.2
Soya, Full Fat, Nature's Harvest, Holland & Barrett*	1oz/28g	111	396	39.0	16.0	20.0	12.0
Soya, Low Fat	1oz/28g	99	352	45.3	28.2	7.2	13.5
Speciality Gluten Free, Doves Farm*	1 Serving/100g	353	353	4.7	85.2	1.8	2.7
Strong, Brown Bread, Allinson*	1 Serving/100g	302	302	14.0	61.0	1.8	6.4
Strong, Brown Bread, Sainsbury's*	1 Serving/100g	320	320	14.0	61.0	1.8	6.4
Strong, Canadian, Waitrose*	1oz/28g	94	337	12.6	68.6	1.4	3.1
Strong, White Bread, Allinson*	1 Serving/100g	330	330	11.5	67.9	1.4	3.7
Strong, White Bread, Tesco*	1 Serving/100g	346	346	11.7	71.6	1.4	3.7
Strong, White Bread, With Kibbled Grains, Allinson*	1 Serving/100g	346	346	11.2	69.7	1.7	4.4
Strong, White, Organic, Waitrose*	1oz/28g	89	319	11.5	64.5	1.7	2.7
Strong, Wholemeal Plain, Waitrose*	1 Serving/100g	311	311	14.5	58.3	2.2	9.0
Very Strong, White Bread, Allinson*	1 Serving/100g	348	348	13.9	69.0	1.8	3.2
White, Bread, Organic, Waitrose*	1oz/28g	69	246	8.8	48.8	0.5	1.8
White, Chapati,	1 Tbsp/20g	67	335	9.8	77.6	0.5	0.0
White, Organic, Waitrose*	1oz/28g	99	355	8.0	77.7	1.3	3.1
White, Plain, Value, Tesco*	1oz/28g	95	341	9.5	70.7	2.2	3.1
White, Wheat, Plain	1oz/28g	95	341	9.4	77.7	1.3	3.1
White, Wheat, Self-Raising	1oz/28g	92	330	8.9	75.6	1.2	3.1
White, Wheat, White, Breadmaking	1oz/28g	95	341	11.5	75.3	1.4	3.1
Wholemeal, Organic, Waitrose*	1oz/28g	89	319	11.0	63.9	2.2	9.0
Wholemeal, Self Raising, Tesco*	1oz/28g	89	317	11.5	62.9	2.2	9.0
Wholemeal, Wheat	1oz/28g	87	310	12.7	63.9	2.2	9.0
FLYING SAUCERS, Co-Op*	1 Sweet/1g	4	370	0.5	90.0	1.0	0.6

F

	Measure INFO/WEIGHT	per Measure KCAL	Nutrition Values per 100g / 100ml				
			KCAL	PROT	CARB	FAT	FIBRE
FLYTE,							
Mars*	1 Bar/45g	196	435	3.6	72.3	14.7	0.0
Snacksize, Mars*	1 Bar/22.5g	98	436	3.8	72.5	14.5	0.0
FOOL,							
Apricot, BGTY, Sainsbury's*	1 Pot/113g	87	77	3.5	8.0	3.4	0.3
Apricot, Fruit, Tesco*	1 Pot/113g	200	177	2.6	16.4	11.2	0.3
Blackcurrant, BGTY, Sainsbury's*	1 Pot/113g	89	79	3.5	10.4	2.6	0.6
Fruit	1oz/28g	46	163	1.0	20.2	9.3	1.2
Fruit, Better for You, Morrisons*	1 Pot/114g	96	84	3.4	10.1	3.4	0.3
Gooseberry, Better For You, Morrison's*	1 Pot/114g	99	87	3.4	10.7	3.4	0.4
Gooseberry, Fruit, BGTY, Sainsbury's*	1 Pot/121g	93	77	2.9	10.0	2.8	0.8
Gooseberry, Fruit, Co-Op*	1 Pot/114g	211	185	3.0	22.0	10.0	1.0
Gooseberry, Fruit, Somerfield*	1 Pot/114g	215	189	3.0	19.0	11.0	0.0
Lemon, Better For You, Morrison's*	1 Pot/114g	96	84	3.4	10.1	3.4	0.3
Lemon, Fruit, BGTY, Sainsbury's*	1 Pot/113g	94	83	3.4	9.7	3.4	0.3
Lemon, Fruit, Shapers, Boots*	1 Pot/113g	105	93	3.8	11.0	3.8	0.0
Raspberry, Fruit, Tesco*	1 Pot/113g	234	207	2.6	23.6	11.3	0.3
Raspberry, Pret A Manger*	1 Pot/140g	188	134	1.7	12.4	8.9	0.4
Rhubarb, Fruit, BGTY, Sainsbury's*	1 Pot/120g	90	75	2.9	9.5	2.8	0.3
Rhubarb, Fruit, Somerfield*	1 Pot/114g	201	176	3.0	16.0	11.0	0.0
Rhubarb, Fruit, Waitrose*	1 Pot/114g	182	160	2.7	11.9	11.3	0.3
Strawberry, Fruit, BGTY, Sainsbury's*	1 Pot/120g	100	83	3.0	11.5	2.8	1.0
Strawberry, Fruit, Co-Op*	1 Pot/114g	188	165	2.0	18.0	9.0	0.8
Strawberry, Fruit, Shapers, Boots*	1 Pot/112g	90	81	3.5	9.2	3.4	0.3
Strawberry, Fruit, Somerfield*	1 Pot/114g	201	176	3.0	16.0	11.0	0.0
FRANKFURTERS,							
Herta*	1 Frankfurter/35g	117	335	12.0	2.0	31.0	0.0
Jumbo, Herta*	1 Frankfurter/80g	236	295	11.7	0.4	27.5	0.0
Jumbo, Marks & Spencer*	1 Frankfurter/94g	277	295	11.7	0.4	27.5	0.0
Real German, Meica*	1 Frankfurter/42g	100	239	12.0	0.5	21.0	0.0
Vegetarian, Tivall*	3 Sausages/90g	220	244	18.0	7.0	16.0	3.0
FRAZZLES, Bacon, Smiths, Walkers*	1 Bag/23g	108	470	8.0	59.0	22.4	0.0
FREEZEPOPS,							
Cola, The Simpsons, Calypso*	1 Freezepop/50ml	15	30	0.0	7.1	0.0	0.0
Orange, The Simpsons, Calypso*	1 Freezepop/50ml	15	30	0.0	7.1	0.0	0.0
Raspberry, The Simpsons, Calypso*	1 Freezepop/50ml	15	30	0.0	7.1	0.0	0.0
FRENCH FRIES,							
Cheese & Onion, Walkers*	1 Bag/22g	94	425	5.4	64.0	16.0	4.2
Fish & Chips, Walkers*	1 Bag/19.0g	79	415	4.2	64.0	16.0	4.3
King Size, Salted, Burger King*	1 Serving/170g	539	317	3.5	42.3	14.7	2.9
Medium, Salted, Burger King*	1 Serving/116g	369	318	3.4	42.2	14.6	3.4
Ready Salted, Walkers*	1 Bag/22g	95	430	5.1	64.0	17.0	4.3
Salt & Vinegar, COU, Marks & Spencer*	1 Bag/25g	88	350	5.1	80.9	1.6	2.3
Salt & Vinegar, Eat Smart, Safeway*	1 Bag/20g	75	375	5.1	80.9	1.6	2.3
Salt & Vinegar, Walkers*	1 Bag/22g	92	420	5.0	63.0	16.0	4.2
Small, Salted, Burger King*	1 Serving/74g	229	310	2.7	41.8	14.8	2.7
Worcester Sauce, Walkers*	1 Bag/22g	92	420	5.1	64.0	16.0	4.2
FRENCH TOAST,							
Asda*	1 Slice/8g	30	381	10.0	74.0	5.0	4.0
Morrisons*	1 Toast/8g	31	393	11.0	72.5	6.6	3.0
Safeway*	1 Slice/8g	31	393	11.0	72.5	6.6	3.0
Tesco*	1 Serving/100g	393	393	11.0	72.5	6.6	3.0
FRIES,							
9/16" Straight Cut Home, Deep Fried, McCain*	1oz/28g	65	233	3.2	32.7	9.9	0.0

F

	Measure INFO/WEIGHT	per Measure KCAL	Nutrition Values per 100g / 100ml				
			KCAL	PROT	CARB	FAT	FIBRE
FRIES,							
9/16" Straight Cut Home, Oven Baked, McCain*	1oz/28g	53	188	3.2	31.5	5.5	0.0
American Style Slim, Iceland*	1 Serving/100g	373	373	6.1	55.8	13.9	7.0
American Style, Frozen, Thin, Tesco*	1 Serving/125g	208	166	2.2	21.1	8.1	1.9
American, 3 Way Cook, Somerfield*	1oz/28g	43	155	3.0	25.0	5.0	0.0
American, Oven, Asda*	1 Serving/180g	432	240	3.4	34.0	10.0	3.0
Bacon, Smiths, Walkers*	1 Bag/25g	126	504	11.7	44.4	31.2	0.0
Cafe Frites, Marks & Spencer*	1 Pack/200g	440	220	3.0	32.7	8.7	2.4
Crinkle, Home, McCain*	1 Serving/135g	248	184	2.3	25.5	9.0	0.0
Crispy French, McCain*	1 Serving/100g	165	165	2.1	24.3	6.6	0.0
Crispy Savoury Seasoning Southern, McCain*	1 Serving/100g	179	179	2.8	26.4	6.9	0.0
Home Oven Chips, McCain*	1oz/28g	53	188	3.2	31.5	5.5	0.0
Home, Frozen, McCain*	1 Serving/100g	141	141	2.0	26.1	4.4	0.0
Home, Oven Cooked, McCain*	1 Serving/100g	202	202	3.2	37.5	6.1	0.0
McDonald's *	1 Regular/78g	207	265	3.8	36.3	11.5	3.6
Medium, Kentucky Fried Chicken*	1 Serving/100g	294	294	3.8	36.4	14.8	3.1
Oven, Straight Cut, Morrisons*	1 Serving/100g	149	149	2.8	24.6	4.3	2.6
Salt & Vinegar, BGTY, Sainsbury's*	1 Bag/15g	50	335	5.5	75.3	1.4	2.7
Scampi, Smiths, Walkers*	1 Bag/27g	134	496	13.0	52.5	26.0	0.0
Southern Spicy Spiral, Deep Fried, McCain*	1oz/28g	58	208	2.7	26.4	10.2	0.0
Southern Spicy Spiral, Oven Baked, McCain*	1oz/28g	46	165	1.7	24.6	6.6	0.0
Southern, Oven Cook, McCain*	1 Serving/80g	146	182	2.7	26.1	8.4	0.0
Southern, Straight Cut, Oven Baked, McCain*	1oz/28g	74	263	4.1	37.1	10.9	0.0
Spicy Curly, Asda*	1 Serving/75g	134	179	2.3	29.0	6.0	2.5
FRISPS,							
Tangy Salt & Vinegar, Frisps*	1 Bag/30g	155	517	5.8	52.2	31.7	4.0
Tasty Cheese & Onion, Frisps*	1 Bag/31g	162	521	6.3	52.4	31.8	4.3
FROMAGE FRAIS,							
0% Fat, Vitalinea*	1 Tbsp/28g	14	50	7.4	4.7	0.1	0.0
Apple Pie, Low Fat, Sainsbury's*	1 Pot/90g	108	120	6.7	17.3	2.6	0.3
Apple Strudel, Safeway*	1 Pot/100g	116	116	6.6	14.8	3.4	0.7
Apricot, Tesco*	1 Pot/100g	77	77	6.5	6.0	3.0	1.3
Apricot, Weight Watchers*	1 Pot/100g	47	47	6.2	5.4	0.1	0.2
Bakewell Tart Flavour, BGTY, Sainsbury's*	1 Pot/100g	54	54	7.6	5.5	0.2	1.1
Banoffee Pie Flavour, Low Fat, Safeway*	1 Pot/100g	135	135	6.8	17.6	4.1	0.2
Banoffee Toffee, Weight Watchers*	1 Pot/100g	64	64	5.7	10.0	0.1	1.1
Black Cherry, Asda*	1 Pot/100g	113	113	4.1	13.0	5.0	0.0
Black Cherry, Good For You, Asda*	1 Pot/100g	54	54	6.0	7.0	0.2	0.0
Blackcurrant, Eat Smart, Safeway*	1 Pot/100g	60	60	7.9	6.1	0.2	0.5
Blackcurrant, Healthy Eating, Tesco*	1 Pot/100g	59	59	7.7	6.5	0.2	0.6
Blackcurrant, Safeway*	1 Pot/100g	121	121	6.7	15.8	3.4	0.9
Blue Parrot Cafe, Sainsbury's*	1 Serving/50g	49	98	6.6	11.0	3.1	0.2
COU, Marks & Spencer*	1 Pot/100g	48	48	7.8	4.5	0.1	0.5
Cherries & Chocolate, Finest, Tesco.*	1 Serving/165g	299	181	5.4	20.1	8.8	0.7
Cherry Pie Flavour, BGTY, Sainsbury's*	1 Pot/100g	54	54	7.6	5.5	0.2	1.1
Chocolate & Orange, Weight Watchers*	1 Pot/100g	64	64	5.7	10.0	0.1	1.1
Chocolate Fudge, Smooth & Creamy, Tesco*	1 Pot/100g	136	136	6.7	13.3	6.2	0.2
Danone*	1 Serving/50g	37	73	7.2	3.9	3.1	0.0
Eat Smart, Safeway*	1 Pot/100g	55	55	7.7	5.1	0.2	1.6
Exotic Fruits, Eat Smart, Safeway*	1 Pot/100g	60	60	7.9	6.6	0.2	0.4
Fabby, Loved By Kids, Marks & Spencer*	1 Pot/42.9g	45	105	6.2	12.3	3.7	0.0
Fruit On The Bottom, Better For You, Morrisons*	1 Pot/100g	66	66	5.6	10.6	0.2	0.0
Fruit, Balanced Lifestyle, Aldi*	1 Pot/100g	52	52	5.4	7.1	0.2	0.7
Fruit, Weight Watchers*	1 Pot/100g	48	48	5.4	6.3	0.1	0.3

F

FROMAGE FRAIS,

INFO/WEIGHT	Measure	per Measure KCAL	KCAL	PROT	CARB	FAT	FIBRE
Good Intentions, Somerfield*	1 Pot/100g	49	49	7.6	4.5	0.1	0.0
Lemon Pie, Low Fat, Sainsbury's*	1 Pot/90g	108	120	6.7	17.3	2.7	0.2
Lemon Sponge Flavour, BGTY, Sainsbury's*	1 Pot/100g	52	52	7.6	5.0	0.2	1.1
Lemon, Balanced Lifestyle, Aldi*	1 Serving/100g	52	52	5.6	6.6	0.3	0.6
Lemon, COU, Marks & Spencer*	1 Serving/100g	50	50	7.3	5.2	0.1	0.3
Mango, Eat Smart, Safeway*	1 Pot/100g	55	55	7.7	5.1	0.2	1.6
Morello Cherries, Perfectly Balanced, Waitrose*	½ Pot/250ml	260	104	2.5	19.1	1.9	1.8
Morrisons*	1 Serving/28g	17	59	9.8	4.8	0.0	0.0
Munch Bunch, Nestle*	1 Pot/42g	50	119	7.6	14.8	2.9	0.0
Natural, Creamy, Co-Op*	1 Pot/200g	204	102	6.1	2.9	7.3	0.0
Natural, French, Virtually Fat Free, Waitrose*	1 Serving/46g	21	46	7.3	3.7	0.2	0.0
Natural, GFY, Asda*	1oz/28g	13	45	8.0	3.3	0.0	0.0
Natural, Healthy Eating, Tesco*	1 Serving/65g	30	46	7.8	3.3	0.2	0.0
Natural, Normandy, BGTY, Sainsbury's*	1 Serving/15g	7	47	7.5	3.9	0.2	0.0
Normandy, Sainsbury's*	1 Serving/25g	29	116	7.7	3.4	8.1	0.0
Orange & Mandarin, Tesco*	1 Pot/100g	75	75	6.5	5.6	3.0	2.3
Peach, BGTY, Sainsburys*	1 Pot/100g	53	53	7.2	5.5	0.2	0.5
Peach, Weight Watchers*	1 Pot/100g	48	48	5.4	6.4	0.1	0.2
Petit Dessert, Co-Op*	1 Pot/60g	74	123	6.3	14.5	4.4	0.0
Petits Filous, Yoplait*	1 Pot/60g	76	127	6.5	14.5	4.7	0.0
Pineapple, Eat Smart, Safeway*	1 Pot/100g	60	60	7.9	6.3	0.2	0.3
Plain	1oz/28g	32	113	6.8	5.7	7.1	0.0
Raspberry & Redcurrant, BGTY, Sainsbury's*	1 Pot/100g	49	49	7.2	4.5	0.2	1.9
Raspberry & Strawberry, Weight Watchers*	1 Pot/100g	48	48	5.4	6.2	0.1	0.3
Raspberry, COU, Marks & Spencer*	1 Pot/100g	49	49	7.8	4.9	0.1	0.4
Raspberry, Eat Smart, Safeway*	1 Pot/100g	50	50	7.6	4.5	0.2	1.8
Raspberry, Healthy Choice, Asda*	1 Pot/100g	41	41	6.0	3.8	0.2	0.0
Raspberry, Healthy Eating, Tesco*	1 Pot/100g	53	53	6.2	6.6	0.2	0.3
Raspberry, Low Fat, Sainsbury's*	1 Pot/90g	96	107	5.8	15.1	2.6	0.1
Raspberry, Muller*	1 Pot/50g	68	135	6.1	13.5	6.3	0.0
Raspberry, Weight Watchers*	1 Pot/100g	49	49	5.3	6.9	0.1	1.2
Real Fruit, Tesco*	1 Pot/100g	54	54	5.6	7.6	0.1	0.1
Red Cherry, Healthy Eating, Tesco*	1 Pot/100g	55	55	6.2	7.2	0.2	0.1
Red Cherry, Tesco*	1 Pot/100g	75	75	6.5	5.5	3.0	2.3
Rhubarb & Crumble, Low Fat, Sainsbury's*	1 Pot/90g	96	107	6.7	14.1	2.6	0.4
Strawberry Tart, Sainsbury's*	1 Pot/100g	54	54	7.6	5.5	0.2	1.1
Strawberry, 99.9% Fat Free, Onken*	1 Serving/50g	46	91	6.9	15.3	0.1	0.0
Strawberry, BGTY, Sainsbury's*	1 Pot/100g	48	48	7.2	4.3	0.2	1.4
Strawberry, Healthy Choice, Asda*	1 Pot/100g	41	41	6.0	3.7	0.2	0.0
Strawberry, Healthy Eating, Tesco*	1 Pot/100g	54	54	6.2	6.8	0.2	0.1
Strawberry, Langley Farm*	1 Pot/125g	189	151	7.0	13.3	7.8	0.0
Strawberry, Low Fat, St Ivel*	1 Pot/100g	69	69	6.9	6.8	1.2	0.0
Strawberry, Puree, Somerfield*	1 Pot/50g	60	120	7.0	14.0	4.0	0.0
Strawberry, Tesco*	1 Pot/100g	75	75	6.5	5.5	3.0	2.5
Strawberry, Weight Watchers*	1 Pot/100g	47	47	5.4	6.2	0.1	0.2
Summer Fruits, Weight Watchers*	1 Pot/100g	48	48	5.4	6.3	0.1	0.4
Toffee & Pecan Pie, Smooth & Creamy, Tesco*	1 Pot/100g	148	148	6.9	14.8	6.8	0.2
Toffee, BGTY, Sainsbury's*	1 Pot/100g	60	60	7.2	7.0	0.3	0.2
Toffee, Weight Watchers*	1 Pot/100g	64	64	5.7	10.0	0.1	1.1
Tropical Fruit, COU, Marks & Spencer*	1 Pot/100g	50	50	7.8	4.5	0.1	0.5
Tropical Fruits, BGTY, Sainsbury's*	1 Pot/100g	54	54	7.3	5.8	0.2	0.3
Vanilla Flavour With Fruit, Thick & Fruity, Weight Watchers*	1 Pot/100g	49	49	5.3	6.9	0.0	1.2
Very Low Fat	1oz/28g	16	58	7.7	6.8	0.2	0.0

F

	Measure INFO/WEIGHT	per Measure KCAL	Nutrition Values per 100g / 100ml				
			KCAL	PROT	CARB	FAT	FIBRE
FROMAGE FRAIS,							
Virtually Fat Free, Safeway*	1 Pot/100g	41	41	6.7	3.2	0.2	0.0
Virtually Fat Free, Tesco*	1 Pot/100g	56	56	5.6	8.2	0.1	0.0
Wildlife, Yoplait*	1 Pot/50g	48	96	7.0	14.0	1.3	0.0
With Cereal, Shape Rise, Danone*	1 Serving/165g	205	124	6.5	23.9	1.3	0.5
With Real Fruit Puree, Nestle*	1 Serving/50g	65	130	7.1	18.9	2.7	0.2
FRUIT,							
A Croquer, McDonald's*	1 Serving/80g	47	59	0.4	13.5	0.4	2.3
Snack Pack, Fresh, Sainsbury's*	1 Serving/120g	54	45	0.1	11.0	0.1	1.3
FRUIT & NUT MIX,							
Exotic, Waitrose*	1 Serving/50g	207	414	9.0	54.6	17.7	4.6
Organic, Waitrose*	1 Pack/100g	489	489	15.0	33.8	32.6	5.4
Papaya Cranberry, WTF, Sainsbury's*	1 Serving/75g	300	400	4.1	63.1	14.6	7.3
TTD, Sainsbury's*	1 Bag/250g	900	360	5.1	49.5	15.7	5.9
FRUIT BAG, Happy Meal, McDonald's*	1 Bag/80g	34	43	0.2	10.0	0.1	1.8
FRUIT BOWL, Sainsbury's*	1oz/28g	12	42	0.6	9.1	0.1	0.1
FRUIT COCKTAIL,							
Fresh & Ready, Sainsbury's*	1 Pack/300g	117	39	0.6	9.0	0.1	1.2
In Apple Juice, Asda*	1/3 Can/80g	40	50	0.3	12.0	0.1	1.6
In Fruit Juice, Morrisons*	1 Can/140g	64	46	0.4	11.0	0.0	0.0
In Fruit Juice, Safeway*	1 Serving/220g	68	31	0.4	7.2	0.0	1.0
In Fruit Juice, Sainsbury's*	1 Serving/198g	97	49	0.3	11.9	0.1	1.3
In Grape Juice, Tesco*	1oz/28g	12	43	0.4	10.0	0.0	1.0
In Juice, Del Monte*	1 Can/415g	203	49	0.4	11.2	0.1	0.0
In Light Syrup, Makes Sense, Somerfield*	½ Can/205g	127	62	0.4	15.0	0.0	1.0
In Light Syrup, Sainsbury's*	½ Can/125g	73	58	0.4	14.0	0.1	1.3
In Syrup, Del Monte*	1 Can/420g	315	75	0.4	18.0	0.1	0.0
In Very Light Syrup, Value,Tesco*	1 Can/410g	123	30	0.4	7.3	0.0	1.0
Juice Drink Sainsbury's*	1 Glass/200ml	94	47	0.2	11.2	0.1	0.1
Safeway*	1 Serving/205g	117	57	0.4	14.0	0.0	1.0
Tropical, Asda*	½ Can/135g	81	60	0.0	15.0	0.0	1.6
Tropical, In Syrup, Sainsbury's*	½ Can/130g	95	73	0.5	17.6	0.1	1.4
Tropical, Morrisons*	½ Can/212g	144	68	0.0	17.0	0.0	0.0
Tropical, Safeway*	½ Can/214g	154	72	0.5	17.6	0.0	1.4
FRUIT COLLECTION, Fresh, Marks & Spencer*	1 Pack/400g	180	45	0.6	10.1	0.2	1.3
FRUIT COMPOTE,							
Apricot & Prune, Yeo Valley*	1 Pot/225g	207	92	0.6	22.3	0.1	1.6
Healthy Eating, Tesco*	1 Pot/140g	113	81	0.9	19.1	0.2	1.6
Orchard Fruits, Good For You, Asda*	1 Pot/180g	113	63	0.5	15.0	0.1	0.0
Organic, Yeo Valley*	1oz/28g	13	47	0.5	11.2	0.0	0.0
FRUIT DESSERT, Sojasun*	1 Pot/135g	105	78	3.5	12.0	1.8	0.0
FRUIT DRINK,							
Alive Tropical Torrent, The Coca Cola Co*	1 Glass/200ml	88	44	0.0	11.0	0.0	0.0
Apple & Blackcurrant, No Added Sugar, Safeway*	1fl oz/30ml	2	8	0.1	1.0	0.0	0.0
Blackcurrant & Apple, Shapers, Boots*	1 Bottle/500ml	10	2	0.0	0.2	0.0	0.0
Five Fruits, Five Alive*	1 Carton/250ml	125	50	0.0	12.0	0.0	0.0
FRUIT FANTASY, Strawberries & Cranberries, Sundora*	1 Serving/25g	70	280	2.5	67.0	0.6	5.4
FRUIT FILLING, Cherry & Amaretto, Asda*	¼ Pack/100g	105	105	0.9	23.0	0.2	0.0
FRUIT GUMS,							
No Added Sugar, Boots*	1 Sweet/1.6g	2	88	0.0	22.0	0.0	0.0
Red & Black, Marks & Spencer*	1 Bag/113g	362	320	5.2	75.8	0.1	0.1
Rowntree's*	1 Pack/48g	164	342	4.7	80.8	0.2	0.0
FRUIT INFUSION, Peach, Lime & Ginger, Marks & Spencer*	1 Serving/250ml	88	35	0.0	8.5	0.0	0.0

F

Measure INFO/WEIGHT	per Measure KCAL	KCAL	PROT	CARB	FAT	FIBRE

FRUIT JUICE,

	Measure INFO/WEIGHT	per Measure KCAL	KCAL	PROT	CARB	FAT	FIBRE
Apple & Mango, Sainsburys*	1 Glass/200ml	108	54	0.3	12.6	0.1	0.1
Multivitamin, Vitafit, Lidl*	1 Glass/200ml	106	53	1.0	12.0	0.0	0.5

FRUIT LOLLY,

Exotic Fruit, Mini, Healthy Living, Tesco*	1 Lolly/31.3g	41	131	1.0	26.4	2.0	1.0
No Added Sugar, Tesco*	1 Lolly/32.4g	26	80	0.1	20.0	0.0	0.1

FRUIT MEDLEY,

Citrus, Somerfield*	1 Serving/80.6g	25	31	0.6	6.9	0.1	0.4
Dried Fruit Mix, Shapers, Boots*	1 Serving/50g	131	262	3.2	61.0	0.6	5.5
Exotic, Co-Op*	1 Serving/120g	54	45	0.6	10.0	0.2	0.0
Exotic, Waitrose*	1 Medley/300g	126	42	0.6	9.5	0.2	1.1
Fresh, Waitrose*	1 Pack/300g	114	38	0.6	8.7	0.1	1.4
In Fresh Orange Juice, Co-Op*	1 Serving/140g	49	35	0.5	9.0	0.0	0.0
Marks & Spencer*	1oz/28g	7	25	0.6	7.1	0.2	1.1
Shapers, Boots*	1 Pack/140g	55	39	0.7	8.6	0.2	1.0
Summer, Waitrose*	1 Bowl/300g	84	28	0.8	5.9	0.1	1.3

FRUIT MIX,

Apricot & Passion Fruit, WTF, Sainsbury's*	½ Pack/125g	374	299	2.7	70.1	0.2	5.1
Tropical Dried, & Coconut Safeway*	1 Pack/50g	185	369	3.0	69.0	9.0	4.3

FRUIT PASTILLES,

Average	1 Tube/33g	108	327	2.8	84.2	0.0	0.0
Co-Op*	1 Sweet/6g	20	337	2.8	81.5	0.0	0.0
Rowntree's*	1 Tube/53g	184	348	4.3	82.9	0.0	0.0
Sainsbury's*	1 Sweet/7g	23	332	3.4	78.7	0.1	0.1
FRUIT PIECES, Mixed In Fruit Juice, Fruiyini, Del Monte*	1 Serving/120g	61	51	0.4	12.0	0.1	0.5
FRUIT RUSH, Rowntrees*	1 Pack/45g	144	319	3.7	75.6	0.2	0.0

FRUIT SALAD,

Autumn, Marks & Spencer*	1 Bowl/400g	220	55	0.4	13.2	0.1	1.8
Chunky, In Grape Juice, Tesco*	1 Serving/135g	63	47	0.4	11.0	0.2	0.8
Classic, Fresh, Marks & Spencer*	1oz/28g	11	40	0.6	8.4	0.1	1.2
Dried, Marks & Spencer*	½ Pack/125g	269	215	1.8	51.4	0.4	5.9
Dried, Nature's Harvest*	½ Pack/125g	231	185	3.1	40.9	1.0	8.0
Dried, Safeway*	1 Serving/50g	109	217	1.7	51.6	0.3	5.1
Exotic, Safeway*	½ Pot/159.6g	75	47	0.6	10.5	0.3	1.1
Exotic, Sainsbury's*	1oz/28g	11	40	0.6	9.1	0.3	1.0
Exotic, Somerfield*	1 Pot/350g	140	40	0.6	9.0	0.2	1.3
Exotic, Tesco*	1 Serving/225g	86	38	0.7	8.4	0.2	1.5
Exotic, Waitrose*	1 Pack/300g	126	42	0.6	9.5	0.2	1.1
Fresh, Asda*	½ Pot/215g	95	44	0.7	10.0	0.1	2.0
Fresh, Golden, Asda*	1 Pot/146.8g	69	47	0.6	11.0	0.1	1.6
Fresh, Marks & Spencer*	1oz/28g	10	36	0.6	9.5	0.2	0.9
Fresh, Morrisons*	1 Pot/180g	77	43	0.7	9.9	0.1	0.0
Fresh, Safeway*	1 Pack/300g	135	45	0.7	10.0	0.2	1.5
Fresh, Sainsbury's*	1 Serving/120g	55	46	0.6	10.5	0.2	1.4
Fresh, Somerfield*	1 Bowl/200g	94	47	0.6	11.0	0.1	1.5
Fresh, Sweet, Ripe & Moist, Tesco*	1 Serving/750g	345	46	0.7	10.6	0.1	1.6
Fresh, Tesco*	1oz/28g	13	45	0.6	10.5	0.1	1.4
Grapefruit & Orange, Fresh, Marks & Spencer*	1 Serving/250g	88	35	0.9	7.4	0.1	1.6
Green, Marks & Spencer*	1 Bowl/400g	200	50	0.6	10.9	0.2	1.2
Homemade	1oz/28g	15	55	0.7	13.8	0.1	1.5
In Fruit Juice, Lisner Selection, Aldi*	1 Pot/400g	316	79	0.5	18.0	0.5	20.0
Luxury, Marks & Spencer*	1oz/28g	11	40	0.6	9.2	0.1	1.1
Melon, Kiwi, Strawbery, Way to Five, Sainsbury's*	1 Pack/245g	74	30	0.8	6.3	0.2	1.3
Mixed, New Improved, Tesco*	1 Pot/225g	79	35	0.8	7.6	0.2	1.2

F

	Measure INFO/WEIGHT	per Measure KCAL	Nutrition Values per 100g / 100ml				
			KCAL	PROT	CARB	FAT	FIBRE
FRUIT SALAD,							
Mixed, Prepared, Sainsbury's*	½ Pack/230g	97	42	0.7	8.9	0.2	1.2
Mixed, Sainsbury's*	1 Bowl/480g	211	44	0.6	10.2	0.1	1.1
Mixed, Tesco*	1 Salad/225g	86	38	0.7	8.3	0.2	1.3
Mixed, Way To Five, Sainsbury's*	1 Pack/430g	168	39	0.7	8.6	0.2	1.2
Pineapple, Mandarin & Grapefruit, Asda*	1 Serving/200g	86	43	0.6	10.0	0.1	0.0
Pret A Manger*	1 Av Pack/300g	120	40	0.5	9.2	0.2	1.2
Seasonal, Asda*	1 Pack/125g	55	44	0.5	10.4	0.1	1.2
Summer, Sainsbury's*	1 Pack/240g	84	35	0.7	7.8	0.2	1.3
Tesco*	1 Serving/200g	70	35	0.8	7.4	0.2	1.4
Tropical, Asda*	1oz/28g	10	36	0.6	8.8	0.2	1.2
Tropical, Fresh, Asda*	1 Pack/400g	164	41	0.7	9.0	0.2	0.0
Tropical, Fresh, Sainsbury's*	1 Pack/230g	104	45	0.7	10.2	0.2	2.0
Tropical, Fruit Snacks, Frozen, Sainsbury's*	1 Serving/175g	79	45	0.7	10.4	0.1	1.6
Tropical, In Light Syrup, Passion Fruit Juice, Tesco*	½ Can/216g	130	60	0.3	14.1	0.1	1.1
Tropical, Marks & Spencer*	1oz/28g	12	44	0.8	9.6	0.3	1.8
Tropical, Tropical Harvest, Aldi*	1 Serving/100g	52	52	0.3	12.8	0.0	1.4
Weight Watchers*	1 Serving/135g	50	37	0.2	9.0	0.1	0.7
FRUIT SELECTION,							
Shapers, Boots*	1 Pack/235g	96	41	0.5	9.2	0.2	0.8
Tray, Fresh, Tesco*	1 Serving/330g	99	30	0.5	6.8	0.1	1.8
FRUIT SNACK TRAY, Fresh, Food To Go, Sainsbury's*	1 Tray/320g	112	35	0.6	7.9	0.1	1.4
FRUIT SPREAD,							
Apricot, Pure, Organic, Whole Earth*	1 Serving/20g	33	167	0.8	40.0	0.4	0.9
High, Blueberry, St Dalfour*	1 Tsp/15g	34	228	0.5	56.0	0.2	2.2
Raspberry, Weight Watchers*	1 Tsp/15g	17	111	0.4	27.1	0.1	0.9
Seville Orange, Weight Watchers*	1 Tsp/15g	17	111	0.2	27.5	0.0	0.3
Strawberry, Weight Watchers*	1 Tsp/15g	17	115	0.2	28.4	0.0	0.4
FRUIT TO GO, Del Monte*	1 Can/113g	80	71	0.0	17.7	0.0	0.0
FRUITIES, Weight Watchers*	1 Serving/2g	3	135	0.0	54.0	0.0	34.0
FU YUNG, Egg	1oz/28g	67	239	9.9	2.2	20.6	1.3
FUDGE,							
All Butter, TTD, Sainsbury's*	1 Pack/125g	536	429	1.3	73.4	14.5	0.0
Average	1oz/28g	123	441	3.3	81.1	13.7	0.0
Butter Tablet, Thorntons*	1oz/28g	116	414	0.9	77.6	11.1	0.0
Butter, Milk, Thorntons*	1 Chocolate/13g	60	462	3.7	68.5	19.2	0.0
Cadbury's*	1 Std Bar/26g	116	445	2.8	72.3	16.3	0.0
Cherry & Almond, Thorntons*	1 Bag/100g	464	464	3.2	70.5	19.1	0.4
Chocolate, Thorntons*	1 Bag/100g	459	459	3.1	69.0	19.1	0.6
Clotted Cream, Marks & Spencer*	1oz/28g	133	474	1.7	67.6	22.1	0.0
Dairy, Co-Op*	1 Sweet/9g	39	430	2.0	76.0	13.0	0.0
Devon, Somerfield*	1 Pack/250g	1060	424	2.0	78.9	11.1	0.0
Double Chocolate Bar, Marks & Spencer*	1 Bar/43g	202	470	4.2	66.9	21.0	0.7
Pure Indulgence, Thorntons*	1 Bar/45g	210	466	1.8	65.9	21.9	0.0
Vanilla, Bar, Marks & Spencer*	1 Bar/43g	205	476	3.7	63.0	23.3	0.4
Vanilla, Thorntons*	1 Bag/100g	465	465	1.8	65.9	21.9	0.0
FUSE, Cadbury's*	1 Std Bar/49g	238	485	7.6	58.2	24.8	0.0
FUSILLI,							
Authentic Italian, Tesco*	1 Serving/100g	354	354	11.5	72.6	1.9	2.7
Bucati, Dry, Sainsbury's*	1 Serving/100g	357	357	12.3	73.1	1.7	2.5
Dried, Napolina*	1oz/28g	99	352	11.5	73.0	1.5	2.2
Dried, Romano*	1 Serving/100g	362	362	12.0	75.0	1.5	0.0
Dried, Waitrose*	1 Serving/120g	452	377	10.8	82.8	0.3	0.0
Egg, Fresh, Waitrose*	1 Serving/125g	361	289	11.4	53.1	3.4	2.1

F

FUSILLI,	Measure INFO/WEIGHT	per Measure KCAL	Nutrition Values per 100g / 100ml				
			KCAL	PROT	CARB	FAT	FIBRE
Fresh, Asda*	1oz/28g	48	170	7.0	31.0	2.0	1.4
Fresh, Cooked, Safeway*	1 Serving/200g	318	159	5.8	30.3	1.6	2.1
Loyd Grossman*	1 Serving/100g	360	360	13.5	73.0	1.5	3.5
Marks & Spencer*	1oz/28g	100	358	13.1	70.2	2.7	2.7
Microwaveable, Dolmio*	1 Serving/220g	299	136	5.3	26.3	1.0	0.0
Organic, Seeds Of Change*	1 Serving/75g	263	350	11.5	75.0	0.3	0.0
Sainsbury's*	1oz/28g	100	357	12.3	73.1	1.7	2.5
Somerfield*	1 Serving/250g	865	346	13.0	69.0	2.0	4.0
Spirals, Fresh, Tesco*	1 Serving/125g	360	288	11.9	51.8	3.7	1.5
Tomato, Weight Watchers*	1 Can/388g	198	51	1.9	10.1	0.4	0.8
Tricolore, Dried, Safeway*	1 Serving/75g	261	348	13.2	70.1	1.7	2.9
Tricolore, Dry, Napolina*	1oz/28g	99	352	11.5	73.0	1.5	2.2
Tricolore, Sainsbury's*	1 Serving/45g	161	357	12.3	73.1	1.7	2.5
Tricolore, Tesco*	1 Serving/60g	211	352	11.0	72.8	1.9	3.0
Tuna, BGTY, Sainsbury's*	1 Pack/400g	304	76	6.0	8.6	2.0	0.5
Twists, Asda*	1 Serving/50g	173	346	12.0	71.0	1.5	3.0
Twists, Tesco*	1 Serving/100g	345	345	13.2	68.5	2.0	2.9
Wholewheat, Italian, Sainsbury's*	1 Serving/90g	284	316	12.7	61.9	2.0	10.0
Wholewheat, Organic, Waitrose*	1 Serving/100g	322	322	13.2	61.7	2.5	9.0
Wholewheat, Safeway*	1oz/28g	90	321	14.4	60.2	2.5	8.4
Wholewheat, Sainsbury's*	1 Serving/50g	158	316	12.7	61.9	2.0	10.0
Wholewheat, Tesco*	1 Serving/100g	335	335	13.0	65.4	2.4	6.8
With Chicken & Courgettes, Sainsbury's*	1 Pack/450g	675	150	8.6	14.6	6.4	0.5

F

	Measure INFO/WEIGHT	per Measure KCAL	Nutrition Values per 100g / 100ml				
			KCAL	PROT	CARB	FAT	FIBRE
GALAXY							
Amicelli, Mars*	1 Serving/13g	66	507	6.2	59.7	27.1	0.0
Caramel, Mars*	1 Bar/49g	239	488	5.3	60.1	25.1	0.0
Chocolate, Mars*	1 Bar/47g	250	532	9.0	56.6	30.0	0.0
Fruit & Hazelnut, Milk, Mars*	1 Bar/47g	235	501	7.1	55.2	28.0	0.0
Liaison, Mars*	1 Bar/48g	233	485	5.4	60.3	24.7	0.0
Ripple, Mars*	1 Bar/33g	169	528	6.9	59.3	29.3	0.0
Swirls, Mars*	1 Bag/150g	747	498	4.9	60.2	26.5	0.0
GAMMON,							
Breaded, Wiltshire, Marks & Spencer*	1oz/28g	39	140	23.6	1.6	4.7	0.0
Honey Roast, Dry Cured, British, TTD, Sainsbury's*	1 Slice/35g	50	142	24.0	3.3	3.6	0.1
Unsmoked, British Steaks, Marks & Spencer*	1 Steak/140g	273	195	29.1	0.3	8.4	0.0
Joint, Irish, With Honey & Mustard Glaze, Tesco*	1 Serving/100g	161	161	18.1	3.2	8.5	0.2
Joint, Lean Only, Boiled	1oz/28g	47	167	29.4	0.0	5.5	0.0
Joint, Smoked, Boneless, Sainsbury's*	1 Serving/100g	208	208	25.0	0.0	12.0	0.0
Joint, With Honey & Mustard Glaze, Tesco*	1 Pack/450g	725	161	18.1	3.2	8.5	0.2
Steaks, Below 5% Fat, Asda*	1 Pack/250g	253	101	19.0	1.0	2.3	0.9
Steaks, Cygnet, Lidl*	1 Steak/170g	277	163	16.4	1.9	9.9	0.0
Steaks, Plate, Smoked, Sainsbury's*	1 Steak/125g	173	138	22.7	0.1	5.2	0.1
Steaks, Plate, Unsmoked, Sainsbury's*	1 Steak/150g	207	138	22.7	0.1	5.2	0.1
Steaks, Prime Cut, Sainsbury's*	1 Serving/250g	380	152	24.8	0.5	5.6	0.1
Steaks, Reduced Salt, Asda*	1 Steak/198g	337	170	22.0	0.2	9.0	0.0
Steaks, Round, Unsmoked, Asda*	1 Steak/125g	126	101	17.0	0.0	3.7	0.0
Steaks, Smoked, Prime, Asda*	1 Steak/250g	280	112	18.0	0.2	4.4	0.0
Steaks, Tendersweet, Lightly Smoked, Sainsbury's*	1 Steak/54g	86	160	27.4	0.1	5.5	0.1
Steaks, Traditional, Marks & Spencer*	1oz/28g	31	110	18.2	0.0	4.3	0.0
Steaks, Unsmoked Prime, Somerfield*	1 Stk Grilled/225g	378	168	24.1	0.2	7.9	0.0
Steaks, Unsmoked, Healthy Eating, Tesco*	1 Serving/110g	100	91	18.6	1.0	1.4	0.0
Steaks, Unsmoked, Prime, Asda*	1 Steak/250g	280	112	18.0	0.2	4.4	0.0
Steaks, Unsmoked, Round, Somerfield*	1 Steak/125g	125	100	16.9	0.0	3.6	0.0
Steaks, With Honey & Mustard, GFY, Asda*	½ Pack/190g	270	142	21.0	4.5	4.4	0.0
GARAM MASALA, Average	1oz/28g	106	379	15.6	45.2	15.1	0.0
GARLIC,							
Powder	1 Tsp/3g	7	246	18.7	42.7	1.2	9.9
Puree	1 Tbsp/18g	61	380	3.5	16.9	33.6	0.0
Puree, Organic, Tesco*	1 Serving/10g	12	119	6.6	22.8	0.2	3.2
Raw	1 Clove/3g	3	98	7.9	16.3	0.6	4.1
GARLIC & HERB, Crust for Cod, Schwartz*	1 Serving/10g	36	359	11.5	72.5	2.6	0.0
GARLIC PUREE, Asda*	1 Tbsp/18g	63	423	2.7	13.0	40.0	6.0
GATEAU,							
Au Fromage Blanc, Ligne et Plaisir*	1 Serving/80g	128	160	8.0	26.0	2.6	0.0
Black Forest, Sara Lee*	1 Serving/80g	221	276	3.6	37.9	12.3	1.2
Black Forest, Tesco*	1 Serving/55g	141	257	3.2	29.9	13.8	0.1
Blackforest, Sainsbury's*	1/8 Gateau/63g	163	259	3.9	27.7	17.1	3.5
Chocolate Layer, Marks & Spencer	1 Serving/86g	278	323	4.2	35.9	18.3	0.9
Chocolate Orange, Co-Op*	1 Slice/97g	320	330	5.0	37.0	18.0	1.0
Coffee, Tesco*	1 Serving/100g	300	300	4.2	32.5	17.0	0.6
Double Chocolate, Sara Lee*	1oz/28g	93	331	5.6	41.3	16.5	0.9
Double Chocolate, Tesco*	1 Serving/45g	124	276	4.4	32.1	14.4	2.2
Double Strawberry, Sara Lee*	1/8 Slice/199g	533	268	3.2	36.2	12.2	0.6
Ice Cream, Chocolate & Vanilla, Iceland*	1 Serving/130g	252	194	3.3	24.1	9.4	0.6
Lemon & Lime, Marks & Spencer*	1 Serving/100g	295	295	3.2	35.0	15.6	0.3
Orange & Lemon, Iceland*	1 Serving/90g	221	245	2.6	33.8	11.0	0.3
Profiterole, TTD, Sainsbury's*	1/6 Gateau/112g	410	365	3.9	26.2	27.2	1.1

G

	Measure INFO/WEIGHT	per Measure KCAL	Nutrition Values per 100g / 100ml				
			KCAL	PROT	CARB	FAT	FIBRE
GATEAU,							
Strawberry, Co-Op*	1 Slice/77g	222	288	5.1	29.2	16.7	1.0
Swiss, Cadbury's*	1/6/60g	228	380	5.2	52.0	16.8	0.9
Toffee Ripple, Sara Lee*	1 Serving/317g	1005	317	4.0	40.2	15.6	0.5
Triple Chocolate, Tesco*	1 Serving/64g	187	292	3.9	31.1	16.9	0.4
GAZPACHO, Average	1oz/28g	13	45	0.8	2.6	3.6	0.6
GELATINE, Average	1oz/28g	95	338	84.4	0.0	0.0	0.0
GEMELLI, Durum Wheat, Tesco*	1 Serving/100g	354	354	13.2	68.5	2.0	2.9
GET DRESSED,							
Classic French, Vinaigrette, Kraft*	1 Tbsp/15ml	6	39	0.1	8.7	0.0	0.5
Classic Italian, Kraft*	1 Serving/25ml	30	120	0.1	5.6	10.3	0.5
Creamy Caesar, Kraft*	1 Serving/66.7g	68	102	2.1	15.0	3.5	0.1
Herb & Garlic, 5% Fat, Kraft*	1 Serving/25ml	29	116	1.3	15.5	5.1	0.2
Honey Mustard, 5% Fat, Kraft*	1 Serving/15ml	20	131	1.3	19.0	5.0	1.2
GET UP & GO, Without Milk, Patrick Holford*	1 Serving/30g	104	347	20.0	53.3	3.3	13.3
GHEE,							
Butter	1oz/28g	251	898	0.0	0.0	99.8	0.0
Palm	1oz/28g	251	897	0.0	0.0	99.7	0.0
Vegetable	1oz/28g	251	895	0.0	0.0	99.4	0.0
Vegetable, Sharwood's*	1oz/28g	251	897	0.0	0.0	99.7	0.0
GHERKINS,							
Drained	1oz/28g	4	14	0.9	2.6	0.1	1.2
In Vinegar, Sainsbury's*	1 Gherkin/36g	5	14	0.9	2.5	0.1	1.2
Sainsbury's*	1 Gherkin/40g	12	30	0.9	6.3	0.1	1.2
Sweet & Sour, Tesco*	1 Serving/100g	34	34	1.0	6.0	0.5	1.2
GIGLIO, Egg, Tesco*	1 Serving/100g	355	355	14.5	66.4	3.5	2.6
GIN,							
37.5% Volume	1 Shot/25ml	52	207	0.0	0.0	0.0	0.0
40% Volume	1 Shot/25ml	56	222	0.0	0.0	0.0	0.0
GINGER,							
Crystallised, Nature's Harvest*	1 Tbsp/15g	50	330	0.3	82.0	0.1	16.0
Fresh	1oz/28g	14	49	1.7	9.5	0.7	0.0
Ground	1 Tsp/2g	5	258	7.4	60.0	3.3	0.0
Root, Raw	1oz/28g	11	38	1.4	7.2	0.6	0.0
Stem, In Sugar Syrup, Sainsbury's*	1oz/28g	76	271	0.2	67.3	0.1	1.4
GINGER ALE,							
American, Low Calorie, Somerfield*	1fl oz/30ml	0	1	0.0	0.0	0.0	0.0
Dry, Sainsbury's*	1 Glass/250ml	95	38	0.1	9.1	0.1	0.1
GINGERBREAD,							
Average	1oz/28g	106	379	5.7	64.7	12.6	1.2
Men, Mini, Marks & Spencer*	1 Biscuit/16.6g	80	470	6.2	63.9	18.6	1.7
GNOCCHI, Fresh, Sainsbury's*	1 Serving/100g	152	152	3.8	33.6	0.3	1.4
Raw, Meat, Fat & Skin	1oz/28g	101	361	16.5	0.0	32.8	0.0
Roast, Meat Only	1oz/28g	89	319	29.3	0.0	22.4	0.0
Roasted, Meat, Fat & Skin	1oz/28g	84	301	27.5	0.0	21.2	0.0
GOOSEBERRIES, Dessert, Raw	1oz/28g	11	40	0.7	9.2	0.3	2.4
GOULASH, Beef, Bistro Range, Tesco*	1 Pack/450g	545	121	7.9	14.6	3.4	0.6
GRANOLA,							
Cranberry & Apple, Good Intentions, Somerfield*	1 Serving/30g	109	363	9.0	71.0	4.8	10.2
Sultana, Crunchy, Organic, Marks & Spencer*	1oz/28g	120	430	8.6	53.9	15.7	6.4
GRAPE & RASPBERRY JUICE, Pressed, Marks & Spencer*	1 Bottle/250ml	138	55	0.4	12.9	0.0	0.1
GRAPE JUICE, White, Sainsbury's*	1 Glass/200ml	132	66	0.1	15.9	0.1	0.1
GRAPEFRUIT,							
Canned, In Juice	1oz/28g	8	30	0.6	7.3	0.0	0.4

G

	Measure INFO/WEIGHT	per Measure KCAL	Nutrition Values per 100g / 100ml				
			KCAL	PROT	CARB	FAT	FIBRE
GRAPEFRUIT,							
Canned, In Syrup	1oz/28g	17	60	0.5	15.5	0.0	0.6
Fresh, Raw	1oz/28g	8	30	0.8	6.8	0.1	1.3
In Syrup, Sainsbury's*	½ Can/250g	188	75	0.5	17.5	0.1	0.4
Medley, Sainsbury's*	1 Serving/75g	43	57	0.4	13.8	0.1	0.3
Raw, Weighed With Peel & Pips	1 Med/340g	68	20	0.5	4.6	0.1	0.9
Ruby Red, In Natural Juice, Tesco*	1 Serving/135g	57	42	0.6	10.0	0.0	0.4
Segments in Juice, Asda*	½ Can/152g	64	42	0.6	10.0	0.0	0.6
Segments, In Grapefruit Juice, John West*	1oz/28g	9	33	0.5	7.0	0.0	0.6
Segments, In Grapefruit Juice, Safeway*	1 Serving/165g	76	46	0.4	11.0	0.0	0.4
Segments, In Grapefruit Juice, Tesco*	1oz/28g	13	46	0.6	10.0	0.0	0.4
Segments, In Juice, Del Monte*	1oz/28g	14	49	0.6	10.9	0.0	0.0
Segments, In Natural Juice, Sainsbury's*	1oz/28g	11	38	0.5	8.7	0.1	0.4
Segments, In Syrup, Sainsbury's*	1oz/28g	20	73	0.5	17.5	0.1	0.4
GRAPEFRUIT & LIME, Quest, Marks & Spencer*	1 Bottle/330ml	53	16	0.0	4.0	0.0	0.0
GRAPEFRUIT JUICE,							
Asda*	1 Glass/200ml	80	40	0.4	9.0	0.1	0.0
Del Monte*	1 Glass/200ml	82	41	0.5	8.8	0.0	0.0
Florida Pink, Somerfield*	1 Glass/200ml	88	44	1.0	10.0	0.0	0.0
Florida Pink, Squeezed, Sainsbury's*	1 Glass/200ml	82	41	0.5	9.2	0.1	0.3
Florida, Marks & Spencer*	1 Glass/200ml	60	30	0.4	7.5	0.0	0.0
Freshly Squeezed, Johnsons*	1 Glass/200ml	64	32	0.7	7.4	0.1	0.0
Golden, Tropicana*	1 Glass/200ml	80	40	0.6	8.0	0.0	0.5
Pure, Sainsbury's*	1 Glass/200ml	82	41	0.4	8.6	0.1	0.1
Pure, Somerfield*	1 Glass/200ml	76	38	1.0	9.0	0.0	0.0
Pure, Tesco*	1 Glass/200ml	82	41	0.4	9.0	0.0	0.0
GRAPES,							
Fresh, Average, Raw	1oz/28g	17	60	0.4	15.4	0.1	0.7
Seedless, Selection Pack, Tesco*	¼ Pack/100g	64	64	0.4	15.4	0.1	0.7
GRATIN,							
Cauliflower, Findus*	1 Pack/400g	340	85	3.5	7.0	5.0	0.0
Creamy Potato, Marks & Spencer*	½ Pack/225g	360	160	2.2	11.9	11.1	0.9
Leek & Carrot, Findus*	1 Pack/400g	440	110	3.5	9.5	6.5	0.0
Potato, Somerfield*	½ Pack/225g	356	158	2.0	11.0	12.0	0.0
Vegetable, Somerfield*	1 Pack/300g	417	139	1.0	5.0	13.0	0.0
GRAVADLAX, Finest, Tesco*	1 Serving/70g	125	178	22.1	0.2	9.9	0.0
GRAVY,							
Beef, Fresh, Sainsbury's*	1 Serving/83ml	45	54	3.1	3.2	3.3	0.5
Beef, Heat Serve, Morrisons*	1 Serving/150g	27	18	0.3	3.9	0.3	0.5
Chicken, Fresh, Marks & Spencer*	1oz/28g	10	35	2.5	5.0	0.1	0.3
For Poultry, Marks & Spencer*	1 Jar/400g	136	34	2.5	5.0	0.4	0.3
Fresh, Somerfield*	1 Pack/300g	69	23	0.0	4.0	1.0	0.0
Granules For Chicken, Dry, Bisto*	1 Serving/4g	15	385	3.2	57.9	15.6	1.4
Granules For Chicken, Made Up, Bisto*	1 Serving/50ml	14	28	0.2	4.4	1.2	0.2
Granules For Chicken, Made Up, SmartPrice, Asda*	1 Serving/100ml	34	34	0.2	3.0	2.3	0.1
Granules For Meat, Made Up, Asda*	1 Serving/100ml	38	38	0.6	4.0	2.4	0.1
Granules For Vegetarian Dishes, Dry Weight, Bisto*	1oz/28g	103	367	2.6	59.5	13.2	1.3
Granules With Onion, Dry, Bisto*	1 Serving/4g	15	365	2.9	56.1	14.3	1.8
Granules for Turkey, Dry, Bisto*	1 Serving/4g	15	367	3.3	53.9	15.3	1.2
Granules, Beef, Dry, Tesco*	1 Serving/6g	29	480	5.5	36.4	34.7	1.5
Granules, Beef, Made Up, Oxo*	1 serving/140ml	27	19	0.6	3.4	0.3	0.0
Granules, Chicken & Hint of Sage & Onion, Dry, Oxo*	3/4 Pint Made/30g	95	316	11.1	54.2	6.1	0.7
Granules, Chicken, Dry, Oxo*	1oz/28g	83	296	11.1	54.2	4.9	0.7
Granules, Chicken, Made Up, Oxo*	1fl oz/30ml	5	18	0.7	3.3	0.3	0.0

G

INFO/WEIGHT	Measure per Measure KCAL		KCAL	PROT	CARB	FAT	FIBRE

GRAVY,

	Measure per Measure			Nutrition Values per 100g / 100ml				
	INFO/WEIGHT	KCAL	KCAL	PROT	CARB	FAT	FIBRE
Granules, Chip Shop Curry, Dry Weight, Bisto*	1 Serving/50ml	234	468	4.3	72.6	17.8	2.7
Granules, Dry, Bisto*	1 Serving/10g	38	384	3.1	56.4	16.2	1.5
Granules, Dry, Value, Tesco*	1oz/28g	111	397	3.2	54.4	18.5	1.0
Granules, Instant, Dry	1oz/28g	129	462	4.4	40.6	32.5	0.0
Granules, Instant, Made Up	1oz/28g	10	34	0.3	3.0	2.4	0.0
Granules, Made Up, Oxo*	1 Serving/150ml	29	19	0.6	3.4	0.3	0.0
Granules, Onion, Dry, Oxo*	1oz/28g	92	328	8.2	62.3	4.8	0.8
Granules, Onion, Made Up, Bisto*	1 Serving/140ml	39	28	0.2	4.2	1.0	0.2
Granules, Onion, Made Up, Oxo*	1fl oz/30ml	6	20	0.5	3.7	0.3	0.0
Granules, Onion, Dry, Morrisons*	1 Serving/25g	124	495	3.4	44.0	34.7	0.0
Granules, Original, Dry, Oxo*	1oz/28g	88	313	10.2	57.2	4.8	1.0
Granules, Vegetable, Dry, Bisto*	1 Serving/4g	15	367	2.6	59.5	13.2	1.3
Granules, Vegetable, Dry, Oxo*	1oz/28g	88	316	8.4	59.5	4.9	0.9
Granules, Vegetable, Dry, Tesco*	½ Pint/20g	94	470	3.8	38.5	33.4	3.7
Granules, Vegetarian, Dry, Bisto*	1 Serving/28g	110	394	2.6	54.9	18.2	1.3
Granules, Vegetarian, Made Up, Bisto*	1 Serving/140ml	39	28	0.2	4.4	1.0	0.0
Instant Mix, Better for You, Morrisons*	1 Serving/25g	80	320	3.5	77.0	0.3	1.2
Mix, Instant, Made Up, BGTY, Sainsbury's*	1fl oz/30ml	10	32	0.3	7.4	0.1	0.1
Onion, Fresh, Asda*	1/6 Pot/77g	30	39	1.7	3.3	2.1	0.4
Onion, Fresh, Somerfield*	1 Pack/300g	195	65	1.0	7.0	4.0	0.0
Onion, Rich, Marks & Spencer*	½ Pack/150g	60	40	2.0	5.9	1.2	0.3
Powder For Pork, Dry, Best, Bisto*	1 Serving/100g	303	303	5.1	62.3	3.7	0.8
Powder, Dry, Tesco*	1 Serving/20g	57	286	7.2	61.0	1.5	2.0
Powder, Sainsbury's*	1 Serving/100ml	15	15	0.4	3.2	0.1	0.1
Roast Beef Flavour, Made Up, Best, Bisto*	1 Serving/50ml	13	26	0.4	5.4	0.4	0.2
Roast Beef, Dry, Schwartz*	1 Pack/27g	90	333	12.7	65.2	2.4	0.0
Roast Chicken, Dry, Schwartz*	1 Pack/26g	95	365	10.2	65.7	6.8	0.0
Roast Turkey, Dry, Schwartz*	1 Serving/6g	21	355	12.0	60.2	7.4	0.0

GREENGAGES,

Raw	1oz/28g	11	41	0.8	9.7	0.1	2.1
Raw, Weighed With Stones	1oz/28g	11	38	0.7	9.2	0.1	2.0

GRILLS,

Cauliflower Cheese, Dalepak*	1 Grill/94g	231	246	4.6	20.0	14.8	2.6
London, Heinz*	1 Can/400g	404	101	7.1	10.9	3.2	3.1
Tikka, Organic, Waitrose*	1 Grill/100g	185	185	6.9	18.5	9.3	3.4
Vegetable, Dalepak*	1 Grill/85g	170	200	5.2	17.2	12.3	3.2
Vegetable, Ross*	1 Grill/114g	252	221	4.3	25.5	11.3	0.9
Vegetable, Tesco*	1 Grill/72.2g	129	179	4.2	18.0	10.0	2.2
GROUSE, Roasted, Meat Only	1oz/28g	36	128	27.6	0.0	2.0	0.0

GUACAMOLE,

Asda*	½ Pot/56.5g	105	184	1.6	4.0	18.0	0.0
Avocado, Reduced Fat, The Fresh Dip Company*	1 Serving/113g	128	113	2.5	6.1	8.7	2.3
Chunky, Marks & Spencer*	1 Serving/50g	65	130	1.5	5.1	11.3	3.7
Chunky, Sainsbury's*	½ Pot/64.9g	120	185	1.6	3.2	18.4	3.8
Doritos*	1 Tbsp/20g	32	159	1.2	2.6	16.0	0.1
Fresh, Sainsbury's*	1oz/28g	59	210	1.8	5.3	20.2	2.5
Fresh, Waitrose*	½ Pot/85.1g	172	202	1.7	3.3	20.2	3.4
GFY, Asda*	1 Pack/113g	144	127	2.8	4.3	11.0	2.2
Reduced Fat, Sainsburys*	½ Pot/65g	86	133	1.5	3.5	12.6	4.0
Reduced Fat, Waitrose*	1 Serving/25g	32	129	3.0	2.7	11.8	4.7
Tesco*	1 Serving/35g	67	190	1.9	4.1	18.4	2.5
Somerfield*	1oz/28g	53	188	2.0	5.0	18.0	0.0

G

	Measure INFO/WEIGHT	per Measure KCAL	Nutrition Values per 100g / 100ml				
			KCAL	PROT	CARB	FAT	FIBRE
GUAVA,							
Canned, In Syrup	1oz/28g	17	60	0.4	15.7	0.0	3.0
Fresh, Raw	1oz/28g	7	26	0.8	5.0	0.5	3.7
Raw, Weighed With Skin & Pips	1oz/28g	7	24	0.7	4.5	0.5	3.3
GUINEA FOWL, Boned & Stuffed, Fresh, FayreGame*	1 Serving/325g	650	200	19.1	3.3	12.1	0.5
GUMBO,							
Cajun Vegetable, Sainsbury's*	1 serving/450g	266	59	1.4	7.7	2.5	1.5
Louisiana Chicken, Perfectly Balanced, Waitrose*	1 Serving/235g	207	88	12.2	3.5	2.8	1.3
GUMS,							
American Hard, Asda*	1 Serving/50g	173	345	0.1	86.0	0.0	0.0
Milk Bottles, Bassett's*	1 Pack/25g	88	353	6.2	78.3	1.6	0.0
Milk Bottles, Milk Flavour, Asda*	1 Pack/100g	369	369	7.0	80.0	2.3	0.4
Percy Pig & Pals, Soft, Marks & Spencer*	1 Sweet/7.6g	28	344	5.8	80.0	0.1	0.0

G

INFO/WEIGHT	Measure per Measure KCAL	KCAL	PROT	CARB	FAT	FIBRE

HADDOCK,

Item	Measure/Weight	KCAL	KCAL	PROT	CARB	FAT	FIBRE
& Chips, Marks & Spencer*	1oz/28g	52	187	7.0	22.6	7.6	2.1
5 Minute Fish, Tesco*	1 Serving/230g	409	178	17.9	1.4	11.2	0.6
Batter, Fried in Blended Oil	1oz/28g	65	232	17.1	10.0	14.0	0.4
Breadcrumbs, Chunky, Marks & Spencer*	1oz/28g	64	230	5.3	12.6	17.1	3.7
Breadcrumbs, Marks & Spencer*	1oz/28g	50	178	13.7	10.8	8.9	1.4
Breaded, Asda*	1 Serving/100g	212	212	13.0	22.0	8.0	3.1
Cheese & Chive Sauce, Healthy Eating, Tesco*	1 Pack/360g	284	79	12.7	2.6	2.0	0.1
Crispy Batter, Iceland*	1 Serving/179g	392	219	15.0	16.0	10.5	1.3
Crumbs, Fried in Blended Oil	1oz/28g	49	174	21.4	3.6	8.3	0.2
Fillets, Battered, Asda*	1 Fillet/100g	241	241	13.0	18.0	13.0	2.5
Fillets, Battered, Marks & Spencer*	1 Fillet/125g	306	245	12.6	16.0	14.6	0.7
Fillets, Boneless, Iceland*	1 Fillet/150g	380	253	17.2	17.1	12.9	1.9
Fillets, Boneless, Scottish, Sainsbury's*	1 Portion/202g	410	203	13.4	16.4	9.3	0.9
Fillets, Breadcrumbs, Scottish, Sainsbury's*	1 Fillet/170g	345	203	13.4	16.4	9.3	0.9
Fillets, Breaded, Scottish, Marks & Spencer*	1 Fillet/128.6g	271	210	12.9	15.2	10.9	1.9
Fillets, Breaded, Tesco*	1 Fillet/142g	251	177	14.3	15.0	6.8	0.9
Fillets, Butter, Smoked, Tesco*	1 Pack/204g	208	102	19.9	0.6	2.1	0.7
Fillets, Cheese & Chive Sauce, Smoked, Seafresh	1 Serving/170g	201	118	14.7	1.2	6.1	0.1
Fillets, Cheese & Parsley Sauce, Smoked, M&S*	1 Pack/190g	200	105	13.7	1.4	5.0	0.4
Fillets, Chunky, Premium, Lidl*	1 Serving/25g	41	165	12.3	12.4	7.3	1.2
Fillets, Chunky, Safeway*	1 Fillet/150g	284	189	14.8	11.2	9.5	1.0
Fillets, Co-Op*	1 Serving/100g	75	75	17.0	0.0	0.6	0.0
Fillets, Crisp Breadcrumbs, Ocean Trader*	1 Fillet/120g	229	191	12.4	14.3	9.4	1.0
Fillets, Crispy Battered, Farmfoods*	1oz/28g	38	137	12.3	14.4	3.4	0.5
Fillets, Fresh, Marks & Spencer*	1 Fillet/113g	90	80	19.0	0.0	0.6	0.0
Fillets, In Cheese Mornay Sauce, Marks & Spencer*	½ Pack/190g	219	115	13.5	1.8	6.1	0.1
Fillets, In Crispy Breadcrumbs, Thistle*	1 Serving/100g	174	174	16.1	9.2	8.8	0.3
Fillets, In Crispy Oven Crumb, Tesco*	1 Fillet/142g	251	177	14.3	15.0	6.6	0.9
Fillets, In Tomato Herb Sauce, BGTY, Sainsbury's*	½ Pack/165g	150	91	12.9	3.6	2.8	0.1
Fillets, Safeway*	1 Pack/326g	293	90	20.8	0.0	0.7	0.0
Fillets, Sainsbury's*	1 Fish/95g	195	205	12.1	15.0	10.3	0.6
Fillets, Smoked, Asda*	1 Fillet/100g	113	113	26.0	0.0	1.0	0.0
Fillets, Smoked, Farmfoods*	1oz/28g	23	81	19.0	0.0	0.6	0.0
Fillets, Smoked, Frozen, Sainsbury's*	1 Fillet/89.7g	87	97	23.4	0.1	0.2	0.8
Fillets, Smoked, Marks & Spencer*	1 Pack/227g	170	75	17.8	0.0	0.1	0.0
Fillets, Smoked, Sainsbury's*	1 Fillet/125g	168	134	18.7	1.1	6.1	0.0
Fillets, Smoked, Steamed, Tesco*	1 Pack/300g	303	101	23.3	0.0	0.9	0.0
Fillets, Smoked, Tesco*	1 Serving/100g	87	87	20.4	0.0	0.6	0.0
Fillets, Somerfield*	1oz/28g	23	81	19.0	0.0	1.0	0.0
Fillets, Tesco*	1 Serving/150g	122	81	19.0	0.0	0.6	0.0
Fillets, Undyed, Smoked, Sainsbury's*	1 Fillet/175g	154	88	22.0	0.5	0.4	0.5
Fillets, in Batter, Youngs*	1 Serving/139.6g	311	222	11.7	14.3	13.3	0.6
Fillets, in Crispy Breadcrumbs, Asda*	1 Fillet/135g	271	201	16.0	14.0	9.0	1.1
Fillets, in Light & Crispy Breadcrumbs, Youngs*	1 Portion/139.8g	274	196	11.4	17.8	8.8	1.1
Fillets, in Light Batter, Ross*	1 Fillet/85g	184	216	11.2	18.4	10.8	1.3
Fillets, in Light Crispy Breadcrumb, Marks & Spencer*	1 Serving/134.2g	255	190	13.8	13.9	9.2	1.4
Fillets, in Oven Crisp Crumb, Morrisons*	1 Fillet/160g	312	195	11.8	19.3	7.9	1.0
Florentine, Eat Smart, Safeway*	1 Serving/250g	200	80	12.0	2.5	1.8	1.3
Florentine, Healthy Eating, Tesco*	1 Pack/370g	303	82	8.2	10.0	1.0	0.5
Flour, Fried in Blended Oil	1oz/28g	39	138	21.1	4.5	4.1	0.2
Grilled	1oz/28g	29	104	24.3	0.0	0.8	0.0
In Batter, Large, Youngs*	1 Serving/100g	310	310	16.4	20.0	18.6	0.8
In Watercress Sauce, GFY, Asda*	1 Pack/400g	268	67	6.0	7.0	1.7	1.4

H

INFO/WEIGHT	Measure	per Measure KCAL	KCAL	PROT	CARB	FAT	FIBRE
HADDOCK,							
Mornay, COU, Marks & Spencer*	1 Pack/200g	160	80	14.0	0.7	2.5	0.3
Mornay, Waitrose*	1 Serving/180g	140	78	14.2	1.9	1.6	0.7
Mornay, With Leek Mash, Eat Smart, Safeway*	1 Pack/369.9g	307	83	7.1	7.9	2.5	1.0
Poached	1oz/28g	32	113	17.7	1.1	4.3	0.0
Portions in Crispy Batter, Safeway*	1 Portion/100g	261	261	12.8	18.7	15.0	1.3
Portions, Breaded, Somerfield*	1 Portion/100g	212	212	12.0	13.0	12.0	0.0
Portions, COU, Marks & Spencer*	½ Pack/136g	170	125	13.5	14.0	1.6	1.3
Portions, Frozen, Tesco*	1 Portion/100g	227	227	12.5	18.0	11.7	0.0
Portions, Safeway*	1 Serving/100g	207	207	12.4	16.7	10.0	1.0
Potato Topped, Cumberland, Marks & Spencer*	1 Pack/300g	390	130	8.2	10.6	6.0	0.4
Rarebit, Smoked, Finest, Tesco*	1 Rarebit/180g	326	181	5.6	19.1	9.2	0.4
Raw	1oz/28g	23	81	19.0	0.0	0.6	0.0
Skinless Fillets, Farmfoods*	1oz/28g	20	73	16.8	0.0	0.6	0.0
Smoked, Poached	1oz/28g	38	134	18.7	1.1	6.1	0.0
Smoked, Raw	1oz/28g	23	81	19.0	0.0	0.6	0.0
Smoked, Steamed	1oz/28g	28	101	23.3	0.0	0.9	0.0
Smoked, Tesco*	1 Serving/150g	152	101	23.3	0.0	0.9	0.0
Smoked, With Cheese & Chive, GFY, Asda	½ Pack/185.7g	195	105	15.0	3.1	3.6	0.3
Steaks, Breaded, Sainsbury's*	1 Steak/97g	210	217	12.3	17.6	10.8	0.8
Steaks, Crispy Batter, Bird's Eye*	1 Steak/145g	307	212	11.0	13.7	12.6	0.5
Steaks, Frozen, Morrisons*	1 Steak/92g	67	73	16.8	0.0	0.6	0.0
Steaks, Morrisons*	1 Serving/170g	126	74	10.7	2.4	2.4	0.3
Steaks, in Butter Sauce, Youngs*	1 Portion/150g	134	89	9.9	4.0	3.7	0.5
Steaks, in Crispy Batter, Morrisons*	1 Portion/100g	241	241	10.9	15.0	15.3	2.1
Steamed	1oz/28g	25	89	20.9	0.0	0.6	0.0
HADDOCK - GOUJONS, Crispy Batter, Marks & Spencer*	1 Serving/100g	250	250	11.7	18.5	14.1	0.8
HAGGIS,							
Neeps & Tatties, Marks & Spencer*	1 Pack/300g	330	110	3.8	12.3	4.8	0.8
Vegetarian, McSween*	1 serving/100g	216	216	6.6	26.8	10.2	2.4
HAKE,							
Breadcrumbs, Marks & Spencer*	1oz/28g	60	215	13.1	11.1	13.5	0.4
Fillets, Sainsbury's*	1 Fillet/85g	86	101	21.1	0.1	1.8	0.1
Grilled	1oz/28g	32	113	22.2	0.0	2.7	0.0
Raw	1oz/28g	26	92	18.0	0.0	2.2	0.0
HAKE - GOUJONS, Marks & Spencer*	1oz/28g	69	245	12.0	21.4	12.6	1.5
HALIBUT,							
Grilled	1oz/28g	34	121	25.3	0.0	2.2	0.0
Poached	1oz/28g	43	154	24.7	1.1	5.7	0.0
Raw	1oz/28g	29	103	21.5	0.0	1.9	0.0
Steamed	1oz/28g	37	131	23.8	0.0	4.0	0.0
HALLOUMI, Total*	1oz/28g	90	320	20.0	0.8	25.0	0.0
HALWA, Average	1oz/28g	107	381	1.8	68.0	13.2	0.0
HAM,							
Applewood Smoked, Dry Cured, Safeway*	1 Slice/28g	37	133	24.8	1.5	3.1	0.0
Applewood Smoked, Safeway*	1 Slice/28g	29	104	19.8	0.2	2.7	0.0
Applewood, Smoked, Slices, Sainsbury's*	1 Slice/17.5g	22	120	22.7	0.9	2.8	0.5
Baked, Danepak*	1 Slice/17g	26	152	18.9	1.4	7.9	0.0
Baked, Organic, Waitrose*	1 Slice/22g	33	149	27.0	0.3	4.4	0.0
Baked, Somerfield*	1oz/28g	43	153	16.0	3.0	9.0	0.0
Bavarian, Asda*	1 Slice/15g	18	121	21.4	0.5	3.7	0.0
Beechwood Smoked, Dry Cure, Somerfield*	1oz/28g	38	135	25.0	2.0	3.0	0.0
Belgian, Sainsbury's*	1 Serving/100g	141	141	19.4	2.0	6.1	0.0
Black Forest, Waitrose*	1 Slice/7.7g	14	181	25.8	0.6	8.4	0.0

HAM,

	Measure INFO/WEIGHT	per Measure KCAL	KCAL	PROT	CARB	FAT	FIBRE
Blossom Honey, Sainsbury's*	1 Pack/140g	172	123	23.2	1.3	2.8	0.5
Boiled, Safeway*	1 Pack/113g	128	113	19.5	1.2	3.4	0.0
Boiled, Waitrose*	1 Slice/12.5g	21	160	21.7	0.0	8.1	0.0
Breaded Wiltshire, Marks & Spencer*	1oz/28g	38	135	23.6	1.0	3.7	0.0
Breaded, Asda*	1 Slice/37g	56	150	24.0	0.9	5.6	3.2
Breaded, Drycure, Asda*	1 Slice/36g	44	122	22.0	2.1	2.8	0.0
Breaded, Traditional Cured, Marks & Spencer*	1oz/28g	41	145	21.8	0.7	5.9	0.0
British Cooked, Somerfield*	1oz/28g	26	94	18.0	1.0	2.0	0.0
British Gammon, Traditional Cured, Marks & Spencer*	1 Slice/30g	39	130	25.4	0.0	3.2	0.0
British Honey Roast, Somerfield*	1oz/28g	27	97	18.0	2.0	2.0	0.0
British, Extra Lean, Marks & Spencer*	1 Slice/11g	10	90	18.0	1.4	1.4	0.0
Brunswick, Sliced, Sainsbury's*	1 Slice/20g	32	160	19.5	0.6	8.8	0.1
Brunswick, Smoked, German, Waitrose*	1 Slice/20g	32	160	19.5	0.6	8.8	0.0
Chargrilled, Wafer Thin, Marks & Spencer*	1 Serving/100g	120	120	21.3	0.5	3.9	0.0
Cooked, For Sandwich, Tesco*	1 Slice/13g	16	124	18.7	1.6	4.8	0.0
Cooked, Healthy Eating, Tesco*	1 Slice/25g	29	117	24.4	0.0	2.2	0.0
Cooked, Sliced, Sainsbury's*	1 Slice/13g	15	115	18.2	0.1	4.7	0.1
Cooked, Sliced, Tesco*	1 Slice/30g	35	118	21.2	0.8	3.3	0.1
Cooked, Spar*	1 Can/198g	232	117	15.8	2.0	5.0	0.0
Cooked, Tesco*	1 Slice/13g	13	97	17.6	0.4	2.8	0.0
Cooked, Thin Sliced, Asda*	1 Slice/12.9g	13	101	18.0	0.7	2.9	0.0
Cooked, Wafer Thin, Budgens*	2 Slices/20g	20	102	16.8	0.8	3.5	0.5
Cooked, Waifos, Denny*	1 Packet/85g	79	93	17.3	1.3	2.0	0.0
Crumbed, Safeway*	1 Slice/28g	32	113	19.5	1.2	3.4	0.0
Crumbed, Wiltshire Cure, Safeway*	1 Slice/32.5g	53	162	23.5	1.0	7.1	0.0
Danish, Marks & Spencer*	1 Slice/11g	10	95	17.7	2.0	1.6	0.0
Danish, Prime Quality, Lean, Marks & Spencer*	1oz/28g	25	90	18.0	0.0	2.0	0.0
Danish, Wafer Thin, Marks & Spencer*	1 Serving/50g	50	100	17.6	1.7	2.9	0.0
Dry Cured, Breaded, Safeway*	4 Slices/115g	156	136	24.8	2.1	3.1	0.0
Dry Cured, Breaded, Sainsbury's*	1 Slice/26g	39	151	21.0	2.3	6.5	0.0
Dry Cured, Breaded, TTD, Sainsbury's*	1 Slice/27g	35	130	21.1	2.5	3.9	0.1
Dry Cured, Carvery, Peppered, Morrisons*	1 Slice/30g	40	132	21.9	2.0	4.1	0.0
Dry Cured, Cooked, Organic, Sainsbury's*	1 Slice/22g	31	141	26.4	1.4	3.3	1.1
Dry Cured, Finest, Tesco*	1 Slice/25g	42	169	25.4	0.0	7.5	0.0
Dry Cured, Mustard, Sainsbury's*	1 Slice/26.1g	40	153	20.2	1.6	7.3	0.1
Dry Cured, Oak Smoked, TTD, Sainsbury's*	1 Slice/27g	32	119	22.5	1.7	2.5	0.1
Dry Cured, Ovenbaked, Asda*	1 Slice/32g	47	147	22.0	3.5	5.0	1.0
Dry Cured, Peppered, Asda*	1 Slice/31g	40	128	22.0	1.7	3.7	0.7
Dry Cured, Peppered, Sainsbury's*	1 Slice/27.1g	38	140	21.2	1.1	5.6	0.1
Dry Cured, Premium Cooked, Plumrose*	1 Slice/20g	28	142	19.9	0.0	7.0	0.0
Dry Cured, Smoked, Finely Sliced, Sainsbury's*	1 Slice/18g	24	135	21.2	1.0	5.1	0.1
Dry Cured, TTD, Sainsbury's*	1 Slice/27g	39	146	20.5	1.6	6.4	0.1
Dry Cured, Thinly Sliced, Somerfield*	½ Pack/59.5g	76	126	22.1	0.1	4.1	0.0
Dry Cured, Wafer Thin, Tesco*	1 Slice/30g	39	130	23.5	0.9	3.6	0.0
Economy, Sainsbury's*	1 Slice/13g	13	102	16.8	0.8	3.6	0.6
English Smoked, Waitrose*	1oz/28g	39	140	21.4	0.0	6.0	0.0
English, Waitrose*	1 Slice/12g	12	97	19.3	0.3	2.5	0.0
Extra Lean, Marks & Spencer*	1 Pack/113g	102	90	18.0	1.4	1.4	0.0
Gammon Joint, Boiled	1oz/28g	57	204	23.3	0.0	12.3	0.0
Gammon Joint, Raw	1oz/28g	39	138	17.5	0.0	7.5	0.0
Gammon Smoked, Dry Cured, Waitrose*	1 Serving/100g	132	132	22.0	0.9	4.4	0.0
Gammon, Asda*	1 Serving/100g	137	137	23.0	0.0	5.0	0.0
Gammon, Cooked, Somerfield*	1oz/28g	45	159	20.0	1.0	8.0	0.0

H

HAM,	INFO/WEIGHT	KCAL	KCAL	PROT	CARB	FAT	FIBRE
Gammon, Honey Roast, Waitrose*	1 Slice/43g	60	139	22.8	0.1	5.3	0.0
Gammon, Oak Smoked, Waitrose*	1 Slice/43g	62	145	24.2	0.0	5.3	0.0
Genuilne Parma, Marks & Spencer*	1 Serving/10g	20	200	30.0	0.0	9.0	0.0
German Black Forest, Safeway*	½ Pack/35g	93	267	27.2	1.3	17.0	0.5
German Black Forest, Sainsbury's*	1 Slice/8g	21	267	27.2	1.3	17.0	0.5
Glazed With Honey & Muscovado Sugar, Waitrose*	1 Slice/21g	25	119	21.3	0.4	3.6	0.0
Great Value, Harris*	1 Slice/10g	10	96	16.3	0.8	3.1	0.0
Honey & Mustard, Wafer Thin, Marks & Spencer*	1 Pack/100g	140	140	20.8	4.6	4.3	0.0
Honey Cured, Wafer Thin, Sainsbury's*	1 Slice/6g	6	108	17.2	2.1	3.4	1.1
Honey Cured, Wafer Thin, TTD, Sainsbury's*	1 Serving/75g	95	126	20.8	1.8	4.0	0.0
Honey Roast, Finely Sliced, Dry Cured, Waitrose*	1 Serving/60g	78	130	22.1	0.8	4.2	0.0
Honey Roast, Bernard Matthews*	1 Slice/21g	24	112	20.4	2.0	2.5	0.0
Honey Roast, Carvery, Courtway*	1 Slice/25g	38	152	21.0	1.5	6.9	0.0
Honey Roast, Co-Op*	1 Slice/23g	28	120	19.0	0.6	5.0	0.0
Honey Roast, Dru Cured, Finely Sliced, Sainsbury's*	1 Slice/18g	24	136	21.4	1.0	5.1	0.1
Honey Roast, Dry Cured, Asda*	1 Slice/31g	42	137	22.0	2.0	4.5	0.5
Honey Roast, Dry Cured, Premium, Co-Op*	1 Slice/33g	41	125	22.0	0.2	4.0	0.0
Honey Roast, Dry Cured, TTD, Sainsbury's*	1 Slice/27g	35	135	21.7	2.6	4.2	0.1
Honey Roast, Dry Cured, Tesco*	1 Slice/25g	33	133	23.5	1.6	3.6	0.0
Honey Roast, English, Waitrose*	1 Slice/12g	13	107	19.9	0.5	2.9	0.0
Honey Roast, Healthy Eating, Tesco*	1 Slice/25g	27	107	22.2	1.7	1.2	0.0
Honey Roast, Lean, Danish, Marks & Spencer*	1 Serving/25g	28	110	19.5	3.1	2.2	0.0
Honey Roast, Mattessons*	1oz/28g	52	187	21.0	3.1	6.5	0.0
Honey Roast, Organic, Waitrose*	1 Slice/45g	63	140	20.6	1.4	5.8	0.0
Honey Roast, Oven Baked, Asda*	1 Slice/31g	42	137	22.0	2.0	4.5	0.5
Honey Roast, Premium, Iceland*	1 Serving/100g	111	111	20.5	1.5	2.6	0.0
Honey Roast, Premium, Safeway*	1 Slice/28g	34	121	19.3	1.8	4.1	0.0
Honey Roast, Safeway*	1 Slice/12g	12	102	17.4	1.7	2.8	0.0
Honey Roast, Sainsbury's*	1 Slice/13g	15	119	18.6	1.7	4.2	0.1
Honey Roast, Sandwich, Tesco*	1 Slice/13g	16	124	18.7	1.6	4.8	0.0
Honey Roast, Slices, Sainsbury's*	1 Slice/13g	14	104	17.4	1.6	3.1	0.0
Honey Roast, TTD, Sainsbury's*	1 Slice/38g	51	135	21.7	2.6	4.2	0.0
Honey Roast, Tesco*	1 Slice/31g	37	120	21.4	1.1	3.3	0.0
Honey Roast, Thin Sliced, Asda*	1 Slice/13g	15	116	19.0	2.9	3.1	1.6
Honey Roast, Thin, Dry Dured, Somerfield*	1 Slice/32g	40	126	21.9	0.4	4.1	0.0
Honey Roast, Wafer Thin, Asda*	1oz/28g	31	112	16.8	3.9	3.2	0.0
Honey Roast, Wafer Thin, Premium, Cut, Safeway*	1 Slice/12g	23	194	23.4	2.6	10.0	0.0
Honey Roast, Wafer Thin, Safeway*	¼ Pack/25g	28	112	16.8	3.9	3.2	0.0
Honey Roast, Wafer Thin, Sainsbury's*	1 Slice/10g	11	113	16.8	5.8	2.5	0.1
Honey Roast, Wafer Thin, Tesco*	1 Serving/25g	27	107	17.1	1.6	3.6	0.0
Honey Roast, Wafer Thin, Waitrose*	1 Slice/10g	10	104	18.7	1.5	2.6	0.0
Honey Roast, Waitrose*	1 Serving/65g	90	139	22.8	0.1	5.3	0.0
Honey Roasted Mustard, Thin Sliced, Asda*	1 Slice/16g	16	103	17.5	3.8	2.0	1.6
Honey Roasted, Morrisons*	1 Slice/30g	47	158	20.9	4.1	6.4	0.5
Honey Roasted, Wafer Thin, Somerfield*	1 Serving/50g	62	124	14.2	5.6	5.0	0.0
Honey, Roast, Prepacked, Waitrose*	1 Slice/17g	20	115	19.7	0.0	4.0	0.0
Italian Dry Cured, Waitrose*	1 Slice/29g	65	223	28.0	0.2	12.0	0.0
Italian Parma, TTD, Sainsbury's*	1 Slice/15g	34	225	28.2	0.1	12.4	0.1
Italian Rostello, Safeway*	1 Serving/60g	78	130	21.0	0.2	5.0	0.0
Joint, Easy Carve, Asda*	1oz/28g	41	146	22.8	1.2	5.9	0.6
Joint, Honey Roast, Asda*	1oz/28g	35	124	23.9	1.7	2.8	0.7
Lean, BGTY, Sainsbury's*	1 Slice/145g	158	109	23.1	1.5	1.2	0.5
Maple Drycure, Asda*	1 Slice/37.1g	53	143	22.0	3.0	4.8	0.0

H

	INFO/WEIGHT	KCAL	KCAL	PROT	CARB	FAT	FIBRE

HAM,

	INFO/WEIGHT	KCAL	KCAL	PROT	CARB	FAT	FIBRE
Mild Cure, Courtway, Aldi*	1 Slice/11g	13	120	16.8	1.6	5.2	0.0
Mild, Cured, Waitrose*	1 Slice/18g	21	114	19.7	0.0	4.0	0.0
Mustard, Thin Sliced, Asda*	1 Slice/13g	13	101	17.0	3.8	2.0	0.0
Norfolk Smoked, Bernard Matthews*	1 Piece/38g	41	108	23.8	0.6	1.0	0.0
Oak Smoked, Asda*	1 Slice/38g	51	134	20.6	1.2	5.2	0.8
Oak Smoked, Waitrose*	1 Slice/18g	24	135	21.1	0.4	5.4	0.0
On The Bone, Breaded, Somerfield*	1oz/28g	45	161	21.0	0.0	9.0	0.0
Organic, Tesco*	1 Slice/42g	76	180	21.2	0.0	10.6	0.4
Oven Baked, Bernard Matthews*	1 Slice/30g	30	101	19.6	1.1	1.9	0.0
Oven Baked, Sliced, Asda*	1 Slice/32g	47	147	22.0	3.5	5.0	1.0
Parma, Extra Special, Asda*	3 Slices/30g	80	267	28.0	0.6	17.0	0.0
Parma, Finest, Tesco*	1 Serving/10g	25	250	31.5	0.5	13.5	0.1
Parma, Marks & Spencer*	1oz/28g	56	200	30.0	0.0	9.0	0.0
Parma, Somerfield*	1oz/28g	63	226	29.0	0.0	12.0	0.0
Parma, The Best, Safeway*	1 Serving/80g	191	239	26.0	0.1	15.0	0.0
Parma, Waitrose*	1 Pack/80g	220	275	26.0	0.1	19.0	0.0
Peppered, Co-Op*	1 Serving/25g	30	120	20.0	0.4	3.6	0.0
Peppered, Thin Sliced, Asda*	1 Slice/12g	12	99	17.0	3.7	1.8	0.0
Princes*	1 Serving/225g	349	155	12.0	1.5	11.0	0.0
Prosciutto di Speck, TTD, Sainsbury's*	1 Slice/12g	26	220	28.4	0.1	11.7	0.1
Prosciutto, Asda*	1 Serving/50g	117	233	29.0	0.0	13.0	0.6
Roast, Wafer Thin, Healthy Eating, Tesco*	½ Pack/50g	48	95	22.0	0.0	0.8	0.0
Safeway*	1 Slice/12g	11	95	17.8	0.7	2.3	0.0
Sandwich, Thin Sliced, Sainsbury's*	1 Pack/180g	162	90	18.9	1.0	1.2	0.5
Scrumpy Cured, Tesco*	1 Slice/34g	60	176	27.2	0.9	7.1	0.0
Slices, Cooked, Sainsbury's*	1 Slice/28g	32	116	18.2	0.1	4.7	0.1
Smoked, Iceland*	1 Slice/24g	30	127	20.6	0.7	4.6	0.0
Smoked, Marks & Spencer*	1 Slice/6g	6	105	19.7	0.2	3.0	0.0
Smoked, Mattessons*	1 Slice/25g	41	165	20.0	3.0	6.8	0.0
Smoked, Safeway*	2 Slices/25g	26	103	17.3	1.8	2.9	0.0
Smoked, Sainsbury's*	1 Slice/12.5g	14	115	18.5	0.1	4.5	0.1
Smoked, Sandwich, Tesco*	1 Slice/28g	35	124	18.7	1.6	4.8	0.0
Smoked, Slices, Sainsbury's*	1 Serving/27g	32	119	22.5	1.7	2.5	0.1
Smoked, Somerfield*	1oz/28g	29	102	17.0	1.0	3.0	0.0
Smoked, Tesco*	1 Slice/31g	36	117	21.7	0.5	3.1	0.0
Smoked, Thin Sliced, Asda*	1 Slice/52	50	96	18.0	2.4	1.6	0.9
Smoked, Thin Sliced, Co-Op*	1 Slice/12g	12	100	18.0	0.7	3.0	0.0
Smoked, Wafer Thin, Asda*	1oz/28g	27	96	16.1	0.8	3.1	0.0
Smoked, Wafer Thin, Sainsbury's*	1 Serving/40g	36	90	16.2	2.0	1.9	0.0
Smoked, Wafer Thin, TTD, Sainsbury's*	1 Slice/5g	6	124	21.3	0.6	4.0	0.1
Smoked, Wafer Thin, Tesco*	1 Serving/50g	53	105	16.6	0.8	3.9	0.0
Tesco*	1 Serving/40g	47	118	21.2	0.8	3.3	0.1
Thick Carved, Finest, Tesco*	1 Serving/75g	89	119	22.8	0.1	3.0	0.0
Thick Cut, Tesco*	1 Serving/85g	119	140	20.6	1.4	5.8	0.0
Thin Sliced, Cooked, Asda*	1 Slice/13g	15	114	20.0	3.8	2.1	0.8
Thin Sliced, Organic, Sainsbury's*	1 Slice/12g	12	100	18.3	1.2	2.4	0.1
Thin Sliced, Sandwich, Bernard Matthews*	1 Slice/14g	13	90	15.0	3.2	1.9	0.0
Thin Sliced, SmartPrice, Asda*	1 Slice/12g	11	92	16.0	0.8	2.7	0.0
Thinly Sliced, Somerfield*	1oz/28g	36	130	15.0	3.0	7.0	0.0
Tinned, Ye Olde Oak*	100g/100g	108	108	12.5	2.0	5.5	0.0
Traditional Cured, Roasted, Marks & Spencer*	1 Slice/28g	42	150	22.6	1.9	5.8	0.0
Traditional Wiltshire Cured, Wafer Thin, Finest, Tesco*	1 Serving/100g	140	140	24.1	0.0	4.8	0.0
Turkey, Smoked, Wafer Thin, Bernard Matthews*	1 Serving/10g	11	112	14.4	3.8	4.4	0.0

H

INFO/WEIGHT	Measure	per Measure KCAL	Nutrition Values per 100g / 100ml				
			KCAL	PROT	CARB	FAT	FIBRE
HAM,							
Wafer Thin, Asda*	1oz/28g	27	95	16.0	0.8	3.1	0.0
Wafer Thin, Bernard Matthews*	1 Slice/45g	42	93	15.7	0.9	2.9	0.0
Wafer Thin, Cooked, Kwik Save*	1 Serving/50g	53	105	15.6	1.4	4.1	0.0
Wafer Thin, Iceland*	1 Slice/9g	8	94	16.4	0.8	2.8	0.0
Wafer Thin, Sainsbury's*	1 Serving/10g	9	93	16.5	2.0	2.1	0.1
Wafer Thin, Tesco*	1 Pack/200g	210	105	16.6	0.8	3.9	0.0
Whisky Oak Smoked, TTD, Sainsbury's*	1 Pack/160g	194	121	21.3	1.3	3.4	0.0
Wiltshire Crumbed, The Best, Safeway*	1 Pack/130g	181	139	24.5	1.0	4.1	0.0
Wiltshire Crumbed, Traditional, Finest, Tesco*	1 Slice/44g	62	140	24.1	0.0	4.8	0.1
HARIBO*,							
American Hard Gums	1 Pack/175g	630	360	0.3	85.5	1.9	0.2
Cola Bottles	1 Sm Pack/16g	57	358	7.7	78.9	1.3	0.3
Cola Bottles, Fizzy	1 Pack/175g	628	359	6.3	78.3	2.3	0.5
Dolly Mixtures	1 Pack/175g	719	411	1.8	90.2	4.8	0.2
Gold Bears	1 Pack/100g	358	358	7.7	78.9	1.3	0.3
Jelly Beans	1 Pack/100g	360	360	3.8	89.2	1.2	0.0
Mint Imperials	1 Pack/175g	695	397	0.4	98.8	0.5	0.1
Starmix	1 Pack/100g	360	360	6.6	79.0	2.0	0.3
Tangfastics	1 Pack/100g	359	359	6.3	78.3	2.3	0.5
Wine Gums	1 Pack/175g	655	374	6.2	85.9	0.6	0.1
HARIBO* MIX,							
Fantasy	1 Sm Pack/100g	360	360	6.6	79.0	2.0	0.3
Horror	1 Sm Pack/100g	360	360	6.6	79.0	2.0	0.3
Kiddies Super	1 Pack/100g	401	401	1.1	95.3	1.7	0.8
Milky	1 Pack/175g	644	368	7.1	79.6	2.3	0.4
HASH,							
Chicken Salsa, Healthy Eating, Tesco*	1 Pack/350g	291	83	4.1	10.6	2.7	1.1
Corned Beef, Asda*	1 Pack/400g	416	104	6.0	12.0	3.6	1.1
Corned Beef, Chilled, Co-Op*	1 Pack/300g	345	115	9.0	5.0	6.0	1.0
Corned Beef, Marks & Spencer*	½ Pack/320g	400	125	9.4	7.2	6.3	1.3
Corned Beef, Morrisons*	1 Serving/100g	82	82	6.3	9.2	2.8	1.1
Corned Beef, Somerfield*	1 Pack/300g	324	108	6.2	8.5	5.5	1.6
Corned Beef, Value, Tesco*	1 Pack/300g	372	124	6.8	12.7	5.1	0.7
Farmhouse, Healthy Eating, Tesco*	1 Serving/300g	264	88	2.2	13.6	2.7	1.1
Vegetable & Lentil, Asda*	1 Pack/289g	254	88	3.2	14.0	2.1	0.0
HASH BROWNS,							
Bird's Eye*	1 Serving/63g	126	200	2.0	21.9	11.6	1.6
Burger King*	1 Hash/102g	318	312	7.2	32.3	19.4	3.8
Deep Fried, McCain*	1oz/28g	69	246	2.0	24.3	15.3	0.0
Farmfoods*	1oz/28g	35	124	2.1	18.2	4.7	2.1
Frozen, McCain*	1 Hash/40g	70	174	3.0	24.0	7.3	0.0
McDonald's*	1 Portion/56g	127	227	2.2	25.3	13.0	3.8
Oven Baked, McCain*	1oz/28g	55	196	1.7	25.5	8.6	0.0
Tesco*	1oz/28g	43	154	2.4	20.0	7.2	1.7
HASLET, Somerfield*	1oz/28g	57	205	15.0	10.0	12.0	0.0
HAZELNUTS,							
Average	10 Whole/10g	65	650	14.1	6.0	63.5	6.5
Chopped, Sainsbury's*	1 Serving/10g	66	660	16.6	5.6	63.5	6.5
Whole, Blanched, Sainsbury's*	1 Serving/50g	330	660	16.6	5.6	63.5	6.5
HEART,							
Ox, Raw	1oz/28g	29	104	18.2	0.0	3.5	0.0
Ox, Stewed	1oz/28g	44	157	27.8	0.0	5.1	0.0
Pig, Raw	1oz/28g	27	97	17.1	0.0	3.2	0.0

H

	Measure INFO/WEIGHT	per Measure KCAL	Nutrition Values per 100g / 100ml				
			KCAL	PROT	CARB	FAT	FIBRE
HEART,							
Pig, Stewed	1oz/28g	45	162	25.1	0.0	6.8	0.0
HERB CUBES,							
Basil, Knorr*	1 Cube/10g	47	472	6.1	35.9	33.8	0.6
Parsley & Garlic, Knorr*	1 Cube/10g	42	422	8.6	35.2	27.4	1.8
HERMESETAS, Hermes*	1 Tsp/0.78	3	387	1.0	96.8	0.0	0.0
HEROES, Miniature, Cadbury's*	3 Sweets/30g	147	490	5.6	59.2	25.6	0.0
HERRING,							
Canned in Tomato Sauce	1oz/28g	54	193	12.8	3.2	14.4	0.0
Dried, Salted	1oz/28g	47	168	25.3	0.0	7.4	0.0
Fillets, Succulent in Olive Oil, Princes*	1 Serving/50g	108	215	20.0	0.0	15.0	0.0
Fillets, in Mustard & Dill Sauce, John West*	1 Can/190g	426	224	11.7	3.7	18.0	0.1
Fillets, in Tomato Sauce, John West*	1 Can/190g	416	219	11.5	4.6	17.2	0.4
Grilled	1oz/28g	51	181	20.1	0.0	11.2	0.0
In Horseradish Sauce, John West*	1oz/28g	64	230	13.0	4.0	18.0	0.0
In Rich Spicy Tomato Sauce, Princes*	1 Can/190g	378	199	11.5	4.5	15.0	0.0
Oatmeal, Fried in Vegetable Oil	1oz/28g	66	234	23.1	1.5	15.1	0.1
Pickled	1oz/28g	59	209	16.7	10.0	11.1	0.0
Raw	1oz/28g	53	190	17.8	0.0	13.2	0.0
Rollmop, With Onion, Asda*	1 Rollmop/65g	89	137	13.2	10.3	4.8	0.8
HIGH LIGHTS,							
Cadbury's*, Made Up	1 Cup/200ml	40	20	1.0	2.5	0.7	0.3
Caffe Latte, Cadbury's*, Made Up	1 Serving/200g	40	20	1.0	2.5	0.7	0.0
Choc Malt Hot Chocolate, Cadbury's*, Made Up	1 Serving/200ml	44	22	1.0	2.5	0.7	0.3
Choc Mint, Cadbury's*, Made Up	1 Serving/200ml	40	20	1.0	2.5	0.7	0.3
Chocolate Drink, Cadbury's, Dry	1 Sachet/10g	36	364	17.1	44.7	13.0	4.6
Chocolate Orange, Cadbury's*, Made Up	1 Serving/200ml	40	20	1.0	2.3	0.7	0.3
Dairy Fudge, Cadbury's*, Made Up	1 Serving/200ml	40	20	1.0	2.8	0.5	0.2
Espresso, Cadbury's*, Made Up	1 Serving/200ml	35	18	1.3	2.0	0.5	0.0
Orange, Cadbury's*, Made Up	1 Serving/200ml	40	20	1.0	2.3	0.7	0.0
Toffee Flavour, Cadbury's*, Made Up	1 Serving/200ml	40	20	1.0	2.6	0.7	0.0
HOKI,							
Fillets, Breaded, Sainsbury's*	1 Serving/135g	248	184	17.7	13.6	6.6	1.2
Grilled	1oz/28g	34	121	24.1	0.0	2.7	0.0
In Breadcrumbs, Youngs*	1 Piece/156g	275	176	14.3	11.7	8.7	0.8
Raw	1oz/28g	24	85	16.9	0.0	1.9	0.0
Steaks, in Crispy Batter, Bird's Eye*	1 Steak/123.1g	320	260	12.4	21.3	13.9	0.8
Steaks, in Crunch Crumb, Bird's Eye*	1 Steak/115.2g	250	217	13.1	17.2	10.6	0.8
HONEY,							
Acacia, Tesco*	1 Tsp/4g	12	307	0.4	76.4	0.0	0.0
Australian Eucalyptus, Finest, Tesco*	1 Tsp/4g	12	307	0.4	76.4	0.0	0.0
Average	1 Tsp/6g	49	288	0.4	76.4	0.0	0.0
Canadian Clover, TTD, Sainsbury's*	1 Tsp/5g	17	339	0.1	84.7	0.1	0.3
Clear, Frank Cooper*	1 Tsp/6g	18	292	0.4	72.6	0.0	0.0
Clear, Safeway*	1 Tbsp/15g	48	322	0.4	80.0	0.0	0.0
Florida Orange, Extra Special, Asda*	1 Tbsp/15g	50	334	0.5	83.0	0.0	0.0
Greek, Waitrose*	1 Tsp/6g	18	307	0.4	76.4	0.0	0.0
Mexican, TTD, Sainsbury's*	1 Tbsp/15g	51	339	0.1	84.7	0.1	0.3
Organic, Marks & Spencer*	1 Tsp/6g	21	355	0.2	88.4	0.1	0.1
Pure & Natural, Morrisons*	1 Tbsp/20g	58	288	0.0	76.4	0.0	0.0
Pure, Clear, Asda*	1 Tbsp/15g	46	306	0.4	79.0	0.0	0.0
Pure, Clear, Blended, Sainsbury's*	1 Tsp/6g	20	331	0.4	82.3	0.1	0.0
Pure, Clear, Chivers*	1 Tsp/6g	19	311	0.6	77.2	0.0	0.0
Pure, Clear, Co-Op*	1 Tbsp/17g	55	322	0.4	80.0	0.0	0.0

H

	Measure INFO/WEIGHT	per Measure KCAL	Nutrition Values per 100g / 100ml				
			KCAL	PROT	CARB	FAT	FIBRE
HONEY,							
Pure, Clear, Organic, Tesco*	1 Dtsp/20g	61	307	0.4	76.4	0.0	0.0
Pure, Clear, Tesco*	1 Serving/27g	84	311	0.4	81.0	0.0	0.0
Pure, Frank Cooper*	1 Tsp/6g	18	292	0.4	72.6	0.0	0.0
Pure, Set, Tesco*	1 Tsp/5g	15	307	0.4	76.4	0.0	0.0
Pure, Set, Waitrose*	1 Tsp/9g	28	307	0.4	76.4	0.0	0.0
Runny, Organic, Sainsbury's*	1 Serving/10g	34	339	0.1	84.7	0.1	0.3
Set, Safeway*	1 Tsps/15g	48	322	0.4	80.0	0.0	0.0
Spanish Orange Blossom, Sainsbury's*	1 Tbsp/15g	51	339	0.1	84.7	0.0	0.3
Tasmanian Leatherwood, TTD, Sainsbury's*	1 Serving/6g	20	339	0.1	84.7	0.1	0.3
HOOCH, * Vodka, (Calculated Estimate)	1 Bottle/330ml	244	74	0.3	5.1	0.0	0.0
HORLICKS,							
Low Fat Instant Powder, Made Up With Water	1 Mug/227ml	116	51	2.4	10.1	0.5	0.0
Malted Chocolate Drink, Light, Horlicks*, Dry	1 Sachet/32g	123	384	13.7	7.3	4.1	1.7
Powder, Made Up With Semi-Skimmed Milk	1 Mug/227ml	184	81	4.3	12.9	1.9	0.0
Powder, Made Up With Skimmed Milk	1 Mug/227ml	159	70	4.3	12.9	0.5	0.0
Powder, Made Up With Whole Milk	1 Mug/227ml	225	99	4.2	12.7	3.9	0.0
HORSERADISH, Raw	1oz/28g	17	62	4.5	11.0	0.3	6.2
HOT CHOCOLATE,							
Caramel Flavoured, Instant, Aldi*, Dry	1 Serving/11g	40	363	18.5	40.6	14.1	8.5
Chocolate Break, Tesco*, Dry	1 Serving/21g	110	524	7.9	58.9	28.5	1.7
Chocolate Time, Safeway*, Dry	1 Serving/30g	123	411	9.4	67.8	11.4	1.8
Drink, Balanced Lifestyle, Camelot, Aldi*, Dry	1 Sachet/11g	40	363	18.5	40.6	14.1	0.5
Galaxy, Mars*, Made Up	1 Mug/28g	115	411	7.0	68.7	12.1	0.0
Instant, BGTY, Sainsbury's*, Dry	1 Sachet/28g	16	56	2.1	10.6	0.6	0.3
Instant, Cadbury's*, Dry	1 Sachet/28g	119	426	10.9	64.2	14.0	2.3
Instant, Good For You, Asda*, Made Up	1 Mug/200ml	106	53	1.8	10.0	0.6	0.4
Instant, Tesco*, Dry	1 Serving/32g	132	414	8.0	68.3	12.1	0.7
Low Calorie, Somerfield*, Dry	1 Sachet/12g	40	330	18.0	48.0	8.0	0.0
Maltesers, Malt Drink, Instant, Mars*, Made Up	1 Serving/220ml	104	47	0.9	7.7	1.4	0.0
Organic, Green & Black's*, Dry	1 Tsp/3g	11	376	7.4	66.8	6.6	0.0
Velvet, Cadbury's*, Dry	1 Serving/28g	136	487	8.6	57.8	24.6	2.0
HOT DOG,							
& Ketchup, McDonald's*	1 Serving/116g	296	255	9.6	25.8	12.6	1.3
American Style, Sainsbury's*	1 Sausage/50g	144	288	13.0	0.5	26.0	0.0
American Style, Tesco*	1 Sausage/75g	164	218	12.7	3.4	17.1	0.0
Big American Style, Princes*	1 Sausage/27g	53	197	8.5	7.0	15.0	0.0
Canned, Ye Olde Oak*	1 Hot Dog/33g	54	165	11.5	5.0	12.0	0.0
Farmfoods*	1 Sausage/50g	84	168	10.0	5.0	12.0	1.0
In Brine, Premium, Ye Olde Oak*	1 Sausage/23g	39	168	11.0	4.0	12.0	1.0
Jumbo, Co-Op*	1 Sausage/75g	169	225	13.0	4.0	18.0	0.0
Lancaster*	4 Sausages/92g	138	150	10.0	4.0	10.5	0.0
Lite, Princes*	1oz/28g	42	150	10.5	5.5	9.5	0.6
Meatfree, Sainsbury's*	1 Sausage/30g	70	235	17.8	4.2	16.4	1.9
Mini, Tesco*	1 Hot Dog/10g	22	218	12.7	3.4	17.1	0.0
Princes*	1 Sausage/23g	42	183	8.0	5.0	14.5	0.0
SmartPrice Asda*	1 Sausage/23g	31	135	10.0	3.5	9.0	0.0
Value, Tesco*	1 Sausage/27g	59	218	12.7	3.4	17.1	0.0
Vegetarian, Tesco*	1 Sausage/30g	81	271	19.0	6.0	19.0	2.0
HOT POT,							
Beef, Apetito*	1 Pack/340g	303	89	5.1	10.3	3.1	1.3
Beef, Ross*	1 Pack/322g	254	79	2.5	9.4	3.5	0.4
Beef, Weight Watchers*	1 Pack/320g	288	90	5.8	10.0	3.0	1.4
Chicken & Cider, Ready Meals, Waitrose*	1 Pack/400g	500	125	6.8	12.9	5.1	1.1

H

	Measure INFO/WEIGHT	per Measure KCAL	Nutrition Values per 100g / 100ml				
			KCAL	PROT	CARB	FAT	FIBRE
HOT POT,							
Chicken, Co-Op*	1 Pack/340g	289	85	6.0	9.0	3.0	0.7
Chicken, Good Choice, Iceland*	1 Pack/400g	276	69	5.0	9.3	1.3	1.0
Chicken, Safeway*	1 Pack/400g	292	73	4.2	10.7	1.5	1.6
Chicken, Sainsbury's*	1 Pack/400g	340	85	5.2	9.9	2.8	1.3
Chicken, Traditional, Pro Cuisine*	1 Pack/400g	208	52	5.8	5.2	0.9	0.0
Chicken, Weight Watchers*	1 Pack/340g	306	90	5.3	11.3	2.6	0.9
Lamb & Vegetable, Asda*	1 Pot/500g	240	48	4.0	7.0	0.4	0.0
Lamb, Heinz*	1 Pack/340g	337	99	4.9	12.7	3.1	1.7
Lamb, Safeway*	½ Pack/225g	218	97	6.9	8.1	4.1	1.3
Lancashire, Asda*	1 Pack/401g	269	67	3.8	10.0	1.3	0.9
Lancashire, Hollands*	1 Serving/250g	340	136	3.6	19.6	4.7	0.0
Lancashire, Safeway*	1 Pack/400g	336	84	8.4	6.6	2.7	1.3
Lancashire, Sainsbury's*	½ Pack/225g	203	90	6.7	9.5	2.8	0.5
Lancashire, Tesco*	½ Pack/225g	205	91	6.0	9.7	3.1	0.5
Minced Beef, Asda*	1 Pack/375g	409	109	7.0	10.0	4.6	1.7
Minced Beef, Classic, Sainsbury's*	1 Pack/450g	491	109	6.1	13.4	3.4	1.0
Minced Beef, Iceland*	1 Pack/500g	505	101	5.5	12.7	3.1	1.3
Minced Beef, Long Life, Sainsbury's*	1 Pack/300g	207	69	3.9	10.0	1.5	0.9
Minced Beef, Mini Favourites, Marks & Spencer*	1 Pack/300g	210	70	5.0	6.4	2.9	2.5
Minced Beef, Sainsbury's*	1 Pack/300g	174	58	3.6	7.0	1.7	2.1
Minced Beef, SmartPrice, Asda*	1 Pack/296g	237	80	3.2	10.0	3.0	1.0
Minced Beef, Tesco*	1 Pack/400g	352	88	3.6	10.6	3.5	1.7
Vegetable, Granovita*	½ Can/210g	202	96	3.0	12.0	4.0	0.0
Vegetable, Ross*	1 Pack/300g	261	87	2.4	11.7	3.5	2.0
Vegetable, Weight Watchers*	1 Pack/335g	228	68	2.6	9.9	1.9	1.5
HOUMOUS,							
30% Less Fat, Asda*	1oz/28g	77	275	8.8	16.4	19.4	2.1
BGTY, Sainsbury's*	1oz/28g	54	192	5.9	15.6	11.8	1.3
Co-Op*	1 Tbsp/25g	91	365	9.0	14.0	30.0	3.0
Fresh, 25% Less Fat, Tesco*	1 Serving/85g	201	236	7.5	12.9	17.2	3.3
Fresh, Dips, Tesco*	1/3 Pot/94g	271	288	6.8	10.7	24.2	3.0
Fresh, Healthy Choice, Safeway*	1oz/28g	74	264	9.1	13.6	19.2	0.0
Fresh, Tesco*	1oz/28g	83	296	7.8	7.9	25.9	3.3
Good For You, Asda*	½ Pot/85g	209	246	9.0	12.0	18.0	4.3
Greek, Somerfield*	1 Serving/50g	152	304	7.6	8.2	26.8	5.5
Lemon & Coriander, Sainsbury's*	½ Pot/85g	247	291	7.0	9.1	25.1	6.0
Light, Morrisons*	½ Pack/85g	200	235	7.4	10.9	18.0	0.0
Low Fat, Safeway*	1 Serving/10g	26	258	9.0	12.8	19.0	3.3
Marks & Spencer*	1oz/28g	87	310	7.1	9.5	27.3	3.3
Mixed Olive, Sainsbury's*	½ Pot/85g	228	268	6.7	8.4	23.1	7.7
Organic, Marks & Spencer*	1 Serving/42g	139	330	6.9	9.1	29.7	3.3
Organic, Tesco*	1 Pot/170g	544	320	6.5	12.3	27.2	2.4
Reduced Fat, Fresh, Tesco*	1oz/28g	66	236	7.5	12.9	17.2	3.3
Reduced Fat, Marks & Spencer*	1oz/28g	67	240	7.5	12.9	17.2	3.3
Reduced Fat, Mediterranean Deli, Marks & Spencer*	1 Serving/75g	158	210	7.5	8.3	16.2	9.3
Reduced Fat, Waitrose*	1oz/28g	67	239	7.7	11.3	18.1	2.6
Roasted Red Pepper, 50% Less Fat, Tesco*	½ Pot/85g	156	184	7.3	10.9	12.4	9.5
Sainsbury's*	1oz/28g	87	312	7.3	8.9	27.5	2.2
Somerfield*	1oz/28g	87	309	8.0	11.0	26.0	0.0
Spicy Red Pepper, Marks & Spencer*	¼ Pot/75g	158	210	7.3	14.8	13.7	2.5
Sun Dried Tomato, Chunky, Tesco*	½ Pot/95g	322	339	6.7	14.0	28.4	3.3
Waitrose*	¼ Pot/74.9g	248	331	7.5	9.2	29.3	3.0
With Crunchy Vegetables, Starbucks*	1 Pot/219g	359	164	4.7	26.4	4.4	2.9

H

	Measure INFO/WEIGHT	per Measure KCAL	Nutrition Values per 100g / 100ml				
			KCAL	PROT	CARB	FAT	FIBRE
HOUMOUS,							
Zorba Delicacies Ltd*	1 Serving/50g	157	313	7.6	10.7	26.6	3.0
HULA HOOPS,							
Barbecue Beef Flavour, Hula Hoops*	1 Bag/34g	170	500	3.9	58.7	27.5	2.4
Beef & Mustard, KP*	1 Bag/50g	260	519	3.9	55.0	31.5	1.8
Cheese & Onion, KP*	1 Bag/34g	179	525	3.9	56.8	31.4	2.2
Cheese Toastie, KP*	1 Bag/34g	178	523	3.4	56.7	31.4	2.0
Minis, Original, KP*	1 Tub/140g	752	537	3.0	52.9	34.8	1.7
Original, KP*	1 Bag/33g	166	504	3.3	58.9	28.1	2.5
Salt & Vinegar, KP*	1 Bag/34g	169	497	3.7	58.4	27.4	2.5
Sizzling Bacon, KP*	1 Bag/34g	175	514	3.2	54.7	31.4	2.1
Totally Cheese Flavour Shoks, KP*	1 Bag/55g	285	519	3.8	54.5	31.8	2.1
HUNGER BREAKS, The Full Monty, Crosse & Blackwell*	½ Can/205g	287	140	8.0	16.3	4.8	4.8

H

ICE CREAM,

INFO/WEIGHT	Measure per Measure KCAL	KCAL	PROT	CARB	FAT	FIBRE
After Eight, Nestle*	1 Serving/55.1g	114	207	3.6	27.1	9.4	0.3
Baileys, Haagen-Dazs*	1oz/28g	73	260	4.5	22.2	17.1	0.0
Banana, Thorntons*	1oz/28g	63	225	4.0	23.8	12.6	0.0
Bananas Foster, Haagen-Dazs*	1 Serving/125ml	260	208	3.2	22.4	12.0	0.0
Banoffee Fudge, Sainsbury's*	1/8 Pot/67g	119	178	2.8	28.7	5.9	0.2
Banoffee, Criminally Creamy, Co-Op*	1oz/28g	66	235	3.0	26.0	13.0	0.1
Belgian Chocolate, Haagen-Dazs*	1oz/28g	89	318	4.6	28.4	20.7	0.0
Berry Nice, Ben & Jerry's*	1 Serving/100g	200	200	0.0	23.0	11.0	0.0
Blocks, Individual Portions, Fredericks Dairies Ltd*	1 Block/65ml	61	94	1.5	11.5	4.9	0.2
Bounty, Mars*	1oz/28g	77	274	3.3	23.8	18.3	0.0
Bournville, Cadbury's*	1 Bar/120g	258	215	3.5	26.0	11.6	0.0
Cappuccino, Thorntons*	1oz/28g	61	218	4.4	20.7	12.9	0.0
Caramel Craze, Organic, Tesco*	1 Serving/100g	253	253	3.3	25.5	15.3	0.0
Caramel, Cadbury's*	1 Serving/65.4ml	169	260	3.2	28.8	15.2	0.0
Caramel, Carte d'Or*	2 Boules/50g	106	212	2.6	30.8	8.7	0.0
Cherrylicious, Tesco*	1 Serving/57.7g	122	210	2.8	37.0	5.6	0.2
Chilli Red, Purbeck*	1 Serving/50g	99	198	4.8	18.7	11.5	0.0
Choc Chip Cookie Dough, Ben & Jerrys*	1 Serving/100g	230	230	3.0	23.0	14.0	0.0
Choc Chip, Cookie Dough, Haagen-Dazs*	1oz/28g	83	296	4.2	27.7	18.8	0.0
Choc Chip, Haagen-Dazs*	1oz/28g	80	286	4.7	24.8	18.7	0.0
Chocolate & Marshmallow, Swirl, BGTY, Sainsbury's*	1 Sm Scoop/40g	69	173	3.9	33.8	2.5	2.8
Chocolate Brownie With Walnuts, Haagen-Dazs*	1 Cup/101g	290	287	5.0	24.8	18.8	0.0
Chocolate Flavour, Soft Scoop, Sainsbury's*	1 Serving/70g	122	174	3.1	23.6	7.5	0.3
Chocolate Fudge Brownie, Ben & Jerry's*	1 Serving/100g	260	260	0.0	31.0	13.0	2.0
Chocolate Fudge Swirl, Haagen-Dazs*	1oz/28g	77	276	4.6	25.6	17.2	0.0
Chocolate Honeycomb, COU, Marks & Spencer*	1 Serving/100ml	150	150	3.5	31.5	2.6	0.7
Chocolate Honeycomb, Co-Op*	1/4 Pot/81g	186	230	4.0	26.0	13.0	0.3
Chocolate Midnight Cookies, Haagen-Dazs*	1oz/28g	81	289	4.9	28.7	17.2	0.0
Chocolate Orange, Deliciously Dairy, Co-Op*	1oz/28g	55	195	4.0	29.0	7.0	0.8
Chocolate Soft Scoop, Asda*	1 Scoop/47g	84	179	3.7	23.0	8.0	0.0
Chocolate, 98% Fat Free, Too Good, Wall's*	1 Spoonful/20ml	15	75	2.2	14.1	1.0	0.2
Chocolate, COU, Marks & Spencer*	1 Serving/140g	231	165	3.9	35.0	2.9	0.8
Chocolate, Dairy, The Best, Safeway*	1 Serving/82.4g	243	296	4.6	28.1	18.3	2.0
Chocolate, Easy Serve, Co-Op*	1oz/28g	46	165	3.0	22.0	7.0	0.3
Chocolate, On Stick, Green & Black's*	1 Stick/100g	214	214	3.7	19.3	13.6	2.1
Chocolate, Organic, Green & Black's*	1 Serving/20g	35	176	3.5	18.6	9.8	1.3
Chocolate, Organic, Iceland*	1oz/28g	58	208	4.9	28.6	8.2	0.0
Chocolate, Organic, Marks & Spencer*	1oz/28g	71	255	5.0	24.0	16.0	1.5
Chocolate, Thorntons*	1oz/28g	67	238	4.6	25.1	12.9	0.0
Chocolate, Weight Watchers*	1 Serving/100ml	92	92	1.8	15.2	2.5	0.5
Chocolatino, Tesco*	1 Serving/100g	243	243	4.4	32.2	10.8	0.6
Chunky Chocolate, Giant, Marks & Spencer*	1 Lolly/89.6g	302	335	4.0	28.0	23.0	2.3
Chunky Monkey, Ben & Jerry's*	1 Serving/100g	280	280	4.0	28.0	17.0	1.0
Coconut, Carte D'or*	1 Serving/100ml	125	125	1.8	14.0	7.1	0.5
Coffee, Finest, Tesco*	1/4 Pot/93g	236	254	4.9	22.5	16.0	0.0
Coffee, Waitrose*	1 Serving/180ml	256	142	3.2	13.2	8.5	0.0
Cookies & Cream, Haagen-Dazs*	1oz/28g	73	262	4.6	22.6	17.0	0.0
Cornish Clotted, Marks & Spencer*	1 Pot/90g	207	230	2.8	21.8	14.5	0.1
Cornish Style, Co-Op*	1oz/28g	53	190	4.0	23.0	9.0	0.1
Cornish Vanilla, Organic, Iceland*	1oz/28g	60	214	4.1	21.4	12.4	0.0
Cornish Vanilla, Soft Scoop, Marks & Spencer*	1oz/28g	56	199	3.9	21.8	10.7	0.2
Cream of Cornish Vanilla, Wall's*	1 Serving/111ml	100	90	1.7	11.0	4.3	0.1
Dairy Cornish, Tesco*	1 Serving/49g	112	228	3.2	24.7	12.3	0.1

ICE CREAM,

	INFO/WEIGHT	KCAL	KCAL	PROT	CARB	FAT	FIBRE
Dairy Milk, Cadbury's*	1 Stick/120ml	286	238	3.5	25.9	14.0	0.0
Dairy Milk, Orange, Cadbury's*	1 Serving/120ml	259	216	3.5	26.0	11.6	0.0
Dairy, Flavoured	1oz/28g	50	179	3.5	24.7	8.0	0.0
Dairy, Pizza Hut*	1 Portion/141.7g	273	192	4.6	23.3	8.9	0.2
Dairy, Vanilla	1oz/28g	54	194	3.6	24.4	9.8	0.0
Dark Toffee, Organic, Green & Black's*	¼ Pot/125ml	193	154	2.8	18.1	7.9	0.1
Demon Chocolate, Marks & Spencer*	1 Serving/79g	208	263	3.7	37.1	11.1	0.6
Double Chocolate, Nestle*	1 Serving/77.5g	250	320	4.8	33.7	18.4	0.0
Dream, Cadbury's*	1 Bar/120ml	264	220	3.6	26.0	11.9	0.0
Dulce De Leche, Bar, Haagan-Daaz*	1 Bar/105g	370	352	3.8	32.3	22.9	0.0
Galaxy, Mars*	1 Bar/60ml	203	339	4.7	29.7	22.4	0.0
Get Fruit, Tropical, Solero*	1 Serving/125ml	163	130	1.6	20.6	4.4	0.4
Heavenly Vanilla, Cadbury's*	1 Serving/250ml	355	142	2.5	12.8	9.3	0.0
Honey, I'm Home, Ben & Jerry's*	1 Serving/100g	260	260	0.0	28.0	15.0	0.0
Honeycomb Harvest, Mackies*	1 Serving/100g	209	209	4.0	25.0	10.0	0.0
Lemon & White Chocolate, Crackpots, Iceland*	1 Serving/100g	202	202	1.7	29.9	8.4	0.3
Lemon Curd Swirl, Duchy Originals*	¼ Pot/101g	247	245	3.7	25.8	14.1	0.0
Lemon Pie, Haagan-Dazs*	1oz/28g	73	262	3.9	24.5	16.3	0.0
Less Than 5% Fat, Asda*	2 Scoops/80g	111	139	2.7	22.0	4.5	0.0
Light Chocolate Ices, Co-Op*	1 Ice/62g	121	195	2.0	18.0	13.0	0.5
Luscious Mint Choc Chip, Morrisons*	1 Serving/50g	99	198	2.9	23.1	10.5	0.7
Magic Maple, Marks & Spencer*	1 Ice Cream/93g	259	278	2.9	39.0	12.3	0.6
Magnum Moments, Wall's*	1 Serving/18ml	58	323	4.0	30.0	20.8	0.0
Mango, 98% Fat Free, Bulla*	1 Serving/70g	94	134	4.2	25.4	1.6	0.0
Maple & Walnut, American, Sainsbury's*	1/8 Pot/68g	121	179	3.1	25.6	7.2	0.2
Maple Brazil, Thorntons*	1oz/28g	66	236	4.1	24.4	13.6	0.0
Mars, Mars*	1 Bar/75g	260	346	5.1	37.2	19.7	0.0
Mince Pie, Finest, Tesco*	¼ Pack/187.5g	478	254	3.9	33.0	11.8	1.1
Mint & Chocolate, Sainsbury's*	1 Serving/80g	154	192	3.4	23.5	9.4	0.4
Mint Choc Chip Soft Scoop, Asda*	1 Serving/46g	86	187	2.9	24.0	9.0	0.3
Mint Choc Chip, Organic, Iceland*	1oz/28g	55	197	4.7	25.8	8.3	0.0
Mint Crisp, Nestle*	1 Serving/75ml	232	309	2.9	25.5	21.9	0.9
Mint Ripple, Good Choice, Iceland*	1 Scoop/50g	59	117	3.0	21.7	2.1	0.1
Mint, Majestic Luxury, Iceland*	1 Serving/79.8g	270	337	3.8	39.3	18.3	1.3
Mint, Thorntons*	1oz/28g	66	237	4.0	25.0	13.4	0.0
Mocha Coffee Indulgence, Sainsbury's*	¼ Pot/82g	178	217	3.2	22.1	12.9	0.1
Monster Mint, Sainsbury's*	1/8 Pot/67g	121	180	3.0	26.3	6.9	0.3
Muddy Pigs, Wall's*	1 Serving/150ml	150	100	1.7	12.1	4.9	0.3
Neapolitan Brick, Co-Op*	1oz/28g	43	155	3.0	20.0	7.0	0.2
Neapolitan Easy Serve, Co-Op*	1oz/28g	42	150	3.0	20.0	7.0	0.2
Neapolitan, Iceland*	1oz/28g	46	164	3.0	21.3	7.4	0.0
Neapolitan, Lidl*	1 Serving/48g	108	226	4.3	29.5	10.0	0.0
Neapolitan, Organic, Iceland*	1oz/28g	55	196	4.2	26.4	8.2	0.0
Neapolitan, Soft Scoop, Asda*	1 Scoop/47g	83	176	3.1	23.0	8.0	0.0
Neapolitan, Soft Scoop, Marks & Spencer*	1 Scoop/65g	120	185	3.8	23.9	8.2	0.1
Neapolitan, Soft Scoop, Sainsbury's*	1 Serving/75g	124	165	2.8	22.8	6.9	0.2
Non-Dairy, Mixes	1oz/28g	51	182	4.1	25.1	7.9	0.0
Non-Dairy, Reduced Calorie	1oz/28g	33	119	3.4	13.7	6.0	0.0
Non-Dairy, Vanilla	1oz/28g	50	178	3.2	23.1	8.7	0.0
Peach Melba, Soft Scoop, Marks & Spencer*	1oz/28g	46	165	2.8	21.4	7.6	0.3
Picnic, Cadbury's*	1 Cone/125ml	258	207	3.4	28.9	9.4	0.3
Praline & Chocolate, Thorntons*	1oz/28g	87	309	4.6	21.3	22.9	0.6
Praline, Green & Black's*	1 Sm Pot/100g	191	191	3.5	20.0	10.8	0.9

ICE CREAM,	INFO/WEIGHT	KCAL	KCAL	PROT	CARB	FAT	FIBRE
Pralines & Cream, Haagen-Dazs*	1oz/28g	77	276	4.2	26.2	17.2	0.0
Rage Chocolate With Caramel Sauce, Treats*	1 Ice Cream/60g	177	295	3.3	30.9	17.5	0.0
Raspberries, Clotted Cream, Waitrose*	1 Tub/500ml	790	158	2.9	18.9	7.9	0.1
Raspberry & Shortcake, Co-Op*	1oz/28g	64	230	3.0	23.0	14.0	0.3
Raspberry Pavlova, Sainsbury's*	1 Serving/100g	202	202	2.7	26.6	9.4	3.3
Raspberry Ripple Brick, Tesco*	1 Serving/48g	71	148	2.6	20.8	6.0	0.2
Raspberry Ripple, Co-Op*	1oz/28g	45	160	3.0	23.0	7.0	0.2
Raspberry Ripple, Organic, Iceland*	1oz/28g	50	180	4.8	22.6	7.8	0.0
Raspberry Ripple, Soft Scoop, Asda*	1 Scoop/46g	75	164	2.5	25.0	6.0	0.0
Raspberry Ripple, Soft Scoop, Tesco*	2 Scoops/50g	79	157	2.5	23.0	6.1	0.2
Raspberry, Easy Serve, Co-Op*	1oz/28g	43	152	2.5	22.3	5.9	0.0
Really Creamy After Dinner Mint, Asda*	1 Serving/100g	191	191	3.4	24.0	9.0	0.4
Really Creamy Chocolate, Asda*	1 Serving/100g	227	227	4.1	28.0	11.0	0.4
Really Creamy Lemon Meringue, Asda*	1 Serving/100ml	100	100	1.8	12.0	5.0	0.1
Really Creamy Toffee, Asda*	1 Serving/120ml	146	122	1.8	17.5	5.0	0.1
Rocky Road, Sainsbury's*	1/8 Pot/67g	137	205	3.8	30.9	7.3	1.0
Rolo, Nestle*	½ Tub/500ml	1180	236	3.4	31.9	10.5	0.2
Rum & Raisin, Organic, Iceland*	1oz/28g	55	195	4.5	28.1	7.2	0.0
Screwball, Asda*	1 Screwball/60g	122	203	3.3	25.0	10.0	1.5
Screwball, Co-Op*	1 Lolly/95g	190	200	2.0	31.0	7.0	0.0
Screwball, Farmfoods*	1 Lolly/72ml	101	177	3.3	27.1	6.1	0.0
Screwball, Morrisons*	1 Screwball/100ml	133	133	2.0	17.0	6.3	0.0
Screwball, Richmond*	1 Screwball/59g	94	160	2.4	25.0	5.7	0.2
Screwball, Safeway*	1 Serving/65g	129	198	3.1	24.5	9.7	0.6
Screwball, Tesco*	1 Screwball/61g	116	190	2.9	25.2	8.6	0.3
Smarties, Nestle*	1 Serving/50g	125	250	3.6	32.3	11.9	0.2
Stem Ginger With Belgian Chocolate, Waitrose*	1 Lolly/109g	255	232	2.9	25.5	13.1	1.7
Sticky Toffee, Cream o' Galloway*	1 Serving/30g	80	266	4.7	28.7	14.7	0.0
Strawberries & Cream, Deliciously Dairy, Co-Op*	1oz/28g	46	165	3.0	24.0	6.0	0.3
Strawberry & Cream, Mivvi, Nestle*	1 Serving/60g	118	196	2.6	29.4	7.6	0.2
Strawberry & Cream, Organic, Sainsbury's*	1 Serving/100g	193	193	3.6	22.6	9.8	0.4
Strawberry Cheesecake, Co-Op*	1/6 Pot/86g	163	190	3.0	29.0	7.0	0.2
Strawberry Cheesecake, Haagen-Dazs*	1oz/28g	74	266	3.9	26.5	16.1	0.0
Strawberry, Fromage Frais, Asda*	1 Pot/46g	87	190	3.7	28.0	7.0	0.3
Strawberry, Get Fruit, Solero*	1 Serving/100ml	120	120	1.5	18.8	4.5	1.3
Strawberry, Haagen-Dazs*	1oz/28g	67	241	4.0	21.5	15.5	0.0
Strawberry, Majestic, Luxury, Iceland*	1 Lolly/100g	281	281	2.7	25.8	18.6	0.1
Strawberry, Thorntons*	1oz/28g	52	185	3.2	22.5	9.3	0.1
Strawberry, Weight Watchers*	1 Pot/57g	81	142	2.5	23.4	3.9	0.2
Tantilising Toffee, COU, Marks & Spencer*	¼ Pot/125ml	125	100	0.6	18.0	2.8	0.0
The Full Vermonty, Ben & Jerry's*	1 Serving/100g	280	280	0.0	27.0	18.0	1.0
Toffee & Biscuit, Weight Watchers*	1 Pot/100ml	93	93	1.5	14.9	2.7	0.1
Toffee & Vanilla, Sainsbury's*	1 Serving/71g	146	205	3.1	26.7	9.5	0.1
Toffee Creme, Haagen-Dazs*	1oz/28g	74	265	4.5	26.7	15.6	0.0
Toffee Fudge, Soft Scoop, Asda*	1 Serving/50g	93	185	2.6	28.0	7.0	0.0
Toffee Ripple, Tesco*	1 Serving/100g	173	173	2.7	24.4	7.2	0.1
Toffee, Deliciously Dairy, Co-Op*	1oz/28g	45	160	3.0	21.0	7.0	0.2
Toffee, Somerfield*	1 Serving/75g	172	229	3.4	33.2	9.2	0.9
Toffee, Thorntons*	1oz/28g	61	218	4.1	24.5	11.6	0.0
Toffee, Too Good To Be True, Wall's*	1fl oz/30ml	23	75	2.2	14.9	0.4	0.1
Totally Toffee, Safeway*	1 Serving/100ml	136	136	1.3	21.1	5.1	0.1
Traditional Cornish Blackberry, Marks & Spencer*	1oz/28g	61	218	2.3	28.0	10.8	0.3
Traditional Cornish Strawberry, Marks & Spencer*	1oz/28g	64	229	2.3	29.7	11.2	0.2

ICE CREAM,

	INFO/WEIGHT	KCAL	KCAL	PROT	CARB	FAT	FIBRE
Traditional, Mackie's*	1 Serving/100ml	196	196	4.1	17.9	11.8	0.0
Triple Chocolate, Safeway*	1 Serving/100g	235	235	3.8	30.0	10.8	0.0
Tropical Fruit Sorbet, Waitrose*	1 Lolly/109.8g	90	82	1.5	14.5	2.0	0.2
Vanilla & Chocolate Swirl, Safeway*	1 Serving/125g	250	200	3.3	26.2	9.1	0.1
Vanilla & Cinnamon, Finest, Tesco*	1 Serving/50g	115	229	3.9	20.2	14.7	0.4
Vanilla & Cinnamon, Spar*	1 Serving/120g	247	206	3.8	28.0	8.6	0.0
Vanilla & Strawberry Swirl, Safeway*	1 Serving/125g	238	190	2.9	27.0	7.5	0.2
Vanilla Bean, Purbeck*	1 Serving/100g	198	198	4.8	18.7	11.5	0.0
Vanilla Brick, Co-Op*	1oz/28g	45	160	3.0	21.0	7.0	0.2
Vanilla Caramel Fudge, Ben & Jerry's*	1 Serving/100g	260	260	4.0	28.0	14.0	0.0
Vanilla Choc Fudge, Haagen-Dazs*	1oz/28g	75	267	4.3	23.5	17.2	0.0
Vanilla Choc Fudge, Tofutti*	1 Tub/500ml	825	165	1.6	20.0	9.0	0.4
Vanilla Dairy, Finest, Tesco*	1 Serving/92g	227	247	4.5	18.0	17.4	0.3
Vanilla Flavour, Budgens*	1oz/28g	45	159	3.0	21.7	6.7	0.1
Vanilla Flavour, Soft Scoop, Sainsbury's*	1 Serving/70g	111	159	3.0	21.7	6.7	0.1
Vanilla With Strawberry Swirl, Mini Tub, Weight Watchers*	1 Mini Tub/57.0g	81	142	2.5	23.4	3.9	0.2
Vanilla, COU, Marks & Spencer*	¼ Pot/79g	111	140	1.7	25.9	2.8	0.8
Vanilla, Carte D'Or*	1 Serving/100ml	110	110	1.6	15.0	4.9	0.2
Vanilla, Criminally Creamy, Co-Op*	1oz/28g	60	215	3.0	18.0	15.0	0.1
Vanilla, Dairy Milk, Cadbury's*	1 Ice/119g	259	216	3.5	26.0	11.6	0.1
Vanilla, Dairy, Organic, Yeo Valley*	1 Serving/100g	206	206	4.9	21.3	11.2	0.0
Vanilla, Deliciously Dairy, Co-Op*	1oz/28g	49	175	3.0	23.0	8.0	0.2
Vanilla, Easy Serve, Co-Op*	1oz/28g	39	140	3.0	18.0	7.0	0.2
Vanilla, Everyday, Co-Op*	1oz/28g	41	145	3.0	18.0	7.0	0.2
Vanilla, Haagen-Dazs*	1oz/28g	70	250	4.5	19.7	17.1	0.0
Vanilla, Light Soft Scoop, 25% Less Fat, Morrisons*	1 Scoop/50g	75	150	2.9	23.2	5.0	0.2
Vanilla, Low Fat, Weight Watchers*	1 Scoop/125ml	75	60	1.1	9.7	1.7	0.1
Vanilla, Organic, Green & Black's*	1 Sm Tub/100ml	164	164	3.5	15.2	9.8	0.1
Vanilla, Organic, Iceland*	1oz/28g	61	217	4.5	22.2	12.2	0.0
Vanilla, Organic, Sainsbury's*	1 Serving/85g	176	207	4.3	20.5	12.0	0.1
Vanilla, Organic, Tesco*	1 Serving/100g	237	237	3.7	16.8	17.2	0.0
Vanilla, Organic, Waitrose*	1 Serving/125g	178	142	2.7	12.4	9.0	0.0
Vanilla, Pizza Express*	1 Serving/100g	119	119	0.9	13.8	6.8	0.0
Vanilla, Really Creamy, Asda*	1 Serving/50g	98	196	3.5	23.0	10.0	0.1
Vanilla, SmartPrice, Asda*	1 Scoop/40g	55	137	2.8	19.0	6.0	0.2
Vanilla, Soft Scoop, 25% Less Fat, Asda*	1oz/28g	42	149	2.9	23.0	5.0	0.0
Vanilla, Soft Scoop, BGTY, Sainsbury's*	1 Serving/75g	104	139	2.7	21.6	4.6	0.2
Vanilla, Soft Scoop, Light, 94% Fat Free, Wall's*	1 Serving/100ml	80	80	1.4	12.4	2.9	0.1
Vanilla, Soft Scoop, Marks & Spencer*	1 Scoop/125ml	225	180	2.9	23.8	8.1	0.1
Vanilla, Soft Scoop, Tesco*	1oz/28g	39	138	2.7	21.6	4.5	0.2
Vanilla, Soft, Non Milk Fat, Waitrose*	1 Serving/125ml	78	62	1.3	8.0	2.7	0.1
Vanilla, Soft-Scoop, Wall's*	2 Scoops/100ml	90	90	1.4	11.2	4.4	0.1
Vanilla, Thorntons*	1oz/28g	63	225	4.9	20.5	13.6	0.0
Vanilla, Too Good to be True, Walls*	1 Serving/50ml	35	70	2.0	14.9	0.4	0.1
Vanilla, Value, Tesco*	1 Serving/56g	75	134	2.7	18.3	5.5	0.2
Vanilla, Wth Vanilla Pods, Sainsbury's*	1 Serving/100g	195	195	3.5	22.5	10.1	0.1
Viennetta, Biscuit Caramel, Walls*	1/6 Serving/58g	183	315	3.3	27.8	20.9	0.0
Viennetta, Cappuccino, Wall's*	1 Serving/75g	191	255	3.5	22.0	17.0	0.0
Viennetta, Chocolate, Wall's*	¼ Pot/80g	200	250	4.1	24.0	15.2	0.0
Viennetta, Forest Fruit, Wall's*	1 Serving/98g	265	270	3.4	27.2	16.2	0.0
Viennetta, Mint, Wall's*	1 Serving/80g	204	255	3.4	23.0	16.6	0.0
Viennetta, Selection Brownie, Wall's*	1 Serving/70g	194	277	4.2	28.5	16.2	0.0
Viennetta, Strawberry Cheesecake Biscuit, Wall's*	1 Serving/100g	305	305	3.5	28.1	20.7	0.0

	Measure INFO/WEIGHT	per Measure KCAL	Nutrition Values per 100g / 100ml				
			KCAL	PROT	CARB	FAT	FIBRE
ICE CREAM,							
Viennetta, Strawberry, Walls*	1 Serving/80g	204	255	3.4	22.1	16.8	0.0
Viennetta, Vanilla, Wall's*	¼ Bar/80gg	204	255	3.3	23.0	16.7	0.0
Virtuous Vanilla & Strawberry, Weight Watchers*	1 Serving/100ml	81	81	1.4	13.3	2.2	0.1
Voluptuous Vanilla, COU, Marks & Spencer*	¼ Pot/125ml	175	140	1.7	25.9	2.8	0.8
White Vanilla Flavour, Soft Scoop, Sainsbury's*	1oz/28g	38	136	2.9	18.8	5.5	0.2
White Vanilla, Soft Scoop, Tesco*	1oz/28g	46	164	3.1	21.8	7.1	0.1
With Cherry Sauce, Tesco*	1 Serving/57.7g	122	210	2.8	37.0	5.6	0.2
Zesty Lemon Meringue, COU, Marks & Spencer*	¼ Pot/73g	120	165	2.6	33.0	2.5	0.5
ICE CREAM BAR,							
Bailey's, Haagen-Dazs*	1oz/28g	86	307	4.1	24.8	21.2	0.0
Caramel, Cadbury's*	1 Bar/64g	188	294	3.7	32.4	16.6	0.0
Choc Chip, Haagen-Dazs*	1oz/28g	90	320	4.3	27.4	21.5	0.0
Chocolate Covered	1oz/28g	90	320	5.0	24.0	23.3	0.0
Chunky Chocolate, Co-Op*	1 Bar/60g	204	340	5.0	35.0	20.0	1.0
Chunky Toffee, Co-Op*	1 Bar/60g	204	340	4.0	34.0	21.0	1.0
Deam, Cadbury's*	1 Serving/118g	260	220	3.6	26.0	11.9	0.0
Feast, Wall's*	1 Bar/60g	190	317	3.3	24.7	22.8	0.0
Peanut, Farmfoods*	1 Bar/60ml	187	360	5.3	36.6	21.4	1.2
Racer, Aldi*	1 Bar/59g	194	328	6.0	34.2	18.6	0.0
Toffee Cream, Haagen-Dazs*	1oz/28g	97	346	4.1	32.2	22.3	0.0
ICE CREAM CONE,							
Average	1 Cone/75g	140	186	3.5	25.5	8.5	0.0
Blackcurrant, GFY, Asda*	1 Cone/67.2g	161	241	3.0	37.0	9.0	0.1
Carousel Wafer Company*	1 Cone/2g	7	342	12.6	65.0	3.7	0.0
Choc 'n' Nut, Farmfoods*	1 Cone/120ml	183	278	5.0	33.0	14.0	1.0
Chocolate & Nut, Co-Op*	1 Cone/110g	307	279	3.9	31.0	15.5	0.6
Chocolate & Vanilla, Good Choice, Iceland*	1 Cone/110ml	161	146	2.7	22.9	6.5	0.8
Chocolate & Vanilla, Marks & Spencer*	1oz/28g	83	295	4.2	31.8	17.0	0.7
Chocolate Flavour, Somerfield*	1 Cone/110ml	329	299	4.0	38.0	15.0	0.0
Chocolate, Marks & Spencer*	1oz/28g	94	335	4.0	28.0	23.0	2.3
Chocolate, Vanilla & Hazelnut, Sainsbury's*	1 Cone/62g	190	306	4.5	33.9	16.9	0.6
Cone, Haagen-Dazs*	1oz/28g	85	303	4.7	25.5	20.3	0.0
Cornetto, GFY, Asda*	1 Cone/67.2g	161	241	3.0	37.0	9.0	0.1
Cornetto, Wall's*	1 Cone/75g	195	260	3.7	34.5	12.9	0.0
Creme Egg, Cadbury's*	1 Cone/115ml	270	235	2.9	29.3	11.6	0.0
Extreme Raspberry, Cornetto, Nestle*	1 Cornetto/88g	220	250	2.5	36.0	10.0	0.2
Flake 99, Cadbury's*	1 Cone/125ml	204	163	2.4	19.6	8.8	0.0
McDonald's*	1 Cone/98g	157	160	4.5	24.4	5.0	0.0
Mini, Tesco*	1 Cone/48g	152	316	4.1	31.5	19.3	0.8
Mint Choc Chip, Iceland*	1 Cone/72g	210	292	3.3	40.4	13.0	1.0
Sticky Toffee, Farmfoods*	1 Cone/120ml	177	272	3.2	36.0	12.8	2.0
Strawberry & Vanilla, Asda*	1 Cone/115ml	193	168	1.8	22.6	7.8	0.1
Strawberry & Vanilla, Farmfoods*	1 Cone/120ml	170	257	3.0	32.0	13.0	2.0
Strawberry & Vanilla, Iceland*	1 Serving/70g	182	260	3.3	37.5	10.8	0.7
Strawberry & Vanilla, Marks & Spencer*	1oz/28g	81	290	4.2	30.9	16.5	0.7
Strawberry & Vanilla, Sainsbury's*	1 Cone/62g	153	247	2.8	36.5	10.0	0.3
Strawberry & Vanilla, Tesco*	1 Cone/70g	194	277	3.0	35.9	13.5	0.3
Strawberry, BGTY, Sainsbury's*	1 Cone/69g	151	219	2.6	37.5	6.5	1.3
Strawberry, Co-Op*	1 Cone/110g	283	257	3.5	33.6	12.1	0.5
Strawberry, Marks & Spencer*	1oz/28g	74	263	3.5	31.1	14.0	0.4
Strawberry, Somerfield*	1 Cone/110g	299	272	3.0	40.0	11.0	0.0
Toffee Flavoured, Somerfield*	1 Cone/110ml	320	291	4.0	39.0	14.0	0.0
Tropical, GFY, Asda*	1 Cone/100g	135	135	2.6	20.0	5.0	0.3

INFO/WEIGHT	Measure per Measure KCAL		Nutrition Values per 100g / 100ml				
			KCAL	PROT	CARB	FAT	FIBRE
ICE CREAM CONE,							
With Flake, McDonald's*	1 Cone/107g	204	191	4.8	27.0	7.2	0.0
ICE CREAM ROLL,							
Artic	1 Portion/70g	140	200	4.1	33.3	6.6	0.0
Basics, Somerfield*	1/6 Roll/110ml	233	212	4.0	35.0	6.0	0.0
Marks & Spencer*	1oz/28g	60	215	3.6	35.2	6.7	0.0
Mini, Cadbury's*	1 Roll/45ml	99	220	3.4	24.3	13.1	0.0
Tesco*	¼ Roll/57g	131	230	3.7	34.5	8.6	0.4
ICE LOLLY,							
Assorted, Farmfoods*	1 Lolly/56ml	35	62	0.0	15.6	0.0	0.0
Assorted, Iceland*	1 Lolly/51g	33	65	0.0	16.2	0.0	0.0
Assorted, Safeway*	1 Lolly/31ml	26	85	0.0	20.9	0.0	0.1
Baby, Tesco*	1 Lolly/32.4g	26	80	0.1	20.0	0.0	0.1
Banana, Whole Milk & Fruit, Mini, BPC, Sainsbury's*	1 Lolly/30ml	34	113	2.7	18.0	3.3	0.0
Blackcurrant Split, Iceland*	1 Lolly/75g	61	81	1.1	12.0	3.2	0.1
Blackcurrant, Dairy Split, Sainsbury's*	1 Lolly/72.7ml	88	121	1.8	20.4	3.6	0.1
Blackcurrant, Real Fruit Juice, Sainsbury's*	1 Lolly/73ml	67	92	0.2	22.8	0.1	0.1
Blackcurrant, Ribena*	1 Lolly/52ml	41	79	0.0	19.2	0.0	0.0
Choc & Almond, Mini, Tesco*	1 Lolly/31g	103	331	4.4	24.8	23.8	0.9
Choc Lime Split, Morrisons*	1 Lolly/73ml	120	164	1.6	20.4	8.4	0.1
Chocolate, Plain, Mini, Tesco*	1 Lolly/31g	94	304	3.1	24.8	21.4	1.2
Chocolate, Pooh Stick, Nestle*	1 Lolly/40g	36	89	2.1	12.9	3.6	0.0
Cider Refresher, Treats*	1 Lolly/70ml	54	77	0.0	19.2	0.0	0.0
Cola Lickers, Farmfoods*	1 Lolly/56ml	37	68	0.0	17.0	0.0	0.0
Elderflower,Tubes, Frozen, Marks & Spencer*	1oz/28g	23	82	0.1	20.5	0.1	0.2
Exotic Fruit, Tesco*	1 Lolly/31.5g	41	131	1.8	26.4	2.0	0.6
Exotic Split, Bars, Marks & Spencer*	1oz/28g	36	127	2.5	25.0	1.9	0.4
Fab, Nestle*	1 Lolly/57g	82	144	0.8	23.7	4.9	0.0
Feast, Chocolate, Mini, Wall's*	1 Lolly/62.9g	195	310	3.4	23.9	21.9	0.0
Frenzy, Farmfoods*	1 Lolly/92ml	235	255	3.1	23.1	16.8	0.6
Fruit Assorted, Basics, Somerfield*	1 Lolly/56ml	32	58	0.0	15.0	0.0	0.0
Fruit Fusion, Mini, Farmfoods*	1 Lolly/45ml	36	79	0.2	19.2	0.1	0.2
Fruit Ices, Made With Orange Juice, Del Monte*	1 Lolly/75ml	79	105	0.5	25.7	0.0	0.0
Fruit Luxury, Mini, Co-Op*	1 Lolly/45g	59	130	2.0	18.0	6.0	0.2
Fruit Split, Asda*	1 Lolly/73.9g	85	115	1.7	19.0	3.6	0.0
Fruit Split, Assorted, Co-Op*	1 Lolly/73g	80	110	1.0	20.0	3.0	0.1
Fruit Split, Better For You, Morrisons*	1 Lolly/72.5g	50	69	1.6	13.9	0.7	0.1
Fruit Splits Assorted, Somerfield*	1 Split/73ml	74	102	0.0	18.0	3.0	0.0
Fruit Splits, Treats*	1 Lolly/75ml	77	103	1.4	17.6	4.1	0.0
Fruit, Assorted, Waitrose*	1 Lolly/73g	59	81	0.0	20.0	0.0	0.1
Fruit, Red, Tesco*	1 Lolly/31.5g	40	128	1.8	25.6	2.0	0.6
Fruity n Freezy, Asda*	1 Lolly/30ml	24	80	0.1	20.0	0.0	0.0
Fruity, Ice Cream, Morrisons*	1 Lolly/73ml	50	69	1.6	13.9	0.7	0.1
Lemon & Lime, Rocket Split, De Roma*	1 Lolly/60ml	65	108	1.0	16.0	4.3	0.2
Lemon & Lime, Mini Bar, Marks & Spencer*	1 Lolly/50g	48	95	0.1	23.6	0.1	0.2
Lemon & Lime, Tubes, Frozen, Marks & Spencer*	1oz/28g	27	95	0.1	23.6	0.1	0.2
Lemonade & Cola, Morrisons*	1 Lolly/55ml	36	65	0.0	16.2	0.0	0.0
Mango & Passion Fruit, TTD, Sainsbury's*	1 Lolly/73ml	76	104	0.2	25.5	0.1	0.6
Mega Truffle, Nestle*	1 Lolly/71.1g	217	305	3.2	28.0	20.1	0.8
Milk Chocolate & Crisped Wheat, Co-Op*	1 Lolly/110g	259	235	3.0	28.0	12.0	0.7
Milk Flavour, Farmfoods*	1 Lolly/50ml	91	182	2.8	20.1	10.1	0.1
Milk, Whole Milk & Fruit, Mini, BPC, Sainsbury's*	1 Lolly/30ml	32	107	3.0	16.7	3.7	0.0
Milky Bar, Nestle*	1 Lolly/45.1g	156	346	4.3	33.2	21.8	0.1
Orange & Lemon Splits, Farmfoods*	1 Lolly/56ml	56	124	1.6	19.8	4.3	0.2

I

ICE LOLLY,	Measure INFO/WEIGHT	per Measure KCAL	Nutrition Values per 100g / 100ml				
			KCAL	PROT	CARB	FAT	FIBRE
Orange Juice, Asda*	1 Lolly/70g	58	83	0.7	20.0	0.0	0.0
Orange Juice, Bar, Marks & Spencer*	1 Lolly/75g	65	86	0.5	21.0	0.0	0.1
Orange Juice, Co-Op*	1 Lolly/73g	51	70	0.4	17.0	0.1	0.1
Orange Juice, Fresh, Eat Smart, Safeway*	1 Lolly/107.1g	75	70	0.4	16.6	0.0	0.1
Orange Juice, Freshly Squeezed, Finest,Tesco*	1 Lolly/80ml	89	111	0.7	27.0	0.0	0.0
Orange Juice, Milfina*	1 Lolly/79.3g	69	87	0.5	23.3	0.0	0.0
Orange Juice, Safeway*	1 Lolly/73ml	62	85	0.7	20.4	0.1	0.0
Orange Juice, Tropicana*	1 Lolly/50g	43	85	0.5	20.7	0.0	0.0
Orange Maid, Nestle*	1 Lolly/73ml	66	91	0.5	21.6	0.0	0.0
Orange, Lidl*	1 Lolly/50g	50	100	0.5	24.4	0.1	0.0
Orange, Real Fruit Juice, Sainsbury's*	1 Lolly/73ml	49	67	0.2	16.5	0.1	0.1
Orange, Real Juice, Sainsbury's*	1 Lolly/72ml	63	88	0.7	21.0	0.1	0.1
Orange, Real Juice, Tesco*	1 Lolly/32g	25	78	0.6	18.7	0.0	0.3
Orange, Tesco*	1 Lolly/77.4g	52	68	0.2	16.8	0.0	0.3
Orange, Water, Iceland*	1 Lolly/75g	74	98	0.2	24.4	0.0	0.2
Pineapple Split, Iceland*	1 Lolly/75g	89	118	1.4	18.5	4.6	0.1
Pineapple, Dairy Split, Sainsbury's*	1 Lolly/72.4ml	84	116	1.8	19.0	3.6	0.1
Pineapple, Real Fruit Juice, Sainsbury's*	1 Lolly/73ml	55	76	0.1	19.0	0.1	0.1
Polar Snappers, Double, Farmfoods*	1 Lolly/60ml	40	66	0.0	16.5	0.0	0.0
Raspberry, Real Fruit Juice, Sainsbury's*	1 Lolly/72g	62	86	0.3	21.0	0.1	0.1
Raspberry, Rocket Split, De Roma*	1 Lolly/60ml	65	108	1.0	16.2	4.3	0.2
Real Fruit Juice, Rocket, Blue Parrot Cafe, Sainsbury's*	1 Lolly/58ml	45	77	0.2	19.1	0.0	0.1
Real Fruit, Dairy Split, Sainsbury's*	1 Lolly/73ml	100	137	2.1	22.8	4.2	0.1
Real Orange, Kids, Tesco*	1 Lolly/31.5g	25	78	0.6	18.7	0.0	0.3
Refresher, Bassett's*	1 Lolly/40g	47	117	2.7	22.2	2.7	0.3
Rocket, Co-Op*	1 Lolly/60g	42	70	0.0	17.0	0.0	0.0
Rolo, Nestle*	1 Lolly/75ml	244	325	3.9	34.9	18.5	0.0
Strawberries 'n' Cream, Tropicana*	1 Lolly/50g	59	117	1.6	25.0	1.2	0.0
Strawberry & Banana, Smoothies, Sainsbury's*	1 Lolly/60g	100	166	1.5	28.0	5.3	0.2
Strawberry & Vanilla, 99% Fat Free, So-Lo, Iceland*	1 Lolly/92g	98	107	2.3	23.5	0.4	2.2
Strawberry Split, Co-Op*	1 Lolly/71ml	75	105	1.0	17.0	3.0	0.1
Strawberry, Dairy Split, Sainsbury's*	1 Lolly/72.9ml	86	118	1.7	19.8	3.6	0.1
Strawberry, Orange & Pineapple, Rocket, Iceland*	1 Lolly/47g	38	81	0.0	20.2	0.0	0.1
Strawberry, So-Lo, Good Choice, Iceland*	1 Lolly/66.4g	84	128	2.4	25.6	1.8	0.1
Strawberry, Whole Milk & Fruit, Mini, BPC, Sainsbury's*	1 Lolly/30ml	32	107	2.7	16.7	3.3	0.0
Traffic Light, Co-Op*	1 Lolly/52g	55	105	0.4	25.0	0.8	0.0
Tropical Fruit, Starburst, Mars*	1 Lolly/93ml	94	101	0.3	24.8	0.1	0.0
Twister, Wall's*	1 Lolly/80ml	76	95	0.6	18.4	1.9	0.0
Vanilla Cream, Covered in White Chocolate, Tesco*	1 Ice Cream/85g	258	303	3.2	29.6	19.1	0.8
Vanilla, Pooh Stick, Nestle*	1 Lolly/40g	34	86	1.9	12.9	3.5	0.0
Wonka Super Sour Tastic, Nestle*	1 Lolly/60ml	84	140	0.0	26.1	3.6	0.0
Zoom, Nestle*	1 Lolly/58.1ml	54	93	0.9	20.6	0.7	0.0
INDIAN BANQUET, For One, COU, Marks & Spencer*	1 Pack/500g	400	80	6.7	10.2	1.2	3.1
INDIAN DAAL, Sainsbury's*	1 Pack/300g	264	88	3.7	8.4	4.4	0.7
INDIAN MEAL							
For One, Good For You, Asda*	1 Serving/495g	644	130	8.0	14.0	4.7	1.0
For One, Healthy Eating, Tesco*	1 Pack/420g	437	104	7.4	14.0	2.1	1.4
INDIAN MENU,							
COU, Marks & Spencer*	1 Pack/550g	413	75	8.4	7.5	1.2	2.1
Meal For Two, Tesco*	1 Serving/537g	811	151	6.3	17.0	6.4	0.8
INDIAN SNACK SELECTION, Safeway*	1 Serving/170g	347	204	4.0	25.8	9.4	1.9
INDIAN TAKEAWAY, Ready Meals, Marks & Spencer*	1oz/28g	42	150	6.7	15.3	7.1	1.5

	Measure	per Measure	Nutrition Values per 100g / 100ml				
	INFO/WEIGHT	KCAL	KCAL	PROT	CARB	FAT	FIBRE
INSTANT WHIP,							
Chocolate Flavour, Bird's*	1oz/28g	109	390	3.8	80.5	5.9	0.7
Strawberry Flavour, Bird's*	1oz/28g	112	400	2.5	85.0	5.4	0.4
IRON BRU, Diet, Barr's*	1 Can/330ml	2	1	0.1	0.1	0.0	0.0

	Measure INFO/WEIGHT	per Measure KCAL	Nutrition Values per 100g / 100ml				
			KCAL	PROT	CARB	FAT	FIBRE
JALFREZI,							
Chicken & Rice, Healthy Eating, Tesco*	1 Pack/420g	483	115	7.9	17.5	1.6	0.3
Chicken With Basmati Rice, Eat Smart, Safeway*	1 Pack/400g	300	75	6.8	8.5	1.0	1.7
Chicken With Pilau Rice, BGTY, Sainsbury's*	1 Pack/450g	432	96	7.0	14.3	1.2	0.8
Chicken With Pilau Rice, GFY, Asda*	1 Pack/445.9g	495	111	8.0	14.0	2.5	1.2
Chicken With Pilau Rice, Patak's*	1 Pack/400g	556	139	9.8	14.7	4.6	0.9
Chicken With Pilau Rice, Perfectly Balanced, Waitrose*	1 Pack/400g	464	116	8.4	15.4	2.3	1.8
Chicken With Pilau Rice, Spar*	1 Pack/400g	472	118	6.7	12.0	4.8	1.2
Chicken With Rice, Sainsbury's*	1 Serving/200g	220	110	7.4	18.3	0.8	1.3
Chicken, Asda*	1 Pack/340g	415	122	10.0	7.0	6.0	1.6
Chicken, Marks & Spencer*	1 Pack/350g	385	110	10.8	4.2	5.7	2.0
Chicken, Medium, Good For You, Asda*	1 Pack/644g	972	151	6.0	22.0	4.3	0.9
Chicken, Sainsbury's*	1 Pack/400g	436	109	12.1	3.4	5.2	1.7
Chicken, Somerfield*	1 Pack/350g	340	97	11.2	2.6	4.6	1.2
Chicken, Tesco*	1 Pack/350g	459	131	11.9	3.8	7.6	1.2
Chicken, Waitrose*	½ Pack/200g	214	107	12.4	2.3	5.3	1.6
Chicken, With Rice, COU, Marks & Spencer*	1 Pack/400g	320	80	9.2	8.3	1.1	1.2
Pilau Rice, Ready Meals, Patak's*	1oz/28g	37	131	7.8	13.5	5.3	0.9
Vegetable, Co-Op*	1 Pack/400g	320	80	1.0	9.0	4.0	2.0
Vegetable, Eastern Indian, Sainsbury's*	1 Pack/400g	208	52	3.4	2.0	3.4	1.7
Vegetable, Take Away Menu For 1, BGTY, Sainsbury's*	1 Pack/148g	43	29	1.8	5.4	0.0	2.3
Vegetable, Waitrose*	1 Pack/400g	256	64	2.2	4.7	4.0	3.7
Vegetable, With Rice, Bird's Eye*	1 Pack/350g	354	101	2.5	20.2	1.1	1.0
JAM,							
Apricot & Peach, 25% Less Sugar, Asda*	1 Tsp/15g	28	184	0.5	45.4	0.1	1.1
Apricot, Baxters*	1 Tsp/15g	32	210	0.0	53.0	0.0	0.8
Apricot, Frank Cooper*	1 Tsp/15g	44	242	0.4	60.1	0.0	0.7
Apricot, Fruit, Asda*	1 Serving/20g	37	183	0.5	45.0	0.5	0.0
Apricot, Grandessa, Aldi*	1 Serving/25g	64	255	0.4	63.0	0.0	0.7
Apricot, Luxury, Baxters*	1 Tsp/15g	38	252	0.0	63.0	0.0	8.0
Apricot, Reduced Sugar, Sainsbury's*	1 Tsp/15g	29	190	0.4	47.0	0.1	0.8
Apricot, Robertsons*	1 Serving/30g	75	249	0.2	61.2	0.0	0.0
Apricot, Sainsbury's*	1 Tsp/15g	40	264	0.3	65.7	0.0	0.8
Apricot, Tesco*	Thin Spread/7g	19	265	0.3	65.0	0.0	0.7
Apricot, Thick, Rhapsodie de Fruit, St Dalfour*	1 Serving/20g	45	227	0.4	56.0	0.3	1.7
Black Cherry, Best, Hartley's*	1 Tsp/20g	49	244	0.4	60.6	0.5	0.0
Black Cherry, Rhapsodie de Fruit, St Dalfour*	2 Tsp/30g	69	230	0.7	56.0	0.3	1.2
Black Cherry, Wilkin & Sons Ltd*	1 Tsp/10g	27	268	0.0	67.0	0.0	0.0
Blackberry, Extra Special, Asda*	1 Tbsp/15.3g	29	190	0.9	45.0	0.7	0.0
Blackcurrant, 25% Less Sugar, Asda*	1 Tsp/15g	27	180	0.5	45.5	0.0	1.8
Blackcurrant, Baxters*	1 Tsp/15g	32	210	0.0	53.0	0.0	1.3
Blackcurrant, Better For You, Morrisons*	1 Serving/10g	20	196	0.6	46.4	0.4	0.0
Blackcurrant, Co-Op*	1 Heaped Tsp/18g	45	250	0.2	63.0	0.0	0.9
Blackcurrant, Diabetic, Stute*	1oz/28g	57	204	0.4	55.0	0.0	2.0
Blackcurrant, Extra, Morrisons*	1 Serving/20g	51	253	0.3	63.0	0.0	2.7
Blackcurrant, Frank Cooper*	1 Tsp/15g	36	243	0.3	60.6	0.0	1.1
Blackcurrant, Hartley's*	1 Serving/42.5g	106	252	0.2	62.8	0.0	0.0
Blackcurrant, Luxury, Baxters*	1 Tsp/15g	38	252	0.0	63.0	0.0	1.4
Blackcurrant, Reduced Sugar, Sainsbury's*	1 Tsp/15g	29	190	0.4	47.0	0.1	1.4
Blackcurrant, Robertson's*	1 Tsp/7g	17	246	0.3	60.5	0.0	0.0
Blackcurrant, Streamline*	1 Serving/20g	38	192	0.6	46.4	0.4	0.0
Blackcurrant, Tesco*	1 Tsp/15g	39	261	0.2	65.0	0.0	1.0
Blackcurrant, Weight Watchers*	1 Tsp/5.7g	6	106	0.2	26.3	0.0	0.9
Blueberry & Blackberry, Baxters*	1 Tsp/15g	38	252	0.0	63.0	0.0	1.2

JAM,

INFO/WEIGHT	per Measure KCAL	KCAL	PROT	CARB	FAT	FIBRE
Country Berries, Luxury, Baxters*	1 Tsp/15g	38	252	0.0	63.0	0.0	1.1
Damson, Extra Fruit, Best, Hartley's*	1 Tsp/5g	12	244	0.2	60.8	0.0	0.0
Damson, Sainsbury's*	1 Serving/25g	40	160	0.4	39.6	0.0	0.4
Fruit With Edible Seeds	1 Tsp/15g	39	261	0.6	69.0	0.0	0.0
Fruits Of The Forest, Extra Special, Asda*	1 Tbsp/15g	29	192	0.9	45.0	0.9	0.0
Golden Peach, Rhapsodie de Fruit, St Dalfour*	2 Tsp/20g	45	227	0.5	56.0	0.1	1.3
Kiwi & Goosberry, 66% Fruit, Asda*	1 Serving/30g	56	187	0.5	45.0	0.5	0.0
Mixed Fruit, Budgens*	1 Tbsp/15g	39	261	0.2	65.0	0.0	0.8
Mixed Fruit, Savers, Safeway*	1 Serving/10g	25	247	0.2	61.0	0.2	0.0
Mixed Fruit, SmartPrice, Asda*	1 Tbsp/15g	36	241	0.2	60.0	0.0	1.0
Mixed Fruit, Value, Tesco*	1 Tsp/5g	13	253	0.2	63.0	0.0	0.8
Original, Hartley's*	1 Tsp/15g	38	252	0.2	62.8	0.0	0.6
Plum, Tesco*	1 Serving/50g	131	261	0.2	64.4	0.0	0.6
Rasberry, Weight Watchers*	1 Tsp/6.3g	7	111	0.4	27.1	0.1	0.9
Raspberry, Asda*	1 Tbsp/15g	39	257	1.0	63.0	0.1	1.0
Raspberry, Baxters*	1 Tsp/15g	38	252	0.0	63.0	0.0	1.2
Raspberry, Classic, Robertson's*	1 Tsp/10g	25	247	0.3	60.8	0.0	0.0
Raspberry, Extra Special, Asda*	1 Tbsp/15.1g	29	192	0.9	45.0	0.9	0.0
Raspberry, Frank Cooper*	1 Tsp/15g	37	247	0.6	60.9	0.1	1.2
Raspberry, Light, Robertson's*	1oz/28g	59	210	0.2	52.3	0.0	0.0
Raspberry, Organic, Marks & Spencer*	1 Serving/4g	10	240	0.6	59.1	0.1	1.5
Raspberry, Reduced Sugar, Asda*	1 Tsp/15g	28	185	0.7	45.0	0.2	0.0
Raspberry, Reduced Sugar, Sainsbury's*	1 Tsp/15g	29	190	0.6	47.0	0.1	1.1
Raspberry, Seedless, Budgens*	1 Tbsp/15g	39	262	0.5	65.0	0.0	0.0
Raspberry, Seedless, Robertson's*	1 Tsp/10g	25	247	0.3	60.8	0.0	0.0
Raspberry, Seedless, Sainsbury's*	1 Tsp/15g	40	264	0.5	65.5	0.0	1.1
Raspberry, Seedless, Tesco*	1 Tsp/15g	38	254	0.5	63.0	0.0	0.0
Raspberry, Somerfield*	1 Tsp/15g	39	261	1.0	64.0	0.0	0.0
Raspberry, St Dalfour*	1 Tsp/15g	34	228	0.7	56.0	0.1	3.0
Raspberry, Streamline*	1 Serving/10g	19	189	0.5	45.6	0.5	0.0
Reduced Sugar	1 Tsp/15g	18	123	0.5	31.9	0.1	0.8
Rhubarb & Ginger, Baxters*	1 Tsp/15g	32	210	0.0	53.0	0.0	0.6
Strawberry & Redcurrant, Reduced Sugar, Streamline*	1 Tbsp/15g	29	192	0.4	46.8	0.3	0.0
Strawberry, 25% Less Sugar, Asda*	1 Tbsp/15g	28	184	0.4	45.5	0.1	0.9
Strawberry, 66% Fruit, Asda*	1 Tbsp/15g	28	187	0.5	45.0	0.5	0.0
Strawberry, Asda*	1 Tbsp/15g	39	257	0.3	64.0	0.0	1.0
Strawberry, Baxters*	1 Tbsp/15g	32	210	0.0	53.0	0.0	5.0
Strawberry, Best, Hartley's*	1 Tbsp/15g	37	244	0.4	60.6	0.0	0.0
Strawberry, Co-Op*	1 Tbsp/15g	39	260	0.3	64.6	0.1	0.6
Strawberry, Extra Special, Asda*	1 Tbsp/15g	28	187	0.5	45.0	0.5	0.0
Strawberry, Frank Cooper*	1 Tbsp/15g	37	248	0.4	61.5	0.0	0.5
Strawberry, Iceland*	1 Tbsp/15g	39	258	0.1	64.0	0.1	0.1
Strawberry, Light, Robertson's*	1 Tbsp/15g	32	210	0.2	52.2	0.0	0.0
Strawberry, Luxury, Baxters*	1 Tbsp/15g	38	252	0.0	63.0	0.0	0.5
Strawberry, Makes Sense, Somerfield*	1 Tsp/7g	18	252	0.3	62.7	0.0	0.6
Strawberry, Morrisons*	1 Tbsp/15g	38	254	0.4	63.0	0.0	0.6
Strawberry, Reduced Sugar, Bonne Maman*	1 Tbsp/15g	28	184	0.5	45.0	0.2	0.0
Strawberry, Reduced Sugar, Sainsbury's*	1 Tbsp/15g	29	190	0.4	47.0	0.1	0.5
Strawberry, Rhapsodie de Fruit, St Dalfour*	1 Tsp/10g	23	227	0.4	56.0	0.1	0.0
Strawberry, Robertson's*	1 Tsp/10g	25	249	0.2	61.2	0.0	0.0
Strawberry, Safeway*	1 Tbsp/15g	39	261	0.3	64.6	0.1	0.6
Strawberry, Sainsbury's*	1 Serving/13g	33	252	0.3	62.7	0.0	0.6
Strawberry, Somerfield*	1 Tsp/15g	39	260	0.0	65.0	0.0	0.0

J

	Measure INFO/WEIGHT	per Measure KCAL	Nutrition Values per 100g / 100ml				
			KCAL	PROT	CARB	FAT	FIBRE
JAM,							
Strawberry, Tesco*	1 Heaped Tsp/20g	53	265	0.3	65.0	0.0	0.6
Strawberry, Weight Watchers*	1 Tsp/6.1g	7	115	0.2	28.4	0.0	0.4
Strawberry, With Extra Fruit, Reduced Sugar, Streamline*	1 Tsp/5g	10	192	0.3	47.1	0.3	0.0
Wild Blackberry Jelly, Baxters*	1 Tsp/15g	32	210	0.0	53.0	0.0	1.2
JAMBALAYA,							
American Style, Tesco*	1 Serving/275g	432	157	7.7	16.0	7.0	0.5
COU, Marks & Spencer*	1 Pack/400g	340	85	6.5	10.8	2.0	0.9
Cajun Chicken, BGTY, Sainsbury's*	1 Pack/400g	364	91	7.7	11.9	1.4	1.1
Marks & Spencer*	1 Pack/480g	552	115	5.8	14.6	3.5	1.2
JELLY,							
Blackberry, Unprepared, Morrisons*	1 Serving/20g	52	261	0.3	65.0	0.0	0.0
Blackcurrant, Made Up, Rowntree's*	¼ Jelly/140ml	100	71	1.4	16.4	0.1	0.0
Blackcurrant, Made Up, Sainsbury's*	¼ Jelly/150g	98	65	1.2	15.1	0.0	0.0
Blackcurrant, Sugar Free, Unprepared, Rowntree's*	1 Pack/24g	73	305	66.5	0.3	0.0	0.4
Crystals, Peach & Pear, Sugar Free, Bird's*	1oz/28g	91	325	64.5	3.3	0.2	0.0
Crystals, Black Cherry, Sugar Free, Bird's*	1oz/28g	92	330	61.0	9.1	0.1	0.0
Crystals, Lemon & Lime, Sugar Free, Bird's*	1oz/28g	92	330	62.5	7.3	0.2	0.0
Fresh Fruit, Marks & Spencer*	1 Pot/175g	131	75	0.2	18.4	0.1	0.3
Fruit Cocktail, Marks & Spencer*	1oz/28g	31	110	0.4	16.4	4.7	0.3
Fruitini, Del Monte*	1 Serving/120g	78	65	0.3	15.3	0.1	0.5
Lemon, Co-Op*, Unprepared	1 Pack/135g	412	305	5.0	71.0	0.0	0.0
Lemon, Somerfield*, Unprepared	1 Pack/135g	393	291	6.0	66.0	0.0	0.0
Lime Flavour, Waitrose*, Unprepared	1 Square/11g	33	296	4.5	69.5	0.0	0.0
Lime, Co-Op*, Unprepared	1 Pack/135g	397	294	5.5	68.1	0.1	1.0
Lime, Made Up, Rowntree's*	¼ Jelly/140ml	100	71	1.4	16.4	0.1	0.0
Lime, Somerfield*, Unprepared	1 Pack/135g	392	290	6.0	66.0	0.0	0.0
Made With Water	1oz/28g	17	61	1.2	15.1	0.0	0.0
Mandarin & Pineapple, Sainsbury's*	1 Pot/125g	95	76	0.2	18.9	0.1	1.2
Mixed Berry, WTF, Sainsbury's*	1 Serving/160g	112	70	0.7	16.3	0.2	1.5
Pots, Orange, Low Sugar, Rowntree's*	1 Pot/115g	7	6	0.1	1.1	0.0	0.5
Raspberry Flavour, Sugar Free, Made Up, Rowntree's*	1 Serving/140ml	13	9	1.9	0.2	0.0	0.0
Raspberry, Co-Op*, Unprepared	1 Pack/135g	402	298	5.5	68.9	0.1	0.0
Raspberry, Unprepared, Rowntree's*	1 Serving/135g	405	300	5.6	67.3	0.4	0.0
Strawberry & Raspberry, Sainsbury's*	½ Pot/280g	230	82	0.2	20.2	0.0	1.2
Strawberry Flavour, Sugar Free, Made Up, Rowntree's*	1 Serving/140ml	14	10	2.1	0.1	0.0	0.0
Strawberry Flavour, Sugar Free, Unprepared, Rowntree's*	1oz/28g	84	300	3.0	64.9	0.4	0.0
Tangerine, Unprepared, Rowntree's*	1 Serving/33g	99	300	5.6	67.3	0.4	0.0
Tropical Fresh Fruit, Eat Smart, Safeway*	1 Serving/185g	120	65	0.6	14.5	0.3	1.1
Tropical Fruit, WTF, Sainsbury's*	1 Serving/160g	144	90	0.3	19.9	1.0	0.9
JELLY BABIES,							
Bassett's*	1 Baby/6g	20	335	4.0	79.5	0.0	0.0
Marks & Spencer*	1 Pack/125g	418	334	5.2	78.0	0.0	0.0
Mini, Waitrose*	1 Bag/125g	370	296	4.3	68.7	0.4	0.0
Somerfield*	1 Sweet/6g	21	343	4.7	80.7	0.0	0.0
Tesco*	1 Baby/6g	20	332	5.3	77.4	0.1	0.1
JELLY BEANS,							
Asda*	1 Bag/100g	364	364	0.1	90.0	0.4	0.2
Marks & Spencer*	1 Bag/113g	407	360	0.1	89.6	0.0	0.0
Rowntree's*	1 Pack/35g	128	367	0.0	91.8	0.0	0.0
JELLY BEARS,							
Co-Op*	1 Sweet/3g	10	325	6.0	76.0	0.1	0.0
JELLY TOTS,							
Rowntree's*	1 Pack/42g	145	346	0.1	86.5	0.0	0.0

J

INFO/WEIGHT	Measure per Measure KCAL	Nutrition Values per 100g / 100ml				
		KCAL	PROT	CARB	FAT	FIBRE
JUICE DRINK,						
Cranberry, Asda*	1/5 Carton/200ml 100	50	0.0	12.0	0.0	0.0
Grape, Apple & Raspberry, Asda*	1 Glass/200ml 90	45	0.2	11.0	0.0	0.0
Orange, Healthy Eating, Tesco*	1 Glass/200ml 56	28	0.3	6.1	0.1	0.0
JUST FRUIT, Shapers, Boots*	1 Pot/140g 60	43	0.6	10.0	0.1	1.5

J

INFO/WEIGHT	Measure per Measure KCAL	Nutrition Values per 100g / 100ml				
		KCAL	PROT	CARB	FAT	FIBRE
KABANOS,						
Polish, Sainsbury's*	1 Kabanos/25g	91	365	23.0	0.1	30.4	0.1
KEBAB,						
BBQ Pork, Sainsbury's*	1 Serving/90g	65	72	11.0	1.4	2.4	0.9
Barbecue Chicken Tikka, Mini, Somerfield*	1oz/28g	38	134	21.0	4.0	4.0	0.0
Cajun Salmon, Tesco*	1 Kebab/75g	100	133	19.8	3.9	4.2	1.3
Chicken & Pineapple, Aldi*	1 Kebab/85g	89	105	13.9	5.3	3.1	0.0
Chicken Mango Flavour, Cooked, Waitrose*	1 Kebab/73g	86	118	24.1	4.5	0.4	0.1
Chicken With Jasmine Rice & Pineapple, ES, Safeway*	1 Pack/380g	380	100	5.8	16.5	1.2	1.2
Chicken With Sweet Chilli Sauce, Finest, Tesco*	½ Pack/175g	242	138	17.9	14.7	0.8	1.2
Chicken With Sweet Chilli Sauce, Marks & Spencer*	1 Serving/165g	228	138	17.9	14.7	0.8	1.2
Chicken, Barbecue, Sainsbury's*	1 Pack/200g	238	119	24.4	1.5	1.7	1.8
Chicken, Honey & Mustard, Marks & Spencer*	1oz/28g	41	145	16.7	8.2	4.8	1.0
Chicken, Mini Fillet, Marks & Spencer*	1 Serving/150g	210	140	20.2	2.0	5.8	0.3
Chicken, Thin Sliced, Heat 'n' Eat, Asda*	½ Pack/50g	92	184	15.0	3.9	12.0	1.1
Chilli & Coriander Chicken Breast, COU, M&S*	½ Pack/200g	200	100	20.6	1.0	1.4	0.0
Chinese Chicken, Mini, Marks & Spencer*	1 Kebab/11g	24	215	19.5	5.1	12.9	0.6
Chinese Salmon, Iceland*	1 Kebab/75g	115	153	23.8	4.1	4.6	1.6
Citrus Tikka Chicken Breast, Sainsbury's*	1 Kebab/61g	79	129	25.6	5.4	0.5	0.9
Citrus Tikka Lamb Kofta, Sainsbury's*	1 Kebab/84g	199	235	18.1	9.8	13.7	2.6
Doner, Heat 'n' Eat Thin Sliced, Asda*	1 Pack/100g	196	196	16.7	8.4	10.6	1.7
Doner, Lidl*	1 Kebab/170g	509	300	14.7	15.3	18.4	0.0
Donner, Iceland*	1 Serving/152.3g	268	176	9.2	24.4	4.7	2.4
Green Pesto Chicken Breast, COU, Marks & Spencer*	1 Serving/200g	160	80	15.1	1.5	1.4	1.0
Green Thai Chicken, Waitrose*	1 Serving/180g	223	124	20.5	1.4	4.0	1.4
Hawaiian Chicken, Mini, Asda*	1 Serving/100g	168	168	21.0	2.9	8.0	0.0
Honey & Mustard Chicken, Sainsbury's*	1 Serving/50g	66	131	24.5	4.3	1.8	0.0
Lamb Kofta With A Mint & Coriander Raita, Safeway*	1 Pack/290g	632	218	16.9	8.4	13.0	1.2
Lamb Kofta, Safeway*	1 Pack/227g	465	205	14.3	5.8	13.4	1.0
Lamb Shami With a Mint Raita Dip, Marks & Spencer*	½ Pack/90g	189	210	12.8	9.7	13.4	3.5
Lamb, Greek Style, Lakeland, Aldi*	1 Serving/100g	196	196	11.8	1.9	15.6	0.0
Lamb, Greek Style, Sainsbury's*	1 Kebab/168g	428	255	17.4	7.7	17.0	2.3
Lamb, Shish, Waitrose*	1 Kebab/55.8g	91	163	16.5	6.8	7.7	1.3
Lamb, With Halloumi Cheese & Olives, Waitrose*	2 Kebabs/150g	246	164	20.0	2.4	8.3	0.2
Mango & Lime Chicken, Waitrose*	1 Serving/180g	275	153	28.2	2.5	3.3	0.3
Mango Salsa Chicken Breast, Sainsbury's*	1 Kebab/60g	85	142	26.3	5.5	1.6	0.6
Pork Sausage, Mini, Grilled, Safeway*	1 Serving/100g	175	175	9.1	3.4	13.5	1.1
Salmon, Hot & Spicy, Tesco*	1 Kebab/75g	89	118	22.0	1.1	2.9	0.0
Shish With Onions & Peppers	1oz/28g	59	212	12.9	3.9	16.2	1.2
Shish in Pitta Bread With Salad	1oz/28g	43	155	13.5	17.2	4.1	1.0
Shish, Marks & Spencer*	1 Serving/100g	185	185	13.8	1.6	13.5	0.6
Spicy Tomato Creole King Prawn, Marks & Spencer*	1 Pack/240g	240	100	14.3	2.9	3.3	0.7
Sticky Barbecue Chicken Thigh, Marks & Spencer*	1 Kebab/100g	160	160	15.6	7.4	7.5	0.8
Sweet Oriental Chicken Breast, COU, Marks & Spencer*	½ Pack/200g	220	110	20.8	4.3	1.0	0.1
Sweetcorn, Tesco*	1 Kebab/130g	74	57	2.0	9.9	1.0	0.9
Tandoori, Marks & Spencer*	1oz/28g	34	120	23.3	1.0	2.5	0.0
Thai Style Chicken, Eat Smart, Safeway*	1 Kebab/85g	85	100	15.3	6.4	1.3	1.4
Tiger Prawn, Asda*	1oz/28g	17	59	14.6	0.0	0.1	0.0
Tikka Chicken, Mini, Somerfield*	1oz/28g	38	134	21.0	4.0	4.0	0.0
Tikka, Mini, Marks & Spencer*	1 Kebab/11g	23	205	18.4	4.0	12.7	0.6
Tomato & Basil Chicken, Eat Smart, Safeway*	1 Kebab/71.5g	82	115	18.0	5.0	2.1	1.5
Vegetable, Asda*	1 Kebab/40g	25	63	1.8	4.5	4.3	2.4
Vegetable, Tesco*	1 Kebab/120g	47	39	1.7	6.8	0.6	1.1
Zesty Lime & Coriander Chicken Breast, M&S*	1 Kebab/100g	125	125	20.8	0.5	4.4	0.4

K

	Measure INFO/WEIGHT	per Measure KCAL	Nutrition Values per 100g / 100ml				
			KCAL	PROT	CARB	FAT	FIBRE
KEDGEREE,							
Average	1oz/28g	48	171	15.9	7.8	8.7	0.1
COU, Marks & Spencer*	1 Pack/370g	426	115	7.9	14.4	2.6	0.8
Perfectly Balanced, Waitrose*	1 Pack/400g	368	92	7.0	10.8	2.3	0.6
Smoked Haddock, Big Dish, Marks & Spencer*	1 Pack/450g	585	130	8.5	13.0	5.0	1.9
KETCHUP,							
BBQ, Heinz*	1 Serving/10g	14	137	1.3	31.3	0.3	0.3
Barbeque, Asda*	1 Tbsp/15g	20	136	0.9	33.0	0.0	0.0
Dip Pot, Burger King*	1 Pot/25g	27	107	1.0	24.7	0.1	0.6
Sachet, Burger King*	1 Sachet/15g	16	107	1.0	24.7	0.1	0.6
Tomato	1oz/28g	32	115	1.6	28.6	0.1	0.9
Tomato, 25% Less Sugar, Asda*	1 Tbsp/10g	7	71	1.6	16.0	0.1	0.0
Tomato, Budgens*	1oz/28g	36	127	2.3	29.2	0.1	0.6
Tomato, Daddies, HP*	1oz/28g	31	110	0.9	26.5	0.3	0.0
Tomato, Frank Cooper*	1 Sachet/12g	14	119	1.0	27.9	0.3	0.6
Tomato, Heinz*	1 Tbsp/15g	16	107	1.0	24.7	0.1	0.6
Tomato, McDonald's*	1 Portion/20g	26	131	1.4	31.2	0.1	0.0
Tomato, No Sugar & Salt, Sainsbury's*	1 Tsp/5g	4	88	1.7	18.4	0.2	0.7
Tomato, Organic, Evernat*	1oz/28g	26	92	1.0	22.0	0.0	0.0
Tomato, Sainsbury's*	1 Tbsp/15g	19	128	0.9	28.7	0.5	1.0
Tomato, SmartPrice, Asda*	1 Tbsp/10g	12	122	0.7	29.0	0.2	0.7
Tomato, Value, Tesco*	1 Tbsp/15ml	21	139	2.3	32.2	0.1	1.4
Wicked Orange, Heinz*	1 Serving/11g	12	108	1.0	24.7	0.1	0.6
KIDNEY,							
Lamb, Fried	1oz/28g	53	188	23.7	0.0	10.3	0.0
Lamb, Raw	1oz/28g	25	91	17.0	0.0	2.6	0.0
Ox, Raw	1oz/28g	25	88	17.2	0.0	2.1	0.0
Ox, Stewed	1oz/28g	39	138	24.5	0.0	4.4	0.0
Pig, Fried	1oz/28g	57	202	29.2	0.0	9.5	0.0
Pig, Raw	1oz/28g	24	86	15.5	0.0	2.7	0.0
Pig, Stewed	1oz/28g	43	153	24.4	0.0	6.1	0.0
KIEV,							
Cheese & Ham, Tesco*	1 Kiev/142.5g	313	219	13.6	12.4	12.8	1.2
Cheese & Mushroom Chicken, Somerfield*	½ Pack/142g	294	207	14.0	15.0	11.0	0.0
Cheese, Smoked Ham & Chicken, Sainsbury's*	1 Kiev/136g	299	220	15.9	12.0	12.8	0.3
Chicken & Garlic Butter, Healthy Living, Tesco*	1 Kiev/142.5g	286	200	14.3	9.9	11.5	0.6
Chicken Breast, Garlic Butter, Sun Valley*	1 Kiev/141g	436	309	13.2	11.8	23.2	0.9
Chicken With Garlic Butter, Tesco*	1 Kiev/125g	343	274	13.7	8.8	20.4	0.7
Chicken, BGTY, Sainsbury's*	1 Kiev/125g	253	202	14.3	11.3	11.1	1.0
Chicken, Bernard Matthews*	1 Kiev/125g	374	299	10.6	13.9	22.3	2.7
Chicken, Better for You, Morrisons*	1 Kiev/134g	304	227	16.1	11.5	13.0	1.0
Chicken, Breaded, Mini, Family, Bernard Matthews*	1 Kiev/23g	46	199	15.7	12.1	9.8	0.0
Chicken, COU, Marks & Spencer*	1 Kiev/150g	188	125	15.8	10.8	1.8	0.5
Chicken, Cheese & Ham, Tesco*	1 Kiev/142g	338	238	16.3	11.3	14.2	0.6
Chicken, Cheesy Bean, Asda*	1 Kiev/94.0g	202	215	12.0	17.0	11.0	1.9
Chicken, Creamy Garlic, Tesco*	1 Kiev/142g	334	235	12.2	9.7	16.4	0.6
Chicken, Creamy Pepper, Safeway*	1 Kiev/133g	306	230	11.9	11.1	15.4	1.1
Chicken, Creamy Pepper, Tesco*	1 Kiev/142g	270	190	12.0	10.0	11.0	2.0
Chicken, Creamy Peppercorn, Sun Valley*	1 Kiev/140g	382	273	13.3	13.5	18.5	0.0
Chicken, Creamy Peppercorn, Tesco*	1 Kiev/141g	303	215	12.8	8.1	14.6	1.5
Chicken, Finest, Tesco*	1 Kiev/237g	460	194	18.0	9.0	9.5	1.0
Chicken, Garlic Butter, Lower Fat, Asda*	1 Kiev/136g	282	207	13.0	14.0	11.0	0.7
Chicken, Garlic Butter, Safeway*	1 Kiev/115g	316	275	13.3	12.5	19.1	1.1
Chicken, Garlic Butter, Somerfield*	1 Kiev/142g	425	299	12.6	8.5	23.9	1.2

K

	Measure INFO/WEIGHT	per Measure KCAL	Nutrition Values per 100g / 100ml				
			KCAL	PROT	CARB	FAT	FIBRE
KIEV,							
Chicken, Garlic, Marks & Spencer*	1 Kiev/150g	375	250	16.5	9.5	16.4	0.5
Chicken, Garlic, Morrisons*	1 Kiev/122g	289	237	14.3	9.8	15.7	0.0
Chicken, Garlic, Safeway*	1 Kiev/147g	413	281	12.9	11.2	20.5	0.9
Chicken, Italian Style, Sainsbury's*	1 Kiev/134.8g	342	253	14.3	12.8	16.1	1.3
Chicken, Maitre Jean-Pierre, Lidl*	1 Pack/284g	781	275	13.3	12.7	19.1	0.0
Chicken, Tesco*	1oz/28g	70	251	16.7	8.8	16.5	1.1
Chicken, Tomato & Mozzarella, Tesco*	1 Kiev/143g	339	237	11.4	7.9	17.7	1.4
Cod & Parsley, Safeway*	1 Kiev/160g	310	194	10.6	17.0	9.2	0.0
Garlic & Parsley Chicken, BGTY, Sainsbury's*	1 Kiev/133g	318	239	15.0	11.7	14.7	1.3
Garlic & Parsley Chicken, Sainsbury's*	1 Kiev/136.4g	426	313	12.0	9.9	25.4	1.0
Garlic & Parsley, TTD, Sainsbury's*	1 Kiev/150g	371	247	15.7	11.1	15.6	0.8
Garlic Chicken, GFY, Asda*	1 Kiev/138.4g	302	219	15.0	15.0	11.0	1.0
Ham & Cheese Chicken, Somerfield*	½ Pack/142g	294	207	14.0	14.0	11.0	0.0
Lemon Butter Chicken, Somerfield*	½ Pack/142g	409	288	12.0	12.0	21.0	0.0
Salmon, Fillet, Tesco*	1 Kiev/160g	376	235	13.3	18.0	12.2	2.5
Tikka Chicken, Asda*	1 Kiev/150g	326	217	15.6	15.6	10.2	0.8
Tikka, Safeway*	1 Kiev/132g	327	248	11.9	10.5	17.5	1.0
Vegetarian, Cheesy Garlic, Meat Free, Sainsbury's*	1 Kiev/123g	263	214	17.3	10.6	11.4	3.0
Vegetarian, Garlic Butter, Tesco*	1 Kiev/142g	462	325	14.4	22.1	19.9	0.8
Vegetarian, Garlic Butter, Tivall*	1 Kiev/125g	366	293	15.1	10.8	21.0	2.6
Vegetarian, Garlic, Safeway*	1 Kiev/142g	423	298	13.2	20.3	18.2	0.7
Vegetarian, Vegetable, Marks & Spencer*	1 Kiev/155g	326	210	4.6	17.8	13.4	2.5
KING PRAWN,							
Creole, With Vegetable Rice, COU, Marks & Spencer*	1 Pack/400g	300	75	4.5	13.3	0.6	0.7
Ginger & Spring Onion, Budgens*	1 Pack/350g	151	43	5.9	2.1	1.2	0.7
With A Spicy Cajun Dip, Sainsbury's*	1 Pack/240g	254	106	14.8	9.1	1.8	1.4
KIPPER,							
Baked	1oz/28g	57	205	25.5	0.0	11.4	0.0
Boil in Bag, Boiled	1oz/28g	66	237	20.0	0.0	17.4	0.0
Fillets, Smoked Scottish, Macrae*	1 Pack/171g	375	219	20.4	0.0	15.1	0.0
Fillets, in Brine, John West*	1 Can/140g	269	192	21.0	0.0	12.0	0.0
Fillets, in Sunflower Oil, John West*	1 Can/140g	321	229	19.0	0.0	17.0	0.0
Grilled	1oz/28g	71	255	20.1	0.0	19.4	0.0
Raw	1oz/28g	64	229	17.5	0.0	17.7	0.0
Smoked, Boned, Tesco*	1 Serving/150g	315	210	17.4	0.0	15.6	0.0
KIT KAT,							
2 Finger, Nestle*	2 Finger Bar/21g	106	506	6.7	60.6	26.3	0.0
4 Fingers, Nestle*	4 Fingers/48g	243	507	6.8	60.2	26.5	1.2
Chunky, Nestle*	1 Bar/55g	283	514	6.5	59.8	27.6	0.0
Chunky, Snack Size, Nestle*	1 Bar/26g	133	513	6.6	60.4	27.2	1.1
Individual Bars, Nestle*	1 Bar/28g	144	513	6.6	60.4	27.2	0.0
Kubes, Nestle*	1 Pack/50g	258	515	5.9	60.9	27.5	1.0
Mini, Nestle*	1 Bar/15g	75	502	7.5	59.4	26.0	0.0
Mint, Nestle*	4 Finger Bar/48g	243	506	6.0	61.4	26.3	1.1
Orange, 2 Finger, Nestle*	2 Finger Bar/20g	101	506	6.7	60.6	26.3	0.0
White, Nestle*	1 Chunky/53g	278	525	8.0	58.3	28.9	0.0
KIWI FRUIT,							
Fresh, Raw	1oz/28g	14	49	1.1	10.6	0.5	1.9
Weighed With Skin	1 Kiwi/60g	25	42	1.0	9.1	0.4	1.6
KOHL RABI,							
Boiled in Salted Water	1oz/28g	5	18	1.2	3.1	0.2	1.9
Raw	1oz/28g	6	23	1.6	3.7	0.2	2.2

	Measure INFO/WEIGHT	per Measure KCAL	Nutrition Values per 100g / 100ml				
			KCAL	PROT	CARB	FAT	FIBRE
KORMA,							
Chicken & Basmati Rice, Tesco*	1 Pot/350g	588	168	4.3	16.9	9.3	2.3
Chicken & Pilau Rice, Asda*	1 Pack/392g	804	205	7.0	24.0	9.0	1.4
Chicken & Pilau Rice, BGTY, Sainsbury's*	1 Pack/450g	513	114	9.0	14.6	2.2	1.2
Chicken & Pilau Rice, GFY, Asda*	1 Pack/400g	600	150	8.0	16.0	6.0	1.3
Chicken & Pilau Rice, Morrisons*	1 Pack/450g	889	198	9.4	15.9	10.7	1.4
Chicken & Pilau Rice, New, BGTY, Sainsbury's*	1 Pack/400g	344	86	8.1	10.8	1.2	1.9
Chicken & Pilau Rice, Somerfield*	1 Pack/340g	687	202	9.0	16.0	11.0	0.0
Chicken & Rice, 95% Fat Free, Bird's Eye*	1 Pack/370g	444	120	6.2	19.6	1.9	1.1
Chicken & Rice, COU, Marks & Spencer*	1 Pack/400g	420	105	8.1	13.7	1.7	0.5
Chicken & Rice, Easy Steam, BGTY, Sainsbury's*	1 Pack/400g	448	112	7.9	17.1	1.3	0.6
Chicken & Rice, Good Choice, Iceland*	1 Pack/400g	464	116	5.8	18.4	2.1	0.8
Chicken & Rice, Healthy Eating, Tesco*	1 Pack/420g	487	116	7.2	17.9	1.8	0.3
Chicken & Rice, Healthy Living, Co-Op*	1 Pack/400g	480	120	8.0	17.0	2.0	1.0
Chicken & Rice, Healthy Living, Tesco*	1 Pack/420g	458	109	7.1	16.1	1.8	1.6
Chicken & Rice, Organic, Tesco*	1 Pack/450g	923	205	6.0	21.5	10.6	0.4
Chicken & Rice, Patak's*	1 Pack/370g	466	126	5.9	15.8	4.8	0.4
Chicken & Rice, Tesco*	1 Pack/450g	594	132	6.8	13.7	5.5	2.6
Chicken & Rice, World Flavours*	1 Pack/500g	705	141	8.7	16.0	4.7	0.0
Chicken Coconut, Sainsbury's*	1 Pack/400g	664	166	13.0	5.3	10.3	1.6
Chicken Meal, BGTY, Restaurant, Sainsbury's*	1 Serving/201g	223	111	15.0	4.0	4.1	1.2
Chicken With Basmati Rice, Eat Smart, Safeway*	1 Pack/380g	399	105	7.0	13.8	1.9	1.5
Chicken With Pilau Rice, Perfectly Balanced, Waitrose*	1 Pack/400g	528	132	8.9	18.3	2.6	1.1
Chicken With Pilau Rice, Safeway*	1 Pack/400g	784	196	7.6	16.9	10.9	2.4
Chicken With Pilau Rice, Sharwood's*	1 Pack/375g	566	151	6.7	15.4	7.0	0.9
Chicken, Eastern Classics*	1 Serving/100g	234	234	9.7	6.0	19.0	2.1
Chicken, Fresh, Chilled, Tesco*	1 Pack/350g	819	234	13.1	6.3	17.4	2.3
Chicken, Indian Meal for 2, Finest, Tesco*	½ Pack/200g	348	174	10.3	6.2	12.0	2.5
Chicken, Indian Takeaway For One, Sainsbury's*	1 Serving/300g	498	166	13.0	5.3	10.3	1.6
Chicken, Indian Takeaway, Iceland*	1 Pack/400g	656	164	11.8	4.5	11.0	1.4
Chicken, Less Than 3% Fat, Bird's Eye*	1 Pack/358g	440	123	6.5	20.4	1.9	0.8
Chicken, Plumrose*	1 Can/392g	431	110	8.0	6.9	5.6	0.0
Chicken, Safeway*	1 Pack/350g	648	185	14.1	8.4	10.6	2.0
Chicken, Sainsbury's*	1 Pack/400g	580	145	14.1	3.3	8.4	0.7
Chicken, Tesco*	1 Pack/350g	620	177	10.8	6.8	11.8	0.6
Chicken, Vegetable Curry & Rice, Tesco*	1 Pack/450g	495	110	7.1	15.2	2.4	1.4
Quorn	1oz/28g	39	140	3.7	16.7	7.0	0.0
Vegetable & Rice, Tesco*	1 Pack/450g	621	138	2.9	18.3	5.9	1.6
Vegetable With Rice, Eat Smart, Safeway*	1 Pack/400g	412	103	3.1	17.5	2.3	1.6
Vegetable, Sainsbury's*	1 Serving/200g	302	151	2.7	6.6	12.6	2.2
KRISPROLLS,							
Cracked Wheat, Original, Pogen*	1 Piece/10g	38	380	12.0	67.0	7.0	9.0
Golden Wheat, Pogen*	1 Serving/10g	41	410	11.0	72.0	8.5	4.0
KULFI, Average	1oz/28g	119	424	5.4	11.8	39.9	0.6
KUMQUATS,							
Canned, In Syrup	1oz/28g	39	138	0.4	35.4	0.5	1.7
Raw	1oz/28g	12	43	0.9	9.3	0.5	3.8

K

	Measure	per Measure	Nutrition Values per 100g / 100ml				
	INFO/WEIGHT	KCAL	KCAL	PROT	CARB	FAT	FIBRE

LAGER,

	Measure INFO/WEIGHT	KCAL	KCAL	PROT	CARB	FAT	FIBRE
Amstel, Heinekin N V*	1 Pint/568ml	227	40	0.5	3.0	0.0	0.0
Becks*	1 Can/275ml	113	41	0.0	3.0	0.0	0.0
Budweiser, Anheuser-Busch*	1 Bottle/330ml	133	40	0.3	2.9	0.0	0.0
Export, Foster's*	1 Pint/568ml	210	37	0.0	2.2	0.0	0.0
Foster's*	1 Pint/568ml	227	40	0.0	3.1	0.0	0.0
French Premier, Somerfield*	1 Bottle/250ml	108	43	0.0	4.0	0.0	0.0
Heineken, Heineken N V*	1 Pint/568ml	256	45	0.5	3.0	0.0	0.0
Low Alcohol	1 Can/440ml	44	10	0.2	1.5	0.0	0.0
Miller Pilsner*	1 Bottle/500ml	150	30	0.3	2.4	0.0	0.0
Organic, Tesco*	1 Bottle/500ml	215	43	0.2	3.5	0.0	0.0
Pills, Holsten*	1 Can/440ml	167	38	0.3	2.4	0.0	0.0
Pilsner, German, Somerfield*	1 Bottle/250ml	73	29	1.0	1.0	0.0	0.0
Premium	1 Can/440ml	260	59	0.3	2.4	0.0	0.0
Premium, Tesco*	1 Can/440	229	52	0.4	4.0	0.0	0.0
Stella Artois*	1 Can/550ml	222	40	0.3	2.9	0.0	0.0

LAMB,

	Measure INFO/WEIGHT	KCAL	KCAL	PROT	CARB	FAT	FIBRE
Average, Trimmed Lean, Raw	1oz/28g	44	156	20.2	0.0	8.3	0.0
Butterflied, Leg, Cook Range, Marks & Spencer*	1 Serving/175g	263	150	18.7	0.4	8.3	0.6
Chops, Asda*	2 Chops/190g	467	246	21.0	0.0	18.0	0.0
Chops, Chump, Somerfield*	1oz/28g	62	222	28.0	0.0	12.0	0.0
Chops, Frozen, Asda*	1/5 Pack/158g	525	332	29.0	0.0	24.0	0.0
Chops, Leg, Bernard Matthews*	1oz/28g	55	196	18.4	0.0	13.6	0.0
Chops, Marks & Spencer*	1oz/28g	56	200	16.9	2.4	13.5	0.0
Chops, Shoulder, Mango & Mint, Waitrose*	1 Chop/250g	555	222	16.7	2.3	16.2	0.5
Chops, Somerfield*	1oz/28g	78	277	18.0	0.0	23.0	0.0
Chump, Topped With Fresh Salsa Verde, Cook!, M&S*	½ Pack/159.4g	254	160	17.6	5.8	7.2	1.5
Diced, BGTY, Sainsbury's*	½ Pack/200g	242	121	20.7	0.1	4.3	0.1
Diced, Healthy Eating, Tesco*	½ Pack/165g	215	130	20.1	0.0	5.5	0.0
Fillet, BGTY, Sainsbury's*	1 Serving/100g	132	132	24.2	0.1	3.9	0.0
In a Pot, Sainsbury's*	1 Pack/450g	554	123	7.6	14.6	3.8	0.7
Leg, Somerfield*	1oz/28g	60	215	26.0	0.0	12.0	0.0
Mince, New Zealand, Sainsbury's*	1 Serving/100g	257	257	21.4	0.0	19.0	0.4
Mince, Premium, Bernard Matthews*	1oz/28g	55	198	17.0	0.9	14.0	0.0
Mince, Raw	1oz/28g	55	196	19.1	0.0	13.3	0.0
Mince, Scottish, Tesco*	1oz/28g	71	254	17.2	0.0	20.4	0.0
Mince, Tesco*	1 Serving/150g	381	254	17.2	0.0	20.0	0.0
Minced, Asda*	1 Serving/100g	198	198	19.0	0.0	13.0	0.0
Minced, Frozen, Morrisons*	1oz/28g	68	242	18.0	0.0	19.0	0.0
Minted, Shoulder Chops, Sainsbury's*	1 Chop/108g	281	260	22.3	10.4	14.4	0.1
Minted, Steaks, Frozen, Asda*	½ Pack/71g	156	220	30.0	4.7	9.0	1.3
Rack, Raw, Lean & Fat	1oz/28g	79	283	17.3	0.0	23.8	0.0
Roast Dinner, Bird's Eye*	1 Pack/340g	357	105	6.6	11.2	3.8	1.4
Shank, White Wine, Garlic & Rosemary Glaze, M&Sr*	1 Pack/325g	455	140	16.4	2.3	7.0	0.1
Shanks in a Rich Balsamic Sauce, Safeway*	½ Pack/705g	1304	185	18.0	3.1	11.0	0.9
Shoulder, Half, Bernard Matthews*	1oz/28g	73	262	15.9	0.0	22.1	0.0
Shoulder, Raw, Lean & Fat	1oz/28g	66	235	17.6	0.0	18.3	0.0
Steak, Asda*	1 Serving/100g	197	197	29.0	0.0	9.0	0.0
Steak, BGTY, Sainsbury's*	1 Serving/125g	185	148	24.1	0.1	5.8	0.1
Steak, Bernard Matthews*	1 Steak/140g	151	108	18.2	0.7	3.6	0.0
Steak, Leg, Boneless, Marks & Spencer*	1 Steak/150g	345	230	28.0	0.0	13.2	0.0
Steak, Leg, Co-Op*	1 Steak/92g	106	115	20.0	0.0	4.0	0.0
Steak, Leg, Grilled, Bernard Matthews*	1 Steak/140g	209	149	23.6	0.3	5.9	0.0
Steak, Leg, Healthy Eating, Tesco*	1 Steak/150g	165	110	20.1	0.0	3.3	0.0

L

	Measure INFO/WEIGHT	per Measure KCAL	Nutrition Values per 100g / 100ml				
			KCAL	PROT	CARB	FAT	FIBRE
LAMB,							
Steak, Leg, Minted, Tesco*	1 Steak/125g	149	119	15.4	2.1	5.4	0.5
Steak, With Redcurrant & Mint Sauce, Asda*	1 Steak/142.8g	327	229	16.0	8.0	13.0	0.0
Stewing, Raw, Lean & Fat	1oz/28g	57	203	22.5	0.0	12.6	0.0
LAMB - ESCALOPE, British, Tesco*	1 Piece/95g	105	110	20.1	0.0	3.3	0.0
LAMB - GRILL STEAK							
Bird's Eye*	1 Grillsteak/71g	170	239	16.5	1.9	18.4	0.7
Minted, Asda*	1 Grillsteak/100g	298	298	28.0	6.0	18.0	0.0
Prime, Asda*	1 Steak/63g	192	304	22.0	2.2	23.0	0.0
LAMB IN,							
Mint Gravy, Sliced, Sainsbury's*	1 Pack/125g	134	107	15.3	2.9	3.8	0.8
Minted Gravy, Shanks, Iceland*	1 Pack/400g	824	206	20.1	1.6	13.2	0.7
LAMB - INDIAN, Fillet, Somerfield*	1 Pack/300g	570	190	17.0	4.0	12.0	0.0
LAMB - KOFTA, Kleftico, Sainsbury's*	1 Pack/401.2g	654	163	13.5	5.5	9.7	0.5
LAMB - MEDITERRANEAN, Shanks, Finest, Tesco*	1 Serving/404g	671	166	15.0	6.6	8.8	2.0
LAMB - MINTED							
Chop, Asda*	1 Serving/113g	312	276	26.0	2.6	18.0	0.0
Grill Sticks, Asda*	1 Stick/57g	133	234	22.0	5.0	14.0	0.3
LAMB - ROAST							
In Gravy, Bird's Eye*	1 Pack/239g	160	67	8.1	3.8	2.2	0.1
Meal, Ready Meals, Marks & Spencer*	1 Pack/340g	459	135	7.5	14.1	5.7	1.5
Minted, In Gravy, Marks & Spencer*	1 Pack/200g	140	70	6.8	6.6	1.5	0.9
LAMB - ROASTED							
Leg, Whole, Medium, Lean	1oz/28g	57	203	29.7	0.0	9.4	0.0
Leg, Whole, Medium, Lean & Fat	1oz/28g	67	240	28.1	0.0	14.2	0.0
Leg, Whole, New Zealand, Chilled, Lean	1oz/28g	58	207	28.8	0.0	10.2	0.0
Leg, Whole, New Zealand, Chilled, Lean & Fat	1oz/28g	64	230	28.0	0.0	13.1	0.0
Leg, Whole, Well Done, Lean	1oz/28g	58	208	31.3	0.0	9.2	0.0
Leg, Whole, Well Done, Lean & Fat	1oz/28g	68	242	29.8	0.0	13.6	0.0
Rack, Lean	1oz/28g	63	225	27.1	0.0	13.0	0.0
Rack, Lean & Fat	1oz/28g	102	363	23.0	0.0	30.1	0.0
Shoulder, Whole, Lean	1oz/28g	61	218	27.2	0.0	12.1	0.0
Shoulder, Whole, Lean & Fat	1oz/28g	83	298	24.7	0.0	22.1	0.0
LAMB - STEWED							
Stewing, Lean	1oz/28g	67	240	26.6	0.0	14.8	0.0
Stewing, Lean & Fat	1oz/28g	78	279	24.4	0.0	20.1	0.0
LAMB WITH,							
Carrot & Swede Mash, Braised, Eat Smart, Safeway*	1 Pack/388g	330	85	7.6	7.4	2.4	1.4
Cherry Tomatoes & Mediterranean Veg, Finest, Tesco*	½ Pack/267g	240	90	7.4	7.9	3.2	0.5
Chunky Vegetables, Braised Shank, Marks & Spencer*	½ Pack/425g	808	190	24.7	2.0	9.0	0.7
Sweet Mint Dressing, Joint, Tesco*	1 Serving/50g	97	193	19.9	1.8	11.8	0.6
LARD, Average	1oz/28g	249	891	0.0	0.0	99.0	0.0
LASAGNE,							
Al Forno, Marks & Spencer*	1 Pack/330g	528	160	9.6	12.3	8.3	1.4
Asda*	1 Pack/378g	427	113	6.0	11.0	5.0	1.1
Asparagus, Marks & Spencer*	1 Pack/360g	414	115	4.7	12.1	5.2	1.2
BGTY, Sainsbury's*	1 Pack/400g	420	105	5.9	15.5	2.2	0.5
Balsamic Onion & Chicken, Marks & Spencer*	1 Pack/375g	563	150	9.5	12.5	6.7	1.5
Beef & Chunky Vegetable, Healthy Living, Tesco*	1 Pack/340g	354	104	5.9	13.8	2.8	1.2
Beef Tomato Bechamel, Healthy Eating, Tesco*	1 Pack/425g	472	111	5.9	12.4	4.2	1.3
Beef, BGTY, Sainsbury's*	1 Pack/400g	340	85	5.3	11.3	2.1	0.6
Beef, Bird's Eye*	1 Pack/384g	515	134	7.0	12.5	6.2	0.7
Beef, Chilled, Safeway*	½ Pack/325g	452	139	7.5	11.8	5.9	1.2
Beef, Eat Smart, Safeway*	1 Pack/380g	380	100	7.6	10.9	2.7	1.3

L

LASAGNE,	Measure INFO/WEIGHT	per Measure KCAL	Nutrition Values per 100g / 100ml				
			KCAL	PROT	CARB	FAT	FIBRE
Beef, Frozen, Co-Op*	1 Pack/340g	388	114	7.5	10.7	4.6	1.4
Beef, Frozen, Findus*	1 Pack/330g	363	110	6.1	11.5	4.2	0.7
Beef, Frozen, Tesco*	1 Pack/400g	492	123	5.7	11.4	6.1	0.7
Beef, Good For You, Asda*	1 Pack/350g	385	110	9.0	14.0	2.0	1.0
Beef, Less Than 5% Fat, Asda*	1 Pack/400g	460	115	5.0	14.0	4.3	0.6
Beef, Morrisons*	1 Pack/400g	596	149	6.3	11.9	8.4	0.3
Beef, Organic, Tesco*	1 Pack/350g	389	111	6.2	11.5	4.5	0.7
Beef, Ready Meals, Waitrose*	1 Pack/325g	471	145	6.7	13.1	7.3	1.4
Beef, Reduced Fat, Waitrose*	1 Pack/325g	345	106	5.5	12.1	4.0	0.8
Beef, Weight Watchers*	1 Pack/300g	297	99	7.4	11.0	2.8	0.7
Better For You, Morrisons*	1 Pack/350g	340	97	7.1	8.6	4.0	0.2
Bird's Eye*	1 Pack/375g	420	112	6.1	11.6	4.6	0.7
Boiled	1oz/28g	28	100	3.0	22.0	0.6	0.9
Bolognese, Co-Op*	1 Pack/500g	758	152	8.1	13.8	7.1	0.0
COU, Marks & Spencer*	1 Pack/360g	324	90	6.9	11.7	1.7	1.0
Chicken, Italian, Sainsbury's*	1 Pack/450g	549	122	8.4	12.6	4.2	0.5
Chicken, Ready Meals, Waitrose*	1 Pack/300g	411	137	6.3	13.0	6.6	0.9
Chicken, Safeway*	1 Pack/400g	420	105	7.2	8.6	4.6	1.1
Classic, Deep Filled, Marks & Spencer*	1 Pack/400g	760	190	10.0	11.2	11.9	0.6
Dried, Napolina*	1oz/28g	99	352	11.5	73.0	1.5	2.2
Extra Special, Asda*	½ Pack/290.9g	416	143	7.0	13.0	7.0	0.3
Family, Marks & Spencer*	¼ Pack/225g	281	125	10.3	6.9	6.2	1.1
Finest, Tesco*	½ Pack/300g	432	144	7.4	13.1	6.9	0.5
Fresh, Findus*	1 Pack/350g	403	115	6.2	11.7	4.5	0.0
GFY, Asda*	1 Pack/410g	328	80	4.8	11.0	1.9	0.2
Good Intentions, Somerfield*	1 Pack/300g	303	101	5.3	13.9	2.7	0.4
Healthy Eating, Tesco*	1 Pack/340g	343	101	5.1	13.4	3.0	0.9
Healthy Living, Tesco*	1 Pack/425g	451	106	5.5	13.5	3.3	1.2
Italia, Marks & Spencer*	1 Pack/400g	640	160	8.2	10.7	9.5	0.8
Italian, Sainsbury's*	1 Pack/450g	639	142	8.7	14.2	5.6	0.6
Italiano, Tesco*	1 Pack/425g	595	140	8.0	12.0	6.7	0.5
Layered, Asda*	1 Pack/300g	444	148	5.0	14.0	8.0	0.3
Lidl*	1 Serving/200g	336	168	8.0	13.7	9.0	0.0
Low Fat, Co-Op*	1 Pack/300g	255	85	6.0	10.0	3.0	1.0
Meat, Somerfield*	1 Pack/600g	768	128	6.0	12.0	6.0	0.0
Mediterranean Vegetable, COU, Marks & Spencer*	1 Pack/360g	306	85	3.4	11.5	2.7	1.4
Mega Value, Tesco*	1 Pack/600g	726	121	4.7	12.2	5.9	0.5
Pizza Hut*	1 Serving/350g	669	191	11.3	17.8	8.3	2.7
Primana, Aldi*	1 Serving/250g	423	169	8.0	14.0	9.0	0.0
Quorn*	1 Pack/300g	249	83	4.1	9.9	3.0	1.3
Quorn, Safeway*	1 Pack/400g	360	90	4.9	10.4	3.2	1.7
Ready Meal, Marks & Spencer*	1 Pack/360g	594	165	11.3	11.7	8.2	1.3
Roasted Mushroom & Spinach, COU, Marks & Spencer*	1 Pack/360g	288	80	5.0	12.1	1.2	1.1
Safeway*	1 Pack/300g	354	118	5.7	11.5	5.5	0.5
Sainsbury's*	1 Pack/300g	339	113	5.2	12.2	4.8	1.3
Salmon & Spinach, Tesco*	1 Pack/400g	292	73	4.9	10.0	1.5	0.8
Sheets, Egg Verdi, Tesco*	1 Serving/50g	177	354	13.0	69.1	2.8	3.0
Sheets, Egg, Italian, Fresh, Sainsbury's*	2 Sheets/85g	150	176	6.7	32.1	2.3	1.5
Sheets, Fresh, Asda*	½ Pack/125g	188	150	6.0	29.0	1.1	0.0
Sheets, Fresh, Somerfield*	1oz/28g	76	270	11.0	56.0	1.0	0.0
Sheets, Fresh, Tesco*	1 Serving/150g	410	273	11.0	50.6	2.9	2.9
Sheets, Italian, Dried, Sainsbury's*	1 Serving/90g	321	357	12.3	73.1	1.7	2.5
Sheets, Organic, Iceland*	2 Sheets/34g	118	348	12.5	69.9	2.0	3.6

L

	Measure INFO/WEIGHT	per Measure KCAL	Nutrition Values per 100g / 100ml KCAL	PROT	CARB	FAT	FIBRE
LASAGNE,							
Sheets, SmartPrice. Asda*	1 Sheet/13g	46	353	11.0	75.0	1.0	3.0
Sheets, Tesco*	1oz/28g	97	346	12.0	72.3	1.0	2.8
Sheets, Uncooked, Co-Op*	1 Sheet/16g	55	345	12.0	72.0	1.0	3.0
Sheets, Value, Tesco*	1oz/28g	95	341	11.0	72.0	1.0	3.0
Sheets, Verdi, No Pre-Cook, Sainsbury's*	1oz/28g	100	357	12.3	73.1	1.7	2.5
Spinach & Cheese, Italian, Sainsbury's*	1 Pack/450g	666	148	6.0	15.5	6.8	0.5
Spinach & Ricotta, Finest, Tesco*	1 Pack/350g	585	167	6.1	11.7	10.6	1.2
Triangles With Chicken, COU, Marks & Spencer*	1 Pack/360g	324	90	7.8	11.9	1.8	1.0
Triple Cheese Spicy Vegetable, The Little Big Food Co.*	1 Pack/360g	472	131	5.8	15.0	5.8	0.8
Value, Tesco*	1 Pack/500g	630	126	4.4	13.7	5.9	0.5
Vegetable	1oz/28g	29	102	4.1	12.4	4.4	1.0
Vegetable, BGTY, Sainsbury's*	1 Pack/400g	286	72	4.8	9.5	1.6	1.4
Vegetable, Eat Smart, Safeway*	1 Pack/380g	266	70	3.5	10.8	1.3	1.4
Vegetable, Findus*	1 Pack/330g	314	95	4.0	13.0	2.5	0.0
Vegetable, Italian Three Layer, Sainsbury's*	1 Pack/450g	554	123	4.8	14.3	5.2	0.5
Vegetable, Italiano, Tesco*	1 Pack/340g	286	84	2.8	11.9	2.8	1.0
Vegetable, Linda McCartney*	1 Pack/320g	374	117	7.0	14.2	3.5	1.9
Vegetable, Low Fat, Co-Op*	1 Pack/300g	195	65	4.0	10.0	2.0	1.0
Vegetable, Luxury Roasted, Safeway*	1 Pack/400g	492	123	3.4	15.8	5.1	1.1
Vegetable, Mediterranean Style, Eat Smart, Safeway*	1 Pack/380g	228	60	3.0	10.1	0.8	1.5
Vegetable, Mediterranean, Linda McCartney*	1 Pack/320g	333	104	3.2	15.8	3.1	1.5
Vegetable, Mediterranean, Waitrose*	1 Pack/351g	397	113	3.7	12.7	5.3	1.0
Vegetable, Morrisons*	1 Pack/400g	464	116	3.8	12.3	5.7	0.7
Vegetable, Somerfield*	1 Pack/298g	185	62	2.5	4.6	3.7	1.4
Vegetable, Two Layered, BGTY, Sainsbury's*	1 Pack/400g	288	72	4.8	9.5	1.6	1.4
Vegetable, Value, Tesco*	1 Pack/500g	410	82	4.1	9.7	3.0	2.3
Vegetable, Weight Watchers*	1 Pack/330g	251	76	3.6	11.8	1.7	0.7
Vegetarian, Tesco*	1 Pack/430g	581	135	5.3	13.6	6.6	1.0
LAVERBREAD, Average	1oz/28g	15	52	3.2	1.6	3.7	0.0
LEEKS,							
Baby, Tesco*	1 Pack/175g	40	23	1.6	2.9	0.5	2.2
Boiled in Salted Water	1oz/28g	6	21	1.2	2.6	0.7	1.7
Boiled in Unsalted Water	1oz/28g	6	21	1.2	2.6	0.7	1.7
Creamed, Frozen, Waitrose*	1 Serving/225g	115	51	1.8	5.5	2.4	0.0
Cut, Farmfoods*	1oz/28g	6	23	1.6	2.9	0.5	2.2
Prepared, Marks & Spencer*	1oz/28g	9	31	1.9	6.0	0.0	3.1
Raw	1oz/28g	6	22	1.6	2.9	0.5	2.2
LEMON, Fresh, Raw	1 Slice/5g	0	7	0.3	1.6	0.0	1.7
LEMON & LIME, Light, Oasis*	1 Bottle/250ml	7	3	0.0	0.2	0.0	0.0
LEMON & MANDARIN, Diet Quest, St Michael*	1 Bottle/330ml	13	4	0.0	1.0	0.0	0.0
LEMON BREEZER, Diet, Bacardi*	1 Bottle/275ml	96	35	0.0	1.2	0.0	0.0
LEMON CURD,							
Asda*	1 Tbsp/15g	44	293	1.0	61.0	5.0	0.2
Average	1 Tbsp/15g	42	283	0.6	62.7	5.0	0.2
Luxury, Sainsbury's*	1 Tbsp/15g	49	329	2.8	60.1	8.6	0.2
Luxury, Waitrose*	1 Tbsp/15g	52	344	3.2	60.1	10.1	0.0
Tesco*	1 Tbsp/15g	45	298	0.6	62.5	4.8	0.0
Waitrose*	1 Tbsp/15g	45	301	0.6	65.3	4.1	0.1
LEMON DRINK, No Added Sugar, Somerfield*	1 Glass/200ml	12	6	0.0	1.0	0.0	0.0
LEMON JUICE,							
Co-Op*	1fl oz/30ml	8	25	0.3	2.0	0.1	0.0
Fresh	1 Tsp/5ml	0	7	0.3	1.6	0.0	0.1

L

	Measure INFO/WEIGHT	per Measure KCAL	Nutrition Values per 100g / 100ml				
			KCAL	PROT	CARB	FAT	FIBRE
LEMON SOLE,							
& Butter, Marks & Spencer*	1oz/28g	49	174	15.1	0.1	12.6	0.0
Breadcrumbs, Marks & Spencer*	1oz/28g	63	225	11.2	17.1	12.7	0.7
Fillets, Chunky Breaded, Tesco*	1 Portion/160g	366	229	10.6	21.1	11.3	0.9
Fillets, Chunky, Boneless, Sainsbury's*	1 Fillet/160g	329	207	12.8	13.5	11.3	1.9
Fillets, In A Light Crispy Crumb, Iceland*	1 Fillet/150g	422	281	15.5	21.8	14.6	0.0
Fillets, Lightly Dusted, Marks & Spencer*	1 Fillet/112.5g	181	160	13.9	10.0	7.7	1.0
Fillets, Marks & Spencer*	½ Pack/110g	193	175	15.1	0.1	12.6	0.0
Fillets, Sainsbury's*	1 Serving/100g	98	98	20.2	0.0	1.7	0.0
Fillets, Tesco*	1 Serving/156g	129	83	17.4	0.0	1.5	0.0
Grilled	1oz/28g	27	97	20.2	0.0	1.7	0.0
Raw	1oz/28g	23	83	17.4	0.0	1.5	0.0
Steamed	1oz/28g	25	91	20.6	0.0	0.9	0.0
in Crumbs, Fried	1oz/28g	60	216	16.1	9.3	13.0	0.4
LEMON SOLE - GOUJONS,							
Boneless, Sainsbury's*	1 Serving/100g	250	250	16.2	20.7	11.4	0.8
Fried in Blended Oil	1oz/28g	105	374	15.5	14.3	28.7	0.0
Marks & Spencer*	1 Serving/100g	235	235	15.0	13.7	13.4	1.2
With Citrus Mayonnaise, Tesco*	1 Serving/250g	610	244	11.7	19.6	13.2	0.8
in Breadcrumbs, Youngs*	1 Serving/150g	339	226	12.2	20.3	10.6	1.1
LEMONADE,							
7-Up, Light, Britvic*	1 Can/330ml	4	1	0.1	0.2	0.0	0.0
Asda*	1 Glass/250ml	83	33	0.0	8.0	0.0	0.0
Cloudy, Diet, Safeway*	1 Can/330ml	7	2	0.0	0.2	0.0	0.0
Cloudy, Diet, Sainsbury's*	1 Can/330ml	7	2	0.1	0.2	0.1	0.3
Cloudy, Sainsbury's*	1 Glass/250ml	118	47	0.1	12.0	0.1	0.1
Diet, Asda*	1 Glass/250ml	3	1	0.0	0.1	0.1	0.0
Diet, Lilt Light, The Coca Cola Co*	1fl oz/30ml	1	3	0.0	0.4	0.0	0.0
Diet, Schweppes*	1 Bottle/500ml	8	2	0.0	0.0	0.0	0.0
Diet, Traditional Style, Sainsbury's*	1 Glass/250ml	8	3	0.1	0.2	0.1	0.1
Diet, Traditional Style, Tesco*	1 Glass/200ml	6	3	0.0	0.8	0.0	0.0
Fresh Squeezed, Marks & Spencer*	1 Bottle/250ml	113	45	0.1	11.8	0.0	0.0
Juice Drink, Asda*	1 Glass/200ml	88	44	0.1	11.0	0.0	0.0
Lime, Safeway*	1 Can/144ml	63	44	0.0	10.6	0.0	0.0
Shapers, Boots*	1 Bottle/500ml	13	3	0.0	0.0	0.0	0.0
Somerfield*	½ Pint/296ml	80	27	0.0	7.0	0.0	0.0
Sprite, Light, Sprite*	1fl oz/30ml	0	2	0.0	0.0	0.0	0.0
Sprite, McDonald's*	1 Regular/251ml	108	43	0.0	10.5	0.0	0.0
Still, Marks & Spencer*	1 Glass/250ml	5	49	0.1	12.9	0.0	0.0
Still, Tesco*	1 Glass/200ml	100	50	0.0	12.0	0.0	0.0
Traditional Style, Tesco*	1 Glass/200ml	100	50	0.0	12.3	0.0	0.0
LEMONCELLO, Asda*	1 Pot/89.3g	191	215	4.6	29.0	9.0	0.2
LENTILS,							
Continental, Dried, Tesco*	1 Serving/50g	146	292	24.4	44.4	1.9	8.9
Green & Brown, Whole, Dried, Boiled in Salted Water	1oz/28g	29	105	8.8	16.9	0.7	3.8
Green & Brown, Whole, Dried, Raw	1oz/28g	83	297	24.3	48.8	1.9	8.9
Green In Water, Sainsbury's*	1 Serving/133g	145	109	8.8	16.9	0.7	3.8
Green, Dried, Tesco*	1 Serving/227g	708	312	20.4	55.6	0.9	10.6
Green, Organic, Evernat*	1oz/28g	87	312	20.4	55.6	0.9	10.6
Green, Tesco*	1 Can/195g	125	64	5.0	10.2	0.4	2.3
Red, Organic, Evernat*	1oz/28g	87	312	23.8	51.3	1.3	4.9
Red, Split, Dried, Boiled in Unsalted Water	1oz/28g	28	100	7.6	17.5	0.4	1.9
Red, Split, Dried, Raw	1oz/28g	89	318	23.8	56.3	1.3	4.9

L

INFO/WEIGHT	Measure per Measure KCAL	KCAL	PROT	CARB	FAT	FIBRE

LETTUCE,

Food	Measure / Weight	per Measure KCAL	KCAL	PROT	CARB	FAT	FIBRE
Average, Raw	1oz/28g	4	14	0.8	1.7	0.5	0.9
Chinese Leaf, Tesco*	1 Serving/200g	36	18	3.5	0.3	0.3	2.6
Hearts Of Tomaine, Sainsbury's*	1oz/28g	4	16	1.0	1.7	0.6	1.2
Iceberg, Herbs, Marks & Spencer*	1oz/28g	4	14	0.8	1.8	0.4	0.8
Iceberg, Morrisons*	1 Serving/100g	13	13	0.7	1.9	0.3	0.0
Iceberg, Prepared, Marks & Spencer*	1oz/28g	4	13	0.7	1.9	0.3	0.6
Iceberg, Shredded, Asda*	1 Serving/100g	13	13	0.7	1.8	0.3	0.6
Iceberg, Shredded, Sainsbury's*	1oz/28g	4	13	0.7	1.8	0.3	0.6
Iceberg, Somerfield*	1oz/28g	4	13	1.0	2.0	0.0	0.0
Iceburg, Crisp & Crunchy, Tesco*	1 Serving/100g	13	13	0.7	1.9	0.3	0.6
Lamb's, Sainsbury's*	1 Serving/25g	4	14	1.9	1.4	0.0	1.0
Lambs, Waitrose*	½ Pack/20g	3	15	0.8	1.7	0.5	0.9
Leafy, Tesco*	1 Serving/20g	3	14	1.2	1.5	0.4	1.9
Romaine, Organic, Tesco*	½ Lettuce/100g	15	15	0.8	1.7	0.5	0.9
Round, Tesco*	1 Serving/100g	15	15	1.0	1.7	0.5	0.0
Sweet Romaine, Safeway*	1 Serving/50g	8	15	0.8	1.7	0.5	0.0

LIME JUICE,

Food	Measure / Weight	per Measure KCAL	KCAL	PROT	CARB	FAT	FIBRE
Cordial, Diluted, Co-Op*	1fl oz/30ml	8	25	0.0	4.0	0.0	0.0
Cordial, Concentrated	1floz/30ml	34	112	0.1	29.8	0.0	0.0
Cordial, Diluted	1 Glass/250ml	55	22	0.0	6.0	0.0	0.0
Cordial, Diluted, Princes*	1fl oz/30ml	8	27	0.0	4.3	0.0	0.0
Fresh	1 Tsp/5ml	0.5	9	0.4	1.6	0.1	0.1
LIMEADE, Sugar Free, Sparkling, Safeway*	1fl oz/30ml	0	1	0.1	0.1	0.1	0.0

LINGUINE,

Food	Measure / Weight	per Measure KCAL	KCAL	PROT	CARB	FAT	FIBRE
Authentic Italian, Tesco*	1 Serving/100g	345	345	13.2	68.5	2.0	2.9
King Prawn, Meal for One, Marks & Spencer*	1 Pack/400g	380	95	6.6	13.1	1.7	2.2
Pomodoro, Marks & Spencer*	1 Pack/300g	360	120	4.1	17.6	3.5	1.2
Sainsbury's*	1 Serving/50g	179	357	12.3	73.1	1.7	2.5
Sun Dried Tomato & Egg, Asda*	1 Serving/200g	324	162	7.0	28.0	2.4	3.9
Tomato & Mushroom, Perfectly Balanced, Waitrose*	1 Pack/350g	294	84	2.2	10.6	3.8	1.0
Vegetable & Ham, BGTY, Sainsbury's*	1 Pack/450g	410	91	4.4	11.7	3.0	0.9
Egg, Fresh, Waitrose*	1 Pack/250g	680	272	11.4	49.4	3.2	5.1
LINSEED, Golden, Organic, Evernat*	1oz/28g	127	452	22.0	6.0	38.0	25.0
LINSEEDS, Chopped, Risetti*	1 Serving/5g	22	448	23.0	38.0	22.0	31.0

LION BAR,

Food	Measure / Weight	per Measure KCAL	KCAL	PROT	CARB	FAT	FIBRE
Mini, Nestle*	1 Bar/16g	80	486	4.6	67.7	21.7	0.0
Nestle*	1 Bar/55g	260	472	4.7	64.5	21.7	0.0
Peanut, Nestle*	1 Bar/49g	256	522	7.1	56.9	29.6	0.0

LIQUEURS,

Food	Measure / Weight	per Measure KCAL	KCAL	PROT	CARB	FAT	FIBRE
Cream	1 Shot/25ml	81	325	0.0	22.8	16.1	0.0
High Strength	1 Shot/25ml	79	314	0.0	24.4	0.0	0.0

LIQUORICE,

Food	Measure / Weight	per Measure KCAL	KCAL	PROT	CARB	FAT	FIBRE
Allsorts, Average	1 Sm Bag/56g	195	349	3.7	76.7	5.2	2.0
Allsorts, Bassett's*	1 Pack/225g	792	352	2.3	75.5	4.5	1.6
Catherine Wheels, Sainsbury's*	1 Wheel/17g	49	286	3.8	67.2	0.3	0.7
Comfits, Marks & Spencer*	1oz/28g	100	357	2.4	86.2	0.3	0.7
Shapes, Average	1oz/28g	78	278	5.5	65.0	1.4	1.9
Panda*	1 Bar/32g	109	340	3.8	78.0	0.5	0.0

LIVER,

Food	Measure / Weight	per Measure KCAL	KCAL	PROT	CARB	FAT	FIBRE
Calves, Fried	1oz/28g	49	176	22.3	0.0	9.6	0.0
Calves, Raw	1oz/28g	29	104	18.3	0.0	3.4	0.0
Calves, With Fresh Sage Butter, Marks & Spencer*	1 Serving/116.7g	211	180	12.8	10.1	10.7	1.5
Calves, With Garlic Butter, Marks & Spencer*	1oz/28g	56	200	13.3	7.3	13.5	0.4

L

	Measure INFO/WEIGHT	per Measure KCAL	Nutrition Values per 100g / 100ml				
			KCAL	PROT	CARB	FAT	FIBRE
LIVER,							
Chicken, Fried	1oz/28g	47	169	22.1	0.0	8.9	0.0
Chicken, Raw	1oz/28g	26	92	17.7	0.0	2.3	0.0
Lamb's With Onions, Marks & Spencer*	1oz/28g	52	185	14.1	6.8	11.3	0.1
Lamb's, Fried	1oz/28g	66	237	30.1	0.0	12.9	0.0
Lamb's, Raw	1oz/28g	38	137	20.3	0.0	6.2	0.0
Lamb's, Tesco*	1 Serving/125g	171	137	20.3	0.0	6.2	0.0
Ox, Raw	1oz/28g	43	155	21.1	0.0	7.8	0.0
Ox, Stewed	1oz/28g	55	198	24.8	3.6	9.5	0.0
Pig's, Raw	1oz/28g	32	113	21.3	0.0	3.1	0.0
Pig's, Stewed	1 Serving/70g	132	189	25.6	3.6	8.1	0.0
LIVER &,							
Bacon With Fresh Mashed Potato, Waitrose*	1 Pack/400g	512	128	6.9	10.2	6.6	0.8
Bacon with Creamy Mash, Good For You, Asda*	1 Pack/385.9g	355	92	7.0	10.0	2.7	1.8
Bacon, British Classics, Tesco*	1 Pack/400g	496	124	10.7	7.1	5.9	0.7
, Marks & Spencer*	1 Serving/200g	250	125	7.6	10.5	6.0	0.9
LIVER SAUSAGE,							
Asda*	1oz/28g	57	204	17.0	2.0	14.2	0.4
Sainsbury's*	1 Slice/13g	27	212	14.4	4.7	15.1	0.5
Sliced, Somerfield*	1 Slice/11g	27	247	14.0	5.0	19.0	0.0
Value, Tesco*	1 Slice/10g	20	200	15.8	6.1	12.5	0.0
LOBSTER,							
Boiled	1oz/28g	29	103	22.1	0.0	1.6	0.0
Breaded Squat With Lemon Mayonnaise Dip, Tesco*	1 Pack/210g	506	241	9.0	19.0	14.4	0.5
Cooked, Asda*	1oz/28g	32	115	22.1	0.0	3.4	0.0
Dressed, John West*	1 Can/43g	45	105	13.0	2.0	5.0	0.0
Dressed, Marks & Spencer*	1oz/28g	76	273	14.3	0.8	23.6	0.1
Half, Marks & Spencer*	1oz/28g	66	235	12.1	2.4	19.6	0.2
LOGANBERRIES, Raw	1oz/28g	5	17	1.1	3.4	0.0	2.5
LOLLIPOPS,							
Assorted Flavours, Asda*	1 Lolly/7g	27	380	0.0	95.0	0.0	0.0
Assorted, Co-Op*	1 Lolly/10g	40	400	0.0	97.0	0.0	0.0
Chupa Chups*	1 Lolly/18g	72	400	0.6	97.2	0.6	0.0
LONGANS, Canned, In Syrup, Drained	1oz/28g	19	67	0.4	17.1	0.3	0.0
LOQUATS, Raw	1oz/28g	8	28	0.7	6.3	0.2	0.0
LUCOZADE,							
Hydro Active, Smithkline Beecham*	1fl oz/30ml	3	10	0.0	2.0	0.0	0.0
Orange Energy Drink, Smithkline Beecham*	1 Bottle/500ml	350	70	0.0	17.2	0.0	0.0
Original, Smithkline Beecham*	1 Bottle/345ml	252	73	0.0	17.9	0.0	0.0
Sport Isotonic Lemon Body Fuel, Smithkline Beecham*	1 Bottle/500ml	140	28	0.0	6.4	0.0	0.0
Sport, Orange, SmithKline Beecham*	1 Bottle/500ml	140	28	0.0	6.4	0.0	0.1
Tropical, SmithKline Beecham*	1 Bottle/380ml	266	70	0.0	17.2	0.0	0.0
LUNCHEON MEAT,							
Pork, John West*	1oz/28g	83	297	13.0	5.0	25.0	0.0
Pork, Slices, Asda*	1oz/28g	78	280	12.9	3.0	24.0	0.0
Pork, Tesco*	1 Slice/14g	40	287	14.0	4.0	23.9	0.0
LYCHEES,							
Canned, In Syrup	1oz/28g	19	68	0.4	17.7	0.0	0.5
Fresh, Raw	1oz/28g	16	58	0.9	14.3	0.1	0.7
In Juice, Amoy*	1oz/28g	13	46	0.4	10.9	0.0	0.0
In Syrup, John West*	½ Can/100g	72	72	0.4	17.7	0.0	0.6
Lotus, In Syrup, Amoy	1oz/28g	19	68	0.4	17.7	0.0	0.0
Raw, Weighed With Skin & Stone	1oz/28g	10	36	0.5	8.9	0.1	0.4

L

	Measure INFO/WEIGHT	per Measure KCAL	Nutrition Values per 100g / 100ml KCAL	PROT	CARB	FAT	FIBRE
M&M'S,							
Mars*	1 Funsize/20g	97	487	4.7	69.6	21.1	0.0
Mini, Mars*	1 Sm Pack/36g	176	489	6.3	63.6	23.2	0.0
Peanut, Mars*	1 Pack/45g	231	514	10.2	57.3	27.1	0.0
Plain, Mars*	1 Pack/48g	240	499	4.1	70.7	20.8	2.1
MACADAMIA NUTS, Salted	6 Nuts/10g	75	748	7.9	4.8	77.6	5.3
MACARONI,							
Authentic Italian, Tesco*	1 Serving/100g	354	354	11.5	72.6	1.9	2.7
Boiled	1oz/28g	24	86	3.0	18.5	0.5	0.9
Dried, Napolina*	1oz/28g	99	352	11.5	73.0	1.5	2.2
Italian, Sainsbury's*	1 Serving/100g	357	357	12.3	73.1	1.7	2.5
Quick Cook, Sainsbury's*	1oz/28g	100	357	12.3	73.1	1.7	2.5
Raw	1oz/28g	97	348	12.0	75.8	1.8	3.1
MACARONI CHEESE,							
Average	1oz/28g	50	178	7.3	13.6	10.8	0.5
BGTY, Sainsbury's*	1 Pack/450g	504	112	5.8	17.2	2.2	1.1
Bettabuy, Morrisons*	1 Serving/205g	229	112	4.3	10.8	5.7	0.4
Bird's Eye*	1 Pack/302g	374	124	4.2	15.6	5.0	0.4
Canned	1oz/28g	39	138	4.5	16.4	6.5	0.4
Chilled, Good For You, Asda*	1 Pack/442.5g	469	106	6.0	14.0	2.9	1.6
Eat Smart, Safeway*	1 Pack/315g	394	125	6.5	19.2	2.1	0.8
Findus*	1 Pack/360g	576	160	6.3	14.3	8.5	0.0
Healthy Eating, Tesco*	1 Pack/340g	252	74	6.6	6.2	2.5	0.6
Heinz*	1 Can/400g	380	95	3.4	9.8	4.7	0.3
Italian, Sainsbury's*	½ Pack/225g	360	160	7.3	15.3	7.7	1.6
Marks & Spencer*	1 Pack/400g	680	170	6.9	12.8	9.9	0.6
New, BGTY, Sainsbury's*	1 Pack/390g	441	113	5.1	18.6	2.0	2.4
Perfectly Balanced, Waitrose*	1 Pack/350g	351	100	6.7	11.4	3.1	0.5
Ross*	1 Pack/300g	327	109	4.2	16.2	3.1	1.3
Tesco*	1 Can/410g	513	125	4.5	10.1	6.3	0.3
Tinned, Sainsbury's*	1 Can/400g	428	107	5.1	12.2	4.2	0.5
Value, Tesco*	1 Pack/300g	489	163	5.7	17.3	7.9	0.7
Waitrose*	1 Pack/350g	466	133	6.8	5.2	9.4	0.0
MACKEREL,							
Arbroath Hot Smoked Scottish, Spink & Sons*	1 Serving/60g	179	298	22.2	0.0	23.2	0.0
Crushed Peppercorns, Smoked, Tesco*	1 Serving/90g	267	297	20.7	0.0	23.8	1.6
Fillets, Honey Roast Smoked, Sainsbury's*	1 Serving/100g	349	349	21.5	4.5	27.3	12.4
Fillets, Hot Smoked, Asda*	1 Serving/170g	580	341	19.0	3.3	28.0	0.6
Fillets, In Brine, Sainsbury's*	1 Can/90g	215	239	20.0	0.1	17.7	0.1
Fillets, In Mustard Sauce, Tesco*	1 Can/120g	274	228	13.9	4.7	17.1	0.0
Fillets, In Spicy Tomato Sauce, Princes*	1 Can/125g	250	200	13.6	4.7	14.1	0.0
Fillets, In Tomato Sauce, Co-Op*	1 Can/125g	219	175	14.0	2.0	12.0	0.0
Fillets, In White Wine & Spices, Connetable*	1 Can/120g	169	141	15.5	1.2	8.2	0.0
Fillets, In a Hot Chilli Sauce, Princes*	1 Serving/100g	296	296	13.3	0.0	27.0	0.0
Fillets, Peppered, Asda*	½ Pack/130g	430	331	22.0	0.0	27.0	0.0
Fillets, Peppered, John West*	½ Pack/62g	184	297	15.7	0.0	26.0	0.0
Fillets, Peppered, Marks & Spencer*	1 Serving/100g	350	350	22.4	0.0	28.7	0.6
Fillets, Peppered, Smoked, Safeway*	1 Fillet/135g	478	354	18.9	0.0	30.9	0.0
Fillets, Peppered, Smoked, Sainsbury's*	1 Serving/106g	388	366	20.8	0.6	31.1	0.1
Fillets, Princes*	1 Can/90g	244	271	19.7	0.0	21.3	0.0
Fillets, Red Pepper & Onion, Smoked, Asda*	1 Serving/90g	319	354	18.0	0.8	31.0	1.2
Fillets, Smoked, Farmfoods*	1oz/28g	99	354	18.9	0.0	30.9	0.0
Fillets, Smoked, Hand Selected, Sainsbury's*	1 Serving/100g	345	345	19.4	0.3	29.6	0.1
Fillets, Smoked, Marks & Spencer*	1oz/28g	80	284	18.1	2.6	22.4	0.1

MACKEREL,	Measure INFO/WEIGHT	per Measure KCAL	Nutrition Values per 100g / 100ml				
			KCAL	PROT	CARB	FAT	FIBRE
Fillets, Smoked, Morrisons*	1 Fillet/100g	298	298	20.3	0.2	24.1	0.6
Fillets, Smoked, Safeway*	1 Serving/95g	336	354	18.9	0.0	30.9	0.0
Fillets, Smoked, Sainsbury's*	1 Serving/100g	386	386	20.1	0.0	34.0	0.1
Fillets, Smoked, Tesco*	1 Serving/100g	297	297	19.7	0.0	24.2	0.0
Fillets, Smoked, Waitrose*	1 Fillet/100g	339	339	20.4	0.3	28.5	0.0
Fillets, Smoked, With Crushed Peppercorns, Waitrose*	1 Can/120g	385	321	18.7	1.6	26.6	0.0
Fillets, Wood Smoked, Princes*	1 Can/80g	125	156	21.0	0.0	8.0	0.0
Fillets, in Brine, Asda*	1 Can/88g	193	219	18.6	0.0	16.1	0.0
Fillets, in Brine, John West*	1 Can/94g	219	233	20.0	0.0	17.0	0.0
Fillets, in Brine, Safeway*	1 Can/125g	301	241	20.4	0.0	17.7	0.0
Fillets, in Brine, Waitrose*	1 Can/125g	278	222	18.2	0.0	16.6	0.0
Fillets, in Curry Sauce, John West*	1oz/28g	65	233	16.0	4.0	17.0	0.3
Fillets, in Green Peppercorn Sauce, John West*	1 Can/125g	329	263	14.0	4.5	21.0	0.1
Fillets, in Mustard Sauce, John West*	1oz/28g	60	215	15.0	5.0	15.0	0.2
Fillets, in Mustard Sauce, Princes*	1 Can/125g	266	213	13.6	6.0	15.0	0.0
Fillets, in Mustard Sauce, Sainsbury's*	1 Can/125g	275	220	14.0	6.0	15.0	0.0
Fillets, in Spicy Tomato Sauce, John West*	1oz/28g	55	198	15.0	3.0	14.0	0.0
Fillets, in Sunflower Oil, John West*	1 Can/94g	244	260	20.0	0.0	20.0	0.0
Fillets, in Tomato Sauce, John West*	1 Can/125g	266	213	17.0	2.5	15.0	0.1
Fillets, in Tomato Sauce, Princes*	1 Can/125g	254	203	13.6	3.3	15.0	0.0
Fillets, in Tomato Sauce, Sainsbury's*	1 Can/125g	204	163	14.0	2.0	11.0	0.1
Fried in Blended Oil	1oz/28g	76	272	24.0	0.0	19.5	0.0
Grilled	1oz/28g	67	239	20.8	0.0	17.3	0.0
Headless Gutted, Somerfield*	1oz/28g	62	220	19.0	0.0	16.0	0.0
In Brine, Skinless & Boneless, Tesco*	1 Can/100g	241	241	20.4	0.0	17.7	0.0
In Tomato Sauce	1oz/28g	58	206	16.4	1.4	15.0	0.0
In Tomato Sauce, Skinless & Boneless, Tesco*	1 Can/125g	240	192	14.1	3.4	13.6	0.0
Peppered, Arbroath Hot Smoked Scottish, Spink & Sons*	1 Serving/60g	182	303	19.7	0.1	24.2	0.0
Raw	1oz/28g	62	220	18.7	0.0	16.1	0.0
Ready to Eat, Morrisons*	1 Portion/100g	298	298	20.3	0.2	24.1	0.6
Smoked	1oz/28g	99	354	18.9	0.0	30.9	0.0
Smoked, Asda*	1 Serving/100g	331	331	22.0	0.0	27.0	0.0
Smoked, Peppered, Morrisons*	1 Serving/100g	296	296	19.9	1.4	23.5	0.6
Steak, in Brine, John West*	1oz/28g	68	243	18.0	0.0	19.0	0.0
Steak, in Tomato Sauce, John West*	1oz/28g	62	221	15.0	2.0	17.0	0.0
In Sunflower Oil, Peppered, Smoked, John West*	1oz/28g	87	311	21.0	0.5	25.0	0.5
In Sunflower Oil, Tesco*	1 Can/125g	333	266	19.7	0.0	20.8	0.0
MADRAS,							
Beef, Tesco*	1 Pack/460g	552	120	5.2	13.1	5.2	1.8
Chicken & Pilau Rice, Asda*	1 Pack/400g	588	147	8.0	13.0	7.0	1.7
Chicken, & Pilau Rice, Somerfield*	1 Pack/340g	496	146	7.0	14.0	7.0	0.0
Chicken, & Rice, Sainsbury's*	1 Pack/461.3g	572	124	5.9	19.6	2.4	0.7
Chicken, Budgens*	1 Pack/350g	553	158	10.7	3.9	11.1	1.8
Chicken, Iceland*	1 Pack/400g	376	94	7.7	4.9	4.8	1.1
Chicken, Indian, Sainsbury's*	1 Pack/400g	636	159	13.3	1.8	10.9	2.6
Chicken, Indian, Tesco*	1 Pack/350g	518	148	11.3	5.6	8.9	1.9
Chicken, Safeway*	1 Pack/350g	469	134	13.4	4.0	7.2	1.8
Chicken, Tesco*	1 Pack/350g	326	93	10.6	3.6	4.1	0.6
Chicken, Vite Fait*	1 Pack/300g	372	124	14.0	3.5	6.0	0.0
Chicken, Waitrose*	1oz/28g	47	168	14.6	3.7	10.5	1.8
MAGIC STARS, Milky Way, Mars*	1 Pack/33.0g	172	522	6.9	58.5	28.9	0.0
MAGNUM,							
Almond, Wall's*	1 Bar/86g	190	221	3.4	19.4	14.4	0.0

INFO/WEIGHT	Measure per Measure KCAL		Nutrition Values per 100g / 100ml				
			KCAL	PROT	CARB	FAT	FIBRE
MAGNUM,							
Caramel & Nuts Bar, Walls*	1 Bar/60g	132	220	4.0	19.0	15.0	0.0
Classic, Snack Size, Wall's*	1 Serving/50g	170	340	4.4	31.6	21.8	0.0
Classic, Wall's*	1 Bar/86g	170	198	2.6	18.4	12.7	0.0
Gluttony, Wall's*	1 Lolly/110ml	425	386	4.5	32.7	26.4	0.0
Greed, Wall's*	1 Bar/110ml	307	279	3.6	29.1	16.4	0.0
White, Wall's*	1 Bar/86g	173	201	2.6	19.4	12.6	0.0
MAKHANI,							
Chicken Tikka & Pilau Rice, BGTY, Sainsbury's*	1 Pack/400g	448	112	8.3	17.5	1.0	1.9
Chicken Tikka, Waitrose*	1 Pack/400g	644	161	13.2	4.2	10.1	1.8
Chicken Tikka, With Pilau Rice, BGTY, Sainsbuy's*	1 Pack/450g	428	95	7.8	12.7	1.4	0.9
Chicken, Sainsbury's*	½ Pack/199.4g	312	157	12.2	2.9	10.7	2.5
MALTESERS,							
Mars*	1 Sm Pack/37g	183	494	10.0	61.4	23.1	0.0
White Chocolate, Mars*	1 Pack/37g	186	504	7.9	61.0	25.4	0.0
MANDARIN ORANGES,							
Canned, In Juice	1oz/28g	9	32	0.7	7.7	0.0	0.3
Canned, In Syrup	1oz/28g	15	52	0.5	13.4	0.0	0.2
In Fruit Juice, Waitrose*	1 Can/295g	112	38	0.6	9.0	0.0	0.0
In Light Syrup, Del Monte*	1 Can/298g	182	61	0.6	13.9	0.1	0.0
Segments, Broken, SmartPrice, Asda*	½ Can/85g	46	54	0.5	13.0	0.0	0.3
Segments, In Fruit Juice, Sainsbury's*	1 Pack/175g	77	44	0.7	10.0	0.1	0.4
Segments, In Mandarin Juice, Co-Op*	½ Can/149g	49	33	0.7	7.6	0.0	0.3
Segments, In Natural Juice, John West*	¼ Can/102g	43	42	0.6	10.0	0.0	0.8
Segments, In Natural Juice, Morrisons*	1 Can/298g	125	42	0.6	10.0	0.0	1.5
Segments, In Natural Juice, Tesco*	½ Can/149g	51	34	0.7	7.7	0.0	0.3
Segments, In Orange Juice, Asda*	½ Can/149g	52	35	0.7	8.0	0.0	0.3
Segments, Spanish, Sainsbury's*	1oz/28g	12	44	0.7	10.0	0.1	0.4
Segments, in Juice, Safeway*	1 Serving/240g	115	48	1.2	10.8	0.0	0.3
Segments, in Light Syrup, Princes*	1 Can /175g	88	50	0.6	12.0	0.1	0.3
Tesco*	1 Serving/150g	59	39	0.9	8.7	0.1	1.2
Without Peel	1 Small/50g	17	34	0.9	8.0	0.1	1.3
MANGE TOUT,							
Boiled in Salted Water	1oz/28g	7	26	3.2	3.3	0.1	2.2
Raw	1oz/28g	9	32	3.6	4.2	0.2	2.3
Safeway*	1 Serving/25g	8	33	3.6	4.2	0.2	0.0
Stir-Fried in Blended Oil	1oz/28g	20	71	3.8	3.5	4.8	2.4
MANGO,							
Chunks, Fully Prepared, Sainsbury's*	½ Pack/125g	76	61	0.7	14.1	0.2	2.6
Fresh, Marks & Spencer*	1 Pack/200g	120	60	0.7	14.1	0.2	2.6
Fresh, Waitrose*	1 Serving/200g	118	59	0.7	14.1	0.2	2.6
Pieces, Freshly Prepared, Waitrose*	1 Serving/100g	59	59	0.7	14.1	0.2	2.6
Pineapple & Passionfruit, Marks & Spencer*	1 Pack/400g	200	50	0.6	10.9	0.2	1.7
Ripe, Canned, In Syrup	1oz/28g	22	77	0.3	20.3	0.0	0.7
Ripe, Raw	1oz/28g	16	57	0.7	14.1	0.2	2.6
Ripe, Raw, Weighed With Skin & Stone	1oz/28g	11	39	0.5	9.6	0.1	1.8
Slices, Amoy*	1 Can/425g	327	77	0.3	20.3	0.0	0.9
Slices, In Syrup, Sainsbury's*	1 Serving/255g	217	85	0.2	20.8	0.1	1.1
TTD, Sainsbury's*	1oz/28g	17	61	0.7	14.1	0.2	2.6
Unripe, Raw	1 Slice/40g	18	46	0.5	11.2	0.2	2.9
MANGO & APPLE JUICE, Copella*	1 Serving/200ml	86	43	0.4	10.1	0.1	0.0
MANGO JUICE, Canned	1 Glass/200ml	78	39	0.1	9.8	0.2	0.0
MARGARINE,							
Average	Thin Spread/7g	52	739	0.2	1.0	81.6	0.0

Measure INFO/WEIGHT	per Measure KCAL	Nutrition Values per 100g / 100ml				
		KCAL	PROT	CARB	FAT	FIBRE
MARGARINE,						
Best For Baking, Asda*	1 Tsp/10g	66	659	0.1	0.5	73.0	0.0
Cooking, Organic, Evernat*	1oz/28g	202	720	0.0	0.0	80.0	0.0
Flora*	1 Serving/8g	42	531	0.0	0.0	59.0	0.0
Low Fat, Asda*	1 Serving/10g	35	346	1.0	0.0	38.0	0.0
Olive, Light, Good For You, Asda*	1 Thin Spread/4g	14	344	0.1	0.5	38.0	0.0
Soya, Granose*	1oz/28g	209	745	0.1	0.1	82.0	0.0
Spread, Clover*	Thin Spread/7g	46	654	0.6	0.2	72.0	0.0
Stork*, Packet	1oz/28g	202	720	0.0	0.1	80.0	0.0
Stork*, Tub	1 Tbsp/14g	92	658	0.1	0.1	73.0	0.0
Sunflower, Granose*	Thin Spread/7g	50	720	0.0	0.0	84.0	0.0
MARINADE,						
Barbecue, COU, Marks & Spencer*	1 Serving/35g	53	150	1.2	35.5	0.2	1.0
Barbecue, In Minutes, Knorr*	1 Pack/110g	337	306	6.2	66.4	1.3	3.4
Chinese, Classic, Sharwood's*	1oz/28g	32	113	1.8	16.1	4.8	1.0
Hot & Spicy Barbecue, Marks & Spencer*	1 Serving/18g	23	130	1.0	31.1	0.3	0.8
Sun Dried Tomato & Basil With Peri-Peri, Nando's*	1 Bottle/270g	319	118	0.1	15.3	9.5	0.8
Thai Coconut, Coriander & Lime, Lea & Perrins*	1oz/28g	45	159	1.3	25.7	6.1	0.0
Tomato & Herb, Lea & Perrins*	1oz/28g	28	100	1.2	24.1	0.5	0.0
White Wine, Garlic & Pepper, Lea & Perrins*	1oz/28g	28	99	0.1	23.7	0.7	0.0
MARJORAM, Dried	1 Tsp/0.6g	3	271	12.7	42.5	7.0	0.0
MARLIN,						
Steaks, Chargrilled, Sainsbury's*	1 Serving/240g	367	153	23.6	0.8	6.1	0.6
Steaks, Raw, Sainsbury's*	1 Steak/110g	109	99	24.3	0.0	0.2	0.0
MARMALADE,						
25% Less Sugar, Asda*	1 Tsp/15g	28	185	0.4	45.6	0.0	0.9
Breakfast Orange, Smartprice, Asda*	1 Tsp/5g	13	257	0.2	64.0	0.0	0.5
Breakfast, Chivers*	1 Tsp/15g	39	260	0.3	64.7	0.0	0.6
Breakfast, Fine Cut, Frank Cooper*	1 Tsp/15g	37	249	0.2	61.9	0.0	0.3
Christmas Orange & Whisky, Marks & Spencer*	1oz/28g	67	240	0.3	59.5	0.2	1.9
Five Fruit, Tesco*	1 Serving/10g	28	278	0.2	68.2	0.1	0.9
Ginger Preserve, Sainsbury's*	1 Tspn/12gm	32	264	0.1	66.0	0.1	0.5
Golden Shred, Light, Robinso'n*	1 Serving/10g	21	210	0.2	52.3	0.0	0.0
Golden Shred, Robertson's*	1 Tsp/15g	38	253	0.2	62.3	0.0	0.0
Grapefruit & Cranberry, Marks & Spencer*	1 Tsp/15g	36	240	0.3	60.3	0.0	1.5
Grapefruit, Fine Cut, Duerr's	1 Tsp/15g	39	261	0.2	65.0	0.0	0.0
Lemon & Lime, Marks & Spencer*	1 Tsp/15g	41	274	0.1	67.9	0.2	0.8
Lemon & Lime, Roses*	1 Tsp/20g	52	260	0.2	64.8	0.0	0.0
Lemon Jelly, No Peel, Tesco*	1 Tsp/15g	39	263	0.1	65.0	0.0	0.4
Lemon Shred, Somerfield*	1 Tsp/15g	39	260	0.0	65.0	0.0	0.0
Lime Shred, Asda*	1 Tbsp/15g	38	253	0.1	63.0	0.1	0.3
Lime Shred, Sainsbury's*	1 Tsp/15g	40	269	0.2	67.0	0.1	0.4
Olde English, Chivers*	1 Tsp/15g	41	276	0.3	68.7	0.0	0.6
Orange & Ginger, Sainsbury's*	1 Tsp/15.1g	40	265	0.2	66.0	0.1	0.4
Orange & Ginger, Thick Cut, Waitrose*	1 Serving/10g	26	262	0.4	65.0	0.0	0.0
Orange & Lemon, Reduced Sugar, Zest*	1 Tsp/6g	12	195	0.3	47.1	0.2	0.0
Orange Jelly, Shredless, Sainsbury's*	1 Tsp/15g	39	261	0.2	65.0	0.1	0.4
Orange Shred, Fine Cut, Jelly, Sainsbury's*	1 Tsp/15g	38	253	0.2	63.0	0.1	0.4
Orange Shred, Fine Cut, Tesco*	1 Tsp/15g	39	263	0.1	65.0	0.0	0.4
Orange, Asda*	1 Serving/28g	52	187	0.5	45.0	0.5	0.0
Orange, ExtraThick Cut, Diabetic, Stute*	1 Tsp/5g	7	144	0.4	37.0	0.0	1.5
Orange, Fine Cut, Asda*	1 Serving/15g	27	182	0.4	45.0	0.0	0.9
Orange, Fine Cut, Crystal, Tiptree, Wilkin & Sons*	1 Tsp/15g	40	268	0.1	67.0	0.0	0.0
Orange, Fresh Fruit, Finest, Tesco*	1 Serving/20g	54	270	0.6	65.2	0.3	0.6

	Measure INFO/WEIGHT	per Measure KCAL	Nutrition Values per 100g / 100ml				
			KCAL	PROT	CARB	FAT	FIBRE
MARMALADE,							
Orange, Henley Thick Cut, English Provender Company*	1 Serving/20g	56	278	0.1	69.6	0.0	0.6
Orange, Lemon & Grapefruit, Baxters*	1 Tsp/15g	38	252	0.0	63.0	0.0	0.1
Orange, Medium Cut, Somerfield*	1 Tsp/15g	39	257	0.0	64.0	0.0	0.0
Orange, Old Times, Tiptree*	1 Tbsp/15g	40	268	0.0	67.0	0.0	0.0
Orange, Reduced Sugar, Diced Cut, Streamline*	1 Tsp/15g	29	192	0.4	47.0	0.3	0.0
Orange, Reduced Sugar, Sainsbury's*	1 Tsp/15g	29	190	0.4	47.0	0.1	0.7
Orange, Seville, Fine Cut, Duerr's*	1 Tsp/14g	37	261	0.2	65.0	0.0	0.0
Orange, Seville, Organic, Waitrose*	1 Serving/12g	31	261	0.3	65.0	0.0	0.7
Orange, Seville, Thick Cut, Organic, Sainsbury's*	1 Tsp/15g	39	261	0.3	65.0	0.1	0.4
Orange, Seville, Thin Cut, Baxters*	1 Tsp/15g	38	252	0.0	63.0	0.0	0.1
Orange, Shredless, Duerr's*	1 Tsp/10g	26	261	0.2	65.0	0.0	0.0
Orange, Shredless, Waitrose*	1 Serving/25g	65	261	0.3	65.0	0.0	0.0
Orange, Thick Cut, Asda*	1 Tbsp/15g	37	249	0.3	62.0	0.0	1.0
Orange, Thick Cut, Co-Op*	1 Tsp/15g	43	285	0.3	70.0	0.2	0.4
Orange, Thick Cut, Duerr's*	1 Serving/15g	39	261	0.2	65.0	0.0	0.0
Orange, Thin Cut, Saver, Safeway*	1 Serving/28g	69	245	0.7	60.0	0.1	0.0
Orange, Value, Tesco*	1 Serving/28g	71	255	0.2	63.1	0.0	0.5
Seville Orange, Fine Cut, Morrisons*	1 Serving/7g	18	261	0.2	65.0	0.0	0.0
Tawny Orange, Tiptree*	1 Tsp/10g	27	268	0.0	67.0	0.0	0.0
Tawny Orange, Wilkin & Sons*	1 Tsp/15g	40	268	0.0	67.0	0.0	0.0
Thick Cut, Somerfield*	1 Tsp/15g	39	260	0.0	65.0	0.0	0.0
Three Fruit, Diabetic, Thursday Cottage*	1 Serving/5g	8	154	0.4	38.0	0.0	1.0
Three Fruits, Fresh Fruit, Sainsbury's*	1 Tsp/15g	38	250	0.0	61.3	0.0	0.0
Traditional Style, Safeway*	1 Serving/10g	27	269	0.3	65.7	0.2	1.0
Weight Watchers*	1 Serving/28g	31	111	0.2	27.5	0.0	0.3
MARMITE, Yeast Extract, Marmite*	1 Tsp/9g	21	234	43.0	14.8	0.4	2.6
MARROW,							
Boiled	1oz/28g	3	9	0.4	1.6	0.2	0.6
Raw	1oz/28g	3	12	0.5	2.2	0.2	0.5
MARS BAR,							
5 Little Ones, Mars*	1 Piece/8g	38	477	4.5	73.6	18.3	0.0
Mars*	1 Std Bar/42g	190	452	4.0	69.6	17.5	0.0
MARSHMALLOW, SQUARES, Rice Krispies, Chewy, Kellogg's*	1 Med Bar/18g	74	410	3.0	78.0	10.0	1.0
MARSHMALLOWS,							
Average	1oz/28g	92	327	3.9	83.1	0.0	0.0
Pink & White, Co-Op*	1 Sweet/7g	24	340	3.0	82.0	0.0	0.0
Princess*	1oz/28g	88	314	3.4	80.0	0.0	0.0
MARZIPAN,							
Bar, Chocolate, Plain, Thorntons*	1 Bar/46g	206	448	5.2	69.1	17.4	2.0
Dark Chocolate, Thorntons*	1 Serving/46g	207	451	5.2	69.4	17.4	2.1
Golden, Waitrose*	1oz/28g	118	420	6.4	67.4	13.9	1.5
Retail	1oz/28g	113	404	5.3	67.6	14.4	1.9
MASALA DAL, Waitrose*	½ Pack/150g	164	109	5.9	12.4	4.0	2.8
MASH POT, Spring Onion & Cheese, Sainsbury's*	1 Pot/274g	170	62	1.4	10.7	1.5	1.8
MAYONNAISE,							
50% Less Fat, Good For You, Asda*	1 Tbsp/10g	32	322	0.8	10.0	31.0	0.0
Aioli, Finest, Tesco*	1 Tsp/5g	20	408	0.8	8.5	41.2	0.0
Average	1 Tsp/11g	80	724	1.9	0.2	79.3	0.0
Dijonnaise, Hellmann's*	1 Tsp/6g	13	210	2.9	5.1	19.7	0.0
Finest, Tesco*	1 Dtsp/22g	155	703	1.1	1.5	77.0	0.0
French Style, BGTY, Sainsbury's*	1 Tbsp/15ml	55	366	0.6	7.5	36.9	0.0
French With Course Ground Mustard, Sainsbury's*	1 Serving/15ml	93	618	0.8	1.7	67.3	0.3
French, Sainsbury's*	1 Tsp/6ml	41	678	1.2	2.4	73.6	1.4

	Measure INFO/WEIGHT	per Measure KCAL	Nutrition Values per 100g / 100ml				
			KCAL	PROT	CARB	FAT	FIBRE
MAYONNAISE,							
Garlic & Herb, Marks & Spencer*	1 Tsp/6g	43	712	3.4	2.4	76.9	0.9
Garlic & Herb, Reduced Calorie, Hellmann's*	1 Serving/25ml	58	233	0.7	13.1	19.3	0.4
Garlic Flavoured, Frank Cooper*	1 Tsp/6g	28	460	2.2	8.8	46.2	0.1
Garlic, Asda*	1 Serving/20g	136	678	1.3	6.0	72.0	0.0
Garlic, Morrisons*	1 Tbsp/15ml	55	365	0.7	8.8	36.0	0.0
Garlic, Waitrose*	1 Tsp/6g	21	346	0.6	8.6	34.3	0.0
Good Intentions, Somerfield*	1 Serving/30g	93	309	0.5	7.4	30.8	0.0
Half Fat, Healthy Choice, Safeway*	1 Tsp/11g	35	319	0.8	10.8	30.3	0.0
Hellmann's*	1 Tsp/11g	79	722	1.1	1.3	79.1	0.0
Lemon, Waitrose*	1 Tsp/8ml	56	694	1.2	1.3	76.0	5.4
Light Dijon, Benedicta*	1 Tbsp/15g	44	292	0.7	6.7	29.2	0.0
Light Squeezable, Hellmanns*	1 Tbsp/15g	44	295	0.7	6.6	29.4	0.0
Light, Morrisons*	1 Tsp/11g	32	287	1.4	8.5	27.5	0.0
Light, BGTY, Sainsbury's*	1 Tsp/11g	33	296	0.5	7.2	29.3	0.0
Light, Hellmann's*	1 Serving/10g	30	299	0.7	6.7	29.8	0.0
Light, Kraft*	1 Serving/25g	61	245	0.6	15.0	20.0	0.0
Light, Organic, Simply Delicious*	1 Tbsp/14g	60	425	1.3	14.5	40.2	0.4
Light, Reduced Calorie, Hellmann's*	1 Serving/15ml	43	285	0.7	6.6	29.4	0.0
Low Fat, Belolive*	1 Serving/15ml	45	298	0.8	11.1	29.0	0.0
Made With Free Range Eggs, Marks & Spencer*	1 Tbsp/15g	108	720	1.1	1.2	78.5	0.0
Mediterranean, Hellmann's*	1 Tsp/11g	79	722	1.1	1.3	79.1	0.0
Mild Dijon Mustard, Frank Cooper*	1 Pot/28g	114	406	3.3	9.3	39.5	0.1
Onion & Chive, BGTY, Sainsbury's*	1 Tbsp/15ml	19	127	2.0	11.8	8.0	0.7
Organic, Evernat*	1 Tsp/11g	83	752	1.3	2.8	81.0	0.0
Organic, Tesco*	1 Tsp/20g	150	749	1.5	2.4	81.5	0.1
Organic, Whole Foods*	1 Tbsp/14g	100	714	0.0	7.1	78.6	0.0
Real, Asda*	1 Serving/10g	72	721	1.3	1.2	79.0	0.1
Real, Hellmann's*	1 Tbsp/15ml	101	676	1.0	1.2	74.0	0.0
Reduced Calorie	1 Tsp/11g	32	288	1.0	8.2	28.1	0.0
Reduced Calorie, Healthy Selection, Somerfield*	1 Tbsp/15ml	49	326	0.8	9.8	31.5	0.0
Reduced Calorie, Hellmann's*	1 Serving/30g	90	299	0.7	6.7	29.8	0.0
Reduced Calorie, Iceland*	1 Tbsp/15ml	48	320	0.8	9.7	31.2	0.0
Reduced Calorie, Tesco*	1 Tbsp/15g	49	326	0.8	9.8	31.5	0.0
Reduced Calorie, Waitrose*	1 Tsp/11g	32	287	1.4	8.5	27.5	0.0
Reduced Fat, Safeway*	1 Tbsp/15ml	48	323	0.8	9.7	31.2	0.0
Reduced Fat, Tesco*	1 Tbsp/15ml	44	292	0.8	7.9	28.6	0.0
Sainsbury's*	1 Tsp/11g	75	686	0.4	1.2	75.4	0.0
Tesco*	1 Serving/28g	203	725	1.3	1.2	79.4	0.0
Value, Tesco*	1 Tbsp/15g	73	488	0.8	5.4	51.4	0.0
Vegetarian, Tesco*	1 Tsp/12g	89	738	1.5	0.8	81.0	0.0
Waitrose*	1 Tbsp/15ml	106	709	1.3	0.8	77.8	0.0
Weight Watchers*	1 Tbsp/15g	42	280	1.0	7.3	27.7	0.7
MCFLURRY,							
Creme Egg, Cadbury, McDonald's*	1 Pack/203g	390	192	4.1	29.9	6.5	0.0
Crunchie, McDonald's*	1 Portion/183g	321	175	4.2	26.1	6.2	0.0
Dairy Milk, McDonalds's*	1 Portion/181g	280	154	4.5	24.3	7.2	0.0
Jammie Dodger, McDonald's*	1 Serving/128g	256	200	3.9	33.6	6.4	0.3
Smarties, McDonald's*	1 Serving/185g	327	177	4.2	26.2	6.2	0.2
MCMUFFIN,							
Bacon & Egg, Double, McDonald's*	1 Pack/226g	573	253	14.7	11.4	16.4	0.8
Bacon & Egg, McDonald's*	1 McMuffin/141g	345	245	14.2	18.5	12.8	1.3
Egg, McDonald's*	1 McMuffin/127g	281	221	12.2	20.4	10.1	1.5
Sausage & Egg, McDonald's*	1 McMuffin/176g	426	242	13.8	14.7	14.1	1.0

	Measure INFO/WEIGHT	per Measure KCAL	Nutrition Values per 100g / 100ml				
			KCAL	PROT	CARB	FAT	FIBRE
MCMUFFIN,							
Scrambled Egg, McDonald's*	1 McMuffin/147g	294	200	10.9	17.5	9.6	1.3
MEAT LOAF,							
Iceland*	1 Serving/150g	332	221	10.8	9.3	15.7	0.9
Somerfield*	1 Pack/454g	867	191	10.0	8.0	13.0	0.0
Turkey & Bacon, Tesco*	1 Serving/225g	401	178	14.7	7.4	9.9	1.1
MEATBALLS,							
Aberdeen Angus In Sauce, Perfectly Balanced, Waitrose*	½ Pack/240g	228	95	10.5	6.5	3.0	1.1
Aberdeen Angus, Waitrose*	3 Meatballs/107g	223	208	20.0	1.0	13.8	0.0
Al Forno, Safeway*	1 Pack/450g	684	152	6.0	16.8	6.8	0.4
Authentic Swedish, Swedish Crown*	1/3 Pack/116g	266	229	14.0	11.0	14.0	0.0
Beef, Asda*	1 Serving/287g	362	126	11.0	7.0	6.0	0.6
Chicken, In Tomato Sauce, Macey's*	½ Can/196g	290	148	7.7	10.4	8.4	0.0
Herby With Pasta & Tomato Sauce, COU, M&S*	1 Pack/300g	360	120	10.4	15.2	1.7	0.9
In Bolognese Sauce, Somerfield*	1 Pack/454g	704	155	7.0	7.0	11.0	0.0
In Gravy, Campbells*	½ Can/205g	164	80	5.6	8.6	2.6	0.0
In Tomato Sauce, Campbell's*	1 Can/410g	340	83	5.4	9.5	2.6	0.0
In a Spicy Tomato Sauce With Spaghetti, COU, M&S*	1 Pack/360g	342	95	6.3	13.5	1.9	1.2
Italian Pork, Al Forno, Sainsbury's*	1 Pack/450g	644	143	6.1	17.6	5.3	1.4
Manhattan Style & Spaghetti, Spicy, Safeway*	1 Pack/450g	540	120	5.7	13.2	4.8	2.0
Marks & Spencer*	1oz/28g	58	208	10.9	10.7	13.5	2.4
Spicy Tomato Sauce & Spaghetti, COU, M&S*	1 Pack/360g	342	95	6.3	13.5	1.9	1.2
Spicy, Marks & Spencer*	1 Pack/400g	540	135	8.8	12.0	6.0	1.4
Swedish, Findus*	½ Pack/100g	230	230	13.0	7.0	17.0	0.0
Swedish, Ikea*	1 Serving/100g	240	240	17.0	4.5	17.0	2.6
Swedish, Sainsbury's*	1 Serving/200g	430	215	14.0	6.0	15.0	2.6
Swedish, Scan*	¼ Pack/88g	189	215	14.0	6.0	15.0	2.6
Turkey, GFY, Asda*	½ Pack/330g	333	101	10.0	7.0	3.7	0.0
MEDAGLIONE,							
Cheese & Red Bell Pepper, Eat Smart, Safeway*	1 Serving/125g	175	140	6.3	21.1	2.9	1.0
Roasted Vegetable & Cheese, Safeway*	½ Pack/125g	297	238	9.3	34.2	7.0	2.7
MELBA TOAST,							
Asda*	1 Toast/5g	20	396	12.0	79.0	3.6	2.8
Buitoni*	1 Serving/33g	130	395	12.1	75.5	4.9	4.6
Co-Op*	1 Slice/3g	11	375	16.0	73.0	2.0	5.0
Dutch, Tesco*	1 Serving/20g	75	377	16.0	73.0	2.3	5.0
Organic, Trimlyne*	1 Pack/28g	109	390	13.0	78.0	2.9	5.5
Original, Van Der Meulen*	1 Slice/3g	12	399	12.8	80.5	2.9	3.9
Safeway*	1 Serving/3g	11	362	12.0	72.0	2.9	3.9
With Sesame, Tesco*	1 Slice/3g	11	370	12.8	61.7	8.0	3.8
MELON,							
Average, Weighed With Skin	1oz/28g	4	16	0.4	3.6	0.1	0.5
Canteloupe, Sainsbury's*	1 Serving/100g	19	19	0.6	4.2	0.1	1.0
Fresh, Average, Raw	1oz/28g	7	24	0.6	5.5	0.1	0.7
Galia, Fresh, Marks & Spencer*	1 Serving/240g	60	25	0.5	5.5	0.1	0.4
Galia, Portions, Somerfield*	1oz/28g	7	25	1.0	6.0	0.0	0.0
Honeydew, Portion, Somerfield*	1oz/28g	8	30	1.0	7.0	0.0	0.0
Just Melon, Shapers, Boots*	1 Pot/139g	39	28	0.6	6.2	0.1	0.6
Kiwi & Strawberry Mixed Fruits, Sainsbury's*	1oz/28g	9	33	0.8	6.3	0.2	1.3
Marks & Spencer*	1 Serving/50g	13	25	0.5	5.6	0.2	0.5
Melon, Pineapple & Strawberry, WTF, Sainsbury's*	1 Pack/245g	86	35	0.6	7.8	0.1	0.9
Mixed, Marks & Spencer*	1 Pot/225g	56	25	0.5	5.6	0.2	0.5
Mixed, Snack Pack, Sainsbury's*	1 Pack/118.5g	32	27	0.1	6.2	0.2	0.5
Orange, Fresh, Marks & Spencer*	1 Serving/240g	48	20	0.6	4.2	0.1	0.1

	Measure INFO/WEIGHT	per Measure KCAL	Nutrition Values per 100g / 100ml				
			KCAL	PROT	CARB	FAT	FIBRE
MELON,							
Pineapple & Strawberry, Fully Prepared, Sainsbury's*	1 Serving/245g	86	35	0.6	7.8	0.1	0.9
Seeds	1oz/28g	163	583	28.5	9.9	47.7	0.0
Slice Selection, Waitrose*	1 Serving/225g	45	20	0.4	4.3	0.1	0.4
Slice, Selection, Tesco*	1 Serving/225g	41	18	0.4	3.9	0.1	0.5
Slices, Fresh, Asda*	1 Pack/500g	80	16	0.4	3.4	0.1	0.0
Water	1 Serving/250g	75	30	0.4	7.0	0.3	0.5
MELON & GRAPE Selection, FTG, Marks & Spencer*	1oz/28g	10	35	0.5	8.6	0.1	0.7
MELON MEDLEY,							
Fresh, Asda*	1 Pack/380g	103	27	0.6	6.0	0.1	0.0
Marks & Spencer*	1 Pot/450g	135	30	0.5	5.6	0.2	0.5
Safeway*	1 Pack/350g	105	30	0.5	6.4	0.2	0.4
Sainsbury's*	1 Pack/290g	81	28	0.6	6.2	0.1	0.6
Salad Bar, Asda*	1oz/28g	7	26	0.6	6.6	0.0	0.7
Tesco*	1 Serving/250g	68	27	0.6	6.0	0.1	0.5
Waitrose*	1 Serving/300g	90	30	0.6	6.7	0.1	0.5
MELT,							
Cheese, Chilli, Fresh, Asda*	1 Melt/29g	87	301	6.0	31.0	17.0	0.0
Cheesy Fish, Young's*	1 Pack/340g	418	123	7.6	8.3	6.6	0.9
Chicken, Salsa, Sainsbury's*	1 Pack/400g	516	129	7.2	10.7	6.4	1.6
Chilli With Spicy Potato Wedges, Asda*	1 Pack/450g	540	120	8.0	12.0	4.4	1.2
Mushroom & Broccoli Potato Wedge, Weight Watchers*	1 Pack/310g	285	92	3.3	12.6	3.1	1.0
Sausage & Bean, Iceland*	1 Pack/400g	588	147	6.5	17.1	5.8	1.6
Toasted Ham & Cheese, McDonald's*	1 Serving/100g	239	239	11.2	30.6	8.0	1.8
Tuna, Go Large, Asda*	1 Roll/175g	509	291	12.0	27.0	15.0	0.0
Tuna, Iceland*	1 Pack/400g	424	106	6.0	11.3	4.2	0.7
Tuna, Marks & Spencer*	1 Pack/218g	621	285	13.0	20.1	17.0	1.0
MERINGUE,							
Average	1oz/28g	106	379	5.3	95.4	0.0	0.0
Chocolate, Waitrose*	1 Meringue/76.8g	342	444	2.6	75.3	14.7	0.5
Coffee Fresh Cream, Asda*	1 Meringue/27.5g	111	396	3.8	57.0	17.0	0.3
Cream, Marks & Spencer*	1 Cake/34.1g	145	425	4.1	52.6	22.2	0.3
Cream, Sainsbury's*	1 Meringue/25g	98	392	3.9	59.0	15.7	0.8
Layered, Tesco*	1/5 Meringue/52g	146	280	3.5	63.2	1.5	1.4
Marks & Spencer*	1 Meringue/12g	47	389	5.2	92.0	0.0	0.0
Mini, Marks & Spencer*	1oz/28g	111	395	6.1	91.6	0.0	0.0
Nests, Asda*	1 Nest/15g	59	390	3.7	93.0	0.3	0.0
Nests, Marks & Spencer*	1 Nest/12g	47	395	6.1	91.6	0.0	0.0
Nests, Safeway*	1 Nest/14.6g	59	391	4.6	92.8	0.2	0.0
Nests, Sainsbury's*	1 Nest/15g	58	387	3.9	92.8	0.0	0.0
Nests, Tesco*	1 Nest/15g	58	388	3.9	92.8	0.1	0.0
Nests, Tropical Fruit, Sainsbury's*	1 Nest/95g	234	246	2.0	42.0	7.8	2.4
Shells, Mini, Asda*	1 Shell/4g	16	388	4.8	92.0	0.1	0.0
Shells, Sainsbury's*	2 Shells/24g	93	387	3.9	92.8	0.0	0.0
Summer Fruits, 90% Fat Free, Sara Lee*	1 Meringue/135g	308	228	2.5	35.7	8.5	2.2
Toffee, Marks & Spencer*	1 Meringue/30g	125	415	4.1	52.2	20.9	0.8
Tropical, Marks & Spencer*	1 Serving/53g	212	400	3.1	37.0	26.9	0.0
MESSICANI, Egg, Marks & Spencer*	1 Serving/100g	355	355	13.9	68.5	2.8	3.0
MIDGET GEMS,							
Marks & Spencer*	1 Bag/113g	367	325	6.3	75.1	0.1	0.0
Smartprice, Asda*	1 Pack/178g	586	329	6.0	76.0	0.1	0.0
MILK,							
Condensed, Skimmed, Sweetened	1oz/28g	75	267	10.0	60.0	0.2	0.0
Condensed, Whole, Sweetened	1oz/28g	93	333	8.5	55.5	10.1	0.0

MILK,

INFO/WEIGHT	Measure	per Measure KCAL	KCAL	PROT	CARB	FAT	FIBRE
Dried Skimmed	1oz/28g	97	348	36.1	52.9	0.6	0.0
Dried Skimmed, Instant, Powder, Tesco*	1oz/28g	100	358	35.0	52.0	1.1	0.0
Dried Whole	1oz/28g	137	490	26.3	39.4	26.3	0.0
Evaporated, Carnation*	1 Serving/85g	136	160	8.2	11.5	9.0	0.0
Evaporated, Full Cream, Waitrose*	1 Tbsp/15ml	24	160	8.2	11.5	9.0	0.0
Evaporated, Light, Carnation*	1 Serving/25g	28	110	7.5	10.5	4.0	0.0
Evaporated, Low Fat, Somerfield*	1oz/28g	31	109	8.0	11.0	4.0	0.0
Evaporated, Safeway*	1 Serving/69g	110	160	8.2	11.5	9.0	0.0
Evaporated, Tesco*	1 Serving/95g	153	161	8.4	11.6	9.0	0.0
Evaporated, Whole	1oz/28g	42	151	8.4	8.5	9.4	0.0
Full Fat, Pasteurised Standardised, Sainsbury's*	1fl oz/30ml	20	68	3.2	4.7	4.0	0.0
Goats, Pasteurised	1fl oz/30ml	18	60	3.1	4.4	3.5	0.0
Goats, Semi-Skimmed, St Helens Farm*	1 Serving/250ml	109	44	3.0	4.3	1.6	0.0
Guernsey, TTD, Sainsbury's*	1 Serving/180ml	135	75	3.6	4.7	4.7	0.0
Half Fat, Marks & Spencer*	1fl oz/30ml	15	49	3.4	5.0	1.7	0.0
Low Fat, Calcia Extra Calcium, Unigate*	1fl oz/30ml	14	45	4.3	6.3	0.5	0.0
Semi Skimmed	1fl oz/28ml	13	46	3.3	5.0	1.6	0.0
Semi Skimmed, Arla*	½ Pint/296ml	145	49	3.4	5.0	1.7	0.0
Semi Skimmed, Asda*	¼ Pint/125ml	61	49	3.4	5.0	1.7	0.0
Semi Skimmed, British Long Life UHT, Sainsbury's*	1 Serving/100ml	49	49	3.4	5.0	1.7	0.0
Semi Skimmed, Budgens*	1 Glass/250ml	123	49	3.3	5.2	1.7	0.0
Semi Skimmed, Co-Op*	1 Serving/100ml	50	50	3.0	5.0	1.7	0.0
Semi Skimmed, Cravendale*	1 Serving/200ml	98	49	3.4	5.0	1.7	0.0
Semi Skimmed, Dairy Crest*	1 Serving/100ml	49	49	3.4	5.0	1.7	0.0
Semi Skimmed, Express*	1 Serving/250ml	123	49	3.4	5.0	1.7	0.0
Semi Skimmed, Fresh 'n' Lo*	1 Glass/200ml	94	47	3.4	4.9	1.6	0.0
Semi Skimmed, Long Life, Tesco*	1 Serving/20ml	10	49	3.4	5.0	1.7	0.0
Semi Skimmed, Low Lactose, Arla*	1 Glass/125ml	56	45	3.4	5.0	1.5	0.0
Semi Skimmed, Morrisons*	1 Serving/50ml	25	49	3.4	5.0	1.7	0.0
Semi Skimmed, Organic, Marks & Spencer*	1 Bottle/568ml	278	49	3.4	5.0	1.7	0.0
Semi Skimmed, Organic, Tesco*	1 Serving/100ml	48	48	3.3	5.0	1.6	0.0
Semi Skimmed, Pasteurised, Robert Wiseman Dairies*	1 Serving/170ml	80	47	3.4	4.9	1.6	0.0
Semi Skimmed, Sainsbury's*	1fl oz/30ml	15	49	3.4	5.0	1.7	0.0
Semi Skimmed, Sommerfield*	1 Serving/50ml	25	49	3.4	5.0	1.7	0.0
Semi Skimmed, Tesco*	1 Glass/200ml	96	48	3.3	5.0	1.6	0.0
Semi Skimmed, Waitrose*	1 Serving/150ml	74	49	3.4	5.0	1.7	0.0
Semi-Skimmed, Organic, McDonald's*	1 Bottle/250ml	123	49	3.4	5.0	1.7	0.0
Skimmed	1fl oz/28ml	9	33	3.3	5.0	0.1	0.0
Skimmed, Budgens*	1 Glass/250ml	88	35	3.4	5.2	0.1	0.0
Skimmed, Co-Op*	1 Serving/100ml	35	35	3.0	5.0	0.1	0.0
Skimmed, Fresh Pasteurised, British, Sainsbury's*	1 Serving/250ml	85	34	3.4	5.0	0.1	0.0
Skimmed, Fresh, Asda*	1 Glass/250ml	85	34	3.4	5.0	0.0	0.0
Skimmed, Fresh, Express*	1 Glass/200ml	68	34	3.4	5.0	0.1	0.0
Skimmed, Long Life British UHT, Sainsbury's*	1 Glass/200ml	70	35	3.4	5.0	0.1	0.0
Skimmed, Long Life UHT, SmartPrice, Asda*	1fl oz/30ml	10	35	3.2	5.2	0.1	0.0
Skimmed, Long Life, Asda*	1 Serving/250ml	85	34	3.4	5.0	0.0	0.0
Skimmed, Long Life, UHT, Safeway*	1 Serving/100ml	34	34	3.4	5.0	0.1	0.0
Skimmed, Marks & Spencer*	1 Serving/100ml	34	34	3.4	5.0	0.1	0.0
Skimmed, Organic, Sainsbury's*	1 Serving/100ml	34	34	3.4	5.0	0.1	0.0
Skimmed, Organic, Tesco*	1 Serving/250ml	85	34	3.3	5.0	0.1	0.0
Skimmed, Powdered, Organic, Evernat*	1oz/28g	96	344	34.0	52.0	0.0	0.0
Skimmed, Tesco*	1 Pint/50ml	17	34	3.3	5.0	0.1	0.0
Skimmed, UHT, Asda*	1floz/30ml	10	34	3.4	5.0	0.1	0.0

MILK,	Measure INFO/WEIGHT	per Measure KCAL	Nutrition Values per 100g / 100ml KCAL	PROT	CARB	FAT	FIBRE
Skimmed, UHT, Tesco*	1 Serving/100ml	34	34	3.3	5.0	0.1	0.0
Skimmed, Unsweetened Condensed, HE, Tesco*	1 Sm Can/205g	221	108	7.5	10.5	4.0	0.0
Soya, Chocolate, So Good*	1 Serving/100ml	71	71	3.0	10.8	1.7	0.0
Soya, Flavoured	1floz/30mls	12	40	2.8	3.6	1.7	0.0
Soya, No Added Sugar, Calcium Enriched, Granose*	1floz/30ml	11	36	3.3	1.9	1.9	0.0
Soya, No Added Sugar, Organic, Granose*	1floz/30ml	10	33	3.3	1.8	1.7	0.0
Soya, Plain	1floz/30ml	10	32	2.9	0.8	1.9	0.0
Soya, So Good*	1fl oz/30ml	15	50	3.4	5.3	1.7	0.0
Soya, Sweetened, Asda*	1fl oz/30ml	14	47	3.3	4.2	1.9	0.0
Soya, Sweetened, Calcium Enriched, Granose*	1floz/30ml	14	45	3.3	4.2	1.9	0.0
Soya, Sweetened, Calcium Enriched, White Wave*	1floz/30ml	14	47	3.3	4.1	1.9	0.0
Soya, Sweetened, Co-Op*	1 Glass/200ml	80	40	3.0	3.0	2.0	1.0
Soya, Sweetened, Safeway*	1fl oz/30ml	12	41	3.3	3.3	1.6	0.2
Soya, Sweetened, Sainsbury's*	1fl oz/30ml	14	45	3.6	2.9	2.1	0.1
Soya, Tesco*	1 Serving/100ml	45	45	3.6	2.9	2.1	1.0
Soya, Unsweetened, Asda*	1fl oz/30ml	11	38	3.3	1.9	1.9	0.0
Soya, Unsweetened, Sainsbury's*	1 Serving/125ml	45	36	3.6	0.6	2.1	0.1
Soya, Unsweetened, UHT, Free From, Sainsbury's*	1 Serving/250ml	80	32	3.3	0.4	1.9	0.2
Soya, Unsweetened, Value, Tesco*	1 Serving/250ml	65	26	2.8	0.2	1.6	0.9
UHT Portions, Kerrygold*	1 Portion/14g	9	66	3.2	4.8	3.9	0.0
Unsweetened, Condensed, Light, Healthy Eating, Tesco*	1 Can/170g	184	108	7.5	10.5	4.0	0.0
Whole, Fresh	1fl oz/28ml	18	66	3.2	4.8	3.9	0.0
Whole, Fresh, Asda*	1 Serving/200ml	128	64	3.2	4.7	3.6	0.0
Whole, Fresh, Organic, Rachel's*	1 Serving/50ml	34	68	3.2	4.7	3.8	0.0
Whole, Organic, Marks & Spencer*	1 Bottle/568ml	386	68	3.2	4.7	4.0	0.0
Whole, Pasteurised, Sainsbury's*	1 Serving/100ml	64	64	3.3	4.7	3.6	0.0
MILK DRINK,							
Chocolate Sterilised Skimmed, Happy Shopper*	1 Bottle/500ml	295	59	3.6	10.4	0.3	0.0
Mars Extra Milk Chocolate Caramel, Mars*	1 Bottle/330g	224	68	3.5	12.1	0.3	0.0
MILK SHAKE,							
Banana Flavour, Frijj*	1 Bottle/500ml	310	62	3.4	10.1	0.8	0.0
Banana Flavour, Mix, Nesquik*	1 Serving/15g	59	395	0.0	97.3	0.5	0.0
Banana Flavour, Shapers, Boots*	1 Bottle/250ml	201	80	5.6	12.8	0.8	1.9
Banana, McDonald's*	1 Regular/336g	396	118	3.2	19.8	3.0	0.0
Banana, Yazoo*	1 Bottle/500ml	325	65	3.1	10.3	1.3	0.0
Chocolate Flavour, BGTY, Sainsbury's*	1 Bottle/500ml	290	58	5.3	8.0	0.5	0.9
Chocolate Flavoured, Fresh, Thick, Frijj*	1 Bottle/500ml	345	69	3.5	11.6	1.0	0.0
Chocolate, Extreme, Frijj*	1 Bottle/500g	425	85	3.9	12.7	2.1	0.0
Chocolate, McDonald's*	1 Regular/336g	403	120	3.4	19.9	3.0	0.0
Measure Up, Asda*	1 Glass/250ml	200	80	6.0	12.0	1.0	2.4
Mount Caramel, Frijj*	1 Bottle/500ml	360	72	3.4	12.7	0.9	0.0
Powder, Made Up With Semi-Skimmed Milk	1 Serving/250ml	173	69	3.2	11.3	1.6	0.0
Powder, Made Up With Whole Milk	1 Serving/250ml	218	87	3.1	11.1	3.7	0.0
Strawberry Flavour, Thick, Low Fat, Frijj*	1 Bottle/250ml	155	62	3.4	10.1	0.8	0.0
Strawberry, McDonald's*	1 Regular/336g	400	119	3.2	20.0	3.0	0.0
Strawberry, Thick, Somerfield*	1 Milkshake/250ml	275	110	4.0	15.0	4.0	0.0
Vanilla Flavour, BGTY, Sainsbury's*	1 Bottle/500ml	230	46	5.3	5.9	0.1	0.4
Vanilla, Frijj*	1 Bottle/500ml	320	64	3.4	10.7	0.8	0.0
Vanilla, McDonald's*	1 Regular/336g	383	114	3.2	18.8	3.0	0.0
MILKY BAR,							
Buttons, Nestle*	1 Mini Bag/16g	87	542	7.6	57.5	31.3	0.0
Choo, Nestle*	1oz/28g	131	468	4.7	73.2	17.6	0.0
Crunchies, Nestle*	1 Pack/30g	168	560	7.0	54.9	34.7	0.0

	Measure INFO/WEIGHT	per Measure KCAL	Nutrition Values per 100g / 100ml				
			KCAL	PROT	CARB	FAT	FIBRE
MILKY BAR,							
Nestle*	1 Bar/12g	65	542	7.6	57.5	31.3	0.0
MILKY WAY,							
Celebrations Chocolate, Mars*	1 Sweet/8g	35	438	0.0	75.0	18.8	0.0
Magic Stars, Mars*	1 Bag/33g	184	557	8.8	51.8	35.0	0.0
Mars*	1 Single Bar/26g	118	454	4.2	72.0	16.6	0.0
MILO, Nestle*	1 Serving/20g	76	380	8.2	72.9	6.0	4.7
MINCEMEAT,							
Average	1oz/28g	77	274	0.6	62.1	4.3	1.3
Organic, Waitrose*	1oz/28g	81	290	0.9	65.8	2.6	2.0
Traditional, Robertson's*	1 Tbsp/7g	49	286	0.6	62.5	3.4	2.5
Traditional, Sainsbury's*	1 Tbsp/23g	65	282	0.9	62.4	3.2	1.4
MINSTRELS, Galaxy, Mars*	1 Pack/42g	206	491	6.0	69.5	21.0	0.0
MINT,							
Dried	1oz/28g	78	279	24.8	34.6	4.6	0.0
Fresh	1oz/28g	12	43	3.8	5.3	0.7	0.0
MINT, JELLY,							
Baxters*	1oz/28g	74	264	0.0	66.0	0.0	0.0
Safeway*	1 Serving/10g	17	174	0.3	41.6	0.0	0.0
Sainsbury's*	1 Serving/10g	27	269	0.1	66.6	0.2	0.3
MINT, MATCHMAKERS, Nestle*	1oz/28g	134	477	5.1	68.7	20.2	0.0
MINTOES, Morrisons*	1 Sweet/8.1g	33	411	0.1	84.4	8.1	0.0
MINTS,							
After Dinner, Dark, Elizabeth Shaw*	1 Chocolate/9g	42	469	2.8	62.5	23.1	0.0
After Dinner, Sainsbury's*	1 Mint/7g	32	456	4.1	62.1	21.2	4.1
After Dinner, Tesco*	1oz/28g	132	471	5.0	70.0	19.0	0.0
After Eight, Nestle*	1 Mint/8g	34	419	2.5	72.4	13.3	0.0
Butter Mintoes, Marks & Spencer*	1 Sweet/9g	35	391	0.0	84.0	6.8	0.0
Clear, Co-Op*	1 Sweet/6g	24	395	0.0	98.0	0.0	0.0
Cool Mint, Smint*	1 Smint/0.2g	0	55	0.6	7.8	1.0	0.0
Cream, Luxury, Thorntons*	1 Chocolate/13g	62	477	4.2	62.3	23.8	2.3
Curiously Strong, Marks & Spencer*	1 Sweet/1g	4	390	0.4	97.5	0.0	0.0
Everton, Co-Op*	1 Sweet/6g	25	410	0.6	92.0	4.0	0.0
Extra Strong, Trebor*	3 Mints/10g	40	396	0.3	98.8	0.0	0.0
Glacier, Fox's*	1 Mint/5g	19	386	0.0	96.4	0.0	0.0
Humbugs, Asda*	1 Sweet/8g	29	362	0.0	86.0	2.0	0.0
Humbugs, Co-Op*	1 Sweet/8g	34	425	0.6	89.9	7.0	0.0
Humbugs, Marks & Spencer*	1 Sweet/9g	37	407	0.6	91.1	4.4	0.0
Humbugs, Thorntons*	1 Sweet/9g	31	340	1.0	87.8	4.4	0.0
Imperials, Co-Op*	1 Sweet/3g	12	395	0.3	98.0	0.2	0.0
Imperials, Marks & Spencer*	1oz/28g	109	391	0.0	97.8	0.0	0.0
Imperials, Sainsbury's*	1 Mint/3g	12	396	0.4	97.9	0.2	0.0
Imperials, Tesco*	1 Mint/3g	12	397	0.6	98.7	0.0	0.0
Mighty, 24-7, Sugar Free, Trebor*	1 Sweet/0.1g	0	277	0.0	94.7	0.0	0.0
Mint Assortment, Marks & Spencer*	1 Sweet/7g	29	414	0.7	85.4	7.7	0.0
Mint Favourites, Bassett's*	1 Sweet/6g	22	367	0.9	77.4	5.9	0.0
Soft, Trebor*	1 Pack/48g	182	380	0.0	94.9	0.0	0.0
MISO, Average	1oz/28g	57	203	13.3	23.5	6.2	0.0
MIXED FRUIT,							
Somerfield*, Dried	1oz/28g	80	285	2.0	68.0	1.0	0.0
Sultanas, Currants, Raisins & Citrus Peel, Asda*, Dried	1 Serving/100g	283	283	2.6	67.0	0.5	1.7
Vine Fruit, Crazy Jack*, Dried	1 Serving/10g	31	309	2.8	74.0	0.3	4.7
MIXED FRUIT PIECES in Orange Jelly, Fruitini*	1 Can/140g	94	67	0.3	15.8	0.1	0.0
MIXED PEEL, Average	1 Tbsp/25g	58	231	0.3	59.1	0.9	4.8

M

INFO/WEIGHT	Measure	per Measure KCAL	Nutrition Values per 100g / 100ml				
			KCAL	PROT	CARB	FAT	FIBRE
MIXED VEGETABLES,							
Canned, Drained, Sainsbury's*	1 Can/200g	114	57	3.0	10.6	0.3	2.3
Canned, Tesco*	1 Can/195g	103	53	2.6	9.2	0.6	27.0
Chunky, Frozen, Sainsbury's*	1 Serving/85g	31	37	2.9	4.7	0.7	3.1
Cooked, Tesco*	1 Serving/100g	27	27	2.3	3.2	0.5	2.3
Farmhouse, Tesco*	1 Serving/80g	32	40	3.6	4.6	0.8	3.0
Fresh, Frozen, Tesco*	1 Serving/75g	36	48	3.0	7.2	0.8	3.2
Freshly Frozen, Iceland*	1 Serving/100g	52	52	3.4	8.3	0.9	3.4
Frozen, Aldi*	1 Serving/100g	34	34	2.8	4.3	0.7	0.0
Frozen, Asda*	1 Serving/100g	53	53	3.1	8.0	0.9	4.0
Frozen, Safeway*	1 Serving/120g	70	58	3.0	9.4	0.9	3.4
Frozen, Sainsbury's*	1 Serving/90g	49	54	2.8	8.4	1.0	3.1
Frozen, Tesco*	1 Serving/100g	49	49	2.9	7.8	0.7	3.2
Frozen, Waitrose*	1 Serving/100g	54	54	3.1	8.7	0.8	3.5
In Water, Straight to Wok, Amoy*	½ Pack/110g	27	25	1.8	3.7	0.3	0.0
Ready To Roast, Asda*	½ Pack/362g	315	87	1.6	13.0	3.2	2.4
Red Peppers & Courgette, Tesco*	1 Pack/250g	68	27	1.7	3.8	0.5	2.0
Sainsbury's*	1 Serving/230g	55	24	2.1	2.5	0.6	0.0
Special, Frozen, Sainsbury's*	1 Serving/80g	54	68	3.4	9.7	1.7	3.2
Straight to Wok, Water Selection, Amoy*	½ Pack/110g	25	23	1.8	3.7	0.3	1.5
MOLASSES, Average	1 Tbsp/20g	53	266	0.0	68.8	0.1	0.0
MONKEY NUTS,							
Roasted, Somerfield*	1oz/28g	111	396	20.0	7.0	32.0	0.0
Roasted, Tesco*	1 Serving/25g	142	566	25.5	3.9	49.8	6.4
MONKFISH,							
Grilled	1oz/28g	27	96	22.7	0.0	0.6	0.0
Raw	1oz/28g	18	66	15.7	0.0	0.4	0.0
Tails, Asda*	1oz/28g	27	96	22.7	0.0	0.6	0.0
MONSTER MUNCH,							
Baked Bean Flavour, Walkers*	1 Pack/25g	120	480	5.5	58.0	25.0	1.4
Flamin' Hot, Walkers*	1 Bag/25g	118	470	7.0	55.0	25.0	1.8
Pickled Onion, Walkers*	1 Bag/25g	120	480	6.0	57.0	25.0	1.7
Roast Beef, Walkers*	1 Pack/25g	119	475	6.6	58.0	24.0	1.5
Spicy, Walkers*	1 Bag/25g	125	500	5.0	55.0	29.0	1.3
MOUSSAKA,							
Beef, BGTY, Sainsbury's*	1 Pack/400g	300	75	6.1	6.8	2.6	1.2
COU, Marks & Spencer*	1 Pack/340g	272	80	5.3	8.5	2.9	1.4
Eat Smart, Safeway*	1 Pack/400g	380	95	5.2	12.6	2.6	1.2
Lamb, Eat Smart, Safeway*	1 Pack/380g	304	80	6.8	4.2	2.7	1.3
Lamb, Finest, Tesco*	1 Pack/330g	521	158	7.7	9.1	10.1	2.0
Lamb, Sainsbury's*	1 Pack/329.1g	497	151	8.4	7.2	9.8	1.0
Perfectly Balanced, Waitrose*	1 Pack/300g	255	85	6.6	7.6	3.1	1.0
Quorn*	1 Pack/400g	364	91	3.6	9.8	4.1	1.2
Ready Meals, Waitrose*	1 Pack/300g	492	164	8.2	10.9	9.7	1.7
Vegetable, Marks & Spencer*	1 Pack/300g	330	110	4.4	11.8	5.2	1.1
Vegetable, Ready Meals, Waitrose*	1oz/28g	38	134	3.7	12.3	7.8	2.3
MOUSSE,							
Aero Chocolate, Nestle*	1 Pot/59g	109	185	5.1	21.0	8.9	0.5
Aero Mint, Nestle*	1 Pot/100g	218	218	4.1	23.6	11.9	0.0
Aero Twist Cappuccino & Chocolate, Nestle*	1 Pot/75g	135	180	4.2	16.8	10.8	0.2
Apricot, Lite, Onken*	1 Pot/150g	156	104	4.6	18.0	1.5	0.3
Banoffee, COU, Marks & Spencer*	1 Pot/70g	102	145	2.9	28.8	2.1	1.5
Black Cherry, Lite, Onken*	1 Pot/150g	156	104	4.6	17.9	1.5	0.3
Blackcurrant, Onken*	1 Pot/150g	210	140	5.2	14.6	6.8	0.0

MOUSSE,	Measure INFO/WEIGHT	per Measure KCAL	KCAL	PROT	CARB	FAT	FIBRE
Cadbury's Flake, Twinpot, St Ivel*	1 Pot/100g	257	257	5.6	27.4	13.9	0.0
Cadbury's Light Chocolate, St Ivel*	1 Pot/64g	79	123	6.2	17.3	3.2	0.0
Caramelised Orange, COU, Marks & Spencer*	1 Pot/70g	91	130	2.8	26.3	1.7	3.4
Chocolate	1 Pot/60g	83	139	4.0	19.9	5.4	0.0
Chocolate & Hazelnut Puree, Onken*	½ Pot/185g	222	120	3.4	19.5	3.1	0.0
Chocolate & Hazelnut, Onken*	1 Pot/125g	173	138	3.3	17.8	6.0	0.0
Chocolate & Mint, COU, Marks & Spencer*	1 Pot/90g	108	120	5.4	17.8	2.6	0.5
Chocolate & Orange, COU, Marks & Spencer*	1 Pot/70g	77	110	5.9	16.0	2.6	0.9
Chocolate & Vanilla, Weight Watchers*	1 Pot/80g	106	132	4.4	22.2	2.8	0.9
Chocolate Orange, Low Fat, Cadbury's*	1 Pot/100g	110	110	5.6	15.1	3.0	0.0
Chocolate With Vanilla Layer, Cadbury's*	1 Pot/100g	162	162	4.8	21.9	6.1	0.0
Chocolate, Asda*	1 Pot/60.9g	127	209	3.8	26.3	9.9	1.1
Chocolate, BGTY, Sainsbury's*	1 Pot/62.5g	78	126	4.0	21.5	2.7	1.1
Chocolate, COU, Marks & Spencer*	1 Pot/70g	81	115	5.8	16.6	2.7	1.0
Chocolate, Eat Smart, Safeway*	1 Pot/62g	81	130	4.1	21.5	2.7	1.1
Chocolate, Good Choice, Iceland*	1 Pot/62.0g	85	137	5.4	22.7	2.7	0.0
Chocolate, Good for You, Asda*	1 Pot/62.5g	85	136	3.8	24.0	2.7	0.0
Chocolate, Healthy Eating, Tesco*	1 Pot/60g	80	134	4.4	23.2	2.6	1.0
Chocolate, Healthy Selection, Low Fat, Somerfield*	1 Pot/60g	81	135	5.3	18.2	4.6	0.0
Chocolate, Iceland*	1 Pot/62g	113	183	4.0	26.3	6.9	0.0
Chocolate, Italian Style, Tesco*	1 Pot/90g	243	270	5.0	32.8	13.2	2.4
Chocolate, Light, Cadbury's*	1 Pot/55g	69	125	6.2	17.5	3.2	0.0
Chocolate, Organic, Evernat*	1oz/28g	83	296	10.1	21.1	19.1	0.0
Chocolate, Pret A Manger*	1 Pot/110g	314	285	2.7	16.9	22.9	1.3
Chocolate, Safeway*	1 Pot/62g	127	205	4.0	25.3	9.8	1.1
Chocolate, Sainsbury's*	1 Pot/62g	122	197	4.0	25.4	8.8	1.1
Chocolate, Somerfield*	1 Pot/60g	115	192	4.3	24.5	8.5	0.0
Chocolate, Tesco*	1 Pot/60g	74	124	4.4	20.8	2.6	1.0
Dream, Cadbury's*	1 Pot/53g	100	189	6.0	22.0	8.0	0.0
Fruit Juice, Shape*	1 Pot/100g	115	115	3.5	18.5	2.8	0.0
Layered Lemon, Co-Op*	1 Pot/100g	140	140	3.0	24.0	3.0	0.2
Layered Strawberry, Co-Op*	1 Pot/100g	120	120	3.0	19.0	3.0	0.2
Lemon Fruit Juice, Shape*	1 Pot/100g	116	116	3.5	18.6	2.8	0.0
Lemon, COU, Marks & Spencer*	1 Pot/70g	81	115	2.9	19.4	2.4	3.5
Lemon, Dessert, Sainsbury's*	1 Pot/62.5g	114	182	3.6	20.7	9.4	0.6
Lemon, Eat Smart, Safeway*	1 Pot/70g	95	135	3.4	23.5	2.7	0.4
Lemon, GFY, Asda*	1 Pot/62.5g	72	114	3.4	19.0	2.7	0.0
Lemon, Healthy Eating, Tesco*	1 Pot/60g	57	95	3.4	14.3	2.7	0.7
Lemon, Less Than 3% Fat, BGTY, Sainsbury's*	1 Pot/62g	59	95	3.4	14.3	2.7	0.7
Lemon, Less Than 3% Fat, Healthy Eating, Tesco*	1 Pot/60g	57	95	3.4	14.3	2.7	0.0
Lemon, Lite, Onken*	1 Pot/150g	156	104	4.6	18.0	1.6	0.0
Lemon, Low Fat, Morrisons*	1 Pot/110g	175	159	3.1	30.5	2.7	0.1
Lemon, Onken*	1 Pot/150g	219	146	5.1	15.8	6.9	0.1
Lemon, Perfectly Balanced, Waitrose*	1 Pot/95g	150	158	3.1	30.2	2.7	0.1
Lemon, Somerfield*	1 Pot/62.5g	114	181	3.5	20.7	9.4	0.6
Lemon, Tesco*	1 Pot/60g	67	111	3.4	18.2	2.7	0.0
Mars, Eden Vale*	1 Pot/110g	215	195	6.0	28.2	6.7	0.7
Milky Way, Mars*	1 Pot/50g	115	229	4.5	20.0	14.5	0.0
Orange & Lemon, Light, Muller*	1 Pot/150g	147	98	4.3	19.3	0.4	0.0
Orange & Nectarine, Shape*	1 Pot/100g	47	47	3.0	4.9	1.9	0.0
Orange Fruit Juice, Shape*	1 Pot/100g	116	116	3.5	18.5	2.8	0.0
Orange, Mango & Lime, Onken*	1 Pot/150g	207	138	5.1	15.3	6.3	0.1
Peach & Passion Fruit, Perfectly Balanced, Waitrose*	1 Pot/95g	118	124	3.5	21.2	2.8	0.5

Measure INFO/WEIGHT	per Measure KCAL	Nutrition Values per 100g / 100ml				
		KCAL	PROT	CARB	FAT	FIBRE
MOUSSE,						
Peach, Onken*	1 Pot/150g	200	133	4.8	13.5	6.6	0.0
Peach, Shape*	1 Pot/100g	43	43	3.0	3.9	1.8	0.1
Pineapple, COU, Marks & Spencer*	1 Pot/70g	84	120	3.3	20.7	2.4	3.5
Pineapple, Lite, Onken*	1 Pot/150g	162	108	4.6	19.0	1.5	0.2
Pineapple, Shape*	1 Pot/100g	43	43	2.9	3.8	1.8	0.1
Plain Chocolate, Low Fat, Nestle*	1 Pot/120g	71	59	2.4	10.4	0.8	0.0
Raspberry Ripple, Economy, Sainsbury's*	1 Serving/50g	39	78	1.3	9.7	3.7	0.3
Raspberry, COU, Marks & Spencer*	1 Pot/70g	81	115	3.0	19.6	2.4	3.9
Raspberry, Lite, Onken*	1 Pot/150g	152	101	4.6	17.3	1.5	1.0
Rhubarb & Vanilla, Onken*	1 Pot/150g	210	140	5.0	15.8	6.3	0.2
Rhubarb, COU, Marks & Spencer*	1 Pot/70g	88	125	2.9	25.7	2.1	4.2
Rhubarb, Lite, Onken*	1 Pot/150g	155	103	4.6	17.8	1.5	0.3
Strawberry Fruity, Organic, Sainsbury's*	1 Pot/125g	129	103	6.2	15.7	3.0	3.6
Strawberry, Asda*	1 Pot/64g	107	167	3.5	18.0	9.0	0.2
Strawberry, Eat Smart, Safeway*	1 Pot/70g	95	135	3.2	24.4	2.7	0.5
Strawberry, Light, Muller*	1 Pot/150g	147	98	4.3	19.4	0.4	0.0
Strawberry, Lite, Onken*	1 Pot/150g	153	102	4.6	17.3	1.6	1.1
Strawberry, Low Fat, Waitrose*	1 Pot/95g	112	118	3.2	20.0	2.8	0.6
Strawberry, Onken*	1 Pot/150g	200	133	4.8	13.5	6.6	0.0
Strawberry, Safeway*	1 Pot/63g	106	168	3.5	17.3	9.4	0.1
Strawberry, Sainsbury's*	1 Pot/63g	106	168	3.4	17.5	9.4	0.1
Strawberry, Shape*	1 Pot/100g	44	44	3.0	4.0	1.8	0.0
Strawberry, Weight Watchers*	1 Pot/90g	124	138	3.0	25.5	2.7	0.5
Summer Fruits, Light, Muller*	1 Pot/149g	143	96	4.3	18.7	0.4	0.0
Tropical Fruits, Light, Muller*	1 Pot/150g	150	101	4.3	20.0	0.4	0.0
Tropical, Eat Smart, Safeway*	1 Pot/90g	122	135	3.3	24.5	2.3	3.2
White Chocolate, Finest, Tesco*	1 Pot/92g	436	474	3.9	30.2	37.5	0.0
MUFFIN,						
Apple, Sultana & Cinnamon, Good For You, Asda*	1 Muffin/50g	134	268	6.0	53.0	3.5	3.9
Average	1 Muffin/57g	161	283	10.1	49.6	6.3	2.0
Blueberry Buster, McVitie's*	1 Muffin/95g	408	429	4.3	49.9	23.6	1.1
Blueberry, American Style, Aldi*	1 Muffin/85g	344	405	4.3	51.2	20.3	0.0
Blueberry, Asda*	1 Muffin/77.3g	272	353	5.0	45.0	17.0	1.3
Blueberry, Marks & Spencer*	1 Muffin/75g	282	376	4.8	52.4	16.4	1.2
Blueberry, Martha White*	1 Muffin/38g	170	447	5.3	73.7	11.8	0.0
Blueberry, Sainsbury's*	1 Muffin/75g	242	322	5.4	46.7	12.6	2.2
Blueberry, Tesco*	1 Muffin/70g	279	398	4.8	39.7	24.4	1.3
Blueberry, Waitrose*	1 Muffin/65g	239	367	4.7	55.2	14.2	1.7
Blueberry, Weight Watchers*	1 Muffin/65g	172	265	6.4	46.9	5.7	2.6
Bran	1 Muffin/57g	155	272	7.8	45.6	7.7	7.7
Bran & Sultana, Weight Watchers*	1 Muffin/60g	144	240	4.5	50.7	2.1	2.3
Buttered With Preserve, McDonald's*	1 Muffin/93g	234	252	5.9	48.1	4.0	2.0
Buttered, McDonald's*	1 Muffin/63g	158	250	8.6	40.7	5.9	2.9
Cafe Latte, Sainsbury's*	1 Muffin/72g	270	375	5.9	43.6	19.7	2.8
Carrot Cake, Entenmanns*	1 Muffin/105g	344	328	5.1	45.8	15.1	3.0
Cheese & Black Pepper, Sainsbury's*	1 Muffin/65g	142	218	12.9	34.6	2.0	1.2
Cheese, Tesco*	1 Muffin/75g	183	244	12.5	38.1	4.6	2.0
Choc Chip, BGTY, Sainsbury's*	1 Muffin/75g	282	376	5.2	51.8	16.4	1.6
Choc Chip, Mini, Weight Watchers*	1 Muffin/15g	47	312	6.6	52.1	8.6	3.1
Chocolate Chip, American Style, Sainsbury's*	1 Muffin/75g	328	437	5.9	52.4	22.7	0.6
Chocolate Chip, Black Friar's*	1 Muffin/50g	218	435	6.0	51.0	23.0	4.0
Chocolate Indulgence, McVitie's*	1 Muffin/75g	254	338	5.8	57.9	9.2	1.3
Chocolate, BGTY, Sainsbury's*	1 Muffin/75g	282	376	5.2	51.8	16.4	1.6

MUFFIN,	Measure INFO/WEIGHT	per Measure KCAL	KCAL	PROT	CARB	FAT	FIBRE
Chocolate, Dairy Cream, Safeway*	1 Muffin/109.7g	430	391	7.3	31.9	26.1	3.1
Chunky Choc n Orange, The Fabulous Bakin Boys*	1 Muffin/40g	154	384	5.0	42.0	22.0	1.0
Chunky Chocolate Chip, McVitie's*	1 Muffin/94g	393	418	5.3	50.6	21.6	0.8
Classic Blueberry, Starbucks*	1 Muffin/129g	438	337	4.4	39.7	17.7	1.4
Dairy Cream Lemon, Safeway*	1 Muffin/110g	409	372	4.4	44.5	19.6	0.0
Double Berry Burst, Entenmann's*	1 Muffin/59g	140	238	4.6	50.1	2.1	1.6
Double Choc Chip, Mini, Asda*	1 Muffin/19g	74	390	6.0	51.0	18.0	0.0
Double Choc Chip, Weight Watchers*	1 Muffin/65g	189	291	6.8	47.2	8.3	3.6
Double Chocolate Chip, Co-Op*	1 Muffin/60g	246	410	6.0	49.0	21.0	3.0
Double Chocolate Chip, Healthier, Tesco*	1 Muffin/72g	272	378	7.0	51.6	16.0	1.4
Double Chocolate Chip, New, Weight Watchers*	1 Muffin/65g	169	260	3.9	52.2	4.0	1.9
Double Chocolate Chip, Sainsbury's*	1 Muffin/72.0g	290	403	4.8	50.0	20.4	1.9
Double Chocolate Chip, Tesco*	1 Muffin/72g	302	419	6.1	48.0	22.5	1.4
Double Chocolate, 95% Fat Free, Entenmann's*	1 Muffin/58g	152	262	2.6	52.3	4.7	1.8
Double Chocolate, Marks & Spencer*	1 Muffin/75g	313	417	5.2	48.7	22.4	1.9
Double Chocolate, Mini, Marks & Spencer*	1 Muffin/30g	131	438	5.7	52.8	22.7	1.2
Double Chocolate, Mini, Tesco*	1 Muffin/28g	116	414	6.3	45.7	23.0	1.4
Double Chocolate, Mini, Weight Watchers*	1 Muffin/15g	45	300	7.0	48.5	8.7	3.5
Double Chocolate, Somerfield*	1 Muffin/70g	298	425	6.8	46.5	23.5	0.0
English, Butter, Tesco*	1 Muffin/67.2g	170	253	11.2	39.8	5.4	2.0
English, Marks & Spencer*	1 Muffin/60g	135	225	11.2	43.7	1.9	2.9
English, Wholewheat, Finest, Tesco*	1 Muffin/70g	98	140	7.6	24.6	1.3	3.7
Galaxy, McVitie's*	1 Muffin/94.0g	358	381	5.1	45.0	20.1	0.0
Lemon & Blueberry, Tesco*	1 Muffin/110g	411	374	4.0	42.4	20.9	1.1
Lemon & Poppy Seed, Entenmann's*	1 Muffin/105g	417	397	5.6	52.8	19.3	2.5
Lemon & Poppy Seed, Marks & Spencer*	1 Muffin/72g	281	390	6.3	46.1	19.8	1.5
Lemon & Sultana, BGTY, Sainsbury's*	1 Muffin/75g	211	281	4.5	55.6	4.5	1.4
Lemon, Boots*	1 Muffin/110g	424	385	3.6	50.0	19.0	1.3
Marks & Spencer*	1 Muffin/56g	126	225	11.2	43.7	1.9	2.9
Mini, Tesco*	1 Muffin/28g	120	428	6.4	50.0	22.6	1.2
Mississipi Mud, Sainsbury's*	1 Muffin/72.1g	274	380	5.2	48.6	18.3	4.2
Mixed Fruit, Low Fat, Abbey Bakery*	1 Muffin/35g	93	267	4.5	55.6	4.5	1.4
Oven Bottom, Asda*	1 Muffin/68g	173	255	10.0	50.4	1.5	2.2
Oven Bottom, Mini, Morrisons*	1 Muffin/42g	107	255	10.0	50.4	1.5	2.2
Oven Bottom, Tesco*	1 Muffin/68g	173	255	10.0	50.4	1.5	2.2
Oven Bottom, Warburton's*	1 Muffin/69g	175	253	10.9	45.8	2.9	0.0
Plain Choc Chip, Tesco*	1 Muffin/72g	302	419	6.2	48.9	22.1	1.1
Plain Chocolate Chip, Sainsbury's*	1 Muffin/75g	313	423	6.4	51.3	21.4	0.6
Plain, Co-Op*	1 Muffin/60g	150	250	13.3	45.0	1.7	1.7
Plain, Iceland*	1 Muffin/100g	173	173	6.5	33.8	1.3	1.5
Premium White, Sainsbury's*	1 Muffin/65g	135	208	8.0	41.4	1.1	2.0
Raspberry Cream, Sainsbury's*	1 Muffin/90g	314	349	3.9	33.8	22.0	1.3
Rolo, Nestle*	1 Muffin/80g	289	361	5.4	44.3	18.0	0.8
Sausage, Egg & Cheese, American Style, Tesco*	1 Muffin/155g	383	247	12.2	19.9	13.2	1.0
Skinny Blueberry, Starbucks*	1 Muffin/129g	306	236	3.7	47.2	3.2	1.7
Skinny Peach & Raspberry, Starbucks*	1 Muffin/120.2g	286	238	5.1	46.5	3.7	1.4
Skinny Sunrise, Starbucks*	1 Muffin/130g	255	194	4.6	36.7	3.0	1.3
Somerfield*	1 Muffin/60g	130	216	12.2	39.3	1.6	1.9
Spiced Fruit, Co-Op*	1 Muffin/60g	159	265	11.0	52.0	2.0	3.0
Spicy Fruit, Sainsbury's*	1 Muffin/63g	140	222	9.6	43.3	1.2	2.7
Sunrise, Starbucks*	1 Muffin/150g	592	395	5.5	40.8	23.1	1.9
Toffee & Pecan, Finest, Tesco*	1 Muffin/127g	551	434	5.4	51.8	22.8	0.9
Toffee Choo Choo, Tesco*	1 Muffin/95g	402	423	6.4	49.1	22.4	1.0

Nutrition Values per 100g / 100ml

	Measure	per Measure	Nutrition Values per 100g / 100ml				
	INFO/WEIGHT	KCAL	KCAL	PROT	CARB	FAT	FIBRE
MUFFIN,							
Toffee Temptation, McVitie's*	1 Muffin/85.5g	295	347	4.7	60.8	9.5	0.8
Vanilla & Choc Chip, GFY, Asda*	1 Muffin/58.5g	151	260	7.0	53.0	2.2	1.6
White Chocolate Chunk Lemon, Mini, Marks & Spencer*	1 Muffin/28g	130	464	6.4	55.4	23.9	2.1
White Chocolate Strawberry, Starbucks*	1 Muffin/142g	583	411	5.7	47.4	22.0	2.3
White, Asda*	1 Muffin/72g	174	242	9.0	48.0	1.6	2.0
White, Finest, Tesco*	1 Muffin/70g	159	227	8.4	45.7	1.2	2.1
White, Marks & Spencer*	1 Muffin/60g	135	225	11.2	43.7	1.9	2.9
White, Safeway*	1 Muffin/63g	142	226	10.3	43.2	1.3	208.0
White, Sainsbury's*	1 Muffin/65g	147	226	10.3	43.2	1.3	2.8
White, Tesco*	1 Muffin/60g	143	238	10.2	42.0	3.2	2.1
White, Waitrose*	1 Muffin/60g	128	213	10.7	39.4	1.4	4.2
Wholemeal, Organic, Waitrose*	1 Muffin/65g	129	198	12.4	32.9	1.9	7.6
Wholemeal, Perfectly Balanced, Waitrose*	1 Muffin/65g	137	211	11.8	36.1	2.2	5.8
Wholemeal, Tesco*	1 Muffin/65g	134	206	11.1	35.9	2.0	5.2
MULBERRIES, Raw	1oz/28g	10	36	1.3	8.1	0.0	0.0
MULLET,							
Grey, Grilled	1oz/28g	42	150	25.7	0.0	5.2	0.0
Grey, Raw	1oz/28g	32	115	19.8	0.0	4.0	0.0
Red, Grilled	1oz/28g	34	121	20.4	0.0	4.4	0.0
Red, Raw	1oz/28g	31	109	18.7	0.0	3.8	0.0
MULTIVITAMINS DRINK, Tropicana*	1fl oz/30ml	16	52	0.5	10.5	0.0	0.1
MUNCHIES,							
Milky Bar, Nestle*	1 Pack/35g	196	560	7.0	54.9	34.7	0.0
Mint, Rowntree, Nestle*	1 Pack/61g	268	433	3.8	67.4	16.5	0.0
Nestle*	1 Pack/52g	255	490	4.7	63.9	24.0	0.0
MUSHROOMS,							
Breaded, Home-Style, Kitchen Range Foods*	1oz/28g	32	113	4.3	23.2	0.4	0.0
Button, Baby, Tesco*	1 Serving/75g	10	13	1.8	0.4	0.5	1.1
Button, Farmfoods*	1oz/28g	6	22	4.0	0.4	0.5	1.1
Button, Organic, Iceland*	1oz/28g	44	157	2.4	0.3	16.2	1.5
Button, Sliced, Sainsbury's*	1 Can/156g	22	14	2.1	0.5	0.5	1.2
Button, Whole, In Salted Water, Tesco*	1 Serving/50g	6	11	1.7	0.6	0.2	1.4
Button, Whole, Sainsbury's*	1 Can/208g	29	14	2.1	0.5	0.5	1.2
Chargrilled, & Pasta, Finest, Tesco*	1 Pot/200g	404	202	5.4	16.7	12.5	1.3
Cheesey, Stuffed, Asda*	½ Pack/145g	131	90	3.4	8.3	4.8	1.7
Chestnut, Tesco*	1 Pack/250g	33	13	1.8	0.4	0.5	1.1
Chinese, Dried, Raw	1oz/28g	80	284	10.0	59.9	1.8	0.0
Closed Cup, Tesco*	1oz/28g	4	13	1.8	0.4	0.5	1.1
Common, Boiled in Salted Water	1oz/28g	3	11	1.8	0.4	0.3	1.1
Common, Canned, Re-Heated, Drained	1oz/28g	3	12	2.1	0.0	0.4	1.3
Common, Fried in Blended Oil	1oz/28g	44	157	2.4	0.3	16.2	1.5
Common, Fried in Butter	1oz/28g	44	157	2.4	0.3	16.2	1.5
Common, Raw	1oz/28g	4	13	1.8	0.4	0.5	1.1
Creamed, Asda*	½ Can/145g	132	91	1.2	8.0	6.0	0.3
Creamed, Chesswood*	1oz/28g	24	86	1.3	9.0	5.0	0.8
Creamed, Tesco*	1oz/28g	19	68	1.3	3.4	5.5	0.3
Dried	1oz/28g	45	159	21.8	4.8	6.0	13.3
Flat, Large, Safeway*	1 Serving/65g	15	23	4.0	0.5	0.5	0.0
Frozen, Sliced, Sainsbury's*	1 Serving/50g	6	12	1.8	0.4	0.3	1.1
Frozen, Tesco*	1oz/28g	4	13	1.8	0.4	0.5	1.1
Garlic	1oz/28g	39	139	2.1	0.6	14.4	1.2
Garlic, Asda*	1 Pack/280g	470	168	5.0	19.0	8.0	1.7
Garlic, Breaded, Asda*	1 Serving/100g	173	173	5.7	17.9	8.8	0.9

MUSHROOMS,	Measure INFO/WEIGHT	per Measure KCAL	Nutrition Values per 100g / 100ml KCAL	PROT	CARB	FAT	FIBRE
Garlic, Breaded, Iceland*	1 Pack/340g	816	240	5.6	18.6	15.9	1.6
Garlic, Fresh, Sainsbury's*	½ Pack/150g	128	85	0.2	8.6	5.5	1.0
Garlic, Marks & Spencer*	1 Serving/100g	95	95	4.0	2.0	8.1	2.8
Garlic, Pizza Hut*	1 Pack/112.2g	217	192	5.9	19.7	9.9	3.4
Garlic, With BBQ Dip, Pizza Hut*	1 Pack/112.2g	264	234	6.2	30.5	10.0	3.4
Garlic, With Sour Cream & Chive Dip, Pizza Hut*	1 Pack/112.2g	429	380	6.4	20.0	30.8	3.4
Oyster, Raw, Finest, Tesco*	1 Serving/28g	6	22	1.6	3.3	0.3	2.6
Oyster, Raw, Unprepared	1oz/28g	2	8	1.6	0.0	0.2	0.0
Porcini, Dried, Merchant Gourmet*	1 oz/28g	36	128	12.3	5.0	6.5	0.0
Raw, Value, Tesco*	1 Serving/28g	4	13	1.8	0.4	0.5	1.1
Shiitake, Cooked	1oz/28g	15	55	1.6	12.3	0.2	0.0
Shiitake, Dried, Raw	1oz/28g	83	296	9.6	63.9	1.0	0.0
Shiitake, Raw, Finest,Tesco*	1 Serving/28g	7	26	2.2	4.4	0.0	1.1
Sliced, Fresh, Frozen, Tesco*	1 Serving/100g	13	13	1.8	0.4	0.5	1.1
Sliced, Frozen, Asda*	1 Serving/28g	3	12	1.8	0.4	0.3	1.1
Sliced, In Salted Water, Tesco*	1 Serving/100g	11	11	1.7	0.6	0.2	1.4
Sliced, in Salted Water, Hartley's*	1 Serving/70g	8	12	2.1	0.0	0.4	1.3
Straw, Canned, Drained	1oz/28g	4	15	2.1	1.2	0.2	0.0
Stuffed With Cheese, Mustard & Herbs, Sainsbury's*	1 Serving/115g	150	130	7.4	6.3	8.3	1.2
Stuffed, Finest, Tesco*	1 Serving/130g	224	172	4.0	7.4	14.0	1.9
Stuffed, With Cheese & Herb Breadcrumbs, Waitrose*	1 Serving/165g	215	130	4.6	16.2	5.2	2.1
MUSSELS,							
Boiled	1 Mussel/7g	7	104	16.7	3.5	2.7	0.0
Canned & Bottled, Drained	1oz/28g	27	98	16.9	3.1	2.1	0.0
Cooked & Shelled, Asda*	1 Pack/175g	186	106	17.0	3.5	2.7	0.0
Garlic Butter Sauce, Cooked, Scottish, Morrisons*	½ Pack/250g	218	87	4.6	3.6	6.0	0.3
Greenshell, New Zealand, Sainsbury's*	1 Serving/60g	74	123	19.2	4.3	2.3	0.1
In Garlic Butter Sauce, Murphys*	½ Pack/225g	162	72	8.1	0.3	4.2	0.0
Raw	1oz/28g	21	74	12.1	2.5	1.8	0.0
Thai Fragrant, Marks & Spencer*	½ Pack/325g	358	110	10.6	4.5	5.7	0.1
Vegetable Oil, Smoked, John West*	1oz/28g	58	207	20.0	7.0	11.0	0.0
White Wine Cream Sauce, Cooked, Scottish, Morrisons*	½ Pack/250g	263	105	9.0	5.4	5.3	0.5
Youngs*	1 Pack/450g	396	88	9.0	5.3	3.5	0.5
MUSTARD,							
American, French's*	1 Tbsp/15g	27	180	6.0	16.0	12.0	0.0
Cajun, Colman's*	1 Tsp/6g	11	187	7.0	23.0	6.5	2.7
Coarse Grain, Frank Cooper*	1 Tsp/6g	12	206	8.9	17.0	11.4	0.0
Colman's*	1 Tsp/5ml	9	188	7.0	19.0	9.3	1.6
Dijon, Asda*	1 Tsp/7g	11	163	7.7	6.6	11.1	0.0
Dijon, Frank Cooper*	1 Tsp/6g	11	179	7.2	10.0	12.3	0.0
Dijon, Marks & Spencer*	1 Tsp/6g	9	153	10.0	7.2	9.5	1.0
Dijon, Organic, Simply Delicious*	1 Serving/10g	17	166	8.2	6.7	10.6	2.6
Dijon, Tesco*	1 Serving/10g	14	141	8.4	6.4	8.2	0.0
English, Colman's*	1 Tsp/10ml	19	188	7.0	19.0	9.3	1.6
English, Frank Cooper*	1 Tsp/6g	11	188	5.7	22.0	8.6	0.2
English, Marks & Spencer*	1 Tsp/6g	14	226	12.6	8.7	15.9	1.0
English, Powder, Colman's*	1 Tsp/5g	26	518	29.0	24.0	34.0	6.2
English, Safeway*	1 Tsp/6g	10	163	6.1	18.3	6.7	0.0
English, With Chillies, Sainsbury's*	1 Tsp/5g	10	204	8.3	18.1	10.9	6.4
French Mild, Colman's*	1 Tsp/6g	6	104	6.3	4.0	7.0	3.8
French, Frank Cooper*	1 Tsp/6g	7	113	4.6	7.0	7.4	0.0
Honey, Colman's*	1 Tsp/6g	12	208	7.4	24.0	8.2	0.0
Mayonnaise, BGTY, Sainsbury's*	1 Tsp/6g	9	146	2.9	13.4	8.8	0.5

	Measure INFO/WEIGHT	per Measure KCAL	Nutrition Values per 100g / 100ml				
			KCAL	PROT	CARB	FAT	FIBRE
MUSTARD,							
Peppercorn, Colman's*	1 Tsp/6g	11	182	8.8	12.0	10.0	4.9
Powder	1 Tsp/3.3g	14	452	28.9	20.7	28.7	0.0
Powder, Made Up	1oz/28g	63	226	14.5	10.4	14.4	0.0
Smooth	1 Level Tsp/8g	11	139	7.1	9.7	8.2	0.0
Sweet Peppers, Colman's*	1 Tsp/6g	13	218	7.9	20.0	11.0	4.9
Tarragon, Tesco*	1 Tbsp/15ml	59	396	0.9	8.6	39.8	0.2
Wholegrain	1 Level Tsp/8g	11	140	8.2	4.2	10.2	4.9
Wholegrain, Colman's*	1 Tsp/6g	10	173	8.5	8.5	11.0	5.9
Wholegrain, Safeway*	1 Tbsp/15g	27	183	8.0	15.2	9.1	0.0
Wholegrain, Sainsbury's*	1 Tsp/5g	7	137	6.5	4.2	10.5	0.0
Wholegrain, Tesco*	1 Tsp/6g	0	153	8.2	8.7	9.5	5.8
MUSTARD & CRESS, Raw	1oz/28g	4	13	1.6	0.4	0.6	1.1

INFO/WEIGHT	Measure per Measure	KCAL	Nutrition Values per 100g / 100ml				
			KCAL	PROT	CARB	FAT	FIBRE
NACHOS,							
American Chilli Beef, Asda*	1 Serving/200g	208	104	10.0	4.7	5.0	0.8
Chicken, Safeway*	½ Pack/170g	352	207	10.3	15.7	11.4	1.8
Chilli, Sainsbury's*	½ Pack/250g	695	278	10.9	29.5	12.9	1.3
Kit, Old El Paso*	½ Pack/260g	598	230	4.0	31.0	10.0	0.0
NASI GORENG,							
Indonesian, Asda*	1 Pack/360g	778	216	7.4	32.3	6.3	1.3
Indonesion, Sainsbury's*	1 Tbsp/15g	24	162	3.3	11.8	11.3	2.1
NECTARINES,							
Fresh, Raw	1oz/28g	11	40	1.4	9.0	0.1	1.2
Weighed With Pips	1 Med/140g	50	36	1.2	8.0	0.1	1.1
NESQUIK,							
Chocolate Flavour, Dry, Nestle*	3 Tsp/15g	57	380	2.5	86.5	2.8	2.2
Strawberry, Dry, Nestle*	1 Serving/10g	39	390	0.0	96.7	0.5	0.0
NIBBLES, Cheese & Ham, Sainsbury's*	½ Pack/50g	257	514	13.1	54.8	27.1	2.6
NIK NAKS,							
Cream 'n' Cheesy, Golden Wonder*	1 Bag/34g	185	545	5.1	56.1	33.4	0.0
Nice 'n' Spicy, Golden Wonder*	1 Bag/34g	185	545	4.7	55.5	33.4	1.0
Rib 'n' Saucy, Golden Wonder*	1 Bag/34g	185	545	5.1	55.7	33.4	1.1
Scampi 'n' Lemon, Golden Wonder*	1 Bag/34g	195	573	5.0	49.6	39.4	1.4
NOODLE BOWL, Szechuan Style Prawn, Tesco*	1 Bowl/400g	376	94	5.5	17.3	0.3	0.9
NOODLES,							
Beef Flavour, Instant, Prepared, Heinz*	1 Pack/384g	257	67	2.1	14.4	0.1	0.6
Char Sui, Cantonese, Sainsbury's*	1 Pack/450g	378	84	6.8	10.5	1.6	1.5
Chicken Flavour, 3 Minute, Dry, Blue Dragon*	1 Pack/85g	403	475	9.3	61.2	21.4	0.0
Chicken Flavour, Dry, Eldorado*	1 Pack/85g	360	423	14.0	61.0	15.0	0.0
Chicken Flavour, Instant, Cooked, Sainsbury's*	1 Pack/335g	409	122	2.7	18.0	4.4	0.1
Chicken Flavour, Instant, Cooked, Asda*	1 Pack/65g	101	155	4.7	23.0	4.9	0.3
Chicken Flavour, Dry, Princes*	1 Pack/85g	395	465	10.0	63.8	18.8	0.0
Chicken, Chinese Style, GFY, Asda*	1 Pack/393g	295	75	6.0	9.0	1.7	0.6
Chicken, Chinese, Asda*	1 Pot/302g	305	101	6.0	16.0	1.4	0.8
Chicken, Dry, Heinz*	1 Serving/85g	257	302	9.5	65.3	0.4	2.7
Chicken, Instant, Prepared, Heinz*	1 Pack/384g	257	67	2.1	14.4	0.1	0.6
Chilli Chicken, GFY, Asda*	1 Pack/415g	461	111	6.0	20.0	0.8	1.0
Chinese, Egg, Medium, Dry, Sharwood's*	1 Serving/65g	223	343	11.0	70.9	1.8	2.5
Chinese, Egg, Thick, Dry, Sharwood's*	1 Serving/100g	343	343	11.0	70.9	1.8	2.5
Chinese, Stir Fry, Sainsbury's*	1 Serving/100g	185	185	6.0	29.5	4.8	1.5
Chow Mein, Chicken Bowl, Uncle Ben's*	1 Pack/330g	307	93	6.1	13.5	1.4	0.0
Chow Mein, Sainsbury's*	1 Pack/125g	136	109	3.9	19.2	1.8	0.8
Chow Mein, Stir Fry, Tesco*	1 Serving/200g	116	58	2.1	9.7	1.2	1.0
Crispy, Blue Dragon*	1 Box/125g	438	350	2.4	84.0	0.5	0.0
Curry, Prepared, Heinz*	1 Pack/85g	58	68	2.1	14.6	0.1	0.6
Curry, Instant, Dry, Heinz*	1 Serving/85g	261	307	9.5	66.4	0.4	2.7
Egg Fried, Cantonese, Safeway*	1oz/28g	29	104	3.4	10.7	5.3	1.1
Egg, Boiled	1oz/28g	17	62	2.2	13.0	0.5	0.6
Egg, Fine Thread, Dry, Marks & Spencer*	1 Serving/63g	221	350	14.3	71.6	0.9	5.1
Egg, Fine, Dry, Sharwood's*	1 Serving/75g	257	343	11.0	70.9	1.8	2.5
Egg, Medium, Asda*	1 Layer/190g	289	152	4.8	31.0	0.8	1.3
Egg, Medium, Dry, Blue Dragon*	1 Sheet/81g	276	341	11.0	70.0	1.9	1.0
Egg, Medium, Sainsbury's*	1 Serving/122.1g	162	133	5.5	25.9	0.7	1.0
Egg, Medium, Dry, Sharwood's*	1 Block/65g	221	340	10.8	70.1	1.8	2.9
Egg, Dry, Raw	1oz/28g	109	391	12.1	71.7	8.2	2.9
Egg, Straight To Wok, Amoy*	½ Pack/75g	113	151	4.2	29.0	2.1	1.3
Egg, Thread, Amoy*	1 Serving/150g	227	151	4.2	29.0	2.1	1.3

	Measure INFO/WEIGHT	per Measure KCAL	Nutrition Values per 100g / 100ml				
			KCAL	PROT	CARB	FAT	FIBRE
NOODLES,							
Egg, Thread, Sharwood's*	1oz/28g	30	107	3.6	21.8	0.6	1.1
Egg, Tossed In Sesame Oil, Asda*	½ Pack/150g	174	116	2.3	11.0	7.0	0.0
Fresh, Tesco*	1 Serving/150g	102	68	2.8	11.4	1.3	0.6
Fried	1oz/28g	43	153	1.9	11.3	11.5	0.5
Instant, Dry, Blue Dragon*	1 Serving/75g	124	165	2.8	25.7	5.7	0.0
Instant, Dry, Sainsburys*	1 packet/100g	392	392	9.4	57.0	14.0	0.2
Japanese Udon, Sainsbury's*	1 Serving/150g	210	140	3.9	27.1	1.8	1.2
Medium, Straight To Wok*	1oz/28g	47	169	6.0	24.5	5.2	0.0
Mung Bean, Dry, Amoy*	1oz/28g	95	341	15.9	66.6	1.2	0.0
Oriental Beef & Sweet Red Pepper, Dry, Colman's*	1 Serving/80g	254	317	4.2	73.4	0.7	5.1
Oriental Style, Break, Asda*	1 Pot/57g	218	382	12.3	80.7	1.2	2.5
Peking Duck, Shapers, Boots*	1 Pack/280g	395	141	7.2	25.0	1.4	1.8
Plain, Boiled	1oz/28g	17	62	2.4	13.0	0.4	0.7
Plain, Raw, Dry	1oz/28g	109	388	11.7	76.1	6.2	2.9
Ramen, With Chilli Beef, Marks & Spencer*	1 Pack/484g	532	110	8.1	11.9	3.6	0.8
Rice, Dry, Amoy*	1oz/28g	101	361	6.5	86.6	1.0	0.0
Rice, Dry, Blue Dragon*	1 Serving/30g	113	376	6.0	88.0	0.0	0.0
Rice, Thai, Dry, Sharwood's*	1 Pack/250g	903	361	6.5	86.8	1.0	2.4
Savoury Vegetable, COU, Marks & Spencer*	1 Pack/450g	270	60	2.9	11.5	0.6	1.2
Singapore, New, Marks & Spencer*	1 Pack/400g	540	135	5.3	14.6	5.9	0.6
Singapore, Sainsbury's*	1 Pack/350g	441	126	3.2	11.9	7.3	2.4
Singapore, Somerfield*	1 Pot/300g	261	87	5.0	15.0	1.0	0.0
Singapore, Tesco*	1 Pack/350g	389	111	6.3	16.8	2.1	0.7
Singapore, Waitrose*	1 Pack/400g	476	119	7.3	12.6	4.4	2.1
Spicy Curry Flavour, Snack, SmartPrice, Asda*	1 Pot/76g	358	471	10.5	65.8	18.4	0.0
Straight to Wok, Amoy*	1 Pack/180g	272	151	4.2	29.0	2.1	1.3
Straight to Wok, New, Amoy*	1 Serving/150g	240	160	5.8	31.7	1.5	0.0
Super, Bacon, Dry, Batchelors*	1 Pack/100g	457	457	9.8	60.9	19.7	3.2
Super, Cheese & Ham, Prepared, Batchelors*	1 Serving/100g	171	171	3.4	22.9	7.3	0.6
Super, Chicken & Ham, Dry, Batchelors*	1 Pack/100g	472	472	9.4	63.2	20.2	1.5
Super, Chicken Flavour, Prepared, Batchelors*	1 Serving/100g	170	170	3.3	22.9	7.3	0.9
Super, Chow Mein Flavour, Prepared, Batchelors*	1 Serving/100g	158	158	3.2	20.9	6.8	1.0
Super, Mild Curry Flavour, Prepared, Batchelors*	1 Serving/100g	157	157	3.2	20.9	6.7	1.0
Super, Mushroom Flavour, Prepared, Batchelors*	1 Serving/100g	157	157	3.2	20.9	6.8	1.0
Super, Spicy Salsa, Dry, Batchelors*	1 Pack/105g	474	451	7.0	63.8	18.6	1.7
Sweet & Sour, BGTY, Sainsbury's*	1 Serving/100g	112	112	2.3	18.6	3.1	0.0
Sweet Chilli, Wok, Findus*	1 Pack/300g	300	100	3.0	20.0	0.5	0.0
Szechuan Beef Flavour, Blue Dragon*	½ Pack/100g	350	350	10.5	72.3	1.2	0.0
Thai Style, Good For You, Asda*	1 Pot/237.9g	226	95	3.0	20.0	0.3	0.8
Thai Style, Sainsbury's*	1 Pack/340g	381	112	3.3	19.4	2.3	0.7
Thai, Waitrose*	1 Pack/300g	357	119	6.8	18.4	2.1	1.7
Udon, New, Amoy*	1 Portion/150g	212	141	4.4	28.8	1.3	0.0
Wholewheat, Blue Dragon*	1 Serving/65g	208	320	12.5	63.0	2.0	8.0
Yaki Soba, Yutaka*	1 Pack/170g	311	183	4.7	35.1	2.2	0.0
NOODLES &, BEAN SPROUTS, Fresh Ideas, Tesco*	1 Pack/250g	310	124	5.4	19.8	2.6	1.9
NOUGAT,							
Almond & Cherry, Marks & Spencer*	1 Sweet/7g	28	405	4.5	76.0	9.1	1.1
Average	1oz/28g	108	384	4.4	77.3	8.5	0.9
Raspberry & Orange Hazelnut, Thorntons*	1 Chocolate/9g	39	433	4.8	60.0	20.0	2.2
NUGGETS,							
Meat Free, Blue Parrot Cafe, Sainsbury's*	1 Nugget/18g	41	228	17.3	12.5	12.1	3.0
Vegetarian, Safeway*	4 Nuggets/80.1g	161	201	16.3	10.5	10.4	3.6

	Measure INFO/WEIGHT	per Measure KCAL	Nutrition Values per 100g / 100ml				
			KCAL	PROT	CARB	FAT	FIBRE
NUT ROAST,							
Average	1oz/28g	99	352	13.3	18.3	25.7	4.2
Courgette & Spiced Tomato, Cauldron Foods*	1 Serving/100g	208	208	11.7	12.5	12.3	4.9
Leek, Cheese & Mushroom, Organic, Cauldron Foods*	½ Pack/143g	343	240	13.2	13.2	14.9	4.1
Lentil	1oz/28g	62	222	10.6	18.8	12.1	3.8
Tomato & Courgette, Organic, Waitrose*	½ Pack/142g	295	208	11.7	12.5	12.3	4.9
Vegetarian, Tesco*	1 Serving/160g	218	136	5.4	11.4	7.6	2.0
NUTMEG, Powder	1 Tsp/3g	16	525	5.8	45.3	36.3	0.0
NUTRI-GRAIN,							
Apple, Kellogg's*	1 Bar/37g	130	350	4.0	68.0	8.0	3.0
Blueberry, Kellogg's*	1 Bar/37g	130	350	4.0	68.0	8.0	3.0
Cappuccino, Kellogg's*	1 Bar/37g	137	370	5.0	66.0	10.0	2.5
Cherry, Kellogg's*	1 Bar/37g	133	360	4.0	68.0	8.0	3.0
Chocolate, Kellogg's*	1 Bar/37g	137	370	4.5	67.0	10.0	3.0
Elevenses Ginger, Kellogg's*	1 Bar/45g	170	378	5.6	66.7	8.9	3.3
Elevenses, Kellogg's*	1 Bar/45g	162	360	5.0	67.0	8.0	3.5
Forest Fruits & Yoghurt Twists, Kellogg's*	1 Bar/37g	133	360	3.5	69.0	8.0	2.0
Mixed Fruits Twists, Kellogg's*	1 Bar/37g	133	360	3.5	69.0	8.0	2.0
Orange, Kellogg's*	1 Bar/37g	137	370	5.0	68.0	9.0	4.0
Strawberry Twists, Kellogg's*	1 Bar/37g	130	350	3.5	69.0	8.0	2.0
Strawberry, Kellogg's*	1 Bar/37g	133	360	4.0	69.0	8.0	3.0
Strawberry, Mini, Kellogg's*	1 Pack/45g	158	350	4.0	69.0	8.0	3.5
Tangy Orange, Kellogg's*	1 Bar/38g	141	370	5.0	68.0	9.0	4.0
NUTS,							
Honey Roasted, Marks & Spencer*	1oz/28g	175	625	18.1	20.5	52.2	5.1
Luxury, Organic, Marks & Spencer*	1oz/28g	179	640	21.1	11.6	56.6	6.1
Mixed	1 Pack/40g	243	607	22.9	7.9	54.1	6.0
Mixed, Chopped, Safeway*	1 Serving/2g	12	588	22.0	10.3	51.0	5.9
Mixed, Chopped, Sainsbury's*	1 Serving/100g	605	605	27.1	9.6	50.9	6.0
Mixed, Chopped, Tesco*	1 Pack/100g	591	591	23.5	10.5	50.6	6.0
Mixed, Feast, Eat Natural*	1 Bar/50g	278	556	18.8	28.0	41.0	0.0
Mixed, Luxury, Unsalted, Somerfield*	1oz/28g	186	663	18.0	10.0	61.0	0.0
Mixed, Natural, Luxury, Tesco*	1oz/28g	179	639	22.6	6.9	57.9	5.6
Mixed, Natures Harvest*	1 Serving/25g	166	662	16.0	5.6	63.9	5.6
Mixed, Roast Salted, Somerfield*	1oz/28g	175	625	24.0	11.0	54.0	0.0
Mixed, Sainsbury's*	1 Bag/200g	1346	673	18.8	4.6	64.5	5.3
Mixed, Unsalted, Sainsbury's*	1 Serving/50g	311	622	18.5	7.2	57.7	8.7
Monkey, Sainsbury's*	1 Serving/100g	564	564	25.6	12.5	46.1	6.2
Natural Assortment, Tesco*	1 Serving/50g	338	676	17.5	6.1	64.6	5.0
Natural, Mixed, Waitrose*	1 Serving/50g	318	635	16.3	18.9	54.9	4.6
Oak Smoke Flavour Selection, Finest, Tesco*	1 Serving/25g	158	633	21.4	11.2	55.8	6.3
Roast Salted, Luxury, KP*	1oz/28g	181	646	21.9	10.1	57.6	5.9
Salted Peanuts & Cashews, Sainsbury's*	¼ Pack/50g	314	627	25.5	12.1	52.3	5.4
Salted, Mixed Roasted, Waitrose*	1 Pack/200g	1252	626	13.7	11.3	58.4	4.4
Salted, Selection, TTD, Sainsbury's*	1 Pack/75g	509	678	16.3	8.9	64.2	7.2
Unsalted, Selection, Sainsbury's*	1 Serving/75g	491	655	14.7	5.0	64.0	6.7
NUTS & RAISINS,							
Mixed	1 Pack/40g	192	481	14.1	31.5	34.1	4.5
Mixed, KP*	1 Serving/50g	273	546	21.4	24.4	40.3	5.2
Mixed, Nature's Harvest*	1 Serving/50g	232	463	12.4	32.9	33.7	3.4
Mixed, Safeway*	1 Serving/50g	264	527	18.6	30.7	36.7	4.8
Mixed, Somerfield*	1oz/28g	159	568	18.0	24.0	45.0	0.0
Mixed, Unsalted, Sainsbury's*	1oz/28g	143	510	16.2	28.0	37.0	4.8

N

	Measure INFO/WEIGHT	per Measure KCAL	Nutrition Values per 100g / 100ml				
			KCAL	PROT	CARB	FAT	FIBRE
OATCAKES,							
Cheese, Nairn's*	1 Cake/8g	38	474	13.8	49.2	24.7	6.2
Fine, Nairn's*	1 Oatcake/7g	32	463	10.9	61.3	19.3	6.0
Highland, Organic, Sainsbury's*	1 Oatcake/12.5g	59	456	10.2	59.8	19.5	5.5
Highland, Walkers*	1 Oatcake/12g	54	451	10.3	56.0	20.6	6.7
Nairn's*	1 Oatcake/10g	45	446	11.0	59.3	18.3	6.6
Organic, Safeway*	1 Oatcake/13g	56	445	11.2	56.7	19.3	6.6
Retail	1oz/28g	123	441	10.0	63.0	18.3	0.0
Rough Scottish, Sainsbury's*	1 Oatcake/11g	51	462	12.3	59.9	19.3	6.5
Rough With Bran, Walkers*	1 Oatcake/13g	59	454	10.2	53.3	22.2	7.8
Rough, Nairn's*	1 Oatcake/11g	48	436	10.6	64.7	18.2	7.2
Rough, Organic, Nairn's*	1 Oatcake/11g	47	428	10.9	57.7	17.0	7.6
Rough, Sainsbury's*	1 Cake/10.6g	51	462	12.3	59.9	19.3	6.5
Rough, Scottish, Tesco*	1 Oatcake/11g	48	434	12.3	54.8	18.4	6.6
Scottish With Cracked Black Pepper, Finest, Tesco*	1 Pack/64g	276	431	11.3	57.6	17.2	9.2
Scottish, Marks & Spencer*	1oz/28g	116	413	9.1	70.0	12.6	8.5
Scottish, Organic, Waitrose*	1 Biscuit/13g	58	447	11.2	57.0	19.4	6.6
Scottish, Paterson's*	1 Cake/12.5g	49	409	11.1	58.6	14.5	8.5
Traditional, Marks & Spencer*	1 Cake/11g	49	445	11.0	59.3	18.3	6.6
Traditional, Rough, Nairn's*	1 Oatcake/11g	47	429	11.7	63.5	17.7	7.8
With Cracked Black Pepper, Walkers*	1 Oatcake/9.5g	39	433	10.4	55.0	19.0	8.5
OATMEAL, Raw	1oz/28g	112	401	12.4	72.8	8.7	6.8
OATS,							
Jumbo, Organic, Evernat*	1oz/28g	117	418	13.0	69.0	9.6	7.4
Jumbo, Organic, Waitrose*	1oz/28g	101	361	11.0	61.1	8.1	7.8
TTD, Sainsbury's*	1 Serving/40g	152	381	9.7	74.7	4.8	0.0
OCEAN,							
Pinks, Asda*	1oz/28g	24	86	10.0	10.0	0.7	0.2
Prawnies, Mini, Asda*	1 Prawnie/11g	9	84	11.0	8.0	0.9	0.5
Snacks, Sainsbury's*	1 Stick/16g	18	113	7.0	21.0	0.1	0.1
Sticks, Sainsbury's*	1 Stick/16g	17	108	7.2	19.7	0.1	0.3
Stix, Farmfoods*	1 Stick/14g	15	110	7.0	20.0	0.2	0.0
OCTOPUS, Raw	1oz/28g	23	83	17.9	0.0	1.3	0.0
OIL,							
Avocado, Olivado*	1 Tsp/5ml	40	802	0.0	0.0	88.0	0.0
Black Truffle Grapeseed, Cuisine Perel*	1 Tbsp/15ml	129	857	0.0	7.1	100.0	0.0
Chilli, Sainsbury's*	1 Tsp/5ml	41	823	0.0	0.0	91.4	0.0
Chilli, Waitrose*	1 Tsp/5ml	41	824	0.0	0.0	91.6	0.0
Chinese Stir Fry, Asda*	1 Tbsp/15ml	123	823	0.0	0.0	91.4	0.0
Coconut	1 Tsp/5ml	45	899	0.0	0.0	99.9	0.0
Corn	1 Tsp/5ml	45	899	0.0	0.0	99.9	0.0
Corn, Mazola*	1 Tsp/5ml	42	830	0.0	0.0	92.0	0.0
Extra Vergine Olio De Oliva, Gentile, Bertolli*	1 Tbsp/15ml	123	820	0.0	0.0	91.0	0.0
Flora*	1 Tsp/5g	45	900	0.0	0.0	100.0	0.0
Grapeseed	1 Tsp/5ml	45	899	0.0	0.0	99.9	0.0
Groundnut, Co-Op*	1 Tsp/5ml	41	824	0.0	0.0	91.6	0.0
Groundnut, Somerfield*	1 Tsp/5ml	41	824	0.0	0.0	92.0	0.0
Hazelnut	1 Tsp/5ml	45	899	0.0	0.0	99.9	0.0
Olive	1 Tbsp/15ml	135	899	0.0	0.0	99.9	0.0
Olive, Central Italian, Sainsbury's*	1 Serving/10ml	82	823	0.1	0.0	91.0	0.0
Olive, Extra Virgin, Asda*	1 Tbsp/15ml	123	819	0.0	0.0	91.0	0.0
Olive, Extra Virgin, Bertolli*	1 Tbsp/15ml	123	820	0.0	0.0	91.0	0.0
Olive, Extra Virgin, Co-Op*	1 Tbsp/15ml	135	900	0.0	0.0	100.0	0.0
Olive, Extra Virgin, Filippo Berio*	1 Tsp/5ml	41	822	0.0	0.0	91.3	0.0

OIL,

INFO/WEIGHT	Measure per Measure KCAL	KCAL	PROT	CARB	FAT	FIBRE
Olive, Extra Virgin, Fruity & Peppery Flavour, Sainsbury's*	1 Tbsp/15ml	123	823	0.1	0.0	91.4	0.0
Olive, Extra Virgin, Mist Spray, Belolive*	1fl oz/30ml	150	500	0.0	0.0	55.0	0.0
Olive, Extra Virgin, Napolina*	1 fl oz/30ml	248	828	0.0	0.0	92.0	0.0
Olive, Extra Virgin, Sainsbury's*	1 Tbsp/15ml	123	823	0.1	0.0	91.4	0.0
Olive, Extra Virgin, Somerfield*	1fl oz/30ml	270	900	0.0	0.0	100.0	0.0
Olive, Extra Virgin, Tesco*	1 Tbsp/10g	90	900	0.0	0.0	100.0	0.0
Olive, Extra Virgin, Waitrose*	1 Tbsp/10ml	82	823	0.0	0.0	91.4	0.0
Olive, Garlic Flavoured, Sainsbury's*	1 Tsp/5ml	41	824	0.0	0.0	91.6	0.0
Olive, Garlic Infused, Tesco*	1 Dtsp/10g	90	900	0.0	0.0	100.0	0.0
Olive, Lemon Flavoured, Sainsbury's*	1 Tbsp/15ml	123	823	0.1	0.0	91.4	0.1
Olive, Light & Mild, Tesco*	1 Tbsp/7.7g	72	900	0.0	0.0	100.0	0.0
Olive, Mild, Sainsbury's*	1 Tbsp/14.9ml	123	823	0.1	0.0	91.4	0.0
Olive, Organic, Marks & Spencer*	1floz/30ml	270	900	0.0	0.0	100.0	0.0
Olive, Pure, Napolina*	1 fl oz/30ml	248	828	0.0	0.0	92.0	0.0
Olive, Safeway*	1 Serving/5ml	41	823	0.0	0.0	91.4	0.0
Olive, Spray, Fry Light*	5 Sprays/1ml	5	498	0.0	0.0	55.2	0.0
Palm	1 Tsp/5ml	45	899	0.0	0.0	99.9	0.0
Peanut	1 Tsp/5ml	45	899	0.0	0.0	99.9	0.0
Rapeseed	1 Tsp/5ml	45	899	0.0	0.0	99.9	0.0
Rapeseed, Lighter Tasting, Goldenfields*	1 Serving/30ml	248	828	0.0	0.0	92.0	0.0
Safflower	1 Tsp/5ml	45	899	0.0	0.0	99.9	0.0
Sesame	1 Tsp/5ml	45	898	0.2	0.0	99.7	0.0
Sesame, Blended, Amoy*	1 Tsp/5ml	44	880	0.0	0.0	100.0	0.0
Sesame, Finest, Tesco*	1 Tsp/3g	27	900	0.0	0.0	100.0	0.0
Sesame, Organic, Evernat*	1 Tsp/5ml	45	900	0.0	0.0	100.0	0.0
Sesame, Pure, Sharwood's*	1 Tsp/5ml	44	881	0.2	0.0	99.7	0.0
Soya	1 Tsp/5ml	45	899	0.0	0.0	99.9	0.0
Stir Fry, Sharwood's*	1fl oz/30ml	269	897	0.0	0.0	99.7	0.0
Sunflower	1 Tsp/5ml	45	899	0.0	0.0	99.9	0.0
Sunflower With Vitamin E, Flora*	1 Serving/5g	45	900	0.0	0.0	100.0	0.0
Sunflower, Flora*	1 Tbsp/15ml	124	826	0.0	0.0	92.0	0.0
Sunflower, Fry Light Spray	1 Spray/0.2ml	1	522	0.0	0.0	55.2	0.0
Sunflower, Mazola*	1 Tsp/5ml	42	830	0.0	0.0	92.0	0.0
Sunflower, Organic, Evernat*	1 Tsp/5ml	45	900	0.0	0.0	100.0	0.0
Sunflower, Pure, Sainsbury's*	1 Tsp/5ml	41	829	0.1	0.0	92.0	0.0
Sunflower, Pure, Tesco*	1oz/28g	252	900	0.0	0.0	100.0	0.0
Toasted Sesame, Sainsbury's*	1 Serving/15ml	124	827	0.1	0.0	91.9	0.0
Ultimate Blend, Udo's Choice*	1 Capsule/1ml	9	900	1.3	0.0	96.8	0.0
Vegetable, Blended, Average	1 Tsp/5ml	45	899	0.0	0.0	99.9	0.0
Vegetable, Iceland*	1 Serving/5g	45	900	0.0	0.0	100.0	0.0
Vegetable, Pure, Sainsbury's*	1 Tbsp/15ml	124	825	0.1	0.0	91.7	0.0
Vegetable, Pure, Tesco*	1fl oz/30ml	270	900	0.0	0.0	100.0	0.0
Vegetable, Safeway*	1 Serving/15ml	124	825	0.0	0.0	91.7	0.0
Walnut	1 Tsp/5ml	45	899	0.0	0.0	99.9	0.0
Wheatgerm	1 Tsp/5ml	45	899	0.0	0.0	99.9	0.0

OKRA,

INFO/WEIGHT	per Measure KCAL	KCAL	PROT	CARB	FAT	FIBRE
Boiled in Unsalted Water	1oz/28g	8	28	2.5	2.7	0.9	3.6
Canned, Drained	1oz/28g	6	21	1.4	2.5	0.7	2.6
Raw	1oz/28g	9	31	2.8	3.0	1.0	4.0
Stir-Fried in Corn Oil	1oz/28g	75	269	4.3	4.4	26.1	6.3

OLIVES,

INFO/WEIGHT	per Measure KCAL	KCAL	PROT	CARB	FAT	FIBRE
Black in Brine, Asda*	1 Can/170g	304	179	0.6	6.0	17.0	4.5
Black, Pitted, In Brine, Safeway*	1 Serving/50g	71	141	1.1	0.1	15.1	2.5

	Measure INFO/WEIGHT	per Measure KCAL	Nutrition Values per 100g / 100ml				
			KCAL	PROT	CARB	FAT	FIBRE
OLIVES,							
Black, Pitted, In Brine, Tesco*	½ Jar/82g	92	112	1.2	3.3	10.5	4.2
Black, Pitted, Sainsbury's*	1 Sm Can/85g	132	155	0.6	0.1	16.9	4.6
Black, Pitted, Somerfield*	1 Olive/3g	4	126	1.0	6.0	11.0	0.0
Black, Sliced, Sainsbury's*	½ Sm Can/43g	55	129	0.6	0.1	14.0	5.1
Black, a la Greque, Waitrose*	1 Serving/28g	78	277	2.0	11.7	24.7	3.2
Finest, Tesco*	1 Serving/50g	100	199	1.3	1.9	20.5	0.0
Green, Piited In Oil, Spanish, Sainsbury's*	1 Pot/90g	107	119	1.1	0.1	12.7	7.5
Green, Pimiento Stuffed, Somerfield*	1 Olive/3g	4	126	1.0	4.0	12.0	0.0
Green, Pitted, Somerfield*	1 Olive/3g	4	147	1.0	1.0	14.0	0.0
Green, Queen, Marks & Spencer*	1oz/28g	34	120	1.4	0.2	12.8	2.4
Green, Spanish Pitted, Waitrose*	1/5 Jar/33g	49	147	1.2	3.9	14.1	2.0
In Brine	1 Olive/3g	3	103	0.9	0.0	11.0	2.9
In Brine, Weighed With Stones	1 Olive/3g	2	82	0.7	0.0	8.8	2.3
Kalamata, Marks & Spencer*	1oz/28g	67	240	1.6	1.4	25.1	1.6
Marinated, Selection, Marks & Spencer*	4 Olives/19.6g	45	225	1.4	3.9	22.6	2.1
Pimento Stuffed, In Brine, Tesco*	1 Serving/25g	38	153	0.8	0.1	16.4	2.1
Sliced, In Brine, Tesco*	1oz/28g	39	141	1.1	0.1	15.1	0.0
OMELETTE,							
Cheese, 2 Egg	1 Omelette/180g	479	266	15.9	0.0	22.6	0.0
Cheese, Findus*	1 Serving/200g	400	200	9.5	14.0	13.0	0.0
Cheese, Great Value, Asda*	1 Omelette/119g	287	239	11.0	3.8	20.0	0.1
Cheese, Tesco*	1 Serving/120g	270	225	11.4	3.7	18.3	0.0
Ham & Mushroom, Farmfoods*	1 Omelette/120g	200	167	8.7	1.8	13.9	0.1
Mushroom & Cheese, Tesco*	1 Omelette/120g	248	207	9.8	1.6	17.9	0.2
Plain, 2 Egg	1 Omelette/120g	229	191	10.9	0.0	16.4	0.0
Spanish	1oz/28g	34	120	5.7	6.2	8.3	1.4
ONION RINGS,							
Battered, Asda*	1 Serving/100g	343	343	3.8	31.0	22.7	1.7
Battered, Sainsbury's*	1 Ring/12g	32	268	3.6	28.9	15.3	2.2
Breadcrumbs, Tesco*	1 Serving/100g	294	294	4.3	34.1	15.6	2.3
Breaded, Iceland*	4 Rings/45g	132	293	4.4	34.2	15.4	2.7
COU, Marks & Spencer*	1oz/28g	95	340	4.7	80.7	1.5	3.7
Large, Burger King*	1 Serving/120g	348	290	4.8	36.4	13.9	3.8
Maize Snacks, Sainsbury's*	½ Pack/50g	240	479	8.5	57.8	23.8	3.9
Marks & Spencer*	1 Pack/40g	186	465	5.2	62.1	21.5	4.3
Oven Crisp Batter, Tesco*	1 Onion Ring/17g	40	236	4.2	24.8	13.3	2.5
Pickled, BGTY, Sainsbury's*	1 Bag/10g	34	340	4.7	77.0	1.5	3.7
Pickled, Better For You, Morrisons*	1 Pack/10g	34	340	5.0	77.0	2.0	4.0
Pickled, COU, Marks & Spencer*	1 Bag/20g	68	340	4.7	80.7	1.5	3.7
Pickled, Healthy Eating, Tesco*	1 Pack/15g	51	340	6.2	74.7	1.8	6.5
Red Mill*	1 Bag/50g	249	498	7.5	58.8	25.9	2.2
Regular, Burger King*	1 Serving/90g	261	290	4.8	36.4	13.9	3.8
Spar**	1 Bag/40g	178	444	7.0	51.4	23.4	3.1
Value, Tesco*	1 Bag/16g	77	482	7.6	58.3	24.3	2.5
ONIONS,							
Baby Spring, Sainsburys*	1 Serving/10g	3	25	2.0	3.0	0.5	1.5
Baked	1oz/28g	29	103	3.5	22.3	0.6	3.9
Boiled in Unsalted Water	1oz/28g	5	17	0.6	3.7	0.1	0.7
Diced, Organic, Iceland*	1 Lge Bag/907g	154	17	0.6	3.7	0.1	0.7
Dried, Raw	1oz/28g	88	313	10.2	68.6	1.7	12.1
Fried in Blended Oil	1oz/28g	46	164	2.3	14.1	11.2	3.1
Fried in Butter	1oz/28g	46	164	2.3	14.1	11.2	3.1
Pickled, Cocktail Silverskin, Drained	1oz/28g	4	15	0.6	3.1	0.1	0.0

	Measure INFO/WEIGHT	per Measure KCAL	Nutrition Values per 100g / 100ml KCAL	PROT	CARB	FAT	FIBRE
ONIONS,							
Pickled, Drained	1 Med Onion/10g	2	24	0.9	4.9	0.2	1.2
Pickled, Silverskin, Haywards*	1oz/28g	3	10	0.4	1.9	0.1	0.4
Pickled, in Sweet Vinegar, Sainsbury's*	1 Serving/50g	17	33	0.6	7.5	0.1	0.7
Raw	1oz/28g	10	36	1.2	7.9	0.2	1.4
Red, Organic, Tesco*	1 Onion/100g	38	38	1.2	7.9	0.2	1.4
Salad, Marks & Spencer*	1 Serving/10g	3	25	2.3	2.9	0.2	1.7
OPTIONS*,							
Choca Mocha Drink	1 Sachet/10g	36	359	14.1	50.1	11.4	7.0
Chocolate Au Lait Drink	1 Sachet/10g	36	355	11.8	54.5	10.0	7.3
Hot Chocolate, Belgian Chocolate, Instant	1 Serving/11g	40	363	12.4	54.9	10.4	7.5
Hot Chocolate, Diet Friendly	1 Sachet/11ml	40	364	14.3	50.6	11.6	7.1
Hot Chocolate, Irish Cream	1 Sachet/10.9g	39	357	13.9	50.0	11.3	8.1
Hot Chocolate, Orange Flavour	1 Serving/11ml	40	364	14.2	50.8	11.6	7.1
Hot Chocolate, Pleasure	1 Sachet/18g	68	377	16.7	48.4	13.0	7.8
Irish Cream Drink	1 Sachet/10g	36	357	13.9	50.0	11.3	8.1
Mint Drink	1 Sachet/10g	36	364	14.3	50.6	11.6	7.1
Outrageous Orange Drink	1 Sachet/10g	36	364	14.2	50.8	11.6	7.1
Toffee Drink	1 Sachet/13g	52	400	10.5	68.9	9.2	0.0
Turkish Delight Drink	1 Sachet/10g	37	365	14.4	50.4	11.7	7.2
ORANGE,							
Burst, Diet, Safeway*	1 Can/330ml	13	4	0.1	0.5	0.1	0.1
Segments, In Natural Juice, Tesco*	1oz/28g	14	50	0.7	11.0	0.0	0.3
Sparkling, Diet, Tesco*	1 Glass/250ml	8	3	0.1	0.5	0.1	0.0
With Cranberry Juice, Marks & Spencer*	1 Bottle/250ml	138	55	0.5	14.0	0.5	1.0
Orange & Acerola, Fruit Juice, Plenty*	1 Glass/200ml	90	45	0.7	9.7	0.1	0.0
Orange & Banana Juice, Asda*	1 Glass/200ml	108	54	0.7	12.0	0.1	0.2
Orange & Cranberry Juice Drink, Ocean Spray*	1fl oz/30ml	14	48	0.0	11.5	0.0	0.0
Orange & Grapefruit Juice, Fresh, Finest, Tesco*	1 Glass/250ml	115	46	0.7	9.6	0.1	0.0
Orange & Grapefruit Juice, Pure, Asda*	1 Glass/200ml	82	41	0.7	9.0	0.0	0.2
Orange & Grapefruit Juice, Pure, Sainsbury's*	1 Glass/250ml	105	42	0.7	9.0	0.1	0.1
Orange & Grapefruit Segments in Juice, Del Monte*	1 Can/411g	197	48	0.6	10.6	0.0	0.0
Orange & Kiwi Fruit Juice, Tropicana*	1 Serving/175ml	90	51	0.5	12.0	0.0	0.0
Orange & Peach, Juice Drink, Somerfield*	1fl oz/30ml	22	72	0.0	11.0	0.0	0.0
Orange & Pineapple Juice, Del Monte*	1 Glass/200ml	96	48	0.5	11.0	0.0	0.0
Orange & Pineapple Juice, Pure, Asda*	1 Glass/120ml	54	45	0.4	10.0	1.0	1.0
Orange & Pink Grapefruit, Fresh, Food to Go, M&S*	1 Pack/250g	100	40	0.9	9.4	0.1	1.4
Orange & Raspberry, Fresh Squeezed, Marks & Spencer*	1 Glass/200ml	96	48	0.7	11.9	0.0	0.0
ORANGE BARLEY WATER, Robinson's*	1oz/28g	28	101	0.3	23.1	0.0	0.0
ORANGE CREAM, Cadbury's*	1 Bar/51g	217	425	2.6	68.6	15.4	0.0
ORANGE DRINK,							
Active Sport, Tesco*	1 Bottle/500ml	135	27	0.0	6.5	0.0	0.0
No Added Sugar, Asda*	1 Glass/250ml	13	5	0.1	0.9	0.0	0.0
Sparkling, Shapers, Boots*	1 Bottle/500ml	15	3	0.1	0.4	0.1	0.0
ORANGE JUICE,							
& Crushed Lychees, Marks & Spencer*	1 Bottle/250ml	100	40	0.5	8.5	0.2	0.7
100% Pure Squeezed, Tesco*	1 Glass/200ml	94	47	1.0	10.4	0.0	0.0
Apple & Passionfruit, Del Monte*	1 Glass/200ml	90	45	0.5	10.1	0.0	0.0
Del Monte*	1 Glass/200ml	88	44	0.6	9.9	0.0	0.0
Florida, Marks & Spencer*	1 Bottle/250ml	85	34	0.5	8.5	0.0	0.0
Florida, Pure Squeezed, Somerfield*	1 Glass/200ml	92	46	1.0	11.0	0.0	0.0
Florida, Pure, Somerfield*	1 Glass/200ml	86	43	1.0	10.0	0.0	0.0
Florida, Smooth, Safeway*	1 Glass/200ml	96	48	0.7	10.7	0.0	0.3
Fresh, Meierienes*	1 Serving/150ml	68	45	0.7	10.4	0.2	0.0

O

	Measure INFO/WEIGHT	per Measure KCAL	Nutrition Values per 100g / 100ml				
			KCAL	PROT	CARB	FAT	FIBRE
ORANGE JUICE,							
Freshly Squeezed, Asda*	1 Glass/200ml	88	44	0.6	10.0	0.0	0.1
Freshly Squeezed, Boots*	1 Glass/200ml	84	42	0.6	9.0	0.1	0.1
Freshly Squeezed, Finest, Tesco*	1 Glass/200ml	92	46	0.8	10.4	0.1	0.1
Freshly Squeezed, Marks & Spencer*	1 Glass/200ml	90	45	0.7	9.8	0.1	0.0
Freshly Squeezed, Morrisons*	1 Bottle/250g	110	44	0.6	9.7	0.1	0.1
Freshly Squeezed, Safeway*	1 Glass/200ml	80	40	0.5	9.1	0.1	0.1
Freshly Squeezed, SunJuice*	1 Bottle/250ml	113	45	0.8	11.4	0.1	0.3
Freshly Squeezed, TTD, Sainsbury's	1 Glass/200ml	98	49	0.6	10.5	0.0	0.4
Freshly Squeezed, Waitrose*	1 Glass/250ml	130	52	0.7	11.8	0.0	0.0
Healthy Living, Tesco*	1 Glass/250ml	70	28	0.3	6.1	0.1	0.0
High Juice, Safeway*	1 Serving/250ml	95	38	0.0	9.1	0.0	0.0
Italian Blood, Del Monte*	1 Glass/250ml	123	49	0.1	12.0	0.0	0.0
Just Juice*	1 Serving/100ml	46	46	0.6	10.4	0.1	0.0
Lidl*	1 Glass/200ml	78	39	0.6	9.0	0.4	0.4
Organic, Evernat*	1 Glass/200ml	86	43	0.7	9.0	0.2	0.2
Pure, Boots*	1 Carton/250ml	115	46	0.5	11.0	0.0	0.0
Pure, Carton, Morrisons*	1 Carton/200ml	84	42	0.6	9.2	0.2	0.0
Pure, Cawston Vale*	1 Can/250ml	118	47	0.5	10.5	0.1	0.0
Pure, Co-Op*	1 Glass/200ml	80	40	0.5	9.0	0.1	0.1
Pure, Florida, Tesco*	1 Glass/250ml	115	46	0.5	10.5	0.0	0.0
Pure, McDonald's*	1 Regular/200ml	94	47	0.7	10.3	0.0	0.1
Pure, Morrisons*	1 Glass/200ml	72	36	0.6	9.0	0.0	0.0
Pure, Organic, Blue Parrot Cafe, Sainsbury's*	1 Carton/250ml	115	46	0.5	10.4	0.1	0.1
Pure, Organic, Waitrose*	1 Serving/328g	154	47	1.0	11.0	0.0	0.0
Pure, Premium, Somerfield*	1 Glass/200ml	88	44	1.0	10.0	0.0	0.0
Pure, Princes*	1 Glass/200ml	84	42	0.5	9.1	0.1	0.1
Pure, Rio D'oro, Aldi*	1 Glass/200ml	80	40	0.2	10.0	0.0	0.0
Pure, Sainsbury's*	1 Glass/200ml	94	47	0.5	10.5	0.1	0.1
Pure, SmartPrice, Asda*	1 Bottle/200ml	90	45	0.5	10.0	0.1	0.1
Pure, Smooth, Tesco*	1 Glass/125ml	58	46	1.0	10.5	0.0	0.0
Pure, Somerfield*	1 Glass/200ml	90	45	1.0	10.0	0.0	0.0
Pure, Tesco*	1 Glass/200ml	92	46	0.5	10.5	0.0	0.0
Pure, Value Tesco*	1 Glass/200ml	86	43	0.6	9.4	0.0	0.0
Pure, Waitrose*	1 Glass/200ml	90	45	0.7	10.0	0.0	0.0
Smooth Style, Tropicana*	1 Carton/250ml	108	43	0.7	9.0	0.0	0.5
Smooth, Asda*	1 Glass/200ml	78	39	0.5	9.0	0.1	0.1
Smooth, Marks & Spencer*	1 Glass/200ml	82	41	0.7	9.1	0.0	0.0
Unsweetened	1 Glass/200ml	72	36	0.5	8.8	0.1	0.1
Unsweetened, Long Life, Economy, Sainsbury's*	1 Glass/200ml	84	42	0.5	9.1	0.2	0.2
With Bits, Asda*	1 Glass/250ml	113	45	0.7	10.0	0.0	0.4
With Calcium, Smooth, Tesco*	1 Glass/250ml	115	46	0.5	10.4	0.0	0.0
With Juicy Bits, 100% Squeezed, Sainsbury's*	1 Serving/150ml	72	48	0.7	10.7	0.1	0.3
With Juicy Bits, Pure Squeezed, Tropicana*	1 Glass/200ml	86	43	0.7	9.0	0.0	0.5
With Mango Puree, Asda*	1 Glass/250ml	115	46	0.6	10.0	0.1	0.4
ORANGES,							
Fresh, Raw	1 Med/160g	59	37	1.1	8.5	0.1	1.7
Weighed With Peel & Pips	1oz/28g	7	26	0.8	5.9	0.1	1.2
ORECCHIETTE, Shells, TTD, Sainsbury's*	1 Serving/50g	184	367	11.5	79.1	0.5	2.0
OREGANO,							
Dried, Ground	1 Tsp/1g	3	306	11.0	49.5	10.3	0.0
Fresh	1oz/28g	18	66	2.2	9.7	2.0	0.0
OVALTINE,							
Hi Malt, Light, Instant Drink	1 Sachet/20g	72	358	9.1	67.1	5.9	2.8

	Measure INFO/WEIGHT	per Measure KCAL	Nutrition Values per 100g / 100ml				
			KCAL	PROT	CARB	FAT	FIBRE
OVALTINE,							
Powder, Made Up With Semi-Skimmed Milk	1 Mug/227ml	179	79	3.9	13.0	1.7	0.0
Powder, Made Up With Whole Milk	1 Mug/227ml	220	97	3.8	12.9	3.8	0.0
OXTAIL,							
Raw	1oz/28g	48	171	20.0	0.0	10.1	0.0
Stewed	1oz/28g	68	243	30.5	0.0	13.4	0.0
OYSTERS,							
Raw	1oz/28g	18	65	10.8	2.7	1.3	0.0
in Vegetable Oil, Smoked, John West*	1oz/28g	64	230	16.0	10.0	14.0	0.0

O

INFO/WEIGHT	Measure	per Measure KCAL	Nutrition Values per 100g / 100ml				
			KCAL	PROT	CARB	FAT	FIBRE
PAELLA,							
Big Dish Chicken & Chorizo, Marks & Spencer*	1 Pack/450g	630	140	7.9	18.4	3.9	1.6
Chicken & Chorizo, Asda*	1 Pack/390g	432	111	9.0	14.1	2.1	2.3
Chicken & Vegetable, Healthy Living, Tesco*	1 Pack/450g	441	98	9.7	11.8	1.3	1.1
Chicken, Healthy Eating, Tesco*	1 Pack/400g	416	104	8.9	15.4	0.8	2.2
Chicken, New, Healthy Eating, Tesco*	1 Pack/370g	329	89	7.2	10.4	2.0	1.2
Chicken, Steam Pack, Healthy Eating, Tesco*	1 Pack/350g	291	83	8.1	11.8	0.4	7.0
Enjoy, Bird's Eye*	1 Pack/500g	620	124	7.7	16.2	3.2	0.6
Seafood, Finest, Tesco*	1 Pack/400g	600	150	6.3	18.9	5.5	2.0
Seafood, Marks & Spencer*	1 Pack/450g	518	115	6.4	13.7	3.8	3.2
Seafood, Sainsbury's*	1 Pack/400g	504	126	8.3	20.3	1.3	0.6
TTD, Sainsbury's*	1 Pack/375g	386	103	8.3	16.9	0.2	3.1
Vegetable, Waitrose*	1 Serving/174g	202	116	2.2	22.7	1.8	1.5
Vesta	1 Paella/160g	558	349	10.9	69.6	2.9	3.0
With Prawns, Chicken, Cod & Salmon, Sainsbury's*	1 Pack/750g	773	103	8.3	16.9	0.2	3.1
PAIN AU CHOCOLAT,							
Marks & Spencer*	1 Pain/60g	210	350	5.9	38.0	19.2	1.6
Tesco*	1 Pain/56g	235	420	7.0	46.5	22.9	1.4
PAK CHOI, Tesco*	1 Serving/100g	11	11	1.0	1.4	0.2	1.2
PAKORA,							
Bhajia, Onion, Fried in Vegetable Oil	1oz/28g	76	271	9.8	26.2	14.7	5.5
Bhajia, Potato Carrot & Pea, Fried in Vegetable Oil	1oz/28g	100	357	10.9	28.8	22.6	6.1
Bhajia, Vegetable, Retail	1oz/28g	66	235	6.4	21.4	14.7	3.6
Potato & Spinach, Mini, Indian Snack Selection, Waitrose*	1 Pakora/21g	56	266	5.4	17.0	19.6	4.5
Sainsbury's*	1 Pakora/55g	166	302	7.3	26.8	18.3	1.1
Spinach, Mini, Indian Snack Selection, Sainsbury's*	1 Pakora/22.1g	48	217	5.3	18.0	13.8	3.4
Vegetable, Indian Selection, Party, Co-Op*	1 Pakora/23g	47	205	6.0	28.0	7.0	4.0
Vegetable, Indian Starter Selection, Marks & Spencer*	1 Pakora/23g	61	265	6.3	19.6	18.1	2.9
Vegetable, Mini, Tesco*	1 Pakora/21g	62	297	5.8	18.0	22.4	3.2
Vegetable, Somerfield*	1 Pakora/15g	46	305	7.0	19.0	23.0	0.0
PANCAKE,							
& Sausage, McDonald's*	1 Portion/262g	671	256	6.1	34.3	10.3	1.1
& Syrup, McDonald's*	1 Pack/209.4g	531	254	2.4	41.9	7.6	0.6
American Style, Large, with Syrup, Tesco*	2 Pancakes/76g	204	268	5.1	54.2	3.4	0.9
Apple & Sultana, Marks & Spencer*	1 Serving/80g	160	200	2.2	30.2	7.9	1.2
Apple, Good For You, Asda*	1 Pancake/85g	114	134	4.2	24.0	2.5	1.0
Aunt Bessie's*	1 Pancake/60g	90	150	6.1	24.6	3.1	1.1
Cherry, GFY, Adsa*	1 Serving/206g	206	100	1.9	18.9	1.8	1.8
Chinatown, Asda*	1 Pancake/10g	34	335	10.9	51.7	9.2	2.4
Chinese Roll, Farmfoods*	1 Roll/88g	125	142	4.3	21.6	4.3	1.0
Chinese Style, Cherry Valley*	1 Pancake/8g	25	310	9.2	54.7	6.0	0.0
Healthy Living, Tesco*	1 Panceake/30g	74	246	7.3	49.9	1.9	1.5
Irish, Marks & Spencer*	1 Pancake/35g	85	243	7.1	53.8	1.4	1.3
Lemon, Marks & Spencer*	1 Pancake/38.3g	89	235	4.5	38.5	7.2	2.8
Maple & Raisin, Marks & Spencer*	1 Pancake/32.7g	89	269	6.5	49.7	5.4	2.2
Mini, Tesco*	1 Pancake/14g	39	277	6.7	50.0	5.6	1.4
Mix, Traditional, Asda*	1 Pack/256g	545	213	6.0	27.0	9.0	1.8
Morello Cherry, Iceland*	1 Pancake/129g	204	158	3.1	29.8	2.9	2.9
Morrisons*	1 Pancake/60g	133	221	8.4	37.3	5.0	1.5
Plain, Sainsbury's*	1 Pancake/63g	144	228	8.4	37.3	5.0	1.5
Raisin & Lemon, Co-Op*	1 Pancake/34g	122	360	8.0	60.0	10.0	2.0
Raisin & Lemon, Safeway*	1 Pancake/35.1g	93	265	5.8	44.5	7.1	1.6
Raisin & Lemon, Sainsbury's*	1 Pancake/35.0g	96	274	5.8	47.8	6.6	2.3
Raisin & Lemon, Tesco*	1 Pancake/36g	99	275	5.8	49.3	6.1	2.7

	Measure INFO/WEIGHT	per Measure KCAL	Nutrition Values per 100g / 100ml				
			KCAL	PROT	CARB	FAT	FIBRE
PANCAKE,							
Sainsburys*	2 Pancakes/92g	256	278	6.1	46.8	7.4	1.8
Savoury, Made With Skimmed Milk	1oz/28g	70	249	6.4	24.1	14.7	0.8
Savoury, Made With Whole Milk	1oz/28g	76	273	6.3	24.0	17.5	0.8
Scotch	1 Pancake/50g	146	292	5.8	43.6	11.7	1.4
Scotch, BGTY, Sainsbury's*	1 Pancake/30g	76	252	5.3	48.5	4.1	1.3
Scotch, Low Fat, Asda*	1 Pancake/32g	87	272	6.0	57.0	2.2	0.0
Scotch, Marks & Spencer*	1 Pancake/34g	95	280	6.5	54.5	4.0	1.6
Scotch, Sainsbury's	1 Pancake/30g	98	337	7.5	54.4	9.9	1.6
Scotch, SmartPrice, Asda*	1 Pancake/35g	107	305	7.0	49.0	9.0	1.4
Sultana & Syrup Scotch, Sainsbury's*	1 Pancake/35g	113	322	6.7	55.2	8.3	1.7
Sultana & Syrup, Asda*	1 Pancake/34g	89	263	5.9	43.7	7.2	1.5
Sultana & Syrup, Iceland*	1 Pancake/35.2g	95	270	5.3	53.0	4.1	1.2
Sweet, Made With Skimmed Milk	1oz/28g	78	280	6.0	35.1	13.8	0.8
Sweet, Made With Whole Milk	1oz/28g	84	301	5.9	35.0	16.2	0.8
Sweet, Raspberry Ripple Sauce, Findus*	1 Pancake/38.1g	80	210	3.9	37.1	4.7	0.9
Syrup, Tesco*	2 Pancakes/60g	175	291	7.0	48.4	7.7	1.9
Toffee Apple, Marks & Spencer*	1 Pancake/88.9g	160	180	2.2	32.6	4.7	1.5
Traditional, Tesco*	1 Pancake/62g	137	221	8.4	35.6	5.0	1.5
Vegetable Roll	1 Roll/85g	185	218	6.6	21.0	12.5	0.0
Warburtons*	1 Serving/28g	64	230	6.3	37.7	6.0	0.0
PANCETTA, Cubetti, Italian, Sainsbury's*	½ Pack/65g	207	318	20.0	0.1	26.4	0.1
PANINI,							
Chicken & Baby Spinach, Costa*	1 Serving/440g	832	189	9.8	32.5	2.5	0.0
Egg & Bacon, Starbucks*	1 Panini/210g	458	218	11.1	22.0	9.5	0.0
Ham & Swiss Cheese, Coffee Republic*	1 Panini/223g	558	250	15.7	20.5	11.7	0.0
Mozarella, Tomato & Pesto, Costa*	1 Panini/209g	487	233	9.6	35.1	7.2	5.0
Mozzarella & Tomato, Coffee Republic*	1 Panini/255g	566	222	11.1	23.6	10.0	0.0
Mozzarella & Tomato, Marks & Spencer*	1 Serving/176g	484	275	11.3	21.3	16.2	2.1
Roasted Vegetables & Cheese, Starbucks*	1 Pack/215g	542	252	8.7	20.6	15.1	0.0
PAPAYA,							
Dried, Sweetened, Tesco*	4 Pieces/25g	59	235	0.4	56.3	0.9	2.9
Pieces, Nature's Harvest*	1 Serving/50g	178	355	0.2	85.4	0.0	2.6
Unripe, Raw	1oz/28g	8	27	0.9	5.5	0.1	1.5
Waitrose*	1 Serving/200g	76	38	0.5	8.8	0.1	1.8
PAPPADS, Green Chilli & Garlic, Sharwood's*	1oz/28g	75	267	19.9	43.3	1.6	9.7
PAPPADUMS, Patak's*	1 Serving/10g	28	275	21.5	43.2	1.9	0.0
PAPPARDELLE,							
Basil, Fresh, Sainsbury's*	1 Serving/240g	281	117	5.0	21.2	1.4	2.0
Chilli, Fresh, Sainsbury's*	1 Serving/250g	303	121	5.7	20.7	1.7	2.0
Cracked Black Pepper, Safeway*	1 Bowl/120g	173	144	5.7	26.5	1.8	1.9
Egg, Italia, Marks & Spencer*	1 Serving/100g	355	355	13.9	68.5	2.8	3.0
Salmon, COU, Marks & Spencer*	1 Pack/358g	340	95	6.3	13.0	1.9	0.8
PAPRIKA, Average	1 Tsp/2g	6	289	14.8	34.9	13.0	0.0
PARATHA, Average	1oz/28g	90	322	8.0	43.2	14.3	4.0
PARCELS,							
Beef Steak, Sainsbury's*	½ Pack/226g	488	216	12.2	6.6	15.6	1.0
Cheese & Ham, Sainsbury's*	1 Pack/250g	445	178	7.4	19.9	7.6	1.5
Chicken & Prosciutto, Sun Dried Tomato, Finest, Tesco*	1 Pack/205g	246	120	18.3	1.8	4.4	0.7
Chilli Beef, Tex Mex Feast, Asda*	1 Parcel/25g	68	270	9.0	27.0	14.0	2.1
Filo, Brie & Cranberry, Tesco*	1 Parcel/22g	82	373	9.5	29.3	24.2	1.5
Filo, Mushroom, Savoury, Creamy, Somerfield*	1oz/28g	86	308	5.0	24.0	21.0	0.0
Italian Tomato & Mozzarella, Fresh, Sainsbury's*	½ Pack/125g	243	194	7.5	23.0	8.0	3.4
Smoked Salmon, Marks & Spencer*	1 Parcel/55g	151	275	15.4	0.7	23.6	0.0

P

INFO/WEIGHT	Measure per Measure KCAL	KCAL	PROT	CARB	FAT	FIBRE
PARCELS,						
Smoked Salmon, Sainsbury's*	1 Pack/115g	269	234	15.8	3.5	17.6	0.2
Smoked Salmon, Tesco*	1 Serving/50g	147	293	16.4	0.0	25.3	0.2
Sun Dried Tomato & Wild Mushrooml, The Best, Safeway*	1 Parcel/181g	483	267	8.8	41.8	7.2	4.2
With Cheese & Sweet Pepper Sauce, Egg, Somerfield*	½ Pack/125g	349	279	12.4	30.7	11.8	2.2
PARMESAN, Flutes, Mini, Safeway*	1 Flute/85g	199	234	8.8	40.1	4.3	1.9
PARMIGIANO REGGIANO, Sainsbury's*	1 Serving/30g	116	388	33.0	0.1	28.4	0.1
PARSLEY,						
Dried	1 Tsp/1.3g	2	181	15.8	14.5	7.0	26.9
Fresh	1oz/28g	10	34	3.0	2.7	1.3	5.0
Thyme & Lemon Stuffing, Paxo*	1 Serving/45g	68	150	4.3	28.4	2.1	2.4
PARSNIP,						
Boiled in Salted Water	1oz/28g	18	66	1.6	12.9	1.2	4.7
Boiled in Unsalted Water	1oz/28g	18	66	1.6	12.9	1.2	4.7
Honey Roasted, Marks & Spencer*	1 Serving/100g	155	155	2.1	30.1	2.8	2.9
Organic, Tesco*	1 Serving/100g	67	67	1.8	12.5	1.1	4.6
Raw	1oz/28g	18	64	1.8	12.5	1.1	4.6
Roast, Asda*	1 Serving/50g	57	113	1.7	18.0	3.8	4.4
Roast, Aunt Bessie's*	1 Serving/125g	206	165	2.2	14.9	10.7	5.1
Roasted, Marks & Spencer*	1 Serving/112g	134	120	1.8	14.3	6.4	0.8
Roasting, Sainsbury's*	4 Parsnips/90g	126	140	2.3	19.8	5.7	6.0
Roasting, Tesco*	1 Parsnip/75g	77	103	1.7	14.5	4.2	4.4
Roasting, Waitrose*	1 Serving/125g	123	98	1.9	12.4	4.5	5.0
Value, Tesco*	1 Serving/150g	101	67	1.8	12.5	1.1	4.6
PARTRIDGE, Roasted, Meat Only	1oz/28g	59	212	36.7	0.0	7.2	0.0
PASANDA,						
Chicken, Marks & Spencer*	½ Pack/150g	240	160	11.3	3.8	10.9	1.3
Chicken, Waitrose*	1oz/28g	52	185	14.8	3.8	12.3	1.1
Chicken, With Pilau Rice, Sharwoods*	1 Pack/376g	538	143	5.8	15.2	6.6	0.8
PASSION FRUIT,						
Raw, Fresh	1 Fruit/15g	5	36	2.6	5.8	0.4	3.3
Weighed With Skin	1oz/28g	6	22	1.7	3.5	0.2	2.0
PASSION FRUIT JUICE, Average	1 Glass/200ml	94	47	0.8	10.7	0.1	0.0
PASTA,						
& Roasted Vegetables, Waitrose*	1oz/28g	43	154	2.4	14.2	9.7	1.0
Blue Cheese, Bacon & Spinach, Marks & Spencer*	1 Pack/400g	640	160	6.5	13.8	8.5	0.7
Cooked, Standard, Buitoni*	1 Serving/100g	129	129	4.8	25.9	0.7	1.2
Dried, Shape, Tesco*	1 Serving/100g	345	345	13.2	68.5	2.0	2.9
Pepper & Tomato, Asda*	1 Serving/250g	340	136	3.2	15.0	7.0	2.4
Tomato & Mascarpone, GFY, Asda*	½ Can/200g	128	64	2.1	9.0	2.2	0.0
Tomato & Pepper, Fireroast, Finest, Tesco*	1 Serving/200g	384	192	3.9	19.4	11.0	1.4
Tomato & Pepper, Good for You, Asda*	1 Pack/400g	344	86	3.1	14.0	1.9	1.1
Tuna & Sweetcorn, Sainsbury's*	1 Pasta/300g	327	109	6.7	14.7	2.6	1.4
Wholewheat, Barilla*	1oz/28g	95	340	13.0	67.5	2.0	6.0
PASTA 'N' SAUCE,						
Cheese, Leek & Ham, Batchelors*	1 Pack/126g	478	379	14.1	68.3	5.5	2.3
Chicken & Mushroom, Batchelors*	1 Pack/126g	455	361	12.4	73.5	2.0	2.7
Chicken & Roasted Garlic Flavour, Batchelors*	½ Pack/60g	223	372	12.6	73.8	2.9	3.4
Creamy Tikka Masala, Batchelors*	1 Pack/122.1g	426	349	12.7	69.5	2.2	4.4
Creamy Tomato & Mushroom, Batchelors*	1 Pack/125g	458	366	13.0	71.0	3.3	3.2
Macaroni Cheese, Batchelors*	1 Pack/115g	435	378	17.2	63.6	6.1	2.8
Mild Cheese & Brocolli, Batchelors*	1 Pack/129g	479	371	13.5	69.0	4.5	2.8
Mushroom & Wine, Batchelors*	1 Pack/132g	498	377	12.0	71.3	4.9	2.5
Tomato & Bacon Flavour, Batchelors*	1 Pack/134g	476	355	13.0	70.0	2.6	3.0

P

INFO/WEIGHT	Measure per Measure KCAL		Nutrition Values per 100g / 100ml				
			KCAL	PROT	CARB	FAT	FIBRE
PASTA 'N' SAUCE,							
Tomato Onion & Herb Flavour, Batchelors*	1 Pack/135g	470	348	13.2	64.5	4.1	5.8
PASTA BAKE,							
Bacon & Leek, Tesco*	1 Pack/450g	774	172	8.1	16.1	8.3	2.0
Bolognese, Italiano, Tesco*	1/3 Pack/284g	409	144	8.7	15.7	5.1	2.3
Cheese & Bacon, Asda*	1 Serving/60g	80	134	2.7	3.8	12.0	0.7
Cheese & Broccoli, Fish Bakes, Bird's Eye*	½ Pack/200g	264	132	12.5	6.1	6.4	0.3
Cheese & Tomato, Tesco*	1 Pack/400g	388	97	3.4	17.8	1.4	1.2
Chicken & Bacon, Tesco*	1oz/28g	46	166	6.9	19.3	6.8	0.5
Chicken & Broccoli, Morrisons*	1 Pack/400g	452	113	6.1	13.3	4.0	0.6
Chicken & Broccoli, Pasta Presto, Findus*	1 Pack/321g	449	140	7.5	12.0	7.0	0.0
Chicken & Broccoli, Safeway*	1 Pack/340g	405	119	8.1	11.7	4.4	1.3
Chicken & Broccoli, Weight Watchers*	1 Bake/305g	290	95	6.0	14.2	1.5	0.9
Chicken & Courgette, Asda*	½ Pack/387.3g	519	134	6.0	14.0	6.0	0.6
Chicken & Roast Mushroom, Healthy Living, Tesco*	1 Pack/390g	413	106	8.6	17.6	0.1	1.3
Chicken & Spinach, Good For You, Asda*	1 Pack/335g	281	84	4.9	10.0	2.7	0.6
Chicken & Spinach, Sainsbury's*	1 Pack/340g	286	84	4.9	10.0	2.7	0.6
Chicken & Sweetcorn, Eat Smart, Safeway*	1 Pack/400g	380	95	6.5	13.0	1.8	1.8
Chicken & Vegetable, Healthy Eating, Tesco*	1 Pack/400g	344	86	6.0	11.8	1.7	0.5
Chicken, Good For You, (400g), Asda*	1 Pack/400g	424	106	6.0	14.0	2.9	0.7
Chicken, Healthy Eating, Tesco*	1 Pack/340g	292	86	7.2	10.9	1.5	0.8
Chicken, Healthy Living, Tesco*	1 Pack/340g	320	94	7.8	12.9	1.3	2.2
Chicken, Italiano, Tesco*	1 Pack/400g	448	112	9.8	10.3	3.5	1.7
Chicken, Morrisons*	1 Pack/401.9g	418	104	7.3	8.6	4.8	0.1
Chicken, Mushroom & Leek, Healthy Eating, Tesco*	1 Pack/450g	468	104	8.6	11.9	2.5	1.4
Chicken, Somerfield*	1 Pack/300g	351	117	8.0	8.0	6.0	0.0
Chicken, Tesco*	1 Pack/400g	448	112	9.8	10.3	3.5	1.7
Chicken, Tesco*	1 Serving/400g	344	86	6.0	11.8	1.7	0.5
Chilli & Cheese, American Style, Tesco*	1 Pack/425g	638	150	6.8	21.8	3.9	1.5
Creamy Ham & Mushroom, Homepride*	1 Pack/425g	489	115	1.8	2.8	10.7	0.0
Creamy Mushroom, Dolmio*	½ Jar/245g	267	109	1.1	5.5	9.2	0.0
Creamy Mushroon, Asda*	¼ Jar/118g	204	173	1.8	3.3	17.0	0.5
Creamy Tomato, Dolmio*	1 Serving/125g	141	113	2.3	8.4	7.2	0.0
Findus*	1 Pack/320g	448	140	7.5	12.0	7.0	0.0
Ham & Broccoli, Asda*	1 Pack/340g	309	91	3.4	10.0	4.1	0.5
Ham & Mushroom, Italiano, Tesco*	1 Pack/425g	646	152	5.8	21.3	4.8	1.7
Italian Bolognese, Asda*	1 Serving/300g	639	213	10.0	14.0	13.0	0.5
Italiano Cheese & Tomato, Tesco*	1 Bake/300g	354	118	3.9	16.1	4.2	1.0
Italiano Chicken, Tesco*	1 Serving/190g	238	125	7.3	13.3	4.7	0.5
Leek & Bacon, Morrisons*	1 Pack/400.7g	553	138	4.8	9.9	9.0	0.2
Meatball, Tesco*	1 Pack/400g	576	144	5.9	19.3	4.8	0.5
Mediterranean Style, Tesco*	1 Pack/450g	423	94	2.9	19.6	0.4	2.0
Penne Mozzarella, Tesco*	1 Pack/340g	408	120	4.7	19.7	2.5	0.6
Pepperoni & Ham, Tesco*	½ Pack/425g	502	118	8.9	19.3	0.6	2.5
Roast Vegetable, Eat Smart, Safeway*	1 Pack/330g	380	115	3.8	19.6	1.9	1.3
Spicy Tomato & Pepperoni, Asda*	1 Pack/440g	431	98	1.1	10.0	6.0	1.2
Spicy Tomato & Pepperoni, Homepride*	1 Jar/450g	324	72	1.5	8.1	3.7	0.0
Sun Dried Tomato, Dolmio*	1 Serving/100ml	83	83	2.2	10.5	3.0	0.0
Tomato & Cheese, Dolmio*	1 Serving/125g	69	55	2.2	8.8	1.2	0.0
Tomato & Herb, Asda*	1 Jar/436g	715	164	1.8	10.0	13.0	1.2
Tomato & Mozzarella, Italiano, Tesco*	1 Pack/340g	418	123	5.5	17.9	3.3	1.0
Tuna & Sweetcorn, Asda*	1 Serving/250g	333	133	5.0	8.0	9.0	0.9
Tuna & Tomato & Fish Sauce, Schwartz*	1 Jar/315g	246	78	2.6	12.1	2.2	0.0
Tuna & Tomato, BGTY, Sainsbury's*	1 Pack/450g	554	123	8.7	12.6	4.2	0.4

P

INFO/WEIGHT	Measure KCAL	per Measure KCAL	PROT	CARB	FAT	FIBRE
PASTA BAKE,						
Tuna, COU, Marks & Spencer*	1 Pack/360g	378	105	8.0	13.4	2.0	1.1
Tuna, Co-Op*	1 Serving/340g	306	90	7.0	12.0	2.0	1.0
Tuna, Eat Smart, Safeway*	1 Pack/345g	345	100	5.7	17.7	0.4	1.3
Tuna, Healthy Eating, Tesco*	1 Pack/340g	258	76	5.4	11.9	0.8	0.5
Tuna, Lean Cuisine*	1 Pack/345.5g	380	110	5.0	16.0	2.5	1.5
Tuna, Safeway*	1 Pack/400g	620	155	8.9	12.0	7.9	1.1
Tuna, Somerfield*	1 Bake/300g	411	137	9.0	10.0	7.0	0.0
Tuna, Tesco*	1oz/28g	36	129	6.9	11.7	6.1	0.9
Vegetable, Asda*	1 Serving/300g	231	77	2.4	9.0	3.5	0.8
Vegetable, Findus*	1 Pack/330.8g	430	130	6.0	13.0	6.5	0.0
Vegetable, Ready Meals, Waitrose*	1oz/28g	44	157	5.9	14.4	8.6	1.0
Vegetable, Tesco*	1 Pack/380g	467	123	5.6	12.6	5.6	1.6
PASTA BREAK,						
Cheese & Ham, Asda*	1 Pot/66g	75	113	3.3	17.0	3.5	0.0
Chicken & Herb, Knorr*	1 Pot/347g	382	110	3.7	16.5	3.3	0.9
Chicken & Mushroom Flavour, Asda*	1 Pot/231g	254	110	2.7	19.0	2.6	0.0
Korma, Asda*	1 Pot/68g	74	109	2.3	19.0	2.6	0.0
PASTA IN, Herb Sauce, Sainsbury's*	1 Pack/420g	441	105	3.5	22.4	0.2	0.8
PASTA QUILLS,						
Cooked, Co-Op*	1 Serving/200g	302	151	5.7	30.2	0.9	1.8
Morrisons*	1 Serving/50g	173	346	12.0	72.3	1.0	0.0
Value, Tesco*	1 Serving/75g	248	330	12.0	71.7	1.5	3.0
PASTA SALAD,						
BBQ Bean, Tesco*	1 Pack/850g	1139	134	3.6	18.5	5.1	1.8
Basil & Parmesan, Tesco*	1 Serving/50g	65	130	4.3	20.2	3.6	0.6
Big Penne, Honey & Mustard Chicken, Marks & Spencer*	1 Pack/380g	646	170	8.1	17.7	7.2	2.6
Carbonara, Waitrose*	1oz/28g	72	257	5.4	8.1	22.6	0.5
Chargrilled Chicken, Italian Style, Fresh, Asda*	1 Pack/200g	318	159	7.0	17.0	7.0	0.4
Chargrilled Chicken, Marks & Spencer*	1 Serving/190g	285	150	9.6	23.6	2.9	1.6
Chargrilled Vegetables & Tomato, Shapers, Boots*	1 Pack/175g	187	107	2.8	17.0	3.1	1.5
Cherry Tomato & Rocket, Healthy Eating, Tesco*	1 Salad/225g	223	99	3.2	15.8	2.5	1.0
Cherry Tomato With Spinach & Pine Nut, M&S*	1 Pack/340g	646	190	5.9	22.1	8.7	0.1
Chicken & Smoked Bacon, Marks & Spencer*	1 Salad/380g	817	215	7.5	19.0	12.3	1.9
Chicken Ceasar, Ginsters*	1 Pack/220g	504	229	7.5	13.6	16.1	0.0
Chicken, Sun Dried Tomato & Basil, HE, Tesco*	1 Serving/190g	215	113	7.6	15.0	2.5	0.9
Crayfish, Rocket & Lemon, Finest, Tesco*	1 Serving/250g	728	291	8.9	28.0	15.9	4.2
Farfalle, Prawns Tomatoes & Cucumber, Sainsbury's*	1 Serving/260g	270	104	4.5	10.9	4.7	0.7
Feta Cheese, Sun Blush Tomatoes, Marks & Spencer*	1 Serving/190g	361	190	5.5	17.2	11.1	2.1
Fire Roasted Tomato, So Good, Somerfield*	½ Pack/100g	199	199	4.4	21.6	10.6	1.5
Garlic Mushroom, Salad Bar, Asda*	1oz/28g	59	212	2.5	12.5	16.9	0.8
Ham & Pineapple, Salad Bar, Asda*	1oz/28g	62	221	3.3	15.6	16.2	1.4
Honey & Mustard Chicken, Marks & Spencer*	1 Serving/190g	304	160	8.7	26.7	2.5	1.5
Honey & Mustard Chicken, Sainsbury's*	1 Pack/260g	447	172	7.3	16.9	8.3	1.4
Italian Style, Asda*	1oz/28g	42	149	3.2	19.1	6.6	1.2
Italian Style, Safeway*	1 Serving/225g	234	104	2.9	17.2	2.6	0.6
Italian Style, Sainsbury's*	1/3 Pot/84g	129	153	3.5	20.5	6.3	1.4
Lime & Coriander Chicken, Marks & Spencer*	1 Serving/190g	371	195	7.6	14.4	12.2	0.6
Mediterranean Chicken, Waitrose*	1 Serving/200g	314	157	7.0	16.9	6.8	2.1
Mediterranean Style, Layered, Waitrose*	1 Pot/275g	190	69	2.6	11.8	1.3	1.0
Mediterranean Tuna, Shapers, Boots*	1 Serving/239g	232	97	6.2	15.0	1.3	0.9
Mediterranean Vegetable & Bean, BGTY, Sainsbury's*	1 Serving/66g	53	80	3.2	12.5	1.9	2.8
Mediterranean, Good Intentions, Somerfield*	1 Pack/250g	290	116	2.8	19.8	2.8	1.1
Mediterranean, Tesco*	1oz/28g	24	87	2.1	9.6	4.5	1.4

P

	Measure INFO/WEIGHT	per Measure KCAL	Nutrition Values per 100g / 100ml KCAL	PROT	CARB	FAT	FIBRE

PASTA SALAD,

	Measure INFO/WEIGHT	per Measure KCAL	KCAL	PROT	CARB	FAT	FIBRE
Mozzarella & Plum Tomatoes, COU, Marks & Spencer*	1 Bowl/255g	204	80	4.6	11.5	1.6	1.7
Mozzarella & Sun Dried Tomato, Waitrose*	1 Serving/150g	312	208	5.8	18.8	12.2	1.3
Pepper, Healthy Eating, Tesco*	1 Salad/210g	139	66	2.4	13.3	0.4	1.0
Prawn Cocktail, Shapers, Boots*	1 Pack/304g	250	82	5.7	11.0	1.7	0.9
Prawn, COU, Marks & Spencer*	1 Pack/274g	260	95	5.1	16.4	1.5	0.9
Prawn, Shapers, Boots*	1 Pot/250g	250	100	4.1	14.0	3.1	0.4
Ready To Eat, Somerfield*	½ Pack/123g	175	142	2.8	17.1	6.9	1.6
Red Pesto, Chicken & Santa Tomatoes, COU, M&S*	1 Serving/270g	285	106	8.1	14.0	2.1	0.6
Roast Chicken & Pesto, Shaker, Sainsbury's*	1 Box/224g	253	113	8.2	12.3	3.4	0.0
Roasted Mushroom, Spinach & Tarragon, Tesco*	1 Pot/200g	216	108	4.3	17.2	2.4	0.8
Roasted Vegetable, Waitrose*	1 Pack/190g	270	142	6.8	18.2	4.6	1.1
Sainsbury's*	½ Pack/160g	235	147	3.2	20.0	6.0	1.5
Salad	1oz/28g	36	127	2.6	13.3	7.4	1.6
Salmon, Marks & Spencer*	1 Serving/380g	817	215	6.8	12.7	15.2	0.7
Spicy Chicken, Geo Adams*	1 Pack/230g	580	252	5.1	14.9	19.1	2.9
Spicy Chilli Pesto, Sainsbury's*	¼ Pot/62.5g	171	272	3.8	20.1	19.6	1.6
Spinach & Nuts, Marks & Spencer*	1oz/28g	64	229	6.9	18.2	15.0	1.6
Succulent King Prawns & Fresh Tomatoes, COU, M&S*	1 Serving/270g	257	95	5.1	16.4	1.5	0.9
Sweetcorn & Pepper, Good For You, Asda*	1 Serving/175g	68	39	1.9	7.0	0.4	0.0
Sweetcorn, Marks & Spencer*	1oz/28g	30	107	2.8	14.9	4.0	1.8
Sweetcorn, Waitrose*	1oz/28g	31	112	6.4	18.9	1.2	1.1
Tiger Prawn, Waitrose*	1 Serving/225g	545	242	5.4	16.7	17.1	0.4
Tomato & Basil Chicken, Marks & Spencer*	1 Serving/279g	446	160	7.0	14.8	7.9	1.8
Tomato & Basil With Red & Green Pepper, Sainsbury's*	¼ Pot/63g	89	141	3.2	16.4	6.9	3.8
Tomato & Basil, Sainsbury's*	1 Serving/250g	383	153	3.5	20.5	6.3	1.4
Tomato & Chargrilled Vegetable, Tesco*	1 Serving/200g	248	124	3.7	18.6	3.9	1.4
Tomato & Mozzarella, Leaf, Shapers, Boots*	1 Pack/185g	356	192	5.1	16.0	12.0	2.5
Tomato & Mozzarella, Waitrose*	1 Pack/225g	380	169	4.3	10.0	12.4	0.6
Tomato & Pepper, Healthy Eating, Tesco*	1 Serving/100g	81	81	2.6	13.9	1.6	1.4
Tomato & Tuna, Snack, Sainsbury's*	1 Serving/200g	238	119	5.3	21.7	1.2	0.0
Tomato, Bacon & Cheese, Ginsters*	1 Pack/220g	381	173	7.4	15.6	9.0	0.0
Torcetti With Avocado, Mozarella Tomatoes, M&S*	1 Pot/190g	200	105	6.9	3.0	7.5	1.7
Torcetti With King Prawns & Tomatoes, COU, M&S*	1 Pack/270g	284	105	5.9	15.1	2.4	2.7
Tuna & Spinach, COU, Marks & Spencer*	1 Pack/270g	257	95	6.8	14.3	1.8	3.8
Tuna & Sweetcorn, COU, Marks & Spencer*	1 Pack/200g	210	105	7.1	18.3	0.9	1.2
Tuna & Sweetcorn, Healthy Eating, Tesco*	1 Pot/200g	230	115	5.7	17.0	2.7	1.3
Tuna & Sweetcorn, Sainsbury's*	1 Serving/100g	111	111	7.1	18.3	1.2	1.2
Tuna Nicoise, Waitrose*	1 Pot/190g	306	161	5.1	14.9	9.0	1.1
Tuna, Eat Smart, Safeway*	1 Pack/220g	220	100	8.0	12.2	1.6	0.5
Tuna, Tesco*	1 Pot/300g	399	133	6.2	10.5	7.3	0.0
Vegetable, Healthy Selection, Somerfield*	1 Pot/200g	180	90	2.8	19.6	0.0	0.7
Vegetable, Somerfield*	1 Salad/200g	288	144	3.0	20.0	6.0	0.0
Wholemeal	1oz/28g	37	131	3.1	13.8	7.5	2.7
Wild Mushroom, TTD, Sainsbury's*	1 Serving/259g	464	179	4.6	16.6	10.5	1.5
With Chargrilled Chicken & Pesto, Marks & Spencer*	1 Serving/190g	295	155	8.0	13.5	7.9	1.3
With Chicken, McDonald's*	1 Serving/190g	266	140	6.6	19.6	3.5	0.2
With Honey & Mustard Chicken, Safeway*	1 Pack/200g	280	140	8.5	18.1	3.7	1.0
With Poached Salmon, Marks & Spencer*	1 Serving/200g	340	170	7.8	16.2	8.4	1.4

PASTA SAUCE,

	Measure INFO/WEIGHT	per Measure KCAL	KCAL	PROT	CARB	FAT	FIBRE
Amatriciana, Fresh, Safeway*	½ Pot/175g	89	51	2.5	5.6	2.1	1.2
Amatriciana, Fresh, Sainsbury's*	½ Pot/153g	69	45	3.5	3.5	1.9	1.3
Amatriciana, Fresh, Sainsbury's*	½ Pot/150g	69	46	3.5	3.6	1.9	1.3
Amatriciana, Good For You, Asda*	½ Pot/175g	88	50	2.3	6.0	1.9	0.0

PASTA SAUCE,

INFO/WEIGHT	Measure per Measure KCAL	KCAL	PROT	CARB	FAT	FIBRE
Amatriciana, Italiano, Tesco*	½ Pot/175g	124	71	4.1	5.3	3.8	0.9
Amatriciana, Tesco*	1 Serving/175g	109	62	2.3	4.0	4.1	0.7
Arrabbiata, BGTY, Sainsbury's*	1 Jar/150g	107	71	1.3	7.6	3.9	0.7
Arrabbiata, Barilla*	1 Serving/100g	47	47	1.5	3.5	3.0	0.0
Arrabbiata, Fresh, Co-Op*	½ Pot/150g	83	55	1.0	5.0	3.0	1.0
Arrabbiata, Fresh, Morrisons*	1 Pot/350g	139	40	1.9	5.4	1.5	0.0
Arrabbiata, Fresh, Safeway*	½ Pot/176g	58	33	1.2	5.1	0.9	1.0
Arrabbiata, Fresh, Tesco*	1 Serving/110ml	29	26	0.7	3.7	0.9	0.9
Arrabbiata, Good For You, Asda*	1 Serving/350g	133	38	1.1	6.0	1.1	0.0
Arrabbiata, Italian, Waitrose*	1 Jar/320g	102	32	1.6	5.6	0.3	0.0
Arrabbiata, Italiano, Tesco*	½ Pot/175g	65	37	1.7	6.1	0.6	1.0
Arrabbiata, Marks & Spencer*	1 Jar/320g	240	75	1.2	6.2	5.3	0.8
Arrabbiata, Sainsbury's*	1oz/28g	13	45	1.4	3.3	2.9	1.6
Aubergine & Pepper, Sacla*	½ Pot/95g	238	250	1.8	5.6	24.5	0.0
Aubergine, Marks & Spencer*	1oz/28g	41	148	1.6	8.4	13.4	3.0
Basil & Oregano For Bolognese, Ragu*	1 Serving/200g	76	38	2.0	7.6	0.0	0.8
Beef Bolognese, Fresh, Asda*	¼ Pot/82g	78	95	4.3	3.4	7.3	0.4
Bolognese With Beef, Tesco*	½ Can/213g	179	84	4.9	5.5	4.7	0.0
Bolognese, Dolmio*	¼ Jar/175g	91	52	1.8	10.3	0.0	0.0
Bolognese, Finest, Tesco*	1 Serving/175g	170	97	7.0	3.8	6.1	0.5
Bolognese, Fresh, Sainsbury's*	½ Pot/150g	120	80	6.0	4.7	4.1	1.2
Bolognese, Fresh, Waitrose*	1 Pot/350g	277	79	5.1	5.3	4.2	0.7
Bolognese, Marks & Spencer*	1 Jar/100g	115	115	7.0	10.8	4.9	1.2
Bolognese, Organic, Seeds Of Change*	1 Jar/530g	313	59	1.5	10.5	1.2	1.2
Bolognese, Original, Asda*	1 Serving/157.5g	73	46	1.4	7.0	1.4	0.8
Bolognese, Original, Light, Dolmio*	1 Serving/125g	44	35	1.6	6.9	0.1	0.0
Bolognese, Original, Sainsbury's*	¼ Jar/136g	90	66	1.9	9.9	2.1	1.3
Bolognese, SmartPrice, Asda*	½ Jar/226g	88	39	0.9	7.0	0.8	0.6
Bolognese, Somerfield*	1 Pack/300g	243	81	3.0	8.0	4.0	0.0
Bolognese, Tesco*	1 Serving/175g	100	57	4.2	4.0	2.6	0.8
Bolognese, Traditional, Ragu	1 Jar/515g	345	67	2.0	9.9	2.1	1.2
Cacciatore, Fresh, Sainsbury's*	½ Pot/150g	152	101	5.4	8.1	5.9	1.5
Carbonara, BGTY, Sainsbury's*	½ Pack/165g	225	136	6.3	23.4	1.9	1.0
Carbonara, Better For You, Morrisons*	1 Serving/30g	26	87	6.1	5.4	4.5	0.0
Carbonara, Dolmio*	1 Serving/150g	224	149	3.4	4.2	13.2	0.0
Chargrilled Vegetable With Extra Virgin Olive Oil, Bertolli*	½ Jar/250g	150	60	2.1	8.7	1.9	2.4
Cheery Tomato & Roasted Pepper, Asda*	1 Jar/171.7g	91	53	1.5	5.0	3.0	2.4
Cheese & Bacon Bake, Homepride*	1oz/28g	27	95	2.0	2.5	8.6	0.0
Cheese & Bacon, Asda*	1 Pack/116g	476	410	13.0	67.0	10.0	2.3
Cheese & Broccoli, Somerfield*	½ Pack/203g	290	143	4.8	16.2	6.5	1.0
Cheese, Fresh, Perfectly Balanced, Waitrose*	½ Pot/175g	144	82	6.1	7.9	2.9	0.5
Cherry Tomato & Basil, Sacla*	1 Serving/96g	90	94	1.2	5.3	7.4	0.0
Chilli With Jalapeno Peppers, Seeds of Change*	1 Jar/350g	322	92	3.6	16.0	1.5	2.2
Chunky Vegetable, Asda*	1 Serving/250g	123	49	1.4	7.0	1.7	1.2
Chunky Vegetables, Somerfield*	1 Jar/525g	226	43	2.0	7.0	1.0	0.0
Cream & Mushroom, Marks & Spencer*	1oz/28g	45	160	1.5	6.6	14.3	0.6
Creamy Mushroom, Chicken Tonight*	¼ Jar/125g	110	88	0.7	2.8	8.2	0.4
Creamy Mushroom, Dolmio*	1 Pack/150g	167	111	1.3	3.7	10.0	0.0
Creamy Mustard, Colman's*	1 Pack/29g	108	374	11.0	46.0	16.0	0.0
Creamy Pepper & Mushroom, Colman's*	1 Pack/25g	82	327	8.1	56.0	9.1	0.0
Creamy Tomato & Bacon Bake, Homepride*	1 Serving/110g	99	90	1.9	6.5	6.3	0.0
Creamy Tomato & Basil, BGTY, Sainsbury's*	½ Jar/250g	173	69	1.7	7.6	3.6	1.0
Creamy Tomato & Herb Bake, Homepride*	1 Jar/455g	464	102	2.0	7.5	7.1	0.0

PASTA SAUCE,

	Measure INFO/WEIGHT	per Measure KCAL	Nutrition Values per 100g / 100ml				
			KCAL	PROT	CARB	FAT	FIBRE
Dolmio*	1 Serving/100g	133	133	4.3	22.5	2.5	0.0
Extra Mushrooms Bolognese, Dolmio*	1 Jar/500g	235	47	1.6	9.3	0.1	0.0
Extra Spicy Bolognese, Dolmio*	1 Serving/250g	133	53	1.7	9.2	1.1	0.0
Fiorentina, Fresh, Sainsbury's*	½ Pot/157g	165	105	3.2	4.3	8.4	0.9
Four Cheese, BGTY, Sainsbury's*	1 Serving/150g	104	69	2.9	5.5	4.0	0.1
Four Cheese, Fresh, Asda*	½ Pot/162g	309	191	5.4	2.2	17.8	0.5
Four Cheese, GFY, Asda*	½ Pot/175g	144	82	4.0	6.3	4.6	0.5
Four Cheese, Loyd Grossman*	1 Jar/350g	476	136	2.6	4.6	11.9	0.0
Four Cheese, Sainsbury's*	1 Serving/150g	296	197	6.6	4.5	17.0	0.8
Garlic & Chilli, Slow Roasted, Seeds of Change*	½ Jar/175g	158	90	1.7	8.7	5.3	2.0
Garlic, Perfectly Balanced, Waitrose*	1 Jar/440g	330	75	2.3	12.7	1.7	2.3
Grilled Vegetables & Balsamic Vinegar, Bertolli*	½ Jar/92.6g	126	135	1.8	6.5	11.3	0.0
Ham & Mushroom, Creamy, Stir & Serve, Homepride*	1 Serving/92g	124	135	1.8	5.5	11.7	0.0
Hot & Spicy, Morrisons*	1 Serving/130g	82	63	1.3	9.3	2.4	1.0
Hot Mixed Peppers Bolognese, Sainsbury's*	1oz/28g	18	66	2.0	9.7	2.1	1.5
Hot Pepper & Mozzarella, Stir Through, Sacla*	½ Jar/95g	229	241	4.7	7.2	21.5	0.0
Italian Cheese, Finest, Tesco*	½ Pot/175g	172	98	4.8	8.4	5.1	0.0
Italian Creamy Mushroom, Stir-in, Safeway*	½ Jar/75g	133	177	4.4	4.5	15.7	1.5
Italian Creamy Porcini Mushroom, Stir In, Sainsbury's*	1 Serving/75g	132	176	4.6	4.1	15.7	1.6
Italian Mushroom, Sainsbury's*	1 Serving/85g	56	66	2.0	9.8	2.1	1.7
Italian Style, Princes*	1 Jar/475g	404	85	1.7	16.0	1.6	1.2
Italian Sun Dried Tomato & Balsamic Vinegar, Sainsbury's*	1 Serving/75g	125	167	2.0	9.7	13.4	1.5
Italian Tomato & Herb, For Pasta, Sainsbury's*	½ Jar/146g	102	70	2.0	11.1	2.0	1.4
Italian Tomato & Mascarpone, Stir In, Sainsbury's*	1 Serving/75g	134	178	2.6	6.9	15.6	0.9
Italian, Tomato, Mushroom & Pancetta, Sainsbury's*	½ Jar/75g	125	167	2.2	6.1	14.9	1.3
Layered Tomato & Mozarella, Finest, Tesco*	1 Jar/160g	232	145	6.6	6.9	10.1	0.7
Leek & Bacon, Safeway*	½ Pot/170.6g	145	85	4.0	5.7	4.9	0.5
Mascarpone, BGTY, Sainsbury's*	1 Serving/120g	379	316	8.6	2.8	30.0	0.0
Mediterrainean Vegetable Pasta, Tesco*	1 Serving/166g	95	57	1.4	9.0	1.7	1.2
Mediterranean Sizzling, Homepride*	1 Serving/96g	83	86	0.9	6.3	6.4	0.0
Mediterranean Tomato, Asda*	1 Jar/500g	285	57	1.5	10.0	1.2	0.0
Mediterranean Vegetable, Organic, Pasta Reale*	1 Pack/300g	183	61	1.0	3.9	4.6	0.3
Mediterranean, BGTY, Sainsbury's*	1oz/28g	23	82	1.9	9.0	4.3	1.4
Mediterranean, Fresh, Waitrose*	1 Pot/350g	214	61	1.4	5.0	3.9	2.4
Mushroom & Garlic, 98% Fat Free, Homepride*	1 Jar/450g	230	51	1.1	8.9	1.4	0.5
Mushroom & Garlic, Deliciously Good, Homepride*	1/3 Jar/147g	109	74	0.9	6.9	4.8	0.3
Mushroom & Garlic, Somerfield*	1 Pack/110g	158	144	4.0	18.0	6.0	0.0
Mushroom & Marsala Wine, Sacla*	½ Pot/85g	165	194	2.2	3.9	18.8	0.0
Mushroom & Mascarpone, Healthy Eating, Tesco*	½ Jar/175g	86	49	2.1	5.3	2.2	0.3
Mushroom, Co-Op*	¼ Jar/125g	75	60	2.0	9.0	2.0	1.0
Mushroom, Colman's*	1 Pack/27g	97	358	14.0	53.0	9.7	0.0
Mushroom, Fresh, Waitrose*	1 Serving/175g	142	81	1.6	5.7	5.7	0.5
Mushroom, Good For You, Asda*	1 Serving/175g	112	64	2.7	7.0	2.8	0.0
Mushroom, Microwaveable, Dolmio*	1 Serving/150g	161	107	1.4	3.8	9.6	0.0
Mushroom, Perfectly Balanced, Waitrose*	1 Jar/440g	330	75	2.6	11.8	1.9	2.2
Mushroom, Sainsbury's*	1 Serving/100g	66	66	2.0	9.8	2.1	1.7
Mushroom, Somerfield*	1 Jar/525g	252	48	2.0	8.0	1.0	0.0
Napoletana, BGTY, Sainsbury's*	½ Pot/151g	71	47	1.2	5.0	2.5	1.3
Napoletana, Fresh, Asda*	1 Pot/330g	135	41	2.2	6.0	1.3	1.4
Napoletana, Fresh, Safeway*	½ Pot/175g	67	38	1.5	6.1	0.8	1.2
Napoletana, Fresh, Waitrose*	1 Serving/175g	82	47	1.3	6.6	1.7	1.0
Napoletana, Good For You, Asda*	1 Serving/175g	58	33	1.0	5.0	1.0	0.0
Napoletana, Morrisons*	1 Serving/175g	82	47	2.6	6.7	1.5	0.0

P

PASTA SAUCE,

INFO/WEIGHT	Measure per Measure KCAL	KCAL	PROT	CARB	FAT	FIBRE
Napoletana, Sainsbury's*	½ Pot/150g	126	84	1.9	6.6	5.6	0.9
Olive & Tomato, Sacla*	1 Serving/95g	87	92	1.3	3.6	8.0	0.0
Olive, Barilla*	1 Serving/100g	92	92	1.5	10.3	5.0	0.0
Onion & Garlic Bolognese, Extra, Dolmio*	1 Serving/125g	66	53	1.7	9.0	1.0	0.0
Onion & Garlic For Bolognese, Ragu*	1 Serving/125g	80	64	2.2	11.4	1.1	1.2
Onion & Garlic, Co-Op*	1 Serving/125g	106	85	2.0	12.0	3.0	0.7
Onion & Garlic, Somerfield*	1 Jar/525g	257	49	2.0	8.0	1.0	0.0
Onion & Garlic, Tesco*	1 Serving/225g	83	37	1.2	7.6	0.3	0.8
Original, Better For You, Morrisons*	1/3 Jar/200g	100	50	1.6	10.6	0.1	1.2
Original, For Bolognese, Ragu*	1 Jar/525g	268	51	1.7	10.7	0.1	1.0
Original, Healthy Eating, Tesco*	1 Jar/455g	155	34	1.2	6.5	0.1	0.8
Pepper & Tomato, Marks & Spencer*	1 Jar/320g	224	70	1.6	6.1	4.2	0.9
Porcini Mushroom & Pepperoni, Asda*	½ Jar/140g	158	113	3.8	11.0	6.0	0.0
Porcini Mushroom Stir In, BGTY, Sainsbury's*	½ Jar/75g	57	76	3.8	5.7	4.2	1.9
Primavera, Fresh, Morrisons*	½ Pot/175g	152	87	2.4	6.1	5.9	0.0
Puttanesca, Marks & Spencer*	1 Jar/320g	256	80	1.5	6.2	5.5	1.9
Puttanesca, Sainsbury's*	1 Serving/110g	132	120	2.0	8.1	8.8	0.0
Puttanesca, The Best, Safeway*	1 Serving/170g	139	82	1.0	5.6	6.2	0.0
Roasted Red Pepper & Tomato, Finest, Tesco*	1 Serving/145g	117	81	1.2	6.8	5.4	2.2
Roasted Vegetable, Microwaveable, Dolmio*	½ Pack/190g	103	54	1.4	7.6	2.0	0.0
Roasted Vegetable, Sainsbury's*	½ Pot/151g	103	68	1.6	6.7	3.9	0.4
Roasted Vegetable, Tesco*	1 Pack/175g	114	65	1.5	8.0	3.0	0.8
Roasted Vegetables & Tuna, BGTY, Sainsbury's*	½ Pot/150g	74	49	3.5	4.5	1.9	3.1
Romano, Aldi*	1 Serving/235g	141	60	1.7	8.8	2.0	1.1
Salsina With Onions & Garlic, Valfrutta*	1 Serving/150g	36	24	1.6	4.5	0.0	1.4
Sliced Mushroom, Tesco*	1 Jar/460g	161	35	1.3	7.0	0.2	0.8
Spicy Italian Chilli, Microwaveable, Dolmio*	1 Sachet/170g	92	54	1.4	7.6	2.0	0.0
Spicy Pepper & Tomato, Sacla*	½ Jar/95g	132	139	1.4	6.8	11.8	0.0
Roasted Garlic, Seeds Of Change*	1 Serving/195g	123	63	1.5	9.7	2.0	1.2
Tomato, Red Pepper, Stir in Sauce for Pasta, Safeway*	½ Jar/75g	48	64	1.6	9.0	2.4	1.1
Spicy With Peppers, Tesco*	1 Jar/455g	177	39	1.2	7.9	0.3	1.1
Spinach & Ricotta, BGTY, Sainsbury's*	1 Serving/150g	74	49	2.7	3.4	2.7	2.2
Spinach & Ricotta, Stir Through, Sacla*	½ Jar/95g	196	206	3.7	3.7	19.6	0.0
Sun Dried Tomato & Basil, Free From, Sainsbury's*	½ Jar/172.2g	124	72	2.9	8.7	2.8	1.5
Sun Dried Tomato & Garlic, Sacla*	1 Serving/95g	177	186	3.0	10.3	14.7	0.0
Sun Dried Tomato & Garlic, The Best, Safeway*	1 Jar/340g	496	146	2.2	6.2	12.5	0.0
Sun Dried Tomato, Asda*	½ Jar/158.7g	165	104	1.9	6.0	8.0	1.5
Sun Dried Tomato, Garlic & Basil, Finest, Tesco*	1 Serving/72.5g	123	168	2.0	6.8	14.8	2.9
Sun Dried Tomato, Marks & Spencer*	1oz/28g	102	363	3.6	12.4	34.9	5.7
Sun Dried Tomato, Stir In, Light, Dolmio*	½ Tub/75g	62	83	1.7	9.8	4.7	0.0
Sun Ripened Tomato & Basil, Dolmio*	1 Serving/150g	117	78	1.3	7.9	4.6	0.0
Sun Ripened Tomato & Basil, Microwaveable, Dolmio*	½ Pack/190g	106	56	1.4	7.9	2.1	0.0
Sweet Pepper, Dolmio*	1 Serving/150g	239	159	1.6	8.8	13.4	0.0
Sweet Red Pepper, Loyd Grossman*	1oz/28g	24	87	1.7	7.3	5.6	1.2
Three Cheeses, Co-Op*	1 Pack/300g	405	135	6.0	6.0	9.0	0.1
Tomato & Aubergine, TTD, Sainsbury's*	1 Serving/150g	107	71	2.1	7.7	3.5	2.0
Tomato & Basil, Bertolli*	1 Serving/250g	118	47	1.5	7.9	1.1	1.6
Tomato & Basil, Dolmio*	1 Serving/170g	95	56	1.4	7.9	2.1	0.0
Tomato & Basil, Loyd Grossman*	½ Jar/175g	152	87	1.7	7.3	5.6	1.2
Tomato & Basil, Organic, Pasta Reale*	1 Pack/300g	216	72	1.0	5.1	5.3	0.4
Tomato & Basil, Organic, Seeds Of Change*	1 Jar/390g	234	60	1.4	8.5	2.2	1.1
Tomato & Chargrilled Vegetable, Loyd Grossman*	1 Serving/150g	134	89	1.8	7.9	5.6	0.9
Tomato & Chilli, Loyd Grossman*	½ Jar/175g	154	88	1.7	7.3	5.7	0.9

P

	Measure INFO/WEIGHT	per Measure KCAL	Nutrition Values per 100g / 100ml				
			KCAL	PROT	CARB	FAT	FIBRE
PASTA SAUCE,							
Tomato & Chilli, Pour Over, Marks & Spencer*	½ Jar/165g	124	75	1.2	6.2	5.3	0.8
Tomato & Chunky Mushroom, Dolmio*	1 Pack/475g	323	68	1.2	7.6	3.7	0.0
Tomato & Herb, Co-Op*	1 Serving/125g	75	60	1.0	9.0	2.0	1.0
Tomato & Herb, Iceland*	1 Serving/100g	59	59	1.4	8.9	2.0	0.7
Tomato & Herb, Marks & Spencer*	1 Jar/500g	400	80	2.6	10.1	3.1	1.7
Tomato & Herb, Organic, Marks & Spencer*	1 Jar/320g	176	55	1.1	6.8	2.6	1.8
Tomato & Herb, Organic, Sainsbury's*	1 Serving/75g	38	51	1.2	6.6	2.0	0.5
Tomato & Herb, Perfectly Balanced, Waitrose*	½ Pot/175g	86	49	1.2	5.3	2.6	0.9
Tomato & Mascarpone, Asda*	1 Serving/175g	210	120	1.6	6.0	10.0	0.0
Tomato & Mascarpone, BGTY, Sainsbury's*	½ Pot/150g	75	50	2.0	3.6	3.0	3.6
Tomato & Mascarpone, Fresh, Sainsbury's*	1 Serving/150g	177	118	2.2	4.2	10.3	1.1
Tomato & Mascarpone, Marks & Spencer*	½ Pack/175g	175	100	3.3	6.6	6.2	0.8
Tomato & Mascarpone, Pasta Reale*	1 Pack/300g	318	106	2.9	5.9	7.9	0.5
Tomato & Mascarpone, Sacla*	½ Jar/95g	161	169	2.2	6.2	15.0	0.0
Tomato & Mascarpone, Tesco*	1 Serving/175g	194	111	2.8	5.4	8.7	0.6
Tomato & Mushroom, Asda*	1 Serving/127g	71	56	1.8	8.0	1.9	1.2
Tomato & Mushroom, Organic, Sainsbury's*	1 Serving/150g	87	58	1.6	7.1	2.6	1.5
Tomato & Olives, La Doria*	1 Jar/90g	76	84	1.2	5.0	6.6	0.0
Tomato & Parmesan, Seeds Of Change*	1 Serving/150g	101	67	2.5	7.8	2.9	1.1
Tomato & Roasted Garlic, Loyd Grossman*	½ Jar/175g	161	92	2.0	8.8	5.5	0.8
Tomato & Smokey Bacon, Dolmio*	1 Pot/150g	240	160	5.5	5.8	13.1	0.0
Tomato & Spicy Sausages, Marks & Spencer*	1 Jar/330g	215	65	4.0	5.5	3.0	0.8
Tomato & Tuna, Loyd Grossman*	½ Jar/175g	154	88	4.4	7.5	4.4	0.8
Tomato & Wild Mushroom, Loyd Grossman*	½ Jar/175g	154	88	2.1	7.4	5.6	1.5
Tomato & Wild Mushroom, Waitrose*	1 Serving/175g	65	37	1.7	6.0	0.7	0.9
Tomato Red Wine Shallots, Bertolli*	½ Jar/250g	113	45	1.7	7.2	1.7	1.5
Tomato With Herbs & Garlic, Italian, Safeway*	1 Serving/120g	73	61	1.9	8.7	2.1	1.3
Tomato With Herbs Buon Appetito, Princes*	1 Jar/475g	214	45	0.7	9.6	0.4	0.0
Tomato With Mushrooms, Italian, Safeway*	½ Jar/235g	146	62	2.0	8.8	2.1	1.9
Tomato With Onions & Garlic, Italian, Safeway*	1 Serving/50g	35	69	2.3	10.2	2.1	1.8
Tomato, Bacon & Mushroom, Asda*	½ Pot/50g	33	66	2.5	6.0	3.6	0.0
Tomato, Basil & Parmesan Stir In, BGTY, Sainsbury's*	1 Serving/75g	69	92	2.9	7.8	5.5	1.0
Tomato, Chilli & Onion, Bertolli*	1 Serving/100g	49	49	1.8	6.7	1.7	1.8
Tomato, Kalamata Olive & Pine Nut, The Best, Safeway*	½ Pot/175g	158	90	1.7	5.0	6.7	1.9
Tomato, Pepper & Herb, Somerfield*	1 Serving/186g	233	125	3.0	17.4	4.8	0.8
Tomato, Roasted Garlic & Mushroom, Bertoli*	1 Jar/500g	255	51	1.9	6.4	2.0	1.5
Tomato, Romano & Garlic, Bertolli*	¼ Jar/181g	127	70	2.9	7.6	3.0	1.7
Traditional, Healthy Choice, Safeway*	1 Jar/475g	257	54	1.8	8.2	1.6	1.3
Traditional, Somerfield*	1 Jar/525g	263	50	2.0	8.0	1.0	0.0
Value, Tesco*	1 Serving/100g	34	34	0.6	6.1	0.8	0.4
Vine Ripened Tomato & Aromatic Basil, Discovery*	1 Serving/125g	161	129	1.8	14.3	7.2	0.0
Vine Ripened Tomato & Black Olive, Bertolli*	½ Jar/92.5g	146	157	2.3	7.3	13.3	0.0
Whole Cherry Tomato & Red Chilli, Sacla*	1 Serving/96g	85	89	1.5	6.2	6.5	0.1
Wild Mushroom & Herb, Seeds Of Change*	1 Serving/190g	103	54	1.6	8.8	1.4	1.2
With Hot Pepper & Cheese, Discovery*	1 Serving/100g	159	159	5.3	5.1	13.0	0.0
PASTA SHAPES,							
Cooked, Tesco*	1 Serving/260g	356	137	5.1	26.3	0.8	1.1
In A Cheese & Broccoli Sauce, Tesco*	1 Serving/84g	317	377	13.1	66.2	6.6	4.1
In Rich Chicken, Garilc & Wine Sauce, Tesco*	1 Pack/110g	393	357	14.0	66.1	4.1	4.2
Postman Pat, HP*	1 Can/410g	279	68	1.8	14.3	0.4	0.7
Scooby Doo, HP*	1 Can/410g	279	68	1.8	14.3	0.4	0.7
Teletubbies, Heinz*	1 Can/400g	244	61	2.0	12.3	0.4	0.6

P

	Measure INFO/WEIGHT	per Measure KCAL	Nutrition Values per 100g / 100ml				
			KCAL	PROT	CARB	FAT	FIBRE
PASTA SHELLS,							
Dry, Morrisons*	1 Serving/125g	443	354	12.0	72.0	2.0	3.0
Egg, Fresh, Waitrose*	1 Serving/125g	345	276	11.6	50.0	2.3	3.9
In Bolognese Sauce, Weight Watchers*	1 Pack/395g	280	71	5.2	9.6	1.3	0.7
PASTA SNACK,							
Chicken & Smoked Bacon, Sainsbury's*	1 Pack/190g	490	258	7.2	14.1	19.2	0.0
Chicken, Morrisons*	1 Pack/250g	285	114	3.3	19.3	2.7	0.0
Ham & Mushroom, Tesco*	1 Pack/300g	618	206	4.2	15.0	14.3	1.1
Tomato & Basil, Healthy Living, Tesco*	1 Pack/200g	116	58	1.8	10.4	1.0	1.0
Tomato & Herb, Morrisons*	1 Pot/247g	247	100	3.1	19.5	1.1	0.0
Tuna Sweetcorn, Tesco*	1 Serving/100g	210	210	5.9	16.9	13.2	1.1
PASTA TWIRLS,							
Asda*	1 Serving/50g	173	346	12.0	71.0	1.5	3.0
Tri-Colour, Sainsbury's*	1 Serving/75g	268	357	12.3	73.1	1.7	2.5
PASTA TWISTS,							
Co-Op*	1oz/28g	97	345	13.0	69.0	2.0	3.0
Morrisons*	¼ Pack/125g	455	364	12.0	72.3	1.0	0.0
Romano, Aldi*	1oz/28g	101	362	12.0	75.0	1.5	2.9
PASTE,							
BBQ Bean, Princes*	1 Serving/33g	35	106	5.7	19.8	0.4	0.0
Beef, Asda*	1 Serving/37g	72	194	17.0	0.1	14.0	0.0
Beef, Princes*	1 Serving/18g	40	220	14.4	5.2	15.8	0.0
Beef, Sainsbury's*	1 Jar/75g	142	189	16.0	1.5	13.2	1.4
Chicken & Ham, Asda*	½ Jar/38g	82	217	14.0	2.1	17.0	0.0
Chicken & Ham, Princes*	1 Jar/100g	233	233	13.6	2.8	18.6	0.0
Chicken & Ham, Sainsbury's*	Thin Spread/9g	14	158	16.0	1.1	10.0	1.1
Chicken & Stuffing, Asda*	½ Jar/35g	71	203	16.0	3.3	14.0	0.0
Chicken & Stuffing, Princes*	1 Jar/100g	229	229	15.7	3.3	17.0	0.0
Chicken, Asda*	Thin Spread/7g	13	184	16.0	0.8	13.0	0.0
Chicken, Princes*	Thin Spread/9g	22	240	12.6	5.6	18.5	0.0
Chicken, Tesco*	1 Serving/12g	30	248	14.8	2.3	20.0	0.1
Chicken, Value, Tesco*	Thin Spread/9g	18	196	15.1	1.8	14.3	0.1
Crab, Classic, Shippam*	1 Jar/35g	48	138	14.1	6.0	6.4	0.0
Crab, Princes*	1 Pot/35g	36	104	13.4	4.8	3.5	0.0
Crab, Tesco*	1 Jar/75g	89	119	14.0	4.6	5.0	0.1
Salmon & Shrimp, Somerfield*	Thin Spread/9g	10	112	17.0	4.0	3.0	0.0
Salmon & Shrimp, Tesco*	1 Jar/75g	83	111	15.1	5.0	3.4	0.1
Salmon, Asda*	1 Serving/53g	76	143	15.0	5.0	7.0	0.0
Salmon, Princes*	1 Serving/30g	59	195	13.5	6.5	12.8	0.0
Sardine & Tomato, Asda*	Thin Spread/9g	11	123	14.0	3.3	6.0	0.0
Sardine & Tomato, Co-Op*	1 Serving/25g	34	135	16.0	3.0	6.0	2.0
Sardine & Tomato, Princes*	1 Jar/75g	110	146	15.4	5.0	7.2	0.0
Sardine & Tomato, Sainsbury's*	1 Mini Pot/35g	60	170	16.9	1.2	10.8	1.3
Sardine & Tomato, Somerfield*	Thin Spread/9g	13	144	15.0	5.0	7.0	0.0
Sun Dried Tomato, Sacla*	1 Serving/10g	40	397	3.0	12.9	37.0	0.0
Tomato, Safeway*	1 Serving/100g	91	91	6.0	18.0	0.0	3.0
Tuna & Mayonnaise, Princes*	1 Pot/75g	158	210	16.6	1.3	15.4	0.0
Tuna & Mayonnaise, Sainsbury's*	1 Tbsp/17g	41	242	19.2	0.6	18.1	1.6
Tuna & Mayonnaise, Somerfield*	Thin Spread/9g	19	209	15.0	2.0	16.0	0.0
Tuna & Mayonnaise, Tesco*	1 Serving/15g	31	209	14.9	2.1	15.7	0.1
Vegetable, Sainsbury's*	1 Serving/17g	26	154	7.4	5.9	11.2	3.4
PASTRAMI,							
American Style, Safeway*	1 Slice/15g	21	140	23.8	2.0	4.1	0.0
American Style, Tesco*	1 Serving/50g	59	117	25.7	0.4	1.4	0.4

P

	Measure INFO/WEIGHT	per Measure KCAL	Nutrition Values per 100g / 100ml				
			KCAL	PROT	CARB	FAT	FIBRE
PASTRAMI,							
Asda*	1 Slice/25g	35	141	24.0	2.0	4.1	0.0
Beef, Wafer Thin, Sainsbury's*	1 Serving/25g	37	146	16.9	1.9	7.9	0.7
Pre- Packed, Asda*	1 Pack/70g	75	107	24.0	0.3	1.1	0.0
Slices, TTD, Sainsbury's*	1 Slice/10g	14	140	23.8	2.0	4.1	0.1
Slices, Waitrose*	1 Slice/10g	12	124	24.3	0.0	3.0	0.0
Turkey, Wafer Thin, Marks & Spencer*	1 Serving/100g	113	113	23.6	1.4	1.6	0.0
Turkey, Wafer Thin, Sainsbury's*	1 Serving/100g	108	108	19.3	3.0	2.1	0.5
Wafer Thin, Marks & Spencer*	1 Pack/75g	101	135	23.5	0.9	4.7	0.1
PASTRY,							
Chinese Flaky	1oz/28g	110	392	5.4	59.3	16.4	0.0
Choux, Cooked	1oz/28g	91	325	8.5	29.8	19.8	1.2
Choux, Raw	1oz/28g	59	211	5.5	19.4	12.9	0.8
Fillo, Asda*	1 Serving/100g	311	311	9.0	62.0	3.0	2.0
Filo, Jus-Rol*	1 Sheet/45g	128	285	8.9	60.0	1.0	0.0
Filo, Sainsbury's*	1 Sheet/33g	104	315	9.2	62.1	4.1	0.8
Flaky, Cooked	1oz/28g	157	560	5.6	45.9	40.6	1.8
Flaky, Raw	1oz/28g	119	424	4.2	34.8	30.7	1.4
Flan Case	1oz/28g	152	544	7.1	56.7	33.6	1.8
Greek	1oz/28g	90	322	4.7	40.0	17.0	0.0
Plain Case, Tesco*	1 Case/200g	966	483	6.3	55.0	28.0	0.9
Puff, Fresh, Sainsbury's*	½ Pack/250g	1113	445	5.4	28.8	34.3	1.3
Puff, Frozen, Jus-Rol*	1 Sheet/213g	846	397	6.1	37.0	25.0	0.0
Puff, Frozen, Raw	1 Shell/47g	175	373	5.7	37.0	23.5	0.0
Puff, Ready Rolled, Jus-Rol*	1 Sheet/240g	998	416	4.2	39.0	27.0	0.0
Shortcrust, Cooked	1oz/28g	146	521	6.6	54.2	32.3	2.2
Shortcrust, Frozen, Jus-Rol*	1 Sheet/225g	1055	469	6.6	41.0	31.0	0.0
Shortcrust, Frozen, Raw	1oz/28g	123	440	4.5	44.3	28.4	1.9
Shortcrust, Raw	1oz/28g	126	449	5.7	46.8	27.9	1.9
Sweet Case, Sainsbury's*	1 Case/230g	1051	457	5.3	56.8	23.2	1.5
Wholemeal, Cooked	1oz/28g	140	499	8.9	44.6	32.9	6.3
Wholemeal, Raw	1oz/28g	121	431	7.7	38.5	28.4	5.4
PASTRY MIX, Short Crust, Somerfield*	1oz/28g	134	479	7.0	49.0	28.0	0.0
PASTY,							
Bite Size Pasties, Food To Go, Sainsburys*	1 Serving/60g	226	377	8.2	31.2	24.4	1.5
Cheese & Onion, Co-Op*	1 Pasty/75g	235	313	9.2	24.5	19.8	1.7
Cheese & Onion, Farmfoods*	1 Pasty/191g	485	254	6.6	25.5	14.0	2.0
Cheese & Onion, Geo Adams*	1 Pasty/150g	420	280	6.9	27.9	15.6	1.1
Cheese & Onion, Sainsbury's*	1 Serving/150g	486	324	7.4	24.5	21.8	1.3
Cheese & Onion, Somerfield*	1 Pasty/145g	419	289	7.0	24.0	18.0	0.0
Chicken & Vegetable, Proper Handmade Cornish*	1 Pasty/255g	671	263	7.4	30.2	13.6	2.4
Cornish Roaster, Ginsters*	1 Pasty/130g	417	321	8.5	29.9	18.6	1.3
Cornish, Asda*	1 Pasty/100g	287	287	7.0	22.0	19.0	1.2
Cornish, BGTY, Sainsbury's*	1 Pasty/135g	308	228	7.7	28.2	9.4	1.6
Cornish, Cheese & Onion, Ginsters*	1 Pasty/130g	511	393	10.4	30.7	25.4	2.3
Cornish, Chicken & Bacon, Ginsters*	1 Pasty/227g	579	255	5.4	25.7	14.5	0.9
Cornish, Co-Op*	1 Pasty/75g	200	267	6.4	23.4	16.4	1.6
Cornish, Marks & Spencer*	1 Pasty/150g	480	320	6.5	27.3	20.3	1.5
Cornish, Mini, Icelands*	1 Pasty/70.3g	214	306	7.0	22.1	21.1	1.2
Cornish, Mini, Marks & Spencer*	1 Pasty/72g	227	315	6.7	21.0	22.6	1.0
Cornish, Mini, Sainsbury's*	1 Pasty/70g	280	400	7.3	28.1	28.7	1.5
Cornish, Mini, Tesco*	1 Pasty/24g	66	274	5.6	23.2	17.7	0.5
Cornish, Morrisons*	1 Pasty/200g	626	313	7.5	29.1	18.5	0.0
Cornish, Original, Ginsters*	1 Pasty/227g	568	250	6.0	19.0	15.8	1.1

	Measure INFO/WEIGHT	per Measure KCAL	Nutrition Values per 100g / 100ml				
			KCAL	PROT	CARB	FAT	FIBRE
PASTY,							
Cornish, Pork Farms*	1 Pasty/250g	673	269	7.7	22.8	16.3	0.0
Cornish, Safeway*	1 Pasty/170g	490	288	7.5	22.6	18.6	1.5
Cornish, SmartPrice, Asda*	1 Pasty/94g	286	304	8.0	32.0	16.0	1.7
Cornish, Tesco*	1 Pasty/150g	467	311	6.8	21.9	21.8	1.6
Cornish, Traditional Style, Geo Adams*	1 Pasty/165g	488	296	7.1	25.4	18.4	1.3
Steak & Onion, Marks & Spencer*	1 Pasty/164g	459	280	8.7	19.2	18.8	1.4
Tandoori & Vegetable, Holland & Barrett*	1 Pack/110g	232	211	4.3	29.4	8.5	1.8
Vegetarian, Cornish, Linda McCartney*	1 Pasty/170g	420	247	5.2	25.5	13.8	1.5
PATE,							
Apricot, Asda*	1 Serving/50g	156	312	12.0	3.0	28.0	0.0
Ardennes, Asda*	1 Serving/50g	143	286	13.9	3.6	24.0	1.3
Ardennes, BGTY, Sainsbury's*	1 Serving/50g	95	189	18.1	2.4	11.9	0.1
Ardennes, Healthy Eating, Tesco*	1 Serving/50g	119	238	16.5	2.6	17.9	1.6
Ardennes, Healthy Living, Tesco*	1 Serving/50g	116	231	14.6	7.7	15.8	1.5
Ardennes, Reduced Fat, Safeway*	1 Serving/50g	97	194	18.5	3.1	11.9	0.1
Ardennes, Reduced Fat, Waitrose*	¼ Pack/42g	94	224	15.4	2.6	16.9	0.5
Ardennes, Safeway*	1 Serving/50g	166	331	12.8	6.0	28.4	0.8
Ardennes, Sainsbury's*	1 Serving/20g	60	299	16.5	2.1	24.9	0.1
Ardennes, Tesco*	1 Tbsp/15g	53	354	13.3	0.5	33.2	1.2
Asparagus, Sainsbury's*	½ Pot/57g	88	153	3.4	5.4	13.1	1.0
Breton Course Country With Apricots, Sainsbury's*	1 Serving/21g	60	285	13.5	7.0	22.5	0.5
Brie & Cranberry, Marks & Spencer*	1 Serving/55g	160	290	7.5	18.9	20.5	0.5
Brussels & Mushroom, 25% Less Fat, Asda*	1 Serving/40g	88	220	14.0	2.7	17.0	0.0
Brussels Style, Quorn*	1 Pack/130g	150	115	10.8	5.7	5.4	3.4
Brussels With Garlic, Asda*	1 Serving/50g	170	340	10.7	4.0	31.3	2.5
Brussels, 25% Less Fat, Morrisons*	¼ Pack/42.5g	107	249	14.2	0.7	20.6	0.0
Brussels, Asda*	1 Serving/50g	175	350	10.7	4.4	32.2	1.7
Brussels, BGTY, Sainsbury's*	1 Serving/50g	137	273	12.6	6.2	22.0	0.1
Brussels, Co-Op*	1 Serving/15g	51	340	11.0	4.0	31.0	2.0
Brussels, Fat Reduced, Somerfield*	1 Serving/50g	96	192	14.0	2.0	14.0	0.0
Brussels, Healthy Eating, Tesco*	1 Serving/28g	66	235	16.4	2.3	17.8	1.9
Brussels, Marks & Spencer*	1 Pot/170g	519	305	13.3	2.8	26.6	1.0
Brussels, Reduced Fat, Asda*	1 Serving/44g	88	199	15.0	2.1	15.0	1.9
Brussels, Reduced Fat, Safeway*	1 Serving/15g	29	193	15.0	3.4	13.3	0.1
Brussels, Reduced Fat, Somerfield*	1 Serving/50g	139	277	14.0	8.0	21.0	0.0
Brussels, Reduced Fat, Waitrose*	1 Serving/40g	92	229	13.2	2.4	18.5	0.5
Brussels, Sainsbury's*	1 Pack/170g	663	390	10.6	1.1	38.2	0.1
Brussels, Sanpareil*	¼ Pack/37g	121	326	13.0	1.0	30.0	0.0
Brussels, Smooth, Safeway*	1 Pack/170g	553	325	11.5	3.9	29.3	1.6
Brussels, Tesco*	1 Serving/28g	92	330	11.0	3.0	30.5	1.1
Brussels, With Forest Mushroom, Co Op*	1 Serving/57g	180	315	12.0	2.0	29.0	1.0
Carrot, Ginger & Spring Onion, Marks & Spencer*	1 Serving/50g	73	145	1.5	9.6	11.0	0.9
Celery, Stilton & Walnut, Waitrose*	1 Pot/115g	294	256	9.0	3.2	23.0	2.2
Chargrilled Vegetable, BGTY Sainsbury's*	½ Pot/57.3g	43	75	4.9	10.8	1.3	2.7
Chick Pea & Black Olive, Cauldron Foods*	1 Pot/113g	203	180	6.2	15.6	10.3	4.5
Chicken & Brandy, Morrisons*	1 Serving/44g	133	303	10.8	4.3	26.9	0.8
Chicken Liver & Brandy, Asda*	1 Serving/50g	177	353	9.0	5.5	32.8	3.2
Chicken Liver & Brandy, Morrow Foods*	1 Serving/28g	50	179	13.6	3.9	12.1	0.5
Chicken Liver Parfait, TTD, Sainsbury's*	1 Serving/20g	72	359	8.0	2.0	35.0	0.5
Chicken Liver With Brandy, Tesco*	1oz/28g	82	293	11.8	3.5	25.8	1.4
Chicken Liver, Marks & Spencer*	1oz/28g	79	281	14.0	1.9	24.1	0.1
Chicken Liver, Organic, Waitrose*	½ Tub/87.5g	205	233	12.6	1.8	18.4	1.4
Coarse Farmhouse, Organic, Sainsbury's*	1 Serving/56g	138	246	13.3	3.7	19.7	0.8

PATE,

	Measure INFO/WEIGHT	per Measure KCAL	KCAL	PROT	CARB	FAT	FIBRE
Coarse Pork Liver With Garlic, Asda*	1 Pack/40g	130	326	13.0	1.0	30.0	0.0
Country Style Coarse, Quorn*	½ Pot/65g	68	104	9.2	7.3	4.2	2.7
Crab, Marks & Spencer*	1oz/28g	63	225	12.1	5.9	17.3	0.0
Crab, Waitrose*	1oz/28g	59	209	14.5	0.5	16.6	0.0
Deli, Quorn*	1oz/28g	32	115	10.8	5.7	5.4	3.4
Duck & Champagne, Luxury, Marks & Spencer*	1oz/28g	106	380	8.3	8.3	35.2	7.8
Duck & Orange, Asda*	1 Serving/40g	94	235	16.0	2.2	18.0	0.0
Duck & Orange, Marks & Spencer*	1oz/28g	88	315	10.6	2.8	29.0	0.5
Duck Liver With Champagne & Truffles, TTD, Sainsbury's*	1 Serving/50g	212	423	8.2	2.5	42.2	0.0
Farmhouse Mushroom, Asda*	1 Serving/50g	126	252	13.0	5.0	20.0	0.7
Farmhouse Style, Finest, Tesco*	1 Serving/28g	83	295	11.9	3.6	25.9	1.0
Farmhouse Style, Marks & Spencer*	¼ Pack/42g	90	215	14.4	1.9	16.9	1.2
Farmhouse With Christmas Ale, Sainsbury's*	1oz/28g	67	239	15.4	1.6	19.1	0.0
Farmhouse With Mushrooms & Garlic, Tesco*	1 Serving/90g	257	285	13.8	0.6	25.3	1.3
Garlic & Herb Yeast, Tartex*	1 Serving/10g	23	230	7.0	10.0	18.0	0.0
Herb, Organic, Suma*	1 Serving/25g	59	234	12.0	6.0	18.0	0.0
Isle of Skye Smoked Salmon, TTD, Sainsbury's*	½ Pot/58g	161	277	16.5	0.8	23.1	0.1
Liver & Bacon, Tesco*	1 Serving/10g	28	276	12.9	4.3	23.0	0.4
Liver & Pork, Healthy Eating, Tesco*	1 Serving/28g	64	229	14.4	8.4	15.3	1.3
Liver Spreading, Somerfield*	1oz/28g	77	275	14.0	3.0	23.0	0.0
Liver, Value, Tesco*	1 Serving/50g	151	302	13.0	4.1	26.0	0.5
Luxury Orkney Crab, Castle MacLellan*	1 Serving/15g	27	178	11.1	9.2	10.7	0.8
Mackerel, Smoked	1oz/28g	103	368	13.4	1.3	34.4	0.0
Mackerel, Tesco*	1 Serving/29g	102	353	14.3	0.5	32.6	0.0
Mediterranean Roast Vegetable, Tesco*	1 Serving/28g	31	112	2.4	4.3	9.4	1.2
Mexican Red Pepper & Wild Chilli Organic Yeast, Tartex*	1 Pot/50g	99	198	6.4	7.0	16.0	0.0
Moroccan Chick Pea, Cauldron Foods*	½ Pack/57.6g	103	177	4.9	9.4	13.3	11.8
Mushroom & Herb, Somerfield*	1oz/28g	81	289	4.0	8.0	27.0	0.0
Mushroom & Tarragon, Cauldron Foods*	1oz/28g	43	155	2.8	5.5	13.5	1.4
Mushroom, BGTY, Sainsbury's*	½ Pot/58g	29	50	4.6	6.7	0.5	3.0
Mushroom, COU, Marks & Spencer*	1oz/28g	17	60	2.9	7.4	1.9	0.9
Mushroom, Marks & Spencer*	1 Pot/115g	224	195	4.2	4.8	17.5	1.3
Mushroom, New, Tesco*	1 Serving/85g	117	138	3.3	9.8	9.5	1.0
Mushroom, Organic, Cauldron Foods*	1oz/28g	33	119	2.8	4.3	10.1	1.0
Mushroom, Sainsbury's*	1oz/28g	47	168	3.1	5.9	15.2	1.3
Mushroom, Tesco*	1oz/28g	42	151	3.2	9.1	11.3	0.9
Poached Salmon & Watercress, Tesco*	1 Serving/25g	60	238	19.2	0.4	17.7	0.2
Pork & Garlic, Somerfield*	1oz/28g	83	295	14.0	3.0	25.0	0.0
Pork & Mushroom, Somerfield*	1oz/28g	95	339	11.0	3.0	31.0	0.0
Pork With Port & Cranberry, Tesco*	1 Serving/28g	83	296	12.1	4.3	25.6	0.6
Pork, With Peppercorns, Tesco*	1 Serving/28g	84	300	12.9	1.4	26.8	0.7
Red Pepper, Marks & Spencer*	1oz/28g	52	185	3.0	6.6	16.2	0.9
Ricotta, Subdried Tomato & Basil, Princes*	1 Jar/110g	343	312	5.2	8.3	28.7	0.0
Roasted Carrot, Ginger & Spring Onion, Marks & Spencer*	1 Serving/50g	73	145	1.5	9.6	11.0	0.9
Roasted Red Pepper & Houmous, Princes*	¼ Jar/27g	32	120	4.6	12.4	5.8	0.0
Roasted Red Pepper, Oven Roasted, Castle MacLellan*	1oz/28g	46	163	3.3	8.2	13.5	0.8
Roasted Vegetable, COU, Marks & Spencer*	1 Pot/115g	86	75	6.2	9.1	1.5	1.4
Salmon, Organic, Marks & Spencer*	1oz/28g	76	270	16.9	0.0	22.5	0.0
Salmon, Smoked, Marks & Spencer*	1oz/28g	74	265	16.9	0.0	22.0	0.0
Scottish Smoked Salmon, Castle MacLellan*	¼ Tub/28g	62	220	13.5	5.6	16.0	0.0
Scottish Smoked Salmon, Marks & Spencer*	1 Serving/30g	81	270	17.0	0.2	22.3	0.0
Smoked Mackerel, Marks & Spencer*	1oz/28g	104	370	13.4	0.7	34.7	0.3
Smoked Mackerel, Sainsbury's*	½ Pot/57g	201	352	15.2	1.9	31.5	0.3

P

	Measure INFO/WEIGHT	per Measure KCAL	Nutrition Values per 100g / 100ml				
			KCAL	PROT	CARB	FAT	FIBRE
PATE,							
Smoked Salmon, Healthy Eating, Tesco*	1 Serving/50g	65	130	17.5	2.6	5.5	0.0
Smoked Salmon, Organic, Waitrose*	1oz/28g	83	296	13.9	2.4	25.6	0.0
Smoked Salmon, Waitrose*	½ Pot/56g	122	217	17.7	1.5	15.6	0.6
Spiced Parsnip & Carrot, Organic, Asda*	½ Pot/58g	63	109	3.7	10.0	6.0	2.6
Spiced Roasted Parsnip & Carrot, Cauldron Foods*	1 Serving/60g	64	107	3.7	9.8	5.9	2.6
Spicy Bean, Princes*	½ Pot/55g	46	84	3.6	16.7	0.3	0.0
Spinach & Soft Cheese, Cauldron Foods*	1 Pack/113g	209	185	5.1	6.8	15.4	2.3
Spinach, Parmesan & Almond, Cauldron Foods*	1/3 Pack/38g	66	173	7.2	6.3	13.2	2.3
Tomato, Lentil & Basil, Cauldron Foods*	1oz/28g	43	154	7.5	15.6	6.8	1.5
Tuna With Butter & Lemon Juice, Sainsbury's*	½ Pot/58g	209	360	19.0	0.1	31.6	0.3
Tuna, Marks & Spencer*	1oz/28g	99	355	18.0	0.0	31.3	0.0
Tuna, Tesco*	1 Pack/115g	332	289	19.8	0.3	23.2	0.2
Vegetable	1oz/28g	48	173	7.5	5.9	13.4	0.0
Vegetable, Cauldron Foods*	1 Pack/112.8g	220	195	9.2	14.1	11.3	4.4
Vegetarian, Mushroom & Tarragon, Waitrose*	1 Serving/30g	47	155	2.8	5.5	13.5	1.4
Vegetarian, Spicy Mexican, Organic, Waitrose*	1 Serving/50g	58	115	6.2	8.6	6.2	3.5
Vegetarian, Spinach, Soft Cheese & Onion, Co-Op*	1oz/28g	48	170	5.0	3.0	15.0	4.0
Vegetarian, Yeast, Wild Mushroom, Grano Vita*	1oz/28g	60	213	10.0	5.0	17.0	0.0
Yeast With Mushrooms, Organic, Tartex*	1oz/28g	56	200	7.0	7.0	16.0	0.0
Yeast With Red & Green Peppers, Vessen*	1 Pot/50g	111	222	6.0	9.0	18.0	0.0
PAVLOVA,							
Bucks Fizz Mini Champagne, Co-Op*	1 Pavlova/19g	62	325	3.0	38.0	18.0	0.5
Mixed Berry, Two, COU, Marks & Spencer*	1 Pavlova/100g	140	140	4.9	27.4	1.8	9.3
Raspberry & Lemon, Asda*	1 Serving/43.4g	101	235	2.8	46.0	4.4	0.5
Raspberry, Co-Op*	1/6 Pavlova/49g	147	300	3.2	44.8	12.0	1.1
Raspberry, Individual, Marks & Spencer*	1 Pavlova/65g	133	205	4.0	41.8	2.4	0.2
Raspberry, Marks & Spencer*	1 Serving/84g	193	230	2.3	33.3	9.6	0.3
Raspberry, Mini, Co-Op*	1 Pavlova/19g	61	320	3.0	56.0	9.0	0.6
Raspberry, Safeway*	1 Serving/53g	163	307	2.9	44.6	13.0	0.5
Raspberry, Sara Lee*	1/6 Slice/55.4g	167	303	2.7	38.5	15.3	1.1
Raspberry, Tesco*	1 Serving/65g	191	294	2.7	41.8	12.9	1.1
Sticky Toffee, Farmfoods*	1/6 Pack/49g	186	380	3.4	47.8	19.5	0.3
Sticky Toffee, Sainsbury's*	1/6 Pack/61g	249	415	3.7	63.1	16.4	0.9
Strawberry & Champagne, Mini, Co-Op*	1 Pavlova/19g	65	340	3.0	40.0	19.0	0.8
Strawberry, COU, Marks & Spencer*	1 Pot/95g	147	155	2.4	30.5	2.4	0.8
Strawberry, Co-Op*	1 Serving/52g	177	340	3.0	50.0	14.0	0.4
Strawberry, Farmfoods*	1/6 Cake/52g	152	292	2.3	36.9	15.0	2.2
Toffee, Co-Op*	1/6 Pavlova/53g	193	365	3.0	52.0	16.0	0.6
Toffee, Mini, Co-Op*	1 Pavlova/18g	69	385	4.0	64.0	13.0	0.0
PAW-PAW,							
Raw, Fresh	1oz/28g	10	36	0.5	8.8	0.1	2.2
Raw, Weighed With Skin & Pips	1oz/28g	8	27	0.4	6.6	0.1	1.7
PEACH, Raw, Fresh	1 Med/110g	36	33	1.0	7.6	0.1	1.5
PEACH & PEAR, Fruit Express, Del Monte*	1 Serving/185g	87	47	0.4	10.8	0.1	0.9
PEACHES,							
& Pears, Pieces In Juice, Fruiti, Sainsbury's*	1 Can/139g	78	56	0.3	13.9	0.1	0.5
Canned, In Juice	1oz/28g	11	39	0.6	9.7	0.0	0.8
Canned, In Syrup	1oz/28g	15	55	0.5	14.0	0.0	0.9
Dried	1oz/28g	61	219	3.4	53.0	0.8	7.3
Halves, Del Monte*	½ Can/207g	101	49	0.5	11.2	0.1	0.0
Halves, In Apple Juice, Asda*	1 Can/234g	117	50	0.5	12.0	0.0	1.0
Halves, In Grape Juice, Safeway*	1 Serving/145g	70	48	0.4	11.7	0.0	1.0
Halves, In Grape Juice, Tesco*	1 Can/410g	180	44	0.5	10.0	0.1	1.0

P

INFO/WEIGHT	Measure	per Measure KCAL	Nutrition Values per 100g / 100ml KCAL	PROT	CARB	FAT	FIBRE
PEACHES,							
Halves, In Syrup, Del Monte*	1 Can/235g	181	77	0.4	18.5	0.1	0.0
In Fruit Juice, John West*	1 Serving/100g	38	38	0.5	9.0	0.0	0.9
In Juice, Del Monte*	1 Can/415g	203	49	0.5	11.2	0.1	0.0
In Juice, Fruitini*	1 Can/140g	77	55	0.4	13.0	0.1	0.0
In Syrup, Del Monte*	1 Can/420g	323	77	0.4	18.5	0.1	0.0
Pieces In Strawberry Jelly, Fruitini*	1 Can/140g	91	65	0.3	15.3	0.1	0.0
Raw, Weighed With Stone	1oz/28g	8	30	0.9	6.8	0.1	1.3
Sliced, Lite, Del Monte*	1 Serving/124g	60	48	0.0	12.0	0.0	0.8
Slices, In Apple Juice, Asda*	1 Can/213g	89	42	0.6	10.0	0.0	0.9
Slices, In Fruit Juice, Del Monte*	½ Can/200g	98	49	0.5	11.2	0.1	0.0
Slices, In Fruit Juice, Sainsbury's*	½ Can/206g	99	48	0.4	11.7	0.1	1.0
Slices, In Fruit Juice, Waitrose*	1 Can/409g	176	43	0.5	10.2	0.0	1.0
Slices, In Grape Juice, Somefield*	1 Can/411g	169	41	0.5	9.7	0.0	0.9
Slices, In Grape Juice, Tesco*	1 Can/250g	110	44	0.5	11.0	0.0	1.0
Slices, In Light Syrup, Sainsbury's*	½ Can/203g	118	58	0.4	14.0	0.1	0.8
Slices, In Light Syrup, Tesco*	1 Serving/135g	90	67	0.4	16.0	0.1	0.8
Slices, In Syrup, Del Monte*	1 Can/227g	175	77	0.4	18.5	0.1	0.0
Slices, in Fruit Juices, Morrisons*	1 Can/225g	104	46	0.4	11.0	0.0	0.0
Slices, in Grape Juice, Co-Op*	1 Sm Can/213g	85	40	0.5	9.9	0.0	1.4
Slices, in Grape Juice, TTD, Sainsbury's*	½ Jar/155g	90	58	0.4	14.0	0.1	0.3
PEANUT BRITTLE, Average	1oz/28g	135	483	8.6	73.8	19.0	2.0
PEANUT BUTTER,							
Creamy, Smooth, Sun Pat*	1 Tsp/15g	93	620	24.0	17.5	50.2	6.1
Crunchy, Asda*	1 Tsp/10g	61	611	28.0	12.0	51.0	6.0
Crunchy, Budgens*	1oz/28g	166	592	23.6	12.5	49.7	6.9
Crunchy, Harvest Spread*	1 Tbsp/25g	148	592	23.6	12.5	49.7	6.9
Crunchy, No Added Sugar, Whole Earth*	1 Tsp/10g	59	592	24.9	10.1	50.2	7.3
Crunchy, Organic, Evernat*	1 Tsp/10g	64	641	29.0	13.0	53.0	7.0
Crunchy, Organic, No Added Sugar, Waitrose*	1 Tbsp/12g	71	592	24.9	10.1	50.2	7.3
Crunchy, Organic, Tesco*	1 Serving/25g	148	592	23.6	12.5	49.7	6.9
Crunchy, Original Style, Whole Earth*	1 Serving/20g	118	592	24.9	10.1	50.2	7.3
Crunchy, Route 66*	1 Tsp/10g	65	648	20.0	13.0	58.0	5.4
Crunchy, Sainsbury's*	1 Tsp/10g	59	594	23.2	12.4	50.2	6.7
Crunchy, Somerfield*	1 Tsp/10g	59	586	24.0	12.0	49.0	6.0
Crunchy, Tesco*	1 Tsp/10g	61	614	27.8	12.0	50.5	6.5
Crunchy, Value, Tesco*	1 Serving/20g	121	606	22.5	11.6	52.2	5.7
Crunchy, Wholenut, Meridian*	1 Tsp/10g	61	612	31.2	12.2	48.7	6.5
Good For You, Asda*	1 Tsp/15g	80	531	28.0	31.0	35.0	0.0
Organic, Essential*	1 Serving/20g	125	623	28.0	13.0	51.0	0.0
Organic, Whole Earth*	1 Serving/5g	30	595	24.6	9.9	50.8	7.1
Original Crunchy, Sun Pat*	1 Tsp/10g	63	630	26.6	12.6	52.8	6.5
Smooth	1 Tsp/10g	62	623	22.6	13.1	53.7	5.4
Smooth, 25% Less Fat, Tesco*	1 Serving/30g	159	529	22.6	30.7	35.1	6.7
Smooth, BGTY, Sainsbury's*	1 Tsp/10g	53	533	22.6	31.7	35.1	6.7
Smooth, Kernel King, Duerr's*	1 Tbsp/15g	89	596	23.3	12.4	50.3	6.8
Smooth, Light, Kraft*	1 Tsp/20g	114	571	16.3	40.1	38.6	0.0
Smooth, Organic, Meridian*	1 Serving/10g	61	612	31.2	12.2	48.7	6.5
Smooth, Somerfield*	1 Tsp/10g	59	592	24.0	11.0	50.0	0.0
Smooth, Sun Pat*	1 Serving/20g	117	585	27.9	14.4	46.3	7.1
Smooth, Tesco*	1 Tsp/10g	61	614	27.8	12.0	50.5	6.5
Stripy, Sun Pat*	1 Tsp/10g	62	617	13.0	35.0	47.0	3.0
Wholegrain	1 Tsp/10g	61	606	24.9	7.7	53.1	6.0
Wholenut, Sainsbury's*	1 Tbsp/15g	90	598	24.2	9.8	51.3	7.0

P

INFO/WEIGHT	Measure per Measure KCAL	Nutrition Values per 100g / 100ml KCAL	PROT	CARB	FAT	FIBRE

PEANUT BUTTER,

	Measure INFO/WEIGHT	per Measure KCAL	KCAL	PROT	CARB	FAT	FIBRE
Wholenut, Tesco*	1 Tsp/5g	30	590	24.9	10.1	50.0	6.3
PEANUTS,							
Chilli, Sainsbury's*	1 Serving/50g	306	612	28.4	7.2	52.2	6.2
Dry Roasted	1oz/28g	165	589	25.5	10.3	49.8	6.4
Dry Roasted, Budgens*	1oz/28g	166	594	23.9	13.7	49.3	6.5
Dry Roasted, KP*	1 Pack/50g	298	596	27.4	8.9	50.1	5.9
Dry Roasted, Sainsbury's*	1 Serving/20g	113	567	26.2	14.3	45.0	6.1
Honey Roasted, KP*	1 Pack/49g	297	607	34.2	15.3	49.9	5.3
Honey Roasted, Waitrose*	1 Bag/200g	1206	603	19.5	31.8	44.2	5.7
Large, Sainsbury's*	1 Serving/10g	60	601	25.6	8.7	51.5	6.9
Organic, Waitrose*	1 Serving/25g	153	610	22.8	11.9	52.4	5.9
Plain	10 Whole/10g	56	564	25.6	12.5	46.1	6.2
Redskin, Organic, Evernat*	1oz/28g	161	574	17.5	18.3	48.0	3.8
Roast Salted, Jumbo, Marks & Spencer*	1oz/28g	174	622	28.5	7.8	53.0	6.2
Roast Salted, Somerfield*	1oz/28g	168	600	29.0	9.0	50.0	0.0
Roasted & Salted	10 Whole/10g	60	602	24.5	7.1	53.0	6.0
Roasted Salted, Brannigans*	1 Pack/50g	311	622	28.5	7.8	53.0	6.2
Roasted, In Shell, Safeway*	1 Serving/50g	295	589	25.5	10.3	49.8	7.4
Salted Roasted, KP*	1 Sm Pack/50g	311	622	28.5	7.8	53.0	6.2
Salted, Budgens*	1oz/28g	166	593	28.1	10.5	48.7	8.6
Salted, Golden Wonder*	1 Bag/50g	303	605	24.4	10.6	51.6	5.8
Salted, Large, Asda*	1 Serving/50g	309	617	28.3	6.6	53.0	6.0
Salted, Roast, Somerfield*	1oz/28g	168	600	29.0	9.0	50.0	0.0
Salted, SmartPrice, Asda*	1 Serving/25g	154	617	28.0	7.0	53.0	6.0
Salted, Sun Valley*	1 Pack/50g	301	602	24.6	7.1	53.0	0.0
Sea Salt, Organic, KP*	1oz/28g	174	622	28.5	7.8	53.0	6.2
Spicy Chilli, Shots, KP*	1 Pack/45g	274	608	28.1	7.7	51.7	6.2
PEANUTS & RAISINS,							
Average	1 Pack/40g	174	435	15.3	37.5	26.0	4.4
Somerfield*	1oz/28g	133	474	19.0	37.0	28.0	0.0
Yoghurt Coated, Nature's Harvest, Holland & Barrett*	1 Pack/100g	465	465	8.9	54.3	25.8	2.0
PEAR JUICE, With A Hint Of Ginger, Pressed, M&S*	1 Glass/250ml	125	50	0.3	11.7	0.1	0.0
PEARL BARLEY,							
Boiled	1oz/28g	34	120	2.7	27.6	0.6	0.0
Raw	1oz/28g	101	360	7.9	83.6	1.7	0.0
PEARS,							
Average, Raw, Weighed with Core	1 Med/170g	68	40	0.3	10.0	0.1	2.2
Canned, In Juice	1oz/28g	9	33	0.3	8.5	0.0	1.4
Canned, In Syrup	1oz/28g	14	50	0.2	13.2	0.0	1.1
Comice, Raw, Weighed with Core	1 Med/170g	56	33	0.3	8.5	0.0	2.0
Conference, Tesco*	1 Fruit/100g	57	57	0.3	13.2	0.3	2.4
Dessert, Safeway*	1 Pear/100g	39	39	0.3	9.2	0.1	0.0
Dried, Marks & Spencer*	1oz/28g	63	225	2.7	53.0	0.5	14.5
Dried, Ready to Eat, Tesco*	1 Serving/100g	189	189	1.4	45.0	0.4	7.1
Dried, Waitrose*	½ Pack/125g	249	199	1.5	47.2	0.5	7.5
Halves, In Fruit Juice, Safeway*	1 Serving/170g	78	46	0.4	11.2	0.0	1.8
Halves, In Grape Juice, Waitrose*	½ Can/205g	100	49	0.3	11.6	0.1	2.0
Halves, In Juice, Somerfield*	1oz/28g	14	49	0.0	12.0	0.0	0.0
Halves, In Light Syrup, Sainsbury's*	1oz/28g	16	56	0.4	13.9	0.1	1.6
Halves, In Light Syrup, Tesco*	1oz/28g	18	65	0.2	15.9	0.0	1.1
Halves, In Natural Juice, Sainsbury's*	1oz/28g	13	45	0.5	10.4	0.1	1.6
Halves, In Syrup, John West*	1oz/28g	18	63	0.4	15.0	0.1	1.6
Halves, Tesco*	1 Serving/100g	35	35	0.3	8.5	0.0	1.4

	INFO/WEIGHT	KCAL	KCAL	PROT	CARB	FAT	FIBRE
PEARS,							
Halves, in Natural Juice, Tesco*	1 Serving/115g	53	46	0.3	11.0	0.0	1.4
In Juice, Del Monte*	1oz/28g	13	45	0.3	10.5	0.1	0.0
Organic, Tesco*	1 Pear/170g	71	42	0.3	10.0	0.1	2.2
Peeled, Raw, Average, Weighed With Skin & Core	1oz/28g	8	29	0.2	7.3	0.1	1.1
Prickly, Raw, Fresh	1oz/28g	14	49	0.7	11.5	0.3	0.0
Quarters, In Fruit Juice, Sainsbury's*	1oz/28g	11	41	0.4	9.7	0.1	1.6
Quarters, In Natural Juice, Tesco*	¼ Can/112g	52	46	0.3	11.0	0.0	1.4
Quarters, in Grape Juice, TTD, Sainsbury's*	½ Jar/157g	89	57	0.0	14.0	0.1	1.5
Red, Tesco*	1 Pear/180g	65	36	0.4	8.3	0.1	2.2
Tinned, Asda*	1 Can/241g	89	37	0.3	9.0	0.0	1.4
William, Raw	1 Med/170g	58	34	0.4	8.3	0.1	2.2
PEAS,							
& Sweetcorn, Fresh, Marks & Spencer*	1oz/28g	21	75	4.8	11.4	1.5	3.0
Boiled in Unsalted Water	1oz/28g	22	79	6.7	10.0	1.6	4.5
Canned, Re-Heated, Drained	1oz/28g	22	80	5.3	13.5	0.9	5.1
Chip Shop Style Mushy, Morrisons*	½ Sm Can/150g	126	84	5.8	13.9	0.4	0.0
Chip Shop Style Mushy, Sainsbury's*	½ Can/150g	114	76	5.2	12.4	0.6	3.1
Dried, Boiled in Unsalted Water	1oz/28g	31	109	6.9	19.9	0.8	5.5
Dried, Raw	1oz/28g	85	303	21.6	52.0	2.4	13.0
Frozen, Asda*	1 Serving/115g	75	65	5.7	8.6	0.9	5.1
Frozen, Bird's Eye*	1 Serving/85g	53	62	4.9	9.0	0.7	4.5
Frozen, Boiled in Salted Water	1oz/28g	19	69	6.0	9.7	0.9	5.1
Frozen, Boiled in Unsalted Water	1oz/28g	19	69	6.0	9.7	0.9	5.1
Frozen, Boiled in Unsalted Water, Tesco*	1 Serving/75g	50	67	5.9	8.9	0.9	5.1
Frozen, Raw	1oz/28g	18	66	5.7	9.3	0.9	5.1
Garden, Bird's Eye*	1 Serving/85g	53	62	4.9	9.0	0.7	4.5
Garden, Canned, Drained, Sainsbury's*	1oz/28g	23	83	5.3	13.5	0.9	5.1
Garden, Canned, No Salt Or Sugar, Sainsbury's*	1 Can/80g	34	43	4.2	5.5	0.5	3.0
Garden, Fresh, Tesco*	1 Serving/250g	215	86	6.9	11.3	1.5	4.7
Garden, Fresh, Waitrose*	1 Serving/190g	163	86	6.9	11.3	1.5	4.7
Garden, Freshly Frozen, Morrisons*	1 Serving/100g	83	83	6.9	11.3	1.5	0.0
Garden, Frozen, Asda*	1 Serving/75g	52	69	6.0	9.0	0.9	5.0
Garden, Frozen, Safeway*	1 Serving/100g	71	71	6.0	9.7	0.9	5.1
Garden, Frozen, Sainsbury's*	1 Serving/80g	55	69	6.0	9.1	0.9	5.1
Garden, Frozen, Tesco*	1 Serving/100g	83	83	6.9	10.4	1.5	4.7
Garden, In Sugared Salted Water, Drained, Tesco*	1 Serving/68g	46	67	5.3	9.4	0.9	5.1
Garden, In Sweetened Salted Water, Safeway*	1 Can/44g	22	50	4.6	7.0	0.3	5.1
Garden, In Water, Asda*	1 Serving/90g	44	49	4.6	7.0	0.3	5.0
Garden, In Water, No Added Sugar or Salt, Morrisons*	1 Can/185g	87	47	4.6	6.5	0.3	0.0
Garden, Marks & Spencer*	1oz/28g	19	67	5.8	10.6	0.4	5.2
Garden, Mint Flavoured, Sainsbury's*	¼ Bag/227g	161	71	6.0	9.7	0.9	5.1
Garden, Minted, Tesco*	1 Serving/50g	42	83	6.9	10.4	1.5	4.7
Garden, Shelled, Tesco*	1 Pack/190g	129	68	6.9	6.6	1.5	4.7
Garden, Tesco*	1oz/28g	19	67	5.3	9.4	0.9	5.1
Garden, Tinned, Asda*	1oz/28g	15	53	4.6	8.0	0.3	5.0
Garden, Tinned, Co-Op*	1 Serving/93g	56	60	5.0	8.0	0.9	6.0
Garden, Young, Marks & Spencer*	1 Serving/100g	70	70	5.8	10.6	0.4	5.2
Giant Marrowfat, Farrows, Batchelors*	1 Can/173g	133	77	5.9	12.3	0.5	4.9
Hand Shelled, Marks & Spencer*	1oz/28g	19	67	5.8	10.6	0.4	5.2
Marrowfat, Asda*	1 Serving/90g	75	83	6.2	13.7	0.4	4.8
Marrowfat, Canned, Drained, Re-Heated,	1oz/28g	28	100	6.9	17.5	0.8	4.1
Marrowfat, Processed, Bigga, Batchelors*	1 Sm Can/160g	106	66	5.6	10.1	0.3	4.0
Marrowfat, Processed, Canned, Co-Op*	1oz/28g	28	99	6.9	16.0	0.8	4.1

	Measure INFO/WEIGHT	per Measure KCAL	Nutrition Values per 100g / 100ml				
			KCAL	PROT	CARB	FAT	FIBRE
PEAS,							
Marrowfat, Processed, In Sugared Salt Water, Tesco*	1 Can/180g	167	93	6.9	14.5	0.8	4.1
Marrowfat, Sainsbury's*	1 Serving/90g	95	105	6.9	17.5	0.8	4.1
Marrowfat, Tesco*	1 Serving/60g	50	83	6.2	13.7	0.4	0.0
Mushy Peas With Vinegar, Chip Shop, Budgens*	1 Can/300g	240	80	5.8	12.5	0.7	1.8
Mushy, Batchelors*	1 Can/415g	320	77	5.2	13.5	0.2	2.7
Mushy, Canned, Re-Heated	1oz/28g	23	81	5.8	13.8	0.7	1.8
Mushy, Chip Shop, Batchelors*	1oz/28g	22	78	4.9	13.8	0.3	3.3
Mushy, Lockwoods*	¼ Pack/113.5g	112	99	8.0	15.9	0.3	0.0
Mushy, Processed, Safeway*	1 Can/300g	255	85	5.8	13.8	0.7	1.8
Mushy, SmartPrice, Asda*	1 Serving/151g	130	86	6.0	14.0	0.7	2.7
Mushy, Somerfield*	1 Serving/100g	80	80	5.9	13.1	0.4	0.0
Mushy, Value, Tesco*	1oz/28g	20	71	5.8	11.3	0.7	1.8
Processed, Canned, Re-Heated, Drained	1oz/28g	28	99	6.9	17.5	0.7	4.8
Processed, Economy, Sainsbury's*	1oz/28g	29	104	6.9	17.5	0.7	4.8
Processed, SmartPrice, Asda*	1oz/28g	24	84	6.0	14.0	0.4	4.8
Processed, Somerfield*	1oz/28g	23	83	6.0	14.0	0.0	0.0
Processed, Sweet Harvest, Aldi*	1oz/28g	23	83	6.2	13.7	0.4	0.0
Processed, Value, Tesco*	½ Can/95g	93	98	6.9	16.0	0.7	0.0
Raw	1oz/28g	23	83	6.9	11.3	1.5	4.7
Small Processed, Batchelors*	1oz/28g	24	87	5.4	15.5	0.4	4.8
Sugar Snap, Boiled in Salted Water	1oz/28g	9	33	3.1	4.7	0.3	1.3
Sugar Snap, Raw	1oz/28g	10	34	3.4	5.0	0.2	1.5
Sugar Snap, Tesco*	1oz/28g	10	35	3.4	5.0	0.2	1.5
Summer Sweet, Green Giant*	3/4 Cup/175ml	107	61	3.4	11.0	0.4	0.0
PEASE PUDDING, Canned, Re-Heated, Drained	1oz/28g	26	93	6.8	16.1	0.6	1.8
PECAN NUTS, Average	3 Nuts/18g	124	689	9.2	5.8	70.1	4.7
PECORINO ROMANO, Tesco*	1 Serving/100g	366	366	28.5	0.0	28.0	0.0
PENNE,							
Arrabbiata, BGTY, Sainsbury's*	1 Pack/450g	414	92	2.9	16.5	1.6	1.9
Chicken & Red Wine, Weight Watchers*	1 Pack/394g	248	63	3.7	10.1	0.7	0.6
Chicken & Tomato, Italian, Sainsbury's*	½ Pack/350g	473	135	7.6	19.0	3.2	1.6
Chilli & Garlic, Asda*	1 Serving/75g	260	346	12.0	71.0	1.5	3.0
Creamy Sun Dried Tomato & Mascarpone, Somerfield*	1 Pack/500g	775	155	5.0	21.0	6.0	0.0
Dried, Napolina*	1oz/28g	99	352	11.5	73.0	1.5	2.2
Dry, Buitoni*	1oz/28g	101	362	12.2	74.4	1.7	2.0
Egg, Asda*	1 Serving/100g	170	170	7.0	31.0	2.0	1.4
Egg, Fresh, Safeway*	1 Bowl/100g	159	159	5.8	30.3	1.6	2.1
Egg, Fresh, Safeway*	¼ Pack/125g	429	343	12.6	65.3	3.5	4.5
Egg, Italiano, Fresh, Tesco*	1 Serving/125g	335	268	10.6	50.3	2.7	2.3
Fresh, Asda*	1oz/28g	50	178	7.0	31.0	2.0	1.4
Fresh, Tesco*	1 Serving/125g	360	288	11.9	51.8	3.7	1.5
Hickory Steak, American, Sainsbury's*	1 Pack/450g	545	121	6.5	19.8	1.8	1.5
Hickory Steak, Asda*	1 Pack/443.0g	660	149	8.0	19.0	4.5	1.1
Italian, Fresh, Sainsbury's*	1 Serving/215g	361	168	7.8	29.4	2.1	1.8
Italian, Sainsbury's*	1 Serving/75g	268	357	12.3	73.1	1.7	2.5
Leek & Bacon, Al Forno, Asda*	½ Pack/300g	531	177	5.0	10.0	13.0	0.5
Marks & Spencer*	1oz/28g	99	355	13.6	68.7	2.9	3.1
Microwaveable, Dolmio*	1 Sachet/220g	299	136	5.3	26.3	1.0	0.0
Nicoise, Sainsbury's*	1 Pack/450g	401	89	2.9	12.4	3.1	1.1
Organic, Sainsbury's*	1 Serving/50g	179	357	12.3	73.1	1.7	2.5
Plain, Dried, Tesco*	1oz/28g	97	345	13.2	68.5	2.0	2.9
Rigate, Buitoni*	1 Serving/120g	422	352	11.2	72.6	1.9	0.0
Rigate, Dried, Safeway*	1 Serving/75g	261	348	13.2	70.1	1.7	2.9

	Measure INFO/WEIGHT	per Measure KCAL	Nutrition Values per 100g / 100ml KCAL	PROT	CARB	FAT	FIBRE
PENNE,							
Rigate, Sainsbury's*	1oz/28g	100	357	12.3	73.1	1.7	2.5
Rigate, Somerfield*	1 Serving/50g	174	348	12.5	69.9	2.0	3.6
Tomato & Basil Sauce, Asda*	½ Pack/314g	185	59	0.8	6.0	3.5	2.0
Tubes, Egg, Fresh, Waitrose*	1 Serving/150g	434	289	11.4	53.1	3.4	1.6
Tuna, Tomato & Olive, Asda*	1 Pack/340g	173	51	4.2	4.2	1.9	0.6
Waitrose*	1 Serving/100g	354	354	11.3	73.1	1.8	2.9
With Chilli & Red Peppers, Asda*	1 Can/400g	224	56	1.3	10.0	1.2	0.6
With Hot Smoked Salmon, Steam Cuisine, M&S*	1 Pack/400g	740	185	9.4	18.6	7.9	2.5
PENNETTE, Tricolore, Sainsbury's*	1 Serving/100g	357	357	12.3	73.1	1.7	2.5
PEPERAMI,							
Hot, Peperami*	1oz/28g	155	554	19.0	2.5	52.0	1.2
Salami Sausage, Peperami*	1oz/28g	150	536	22.0	1.7	49.0	0.1
PEPPER,							
Black, Freshly Ground	1 Tsp/2g	5	226	10.9	64.8	3.3	0.0
Cayenne, Ground	1 Tsp/1.8g	6	318	12.0	31.7	17.3	0.0
PEPPERMINT CREAM, Fry's*	1 Bar/51g	217	425	2.6	68.8	15.4	0.0
PEPPERONI,							
American Style, Tesco*	1 Piece/5g	19	387	20.0	3.2	32.7	0.0
Asda*	1 Slice/6g	24	405	22.0	6.6	32.3	0.0
Ready to Eat, Sainsbury's*	1 Serving/25g	94	376	24.9	0.1	30.7	0.1
Spicy Italian, Marks & Spencer*	1 Pack/50g	158	316	20.9	1.1	25.3	0.0
Tomato Spicy, Stir In, Dolmio*	1oz/28g	41	147	3.4	7.9	11.5	0.0
PEPPERS,							
Capsicum, Chilli, Green, Raw	1oz/28g	6	20	2.9	0.7	0.6	0.0
Capsicum, Chilli, Red, Raw	1oz/28g	7	26	1.8	4.2	0.3	0.0
Capsicum, Green, Boiled in Salted Water	1oz/28g	5	18	1.0	2.6	0.5	1.8
Capsicum, Green, Raw	1oz/28g	4	15	0.8	2.6	0.3	1.6
Capsicum, Red, Boiled in Salted Water	1oz/28g	10	34	1.1	7.0	0.4	1.7
Capsicum, Red, Raw	1oz/28g	9	32	1.0	6.4	0.4	1.6
Capsicum, Yellow, Raw	1oz/28g	7	26	1.2	5.3	0.2	1.7
Fresh, Value, Tesco*	1 Serving/10g	2	16	0.8	2.6	0.3	1.6
Green, Filled, Tesco*	1 Pepper/150g	117	78	2.6	9.0	3.5	0.7
Jalapeno, Co-Op*	1oz/28g	74	265	5.0	31.0	13.0	0.9
Jalapeno, Flamin' Hot, Kitchen Range Foods*	1oz/28g	62	223	4.6	22.9	12.7	0.0
Mixed, Organic, Iceland*	1oz/28g	8	28	1.1	5.1	0.4	1.8
Mixed, Sliced, Asda*	1 Serving/100g	28	28	1.1	4.9	0.4	1.8
Mixed, Sliced, Farmfoods*	1oz/28g	7	24	0.9	4.3	0.4	1.6
Mixed, Sliced, Ready, Frozen, Tesco*	1 Serving/28g	7	25	1.0	4.6	0.3	1.6
Red, Filled, Marks & Spencer*	1 Serving/115g	86	75	2.9	11.1	2.4	1.5
Roasted Red & Yellow, in Oil, Marks & Spencer*	1 Serving/40g	34	85	1.1	4.4	6.9	3.5
Stuffed With Rice	1oz/28g	24	85	1.5	15.4	2.4	1.3
Stuffed With Vegetables, Cheese Topping	1oz/28g	31	111	3.4	9.8	6.7	1.5
Stuffed, Fresh, Asda*	1 Pepper/150g	144	96	3.8	9.0	5.0	1.2
Stuffed, Perfectly Balanced, Waitrose*	1 Pack/300g	243	81	3.0	11.8	2.4	1.3
Stuffed, Sainsbury's*	1 Serving/137g	169	123	3.3	11.8	6.9	1.0
Yellow, Stuffed, Italian, Ready to Roast, Sainsbury's*	1 Pack/136g	144	106	5.3	9.9	5.0	1.3
PERNOD, 19% Volume	1 Shot/50ml	65	130	0.0	0.0	0.0	0.0
PESHWARI NAAN, Indian Meal for 2, Finest, Tesco*	½ Pack/200g	612	306	8.3	48.3	8.9	5.2
PETIT POIS,							
& Baby Carrots, Safeway*	1 Can/138g	57	41	2.5	7.4	0.0	1.0
& Baby Onions, Marks & Spencer*	1oz/28g	14	50	2.8	9.5	1.7	3.4
Canned, Drained	1 Serving/65g	29	45	5.2	4.9	0.6	4.3
Fresh Frozen, Tesco,*	1 Serving/100g	48	48	5.0	5.5	0.9	4.5

	Measure INFO/WEIGHT	per Measure KCAL	Nutrition Values per 100g / 100ml				
			KCAL	PROT	CARB	FAT	FIBRE
PETIT POIS,							
Frozen, Boiled in Salted Water	1 Serving/65g	32	49	5.0	5.5	0.9	4.5
Frozen, Boiled in Unsalted Water	1 Serving/65g	32	49	5.0	5.5	0.9	4.5
Frozen, Sainsbury's*	1 Serving/80g	40	50	5.0	5.4	0.9	4.5
PHEASANT,							
Roasted, Meat Only	1oz/28g	62	220	27.9	0.0	12.0	0.0
Roasted, Meat Only, Weighed With Bone	1oz/28g	32	114	14.5	0.0	6.2	0.0
PICCALILLI,							
Haywards*	1 Serving/28g	18	66	1.4	13.9	0.5	0.0
Marks & Spencer*	1 Tbsp/15g	11	70	1.9	13.5	1.2	1.1
Morrisons*	1 Tsp/10g	7	72	1.7	14.7	0.7	0.0
Safeway*	1 Serving/10g	8	75	1.6	15.0	0.7	0.6
Sainsbury's*	1 Dtsp/15g	9	60	1.8	11.9	0.6	0.7
Sweet, Asda*	1 Tbsp/15g	17	112	0.5	27.0	0.2	0.6
Sweet, Somerfield*	1 Tsp/10g	11	107	1.0	24.0	1.0	0.0
PICKLE,							
Branston, Crosse & Blackwell*	1 Tsp/10g	14	140	0.7	34.2	0.3	1.3
Brinjal, Patak's*	1 Tsp/16g	57	355	2.1	36.5	24.4	0.9
Chilli Tomato, Patak's*	1oz/28g	27	95	2.5	16.0	3.2	1.5
Chilli, Branston*	1 Tsp/16g	21	130	0.7	30.0	0.7	1.5
Chilli, Patak's*	1 Tsp/16g	49	305	4.1	1.4	33.7	0.0
Garlic, Patak's*	1 Tsp/16g	43	267	3.6	21.3	18.5	1.6
Lime, Hot, Asda*	1 Dtsp/10g	12	123	2.2	6.0	10.0	1.0
Lime, Hot, Patak's*	1 Tsp/16g	30	186	2.6	4.2	18.7	0.3
Lime, Marks & Spencer*	1 Tsp/16g	34	215	0.8	42.5	4.8	2.4
Lime, Oily	1oz/28g	50	178	1.9	8.3	15.5	0.0
Lime, Sharwood's*	1 Tsp/16g	24	152	2.2	15.0	9.3	2.9
Mango, Hot, Patak's*	1 Tsp/16g	42	265	2.3	8.0	25.7	1.9
Mild Mustard, Heinz*	1 Tbsp/10g	13	129	2.2	25.7	1.3	0.9
Original, Tesco*	1 Tsp/25g	33	132	0.8	30.4	0.2	1.1
Ploughman's, Heinz*	1 Tbsp/10g	12	117	0.8	26.7	0.2	0.9
Sandwich, Branston*	1 Tsp/10g	14	140	0.7	34.2	0.3	1.3
Sandwich, Somerfield*	1 Tsp/10g	15	150	1.0	36.0	0.0	0.0
Smooth, Branston*	1 Serving/13g	18	139	0.6	34.0	0.1	1.4
Spicy, Branston*	1 Heaped Tsp/15g	21	140	0.7	34.7	0.3	1.3
Sweet	1 Tsp/10g	14	141	0.6	36.0	0.1	1.2
Sweet Harvest, Asda*	1 Serving/25g	39	154	0.8	37.0	0.3	0.8
Sweet, Budgens*	1 Tsp/10g	14	141	0.8	34.0	0.2	0.0
Sweet, Frank Cooper*	1 Pot/20g	21	104	0.5	25.3	0.1	0.8
Sweet, Hartley's*	1 Tsp/16g	7	140	0.5	36.2	0.0	0.0
Tangy, Sandwich, Heinz*	1 Tsp/10g	13	134	0.7	31.4	0.2	0.9
Tomato, Tangy, Heinz*	1 Tsp/10g	10	102	2.0	22.0	0.3	1.5
PICKLES,							
Dill, Cucumbers, Safeway*	1oz/28g	5	19	0.9	3.5	0.2	0.0
Mixed, Salad Bar, Asda*	1oz/28g	11	40	0.5	9.2	0.1	0.0
Red Cabbage In Vinegar, Healthy Selection, Somerfield*	1oz/28g	4	13	1.0	2.0	0.0	0.0
Red Cabbage, Asda*	1 Serving/50g	16	32	1.6	6.0	0.1	0.0
PICNIC, Cadbury's*	1 Bar/48g	228	475	7.5	58.3	23.6	0.0
PIE,							
Admiral's, Ross*	1 Pie/340g	357	105	4.8	10.9	4.6	0.7
Admiral, Youngs*	1 Serving/250g	263	105	4.8	10.6	4.6	0.7
Apple & Blackberry, Lattice Topped, BGTY, Sainsbury's*	¼ Serving/100g	256	256	2.8	44.4	7.5	3.1
Apple & Blackberry, Shortcrust, Marks & Spencer*	1 Serving/142g	469	330	4.3	50.2	12.5	1.1
Apple & Blackberry, Somerfield*	¼ Pie/106g	280	264	4.0	36.0	12.0	0.0

PIE,

INFO/WEIGHT	Measure per Measure	KCAL	Nutrition Values per 100g / 100ml				
			KCAL	PROT	CARB	FAT	FIBRE
Apple & Blackberry, Tesco*	1 Serving/106g	287	271	4.2	38.4	11.2	1.7
Apple & Blackcurrant, Mr Kipling*	1 Pie/66g	220	334	3.4	51.0	12.9	0.0
Apple Meringue, Frozen, Sara Lee*	1/6 Slice/74g	179	242	2.7	37.9	8.8	1.5
Apple Slice, Colonels Pies, Kentucky Fried Chicken*	1 Slice/113g	310	274	1.7	38.9	12.3	0.0
Apple, American, Iceland*	1 Portion/92g	258	280	4.8	39.2	11.6	2.2
Apple, Cooked, Speedibake*	1 Serving/120g	340	283	3.4	38.5	12.8	1.5
Apple, Deep Filled, Iceland*	1 Portion/116g	332	286	2.5	39.2	13.2	1.1
Apple, Deep Filled, Sainsbury's*	1/4 Pie/137g	374	273	3.8	35.6	12.8	1.6
Apple, Family, Morrisons*	1/6 Pie/116g	326	281	3.1	39.9	12.1	3.1
Apple, Individual, Somerfield*	1 Pie/47.2g	178	379	3.5	53.2	16.9	1.3
Apple, McDonald's*	1 Pie/78g	225	289	2.8	33.2	16.1	1.4
Apple, McVitie's*	1 Slice/117g	316	270	3.0	39.0	11.0	2.0
Apple, Pastry Top & Bottom	1oz/28g	74	266	2.9	35.8	13.3	1.7
Apple, Puff Pastry, Marks & Spencer*	1 Pie/135g	338	250	2.4	31.3	12.7	1.0
Apple, Safeway*	1 Serving/80g	241	301	3.3	45.5	11.8	0.0
Apple, Sainsbury's*	1/6/118g	314	266	3.4	37.1	11.5	0.6
Apple, SmartPrice, Asda*	1 Serving/47g	178	379	3.5	53.0	17.0	1.3
Apple, Tesco*	1 Pie/47g	191	406	3.3	59.4	17.2	1.5
Apple, Value, Tesco*	1 Pie/47g	179	381	3.4	53.2	17.0	1.3
Apricot Fruit, GFY, Asda*	1 Serving/52g	162	311	3.3	52.0	10.0	0.0
Banoffee Cream, American Dream, McVitie's*	1 Portion/70g	277	396	4.3	36.7	25.5	0.8
Banoffee, Shape*	1 Serving/120g	175	146	3.3	28.0	2.3	0.5
Banoffee, Tesco*	1 Pie/112g	381	340	3.7	45.4	15.9	1.2
Beef Steak, Aberdeen Angus, Top Crust, Waitrose*	1/2 Pie/280g	476	170	10.0	13.4	8.6	4.1
Beef, Sainsbury's*	1 Pie/209.8g	536	255	10.3	21.2	14.3	2.0
Blackberry & Apple, Sara Lee*	1 Serving/100g	272	272	2.9	34.0	13.9	0.0
Blackcurrant, Deep Filled, Sainsbury's*	1 Slice/137g	440	321	5.8	42.6	14.1	2.2
Blackcurrant, Shortcrust, Marks & Spencer*	1 Pie/142g	412	290	3.9	45.6	10.1	1.3
Bramley Apple & Blackberry, Marks & Spencer*	1/4 Pie/146g	380	260	3.4	39.8	9.9	1.3
Bramley Apple & Custard, Lattice Topped, Mr Kipling*	1 Pie/64g	217	339	3.6	48.3	14.6	1.1
Bramley Apple, Co-Op*	1 Serving/110g	242	220	2.0	41.0	5.0	1.0
Bramley Apple, Deep Filled, Mr Kipling*	1 Pie/66g	220	333	3.4	50.7	13.0	1.3
Bramley Apple, Deep Filled, Sainsbury's*	1/6 Pie/120g	329	274	3.7	38.0	11.9	1.9
Bramley Apple, Individual, Mr Kipling*	1 Pie/66g	220	334	3.4	51.0	13.0	0.0
Bramley Apple, Marks & Spencer*	1 Pie/55g	184	335	2.9	57.6	11.7	1.6
Bramley Apple, Reduced Fat, Asda*	1 Pie/56g	176	314	3.3	55.1	9.4	1.3
Bramley Apple, Rowan Hill Bakery, Lidl*	1 Pie/64g	216	337	3.6	51.5	13.0	1.4
Bramley Apple, Somerfield*	1/6 Pie/70.2g	193	275	3.5	34.0	12.8	2.4
Bramley Apple, Tesco*	1/8 Slice/87g	224	257	3.8	37.4	10.2	1.7
Buffet Pork, Farmfoods*	1 Pie/65g	252	388	8.8	28.2	26.7	1.0
Cheese & Pickle Pork, Mini, Tesco*	1 Pie/49g	191	389	9.2	29.3	26.1	1.2
Cherry, Deep Filled, Somerfield*	1/6 Pie/90g	259	288	3.0	41.0	12.0	0.0
Cherry, Shortcrust, Marks & Spencer*	1 Pie/142g	412	290	3.6	43.4	10.9	0.8
Chicken & Asparagus, McDougalls*	1 Serving/170g	490	288	8.0	19.0	20.0	0.9
Chicken & Bacon, Filo Pastry, Finest, Tesco*	1 Serving/160g	362	226	11.3	18.9	11.7	1.7
Chicken & Broccoli Lattice, Sainsbury's*	1/2 Pie/192g	520	271	9.3	22.4	16.0	0.9
Chicken & Broccoli, Potato Top, Asda*	1 Pack/400g	319	80	5.3	10.8	1.8	0.7
Chicken & Broccoli, COU, Marks & Spencer*	1 Pack/300g	240	80	6.8	8.9	2.0	1.5
Chicken & Broccoli, Eat Smart, Safeway*	1 Pack/400g	320	80	6.9	8.5	2.0	1.2
Chicken & Broccoli, Good Intentions, Somerfield*	1 Pack/400g	304	76	6.1	9.3	1.6	0.5
Chicken & Broccoli, Good for You, Asda*	1 Pack/400g	340	85	7.0	9.0	2.3	0.5
Chicken & Broccoli, Healthy Eating, Tesco*	1 Pack/400g	312	78	6.0	10.2	1.5	1.0
Chicken & Broccoli, Healthy Living, Tesco*	1 Pack/450g	387	86	5.4	9.9	2.7	0.7

P

PIE,

	Measure INFO/WEIGHT	per Measure KCAL	Nutrition Values per 100g / 100ml				
			KCAL	PROT	CARB	FAT	FIBRE
Chicken & Broccoli, Lattice, Tesco*	½ Pie/200g	496	248	8.5	18.9	15.4	2.1
Chicken & Gravy, Deep Fill, Asda*	1 Serving/130g	342	263	9.0	23.0	15.0	0.9
Chicken & Ham, Deep Filled, Somerfield*	¼ Pie/138g	348	252	11.0	21.0	14.0	0.0
Chicken & Ham, Morrisons*	¼ Pie/115.1g	267	232	8.7	22.5	11.9	0.8
Chicken & Ham, Safeway*	1 Pie/134.7g	385	285	9.2	23.0	17.4	1.3
Chicken & Ham, Sainsbury's*	1 Pie/128g	461	360	11.0	28.5	22.4	2.0
Chicken & Ham, Tesco*	1 Serving/113g	293	259	9.4	20.2	15.6	1.2
Chicken & Mushroom, Asda*	1 Pie/ 150g	444	296	7.7	25.4	18.2	1.0
Chicken & Mushroom, Farmfoods*	1 Pie/110g	271	246	5.6	22.4	14.9	0.9
Chicken & Mushroom, Fray Bentos*	1 Pie/475g	770	162	6.7	11.6	9.9	0.0
Chicken & Mushroom, Individual, Co-Op*	1 Pie/149g	465	312	8.6	24.5	19.9	1.2
Chicken & Mushroom, Morrisons*	1 Serving/100g	261	261	7.6	22.9	15.4	0.9
Chicken & Mushroom, Puff Pastry, Sainsbury's*	1 Pie/150g	450	300	7.8	29.6	16.7	0.9
Chicken & Mushroom, Shortcrust, Somerfield*	¼ Pie/125g	410	328	6.2	24.7	22.7	1.2
Chicken & Mushroom, Tesco*	1 Pie/150g	449	299	8.6	22.4	19.4	1.7
Chicken & Vegetable, Asda*	1 Pie/130.7g	329	251	8.0	21.0	15.0	1.4
Chicken & Vegetable, Farmfoods*	1 Pie/128g	384	300	7.2	25.4	18.8	1.4
Chicken & Vegetable, Freshbake*	¼ Pie/114g	298	261	6.2	23.2	15.9	1.1
Chicken & Vegetable, Kids, Tesco*	1 Serving/235g	235	100	5.9	9.1	4.5	0.7
Chicken & Vegetable, Microbake, Freshbake*	1 Pie/100g	348	348	10.2	40.8	16.1	1.8
Chicken & Vegetable, Perfectly Balanced, Waitrose*	1 Serving/375g	285	76	5.1	10.8	1.4	1.3
Chicken & Vegetable, Potato Topped, Somerfield*	1 Pack/350g	270	77	3.7	8.8	3.0	2.0
Chicken & Vegetable, Value, Tesco*	1 Pie/150g	378	252	5.5	19.7	16.8	1.0
Chicken Cottage, Tesco*	1 Pack/400g	324	81	5.9	11.5	1.3	0.8
Chicken, Aunt Bessie's*	¼ Pie/200g	452	226	9.5	22.3	11.0	1.3
Chicken, Bacon & Cheese, Lattice, Bird's Eye*	1 Lattice/157g	403	257	10.4	17.0	16.4	1.1
Chicken, Bird's Eye*	1 Pie/158g	414	262	7.2	23.1	15.6	1.3
Chicken, Broccoli & White Wine, Waitrose*	1 Serving/200g	605	303	12.6	17.7	20.3	2.3
Chicken, Cheese & Brocolli Lattice, Bird's Eye*	1 Lattice/150g	380	253	10.3	18.4	14.8	1.0
Chicken, Eat Smart, Safeway*	1 Pack/400g	340	85	8.2	9.0	1.7	1.2
Chicken, Individual Shortcrust, Asda*	1 Pie/175g	534	305	10.0	28.0	17.0	1.0
Chicken, Individual, Bird's Eye*	1 Pie/155g	473	305	8.7	25.6	18.6	1.9
Chicken, New Gate, Lidl*	1 Pie/142g	358	252	6.1	23.1	16.6	1.0
Chicken, Short Crust, Marks & Spencer*	1 Pie/170g	510	300	9.7	26.2	17.4	1.7
Chocolate, Mini, Waitrose*	1 Pie/24.0g	109	455	5.3	51.4	25.3	1.7
Cod & Prawn, Marks & Spencer*	1oz/28g	43	155	10.6	8.7	8.9	0.7
Cod & Smoked Haddock, COU, Marks & Spencer*	1 Serving/300g	195	65	6.8	6.2	1.3	1.4
Cottage, Aberdeen Angus, Waitrose*	1 Pie/350g	340	97	5.3	11.0	3.5	0.9
Cottage, Asda*	1 Pie/300g	258	86	4.3	11.0	2.8	0.9
Cottage, Classic British, Sainsburys*	1 Pack/450g	500	111	6.3	11.1	4.6	0.6
Cottage, Eat Smart, Safeway*	1 Pack/388g	310	80	5.5	8.7	2.3	1.9
Cottage, Fresh, Marks & Spencer*	1 Pie/400g	460	115	6.8	9.9	5.6	0.6
Cottage, Frozen, Asda*	1 Serving/121g	146	121	4.8	12.0	6.0	0.6
Cottage, Good For You, Asda*	1 Pack/414g	302	73	6.0	9.0	1.4	1.3
Cottage, Good Intentions, Somerfield*	1 Serving/300g	261	87	6.2	11.0	2.0	1.2
Cottage, Healthy Eating, Tesco*	1 Pie/450g	347	77	4.7	9.9	2.0	0.7
Cottage, Healthy Living, Co-Op*	1 Pack/400g	340	85	5.0	11.0	2.0	1.0
Cottage, Healthy Living, Tesco*	1 Pack/400g	356	89	5.4	10.7	2.7	1.9
Cottage, Iceland*	1 Pack/400g	468	117	5.1	13.6	4.7	0.7
Cottage, Large, Tesco*	1 Pack/475g	575	121	5.5	10.8	6.2	0.5
Cottage, Luxury, Marks & Spencer*	½ Pack/310g	403	130	7.7	9.5	6.9	1.6
Cottage, Meal for One, Marks & Spencer*	1 Pack/445g	356	80	4.7	7.1	3.7	1.2
Cottage, Meatfree, Sainsbury's*	1 Pack/400g	364	91	4.4	11.7	3.0	0.7

PIE,

	Measure INFO/WEIGHT	per Measure KCAL	KCAL	PROT	CARB	FAT	FIBRE
			Nutrition Values per 100g / 100ml				
Cottage, Mega, Tesco*	1 Pie/500g	470	94	4.1	11.6	3.5	0.7
Cottage, Quorn*	1 Pie/300g	213	71	2.7	10.7	1.9	1.3
Cottage, Quorn, Sainsburys*	1 pack/450g	329	73	3.0	10.2	2.2	1.8
Cottage, Safeway*	1 Pack/450g	486	108	6.0	9.4	5.2	1.1
Cottage, Sainsbury's*	1 Pack/300g	207	69	3.8	10.4	1.4	1.2
Cottage, SmartPrice, Asda*	1 Pie/159g	149	94	3.1	12.0	3.7	0.7
Cottage, Tesco*	1 Pie/300g	300	100	3.3	12.5	4.1	0.5
Cottage, Weight Watchers*	1 Pack/320g	230	72	3.8	11.3	1.2	0.5
Creamy Mushroom, Quorn, Sainsbury's*	1 Pie/134g	355	265	5.1	24.7	16.2	1.9
Cumberland Fish, Healthy Eating, Tesco*	1 Pack/450g	378	84	6.0	10.0	2.2	0.8
Cumberland, Asda*	1 Serving/300g	336	112	6.0	12.0	4.4	0.9
Cumberland, British Classics, Tesco*	1 Pack/500g	490	98	5.2	8.2	4.9	1.3
Cumberland, Healthy Living, Tesco*	1 Pie/500g	430	86	4.5	10.8	2.7	1.2
Cumberland, Marks & Spencer*	1 Pie/195g	312	160	6.9	10.1	10.4	1.1
Cumberland, Tesco*	1 Pie/500g	575	115	6.3	10.9	5.1	1.3
Dutch Apple, Burger King*	1 Pie/113g	339	300	1.7	46.0	12.3	0.8
Festive, BGTY, Sainsbury's*	1 Pie/58g	222	383	6.2	69.9	8.7	2.6
Fish	1 Serving/250g	263	105	8.0	12.3	3.0	0.7
Fish With Cheese, Ross*	1 Pack/300g	321	107	4.7	12.0	4.5	0.8
Fish With Vegetables, Ross*	1 Pack/300g	255	85	4.4	10.2	2.9	1.3
Fish, Asda*	1 Pack/338g	372	110	6.0	11.0	4.7	1.3
Fish, Better for You, Morrisons*	1 Pack/350g	301	86	5.0	10.0	2.9	0.9
Fish, Co-Op*	1 Pack/400g	380	95	4.0	12.0	4.0	0.9
Fish, Creamy, Finest, Tesco*	1 Serving/300g	438	146	10.3	5.7	9.1	0.8
Fish, GFY, Asda*	1 Pack/356.4g	360	101	6.0	14.0	2.3	0.9
Fish, Good Intentions, Somerfield*	1 Pack/400g	284	71	5.2	10.2	1.0	0.5
Fish, Healthy Living, Tesco*	1 Pack/400g	316	79	4.0	10.8	2.2	1.7
Fish, Luxury With Cheddar Mashed Potato, Sainsbury's*	½ Pack/301g	394	131	7.0	9.2	7.4	0.7
Fish, Luxury, Cafe Culture, Marks & Spencer*	1 Pack/660g	627	95	7.1	7.8	4.0	1.1
Fish, Luxury, Marks & Spencer*	1 Pack/300g	330	110	7.3	7.6	5.6	1.5
Fish, Mashed Potato Topped, Asda*	¼ Pie/257g	306	119	6.0	8.0	7.0	0.5
Fish, Spar*	1 Pack/400g	460	115	5.4	12.9	4.6	1.5
Fish, Topped With Potato, Good For You, Asda*	1 Pack/450g	414	92	6.0	9.0	3.6	1.1
Fisherman's, Asda*	1 Serving/300g	429	143	7.0	13.0	7.0	0.0
Fisherman's, Chilled, Co-Op*	1 Pie/300g	345	115	4.0	11.0	6.0	0.7
Fisherman's, Healthy Eating, Tesco*	1 Pie/400g	308	77	5.1	9.2	2.2	1.3
Fisherman's, Healthy Options, Asda*	1 Pie/406g	337	83	5.0	10.0	2.5	0.9
Fisherman's, Morrisons*	1 Serving/300g	246	82	3.8	9.5	3.3	1.0
Fisherman's, Nisa Heritage*	1 Serving/550g	589	107	5.2	9.0	5.6	0.2
Fisherman's, Sainsbury's*	1 Pack/300g	195	65	3.9	9.7	1.2	1.2
Fisherman's, Tesco*	1 Pie/300g	390	130	7.0	12.3	5.9	1.2
Fisherman's, Youngs*	1 Pack/375g	499	133	6.2	11.2	7.0	0.8
Fruit, Pastry Top & Bottom	1oz/28g	73	260	3.0	34.0	13.3	1.8
Gala, Tesco*	1 Serving/70g	241	344	10.6	24.5	25.2	0.0
Haddock & Broccoli, Marks & Spencer*	1 Serving/250g	263	105	8.1	9.3	4.0	0.5
Haddock Cumberland, Marks & Spencer*	1 Pie/300g	390	130	8.2	10.6	6.0	0.4
Haddock, Eat Smart, Safeway*	1 Pack/400g	300	75	5.2	10.0	1.4	1.0
Key Lime, Sainsbury's*	¼ Pie/80g	280	350	4.2	51.8	14.0	0.7
Lamb Shepherd's, Waitrose*	1 Pie/350g	448	128	7.1	10.5	6.4	1.0
Lemon Meringue, 90% Fat Free, Sara Lee*	1/6 Slice/75g	204	273	2.4	46.1	8.9	0.9
Lemon Meringue, I Need A, Marks & Spencer*	1 Pot/105g	221	210	2.1	23.3	12.0	2.6
Lemon Meringue, Lyons*	1 Serving/100g	310	310	0.0	45.9	14.4	0.0
Lemon Meringue, Marks & Spencer*	1/6 Pie/78g	215	275	3.9	40.4	11.0	0.8

P

PIE,	Measure INFO/WEIGHT	per Measure KCAL	Nutrition Values per 100g / 100ml KCAL	PROT	CARB	FAT	FIBRE
Lemon Meringue, Mr Kipling*	1 Cake/51g	184	360	2.9	59.9	12.1	3.0
Lemon Meringue, Tesco*	1 Pie/385g	989	257	4.0	43.7	7.3	0.5
Lemon Meringue, Weight Watchers*	1 Serving/85g	161	189	2.4	43.1	0.5	0.6
Mariner's, Ross*	1 Pie/340g	435	128	5.0	13.9	5.9	1.0
Mashed Potato Topped Cumberland, Marks & Spencer*	1/3 Pack/300g	360	120	5.8	9.6	5.9	1.0
Meat & Potato, Shortcrust, Co-Op*	¼ Pie/137g	403	294	7.3	23.3	19.1	1.4
Meat & Potato, Value, Tesco*	1 Pie/95g	274	288	6.9	23.8	18.4	3.5
Meat, Freshbake*	1 Pie/48.6g	153	313	6.6	23.2	21.6	1.0
Mince, Christmas, Sainsbury's*	1 Pie/37g	147	397	4.5	58.0	16.3	2.6
Mince, Deep Filled, Tesco*	1 Pie/57g	215	376	3.9	57.8	14.3	1.6
Mince, Deep, Sainsbury's*	1 Pie/67g	240	358	3.5	55.0	13.8	1.4
Mince, Finest, Tesco*	1 Pie/61g	234	384	4.3	59.9	14.1	2.7
Mince, Free From Tesco*	1 Pie/60g	188	314	2.0	58.4	8.0	4.8
Mince, Individual	1 Pie/48g	203	423	4.3	59.0	20.4	2.1
Mince, Lattice, Marks & Spencer*	1 Pie/51g	204	400	4.4	58.0	16.8	4.1
Mince, Luxury, Deep Filled, Marks & Spencer*	1 Pie/65g	234	360	4.3	55.0	13.8	3.8
Mince, Merry, Mr Kipling*	1 Pie/62g	234	376	3.7	59.2	13.8	1.5
Mince, Mini, Waitrose*	1 Pie/30g	150	501	5.7	51.3	30.3	1.7
Mince, Mr Kipling*	1 Pie/62g	231	372	3.8	56.8	14.4	1.5
Mince, Safeway*	1 Pie/55g	213	388	3.9	58.8	15.2	1.6
Mince, Tesco*	1 Pie/47g	180	383	3.9	54.7	16.5	1.5
Minced Beef & Onion, Aberdeen Angus, Somerfield*	1 Serving/240g	732	305	8.6	25.8	18.6	1.0
Minced Beef & Onion, Bird's Eye*	1 Pie/145g	419	289	7.1	26.3	17.3	0.7
Minced Beef & Onion, Dennys*	1 Sm Pie/140g	288	206	6.1	17.3	14.1	0.0
Minced Beef & Onion, Farmfoods*	1 Pie/128g	378	295	7.3	24.4	18.7	1.0
Minced Beef & Onion, Sainsbury's*	1 Pie/150g	410	273	6.8	27.8	15.0	0.9
Minced Beef & Onion, Tesco*	1 Pie/150g	455	303	5.7	27.4	19.0	1.7
Minced Steak, Aberdeen Angus, Sainsbury's*	1/3 Pie/174g	527	303	8.8	27.0	17.8	1.0
Mississippi Mud, Tesco*	1 Serving/104g	399	384	5.3	33.1	25.6	1.8
Moroccan Filo, Marks & Spencer*	1 Serving/130g	215	165	5.5	22.8	5.9	1.6
Mushroom & Parsley Potato, Waitrose*	1 Pack/350g	347	99	2.5	10.9	5.0	1.2
Ocean With Cod, Weight Watchers*	1 Pack/295g	251	85	5.4	10.0	2.6	0.8
Ocean With White Fish, Weight Watchers*	1 Pack/295g	224	76	4.8	10.6	1.6	0.5
Ocean, BGTY, Sainsbury's*	1 Pack/350g	270	77	5.4	10.5	1.5	1.1
Ocean, Marks & Spencer*	1 Pie/650g	532	95	8.2	7.6	3.5	0.9
Ocean, Youngs*	1 Serving/187.5g	250	133	6.2	11.2	7.0	0.8
Pork & Egg, Marks & Spencer*	¼ Pie/108g	379	351	9.7	19.8	25.9	0.8
Pork & Kentish Cider With Mustard Mash, COU, M&S*	1 Pack/300g	240	80	6.7	9.0	1.8	1.4
Pork & Pickle, Bowyers*	1 Pie/150g	576	384	10.0	26.3	27.3	0.0
Pork & Pickle, Pork Farms*	1 Pie/50g	185	370	8.5	30.1	24.0	0.0
Pork, Buffet, Bowyers*	1 Pie/60g	217	362	10.4	24.9	24.5	0.0
Pork, Crusty Bake, Mini, Sainsbury's*	1 Pie/43g	165	384	11.5	26.0	26.0	1.5
Pork, Crusty Bake, Sainsbury's*	1 Pie/75g	293	390	10.5	27.0	26.7	1.0
Pork, Geo Adams*	1 Pie/125g	488	390	11.8	23.1	27.8	0.9
Pork, Melton Mowbray, Cured, Marks & Spencer*	1 Pie/290g	1044	360	10.1	25.9	24.5	1.0
Pork, Melton Mowbray, Lattice, Sainsbury's*	1 Serving/100g	342	342	10.8	21.7	23.6	1.2
Pork, Melton Mowbray, Medium, Somerfield*	¼ Pie/70g	275	393	11.0	27.0	27.0	0.0
Pork, Melton Mowbray, Mini, Co-Op*	1 Pie/49g	189	385	11.0	24.0	27.0	2.0
Pork, Melton Mowbray, Mini, Morrisons*	1 Pie/50.1g	197	393	10.9	31.3	24.9	0.9
Pork, Melton Mowbray, Mini, Tesco*	1 Pie/50g	196	392	12.6	20.8	28.7	2.9
Pork, Melton Mowbray, Safeway*	1 Pie/50g	197	393	10.9	31.3	24.9	0.9
Pork, Melton Mowbray, Small, Somerfield*	½ Pie/64g	237	371	12.0	30.0	23.0	0.0
Pork, Melton Mowbray, Tesco*	1 Sm Pie/148g	679	459	10.0	29.0	33.7	1.3

P

PIE,

INFO/WEIGHT	per Measure KCAL	KCAL	PROT	CARB	FAT	FIBRE
Pork, Melton, Mini, Marks & Spencer*	1oz/28g	112	400	10.8	28.4	27.3	1.2
Pork, Melton, Mini, Pork Farms*	1 Pie/50g	200	399	8.9	26.2	29.2	0.0
Pork, Mini, Tesco*	1 Pie/45g	162	359	10.2	25.9	23.8	1.0
Pork, Somerfield*	1 Pie/110g	442	402	11.0	24.0	29.0	0.0
Potato & Meat, Farmfoods*	1 Pie/158g	416	263	5.4	22.0	17.0	1.0
Quorn & Mushroom, Tesco*	1 Pie/141g	378	268	5.3	23.8	16.8	1.3
Quorn & Vegetable	1oz/28g	52	186	6.9	14.7	11.5	2.0
Quorn Cottage, Safeway*	1 Pack/400g	260	65	3.5	10.0	1.1	2.0
Quorn, Creamy Mushroom, Quorn*	1 Pie/134g	355	265	5.1	24.7	16.2	1.9
Rhubarb, Sara Lee*	1 Serving/89.6g	225	250	2.9	28.7	13.8	1.3
Roast Chicken & Broccoli, Marks & Spencer*	1 Serving/320g	272	85	8.1	8.8	1.9	1.3
Roast Chicken & Ham, Deep Filled, Sainsbury's*	1 Pie/210g	594	283	8.0	23.0	17.7	1.0
Roast Chicken & Mushroom, Luxury, Marks & Spencer*	½ Pie/275g	880	320	9.9	20.0	22.5	1.0
Roast Chicken, COU, Marks & Spencer*	1 Pack/300g	240	80	7.3	9.1	1.3	1.2
Roast Chicken, Marks & Spencer*	1/3 Pack/183g	503	275	8.5	25.7	15.4	1.0
Roast Chicken, Sainsbury's*	1/3 Pie/173g	535	311	10.5	27.2	17.8	0.9
Salmon & Broccoli Lattice Bar, Asda*	1/3 Bar/133g	360	271	6.0	28.0	15.0	0.8
Salmon & Broccoli, Bird's Eye*	1 Pie/351g	449	128	6.6	11.4	6.2	0.7
Salmon & Broccoli, Filo Pastry, Finest, Tesco*	1 Pie/170g	386	227	7.9	18.9	13.3	2.1
Salmon & Broccoli, Premium, Tesco*	1 Serving/170g	425	250	6.1	17.7	17.2	0.7
Salmon Cottage, Sainsbury's*	1 Pack/300g	219	73	4.6	10.4	1.4	1.3
Salmon, Value, Tesco*	1 Pack/300g	312	104	4.5	11.3	4.5	1.0
Sausage & Onion, Tesco*	1 Pack/300g	333	111	2.3	11.7	6.1	0.5
Scotch, Co-Op*	1 Pie/132g	408	309	7.3	27.3	18.9	1.5
Scotch, Farmfoods*	1 Pie/151g	430	285	7.8	26.8	16.3	1.2
Scottish Steak, Topcrust Puff Pastry, Marks & Spencer*	1 Portion/240g	432	180	13.1	12.1	8.5	0.7
Shepherd's With Lamb, Weight Watchers*	1 Pack/320g	234	73	3.8	11.6	1.2	0.5
Shepherd's, Asda*	1 Pie/153g	193	126	5.0	13.0	6.0	0.8
Shepherd's, BGTY, Sainsbury's*	1 Pack/300g	225	75	3.6	10.2	2.2	1.7
Shepherd's, Baked Bean Cuisine, Heinz*	1 Pie/340g	299	88	4.1	11.6	2.8	1.5
Shepherd's, British Classics, Tesco*	1 Pack/500g	715	143	4.8	10.5	9.1	1.4
Shepherd's, COU, Marks & Spencer*	1 Pack/300g	210	70	5.2	8.6	1.3	1.6
Shepherd's, Classic British, Sainsbury's*	1 Pack/450g	500	111	6.6	10.8	4.6	0.7
Shepherd's, Frozen, Tesco*	1 Pack/400g	508	127	4.2	11.7	7.1	1.0
Shepherd's, Great Value, Asda*	1 Pack/400g	376	94	4.7	12.0	3.0	0.6
Shepherd's, Healthy Choice, Safeway*	1 Pack/333g	333	100	6.3	10.7	3.5	0.9
Shepherd's, Iceland*	1 Serving/170g	224	132	5.4	14.7	5.6	0.8
Shepherd's, Marks & Spencer*	1 Pack/400g	380	95	5.3	9.7	3.9	1.4
Shepherd's, Safeway*	1 Serving/200g	200	100	7.5	7.5	4.4	1.4
Shepherd's, Sainsbury's*	1 Pie/300g	225	75	3.6	10.2	2.2	1.7
Shepherd's, Tesco*	1 Pie/400g	380	95	6.0	10.5	3.2	0.7
Shepherd's, Welsh Hill Lamb, Marks & Spencer*	½ Pack/310g	295	95	5.4	10.2	3.5	1.5
Smoked Haddock, Eat Smart, Safeway*	1 Pack/400g	376	94	8.1	10.1	2.4	1.2
Steak & Ale, Budgens*	1 Pack/225g	583	259	7.2	19.5	16.9	0.9
Steak & Ale, Deep Filled, Somerfield*	1 Pie/200g	550	275	12.0	22.0	16.0	0.0
Steak & Ale, Fray Bentos*	1 Pie/425g	697	164	7.6	13.0	9.1	0.0
Steak & Ale, Pub Style, Co-Op*	1 Pie/250g	538	215	9.0	17.0	12.0	2.0
Steak & Gravy, Somerfield*	1oz/28g	67	239	13.0	23.0	11.0	0.0
Steak & Kidney, Bird's Eye*	1 Pie/146g	419	287	7.5	24.4	17.7	1.7
Steak & Kidney, Family, Co-Op*	1/6 Pie/87g	278	320	9.0	26.0	20.0	0.9
Steak & Kidney, Family, Iceland*	1/3 Pie/225g	502	223	10.2	16.3	13.0	2.1
Steak & Kidney, Individual	1 Pie/200g	646	323	9.1	25.6	21.2	0.9
Steak & Kidney, Morrisons*	1 Serving/142g	351	247	8.1	21.8	14.1	0.0

	Measure INFO/WEIGHT	per Measure KCAL	Nutrition Values per 100g / 100ml				
			KCAL	PROT	CARB	FAT	FIBRE
PIE,							
Steak & Kidney, Premium, Tesco*	1 Serving/170g	428	252	9.9	18.3	15.5	1.2
Steak & Kidney, Puff Pastry, Sainsbury's*	1 Pie/150g	423	282	8.2	26.9	15.7	0.9
Steak & Kidney, Shortcrust Pastry, Classic, Sainsbury's*	1/3 Pie/174g	515	296	10.2	26.5	16.6	0.8
Steak & Kidney, Tinned, Fray Bentos*	½ Pie/212g	346	163	8.2	12.9	8.8	0.0
Steak & Mushroom, Asda*	1 Pack/300g	270	90	5.0	10.0	3.3	0.7
Steak & Mushroom, Bird's Eye*	1 Pie/142g	389	274	7.5	22.7	17.0	2.0
Steak & Mushroom, Co-Op*	1 Pie/454g	1158	255	9.0	20.0	15.0	1.0
Steak & Mushroom, Deep Fill, Asda*	1/3 Pie/175g	476	272	11.0	21.0	16.0	1.1
Steak & Mushroom, Family, Iceland*	¼ Pie/164g	366	223	10.5	15.4	13.3	2.9
Steak & Mushroom, Healthy Eating, Tesco*	1 Serving/200g	380	190	10.5	24.2	5.7	1.9
Steak & Mushroom, McDougalls*	1 Pack/340g	779	229	9.0	10.0	17.0	1.0
Steak & Mushroom, Sainsbury's*	¼ Pie/130g	372	286	8.6	26.0	16.4	1.0
Steak & Onion, Farmfoods*	1 Pie/127g	382	301	6.0	26.4	19.1	1.0
Steak & Red Wine, Puff Pastry, Pub, Sainsbury's*	1 Pie/240g	497	207	7.2	16.8	12.3	2.1
Steak, Asda*	1 Pie/150g	453	302	9.2	25.1	18.3	1.0
Steak, Au Gratin, Tesco*	1 Pack/450g	594	132	8.7	10.7	6.0	1.1
Steak, Classic British, Shortcrust Pastry, Sainsbury's*	¼ Pie/130g	519	299	9.9	27.1	16.8	0.9
Steak, Marks & Spencer*	1oz/28g	64	230	10.0	19.0	12.7	1.2
Steak, Puff Pastry, Deep Filled, Somerfield*	½ Pie/275g	715	260	10.0	23.7	13.9	0.8
Steak, Safeway*	¼ Pie/130g	381	293	9.4	27.4	16.2	1.1
Steak, Short Crust, Sainsbury's*	¼ Pie/131g	392	299	9.9	27.1	16.8	0.9
Steak, Shortcrust Pastry, Tesco*	1/3 Pie/300g	693	231	10.7	21.9	11.2	1.0
Steak, Tesco*	1 Serving/205g	556	271	7.2	23.3	16.5	1.4
Strawberry Creme, Slice, Kentucky Fried Chicken*	1 Slice/78g	279	358	5.4	41.0	19.2	2.5
Summer Fruits, Orchard Tree, Aldi*	1/8 Pie/75g	242	323	3.0	46.6	13.8	1.2
Tuna & Sweetcorn, Healthy Living, Tesco*	1 Pack/450g	392	87	7.1	8.6	2.7	2.0
Turkey & Ham, Farmfoods*	1 Pie/147g	404	275	8.6	26.5	14.9	1.4
Turkey & Ham, Shortcrust, Marks & Spencer*	1/3 Pie/183g	494	270	11.9	19.5	15.9	1.0
Vegetable & Cheddar Cheese, Waitrose*	1 Pie/210g	475	226	4.9	17.8	15.0	1.2
Vegetable & Cheese, Asda*	1 Pie/131g	346	264	6.0	24.0	16.0	1.8
Vegetable, Healthy Eating, Tesco*	1 Pack/450g	360	80	2.7	11.1	2.7	0.8
Vegetarian, Deep Country, Linda McCartney*	1 Pie/176g	444	252	6.8	27.6	13.3	1.4
Vegetarian, Shepherd's, Linda McCartney*	1 Pack/340g	317	93	4.6	13.9	2.1	1.6
Vegetarian, Vegetable Cumberland, Marks & Spencer*	½ Pack/211.1g	190	90	2.8	13.4	2.6	1.6
Welsh Lamb, Sainsbury's*	¼ Pie/120g	290	242	9.1	19.2	14.3	0.8
West Country Chicken, Sainsbury's*	1 Serving/240g	614	256	11.9	17.1	15.6	2.1
PIE FILLING,							
Apple, Sainsbury's*	1 Serving/75g	67	89	0.1	22.1	0.1	1.0
Black Cherry, Fruit, Sainsbury's*	1 Serving/100g	73	73	0.3	17.7	0.1	0.3
Blackcurrant, Fruit, Sainsbury's*	1 Serving/100g	82	82	0.4	20.0	0.1	1.6
Cherry	1oz/28g	23	82	0.4	21.5	0.0	0.4
Fruit	1oz/28g	22	77	0.4	20.1	0.0	1.0
Lemon, Sainsbury's*	1 Sachet/280g	218	78	0.1	18.6	0.4	0.0
Summer Fruits, Fruit, Tesco*	1 Can/385g	377	98	0.4	24.1	0.0	0.9
PIGEON,							
Roasted, Meat Only	1oz/28g	52	187	29.0	0.0	7.9	0.0
Roasted, Meat Only, Weighed With Bone	1oz/28g	25	88	13.6	0.0	3.7	0.0
PIKELETS,							
Less Than 2% Fat, Marks & Spencer*	1 Pikelet/35g	70	200	7.3	39.1	1.3	1.6
Tesco*	1 Pikelet/35g	68	193	5.8	40.9	0.7	1.7
PILAF,							
Forest Mushroom & Pine Nut, Bistro, Waitrose*	1 Serving/225g	338	150	7.0	15.8	6.5	1.5
With Tomato	1oz/28g	40	144	2.5	28.0	3.3	0.4

P

	Measure INFO/WEIGHT	per Measure KCAL	Nutrition Values per 100g / 100ml				
			KCAL	PROT	CARB	FAT	FIBRE
PILCHARDS,							
Canned in Tomato Sauce	1oz/28g	40	144	16.7	1.1	8.1	0.0
Fillets, In Virgin Olive Oil, Glenryck*	1 Serving/92g	223	242	23.3	2.0	15.7	0.0
In Brine, Pacific, Glenryck*	½ Can/77g	110	143	22.3	0.0	6.0	0.0
In Brine, Princes*	1 Serving/155g	229	148	19.0	0.0	8.0	0.0
In Tomato Sauce, Princes*	1 Serving/78g	105	135	16.0	2.5	6.8	0.0
in Tomato Sauce, Glenryck*	1oz/28g	32	114	16.7	2.3	4.3	0.0
in Tomato Sauce, John West*	1oz/28g	40	144	16.7	1.0	8.1	0.0
PIMMS, 19% Volume	1fl oz/30ml	44	146	0.0	0.0	0.0	0.0
PINE NUTS,							
Average	1oz/28g	193	688	14.0	4.0	68.6	1.9
Kernals, Tesco*	1 Serving/20g	140	699	16.5	4.0	68.6	1.9
PINEAPPLE,							
& Papaya, Dried, Garden Gang, Asda*	1 Pack/50g	142	283	2.8	64.0	1.7	8.0
Canned, In Juice	1oz/28g	13	47	0.3	12.2	0.0	0.5
Canned, In Syrup	1oz/28g	18	64	0.5	16.5	0.0	0.7
Chunks, Fresh Ideas, Tesco*	1 Pack/200g	88	44	0.4	10.1	0.2	1.3
Chunks, Fresh, Necta*	1 Pot/340g	214	63	0.4	15.0	0.1	0.0
Chunks, Fruit Express, Del Monte*	1 Pot/130g	85	65	0.4	15.0	0.1	0.0
Chunks, In Juice, Somerfield*	1oz/28g	17	61	0.0	15.0	0.0	0.0
Chunks, In Light Syrup, Somerfield*	1oz/28g	21	75	0.0	18.0	0.0	0.0
Chunks, In Pineapple Juice, Asda*	1 Can/272g	133	49	0.3	12.0	0.1	0.0
Chunks, In Pineapple Juice, St Michael*	1 Serving/115g	63	55	0.5	12.2	0.2	0.5
Chunks, Sainsbury's*	¼ Pack/84g	37	44	0.0	10.1	0.2	1.2
Crushed, Del Monte*	1 Serving/28g	14	50	0.4	12.2	0.1	0.4
Cubes, Tesco*	1 Can/259g	130	50	0.3	12.2	0.0	0.5
Dried, Tesco*	1 Serving/15g	35	230	0.4	52.9	1.9	1.7
Fresh, Marks & Spencer*	1 Pack/260g	117	45	0.4	10.1	0.2	1.2
Fresh, Raw	1oz/28g	11	41	0.4	10.1	0.2	1.2
Fresh, Waitrose*	1 Serving/250g	110	44	0.4	10.1	0.2	1.2
Golden, Asda*	½ Pot/100g	43	43	0.4	10.0	0.2	1.2
In Own Juice, Del Monte*	1 Can/432g	281	65	0.4	15.0	0.1	0.0
Organic, Waitrose*	1oz/28g	12	44	0.4	10.1	0.2	1.2
Pieces, In Juice, Princes*	1 Can/227g	114	50	0.3	12.2	0.0	0.5
Pieces, In Natural Juice, Sainsbury's*	1 Can/140g	85	61	0.4	14.7	0.1	0.7
Pieces, In Natural Juice, Tesco*	1oz/28g	15	52	0.3	12.0	0.0	0.5
Pieces, In Own Fruit Juice, Safeway*	1 Serving/170g	83	49	0.3	12.0	0.0	1.4
Pieces, In Pineapple Juice, Fruitime, Tesco*	1 Can/140g	84	60	0.3	14.0	0.0	0.5
Pieces, Somerfield*	1 Serving/79.5g	35	44	0.4	10.1	0.2	1.2
Rings, In Pineapple Juice, John West*	1 Can/106g	43	41	0.3	10.0	0.0	0.7
Rings, Safeway*	1 Serving/25g	17	68	0.5	16.5	0.0	0.7
Rings, Sainsbury's*	1 Serving/50g	22	44	0.4	10.1	0.2	1.2
Rings, in Fruit Juice, Safeway*	1 Can/224g	121	54	0.4	13.0	0.0	0.9
Slices, Fully Prepared, Sainsbury's*	1 Pot/250g	110	44	0.4	10.1	0.2	1.2
Slices, Gold, Del Monte*	1 Serving/200g	82	41	0.4	9.6	0.2	1.2
Slices, In Fruit Juice, Waitrose*	½ Can/67g	34	50	0.5	12.2	0.0	0.5
Slices, In Natural Juice, Sainsbury's*	½ Can/216g	132	61	0.4	14.7	0.1	0.7
Slices, In Natural Juice, Tesco*	1 Slice/56g	28	50	0.3	12.2	0.0	0.5
Slices, In Pineapple Juice, Asda*	½ Can/216g	106	49	0.3	12.0	0.0	0.0
Slices, In Syrup, Sainsbury's*	1 Serving/60g	37	62	0.4	15.0	0.0	1.3
Slices, in Juice, Co-Op*	1 Can/220g	110	50	0.3	12.3	0.0	0.9
PINEAPPLE & COCONUT Juice, Sainsbury's*	1 Glass/250ml	128	51	0.4	11.9	0.1	0.1
PINEAPPLE JUICE,							
Asda*	1 Glass/250ml	125	50	0.3	11.6	0.1	0.3

P

	Measure INFO/WEIGHT	per Measure KCAL	Nutrition Values per 100g / 100ml				
			KCAL	PROT	CARB	FAT	FIBRE
PINEAPPLE JUICE,							
Del Monte*	1 Glass/200ml	104	52	0.4	12.0	0.0	0.0
Fresh Squeezed, Marks & Spencer*	1 Glass/250ml	75	30	0.2	8.8	0.0	0.6
Pure, Asda*	1 Glass/200ml	100	50	0.3	11.6	0.1	0.0
Pure, Princes*	1 Glass/200ml	94	47	0.3	10.8	0.1	0.0
Pure, Sainsbury's*	1 Glass/200ml	106	53	0.4	12.3	0.1	0.1
Pure, Tesco*	1 Serving/100ml	54	54	0.3	12.4	0.1	0.0
Pure, Waitrose*	1 Glass/200ml	106	53	0.3	12.4	0.0	0.0
Unsweetened	1 Glass/200ml	82	41	0.3	10.5	0.1	0.0
PINEAPPLE PIECES, Yoghurt Coated, Holland & Barrett*	1 Pack/100g	344	344	2.1	46.8	19.3	0.6
PINK GRAPEFRUIT, In Natural Juice, Waitrose*	1 Serving/100g	32	32	0.6	7.3	0.0	0.4
PINK GRAPEFRUIT JUICE,							
Freshly Squeezed, Marks & Spencer*	1 Glass/200ml	70	35	0.5	7.8	0.1	0.0
Ocean Spray*	1 Glass/200ml	84	42	0.3	9.7	0.0	0.0
Sainsbury's*	1 Glass/200ml	82	41	0.5	9.2	0.1	0.3
Tropicana*	1 Glass/250ml	100	40	0.6	8.0	0.0	0.5
PISTACHIO NUTS,							
Golden Wonder*	1 Bag/40g	246	615	21.1	7.8	55.5	5.5
Iran, Sainsbury's*	1 Serving/15g	90	601	17.9	8.2	55.4	6.1
Marks & Spencer*	1 Pack/125g	763	610	22.5	10.2	52.8	10.7
Roast Salted, KP*	1oz/28g	176	630	20.8	11.9	55.5	6.0
Roasted & Salted	10 Nuts/8g	48	601	17.9	8.2	55.4	6.1
Roasted & Salted, Sainsbury's*	1 Serving/50g	312	625	21.2	11.2	55.1	6.2
Roasted & Salted, Waitrose*	1 Serving/25g	144	576	18.5	8.2	52.1	6.1
Unsalted, Roasted, KP*	1oz/28g	179	640	20.8	14.2	55.5	6.0
Whole. Shelled, Sainsbury's*	1 Serving/25g	151	602	20.7	7.5	54.3	6.0
PIZZA,							
American Hot, Chicargo Town*	1 Pizza/170g	445	262	8.2	30.8	11.8	0.9
American Hot, Pizza Express*	½ Pizza/264g	517	196	10.6	26.8	5.1	1.1
American Hot, Pizza Express, Sainsbury's*	½ Pizza/147g	281	191	9.9	28.2	4.4	1.4
BBQ Chicken Stuffed Crust, Asda*	½ Pizza/245g	613	250	13.0	27.0	10.0	2.7
BBQ Chicken, Chicago Town*	1 Pizza/172.4g	373	217	7.0	30.9	7.3	1.0
BBQ Chicken, Thin & Crispy, Sainsbury's*	½ Pizza/147g	384	261	13.8	33.1	8.2	1.6
BBQ Chicken, Thin & Crispy, Tesco*	1 Serving/165g	355	215	11.9	31.6	4.5	1.2
BBQ Chicken, Weight Watchers*	1 Pizza/224g	412	184	11.5	26.5	3.5	2.7
Bacon & Mushroom Pizzeria, Sainsbury's*	1 Pizza/355g	880	248	11.7	34.5	7.0	3.7
Bacon & Mushroom, Deep Pan, Big Bite, Goodfella's*	¼ Pizza/104g	241	232	11.3	27.3	8.6	3.6
Bacon & Mushroom, Stone Bake, Marks & Spencer*	1 Pizza/375g	750	200	9.9	27.2	6.4	1.6
Bacon & Mushroom, Thin & Crispy, Sainsbury's*	½ Pizza/150g	396	264	12.9	29.2	10.6	1.7
Bacon & Mushroom, Thin & Crispy, Somerfield*	¼ Pizza/81g	189	233	11.0	24.0	10.0	0.0
Bacon, Mushroom & Tomato, Stonebaked, Tesco*	1 Serving/173g	351	203	9.9	24.1	7.4	2.0
Balsamic Roast Vegetable & Mozzarella, Sainsbury's*	½ Pizza/200g	444	222	8.5	29.4	7.8	2.4
Bistro Caramelised Onion, Feta & Rosemary, Waitrose*	½ Pizza/229.9g	607	264	8.6	26.1	13.9	2.4
Bistro Cheese & Tomato, Waitrose*	½ Pizza/205g	488	238	10.0	27.6	9.7	1.2
Bistro Salami & Pepperoni, Waitrose*	½ Pizza/190g	492	259	12.9	28.8	10.2	1.5
Cajun Chicken, BGTY, Sainsbury's*	½ Pizza/165g	363	220	11.0	36.0	3.6	1.7
Cajun Chicken, Sainsbury's*	½ Pizza/146g	285	195	12.9	31.8	1.8	2.6
Cajun Style Chicken, Stonebaked, Tesco*	1 Pizza/561g	1318	235	11.9	24.8	9.8	1.4
Capricciosa, Pizza Express*	1 Serving/300g	753	251	13.6	29.1	9.8	0.0
Caprina, Pizza Express*	1 Pizza/300g	635	212	8.0	31.0	7.3	0.0
Charged Up Chilli Beef, Goodfella's*	½ Pizza/357g	857	240	12.8	26.4	9.2	1.6
Chargrilled Chicken & Bacon Pizzeria, Sainsbury's*	½ Pizza/181g	554	306	12.8	35.4	12.6	1.2
Chargrilled Chicken & Vegetable, Good For You, Asda*	½ Pizza/166g	355	214	13.0	36.0	2.0	2.0
Chargrilled Chicken & Vegetable, Low Fat, Bertorelli*	1 Pizza/180g	439	244	14.2	39.3	4.4	2.3

PIZZA,

INFO/WEIGHT	Measure per Measure	KCAL	Nutrition Values per 100g / 100ml				
			KCAL	PROT	CARB	FAT	FIBRE
Chargrilled Chicken, Iceland*	1 Pizza/381g	804	211	12.3	25.4	6.7	2.0
Chargrilled Chicken, Thin & Crispy, Asda*	1 Serving/185g	387	209	9.0	32.0	5.0	1.6
Chargrilled Vegetable, COU, Marks & Spencer*	1 Pizza/294g	397	135	6.0	23.4	2.4	1.9
Chargrilled Vegetable, Eat Smart, Safeway*	1 Pizza/206g	361	175	10.2	27.6	2.1	2.6
Chargrilled Vegetable, Frozen, BGTY, Sainsbury's*	1 Pizza/290g	548	189	10.2	26.7	4.6	3.0
Chargrilled Vegetable, Healthy Eating, Tesco*	½ Pizza/143g	320	224	10.4	39.6	2.7	1.1
Cheese & Tomato French Bread, Findus*	1 Piece/143g	336	235	9.1	32.2	7.7	1.5
Cheese & Tomato Slice, Ross*	1 Slice/77g	148	192	6.5	22.2	8.6	2.0
Cheese & Tomato Thin & Crispy, Stonebaked, Tesco*	1 Pizza/155g	355	229	11.6	28.1	7.8	1.3
Cheese & Tomato, 9.5", Domino's Pizza*	1 Slice/52g	125	241	12.8	34.9	5.6	3.2
Cheese & Tomato, Basics, Somerfield*	1 Serving/80g	194	242	9.7	35.1	7.0	1.9
Cheese & Tomato, Big Value, Ross*	1 Pizza/716g	1446	202	7.8	32.2	4.7	2.7
Cheese & Tomato, Blue Parrot Cafe, Sainsbury's*	¼ Pizza/87.5g	218	248	12.7	29.5	8.8	1.2
Cheese & Tomato, Deep & Crispy, Safeway*	1 Pizza/510g	1214	238	10.2	33.3	7.1	1.5
Cheese & Tomato, Deep Pan, Goodfella's*	¼ Pizza/102.4g	258	253	11.5	29.6	10.5	3.7
Cheese & Tomato, Deep Pan, Sainsbury's*	1 Pizza/182g	470	258	11.7	33.1	8.7	1.9
Cheese & Tomato, Eat Smart, Safeway*	1 Pizza/165g	355	215	11.5	40.1	0.7	1.9
Cheese & Tomato, Economy, Sainsbury's*	1 Pizza/60g	142	237	11.2	34.1	6.2	1.8
Cheese & Tomato, French Bread, Co-Op*	1 Pizza/135g	270	200	9.0	27.0	6.0	2.0
Cheese & Tomato, Healthy Eating, Tesco*	1 Serving/100g	211	211	11.9	35.5	2.4	1.6
Cheese & Tomato, Italiano Range, Tesco*	1 Pizza/380g	969	255	11.4	31.7	9.2	3.3
Cheese & Tomato, Light & Crispy Slices, M&S*	1 Slice/52g	120	230	9.4	30.3	7.8	1.9
Cheese & Tomato, Micro, McCain*	1 Slice/135g	420	311	11.7	29.5	16.2	0.0
Cheese & Tomato, Mini, Marks & Spencer*	1 Pizza/95g	233	245	10.0	38.7	5.8	1.6
Cheese & Tomato, Morrisons*	1 Serving/143g	204	143	7.0	19.0	4.3	0.7
Cheese & Tomato, Sainsbury's*	1 Pizza/247g	706	286	13.7	35.4	9.9	2.4
Cheese & Tomato, Small, Tesco*	1 Pizza/102g	226	222	9.5	31.9	6.3	1.2
Cheese & Tomato, SmartPrice, Asda*	1 Pizza/125g	356	285	13.0	38.0	9.0	0.0
Cheese & Tomato, Square, Sainsbury's*	1 Square/160g	435	272	14.0	37.6	7.3	2.1
Cheese & Tomato, Stone Baked, Co-Op*	1 Pizza/325g	699	215	10.0	26.0	8.0	3.0
Cheese & Tomato, Stonebaked, Organic, Co-Op*	1 Pizza/330g	677	205	9.0	26.0	7.0	4.0
Cheese & Tomato, Stonebaked, Safeway*	½ Pizza/190g	437	230	12.0	32.3	5.9	1.5
Cheese & Tomato, Stonebaked, Thin & Crispy, Tesco*	½ Pizza/161g	388	241	11.6	29.4	8.6	2.1
Cheese & Tomato, Thin & Crispy, Asda*	1 Pizza/366g	827	226	11.0	23.0	10.0	2.0
Cheese & Tomato, Thin & Crispy, Carlos*	1 Pizza/155g	405	261	11.4	35.0	8.4	1.2
Cheese & Tomato, Thin & Crispy, Morrisons*	1 Pizza/335g	787	235	11.6	27.4	8.7	0.0
Cheese & Tomato, Thin & Crispy, Organic, Tesco*	½ Pizza/147g	369	251	10.6	30.1	9.8	1.3
Cheese & Tomato, Thin & Crispy, Sainsbury's*	1 Serving/135g	329	244	11.4	26.0	11.1	1.5
Cheese & Tomato, Thin & Crispy, Stonebaked, Tesco*	1/3 Pizza/212g	509	240	10.1	29.2	9.2	1.4
Cheese & Tomato, Thin & Crispy, Waitrose*	½ Pizza/118g	245	208	9.2	25.0	7.9	1.3
Cheese & Tomato, Value, Tesco*	1 Serving/140g	319	228	10.0	28.7	8.1	2.4
Cheese Feast, Big Fill, Somerfield*	1 Pizza/430g	1135	264	13.0	28.0	11.0	0.0
Cheese Feast, Deep Pan, Asda*	½ Pizza/210g	500	238	11.4	26.7	9.5	1.1
Cheese Suprema, Freschetta, Schwan's*	½ Pizza/150g	392	261	12.4	32.4	9.3	1.8
Cheese Supreme, New Recipe, Goodfella's*	¼ Pizza/102g	269	264	12.3	31.2	10.0	2.2
Cheese Triple, Chicago Town*	1 Serving/170g	418	246	9.9	27.6	10.7	0.0
Cheese, Onion & Garlic, Pizzeria, Waitrose*	½ Pizza/245.2g	684	279	10.8	29.8	11.8	2.5
Cheese, Thin & Crispy, Goodfella's*	1 Serving/275g	729	265	15.7	27.6	10.1	1.8
Cheesefeast, Deep & Crispy 12", Takeaway, Iceland*	1 Slice/132g	342	259	13.1	32.8	8.4	1.5
Chesse & Tomato, Kids Crew, Iceland*	1 Pizza/89.9g	204	227	9.6	32.4	6.5	1.2
Chicken & Bacon, Loaded, Tesco*	1 Serving/258g	622	241	12.8	25.4	9.8	1.9
Chicken & Maple Bacon Carbonara, Asda*	½ Pizza/195g	484	248	11.0	33.0	8.0	2.2
Chicken & Red Pepper Tapenade, TTD, Sainsbury's*	¼ Pizza/39.0g	103	264	12.3	25.5	12.5	2.1

PIZZA,	Measure INFO/WEIGHT	per Measure KCAL	KCAL	PROT	CARB	FAT	FIBRE
Chicken & Red Pepper, Healthy Eating, Tesco*	1 Pizza/260g	608	234	12.7	40.1	2.5	0.7
Chicken & Spinach, Eat Smart, Safeway*	1 Pizza/165g	322	195	19.0	24.0	2.1	2.5
Chicken & Sweetcorn, Stonebaked, Tesco*	1 Serving/177g	354	200	11.9	26.0	5.4	2.0
Chicken & Vegetable, Stone Baked, GFY, Asda*	½ Pizza/160.8g	349	217	13.0	36.0	2.3	1.7
Chicken Provencal, Goodfellas*	½ Pizza/142.5g	389	272	13.7	25.9	12.6	2.1
Chicken Salsa, Healthy Choice, Safeway*	½ Pizza/177g	437	246	13.3	40.9	3.2	1.6
Chicken Salsa, Healthy Eating, Tesco*	½ Pizza/169g	313	185	13.0	30.3	1.3	1.5
Chicken Salsa, Healthy Living, Tesco*	½ Pizza/169g	313	185	13.0	30.3	1.3	1.5
Chicken Salsa, Thin Crust, Healthy Selection, Budgens*	½ Pizza/163g	295	181	10.5	30.5	1.9	1.4
Chicken Supreme, Medium Pan, Pizza Hut*	½ Pizza/300g	810	270	13.0	29.0	12.0	2.0
Chicken, Thin & Crispy, Somerfield*	½ Pizza/159g	356	224	11.1	29.0	7.1	2.9
Chilli Beef, Stone Bake, Marks & Spencer*	1 Pizza/395g	790	200	9.6	26.7	5.8	1.9
Chorizo & CherryBell Peppers, TTD, Sainsbury's*	½ Pizza/194.7g	589	302	13.8	33.0	12.8	2.2
Cream Cheese & Pepperonata, Calzone, Waitrose*	½ Pizza/165g	383	232	7.0	29.4	9.6	1.5
Deep South, Chicago Town*	1 Pizza/171g	363	212	6.9	30.0	7.1	0.0
Delicata Four Season Ultra Thin, TTD, Sainsbury's*	½ Pizza/168g	445	265	13.3	24.3	12.9	2.3
Delicata Mushroom & Onion Ultra Thin, TTD, Sainsbury's*	½ Pizza/165g	507	307	12.0	28.7	16.0	2.6
Deluxe, 9.5", Domino's Pizza*	1 Slice/66g	171	259	12.8	29.1	10.1	2.4
Double Cheese, Chicago Town*	1 Pizza/405g	932	230	11.7	30.6	6.7	0.0
Double Cheese, Square Snacks, Food Explorer, Waitrose*	1 Pizza/145.5g	415	286	12.4	40.2	7.5	1.9
Fajita Chicken, COU, Marks & Spencer*	1 Pizza/255g	434	170	9.9	25.5	2.4	1.2
Fajita Vegetable, BGTY, Sainsbury's**	1 Pizza/214g	366	171	8.9	30.8	1.4	2.9
Fingers & Curly Fries, Marks & Spencer*	1 Pack/211.8g	360	170	7.9	22.9	4.9	1.6
Fingers, McCain*	1 Finger/33g	76	230	11.8	28.9	7.5	0.0
Fire Roasted Pepper, Sainsbury's*	1 Pizza/344g	605	176	5.3	35.3	1.5	1.6
Five Cheese & Pepperoni, Deep & Crispy, Waitrose*	1/3 Pizza/200g	560	280	11.7	32.3	11.6	1.3
Flamed Chicken & Vegetables, BGTY, Sainsbury's*	1 Pizza/260g	660	254	14.2	39.3	4.4	2.3
Flamin' Hot, Deep Dish, Chicago Town*	1 Pizza/170g	454	267	8.6	31.1	12.0	0.0
Focaccia Goats Cheese & Caramelised Onion, Sainsbury's*	1 Pizza/186g	543	292	8.6	34.1	13.5	1.9
Focaccia Tomato & Black Olive, TTD, Sainsbury's*	½ Pizza/222g	515	232	9.3	28.7	8.9	2.9
Four Cheese & Tomato, Pizzatilla, Marks & Spencer*	1 Serving/69.3g	224	324	10.5	26.0	19.9	1.5
Four Cheese Tomato, Safeway*	1 Serving/125g	318	254	12.8	36.8	6.1	1.7
Four Cheese, Deep Pan, Tesco*	½ Pizza/253g	741	293	14.6	33.6	11.1	1.5
Four Cheese, Freschetta, Schwan*	¼ Slice/75g	205	273	11.3	34.8	9.8	1.4
Four Cheese, Marks & Spencer*	1oz/28g	67	240	13.2	30.3	7.5	1.2
Four Cheese, Thin Crust, Tesco*	½ Pizza/142g	386	272	14.5	31.8	9.6	1.8
Four Cheese, Weight Watchers*	1 Pizza/186g	400	215	10.8	34.9	3.8	1.6
Four Seasons, Pizza Express*	1 Serving/300g	720	240	11.6	29.2	9.6	0.0
French Bread, Blue Parrot Cafe, Sainsbury's*	1 Pizza/132g	271	205	10.7	30.8	4.3	1.3
Full House, 9.5", Domino's Pizza*	1 Slice/74g	183	247	12.5	25.5	10.5	1.8
Funghi, Pizzaroma, Safeway*	½ Pizza/205g	506	247	10.8	29.3	9.6	2.9
Garlic & Mushroom, Asda*	½ Pizza/241g	696	289	10.0	24.0	17.0	1.6
Garlic & Mushroom, Thin & Crispy, Sainsbury's*	1 Pizza/260g	829	319	11.1	31.2	16.6	1.7
Garlic Chicken & Spinach, Perfectly Balanced, Waitrose*	½ Pizza/172g	351	204	13.3	30.8	3.1	2.3
Garlic Chicken, Deep Pan, Sainsbury's*	½ Pizza/214g	464	217	11.2	28.3	6.5	3.3
Garlic Mushroom & Mascarpone, Pizzaria, Waitrose*	½ Pizza/195.2g	486	249	9.3	31.6	9.5	0.5
Garlic Mushroom, BGTY, Sainsbury's*	½ Pizza/123g	262	213	11.6	37.2	2.0	2.7
Garlic Mushroom, Ciabatta Style, Stonebake, Goodfella's*	½ Pizza/186.6g	475	254	10.0	27.9	12.3	2.2
Garlic Mushroom, Classico, Tesco*	½ Pizza/207.5g	415	200	10.0	24.9	6.7	2.6
Garlic Mushroom, Italian Style, Somerfield*	½ Pizza/175g	460	263	9.0	33.0	10.0	0.0
Garlic Mushroom, Safeway*	½ Pizza/155g	482	311	9.4	39.2	12.9	1.7
Garlic Mushroom, Tesco*	1 Pizza/425g	829	195	9.3	21.6	8.0	5.3
Grilled Pepper, Weight Watchers*	1 Pizza/220g	392	178	10.0	29.3	2.3	1.8

P

INFO/WEIGHT	Measure	per Measure KCAL	Nutrition Values per 100g / 100ml KCAL	PROT	CARB	FAT	FIBRE
Ham & Cheese, Chunky, Asda*	1 Serving/90g	211	234	12.0	39.0	3.3	4.7
Ham & Cheese, Mini, Tesco*	1 Serving/92g	228	248	13.6	31.3	7.6	3.2
Ham & Cheese, Ultra Thin, Sodebo*	1 Pizza/200g	400	200	11.3	29.1	4.3	0.0
Ham & Mushroom Calzone, Waitrose*	½ Pizza/145g	363	250	10.0	31.6	9.3	1.6
Ham & Mushroom Slices, Farmfoods*	1 Slice/89g	170	191	8.0	34.0	2.6	0.9
Ham & Mushroom, BGTY, Sainsbury's*	½ Pizza/158g	291	184	10.2	26.4	4.2	2.9
Ham & Mushroom, COU, Marks & Spencer*	1 Pack/245g	392	160	9.2	25.7	2.4	1.3
Ham & Mushroom, Deep & Crispy, Tesco*	1 Serving/210g	420	200	9.7	29.2	4.9	1.1
Ham & Mushroom, Deep Pan, Waitrose*	½ Pizza/219.9g	453	206	10.9	26.6	6.2	1.0
Ham & Mushroom, Healthy Eating, Tesco*	1 Pizza/252g	491	195	10.4	35.6	1.2	2.0
Ham & Mushroom, New, BGTY, Sainsbury's*	1 Pizza/248g	526	212	12.1	37.8	1.4	2.9
Ham & Mushroom, Stone Baked, Goodfella's*	½ Pizza/175g	439	251	9.6	27.6	11.4	1.2
Ham & Mushroom, Stonebaked, Stateside Foods*	¼ Pizza/101g	225	223	9.9	31.9	6.2	1.4
Ham & Mushroom, The Italian, Medium 12", Pizza Hut*	1 Slice/96g	270	281	13.6	35.4	10.6	2.6
Ham & Mushroom, Thin & Crispy, Asda*	1 Pizza/360g	760	211	11.0	26.0	7.0	2.4
Ham & Mushroom, Thin & Crispy, Somerfield*	½ Pizza/170g	357	210	10.8	24.0	7.9	1.0
Ham & Mushroom, Thin & Crispy, Tesco*	1 Serving/166g	349	210	13.0	23.9	6.9	2.4
Ham & Onion, Tesco*	1 Serving/181g	453	250	11.8	29.0	9.6	2.2
Ham & Pineapple, American Deep Pan, Sainsbury's*	1 Pizza/412g	1001	243	10.5	32.6	7.8	1.7
Ham & Pineapple, Chicago Town*	1 Pizza/435g	866	199	10.0	29.7	4.5	0.0
Ham & Pineapple, Deep Dish, Chicago Town*	1 Serving/170g	403	237	8.0	26.1	11.2	0.0
Ham & Pineapple, Deep Pan, American, Goodfella's*	1 Pizza/445g	1095	246	14.7	26.7	9.6	1.6
Ham & Pineapple, Deep Pan, American, Stateside Foods*	1 Serving/200g	412	206	9.7	34.2	3.4	1.6
Ham & Pineapple, Deep Pan, Ciabatta, Iceland*	½ Pizza/185g	440	238	11.6	30.3	7.8	0.8
Ham & Pineapple, Deep Pan, Tesco*	1 Pizza/217g	399	184	9.8	29.8	2.9	1.9
Ham & Pineapple, Eat Smart, Safeway*	1 Serving/151g	279	185	13.6	27.2	2.4	2.5
Ham & Pineapple, Healthy Eating, Tesco*	1 Serving/169g	343	203	11.9	35.4	1.5	1.3
Ham & Pineapple, Light & Crispy Slices, M&S*	1 Slice/58g	116	200	9.7	29.1	5.1	1.6
Ham & Pineapple, Loaded, Tesco*	½ Pizza/265g	557	210	11.3	28.7	5.5	1.4
Ham & Pineapple, Stone Bake, Marks & Spencer*	1 Pizza/345g	690	200	10.1	28.3	5.7	1.6
Ham & Pineapple, Stonebaked, Tesco*	1 Serving/171g	363	212	11.5	27.1	6.4	1.9
Ham & Pineapple, Thin & Crispy Italian Morrisons*	1 Pizza/375g	746	199	10.2	24.9	6.1	0.0
Ham & Pineapple, Thin & Crispy, Good Choice, Iceland*	1 Pizza/600g	1338	223	11.7	33.1	4.9	1.7
Ham & Pineapple, Thin & Crispy, Goodfella's*	1 Serving/163g	333	204	10.6	22.8	7.8	2.4
Ham & Pineapple, Thin & Crispy, Iceland*	1 Serving/110g	285	259	9.9	29.2	11.4	1.3
Ham & Pineapple, Thin & Crispy, Safeway*	½ Pizza/182g	455	250	13.6	29.9	7.9	4.0
Ham & Pineapple, Thin & Crispy, Sainsbury's*	1 Pizza/305g	824	270	13.5	29.8	10.7	1.7
Ham & Pineapple, Thin & Crispy, Somerfield*	½ Pizza/192g	405	211	10.7	21.5	9.1	2.4
Ham & Pineapple, Thin & Crispy, Waitrose*	1 Pizza/220g	616	280	12.8	33.3	9.6	2.2
Ham & Roast Onion, Classico, Italiano, Tesco*	1 Pizza/181.5g	455	250	11.8	29.0	9.6	2.2
Ham, Mushroom & Tomato, BGTY, Sainsbury's*	½ Pizza/150g	307	206	11.8	30.4	4.1	1.2
Hawaiian, Healthy Living, Tesco*	½ Pizza/175g	301	172	7.5	30.0	2.5	2.9
Hawaiian, Medium Pan, Pizza Hut*	1 Slice/96g	241	251	12.6	29.2	9.3	1.4
Hawaiian, Thin Crust, Tesco*	½ Pizza/205g	398	194	8.4	28.3	5.3	2.1
Hickory Steak, Marks & Spencer*	1 Pizza/400g	820	205	9.9	25.7	6.7	1.4
Honey Roast Salmon & Broccoli, BGTY, Sainsbury's*	1 Serving/280g	613	219	10.2	34.4	4.5	3.5
Hot & Spicy Meat Feast, Thin & Crispy, Tesco*	½ Pizza/160g	443	277	12.4	25.8	13.8	1.5
Hot & Spicy Pepperoni, Stuffed Crust, Asda*	1 Pizza/245g	666	272	13.9	26.5	12.2	2.4
Hot & Spicy, Deep Dish, Chicago Town*	1 Pizza/177g	434	245	8.6	30.4	9.9	0.9
Hot & Spicy, Deep Dish, Schwan's*	1 Pizza/170g	423	249	9.1	27.6	11.4	0.0
Hot & Spicy, Thin & Crispy, Somerfield*	1 Pizza/305g	918	301	12.0	25.0	17.0	0.0
Hot Chicken, Stone Bake, Marks & Spencer*	1 Pizza/380g	798	210	11.5	25.1	6.8	1.3
Italian Bacon, Mushroom & Parmesan, Marks & Spencer*	1 Pizza/315g	819	260	10.1	27.0	12.3	0.9

P

PIZZA,

INFO/WEIGHT	Measure	per Measure KCAL	KCAL	PROT	CARB	FAT	FIBRE
Italian Cheese & Ham, The Little Big Food Company*	1 Pizza/95g	236	248	11.0	36.3	6.6	1.0
Italian Meat Feast, Thin & Crispy, Waitrose*	1 Pizza/182g	477	262	10.7	26.5	12.6	1.8
Italian Meat, So Good, Somerfield*	½ Pizza/200g	468	234	14.0	32.4	5.4	2.4
Italian Meats, Finest, Tesco*	½ Pizza/217g	449	207	13.6	29.4	3.9	1.3
Italian Mozzarella & Black Forest Ham, Asda*	¼ Pizza/110g	227	206	10.0	28.0	6.0	2.7
La Reine, Pizza Express, Sainsbury's*	½ Pizza/155g	361	233	12.3	29.8	7.2	1.9
La Reine, Takeaway, Pizza Express*	¼ Pizza/138g	324	235	12.4	30.0	7.3	1.9
Leek & Rosemary, Prince Carlo, Pizza Express*	1 Pizza/400g	708	177	8.0	24.5	6.0	0.0
Loaded Cheese, Goodfella's*	1 Pizza/417g	1055	253	11.5	28.9	10.2	3.6
Margherita Cheese & Tomato, San Marco*	½ Pizza/200g	454	227	10.7	29.8	7.2	1.2
Margherita, Classico, Tesco*	1 Serving/150g	383	255	11.4	31.7	9.2	3.3
Margherita, Finest, Tesco*	1 Serving/207g	441	213	11.0	30.5	5.2	1.2
Margherita, Healthy Living, Tesco*	1 Serving/165g	300	182	8.4	29.7	3.3	3.1
Margherita, Italian Stone Baked, Somerfield*	1 Pizza/290g	554	191	10.0	22.0	7.0	0.0
Margherita, Italian Style, Somerfield*	½ Pizza/190g	424	223	10.0	32.0	6.0	0.0
Margherita, Italiano, Tesco*	1 Serving/172.5g	336	194	9.5	30.1	4.0	2.5
Margherita, Medium Pan, Pizza Hut*	1 Slice/85g	239	281	12.7	31.1	11.8	2.1
Margherita, Pizza Express*	½ Pizza/135g	263	195	10.2	30.5	3.6	1.4
Margherita, Pizza Express*	1 Pizza/269.7g	527	195	10.2	30.5	3.6	1.4
Margherita, Pizza Express, Sainsbury's*	½ Pizza/243.2g	484	199	10.2	31.8	3.4	1.5
Margherita, Pizzeria, Sainsbury's*	½ Pizza/165g	450	273	13.9	34.5	8.8	2.9
Margherita, Stone Baked, Good For You, Asda*	¼ Pizza/73g	158	217	11.0	39.0	1.9	1.8
Margherita, Stone Baked, Goodfella's*	1 Slice/36g	95	263	10.9	31.9	11.4	7.6
Margherita, Stonebaked Ciabatta, Goodfella's*	½ Pizza/149.5g	405	270	11.3	32.8	11.5	2.6
Margherita, Stuffed Crust Original, Pizza Hut*	1 Slice/125.3g	330	262	14.9	28.5	9.8	1.0
Margherita, The Italian, Medium, Pizza Hut*	1 Slice/95g	292	307	15.2	39.5	10.8	2.3
Margherita,, So Good, Somerfield*	½ Pizza/220.2g	513	233	9.9	29.5	8.4	2.2
Marinated Tomato & Mascarpone, Piccadella, Tesco*	1 Pizza/260g	634	244	6.4	31.6	10.2	2.2
Massive On Meat, Deep Pan, Goodfella's*	1 Serving/106g	259	244	10.4	30.6	8.9	3.0
Meat Feast, American Style, Sainsbury's*	½ Pizza/263g	642	244	12.6	26.2	9.9	2.9
Meat Feast, Asda*	¼ Pizza/100g	316	316	14.0	38.0	12.0	2.0
Meat Feast, Big Fill, Somerfield*	1 Pizza/455g	1019	224	11.0	26.0	8.0	0.0
Meat Feast, Deep & Crispy, Iceland*	1/6 Pizza/136g	345	254	11.2	33.7	8.3	2.0
Meat Feast, Deep Pan, Asda*	½ Pizza/214g	482	225	10.0	26.0	9.0	1.2
Meat Feast, Loaded, Deep Pan, Tesco*	½ Pizza/282g	776	275	12.0	26.1	13.6	1.9
Meat Feast, Medium Pan, Pizza Hut*	1 Slice/114g	324	284	14.6	24.4	14.2	0.9
Meat Feast, The Italian, 12", Pizza Hut*	1 Slice/113g	341	302	15.4	30.3	14.3	2.3
Meat Feast, Thin & Crispy, Safeway*	½ Pizza/179.2g	430	240	12.0	27.2	9.2	4.8
Meat Feast, Thin & Crispy, Somerfield*	½ Pizza/164.8g	413	250	12.4	25.7	10.8	3.2
Meaty, The Edge, Pizza Hut*	1 Slice/64g	207	323	16.6	23.3	18.2	0.0
Mediterranean Vegetable, Good Intentions, Somerfield*	1 Pizza/375.2g	604	161	7.3	30.2	1.2	1.7
Mediterranean Vegetable, Morrisons*	1/6 Slice/80.8g	156	193	8.6	25.8	6.2	3.5
Mediterranean Vegetable, Pizzeria, Sainsbury's*	1 Serving/211.3g	430	204	8.4	28.7	6.2	2.4
Mexican Chicken, COU, Marks & Spencer*	1 Pizza/248g	384	155	10.3	25.0	2.0	2.0
Mexican Style, Morrisons*	½ Pizza/180g	437	243	13.7	26.0	9.4	2.0
Micro, McCain*	½ Serving/133g	388	292	12.4	26.9	15.0	0.0
Mighty Meaty, 9.5", Domino's Pizza*	1/6 Pizza/71g	177	249	13.9	25.5	10.2	2.8
Mixed Grill, 9.5", Domino's Pizza*	1 Slice/75g	178	237	12.0	26.2	9.3	2.3
Mozzarella & Tomato, Gluten Free, Dietary Specials*	1 Pizza/320g	646	202	6.7	33.1	4.7	1.3
Mozzarella & Cherry Tomato, Stonebaked, Safeway*	½ Pizza/262.5g	618	235	10.6	30.3	7.8	3.5
Mozzarella, Lidl*	1 Serving/175g	436	249	10.1	22.7	13.1	0.0
Mozzarella, Provolone, Cheese & Tomato, M&S*	1 Slice/50g	113	225	11.5	24.8	8.8	1.0
Mushroom & Roasted Onion, Waitrose*	½ Pizza/187.4g	402	215	9.8	28.9	6.7	1.3

P

PIZZA,

INFO/WEIGHT	Measure	per Measure KCAL	KCAL	PROT	CARB	FAT	FIBRE
Mushroom & Three Cheese, PB, Waitrose*	½ Pizza/158g	314	199	9.0	34.1	3.0	2.2
Mushroom, Pizza Express*	1 Pizza/400g	627	157	7.5	21.9	5.2	0.0
Napoletana, TTD, Sainsbury's*	1 Pizza/374g	1070	286	11.1	28.5	12.2	2.0
Napoli Ham & Mushroom, San Marco*	½ Pizza/219g	449	205	10.0	27.5	6.1	2.8
Pepperonata, Delicata, Sainsbury's*	1 Pizza/330g	917	278	12.9	24.3	14.4	2.6
Pepperoni & Jalapeno Chill, Asda*	1 Pizza/277g	742	268	10.0	39.0	8.0	1.8
Pepperoni & Onion, 9", Sainsbury's*	½ Pizza/207g	615	297	13.4	31.7	13.0	1.9
Pepperoni Bacon, Primo*	½ Pizza/111g	360	324	10.5	42.5	13.1	0.0
Pepperoni Passion, 9.5", Domino's Pizza*	1 Slice/65g	186	286	13.6	31.5	11.6	1.4
Pepperoni, American Style Deep Pan, Co-Op*	1 Pizza/395g	988	250	12.0	28.0	10.0	1.0
Pepperoni, Chicago Town*	1 Sm Pizza/170g	471	277	11.5	28.8	12.9	0.0
Pepperoni, Chilli & Vegetable, Fresh, Tesco*	1 Pizza/260g	660	254	9.5	35.1	8.4	1.7
Pepperoni, Classico, Tesco*	½ Pizza/205g	586	286	11.6	27.3	14.5	1.9
Pepperoni, Deep & Crispy, Iceland*	1 Serving/175g	490	280	11.9	31.1	12.0	1.8
Pepperoni, Deep & Crispy, Tesco*	1 Pizza/375g	881	235	10.1	31.8	7.5	1.2
Pepperoni, Deep Filled, Chicago Town*	1 Serving/202.3g	620	307	11.5	28.0	16.6	1.3
Pepperoni, Deep Pan, Farmfoods*	½ Pizza/202g	491	243	8.3	28.8	10.5	2.0
Pepperoni, Deep Pan, Goodfella's*	¼ Slice/109g	294	270	12.7	28.9	11.6	1.6
Pepperoni, Deep Pan, Morrisons*	1/6 Pizza/75.7g	194	255	8.6	27.9	12.1	1.9
Pepperoni, Deep Pan, Safeway*	½ Pizza/198g	558	283	13.9	28.9	12.4	2.5
Pepperoni, Deluxe, American Deep Pan, Sainsbury's*	1 Pizza/424g	1077	254	13.3	28.7	9.5	2.7
Pepperoni, Extra, Chicago Town*	1 Pizza/460g	994	216	9.6	27.7	7.4	0.0
Pepperoni, Feast, Deep Dish, Schwan's*	1 Pizza/435g	1188	273	9.9	26.3	14.2	0.0
Pepperoni, Freschetta, Schwan's*	1 Pizza/310g	846	273	10.8	31.6	11.5	0.0
Pepperoni, Goodfella's*	1 Pizza/337g	900	267	13.2	26.3	12.9	1.7
Pepperoni, Individual, Chicago Town*	1 Pizza/168g	496	295	9.9	30.9	14.6	0.8
Pepperoni, Italian Style, Somerfield*	1 Pizza/380g	920	242	11.0	32.0	8.0	0.0
Pepperoni, Italian, Thin & Crispy, Morrisons*	1 Pizza/365g	843	231	11.1	25.0	9.6	0.0
Pepperoni, Italiano Classico, Tesco*	1 Pack/419g	1060	253	11.6	26.1	11.4	2.4
Pepperoni, Italiano Style, Tesco*	1 Serving/215g	495	230	9.3	28.4	8.8	2.4
Pepperoni, Micro, McCain*	1 Serving/135g	405	300	12.1	26.5	16.2	0.0
Pepperoni, Oven Rising, Safeway*	1 Serving/95g	259	273	8.2	39.9	9.0	1.9
Pepperoni, Pizza Outler*	1 Slice/100g	410	410	19.0	45.0	17.0	3.0
Pepperoni, Pizzeria, Sainsbury's*	½ Pizza/197g	528	268	12.5	34.7	8.8	1.3
Pepperoni, Stateside Foods*	½ Pizza/370g	988	267	12.2	32.3	9.8	1.4
Pepperoni, Stone Baked, Carlos*	1 Pizza/330g	832	252	13.0	23.0	12.0	0.0
Pepperoni, Stone Baked, Pizzaroma, Safeway*	½ Pizza/178.4g	479	269	12.9	30.6	10.6	2.2
Pepperoni, Stonebaked, Goodfella's*	½ Pizza/181g	503	278	11.9	27.4	14.4	2.4
Pepperoni, The Insider, Pizza Hut*	1 Slice/137g	360	263	12.4	25.5	12.4	1.5
Pepperoni, Thin & Crispy Goodfella's*	1 Pizza/593g	1595	269	13.8	26.9	11.8	2.3
Pepperoni, Thin & Crispy, Co-Op*	1 Pizza/270g	689	255	11.0	26.0	11.0	1.0
Pepperoni, Thin & Crispy, Safeway*	½ Pizza/133.1g	394	296	11.8	33.9	12.6	1.5
Pepperoni, Thin & Crispy, Sainsbury's*	½ Pizza/132g	395	299	13.7	27.0	15.1	5.1
Pepperoni, Thin & Crispy, Tesco*	¼ Pizza/132g	379	287	11.5	30.3	13.3	2.3
Pepperoni, Thin & Crispy, Waitrose*	½ Pizza/225g	581	258	11.0	25.7	12.3	1.2
Pleasure With Fire Roasted Vegetables, Heinz*	½ Pizza/200g	418	209	9.5	24.8	8.0	2.4
Pork, American Style Tennesse BBQ, Asda*	1 Pizza/248.7g	563	226	11.0	32.0	6.0	2.5
Prosciutto & Fresh Rocket, TTD, Sainsbury's*	½ Pizza/164.2g	541	330	11.9	39.9	13.6	2.5
Prosciutto & Mascarpone, Safeway*	½ Pizza/200g	522	261	12.3	29.8	10.3	2.2
Prosciutto Con Funghi, Lidl*	½ Pizza/200g	454	227	9.5	31.5	7.0	0.0
Prosciutto, Classico, Tesco*	½ Pizza/205g	461	225	11.7	33.6	4.9	2.5
Prosciutto, Italian Style, Co-Op*	½ Pizza/183g	421	230	13.0	29.0	7.0	3.0
Prosciutto, Pizzaria, Sainsbury's*	1 Pizza/325g	806	248	11.4	34.7	7.1	3.2

P

PIZZA,

Measure INFO/WEIGHT	per Measure KCAL	KCAL	PROT	CARB	FAT	FIBRE
		Nutrition Values per 100g / 100ml				
Quattro Formaggi Pizzeria, Sainsbury's*	½ Pizza/175g	490	280	12.8	30.8	12.1	2.5
Quattro Formaggio, Tesco*	½ Pizza/219g	572	261	12.5	27.0	11.4	2.3
Roasted Vegetable & Goats Cheese, Safeway*	½ Pizza/200g	454	227	9.9	30.8	7.1	2.7
Roasted Vegetable, For One, GFY, Asda*	1 Pizza/96.0g	190	198	9.0	32.0	3.8	1.5
Roasted Vegetable, Italian Style, Stone Baked, Safeway*	1 Serving/185g	339	183	8.6	31.1	2.7	1.5
Roasted Vegetable, Wood Fired, Pizzaroma, Safeway*	½ Pizza/175g	350	200	7.9	27.0	6.3	5.1
Salami & Ham, Pizzeria, Waitrose*	½ Pizza/205g	443	216	10.1	28.7	6.7	1.8
Salami Con Mozarella, Lidl*	½ Pizza/200g	534	267	9.9	31.5	11.2	0.0
Salami, Lidl*	1 Pizza/350g	854	244	8.1	29.4	9.2	0.0
Salami, Ultra Thin Italian, Tesco*	1 Serving/263g	692	263	12.0	31.9	9.7	1.0
Sicilian, Premium, Co-Op*	1 Pizza/600g	1320	220	9.0	27.0	8.0	2.0
Simply Cheese, Goodfella's*	¼ Pizza/81.9g	226	276	16.3	22.5	13.4	1.9
Slice Selection, Marks & Spencer*	1 Serving/52g	120	230	9.4	30.3	7.8	1.9
Smoked Ham & Mushroom, Thin & Crispy, Co-Op*	1 Pizza/400g	792	198	9.0	30.3	4.5	1.7
Smoked Ham & Peppers, Healthy Living, Tesco*	1 Serving/282g	386	137	8.7	21.1	2.0	1.8
Smoked Ham & Pineapple, Deep Pan, Co-Op*	1 Pizza/395g	1142	289	11.6	36.7	10.6	1.7
Smoked Ham & Pineapple, Weight Watchers*	1 Pizza/241g	429	178	10.3	27.6	2.9	1.5
Spicy Beef, Goodfella's*	½ Pizza/147.5g	392	265	12.4	26.5	12.1	2.2
Spicy Chicken, Iceland*	1 Pizza/345g	797	231	13.4	29.9	6.6	1.5
Spicy Chicken, Micro, McCain*	1 Pizza/133g	388	292	12.4	26.9	15.0	0.0
Spicy Pepperoni, Tesco*	1 Pizza/380g	756	199	8.9	27.7	5.8	2.6
Spicy Vegetable Nacho, GFY, Asda*	1 Pizza/282.7g	637	225	10.0	36.0	4.5	3.3
Spicy Vegetable, Italian Style, Stateside Foods*	1 Pizza/361g	834	231	9.5	29.2	8.5	3.9
Spicy Vegetable, Low Fat, Bertorelli*	1 Pizza/180g	243	135	6.0	23.4	2.4	1.9
Spinach & Bacon, Thin & Crispy, Marks & Spencer*	1 Pizza/290g	740	255	10.6	26.8	12.1	1.0
Spinach & Goats Cheese, BGTY, Sainsbury's*	½ Pizza/160g	304	190	6.8	31.8	3.9	2.4
Spinach & Ricotta, BGTY, Sainsbury's*	1 Pizza/265g	535	202	10.4	34.4	2.5	2.6
Spinach & Ricotta, Classico, Tesco*	1 Pizza/208g	437	210	8.6	27.3	7.3	2.0
Spinach & Ricotta, Extra Special, Asda*	1 Pizza/400g	940	235	9.0	34.0	7.0	1.9
Spinach & Ricotta, GFY, Asda*	1 Pizza/160g	375	234	8.8	40.0	4.4	1.8
Spinach & Ricotta, Healthy Living, Tesco*	1 Pizza/304g	429	141	8.3	21.1	2.6	1.9
Spinach & Ricotta, Pizzaroma, Safeway*	1 Pizza/420g	1042	248	10.9	31.4	8.8	3.6
Spinach & Ricotta, Pizzeria, Sainsbury's*	1 Pizza/390g	1002	257	11.4	30.8	10.7	2.1
Spinach With Bacon & Mushroom, Good For You, Asda*	1 Serving/270g	618	229	13.0	34.0	4.5	2.6
Steak, Stone Bake, Marks & Spencer*	1 Pizza/400g	820	205	9.9	25.7	6.7	1.4
Sunblushed Tomato & Mascarpone, Pizzadella, Tesco*	1 Serving/275g	894	325	8.5	36.7	16.0	1.5
Super Supreme, Family, Chicago Town*	¼ Pizza/225g	527	234	9.6	24.5	10.8	0.0
Supreme, Deep Dish, Individual, Chicago Town*	1 Pizza/170g	456	268	9.2	30.8	12.0	1.0
Supreme, Deep Pan, Safeway*	1 Serving/189g	450	238	10.8	27.0	9.6	4.7
Supreme, Medium Pan, Pizza Hut*	1 Slice/105.7g	292	275	12.6	25.1	13.8	1.2
Supreme, Square To Share, Farmfoods*	1 Serving/93g	196	211	10.7	22.9	8.6	1.1
Supreme, The Italian, Medium, Pizza Hut*	1 Slice/106g	297	280	13.0	33.4	11.4	2.1
Sweet Chilli Chicken, BTGY, Sainsbury's*	½ Pizza/138g	276	200	13.0	33.2	1.7	2.1
Sweet Chilli Chicken, Stonebaked, Goodfella's*	½ Pizza/170g	423	249	12.9	22.3	12.1	3.0
Tandoori Hot, 9.5", Domino's Pizza*	1 Slice/67g	137	205	12.2	27.8	5.2	2.8
The Big Cheese, Deep Pan, Goodfella's*	1/6 Pizza/118g	295	250	12.2	25.9	10.8	1.1
The Big Eat Meat X-Treme, Deep Pan, Goodfella's*	½ Pizza/352g	806	229	11.6	27.1	8.2	3.6
The Works, The Edge, Pizza Hut*	1 Slice/64g	161	252	12.9	22.0	12.5	0.0
Three Cheese Calzone, Waitrose*	1 Calzone/265g	747	282	10.4	33.0	12.0	1.4
Three Cheeses & Tomato, Stonebaked, Co-Op*	1 Pizza/415g	888	214	10.0	25.2	8.1	1.5
Three Meat, Thin & Crispy, Sainsbury's*	½ Pizza/147g	344	234	12.5	23.4	10.7	1.3
Tomato & Cheese French Bread, Farmfoods*	1 Pizza/89g	164	184	5.6	9.9	13.5	1.2
Tomato & Cheese, Ross*	1 Pizza/81g	181	224	7.4	31.5	7.6	2.5

P

	Measure INFO/WEIGHT	per Measure KCAL	Nutrition Values per 100g / 100ml				
			KCAL	PROT	CARB	FAT	FIBRE
PIZZA,							
Tomato & Cheese, Savers, Safeway*	1 Pizza/140g	371	265	9.5	38.4	8.1	3.0
Tomato & Cheese, Snack Size, Farmfoods*	1 Pizza/89g	164	184	5.6	9.9	13.5	1.2
Tomato & Cheese, Stone Bake, Marks & Spencer*	1 Pizza/340g	782	230	10.8	30.1	8.4	1.6
Tomato & Cheese, Thin & Crispy, Marks & Spencer*	1 Pizza/300g	705	235	11.0	27.7	9.4	1.2
Tomato & Red Pepper, Perfectly Balanced, Waitrose*	½ Pizza/163g	313	192	6.6	38.1	1.5	1.9
Tomato & Ricotta, Waitrose*	½ Pizza/207.5g	443	214	7.8	25.7	8.9	2.2
Tomato, Aubergine & Spinach, Pizzeria, Waitrose*	½ Pizza/193g	403	209	7.8	35.4	4.0	3.6
Tomato, Basil & Garlic, Weight Watchers*	1 Serving/198.0g	394	199	10.9	30.2	3.8	2.9
Tomato, Mushroom & Bacon, Deep Pan, Co-Op*	1 Pizza/420g	882	210	9.0	25.0	8.0	2.0
Triple Cheese, Deep Dish, Chicago Town*	1 Serving/170g	418	246	9.9	27.6	10.7	0.0
Triple Cheese, Deep Pan, Morrisons*	1/6 Pizza/74.7g	199	265	10.4	28.2	12.3	1.9
Tuna & Caramelised Red Onion, COU Marks & Spencer*	1 Pizza/245g	429	175	9.6	26.7	2.3	1.2
Tuna Sweetcorn, BGTY, Sainsbury's*	1 Pizza/304g	602	198	13.5	31.7	1.9	2.7
Turkey Tikka With Indian Sauce, Bernard Matthews*	½ Pizza/165g	335	203	10.1	31.0	4.3	0.0
Tuscan Vegetable & Mozzarella, WTF, Sainsbury's*	1 Pizza/317g	552	174	5.7	26.6	5.0	2.3
Ultimate Meat Feast, Sainsbury's*	1 Pizza/465g	1302	280	13.5	35.1	10.3	1.7
Veg-a-Roma Without Cheese, Domino's Pizza*	1 Sm Pizza/354g	712	201	8.4	33.4	3.8	2.7
Vegetable Supreme, Safeway*	¼ Pizza/170g	352	207	10.4	25.9	6.9	2.9
Vegetable, Asda*	1 Pizza/368.7g	554	150	7.0	24.0	2.9	3.4
Vegetable, COU, Marks & Spencer*	1 Pizza/294g	397	135	6.4	23.2	2.4	1.9
Vegetable, Deep Pan, Co-Op*	1 Pizza/425g	829	195	8.0	25.0	7.0	2.0
Vegetable, Healthy Living, Tesco*	1 Serving/200g	302	151	8.1	23.5	2.7	4.4
Vegetable, Thin & Crispy, Iceland*	½ Pizza/200g	442	221	8.3	23.2	10.6	1.7
Vegetarian, Original Medium, Pizza Hut*	1 Slice/93.5g	227	241	11.2	28.0	9.4	1.9
Vegetarian, Supreme, 9.5", Domino's Pizza*	1 Slice/71g	137	193	10.8	27.0	4.6	2.4
Vegetarian, Weight Watchers*	1 Serving/100g	400	400	18.0	69.0	5.0	2.0
Veggie, The Edge, Pizza Hut*	1 Slice/60g	137	228	11.4	24.6	9.3	0.0
Veneziana, Pizza Express*	1 Pizza/300g	614	205	8.8	30.9	6.2	0.0
PIZZA BASE,							
Deep Pan, Napolina*	1 Base/260g	757	291	7.9	58.0	3.0	0.2
Gluten Free, Glutafin*	1 Base/110g	278	253	3.0	49.0	5.0	4.5
Italian, Sainsbury's*	1 Base/150g	452	301	7.6	57.0	4.8	1.5
Mini, Napolina*	1 Base/75g	218	291	7.9	58.0	3.0	0.2
Thin & Crispy, 9", Sainsbury's*	½ Pizza/70.1g	176	251	8.4	47.3	3.1	4.4
Thin & Crispy, Napolina*	1 Base/150g	437	291	7.9	58.0	3.0	0.2
Thin & Crispy, Safeway*	1 Base/140g	393	281	9.0	54.0	3.2	2.4
Thin & Crispy, Sainsbury's*	1 Base/140g	421	301	9.9	62.8	1.1	1.1
PIZZA BASE MIX,							
Morrisons*	1 Serving/77g	313	407	12.7	77.9	5.0	3.6
Sainsbury's*	1 Pack/145g	486	335	12.8	62.3	3.8	2.9
PLAICE,							
& Prawns in Breadcrumbs, Aldi*	1 Serving/100g	212	212	8.6	25.4	8.4	0.0
Breaded, Asda*	1 Serving/150g	351	234	15.0	12.0	14.0	0.5
Filled With Prawns & Garlic, Somerfield*	1 Plaice/171g	366	214	12.0	14.8	11.9	0.7
Filles, Extra Trimmed, Sainsbury's*	1 Fillet/150g	144	96	20.1	0.0	1.7	0.0
Fillets, Breaded, Asda*	1 Serving/150g	389	259	9.0	22.0	15.0	1.4
Fillets, Breaded, Chunky, Boneless, Tesco*	1 Fillet/160g	318	199	11.6	17.0	9.4	0.9
Fillets, Breaded, Marks & Spencer*	1 Fillet/125.6g	271	215	11.1	15.3	12.4	1.0
Fillets, Breaded, Waitrose*	1 Fillet/150g	291	194	13.2	9.9	11.3	0.3
Fillets, Chunky, Sainsbury's*	1 Fillet/160g	328	205	12.6	16.6	9.8	0.5
Fillets, Florentine, Sainsbury's*	½ Pack/180g	222	123	11.7	2.7	7.3	0.7
Fillets, In Crispy Breadcrumbs, Somerfield*	1 Serving/150g	290	193	12.0	17.0	8.6	1.4
Fillets, In Crispy Breadcrumbs, Whole, Sainsbury's*	1 Fillet/333g	839	252	14.9	16.5	14.0	0.1

	Measure INFO/WEIGHT	per Measure KCAL	Nutrition Values per 100g / 100ml				
			KCAL	PROT	CARB	FAT	FIBRE
PLAICE,							
Fillets, Somerfield*	1oz/28g	22	79	17.0	0.0	1.0	0.0
Fillets, Tesco*	1 Serving/100g	79	79	16.7	0.0	1.4	0.0
Fillets, in Breadcrumbs, Safeway*	1 Serving/160g	349	218	13.2	15.8	11.3	1.4
Fillets, in Crispy Crumb, Safeway*	1 Fillet/160g	352	220	13.2	15.8	11.3	1.4
Grilled	1oz/28g	27	96	20.1	0.0	1.7	0.0
In Batter, Fried in Blended Oil	1oz/28g	72	257	15.2	12.0	16.8	0.5
In Crumbs, Fried in Blended Oil	1oz/28g	64	228	18.0	8.6	13.7	0.2
Raw	1oz/28g	22	79	16.7	0.0	1.4	0.0
Steamed	1oz/28g	26	93	18.9	0.0	1.9	0.0
With Mushrooms & Prawns, Sainsbury's*	1 Serving/170g	354	208	12.0	15.9	10.7	1.7
With Spinach & Ricotta Cheese, Whole, Sainsbury's*	1 Fillet/159g	334	210	11.6	17.2	10.5	0.8
PLAICE - GOUJONS,							
Baked	1oz/28g	85	304	8.8	27.7	18.3	0.0
Fried in Blended Oil	1oz/28g	119	426	8.5	27.0	32.3	0.0
PLANTAIN,							
Boiled in Unsalted Water	1oz/28g	31	112	0.8	28.5	0.2	1.2
Raw	1oz/28g	33	117	1.1	29.4	0.3	1.3
Ripe, Fried in Vegetable Oil	1oz/28g	75	267	1.5	47.5	9.2	2.3
PLUMS,							
Average, Raw, Weighed With Stones	1oz/28g	10	34	0.5	8.3	0.1	1.5
Average, Stewed Without Sugar	1oz/28g	8	30	0.5	7.3	0.1	1.3
Fresh, Raw	1oz/28g	10	36	0.6	8.8	0.1	1.6
Safeway*	1 Serving/68g	26	38	0.6	8.7	0.1	1.6
Soft Dried, Blue Parrot Cafe, Sainsbury's*	1 Pack/50g	119	237	2.6	55.6	0.5	7.1
POLENTA,							
Organic, Kallo*	1 Serving/150g	543	362	8.5	78.0	1.8	0.0
Ready Made, Italfresco*	1 Serving/100g	72	72	1.6	15.7	0.3	0.0
POLO,							
Citrus Sharp, Nestle*	1 Tube/34g	134	393	0.0	96.6	1.0	0.0
Mints, Original, Nestle*	1 Mint/2g	8	404	0.0	98.9	1.1	0.0
Smoothies, Nestle*	1 Sweet/4g	16	408	0.1	86.9	6.8	0.0
Spearmint, Nestle*	1 Tube/35g	139	397	0.0	96.6	1.1	0.0
POLO FRUITS, Nestle*	1 Tube/37g	142	383	0.0	96.0	0.0	0.0
POMEGRANATE,							
Raw, Fresh	1oz/28g	14	51	1.3	11.8	0.2	3.4
Weighed With Skin	1oz/28g	9	33	0.9	7.7	0.1	2.2
POP TARTS,							
Chocolate, Kellogg's*	1 Pop Tart/50g	200	400	6.0	67.0	11.0	2.5
Cream Cheese & Cherry Swirl, Kellogg's*	1 Serving/62g	250	403	3.2	59.7	17.7	1.0
Frosted Brown Sugar Cinnamon, Kellogg's*	1 Serving/50g	210	420	6.0	68.0	14.0	2.0
Strawberry Sensation, Kellogg's*	1 Pop Tart/50g	195	390	4.0	69.0	11.0	2.0
POPCORN,							
Butter Flavour, Microwave, Popz*	1 Serving/100g	504	504	7.0	51.5	30.0	9.2
Butter Toffee, Tesco*	1 Pack/350g	1418	405	2.2	81.7	7.7	4.3
Butter, Microwave, Act 11*	1 Bag/90g	425	472	9.0	69.0	18.0	9.0
Chocolate Toffee, Mini Bites, Marks & Spencer*	1 Bite/9g	44	490	4.9	68.4	22.1	1.2
Plain	1oz/28g	166	593	6.2	48.7	42.8	0.0
PlayTime Popcorn, Salt, Sold at Cinema	1 Serving/100g	519	519	8.3	45.9	33.6	0.0
Popping Corn, Organic, Evernat*	1oz/28g	165	588	6.2	44.4	42.8	6.6
Ready Salted, Microwave, Popz*	1 Serving/20g	101	504	7.0	51.5	30.0	9.2
Salted, Blockbuster*	1 Bowl/25g	121	482	8.2	57.8	24.3	5.5
Sweet, Blockbuster*	1 Serving/100g	470	470	6.2	67.2	17.9	6.0
Sweet, Butterkist*	1 Serving/100g	391	391	4.9	76.2	7.4	0.0

INFO/WEIGHT	Measure	per Measure KCAL	Nutrition Values per 100g / 100ml				
			KCAL	PROT	CARB	FAT	FIBRE
POPCORN,							
Sweet, Microwave, Cinema, Popz*	1 Bag/85g	420	494	6.0	60.0	25.5	8.2
Toffee, 90% Fat Free, Butterkist*	1 Pack/35g	142	406	2.8	77.7	9.3	0.0
Toffee, Blockbuster*	¼ Pack/50g	221	441	2.2	77.4	13.7	2.9
Toffee, Sainsbury's*	1 Pack/100g	423	423	2.6	80.8	9.9	1.5
Vanilla, Cinema Sweet Microwave, Act II*	½ Pack/50g	234	468	9.0	71.0	16.0	12.0
POPPADUMS,							
Fried in Vegetable Oil	1oz/28g	103	369	17.5	39.1	16.9	0.0
Marks & Spencer*	1 Poppadum/9g	42	467	17.4	39.3	26.6	8.4
Mercifully Mild, Phileas Fogg*	1 Serving/30g	150	499	14.8	36.8	32.6	6.0
Mildly Spiced, Sharwood's*	1 Poppadum/12g	58	444	18.4	35.5	25.3	10.5
Mini, Sainsbury's*	½ Pack/50g	249	498	14.9	36.9	32.3	7.6
Plain, Asda*	1 Poppadum/9g	44	484	18.0	40.0	28.0	0.0
Plain, Indian To Go, Sainsbury's*	1 Poppadum/8.4g	32	405	18.4	43.4	17.5	9.0
Plain, Waitrose*	1 Serving/9g	37	408	21.0	39.3	18.6	9.1
Spicy, COU, Marks & Spencer*	1 Pack/26g	85	325	23.5	51.9	2.4	8.1
POPPETS*,							
Chocolate Raisins	1 Box/100g	409	409	4.8	66.0	14.0	0.0
Mint Cream	1oz/28g	119	424	2.0	75.0	13.0	0.0
Peanut	1 Box/100g	544	544	16.4	37.0	37.0	0.0
Toffee, Milk Chocolate	1 Box/100g	484	484	4.6	67.0	22.0	0.0
POPPY SEEDS, Asda*	1 Serving/2g	11	556	21.0	19.0	44.0	0.0
PORK,							
BBQ, Chunky, Tesco*	1 Pack/170g	226	133	23.3	4.6	2.4	0.2
Char Sui in Cantonese Sauce, Asda*	1 Pack/360g	623	173	9.8	28.4	2.2	0.5
Char Sui, Takeaway, Iceland*	1 Pack/400g	412	103	7.9	12.5	2.4	1.2
Chinese, Steaks, Shoulder, Sainsbury's*	1 Steak/100g	243	243	28.6	1.6	13.6	1.1
Chop, Asda*	1 Chop/180g	468	260	29.0	0.0	16.0	0.0
Chop, Basted, Asda*	1 Serving/100g	158	158	26.0	0.0	6.0	1.1
Chops, Shoulder, Sainsbury's*	1 Serving/150g	348	232	25.9	0.0	14.3	0.0
Diced, Healthy Eating, Tesco*	1 Serving/75g	83	110	21.3	0.0	2.7	0.0
Fillet, BGTY, Sainsbury's*	½ Pack/175g	256	146	30.9	0.1	2.5	0.1
Joint With Herbes de Provence, Sainsbury's*	¼ Joint/200g	302	151	19.2	0.1	8.2	0.6
Joint With Leek & Cheese Stuffing, Sainsbury's*	1 Serving/100g	231	231	31.0	3.0	10.5	1.1
Leg, Diced, Waitrose*	1oz/28g	30	108	22.8	0.0	0.8	0.0
Leg, Joint, Marks & Spencer*	¼ Pack/125g	138	110	19.9	0.4	3.1	0.0
Lemon & Thyme, TTD, Sainsbury's*	1 Serving/67g	159	238	19.8	5.6	15.2	0.3
Loin, Joint, Raw, Lean & Fat	1oz/28g	69	246	19.3	0.0	18.8	0.0
Loin, Oak Smoked, Sainsbury's*	1 Slice/12.5g	21	163	24.0	0.9	7.0	0.1
Loin, Steak, Fried, Lean	1oz/28g	53	191	31.5	0.0	7.2	0.0
Loin, Steak, Fried, Lean & Fat	1oz/28g	77	276	27.5	0.0	18.4	0.0
Loin, Steak, Marks & Spencer*	1 Serving/125g	281	225	19.9	0.0	16.1	0.0
Loin, Steak, Raw, Lean & Fat	1oz/28g	63	225	19.9	0.0	16.1	0.0
Loin, Steak, Sainsbury's*	1 Serving/74g	167	225	26.1	0.3	13.3	0.8
Lunch Tongue, Tesco*	1 Serving/125g	228	182	20.4	0.8	10.8	0.0
Medaliions, Healthy Eating, Tesco*	1 Serving/113.5g	125	110	21.3	0.0	2.7	0.0
Mince, Extra Lean, BGTY, Sainsbury's*	1 Serving/227g	320	141	19.3	0.1	7.1	0.6
Mince, Healthy Eating, Tesco*	1 Pack/400g	444	111	20.2	0.7	3.0	0.0
Mince, Raw	1oz/28g	46	164	19.2	0.0	9.7	0.0
Oven Roast, Asda*	1oz/28g	32	114	22.3	0.0	2.8	0.0
Ribsters, Quorn*	2 Ribsters/83.9g	99	118	15.9	4.8	3.9	2.8
Steak, Raw, Lean	1oz/28g	34	120	22.4	0.0	3.4	0.0
Steak, Raw, Lean & Fat	1oz/28g	47	169	21.0	0.0	9.4	0.0
Steaks, With Honey & Mustard Sauce, Tesco*	½ Pack/160g	258	161	16.3	7.3	7.4	1.4

P

	Measure INFO/WEIGHT	per Measure KCAL	Nutrition Values per 100g / 100ml				
			KCAL	PROT	CARB	FAT	FIBRE
PORK,							
Strips, Stir Fry, Healthy Eating, Tesco*	1 Pack/300g	330	110	21.3	0.0	2.7	0.0
Tongue, Lunch, Asda*	1 Slice/21g	37	175	21.4	1.5	9.3	0.0
Tongue, Lunch, Sainsbury's*	1 Slice/15.5g	31	193	19.2	1.8	12.1	0.0
Trimmed, Lean, Raw	1oz/28g	34	123	21.8	0.0	4.0	0.0
PORK &,							
Chestnut Stuffing, Marks & Spencer*	1oz/28g	64	230	5.3	12.6	17.1	3.7
Ham, Chopped, Spam*	1 Serving/100g	296	296	14.5	3.2	24.2	0.0
PORK - CHINESE, Steak, Asda*	1 Serving/250g	508	203	22.0	4.0	11.0	1.3
PORK - ESCALOPE,							
BGTY, Sainsbury's*	½ Pack/200g	274	137	31.1	0.0	1.4	0.0
British, Healthy Eating, Tesco*	1 Escalope/125g	138	110	21.3	0.0	2.7	0.0
GFY, Asda*	1 Escalope/120g	182	152	31.0	0.0	3.1	0.0
PORK - GRILLED,							
Steak, Lean	1oz/28g	47	169	33.9	0.0	3.7	0.0
Steak, Lean & Fat	1oz/28g	55	198	32.4	0.0	7.6	0.0
PORK - HONEY ROAST, Loin, Sainsbury's*	1 Slice/12g	20	165	23.6	2.7	6.6	0.1
PORK - HOT & SPICY, Steak, Shoulder, Waitrose*	1 Steak/100g	207	207	19.5	1.3	13.7	0.0
PORK - MEDALLIONS, Loin, BGTY, Sainsbury's*	1 Pack/220g	142	129	27.2	0.0	2.2	0.8
PORK - ROAST,							
Cured, British, Loin, Marks & Spencer*	1 Slice/10g	14	140	25.2	0.7	4.4	0.0
Dinner, Bird's Eye*	1 Pack/362g	340	94	7.5	10.9	2.3	1.4
Loin, Joint, Lean	1oz/28g	51	182	30.1	0.0	6.8	0.0
Loin, Joint, Lean & Fat	1oz/28g	71	253	26.3	0.0	16.4	0.0
Loin, Stuffed, Marks & Spencer*	1 Slice/12g	22	180	24.4	2.4	7.9	0.0
PORK - ROULADE, Tenderloin, Waitrose*	1 Pack/171g	282	165	18.4	5.9	7.5	1.8
PORK - SLICES,							
Roast, Co-Op*	1 Slice/30g	38	125	22.0	0.0	4.0	0.0
Roast, Safeway*	1 Slice/28g	40	142	23.4	0.9	5.0	0.0
PORK - SMOKED, Cured, Loin, Marks & Spencer*	1oz/28g	43	155	18.1	0.0	9.1	0.0
PORK - STEWED,							
Mince	1oz/28g	53	191	24.4	0.0	10.4	0.0
Steak, Lean	1oz/28g	49	176	33.6	0.0	4.6	0.0
Steak, Lean & Fat	1oz/28g	56	199	31.0	0.0	8.3	0.0
PORK SCRATCHINGS,							
KP*	1 Pack/20g	125	624	47.3	0.5	48.1	0.5
Tavern Snacks*	1 Pack/30g	187	624	47.3	0.5	48.1	0.5
PORK WITH,							
Sage & Onion Stuffing, Joint, BGTY, Sainsbury's*	1 Serving/150g	246	164	29.5	3.3	3.6	1.3
Sage, Onion & Lemon Stuffing, Joint, Sainsbury's*	1 Serving/260g	699	269	27.4	2.2	16.7	1.4
PORT, Average	1 Serving/50ml	79	157	0.1	12.0	0.0	0.0
POT NOODLE*,							
Beef & Tomato	1 Pot/90g	382	424	10.7	60.3	15.5	3.7
Chow Mein	1 Pot/89g	385	433	11.6	60.5	16.0	2.7
Nice'n'Spicy	1 Pot/87g	380	437	9.7	61.5	16.9	2.7
Spicy Curry	1 Pot/89g	379	426	9.8	61.5	15.6	3.0
Sweet & Sour	1 Pot/86g	376	437	9.4	63.2	16.2	2.7
POT RICE,							
Chicken & Sweetcorn, Pot Rice*	1 Pot/68g	243	357	13.1	65.8	4.6	4.0
Chicken Curry, Pot Rice*	1 Pot/74g	253	342	11.0	67.2	2.3	3.3
POT AU CHOCOLAT, COU, Marks & Spencer*	1 Serving/120g	168	140	5.6	26.4	2.1	1.1
POTATO,							
Boulangere, Marks & Spencer*	½ Pack/225g	180	80	2.8	15.9	0.9	0.9
Hasselback, Sainsbury's*	½ Pack/149g	155	104	1.9	22.0	0.9	2.9

P

	Measure INFO/WEIGHT	per Measure KCAL	Nutrition Values per 100g / 100ml				
			KCAL	PROT	CARB	FAT	FIBRE
POTATO,							
New, Butter & Parsley & Chives & Mint, Marks & Spencer*	1 Sm Pack/180g	162	90	1.4	12.8	3.5	1.3
Simply Mash, COU, Marks & Spencer*	½ Pack/225g	169	75	1.5	12.1	2.2	1.6
POTATO - BAKE,							
Cheese & Bacon, Homepride*	1 Serving/210g	277	132	1.6	3.2	12.5	0.0
Cheese & Onion, Tesco*	1 Pack/400g	376	94	2.4	10.0	4.9	1.0
Garlic & Herb, Homepride*	1 Serving/100g	148	148	0.7	4.2	14.2	0.0
POTATO - BAKE MIX,							
Creamy Cheddar Cheese, Colman's*	1 Pack/45g	189	420	11.5	34.8	26.0	9.6
Ham & Leek, Colman's*	1 Pack/44g	181	412	9.9	40.4	24.0	2.1
POTATO - BAKED,							
Chicken & Mushroom, Homepride*	1 Serving/105g	128	122	2.3	1.9	11.7	0.0
Healthy Eating, Tesco*	1 Potato/200g	222	111	3.5	19.7	2.0	1.9
Leek & Cheese, Marks & Spencer*	1 Serving/206g	206	100	3.8	13.4	3.1	3.2
Safeway*	1 Serving/200g	230	115	4.6	10.3	6.2	2.5
Tesco*	1 Serving/175g	138	79	2.0	17.3	0.2	1.3
Waitrose*	1 Serving/100g	157	157	3.0	17.9	8.1	1.5
With Bacon, Finest, Tesco*	1 Pack/400g	484	121	3.7	15.1	5.2	0.9
With Cheddar Cheese, COU, Marks & Spencer*	1 Potato/164g	164	100	2.9	17.3	1.9	2.0
With Cheddar Cheese, Farmfoods*	1 Potato/143g	196	137	4.7	21.0	3.8	1.9
With Cheese, Healthy Eating, Tesco*	1 Potato/200g	222	111	3.5	19.7	2.0	1.9
With Cheese, Safeway*	1 Serving/100g	119	119	4.7	10.6	6.4	2.6
With Cheese, Tesco*	1 Pack/400g	448	112	2.7	18.7	2.9	1.0
With Chilli Con Carne, Eat Smart, Safeway*	1 Serving/300g	225	75	6.1	8.9	1.3	1.9
With Chilli, COU, Marks & Spencer*	1 Pack/300g	270	90	6.0	11.0	2.1	1.2
With Tuna & Sweetcorn, COU, Marks & Spencer*	1 Pack/300g	270	90	5.1	12.8	1.8	1.4
POTATO - BOMBAY,							
Asda*	½ Can/196.0g	198	101	2.0	12.0	5.0	1.1
Canned, Tesco*	1 Can/400g	296	74	1.6	11.9	2.2	0.7
Eat Smart, Safeway*	1 Serving/225g	124	55	1.3	7.3	1.9	2.3
Indian Takeaway For 1, Sainsbury's*	1 Serving/200g	202	101	1.8	11.8	5.2	1.7
Marks & Spencer*	1 Pack/300g	300	100	1.5	12.1	4.8	1.6
Meal Solutions, Co-Op*	1 Pack/300g	210	70	1.0	8.0	4.0	2.0
Mild, Flavour Of India, Sainsbury's*	½ Can/200g	166	83	2.0	13.0	2.5	1.4
Sainsbury's*	1 Pack/300g	303	101	1.8	11.8	5.2	1.7
Tesco*	1 Pack/350g	413	118	1.8	13.5	6.4	1.1
Waitrose*	1 Pack/300g	246	82	1.6	9.3	4.3	2.2
POTATO - CAKES,							
Asda*	1 Cake/70.4g	118	169	2.4	37.0	1.3	1.0
Fried in Vegetable Oil	1oz/28g	59	210	3.9	31.4	8.5	1.6
Rosti, Marks & Spencer*	1 Serving/100g	140	140	1.5	16.8	7.5	1.8
Sainsbury's*	1 Cake/65g	114	176	4.3	36.2	1.6	3.2
Toasted, Tesco*	1 Cake/58g	116	200	4.4	40.5	2.3	2.2
Warburton's*	1 Cake/45g	119	264	5.9	38.6	9.6	0.0
POTATO - CREAMED, With Cabbage, Asda*	1 Pack/350g	256	73	1.3	11.0	2.6	0.0
POTATO - FARLS, Marks & Spencer*	1 Farl/55g	79	144	4.2	33.8	0.4	4.7
POTATO - FRIED, Crispy, Marks & Spencer*	1 Pack/400g	660	165	2.0	22.6	7.1	1.4
POTATO - FRITTERS,							
Crispy, Bird's Eye*	1 Fritter/20g	29	145	2.0	16.3	8.0	1.2
With Sweetcorn, Marks & Spencer*	1 Pack/135g	304	225	4.4	24.1	12.6	2.3
POTATO - INSTANT,							
Mash, SmartPrice, Dry, Asda*	½ Pack/60g	209	349	8.0	78.0	0.5	7.0
Mashed, Good Choice, Made Up, Iceland*	1 Serving/100g	69	69	1.7	15.3	0.1	1.8
Mashed, Made Up With Water, Smash*	1 Serving/160g	96	60	1.4	13.2	0.2	0.6

P

	Measure INFO/WEIGHT	per Measure KCAL	Nutrition Values per 100g / 100ml				
			KCAL	PROT	CARB	FAT	FIBRE
POTATO - INSTANT,							
Mashed, Made Up, Safeway*	1 Pack/669.7g	442	66	1.3	15.0	0.1	0.8
Mashed, Made Up Sainsbury's*	1 Serving/210g	151	72	2.4	15.0	0.3	1.9
Powder, Made Up With Water	1 Serving/180g	103	57	1.5	13.5	0.1	1.0
POTATO - JACKET,							
Baked Bean & Sausage, Asda*	1 Pack/300g	447	149	5.0	25.0	3.2	2.7
Beef Chilli, Asda*	1 Pack/300g	372	124	5.0	22.0	1.8	2.1
Cheese & Beans, Somerfield*	1 Pack/338.9g	305	90	4.1	13.8	2.0	2.2
Cheese & Butter, Tesco*	1 Potato/200g	214	107	4.2	14.6	3.5	1.0
Cheese Filled, Farmfoods*	2 Halves/255g	349	137	4.7	21.0	3.8	1.9
Cheesy, GFY, Asda*	1 Serving/155g	129	83	2.6	16.0	1.0	2.1
Con Carne, Somerfield*	1 Pack/340g	319	94	5.5	10.3	3.4	1.2
Creamy Mushroom, Asda*	1 Serving/100g	124	124	3.5	22.0	2.4	1.7
Halves, Marks & Spencer*	1 Serving/250g	188	75	2.0	14.2	1.1	1.7
Spicy Chilli Con Carne, Spar*	1 Pack/340g	265	78	3.4	12.4	1.6	1.5
Tuna & Sweetcorn, Deep Filled, Marks & Spencer*	1 Pack/300g	270	90	4.9	13.1	2.2	1.2
Tuna & Sweetcorn, Somerfield*	1 Pack/340g	333	98	3.2	12.5	3.9	1.0
With Baked Beans & Mozzarella, Eat Smart, Safeway*	1 Pack/283g	255	90	5.8	12.8	1.4	2.3
With Cheese Mash, Good For You, Asda*	1 Potato/200g	194	97	2.9	17.0	1.9	0.0
With Cheese, Safeway*	1 Potato/200g	165	83	2.1	16.3	0.9	2.1
With Chicken Tikka, COU, Marks & Spencer*	1 Serving/300g	240	80	5.4	10.9	1.6	1.3
With Chilli Con Carne, COU, Marks & Spencer*	1 Potato/300g	270	90	6.0	11.0	2.1	1.2
With Chilli Con Carne, Eat Smart, Safeway*	1 Pack/300g	225	75	6.1	8.9	1.3	1.9
With Chilli Con Carne, Pro Cuisine*	1 Pack/340g	347	102	4.6	18.7	1.0	0.0
With Chilli, BGTY, Sainsbury's*	1 Pack/350g	319	91	5.3	14.3	1.4	1.2
With Garlic Butter Filling, Morrisons*	1 Potato/210g	239	114	1.7	13.6	5.9	0.9
With Garlic Butter, Mini, Safeway*	1 Pack/450g	495	110	1.8	14.6	4.6	2.4
With Garlic Mushrooms, BGTY Sainsbury's*	1 Pack/350g	263	75	2.3	14.4	0.9	1.2
With Garlic Mushrooms, Eat Smart, Safeway*	1 Pack/300g	210	70	2.7	8.1	2.7	1.6
Garlic, Mini, Asda*	1 Serving/65g	59	91	2.2	13.0	3.3	0.0
With Herb & Rock Salt Seasoning, Marks & Spencer*	1 Pack/500g	375	75	2.0	14.2	1.1	1.7
With Spicy Mushroom & Onion, Marks & Spencer*	1 Pack/300g	210	70	2.2	13.9	0.8	1.2
With Tuna & Sweetcorn, BGTY, Sainsbury's*	1 Pack/350g	361	103	6.5	13.2	2.7	1.3
With Tuna & Sweetcorn, COU, Marks & Spencer*	1 Pack/300g	270	90	5.1	12.8	1.8	1.4
With Tuna & Sweetcorn, Eat Smart, Safeway*	1 Pack/300g	240	80	5.3	10.3	1.9	1.4
POTATO - MASH,							
Bacon & Spring Onion, Finest, Tesco*	½ Pack/200g	214	107	4.3	10.8	5.2	1.6
Cabbage & Spring Onion, COU, Marks & Spencer*	1 Serving/225g	180	80	1.7	11.8	2.5	1.9
Cabbage & Spring Onion, Sainsbury's*	½ Pack/225g	279	124	2.0	14.8	6.3	1.1
Carrot & Swede, Sainsbury's*	½ Pack/225g	230	102	1.9	11.7	5.3	1.5
Cheddar, Tesco*	1 Pack/500g	555	111	2.7	13.0	5.4	1.0
Creamy, Finest, Tesco*	½ Pack/250g	373	149	2.0	12.4	10.1	1.2
Fresh, Tesco*	1 Pack/400g	368	92	2.1	11.1	4.4	1.9
Fresh, With Butter, Sainsbury's*	½ Pack/225g	290	129	1.5	15.4	6.8	1.1
Leek & Cheese, COU, Marks & Spencer*	½ Pack/225g	180	80	3.0	12.0	2.1	1.3
Maris Piper With Cream & Butter, Marks & Spencer*	½ Pack/200g	180	90	1.1	12.9	3.6	0.4
Maris Piper, Sainsbury's*	1 Serving/225g	290	129	1.5	15.4	6.8	1.1
Mustard, With Caramelised Onions, Finest, Tesco*	1 Serving/200g	232	116	2.6	16.0	4.6	1.8
Olive Oil, Healthy Eating, Tesco*	1 Serving/100g	90	90	2.1	15.5	2.2	0.9
Sun Dried Tomato & Basil, COU, Marks & Spencer*	1 Serving/170g	128	75	1.0	14.4	1.5	1.2
Tesco*	½ Pack/200g	184	92	2.1	11.1	4.4	1.9
With Leeks, Creamy, Bird's Eye*	1 Pack/300g	300	100	2.0	7.3	7.0	0.8
POTATO - MASHED,							
Asda*	1 Serving/175g	159	91	1.8	16.0	2.2	1.1

INFO/WEIGHT	Measure per Measure KCAL	KCAL	PROT	CARB	FAT	FIBRE

	Measure INFO/WEIGHT	per Measure KCAL	Nutrition Values per 100g / 100ml			
			KCAL	PROT	CARB	FAT	FIBRE

POTATO - MASHED,

	Measure INFO/WEIGHT	per Measure KCAL	KCAL	PROT	CARB	FAT	FIBRE
Creamy, Fresh, Waitrose*	1 Serving/200g	164	82	1.9	14.2	1.9	1.1
Fresh, Sainsbury's*	½ Pot/200g	192	96	2.0	14.6	2.8	1.0
Frozen, Aunt Bessie's*	1 Serving/250g	288	115	1.9	14.3	5.1	1.3
Frozen, Good Choice, Iceland*	1 Serving/200g	138	69	1.7	15.3	0.1	1.8
Frozen, Sainsbury's*	1/3 Pack/228g	249	109	1.7	13.4	5.4	2.3
Good For You, Asda*	½ Pack/200g	176	88	1.9	17.0	1.4	0.0
Homestyle, Aunt Bessie's*	1 Serving/200g	230	115	1.9	14.3	5.1	1.3
Spring Onion, Iceland*	1 Serving/230g	209	91	2.0	14.0	3.0	3.0
With Butter, Old	1oz/28g	29	104	1.8	15.5	4.3	1.1
With Fried Onion, Smash*	½ Pack/269g	191	71	1.6	13.4	1.3	0.7
With Margarine, Old	1oz/28g	29	104	1.8	15.5	4.3	1.1

POTATO - ROAST,

	Measure INFO/WEIGHT	per Measure KCAL	KCAL	PROT	CARB	FAT	FIBRE
BGTY, Sainsbury's*	1 Serving/100g	145	145	2.2	23.9	4.5	2.0
Baby, Finest, Tesco*	½ Pack/150g	149	99	3.6	15.1	2.7	1.4
COU, Marks & Spencer*	½ Pack/150g	158	105	2.2	18.1	2.6	3.3
Crispy, Aunt Bessie's*	1 Serving/83g	154	185	2.3	22.9	9.3	1.8
Crispy, Cooked, Marks & Spencer*	1 Serving/85g	94	110	1.6	21.2	2.1	1.2
Deep Fried, McCain*	1oz/28g	47	167	3.0	22.5	7.2	0.0
Frozen, Asda*	1 Serving/100g	188	188	2.6	22.0	10.0	0.8
Garlic, Somerfield*	1 Pack/320g	422	132	2.0	20.0	5.0	0.0
Good Choice, Iceland*	1 Serving/100g	143	143	2.7	29.5	1.6	1.5
Home Roasts, Crispy, McCain*	1 Serving/75g	95	126	2.2	23.6	3.6	0.0
Marks & Spencer*	½ Pack/150g	180	120	2.4	19.9	3.2	2.8
Oven Baked, McCain*	1oz/28g	31	109	2.6	21.6	1.4	0.0
Pepper & Basil Layer, Safeway*	1 Pack/260g	195	75	1.7	8.8	3.4	1.9
Traditional, Iceland*	1 Serving/100g	182	182	3.3	27.8	6.4	1.8
¼ Cut, Deep Fried, McCain*	1oz/28g	45	161	3.1	22.5	6.5	0.0
¼ Cut, Oven Baked, McCain*	1oz/28g	42	149	3.5	25.9	3.5	0.0

POTATO - SAUTE,

	Measure INFO/WEIGHT	per Measure KCAL	KCAL	PROT	CARB	FAT	FIBRE
Deep Fried, McCain*	1oz/28g	47	167	2.6	23.3	7.0	0.0
Oven Baked, McCain*	1oz/28g	56	199	4.4	36.9	3.8	0.0

POTATO - SKINS,

	Measure INFO/WEIGHT	per Measure KCAL	KCAL	PROT	CARB	FAT	FIBRE
Cheddar & Bacon Snack Chips, T.G.I. Friday's*	1 Serving/28g	42	150	0.0	17.0	9.0	1.0
Cheese & Bacon, Tesco*	1 Serving/95g	241	254	9.2	19.5	15.5	3.0
Loaded, American, Asda*	1 Serving/78.4g	293	375	15.0	27.0	23.0	2.4
Loaded, Cheese & Bacon, Bird's Eye*	2 Skins/120g	236	197	6.6	21.6	9.3	2.1
Loaded, Healthy Eating, Tesco*	1 Serving/340g	425	125	7.7	17.9	2.5	0.6
Loaded, New York Style, Tesco*	1 Burger/35g	89	254	9.2	19.5	15.5	3.0
Loaded, With Cheese & Bacon, Asda*	1 Serving/253.2g	314	124	6.0	16.0	4.0	2.3
Loaded, With Soured Cream, Marks & Spencer*	½ Pack/150g	308	205	9.1	15.8	11.9	0.9

POTATO - SLICES,

	Measure INFO/WEIGHT	per Measure KCAL	KCAL	PROT	CARB	FAT	FIBRE
Crispy, Marks & Spencer*	1oz/28g	55	195	3.2	20.2	11.3	2.8
Garlic & Herb, Heinz*	1oz/28g	23	82	1.7	10.2	3.9	0.7

POTATO - SMILES,

	Measure INFO/WEIGHT	per Measure KCAL	KCAL	PROT	CARB	FAT	FIBRE
Deep Fried, McCain*	1oz/28g	64	227	3.7	31.3	9.7	0.0
Oven Baked, McCain*	1oz/28g	62	220	3.9	31.9	8.6	0.0

POTATO - WAFFLES,

	Measure INFO/WEIGHT	per Measure KCAL	KCAL	PROT	CARB	FAT	FIBRE
Bird's Eye*	1 Waffle/56g	94	167	2.0	20.7	8.5	1.5
Frozen, Grilled, Asda*	1 Waffle/57g	104	183	2.0	21.0	10.1	1.7
Mini, Sainsbury's*	1 Waffle/11g	27	242	2.8	20.1	16.7	1.0
Mini, Baked, McCain*	1oz/28g	62	221	3.9	32.0	8.6	0.0
Tesco*	1 Waffle/56g	97	174	2.4	23.8	7.7	0.8

P

POTATO - WEDGES,	Measure INFO/WEIGHT	per Measure KCAL	KCAL	PROT	CARB	FAT	FIBRE
& Dip, Marks & Spencer*	1 Pack/450g	698	155	2.5	20.4	7.4	1.8
BBQ Flavour, Asda*	1 Serving/100g	185	185	2.9	23.0	9.0	1.7
BGTY, Sainsbury's*	½ Pack/190g	179	94	3.0	16.4	1.8	3.4
Baked, GFY, Asda*	1 Pack/450g	630	140	2.2	23.0	4.4	1.9
Bombay With Yoghurt & Mint Dip, Healthy Living, Tesco*	1 Serving/170g	139	82	1.3	14.5	2.1	0.9
Chunky, McCain*	10 Wedges/175g	242	138	2.4	23.3	4.7	0.0
Domino's Pizza*	1 Serving/198g	428	216	4.1	30.3	8.7	0.0
Frozen, Tesco*	1 Serving/200g	262	131	2.0	22.4	3.7	1.8
Garlic & Herb, COU, Marks & Spencer*	1 Pack/300g	300	100	2.3	16.4	2.6	3.2
Garlic & Herb, Kitchen Range Foods*	1oz/28g	42	151	1.6	18.5	7.8	0.0
Hot & Spicy With Salsa Dip, Healthy Living, Tesco*	1 Serving/170g	112	66	1.1	12.4	1.3	1.4
Hot & Spicy, Frozen, Sainsbury's*	1 Serving/70g	98	140	2.8	23.7	3.8	2.0
In BBQ Sauce, Micro, McCain*	1 Box/200g	234	117	2.2	23.5	2.4	0.0
McDonald's	1 Portion/176g	368	208	3.3	26.1	10.1	2.2
Micro, Tesco*	1 Pack/100g	170	170	2.6	24.5	6.8	2.3
New York Style, Healthy Eating, Tesco*	½ Pack/125g	124	99	2.3	16.4	2.7	1.3
Oven Baked, Waitrose*	1oz/28g	46	165	2.4	29.2	4.3	2.1
Savoury, McCain*	1 Serving/200g	300	150	2.9	22.7	6.2	0.0
Savoury, Waitrose*	1/3 Bag/250g	350	140	2.3	22.9	4.3	1.9
Sour Cream & Chives, McCain*	1 Serving/100g	132	132	2.4	24.0	4.1	0.0
Southern Fried Style, Tesco*	1 Serving/155g	233	150	3.0	14.1	9.1	2.0
Southern Fried, Asda*	1 Serving/188g	263	140	2.9	23.0	4.0	1.8
Spicy, Asda*	1 Serving/100g	145	145	1.8	21.8	5.7	2.1
Spicy, & Garlic Dip, Linda McCartney*	1 Pack/300g	366	122	2.6	15.3	5.6	3.1
Spicy, American Style, Sainsbury's*	½ Pack/155.7g	190	122	3.0	20.1	3.3	3.5
Spicy, Deep Fried, McCain*	1oz/28g	52	187	3.6	27.3	8.1	0.0
Spicy, Marks & Spencer*	½ Pack/225g	349	155	2.4	21.8	6.5	1.3
Spicy, Occasions, Sainsbury's*	1 Serving/100g	144	144	2.5	23.7	4.3	0.4
Spicy, Oven Baked, McCain*	1oz/28g	61	219	4.2	34.8	8.4	0.0
Spicy, Simple Solutions, Tesco*	1 Serving/150g	141	94	4.6	12.2	3.0	1.4
With Broccoli & Mozzarella Cheese, Weight Watchers*	1 Pack/320g	294	92	3.1	13.3	3.0	1.0
With Garlic & Herb, Ready to Roast, Sainsbury's*	½ Pack/150g	239	159	2.4	25.7	5.2	2.1
With Soured Cream & Chive Dip, Safeway*	1 Pack/450g	639	142	3.1	22.1	4.6	2.1
POTATO CHIPS,							
Ready Salted, Sainsbury's*	¼ Pack/33g	174	526	5.6	51.7	33.0	3.8
Reduced Fat, Cape Cod*	1 Bag/140g	664	474	7.9	53.5	25.4	6.4
POTATOES,							
Anya, Sainsbury's*	1 Serving/100g	80	80	1.4	19.7	0.1	1.0
Baked, Flesh & Skin	1 Med/180g	245	136	3.9	31.7	0.2	2.7
Baked, Flesh Only	1 Med/160g	123	77	2.2	18.0	0.1	1.4
Baking, Tesco*	1 Potato/200g	158	79	2.0	17.3	0.2	1.3
British White, Tesco*	1 Serving/100g	79	79	2.1	17.2	0.2	1.3
Charlotte, Baby, Tesco*	1 Serving/184g	136	74	1.7	16.1	0.3	10.0
Charlotte, Sainsbury's*	1 Serving/100g	80	80	1.4	19.7	0.1	1.0
Crispy, With Smoked Bacon & Rosemary, Sainsbury's*	½ Pack/200g	282	141	4.2	16.2	6.6	1.9
Dauphinois, Sainsbury's*	½ Can/200g	176	88	1.8	10.9	4.1	0.6
Dauphinoise, Finest, Tesco*	1 Serving/200g	332	166	2.2	14.7	10.9	0.8
Dauphinoise, Waitrose*	½ Pack/210g	355	169	2.2	10.8	13.0	2.2
Desiree, Safeway*	1 Serving/200g	146	73	2.1	15.7	0.2	0.0
Garlic, Tapas Selection, Sainsbury's*	1 Serving/22g	49	224	2.6	10.4	19.1	0.7
Hasselback, Asda*	1 Serving/175g	182	104	1.9	22.0	0.9	2.9
Jacket Wedges, Sainsbury's*	1 Serving/100g	151	151	3.0	27.3	3.3	2.6
Jersey Royal, Asda*	1 Can/186g	108	58	1.3	13.0	0.1	2.1

P

INFO/WEIGHT	Measure	per Measure KCAL	Nutrition Values per 100g / 100ml KCAL	PROT	CARB	FAT	FIBRE
POTATOES,							
Jersey, New, Canned, Sainsbury's*	1 Can/191g	128	67	1.5	15.1	0.1	0.8
King Edward, Roast, Sainsbury's*	1oz/28g	50	179	2.6	20.7	9.5	0.8
Lemon & Rosemary, Finest, Tesco*	½ Pack/200g	200	100	2.1	14.7	3.7	2.0
New, Boiled in Salted Water	1oz/28g	21	75	1.5	17.8	0.3	1.1
New, Boiled in Unsalted Water	1oz/28g	21	75	1.5	17.8	0.3	1.1
New, Canned, Re-Heated, Drained	1oz/28g	18	63	1.5	15.1	0.1	0.8
New, Chipped, Fried in Corn Oil	1oz/28g	64	228	4.4	33.3	9.5	1.7
New, Crushed, The Best, Safeway*	1 Pack/400g	440	110	2.2	12.6	5.2	1.3
New, Garlic & Herb, Co-Op*	1 Serving/100g	115	115	1.0	15.0	5.0	2.0
New, In Herbs & Butter, Asda*	1 Pack/590g	637	108	1.6	17.0	3.3	1.2
New, Tinned, Sainsbury's*	1 Tin/359.9g	241	67	1.5	15.1	0.1	0.8
New, Tinned, SmartPrice, Asda*	1 Serving/100g	56	56	1.3	13.0	0.1	2.1
New, in Salt Water, Value, Tesco*	1 Can/345g	217	63	1.7	13.8	0.1	0.8
New, in Salted Water, Hartley's*	1 Pack/172g	98	57	1.3	12.6	0.1	0.8
New, in Skins, Boiled in Salted Water	1oz/28g	18	66	1.4	15.4	0.3	1.5
New, in Skins, Boiled in Unsalted Water	1oz/28g	18	66	1.4	15.4	0.3	1.5
New, in a Herb Marinade, Tesco*	¼ Pack/150g	152	101	1.3	13.0	4.9	1.5
Old, Average, Raw	1oz/28g	21	75	2.1	17.2	0.2	1.3
Old, Boiled in Salted Water	1oz/28g	20	72	1.8	17.0	0.1	1.2
Old, Boiled in Unsalted Water	1oz/28g	20	72	1.8	17.0	0.1	1.2
Old, Roast in Blended Oil	1oz/28g	42	149	2.9	25.9	4.5	1.8
Old, Roast in Lard	1oz/28g	42	149	2.9	25.9	4.5	1.8
Ramano Red, Waitrose*	1 Serving/190g	139	73	2.1	15.7	0.2	1.3
Red, Sainsbury's*	1 Serving/300g	216	72	1.8	17.0	0.1	1.2
Roasting, Ovenbaked, Iceland*	1 Serving/150g	192	128	2.1	21.2	3.9	1.9
Rosemary & Garlic, Waitrose*	1 Serving/150g	237	158	3.8	30.7	2.2	2.9
Rosemary, Ready to Bake, Marks & Spencer*	½ Pack/150g	150	100	3.0	16.0	2.4	1.4
POTATOES WITH,							
Butter & Herbs, Baby, Sainsbury's*	¼ Pack/141g	135	96	1.4	14.7	3.5	1.5
Butter, Parsley, Chives & Mint, New, Marks & Spencer*	1 Serving/100g	80	80	1.6	9.7	3.7	1.5
Garlic & Rosemary, Roasted, Safeway*	½ Pack/175g	263	150	2.6	21.9	5.7	2.7
Herb Butter, Baby, Safeway*	1 Serving/200g	158	79	1.4	15.6	1.2	1.4
Parsley Butter, New, TTD, Sainsbury's*	1 Serving/150g	126	84	2.2	13.3	2.4	1.0
Sunblush Tomato, New, Marks & Spencer*	1 Pack/385g	347	90	1.6	17.2	1.8	1.3
POUSSIN, Raw, Meat & Skin	1oz/28g	57	202	19.1	0.0	13.9	0.0
POWERADE, Ice Storm, The Coca Cola Co*	1 Bottle/500ml	120	24	0.0	6.0	0.0	0.0
PRAWN BHUNA, Tandoori, Indian, Sainsbury's*	½ Pack/200g	152	76	5.5	4.5	4.0	1.7
PRAWN COCKTAIL,							
BGTY, Sainsbury's*	1oz/28g	45	160	7.5	2.3	13.4	0.5
Better For You, Morrisons*	1 Serving/100g	149	149	4.7	9.7	10.3	0.1
COU, Marks & Spencer*	1oz/28g	24	85	11.6	4.9	2.2	0.5
Light, Asda*	1oz/28g	45	160	9.9	4.8	11.2	0.0
Marks & Spencer*	1oz/28g	97	345	8.7	3.0	33.1	1.2
Reduced Fat, Marks & Spencer*	1oz/28g	43	152	9.1	2.9	11.6	1.1
Reduced Fat, Tesco*	1 Serving/200g	304	152	7.6	6.5	10.6	0.4
Safeway*	½ Pot/100g	373	373	7.6	3.4	36.5	0.2
Sainsbury's*	1 Serving/200g	706	353	7.9	2.7	34.5	0.5
Tesco*	1 Tub/200g	834	417	7.3	3.5	41.5	0.1
PRAWN CRACKERS,							
Asda*	1 Serving/25g	134	535	2.0	53.0	35.0	0.0
Marks & Spencer*	1 Pack/15g	83	550	3.0	62.3	32.0	0.0
Sainsbury's*	1 Cracker/3g	16	537	2.4	60.4	31.7	0.8
Tesco*	1/3 Pack/20g	114	568	3.7	44.0	41.9	0.5

P

	Measure INFO/WEIGHT	per Measure KCAL	Nutrition Values per 100g / 100ml				
			KCAL	PROT	CARB	FAT	FIBRE
PRAWN CRACKERS,							
Uncooked, Sharwood's*	1oz/28g	136	487	0.7	52.7	29.7	1.7
PRAWN CREOLE, Spicy, BGTY, Sainsbury's*	1 Pack/400g	436	109	4.2	20.9	0.9	0.4
PRAWN GULNARI, With Rice, COU, Marks & Spencer*	1 Pack/400g	400	100	4.0	18.7	0.8	1.6
PRAWN MASALA, King, Waitrose*	1 Pack/350g	385	110	7.1	3.8	7.4	1.8
PRAWN TOAST,							
Chinese Snack Selection, Mini, Tesco*	1 Toast/11g	36	330	9.4	18.8	24.2	1.9
Dim Sum Selection, Sainsbury's*	1 Toast/8g	23	283	9.9	19.2	18.5	2.0
Sesame, Occasions, Sainsbury's*	1 Toast/12.0g	34	283	9.9	19.2	18.5	2.0
Waitrose*	1 Toast/21g	47	223	9.7	7.4	17.2	5.8
PRAWNS,							
Batter Crisp, Lyons*	1 Pack/160g	350	219	8.0	18.2	12.7	1.1
Black Tiger, Raw, Asda*	1oz/28g	20	71	17.4	0.0	0.1	0.0
Boiled	1 Prawn/3g	3	99	22.6	0.0	0.9	0.0
Chilli & Coriander, Marks & Spencer*	1 Serving/70g	67	95	17.9	0.6	2.2	0.6
Chilli, Battered, Marks & Spencer*	1oz/28g	63	225	7.2	23.8	11.5	0.5
Chilli, Marks & Spencer*	1oz/28g	22	79	17.9	0.6	0.5	0.6
Chinese, Oriental Express*	1 Serving/320g	218	68	3.2	13.8	0.6	1.9
Cold Water, Finest, Tesco*	1oz/28g	18	66	14.3	0.1	0.2	0.1
Cooked & Peeled, Asda*	1 Serving/100g	72	72	16.0	0.0	0.9	0.0
Cooked & Peeled, Frozen, Tesco*	1 Serving/100g	99	99	22.6	0.0	0.9	0.0
Cooked & Peeled, Somerfield*	1oz/28g	18	66	14.0	0.0	1.0	0.0
Cooked & Peeled, Tesco*	1 Serving/75g	54	72	15.6	1.0	0.6	0.1
Dried	1oz/28g	79	281	62.4	0.0	3.5	0.0
Extra Large, Frozen, North Atlantic, TTD, Sainsbury's*	1 Serving/106g	82	77	17.0	0.1	1.0	0.1
Extra Large, Marks & Spencer*	1oz/28g	27	97	21.0	0.2	1.4	0.0
Filo & Breaded Wrapped, Marks & Spencer*	1 Serving/19g	45	235	9.5	20.4	13.0	1.4
Fresh, Asda*	1 Serving/200g	176	88	21.0	1.0	0.1	0.0
Fresh, Value, Tesco*	1 Serving/80g	79	99	22.6	0.0	0.9	0.0
Honduran King, Marks & Spencer*	1 Pack/140g	112	80	18.2	0.0	1.0	0.5
Hot & Spicy, Lyons*	1oz/28g	89	318	11.0	26.1	18.9	2.8
Icelandic, Waitrose*	1 Pack/100g	107	107	22.6	0.0	1.8	0.0
In Creamy Garlic Sauce, Youngs*	1 Serving/158g	261	165	8.5	0.3	14.5	0.0
In Red Thai Curry Sauce, Youngs*	1 Pack/255g	197	77	4.8	6.5	3.4	0.8
King With Creamy Lime Dip, Waitrose*	1 Pot/230g	518	225	15.8	0.8	17.7	0.2
King, Chilli & Coriander, Sainsbury's*	1 Pack/140g	133	95	13.8	0.5	4.2	0.5
King, Extra Large, Sainsbury's*	10 Prawns/70g	53	76	14.9	1.4	1.2	0.3
King, Frozen, Tesco*	1 Bag/200g	106	53	12.6	0.0	0.3	0.0
King, In Filo, Finest, Tesco*	1 Prawn/20g	38	189	13.0	27.8	2.9	1.6
King, Japanese Noodle Box, Marks & Spencer*	1 Pack/300g	330	110	5.8	16.0	2.7	1.6
King, Jumbo, Marks & Spencer*	1 Serving/80g	56	70	13.9	0.0	1.8	0.0
King, Large, Honduran, Marks & Spencer*	1 Pack/140g	98	70	15.1	0.2	0.9	0.0
King, Marks & Spencer*	1oz/28g	19	68	15.2	0.0	0.8	0.0
King, Peeled, Marks & Spencer*	1oz/28g	19	69	15.1	0.2	0.9	0.0
King, Premium Quality, Lyons*	1 Serving/100g	69	69	15.3	0.0	0.9	0.5
King, Tiger, Cooked & Peeled, Tesco*	½ Pack/125g	96	77	17.5	0.3	0.6	0.0
North Atlantic, Farmfoods*	1oz/28g	17	60	14.0	0.0	0.4	0.0
North Atlantic, Marks & Spencer*	½ Pack/100g	95	95	20.0	0.0	1.6	0.0
Peeled, Frozen, Youngs*	1 Serving/100g	68	68	15.9	0.0	0.5	0.0
Peeled, North Atlantic, Safeway*	1 Serving/60g	38	63	14.8	0.0	0.4	0.0
Peeled, Sainsbury's*	1 Serving/125g	85	68	16.0	0.1	0.4	0.1
Peeled, Youngs*	1oz/28g	28	99	22.6	0.0	0.9	0.0
Raw, Weighed Whole With Shell	1oz/28g	21	76	17.6	0.0	0.6	0.0
Small, Sainsbury's*	1oz/28g	22	77	17.0	0.1	1.0	0.1

P

	Measure INFO/WEIGHT	per Measure KCAL	Nutrition Values per 100g / 100ml				
			KCAL	PROT	CARB	FAT	FIBRE
PRAWNS,							
Sweet & Sour, Cantonese, Easy Steam, Sainsbury's*	1 Pack/400g	424	106	4.3	16.8	2.4	3.0
Sweet Chilli Sauce, Asda*	1 Pack/360g	500	139	4.1	15.0	6.9	0.3
Sweet Chilli, With Rice, Tesco*	1 Pack/460g	488	106	2.4	19.2	2.2	0.5
Thai, Marks & Spencer*	1oz/28g	29	103	5.2	13.6	3.1	1.3
Tiger, Cooked & Peeled, Somerfield*	1 Pack/180g	122	68	15.0	0.0	1.0	0.0
Tiger, Jumbo, Asda*	1 Serving/50g	33	65	14.0	0.0	1.0	0.0
Tiger, Jumbo, Sainsbury's*	1 Serving/250g	168	67	14.9	0.1	0.8	0.0
Tiger, Marks & Spencer*	1oz/28g	19	69	15.1	0.2	0.9	0.0
Tiger, Raw, Safeway*	1 Serving/100g	67	67	14.9	0.0	0.8	0.0
Tiger, Sainsbury's*	1 Pack/250g	168	67	14.9	0.1	0.8	0.1
Tiger, Tesco*	1oz/28g	19	67	14.5	0.0	1.0	0.0
Value, Tesco*	½ Pack/175g	126	72	15.6	1.0	0.6	0.1
PRETZELS,							
American Style, Salted, Sainsbury's*	1 Serving/50g	191	381	9.6	81.8	4.0	5.2
Lightly Salted, Tesco*	1 Serving/25g	99	395	9.3	73.4	7.1	5.5
Marks & Spencer*	1 Serving/100g	375	375	10.4	73.7	4.2	4.7
Mini, Eat Smart, Safeway*	1 Bag/25g	90	360	9.6	79.7	2.5	5.5
New York Style, Salted, Mini, Shapers, Boots*	1 Serving/25g	94	375	10.0	79.0	2.1	4.2
New York Style, Shapers, Boots*	1 Bag/24g	94	391	11.0	81.0	2.5	3.8
Salt & Cracked Black Pepper, COU, Marks & Spencer*	1 Pack/25g	95	380	9.7	83.3	2.4	2.7
Salted, Safeway*	1 Serving/50g	192	383	10.3	76.0	4.2	4.6
Sea Salt & Black Pepper, Tesco*	1 Serving/50g	192	383	10.6	76.7	3.7	2.3
Sea Salt & Cracked Black Pepper, Sainsbury's*	1 Serving/50g	191	381	9.5	79.0	4.0	3.8
Snacks, The Fabulous Bakin Boys*	1 Pack/24g	96	401	9.0	79.5	4.9	2.5
Sour Cream & Onion, Marks & Spencer*	1 Pack/150g	683	455	11.0	70.9	14.5	0.7
Sour Cream & Onion, Tesco*	1 Serving/25g	114	457	8.4	67.7	17.0	2.3
With Sea Salt, Giant, Marks & Spencer*	1 Pretzel/8g	31	390	9.7	77.3	6.8	5.4
PRINGLES,							
Barbecue, Pringles*	1 Serving/50g	267	533	4.9	48.0	36.0	5.1
Cheese & Onion, Pringles*	1 Serving/50g	266	532	4.5	47.0	36.0	4.9
Curry, Pringles*	1 Serving/50g	266	531	5.2	46.0	36.0	3.4
Hot & Spicy, Pringles*	1 Serving/50g	273	546	5.0	49.0	37.0	3.3
Original, Pringles*	1 Serving/50g	274	547	4.7	47.0	38.0	5.1
Paprika, Pringles*	1 Serving/50g	268	535	5.7	46.0	36.0	5.0
Pizza, Pringles*	1 Serving/50g	268	536	5.1	43.0	37.0	4.8
Salt & Vinegar, Pringles*	1 Serving/50g	265	530	4.5	47.0	36.0	4.8
Sour Cream & Onion, Pringles*	1 Serving/50g	270	539	5.3	46.0	37.0	4.9
Sour Cream & Onion, Light, Pringles*	1 Serving/50g	233	466	5.4	56.0	25.0	4.6
PROBIOTIC DRINK, Orange, Health, Tesco*	1 Serving/100g	67	67	1.5	13.4	0.9	1.3
PROFITEROLES,							
Classic French, Sainsbury's*	1 Serving/90g	284	316	6.6	33.7	17.2	0.1
Dairy Cream, Co-Op*	¼ Pack/70g	242	345	6.0	24.0	25.0	0.5
Somerfield*	1 Serving/100g	273	273	5.0	31.0	14.0	0.0
Stack, Sainsbury's*	¼ Pack/74g	301	407	5.4	38.3	25.8	2.1
PROVAMEL*,							
Alpro Soya, Caramel Flavoured Soya Dessert	1 Pot/125g	103	82	3.0	13.7	1.7	0.3
Alpro Soya, Chocolate Flavoured Soya Dessert	1 Pot/125g	110	88	3.0	13.8	2.3	0.9
Alpro Soya, Peach Dessert	1 Pot/125g	109	87	3.8	12.4	2.2	0.3
Alpro Soya, Vanilla Flavoured Dessert	1 Pot/125g	100	80	3.0	13.0	1.8	0.0
Black Cherry Yofu	1 Pot/125g	106	85	3.7	12.9	2.1	1.2
Chocolate Dessert	1 Pot/100g	105	105	1.2	10.2	6.6	0.0
Chocolate Soya Dessert	1 Pot/125g	116	93	3.0	14.9	2.3	1.3
Fruits Of The Forest Soya Dessert	1 Serving/125g	98	78	3.0	11.9	1.8	0.3

P

	Measure INFO/WEIGHT	per Measure KCAL	Nutrition Values per 100g / 100ml				
			KCAL	PROT	CARB	FAT	FIBRE
PROVAMEL*,							
Hazelnut Soya Dessert	1 Pot/125g	126	101	3.0	16.0	2.8	1.2
Peach & Mango Yofu, Organic	1 Pot/125g	116	93	3.7	14.7	2.1	1.2
Peach & Pear Flavour Yofu, Junior	1 Pot/125g	105	84	3.8	12.4	2.2	0.0
Peach Yofu	1 Pot/125g	109	87	3.8	13.3	2.1	1.2
Red Cherry Yofu, Organic	1 Pot/125g	116	93	3.7	14.8	2.1	1.2
Soya Alternative To Milk	½ Pint/284ml	102	36	3.6	0.6	2.1	1.2
Soya Alternative To Milk, Calcium & Vitamins	1 Carton/250ml	113	45	3.6	2.9	2.1	1.0
Soya Alternative To Milk, No Added Sugar Or Salt	1 Carton/500ml	180	36	3.6	0.6	2.1	1.0
Soya Alternative To Milk, Organic	1 Carton/500ml	255	51	3.6	4.3	2.1	1.0
Soya Dream	1 Carton/250ml	445	178	3.0	1.7	17.7	1.1
Soya Milk, Chilled	1 Serving/100ml	46	46	3.7	2.8	2.1	0.3
Soya Milk, Unsweetened, Organic	1 Serving/100ml	36	36	3.7	0.4	2.1	0.3
Strawberry & Banana Flavour Yofu, Junior	1 Pot/125g	106	85	3.8	12.7	2.2	0.0
Strawberry Flavour Soya Alternative To Milk	1 Carton/250ml	160	64	3.6	7.7	2.1	1.2
Strawberry Yofu	1 Pot/125g	106	85	3.8	12.6	2.1	1.3
Vanilla Flavour Yofu	1 Pot/125g	96	77	4.1	10.0	2.3	1.3
Vanilla Soya Dessert	1 Pot/125g	108	86	3.0	14.4	1.8	1.0
Yofu, Organic	1oz/28g	15	53	4.5	2.8	2.6	1.5
Yoghurt, Peach, Alpro Soya	1 Pot/125g	109	87	3.8	12.4	2.2	0.3
PROVENCALE,							
Cabillaud à la, Weight Watchers*	1 Pack/380g	327	86	5.1	10.3	2.7	0.0
Chicken & Pasta, Easy Steam, BGTY, Sainsbury's*	1 Pack/400g	412	103	8.4	15.8	0.7	1.2
Chicken, Steam Cuisine, Marks & Spencer*	1oz/28g	34	120	9.6	12.7	3.8	1.4
Cod, Cote Table*	1 Serving/281g	185	66	8.6	3.4	2.0	0.0
King Prawn & Mushroom, Marks & Spencer*	½ Pack/185g	120	65	7.2	3.9	2.5	0.9
Mushroom, Fresh, COU, Marks & Spencer*	½ Pack/150g	60	40	2.6	4.1	1.5	1.8
Prawn & Mushroom With Pasta, COU, Marks & Spencer*	1 Pack/400g	360	90	5.9	15.7	0.5	0.0
Ratatouille, Tesco*	½ Can/195g	72	37	1.1	4.2	1.8	0.9
Ratatouille, Waitrose*	½ Can/195g	107	55	1.5	7.8	2.1	0.8
PRUNE JUICE, Pure, Tesco*	1 Glass/250ml	180	72	0.7	16.8	0.1	1.2
PRUNES,							
Agen, Snack Pack, Marks & Spencer*	1 Pack/50g	98	195	1.4	46.7	0.3	4.1
Breakfast, In Fruit Juice, Sainsbury's*	1 Serving/130g	113	87	1.1	20.7	0.1	1.1
California, Stoned, Ready to Eat, Sunsweet*	5 Prunes/40g	92	230	2.6	54.4	0.3	7.2
Californian, In Syrup, Safeway*	1 Serving/104g	98	94	0.8	22.4	0.1	1.9
Californian, Tesco*	1 Serving/30g	45	149	2.5	33.9	0.4	5.7
Canned In Juice	1oz/28g	22	79	0.7	19.7	0.2	2.4
Canned In Syrup	1oz/28g	25	90	0.6	23.0	0.2	2.8
Dried Fruit, Ready To Eat, Tesco*	6 Prunes/50g	75	149	2.5	33.9	0.4	5.7
Dried, Marks & Spencer*	1oz/28g	68	244	2.3	62.3	0.1	4.2
French, Waitrose*	1 Serving/40g	60	149	2.5	33.9	0.4	5.7
In Apple Juice, Tesco*	1 Can/213g	198	93	0.7	22.0	0.2	2.4
Large, Waitrose*	1oz/28g	47	169	2.8	38.4	0.5	6.5
Pitted, Organic, Waitrose*	1oz/28g	47	169	2.8	38.4	0.5	6.5
Raw, Fresh	1oz/28g	45	160	2.8	38.4	0.5	6.5
Ready To Eat, Sainsbury's*	1 Serving/75g	112	149	2.5	33.9	0.4	5.7
Stewed With Sugar	1oz/28g	29	103	1.3	25.5	0.2	3.1
Stewed Without Sugar	1oz/28g	23	81	1.4	19.5	0.3	3.3
Sweet, Pitted, Stoneless, Asda*	1 Pack/50g	75	149	2.5	34.0	0.3	6.0
Vanilla, Sainsbury's*	1 Serving/27g	47	175	2.9	42.2	0.9	6.2
With Stones, Ready to Eat, Tesco*	1 Serving/50g	64	128	2.1	29.2	0.3	4.9
PUDDING,							
Apple & Custard, Sainsbury's*	1 Serving/115g	132	115	5.4	19.0	1.9	0.1

PUDDING,	Measure INFO/WEIGHT	per Measure KCAL	KCAL	PROT	CARB	FAT	FIBRE
Blackberry & Bramley Apple, Marks & Spencer*	¼ Pudding/152g	365	240	3.3	38.2	8.2	2.0
Butterscotch, Instant, Fat Free, Jello*	1 Serving/7.5g	27	333	1.3	78.7	1.3	0.0
Chocolate Marks & Spencer*	1 Serving/105g	401	382	6.2	40.7	21.6	1.1
Chocolate Sponge, Healthy Eating, Tesco*	1 Pudding/102g	197	191	4.4	34.7	3.8	0.9
Chocolate With Chocolate Sauce, BGTY, Sainsbury's*	1 Pudding/110g	161	146	3.5	28.6	1.9	2.3
Chocolate With Chocolate Sauce, Heinz*	¼ Can/77g	213	277	2.1	47.2	8.8	0.8
Chocolate, BGTY, Sainsbury's*	1 Pudding/110g	293	266	4.7	51.5	4.7	0.6
Chocolate, Delice*	1 Pot/100g	136	136	2.5	18.9	5.4	0.0
Chocolate, GFY, Asda*	1 Pudding/124g	274	221	4.4	42.0	3.9	2.7
Chocolate, Perfectly Balanced, Waitrose*	1 Pot/105g	196	187	3.8	36.0	3.1	0.8
Creamy Brioche With Apricot Compote, Co-Op*	1 Pack/230g	391	170	6.0	22.0	6.0	0.9
Creme aux Oeufs a la Vanille, Weight Watchers*	1 Pot/100g	116	116	4.8	17.0	3.2	0.0
Creme aux Oeufs au Chocolat, Weight Watchers*	1 Pot/100g	136	136	4.7	19.7	4.3	0.0
Eve's, 5% Fat, Marks & Spencer*	1 Pudding/223g	323	145	3.0	23.5	4.4	0.6
Eve's, BGTY, Sainsbury's*	1 Pudding/145g	164	113	2.2	23.4	1.2	0.7
Eve's, Eat Smart, Safeway*	1 Pudding/87g	131	150	2.3	30.6	1.8	0.9
Eve's, Marks & Spencer*	1 Serving/118g	254	215	2.7	32.3	8.3	0.4
Eve's, With Custard, Less Than 5% Fat, M&S*	1 Pudding/205g	318	155	3.4	24.7	4.6	0.7
Eve's, With Custard, Snack, Marks & Spencer*	1 Serving/230g	437	190	3.2	22.6	9.2	0.7
Forest Fruit Sponge, Eat Smart, Safeway*	1 Pot/88.2g	150	170	4.2	33.5	1.8	2.6
Jam Roly Poly & Custard, Co-Op*	1 Serving/105g	263	250	3.0	44.0	7.0	0.8
Lemon Sponge With Lemon Sauce, Eat Smart, Safeway*	1 Pudding/90g	135	150	2.2	29.0	2.6	1.4
Lemon, BGTY, Sainsbury's*	1 Serving/100g	151	151	2.9	31.0	1.9	0.5
Lemon, Marks & Spencer*	1 Pudding/105g	328	312	4.3	39.4	15.2	2.3
Lemon, Perfectly Balanced, Waitrose*	1 Serving/105g	212	202	3.4	41.7	2.4	0.6
Lemon, Sainsbury's*	1 Pudding/110g	304	276	3.4	41.4	10.8	0.6
Macaroni, Creamed, Ambrosia*	1 Can/425g	374	88	3.6	14.6	1.7	0.3
Spotted Dick, Asda*	1 Serving/105g	282	269	2.9	34.3	13.3	1.3
Spotted Dick, Sainsbury's*	¼ Pudding/82g	270	329	4.1	50.9	12.1	1.6
Sticky Toffee & Sticky Toffee Sauce, BGTY, Sainsbury's*	1 Serving/130g	319	245	5.0	49.3	4.1	2.2
Sticky Toffee, Co-Op*	¼ Pudding/100g	355	355	3.0	40.0	20.0	0.7
Sticky Toffee, Farmfoods*	¼ Pudding/186g	627	337	4.1	65.7	6.4	0.3
Sticky Toffee, Marks & Spencer*	1 Pudding/105g	337	321	3.5	51.9	11.0	1.1
Sticky Toffee, Tesco*	1 Serving/110g	287	261	3.3	31.8	13.4	0.7
Sticky Toffee, With Custard, Somerfield*	1 Pack/245g	576	235	3.0	38.0	8.0	0.0
Strawberry Jam With Custard, Farmfoods*	1 Serving/145g	525	362	3.2	35.5	23.9	0.9
Summer Fruits, Co-Op*	1 Pack/260g	273	105	1.0	25.0	0.2	1.0
Summer Fruits, Tesco*	1 Serving/100g	72	72	1.3	16.3	0.2	2.9
Summer Pudding, BGTY, Sainsbury's*	1 Pot/110g	223	203	3.2	40.9	4.6	2.4
Summer Pudding, Healthy Eating, Tesco*	1 Serving/100g	89	89	1.9	19.1	0.6	2.2
Summer Pudding, Safeway*	1 Pudding/135g	196	145	2.5	32.9	0.4	3.1
Summer Pudding, Waitrose*	1 Pot/120g	125	104	2.0	23.1	0.4	1.4
Summerfruit, Healthy Eating, Tesco*	1 Pudding/100g	72	72	1.3	16.3	0.2	2.9
Syrup Sponge, Iceland*	1 Serving/72.8g	228	312	5.1	54.1	8.4	0.9
Syrup, Individual, Co-Op*	1 Pudding/170g	604	355	3.0	38.0	21.0	1.0
Syrup, Marks & Spencer*	1 Serving/105g	370	352	3.9	61.7	10.0	0.8
Treacle Sponge, Heinz*	1 Serving/160g	445	278	2.5	48.9	8.1	0.6
PULSES, Mixed In Water, Sainsbury's*	½ Can/120g	131	109	8.7	13.6	2.2	4.6
PUMPKIN,							
Boiled in Salted Water	1oz/28g	4	13	0.6	2.1	0.3	1.1
Raw	1oz/28g	4	13	0.7	2.2	0.2	1.0
Seeds	1oz/28g	159	569	24.4	15.2	45.6	5.3
Seeds, Organic, Evernat*	1oz/28g	158	565	24.4	15.2	45.6	5.3

P

	Measure INFO/WEIGHT	per Measure KCAL	Nutrition Values per 100g / 100ml				
			KCAL	PROT	CARB	FAT	FIBRE
QUALITY STREET,							
Nestle*	1 Serving/25g	117	466	4.0	66.0	20.7	0.8
QUAVERS,							
Cheese, Walkers*	1 Bag/16g	82	515	3.0	61.0	29.0	1.2
Prawn Cocktail, Walkers*	1 Bag/16g	82	510	2.6	61.0	28.0	1.2
Salt & Vinegar, Walkers*	1 Bag/16g	80	500	2.3	58.0	29.0	1.1
Streaky Bacon, Walkers*	1 Pack/19.6g	103	515	2.2	62.0	29.0	1.3
QUICHE,							
Asparagus & Cheese, Safeway*	¼ Quiche/100g	260	260	7.5	18.2	17.4	1.4
Baby Spinach & Gruyere, Sainsbury's*	¼ Quiche/93g	228	245	7.4	15.1	17.2	1.0
Bacon & Cheese, Pork Farms*	1 Pack/120g	378	315	11.1	20.8	20.0	0.0
Bacon & Leek, Asda*	¼ Quiche/109g	311	285	9.0	15.0	21.0	0.8
Bacon & Tomato, Good Intentions, Somerfield*	1 Serving/145g	255	176	5.7	5.1	14.8	0.1
Bacon & Tomato, Safeway*	¼ Quiche/100g	287	287	8.6	20.3	19.0	1.4
Bacon, Leek & Mushroom, Marks & Spencer*	¼ Quiche/100g	250	250	8.7	14.2	17.9	2.1
Brie & Smoked Bacon, Asda*	¼ Quiche/90g	249	277	8.9	17.8	18.9	1.0
Broccoli & Cheddar Cheese, Safeway*	1 Pack/300g	813	271	7.7	19.8	17.9	1.9
Broccoli & Stilton, Mini, Sainsbury's*	1 Quiche/14g	52	369	8.8	35.2	21.4	3.3
Broccoli, Extra Value, Tesco*	1 Serving/125g	341	273	10.0	15.1	19.2	0.8
Broccoli, Healthy Eating, Tesco*	1 Quiche/175g	308	176	6.7	21.5	7.0	1.4
Broccoli, Tesco*	1 Quiche/175g	340	194	7.0	20.9	9.2	1.4
Broccoli, Tomato & Cheese, BGTY, Sainsbury's*	1 Quiche/390g	632	162	6.4	15.7	8.2	1.3
Broccoli, Tomato & Cheese, Sainsbury's*	1 Serving/125g	274	219	6.1	15.5	14.7	1.3
Cheddar Cheese & Onion, Safeway*	¼ Quiche/100g	293	293	8.3	21.6	19.3	1.5
Cheese & Bacon, Healthy Eating, Tesco*	1 Serving/155g	307	198	9.1	19.9	9.1	1.4
Cheese & Bacon, SmartPrice, Asda*	¼ Quiche/82g	208	257	6.0	20.0	17.0	0.7
Cheese & Bacon, Tesco*	¼ Quiche/100g	324	324	10.5	16.4	24.0	1.7
Cheese & Broccoli, Good Intentions, Somerfield*	1 Quiche/145g	409	282	6.9	27.7	15.9	1.8
Cheese & Chive, Healthy Eating, Tesco*	1 Serving/86g	169	197	10.4	22.1	7.4	1.2
Cheese & Ham, Basics, Somerfield*	¼ Quiche/81g	187	231	7.0	20.1	13.6	0.7
Cheese & Ham, Sainsbury's*	1 Serving/100g	266	266	9.3	14.4	19.0	1.2
Cheese & Ham, Somerfield*	1 Quiche/325g	835	257	7.0	18.0	18.0	0.0
Cheese & Mushroom, Budgens*	½ Quiche/170g	474	279	7.8	18.4	19.3	1.4
Cheese & Onion, Better For You, Morrisons*	1 Serving/100g	212	212	10.1	20.2	10.2	1.4
Cheese & Onion, Marks & Spencer*	1 Slice/100g	250	250	8.2	16.1	17.2	1.5
Cheese & Onion, Morrisons*	¼ Quiche/112g	364	325	10.1	20.3	22.6	1.1
Cheese & Onion, Reduced Fat, Safeway*	¼ Flan/100g	212	212	9.6	20.8	10.0	1.5
Cheese & Onion, Safeway*	1 Serving/310g	797	257	7.2	25.2	14.2	0.0
Cheese & Onion, Sainsbury's*	1 Quiche/390g	956	245	8.0	15.0	17.0	0.9
Cheese & Onion, Somerfield*	1 Quiche/300g	696	232	8.0	14.0	16.0	0.0
Cheese & Onion, Tesco*	1 Serving/90g	230	256	8.2	18.1	16.8	2.5
Cheese & Onion, Value, Tesco*	½ Quiche/200g	526	263	8.6	16.1	18.2	0.7
Cheese & Onion, Waitrose*	1 Serving/85g	182	214	6.4	13.9	14.8	3.6
Cheese & Tomato, Asda*	¼ Quiche/105g	274	261	8.0	19.0	17.0	0.9
Cheese & Tomato, Marks & Spencer*	1 Serving/100g	230	230	7.7	15.1	15.6	1.6
Cheese & Tomato, Morrisons*	½ Quiche/64g	195	304	7.3	22.8	20.5	1.0
Cheese & Tomato, Somerfield*	1 Quiche/135g	416	308	10.0	23.0	19.0	0.0
Cheese & Tomato, Tesco*	1 Serving/100g	274	274	7.5	18.3	19.0	1.4
Cheese Potato & Onion, Safeway*	1/3 Quiche/115g	361	314	8.8	24.1	20.3	1.5
Cheese, Broccoli & Tomato, Nisa Heritage*	1 Serving/85g	234	275	7.3	17.5	19.5	1.4
Cheese, Onion & Chive, Healthy Eating, Tesco*	1 Slice/100g	202	202	10.9	21.2	8.2	1.3
Cheese, Onion & Chive, SmartPrice, Asda*	¼ Quiche/83g	213	257	6.0	20.0	17.0	0.7
Chicken & Basil, Finest, Tesco*	1 Serving/134g	381	284	9.3	19.8	18.6	1.3
Chicken, Bacon & Mushroom, Asda*	1 Quiche/425g	1131	266	9.0	17.0	18.0	0.8

QUICHE,

INFO/WEIGHT	Measure per Measure KCAL	KCAL	PROT	CARB	FAT	FIBRE
Cumberland Sausage & Onion, Sainsbury's*	1 Serving/180g 486	270	7.0	18.8	18.5	1.3
Cumberland Sausage, Tesco*	1 Serving/100g 237	237	7.3	17.7	15.2	2.2
Davidstow Cheddar Cheese & Caramelised Onion, Asda*	1/3 Quiche/116.5g 369	315	7.0	20.0	23.0	1.0
Egg, Bacon & Cheese, Iceland*	1 Serving/90g 299	332	7.7	23.5	23.0	1.9
Gammon, Leek & Cheddar Cheese, Somerfield*	1/4 Quiche/95g 251	264	7.6	19.9	17.1	0.9
Garlic Mushroom, Asda*	1/4 Quiche/105g 273	260	7.0	22.0	16.0	0.7
Goats Cheese & Red Pepper, Tesco*	1 Serving/87g 271	312	5.8	19.2	23.6	0.9
Ham & Mustard, Good For You, Asda*	1 Quiche/155g 327	211	9.0	19.0	11.0	3.9
Ham & Soft Cheese, Tesco*	1/4 Quiche/100g 280	280	7.4	17.5	20.1	1.9
Ham & Tomato, Marks & Spencer*	1/2 Pack/200g 440	220	8.1	12.4	15.5	2.9
Ham, Cheese & Chive, Good For You, Asda*	1 Serving/78g 186	239	8.0	27.0	11.0	1.0
Leek & Sweet Potato, Waitrose*	1/2 Quiche/200g 440	220	5.3	17.0	14.5	2.3
Leek, Cheese & Chive, Sainsbury's*	1/3 Quiche/125g 293	234	7.1	14.9	16.2	1.3
Lorraine, Asda*	1 Serving/106g 318	300	9.0	21.0	20.0	2.3
Lorraine, BGTY, Sainsbury's*	1 Serving/128g 273	213	10.9	17.7	10.9	0.7
Lorraine, Budgens*	1 Pack/180g 520	289	8.2	25.6	17.1	0.8
Lorraine, Co-Op*	1/3 Quiche/108g 313	290	11.0	20.0	21.0	3.0
Lorraine, Finest, Tesco*	1 Serving/100g 330	330	8.4	17.5	25.1	1.5
Lorraine, Healthy Eating, New Improved Recipe, Tesco*	1/4 Quiche/100g 202	202	13.0	20.9	7.4	1.3
Lorraine, Healthy Living, Tesco*	1 Serving/200g 404	202	13.0	20.9	7.4	1.3
Lorraine, Quiche Selection, Marks & Spencer*	1 Slice/56g 160	285	12.8	12.3	20.6	2.1
Lorraine, Reduced Fat, Safeway*	1/4 Quiche/100g 231	231	11.0	18.9	12.4	1.4
Lorraine, Sainsbury's*	1/3 Quiche/128g 341	265	9.3	14.4	19.0	0.9
Lorraine, Somerfield*	1/4 Quiche/87g 260	299	10.1	17.1	21.1	0.7
Lorraine, TTD, Sainsbury's*	1/3 Pie/158g 482	305	10.2	15.1	22.7	0.9
Lorraine, Tesco*	1 Serving/81g 262	324	9.8	18.4	23.5	0.8
Mediterranean Vegetable, BGTY, Sainsbury's*	1 Quiche/180g 392	218	8.2	18.8	12.2	1.3
Mediterranean Vegetable, Sainsbury's*	1 Serving/200g 482	241	6.3	14.6	17.5	2.2
Mediterranean, Good For You, Asda*	1 Serving/25g 54	217	9.0	25.0	9.0	2.4
Mushroom Medley, Waitrose*	1/4 Quiche/100g 222	222	6.4	15.0	15.2	2.9
Mushroom, Bacon & Leek, Marks & Spencer*	1 Pack/170g 425	250	8.7	13.4	18.1	1.6
Mushroom, Marks & Spencer*	1/4 Quiche/100g 235	235	6.1	14.6	16.7	2.8
Mushroom, Sainsbury's*	1/3 Quiche/125g 283	226	7.1	15.9	14.9	1.2
Mushroom, Somerfield*	1/4 Quiche/82g 212	258	9.0	20.0	16.0	0.0
Red Pepper, Goats Cheese & Spinach, Waitrose*	1 Serving/100g 218	218	6.5	15.8	14.3	2.6
Roast Sweet Potato, Carrot & Corriander, Asda*	1/2 Quiche/207.5g 524	252	7.0	20.0	16.0	1.0
Salmon & Asparagus, Healthy Eating, Tesco*	1 Quiche/345g 621	180	7.5	20.2	7.7	1.2
Salmon & Broccoli, Asda*	1/4 Quiche/106g 289	273	10.0	20.0	17.0	2.6
Salmon & Broccoli, Budgens*	1/2 Quiche/187g 539	288	11.2	17.7	19.1	0.6
Salmon & Broccoli, Tesco*	1 Serving/133g 355	267	8.8	17.0	18.0	1.8
Salmon & Spinach, Sainsbury's*	1/3 Quiche/125g 318	254	8.2	15.9	17.5	1.0
Sausage & Onion, Sainsbury's*	1 Serving/100g 287	287	7.1	19.7	20.0	1.2
Spinach & Ricotta, Safeway*	1/4 Quiche/85g 193	227	7.9	22.6	11.7	1.7
Spinach Ricotta Cheese & Red Pepper, Safeway*	1 Serving/120g 304	253	6.2	20.2	16.4	1.2
Spinach, Ricotta & Gruyere Slice, Somerfield*	1 Slice/130g 348	268	7.0	15.0	20.0	0.0
Summer Vegetable, Marks & Spencer*	1/4 Quiche/100g 225	225	4.9	14.5	16.5	1.7
Sunblush Tomato, Basil & Mozzarella, Somerfield*	1/4 Quiche/88g 221	251	7.7	17.9	16.5	1.0
Sweet Cherry Pepper & Fontal Cheese, Finest, Tesco*	1/4 Slice/100g 293	293	6.7	16.9	22.1	0.9
Three Cheese & Onion, Good For You, Asda*	1 Serving/73g 188	258	10.0	23.0	14.0	3.1
Tomato & Cheese, Sainsbury's*	1/3 Quiche/133g 374	281	7.9	20.9	18.4	1.5
Tomato Cheese & Courgette, Good For You, Asda*	1 Serving/155g 333	215	7.0	22.0	11.0	3.3
Tomato, Broccoli & Cheese, Sainsbury's*	1 Serving/180g 437	243	6.7	19.6	15.3	1.5
Tomato, Cheese & Courgette, Asda*	1 Quiche/100g 333	333	11.0	34.0	17.0	5.0

Q

INFO/WEIGHT	per Measure KCAL	KCAL	PROT	CARB	FAT	FIBRE
QUICHE,						
Tomato, GFY, ASDA*	¼ Quiche/50g	94	188	8.0	21.0	8.0	0.8
Tomato, Mushroom & Bacon, Sainsbury's*	1 Serving/187g	447	239	7.5	15.2	16.5	1.1
Tuna, Tomato & Basil, Asda*	1 Serving/125g	305	244	9.0	16.0	16.0	1.5
Vegetable, Tesco*	1 Serving/100g	257	257	6.9	17.5	17.7	1.5
QUICK SNACK,						
Chicken & Mushroom Flavour, Value Tesco*	1 Pot/80g	274	342	14.9	60.6	4.5	7.0
Rice, Chilli, Sainsbury's*	1 Pack/280g	241	86	2.5	18.6	0.2	0.0
QUINCES, Average	1oz/28g	7	26	0.3	6.3	0.1	0.0
QUINOA, Average	1oz/28g	87	309	13.8	55.7	5.0	0.0
QUORN,						
Chunky Pieces	1 Serving/87g	90	103	14.0	5.8	2.6	6.0
Myco-Protein	1oz/28g	24	86	11.8	2.0	3.5	4.8
QUORN - GOUJONS, With Chunky Salsa Dip, Quorn*	1oz/28g	57	204	10.4	17.0	10.5	3.0
QUORN BALLS,						
Swedish Style, In Chunky Tomato & Basil Sauce, Quorn*	1 Pack/400g	296	74	8.2	5.0	2.3	2.0
Swedish Style, Quorn*	3 Balls/50g	72	144	22.0	5.4	3.8	3.2
QUORN DELI,						
Chicken Style, Slices, Quorn*	3 Slices/33g	36	108	16.9	4.0	2.7	3.2
Ham Flavour, Quorn*	1 Slice/20g	26	130	19.3	6.1	3.1	3.1
Ham, Wafer Thin, Quorn*	1 Serving/18g	23	130	19.3	6.1	3.1	3.1
Turkey Flavour With Stuffing, Quorn*	1 Slice/13g	13	102	13.7	8.3	1.5	4.5
QUORN ESCALOPES, Garlic & Herb, Quorn*	1 Escalope/140g	293	209	8.9	16.9	11.8	3.8
QUORN FILLETS,						
Cajun Spice, Quorn*	1 Serving/100g	176	176	10.9	14.7	8.2	3.4
Chargrilled Tikka Style, Mini, Quorn*	½ Pack/85g	110	129	12.5	14.4	2.4	5.0
Chinese Style Char Grilled, Mini, Quorn*	1 Serving/85g	115	135	12.1	15.6	2.7	4.7
Garlic & Herb, Quorn*	1 Fillet/100g	198	198	10.7	16.7	9.8	4.1
Hot & Spicy, Quorn*	1 Fillet/100g	176	176	10.9	14.7	8.2	6.4
In Breadcrumbs, Quorn	1 Fillet/94g	184	196	11.0	14.2	10.6	3.8
In White Wine & Mushroom Sauce, Quorn*	1 Pack/325g	247	76	6.3	6.0	3.0	2.1
In a Mediterranean Marinade, Quorn*	1 Fillet/80g	90	112	12.5	8.8	3.0	4.0
Lemon & Black Pepper, Quorn*	1 Fillet/100g	195	195	11.6	17.2	8.9	3.3
Lemon & Pepper, Sainsbury's*	1 Fillet/100g	198	198	11.6	16.9	9.3	3.8
Oriental, Sainsbury's*	1 Serving/294g	353	120	4.0	24.6	0.6	1.8
Provencale, Morrisons*	1 Serving/165g	94	57	5.4	5.8	1.4	1.1
Quorn*	2 Fillets/102g	88	86	13.1	4.9	1.5	4.9
Thai, Quorn*	1 Serving/79.4g	85	107	14.9	6.1	2.5	3.6
With A Crispy Seasonal Coating, Quorn*	1 Fillet/100g	197	197	8.8	18.4	9.8	3.0
QUORN GRILLS, Lamb Flavour, Quorn*	1 Grill/90g	104	116	11.4	10.4	3.2	4.2
QUORN MINCE, Quorn*	1 Pack/300g	273	91	15.0	1.4	2.8	4.9
QUORN NUGGETS,						
Quorn*	1 nugget/20g	38	191	10.6	15.7	9.5	3.5
Southern Style, Quorn*	1 Nugget/20g	39	197	12.1	15.7	9.5	3.5
QUORN PIECES,						
Quorn*	1 Pack/300g	276	92	14.0	1.8	3.2	4.8
QUORN SLICES, With Sage & Onion Stuffing, Quorn*	¼ Pack/70g	47	67	7.5	4.9	1.9	3.0
QUORN STEAKS,						
Peppered, Quorn*	1 Steak/98.2g	107	109	11.4	7.4	3.8	4.0
Peppered, Sainsbury's*	1 Steak/95g	124	130	11.9	11.9	4.2	4.5

Measure · Nutrition Values per 100g / 100ml

INFO/WEIGHT	Measure	per Measure KCAL	Nutrition Values per 100g / 100ml				
			KCAL	PROT	CARB	FAT	FIBRE
RABBIT,							
Raw, Meat Only	1oz/28g	38	137	21.9	0.0	5.5	0.0
Stewed, Meat Only	1oz/28g	32	114	21.2	0.0	3.2	0.0
RADDICCIO, Raw	1oz/28g	4	14	1.4	1.7	0.2	1.8
RADIATORE,							
Sainsbury's*	1 Serving/75g	268	357	12.3	73.1	1.7	2.5
Somerfield*	1oz/28g	97	346	13.0	69.0	2.0	0.0
RADISH,							
Red, Raw	1oz/28g	3	12	0.7	1.9	0.2	0.9
Sainsbury's*	1 Pack/150g	18	12	0.7	1.9	0.2	0.9
White/Mooli, Raw	1oz/28g	4	15	0.8	2.9	0.1	0.0
RAISINS,							
Average	1 Tbsp/30g	82	272	2.1	69.3	0.4	2.0
Californian, Organic, Evernat*	1 Serving/65g	188	289	2.1	69.3	0.4	2.0
Californian, Seedless, Safeway*	1 Pack/14g	44	316	3.3	77.5	0.4	0.0
Californian, Seedless, Sainsbury's*	1oz/28g	91	326	3.0	71.4	0.7	5.9
Californian, Sun Dried, Sun-Maid*	1 Pack/42g	128	304	3.0	71.4	0.7	5.8
Jumbo, Juicy, Asda*	1 Serving/50g	144	288	2.1	69.0	0.4	4.0
Milk Chocolate, Tesco*	1 Lge Bag/227g	933	411	4.8	63.3	15.4	0.9
Pocket Snack, Sundora*	1 Serving/50g	116	231	1.7	55.4	0.3	1.8
Seedless, Asda*	1 Serving/25g	72	288	2.1	69.0	0.4	2.0
Seedless, Somerfield*	1oz/28g	92	330	3.0	77.0	1.0	0.0
Seedless, Tesco*	1 Serving/10g	27	265	1.1	64.1	0.5	6.8
Snack Pack, Blue Parrot Cafe, Sainsbury's*	1 Pack/14g	40	289	2.1	69.3	0.4	2.0
Sun Dried, Organic, Crazy Jack*	1 Serving/100g	289	289	2.1	69.3	0.4	1.0
Sun Dried, Seedless, Somerfield*	1 Serving/28g	86	307	2.6	73.3	0.4	2.0
Yoghurt Coated, Holland & Barrett*	1 Bag/100g	404	404	2.6	66.6	16.5	1.0
RAISINS & SULTANAS,							
Jumbo, Marks & Spencer*	1 Pack/50g	133	265	2.4	62.4	0.5	2.6
Jumbo, Safeway*	1 Pack/250g	773	309	2.4	73.1	0.8	5.7
RAITA,							
Plain	1oz/28g	46	166	2.6	5.5	15.3	0.0
RASPBERRIES,							
Canned, In Syrup	1oz/28g	25	88	0.6	22.5	0.1	1.5
Fresh, Raw	1oz/28g	7	25	1.4	4.6	0.3	2.5
Fresh, Tesco*	1 Pack/125g	34	27	1.4	4.6	0.3	2.5
Frozen, Asda*	1 Serving/100g	26	26	1.4	4.5	0.3	2.5
In Apple Juice, Asda*	½ Can/145g	48	33	0.9	7.0	0.2	1.5
In Fruit Juice, Waitrose*	1 Serving/142g	47	33	0.9	6.8	0.2	1.5
RASPBERRY JUICE, Cooler With Mint, Sainsbury's*	1 Serving/250ml	63	25	0.1	6.0	0.1	0.1
RATATOUILLE,							
Chicken, Finest, Tesco*	1 Pack/550g	407	74	7.8	5.9	2.1	0.0
Ratatouille, Sainsbury's*	½ Can/190g	80	42	0.8	5.7	1.8	1.0
Safeway*	1 Serving/200g	78	39	1.0	3.0	2.5	1.6
Sainsbury's*	1 Pack/300g	99	33	1.5	5.5	0.6	1.6
Vegetable, Marks & Spencer*	1 Pack/300g	135	45	2.3	2.5	3.0	2.1
RAVIOLI,							
Amatriciana, TTD, Sainsbury's*	1 Serving/125g	390	312	16.6	33.3	12.5	3.5
Asparagus & Ham, Healthy Eating, Tesco*	½ Pack/125g	203	162	8.2	26.5	2.6	0.6
Asparagus, Waitrose*	1 Serving/150g	303	202	10.5	26.4	6.0	2.0
Basil & Parmesan, Organic, Sainsbury's*	½ Pack/192g	290	151	7.4	21.1	5.2	2.1
Beef, Chef Boyardee*	1 Can/100g	190	190	6.0	31.0	5.0	2.0
Beef, Fresh, Safeway*	1 Serving/137g	352	257	10.0	39.4	6.6	3.0
Blue Cheese & Bacon, Safeway*	½ Pack/125g	288	230	10.5	24.9	9.6	1.6

R

RAVIOLI,

	Measure INFO/WEIGHT	per Measure KCAL	KCAL	PROT	CARB	FAT	FIBRE
Cheese & Asparagus, Waitrose*	1 Serving/100g	242	242	12.6	31.7	7.2	2.4
Cheese & Sun Dried Tomato, Co-Op*	½ Pack/125g	356	285	12.0	38.0	9.0	2.0
Cheese & Tomato, Fresh, Organic, Tesco*	1 Serving/125g	343	274	12.5	30.8	11.2	1.1
Cheese & Tomato, Heinz*	1 Can/410g	332	81	2.7	14.1	1.5	0.6
Cheese, Garlic, & Herb, Safeway*	½ Pack/125g	263	210	9.1	26.5	7.6	2.0
Cheese, Tomato & Basil, Italiano, Tesco*	½ Pack/125g	304	243	13.6	24.1	10.2	0.5
Chicken & Mushroom, Finest, Tesco*	½ Pack/125g	268	214	11.6	25.8	7.1	1.1
Chicken & Rosemary, Perfectly Balanced, Waitrose*	½ Pack/125g	266	213	14.9	30.4	3.5	2.1
Chicken & Tomato, Perfectly Balanced, Waitrose*	1 Serving/125g	265	212	13.5	33.4	2.7	2.8
Feta Cheese, Marks & Spencer*	1 Serving/100g	195	195	9.1	20.5	8.5	1.3
Five Cheese, Weight Watchers*	1 Pack/330g	271	82	3.2	11.1	2.8	0.8
Florentine, Weight Watchers*	1 Serving/241g	220	91	3.7	14.1	2.1	1.2
Four Cheese, Good Intentions, Somerfield*	1 Pack/353g	367	104	4.1	14.0	3.5	1.7
Four Cheese, Italia, Marks & Spencer*	1 Pack/360g	432	120	6.7	13.1	4.6	1.0
Free Range Duck, TTD, Sainsbury's*	½ Pack/161g	314	195	11.5	21.0	7.3	2.3
Fresh, Pasta Reale*	1 Serving/150g	459	306	13.1	53.3	5.9	0.0
Garlic & Herb, Italiano, Tesco*	1 Serving/100g	318	318	11.1	39.1	13.0	2.6
Goat's Cheese & Pesto, Asda*	½ Pack/150g	204	136	6.0	20.0	3.6	0.0
In Tomato Sauce, Carlini, Aldi*	1 Can/400g	324	81	3.1	15.0	1.0	0.5
In Tomato Sauce, Heinz*	1 Can/410g	299	73	2.6	13.0	1.1	0.6
In Tomato Sauce, Meat Free, Heinz*	1 Can/410g	308	75	2.4	14.4	0.8	0.5
In Tomato Sauce, Tesco*	1 Can/400g	276	69	2.7	14.2	0.1	1.3
Meat, Italian, Fresh, Asda*	½ Pack/150g	261	174	8.0	26.0	4.2	0.0
Meditteranean Vegetable, Healthy Eating, Tesco*	1 Serving/125g	199	159	6.7	27.2	2.6	0.9
Mozzarella Tomato & Basil, Tesco*	1 Serving/125g	304	243	13.6	24.1	10.2	0.5
Mushroom & Mascarpone, The Best, Safeway*	1 Pack/175g	466	266	9.9	31.8	11.0	1.0
Mushroom, Fresh, Budgens*	1 Pack/250g	485	194	7.7	28.8	6.0	1.7
Mushroom, Italian, Fresh, Somerfield*	½ Pack/125g	336	269	10.8	34.4	9.8	1.8
Mushroom, Italiano, Tesco*	1 Serving/125g	333	266	10.4	27.0	12.9	3.0
Mushroom, Safeway*	½ Pack/125g	243	194	7.5	25.5	6.9	1.8
Mushroomi, Tesco*	½ Pack/125g	333	266	10.4	27.0	12.9	3.0
Prosciuttoi, Ready Meal, Marks & Spencer*	1 Pack/100g	195	195	13.3	17.0	8.1	1.0
Red Onion & Brunello Wine, TTD, Sainsbury's*	1 Serving/125g	235	188	7.5	23.0	7.3	2.5
Rich Beef & Red Wine, Morrisons*	1 Serving/150g	396	264	12.1	40.6	7.2	3.0
Roast Garlic & Herb, Tesco*	½ Pack/125g	343	274	12.8	31.1	10.9	1.1
Roasted Pepper, Marks & Spencer*	1 Pack/400g	540	135	5.4	11.0	7.7	1.1
Roasted Vegetable, Asda*	½ Pack/150g	218	145	6.0	29.0	0.5	0.0
Smartprice, Asda*	1 Can/400g	272	68	2.7	14.0	0.1	1.3
Smoked Ham, Bacon & Tomato, Italiano, Tesco*	1 Can/125g	303	242	10.8	32.3	7.7	2.9
Spinach & Ricotta, Waitrose*	1 Serving/125g	309	247	10.5	35.0	7.2	1.9
Sweet Pepper & Chilli, Tesco*	½ Pack/125g	324	259	12.5	27.1	11.2	2.7
Tomato Cheese & Meat, Sainsbury's*	1 Serving/125g	314	251	12.4	21.4	12.9	2.2
Vegetable In Tomato Sauce, Italiana, Weight Watchers*	1 Can/385g	266	69	1.7	11.0	2.1	0.5
Vegetable, Morrisons*	1 Can/400g	276	69	2.4	13.9	0.4	0.0
Vegetable, Sainsbury's*	1 Can/400g	328	82	2.6	16.3	0.7	0.7
Vegetable, Tesco*	½ Can/200g	164	82	2.6	16.3	0.7	0.7
Wild Mushroom, Al Forno, TTD, Sainsbury's*	1 Pack/300g	459	153	7.0	14.0	7.7	1.2

RED BULL

	Measure INFO/WEIGHT	per Measure KCAL	KCAL	PROT	CARB	FAT	FIBRE
Regular	1 Can/250ml	113	45	0.0	11.3	0.0	0.0
Sugar Free*	1 Can/250ml	8	3	0.0	1.0	0.0	0.0

RED GRAPE JUICE,

	Measure INFO/WEIGHT	per Measure KCAL	KCAL	PROT	CARB	FAT	FIBRE
Safeway*	1 Serving/120ml	77	64	0.1	15.5	0.0	0.0
Sainsbury's*	1 Glass/200ml	138	69	0.1	16.6	0.0	0.0

R

	Measure INFO/WEIGHT	per Measure KCAL	Nutrition Values per 100g / 100ml				
			KCAL	PROT	CARB	FAT	FIBRE
RED GRAPES,							
Shapers, Boots*	1 Bag/120g	84	70	0.5	18.0	0.1	0.8
REDCURRANT JELLY,							
Average	1oz/28g	67	240	0.3	63.8	0.0	0.0
Baxters*	1oz/28g	73	260	0.0	65.0	0.0	0.0
REDCURRANTS, Raw	1oz/28g	6	21	1.1	4.4	0.0	3.4
REHYDRATION DRINK, Citrus, Low Calorie, Shapers, Boots*	1 Bottle/500ml	10	2	0.1	0.1	0.1	0.0
RELISH,							
Barbeque, Sainsbury's*	1 Serving/50g	50	100	1.0	19.3	2.1	1.1
Caramelised Onion & Chilli, Marks & Spencer*	1 Serving/20g	47	235	1.4	55.1	1.1	1.0
Caramelised Red Onion, Tesco*	1 Serving/10g	28	280	0.6	69.1	0.1	0.7
Hamburger, Bick's*	1oz/28g	27	96	1.3	22.3	0.2	0.0
Onion, Marks & Spencer*	1oz/28g	46	165	1.0	32.1	3.0	1.1
Salsa, Waitrose*	1oz/28g	21	74	2.1	14.7	0.2	2.0
Sweetcorn, Bicks*	1 Tbsp/22g	23	103	1.3	24.3	0.2	0.0
Sweetcorn, Safeway*	1 Serving/50g	69	137	1.0	32.4	0.4	0.5
Tomato & Chilli Texan Style, Tesco*	1 Tbsp/14g	20	140	1.7	32.0	0.1	1.1
Tomato, Marks & Spencer*	1oz/28g	36	130	1.8	30.2	0.3	1.5
REVELS, Mars*	1 Sm Bag/35g	173	495	6.2	65.6	23.1	0.0
RHUBARB,							
Fresh, Raw	1oz/28g	2	7	0.9	0.8	0.1	1.4
No Added Sugar, Asda*	¼ Can/133g	8	6	0.8	0.7	0.0	1.3
Stewed With Sugar	1oz/28g	13	48	0.9	11.5	0.1	1.2
Stewed Without Sugar	1oz/28g	2	7	0.9	0.7	0.1	1.3
RIBENA*,							
Apple Juice Drink	1 Carton/287ml	132	46	0.0	11.1	0.0	0.0
Blackcurrant Juice Drink	1 Carton/288ml	164	57	0.0	14.0	0.0	0.0
Blackcurrant Juice Drink, Toothkind	1 Carton/288ml	12	4	0.0	0.7	0.0	0.0
Blackcurrant, Diluted With Water	1 Serving/180ml	81	45	0.0	11.0	0.0	0.0
Light	1 Bottle/288ml	63	22	0.0	5.2	0.0	0.0
Orange Tropical Juice Drink, Toothkind	1 Carton/288ml	9	3	0.0	0.6	0.0	0.0
Strawberry Juice Drink, Toothkind	1 Carton/288ml	12	4	0.0	0.7	0.0	0.0
RIBS,							
Barbecue, American Style, Tesco*	1 Serving/250g	595	238	25.0	11.5	10.2	0.3
Chinese King, Farmfoods*	1 Rib/79g	185	234	11.9	4.0	19.0	1.5
In Spicy BBQ Sauce, Asda*	1 Pack/360g	842	234	19.8	7.6	13.8	0.0
Pork, BBQ, Sainsbury's*	1 Rib/60g	188	314	28.5	3.8	20.5	0.1
Pork, Barbecue, Mini, Waitrose*	1 Serving/100g	225	225	19.7	4.6	14.2	0.0
Pork, Chinese Style, Grilled, Safeway*	1 Serving/100g	309	309	24.8	6.2	20.5	0.0
Pork, Chinese Style, Jumbo, Sainsbury's*	1oz/28g	82	293	27.3	4.2	18.6	0.1
Pork, Rib Rack, Smokey Barbecue, Farmfoods*	1oz/28g	83	296	15.3	5.7	23.5	0.6
Pork, Single, BBQ, Asda*	1oz/28g	58	206	23.7	3.5	10.7	0.0
Pork, Spare, Chops, Braised, Lean	1oz/28g	60	213	30.5	0.0	10.1	0.0
Pork, Spare, Chops, Braised, Lean & Fat	1oz/28g	69	247	28.1	0.0	15.0	0.0
Pork, Spare, Chops, Raw, Lean & Fat	1oz/28g	52	186	18.5	0.0	12.4	0.0
Pork, Spare, Steaks, Raw, Lean & Fat	1oz/28g	47	168	18.7	0.0	10.4	0.0
RICCOLI, Egg, Fresh, Waitrose*	1oz/28g	81	289	11.4	53.1	3.4	2.1
RICE,							
& Wild Rice, Safeway*	1 Serving/75g	194	259	6.0	57.8	0.4	0.5
American Brown, Waitrose*	1 Serving/50g	173	345	6.7	73.2	2.8	1.9
American Easy Cook, Dry Weight, Sainsbury's*	1 Serving/50g	179	358	6.8	76.6	2.6	0.8
American Easy Cook, Long Grain, Veetee*	1 Serving/80g	285	356	8.1	78.8	0.9	0.0
Arborio Risotto, Asda*	1 Serving/125g	438	350	7.0	78.0	1.1	0.0
Arborio Risotto, Sainsbury's*	1 Serving/120g	419	349	7.0	78.5	0.8	1.4

R

RICE,

INFO/WEIGHT	Measure per Measure KCAL	Nutrition Values per 100g / 100ml KCAL	PROT	CARB	FAT	FIBRE
Arborio, Tesco*	1 Serving/80g	277	346	7.4	78.3	0.4	1.1
BBQ & Spicy, Marks & Spencer*	1 Pack/250g	463	185	6.1	23.7	7.2	1.2
Balti, Break, Asda*	1 Serving/60g	209	348	13.3	70.0	1.7	0.0
Basmati, & Wild, Easy Cook, Tilda*	1oz/28g	98	349	9.4	77.0	0.4	0.9
Basmati, & Wild, Marks & Spencer*	1 Pack/180g	189	105	2.8	22.5	0.4	1.2
Basmati, Boil In Bag, Tesco*	½ Bag/60g	212	353	7.4	79.8	0.5	0.4
Basmati, Boil in the Bag, Asda*	1 Serving/62g	221	357	10.0	76.0	1.4	0.4
Basmati, Brown, Asda*	1 Serving/50g	181	362	10.0	71.0	4.0	2.3
Basmati, Brown, Cooked, Tilda*	1 Serving/100g	154	154	31.9	4.1	1.2	1.9
Basmati, Brown, Tesco*	1 Serving/50g	176	351	9.4	73.0	2.4	2.3
Basmati, Brown, Tilda*	1oz/28g	97	347	9.2	71.4	2.7	1.9
Basmati, Cooked, Sainsbury's*	1 Serving/150g	191	127	2.6	28.6	0.2	0.1
Basmati, Easy Cook, Patak's*	1 Serving/40g	121	302	6.2	67.8	0.6	0.6
Basmati, Easy Cook, Tesco*	1 Serving/50g	178	356	8.1	79.8	0.5	0.4
Basmati, Easy Cook, Tilda*	1oz/28g	98	349	8.5	78.4	0.1	0.4
Basmati, Easy Cook, Uncle Ben's*	1 Serving/63g	216	343	9.0	76.0	0.6	1.9
Basmati, Express, Uncle Ben's*	½ Pack/125g	173	138	2.8	29.9	1.3	0.0
Basmati, Indian, Tesco*	1 Serving/56g	194	347	8.4	76.1	0.9	0.1
Basmati, Pilau, Rizazz, Tilda*	1 Serving/125g	183	146	2.5	28.7	2.4	0.0
Basmati, Pure, Cook in the Bag, Tilda*	1 Serving/50g	174	348	8.6	77.6	0.4	0.4
Basmati, Pure, Rizazz, Tilda*	1 Bag/250g	383	153	2.6	30.2	2.4	0.0
Basmati, Sainsbury's*	1 Serving/50g	176	352	7.4	80.0	0.3	0.2
Basmati, Somerfield*	1 Serving/100g	343	343	9.3	75.4	0.5	1.6
Basmati, Spicy Mexican, Tilda*	1 Serving/125g	188	150	2.9	28.1	2.9	0.5
Basmati, Steamed, Sainsbury's*	1 Serving/250g	298	119	3.6	25.9	0.1	1.5
Basmati, Thai Lime & Coriander, Tilda*	½ Pack/125g	185	148	2.4	28.4	2.8	0.1
Basmati, Tilda*	1oz/28g	97	348	8.6	77.6	0.4	0.4
Basmati, Value, Tesco*	1oz/28g	98	350	7.0	79.4	0.5	0.4
Basmati, White, Marks & Spencer*	1 Serving/75g	254	339	8.8	74.4	0.7	4.4
Basmati, White, Raw	1oz/28g	101	359	7.4	79.8	0.5	0.0
Brown, American Easy Cook, Safeway*	1 Serving/75g	262	349	6.9	74.0	2.8	1.9
Brown, American Easy Cook, Tilda*	1oz/28g	99	352	8.1	75.1	2.1	1.9
Brown, American, Asda*	1 Serving/75g	273	364	9.0	74.0	3.5	0.0
Brown, American, Easy Cook, Tesco*	1 Serving/100g	349	349	6.9	74.0	2.8	1.9
Brown, American, Easy Eook, Asda*	1 Serving/50g	175	349	7.0	74.0	2.8	1.9
Brown, American, Wholegrain, Dry, Sainsbury's*	1 Serving/50g	173	346	6.8	71.6	2.8	2.6
Brown, Boil In The Bag, Safeway*	1 Bag/125g	434	347	8.0	72.0	3.0	3.3
Brown, Boil in The Bag, Cooked, Sainsbury's*	½ Bag/170g	218	128	2.6	27.0	1.1	1.2
Brown, Boiled	1oz/28g	39	141	2.6	32.1	1.1	0.8
Brown, Long Grain, Organic, Crazy Jack*	1 Serving/100g	377	377	6.7	81.0	2.8	1.9
Brown, Raw	1oz/28g	100	357	6.7	81.3	2.8	1.9
Brown, Wholegrain, Dry, Sainsbury's*	1 Serving/40g	135	338	6.8	71.5	2.8	2.5
Brown, Wholegrain, Tesco*	1 Serving/50g	173	346	8.1	71.7	3.0	3.4
Carnaroli Risotto, Tesco*	1 oz/28g	99	352	7.6	77.2	1.4	1.2
Chinese Savoury, Batchelors*	1 Serving/50g	177	354	9.9	73.1	2.4	2.8
Chinese Style, Express, Uncle Ben's*	1 Pack/250g	338	135	3.1	27.3	1.5	0.0
Coconut & Lime, Asda*	1 Pack/360g	695	193	4.5	32.7	4.9	0.9
Coconut, Marks & Spencer*	½ Pack/124g	217	175	3.1	31.8	4.0	0.3
Coriander & Herbs, Batchelors*	1/3 Pack/76g	280	369	7.9	79.6	3.5	5.0
Egg Fried, Asda*	1oz/28g	43	152	4.2	23.4	4.4	1.8
Egg Fried, Cantonese, Sainsbury's*	½ Pot/260g	465	179	4.0	27.4	8.0	1.3
Egg Fried, Chinese Style, Tesco*	1 Portion/250g	418	167	4.4	27.9	4.2	0.7
Egg Fried, Chinese Takeaway, Iceland*	1 Pack/340g	466	137	2.8	26.1	2.4	0.6

R

	Measure INFO/WEIGHT	per Measure KCAL	Nutrition Values per 100g / 100ml				
			KCAL	PROT	CARB	FAT	FIBRE
RICE,							
Egg Fried, Chinese Takeaway, Tesco*	1 Serving/200g	250	125	4.7	23.3	1.5	1.8
Egg Fried, Chinese, Sainsbury's*	1 Pack/200g	350	175	4.5	27.8	5.1	1.2
Egg Fried, Express, Uncle Ben's*	1 Pack/250g	440	176	4.1	30.5	4.2	0.0
Egg Fried, Marks & Spencer*	1 Pack/200g	420	210	4.1	32.4	7.0	0.3
Egg Fried, New, Tesco*	1 Serving/250g	365	146	4.0	23.9	3.8	3.1
Egg Fried, Oriental Express*	1 Pack/425g	531	125	4.0	22.2	2.3	1.3
Egg Fried, Original, Asda*	1 Pack/250g	425	170	4.0	25.0	6.0	1.6
Egg Fried, Rizazz, Tilda*	1 Pack/250g	358	143	3.3	25.4	3.1	0.0
Egg Fried, Safeway*	1 Serving/180g	351	195	4.9	34.8	4.0	0.7
Egg Fried, Somerfield*	1 Pack/200g	298	149	7.2	25.0	2.2	1.1
Egg Fried, Tesco*	1 Pack/250g	313	125	4.7	23.3	1.5	1.8
Egg Fried, Waitrose*	1 Pack/300g	426	142	3.0	20.6	5.2	1.0
Egg, Chinese Style, Morrisons*	1 Serving/250g	285	114	2.1	16.8	4.8	0.7
Fried, Chicken, Chinese Takeaway, Iceland*	1 Pack/340g	510	150	6.5	20.7	4.6	0.6
Fried, Duck, Chicken & Pork Celebration, Sainsbury's*	1 Pack/450g	545	121	7.9	14.2	3.6	1.5
Garlic & Butter Flavoured, Batchelors*	1 Serving/50g	175	350	8.0	79.8	2.8	5.0
Golden Savoury, Cooked, Tesco*	1 Serving/178g	219	123	3.0	25.0	1.0	1.0
Golden Savoury, New Improved Flavour, Batchelors*	1 Pack/120g	439	366	9.3	78.9	1.5	4.5
Golden Vegetable, Express, Uncle Ben's*	1 Pack/250g	350	140	2.9	28.2	1.8	0.0
Imperial Red, Merchant Gourmet*	1oz/28g	85	305	8.6	61.2	2.5	8.6
Italian, Easy Cook, Tesco*	1 Serving/75g	260	347	7.0	77.6	0.9	0.4
Italian, Risotto, Marks & Spencer*	1oz/28g	94	336	6.8	76.0	0.5	2.6
Long Grain	1oz/28g	90	320	8.0	74.4	0.9	3.9
Long Grain, & Wild, American, Sainsbury's*	1 Serving/75g	231	308	6.2	69.0	0.8	2.0
Long Grain, & Wild, Asda*	1 Serving/75g	272	363	9.0	77.0	2.1	0.0
Long Grain, & Wild, Cooked, Tesco*	1 Serving/200g	300	150	3.0	31.8	1.3	0.2
Long Grain, American Easy Cook, Somerfield*	1 Serving/100g	350	350	7.6	77.6	1.0	1.5
Long Grain, American Easy Cook, Tesco*	1 Serving/75g	260	347	7.0	77.6	0.9	0.4
Long Grain, American Easy Cook, Tilda*	1oz/28g	99	355	7.6	79.9	0.6	0.4
Long Grain, American, Asda*	1 Serving/70g	252	360	7.0	81.0	0.9	0.4
Long Grain, American, Boil in Bag, Cooked, Sainsbury's*	½ Bag/169g	221	131	2.7	29.6	0.2	0.2
Long Grain, American, Co-Op*	1 Serving/50g	175	350	8.0	77.0	1.0	1.0
Long Grain, American, Cooked, Sainsbury's*	½ Pack/138g	214	155	3.4	27.9	3.3	0.3
Long Grain, American, Morrisons*	1oz/28g	99	354	6.6	79.7	0.8	0.0
Long Grain, American, Safeway*	1 Serving/75g	263	351	6.5	79.0	1.0	0.5
Long Grain, American, Tilda*	1oz/28g	99	353	7.7	79.2	0.6	0.4
Long Grain, Basics, Somerfield*	1oz/28g	97	348	7.5	76.9	1.2	0.6
Long Grain, Boil in the Bag, Asda*	1 Serving/62g	221	357	8.0	79.0	1.0	0.6
Long Grain, Express, Uncle Ben's*	1 Pack/250g	360	144	2.6	31.1	1.0	0.0
Long Grain, Uncle Ben's*	1oz/28g	94	337	7.4	76.0	0.4	1.8
Long Grain, Value, Tesco*	1 Serving/50g	174	347	7.0	77.6	0.9	0.4
Long Grain, White, Frozen, Microwavable, Sainsbury's*	1 Sachet/200g	210	105	2.7	22.4	0.5	1.1
Mediterranean Tomato, Rizazz, Tilda*	½ Pack/125g	194	155	2.7	28.6	3.3	0.0
Mexican Style, Old El Paso*	1 Serving/75g	268	357	9.0	78.0	1.0	0.0
Mexican, Ready Meals, Waitrose*	1 Pack/300g	432	144	2.6	27.8	2.5	0.5
Mushroom & Coconut, Organic, Waitrose*	1 Pack/300g	474	158	3.7	24.5	5.0	1.4
Mushroom Savory, Bettabuy, Morrisons*	1 Serving/128.4g	131	102	2.3	21.5	0.8	0.0
Pilau, 3 Colour Indian, Sainsbury's*	1 Pot/520g	1175	226	3.9	33.7	8.4	0.6
Pilau, Batchelors*	1/3 Pack/76g	280	369	7.9	79.6	3.5	5.0
Pilau, Bengali, Sainsbury's*	1 Pack/200g	330	165	4.2	26.5	4.7	2.2
Pilau, Express, Uncle Ben's*	½ Pack/125g	211	169	3.1	31.0	3.6	0.0
Pilau, Indian Mushroom, Sainsbury's*	1 Serving/100g	119	119	3.0	21.3	2.4	1.9
Pilau, Indian Takeaway For 1, Sainsbury's*	1 Serving/201g	334	166	4.1	32.1	2.4	0.5

R

RICE,	Measure INFO/WEIGHT	per Measure KCAL	Nutrition Values per 100g / 100ml				
			KCAL	PROT	CARB	FAT	FIBRE
Pilau, Sharwood's*	1oz/28g	99	354	9.0	76.8	1.2	1.8
Pilau, Takeaway Menu For 1, BGTY, Sainsbury's*	1 Pack/151g	227	150	4.8	32.8	0.0	1.7
Saffron, Sainsbury's*	½ Pack/299g	368	123	2.2	26.9	0.7	0.0
Savoury, Beef, Batchelors*	½ Pack/62g	222	358	9.4	74.9	2.3	3.2
Savoury, Chicken, Batchelors*	1 Pack/124g	443	357	9.9	74.5	2.2	2.9
Savoury, Mild Curry, Batchelors*	½ Pack/61g	217	355	8.4	76.0	1.9	1.8
Savoury, Mixed Vegetable, Tesco*	1 Serving/63g	219	347	8.8	71.1	3.0	6.4
Savoury, Mushroom & Pepper, Cooked, Morrisons*	1 Serving/200g	204	102	2.3	21.5	0.8	0.0
Savoury, Mushroom, Batchelors*	1 Sachet/122g	439	360	10.9	74.3	2.1	2.5
Savoury, Paella, Tesco*	1 Serving/60g	220	367	8.4	72.7	4.7	4.5
Savoury, Spicy Mexican Style, Tesco*	1 Serving/164g	584	356	9.0	69.9	4.5	6.0
Savoury, Sweet & Sour, Batchelors*	1 Serving/135g	419	310	9.4	75.6	2.1	3.1
Savoury, Tandoori, Batchelors*	1 Serving/120g	430	358	10.3	73.5	2.5	3.0
Savoury, Vegetable, Co-Op*	½ Pack/60g	210	350	9.0	76.0	1.0	3.0
Spanish Paella, Sainsbury's*	1 Serving/100g	349	349	7.0	78.5	0.8	1.4
Spanish Paella, Special Recipe, Sainsbury's*	1 Pack/125g	134	107	2.1	22.5	0.9	0.2
Special Fried, Asda*	1oz/28g	42	149	5.4	21.0	4.9	1.5
Special Fried, Marks & Spencer*	1 Pack/450g	923	205	6.2	27.2	7.8	0.5
Special Fried, Somerfield*	1 Pack/200g	316	158	5.0	25.0	4.0	0.0
Special Fried, Tesco*	1 Pack/250g	333	133	7.6	17.6	3.6	1.7
Sticky Thai, Safeway*	1 Pack/200g	260	130	2.5	25.6	1.8	1.4
Sweet & Sour Savoury, Cooked, Asda*	½ Pack/126g	154	122	2.5	26.0	0.9	3.0
Sweet & Sour, Rice Bowl, Uncle Ben's*	1 Pack/350g	364	104	5.2	19.5	0.6	0.0
Thai, Chicken, Enjoy, Bird's Eye**	1 Pack/500g	535	107	6.9	13.2	3.0	0.7
Thai, Fragrant, Asda*	1 Serving/75g	264	352	7.0	79.0	0.9	0.0
Thai, Fragrant, Tesco*	1 Serving/75g	262	349	7.3	79.1	0.4	0.8
Thai, Jasmine, Tilda*	1oz/28g	97	348	7.1	79.5	0.2	0.4
Thai, Marks & Spencer*	1oz/28g	96	342	6.9	78.0	0.3	2.3
Thai, Sticky, Sainsbury's*	1 Serving/100g	132	132	2.3	26.1	2.0	0.3
Tomato & Basil, Express, Uncle Ben's*	1 Pack/250g	450	180	3.9	31.5	4.3	0.0
Valencia For Paella, Asda*	1 Serving/125g	435	348	6.0	79.0	0.8	0.0
Vegetable Pilau, Express, Uncle Ben's*	1 Pack/250g	445	178	3.4	33.8	3.2	0.0
Vegetable, Frozen, Tesco*	1 Serving/100g	105	105	4.0	20.8	0.6	1.1
Vegetable, Original, Bird's Eye*	1oz/28g	29	105	4.0	20.8	0.6	1.1
White, American Easy Cook, Cooked, Safeway*	1 Serving/180g	243	135	2.8	28.3	1.3	0.1
White, Boil in Bag, Sainsbury's*	1 Serving/169g	221	131	2.7	29.6	0.2	0.2
White, Easy Cook, Asda*	1 Serving/50g	178	356	7.0	79.0	0.9	0.4
White, Easy Cook, Italian, Sainsbury's*	1 Serving/50g	179	358	6.8	76.6	2.6	0.8
White, Flaked, Raw	1oz/28g	97	346	6.6	77.5	1.2	0.0
White, Fried	1oz/28g	37	131	2.2	25.0	3.2	0.6
White, Glutinous, Boiled	1oz/28g	18	65	1.7	14.7	0.3	0.0
White, Glutinous, Raw	1oz/28g	101	359	8.4	74.9	1.6	0.0
White, Microwaveable, Safeway*	1 Sachet/200g	210	105	2.7	22.4	0.5	1.1
White, Polished, Boiled	1oz/28g	34	123	2.2	29.6	0.3	0.2
White, Polished, Raw	1oz/28g	101	361	6.5	86.8	1.0	0.5
White, Red & Wild, Merchant Gourmet*	1 Sachet/125g	430	344	7.5	71.8	3.0	3.1
Wholegrain, Uncle Ben's*	1 Serving/65g	226	347	8.4	73.0	2.4	3.4
Yellow, Ready Cooked, Tesco*	1oz/28g	32	113	2.7	27.1	1.3	0.1
RICE & RED Kidney Beans, Average	1oz/28g	49	175	5.6	32.4	3.5	2.5
RICE BITES, Cheese & Onion Flavour, Asda*	1 Pack/30g	137	456	7.0	71.0	16.0	0.2
RICE BOWL,							
Chicken & Mushroom, Sharwood's*	1 Pack/350g	392	112	4.8	17.1	2.7	0.7
Chicken Tikka Masala, Uncle Bens*	1 Serving/350g	382	109	5.9	15.9	2.4	0.0

R

INFO/WEIGHT	Measure	per Measure KCAL	Nutrition Values per 100g / 100ml				
			KCAL	PROT	CARB	FAT	FIBRE
RICE BOWL,							
Free From, Sainsbury's*	1 Serving/182g	146	80	1.6	17.1	0.6	1.4
Honey BBQ Chicken, Uncle Ben's*	1 Pack/350g	420	120	5.4	23.1	0.6	0.0
RICE CAKES,							
Apple & Cinnamon Flavour, Kallo*	1 Cake/11g	41	376	6.2	83.1	2.2	3.9
Bacon, Asda*	1 Cake/9g	42	462	8.0	67.0	18.0	0.0
Black & White Sesame, Clearspring*	1 Cake/8g	31	385	7.4	82.2	2.9	0.0
Caramel Flavour, Kallo*	1 Cake/9.9g	38	383	6.2	78.9	4.8	3.9
Caramel Flavour, Tesco*	1 Cake/35g	133	379	5.5	82.7	2.9	0.9
Chocolate Flavour, Happy Shopper*	2 Portions/33.3g	155	469	5.1	69.9	18.8	2.4
Co-Op*	1 Cake/20g	80	402	8.0	84.0	3.1	0.0
Dark Chocolate, Organic, Kallo*	1 Cake/12g	57	471	6.8	57.2	24.1	7.4
Honey, Puffed, Kallo*	1 Serving/50g	182	364	7.0	80.0	2.0	6.7
Lightly Salted, Thick Slice, Low Fat, Kallo*	1 Cake/8g	30	372	8.0	78.7	2.8	5.1
Low Fat, Kallo*	1 Cake/10g	38	375	6.2	83.1	2.2	3.9
Milk Chocolate, Kallo*	1 Cake/15g	77	511	6.5	56.2	28.7	3.5
Oat, Kallo*	1 Slice/7.7g	28	351	10.6	75.3	5.5	9.1
Oat, Lightly Salted, Thick Slice, Kallo*	1 Cake/7.6g	28	356	10.6	75.0	5.5	9.0
Rice Bites, Asda*	1 Cake/8.8g	42	466	8.0	68.0	18.0	0.0
Ryvita*	1 Cake/7g	28	395	8.8	82.1	3.4	1.3
Salt 'n' Vinegar, Jumbo, Tesco*	1 Cake/8.8g	28	306	8.4	62.5	7.5	6.0
Savoury With Yeast Extract, Kallo*	1 Slice/11g	40	364	12.7	72.0	2.8	4.7
Savoury, Kallo*	1 Cake/8g	28	355	14.2	67.5	3.2	4.4
Sesame, Ryvita*	1 Slice/7.3g	28	396	8.2	82.3	3.8	1.3
Slightly Salted, Thick Slice, Organic, Kallo*	1 Cake/8g	30	372	8.0	78.7	2.8	5.1
Thin Slice, Organic, Kallo*	1 Cake/5g	19	372	8.0	78.7	2.8	5.1
Thin Slice, Organic, Waitrose*	1 Cake/6g	23	391	9.0	81.3	3.3	3.8
Wholegrain, No Added Salt, Thick Slice, Organic, Kallo*	1 Cake/9g	33	365	7.6	80.0	3.1	3.4
With Sesame, Organic, Evernat*	1 Cake/4g	15	368	8.5	74.5	4.0	0.0
With Sesame, Organic, Kallo*	1 Cake/7.5g	30	373	8.0	78.0	3.2	5.4
With Sesame, Thick Sliced, No Added Salt, Kallo*	1 Cake/10g	37	373	8.0	78.0	3.2	5.4
RICE CRACKERS,							
Choco Noir, Bonvita*	1 Cracker/18g	79	440	6.8	64.0	18.5	0.0
Japanese, Apollo*	1 Pack/75g	297	396	9.6	78.8	4.7	0.9
Japanese, Mini, Sunrise*	1 Serving/50g	180	360	7.0	83.0	0.0	7.0
Thin, Blue Dragon*	3 Crackers/5g	20	395	6.1	84.4	3.7	0.0
RICE PUDDING,							
50% Less Fat, Asda*	½ Can/212g	170	85	3.3	16.2	0.8	0.2
Apple, 99% Fat Free, Mullerice, Muller*	1 Pot/150g	125	83	3.5	15.3	0.9	0.0
BGTY, Sainsbury's*	½ Can/212g	180	85	3.3	16.2	0.8	0.2
Caramel, Mullerice, Muller*	1 Pot/200g	210	105	3.5	17.4	2.4	0.0
Clotted Cream, Marks & Spencer*	1 Pudding/185g	431	233	3.0	19.2	16.6	0.2
Creamed With Sultanas & Nutmeg, Ambrosia*	½ Can/200g	210	105	3.2	16.6	2.9	0.1
Creamed, Asda*	1 Serving/215.4g	196	91	3.2	16.0	1.6	0.0
Creamed, Canned, Ambrosia*	1 Can/425g	383	90	3.1	15.2	1.9	0.0
Creamed, Co-Op*	1 Can/170g	153	90	3.0	16.0	1.5	0.0
Creamed, Healthy Eating, New, Tesco*	1 Can/215g	146	68	3.6	11.4	0.9	0.0
Creamed, Low Fat, Ambrosia*	1 Serving/150g	129	86	3.3	16.1	0.9	0.0
Creamed, Morrisons*	1 Can/212g	189	89	3.1	15.7	1.6	0.0
Creamed, Pot, Ambrosia*	1 Pot/150g	152	101	3.2	16.5	2.5	0.0
Creamy Rice With Tropical Crunch, Ambrosia*	1 Pack/210g	307	146	3.6	23.4	4.2	0.6
Creamy Rice, Shape*	1 Serving/175g	149	85	3.5	15.4	1.0	0.4
Creamy With Strawberry Crunch, Ambrosia*	1 Pack/205g	297	145	3.9	23.0	4.2	0.7
Eat Smart, Safeway*	1 Serving/212g	138	65	3.4	10.3	0.8	0.0

R

INFO/WEIGHT	Measure	per Measure KCAL	Nutrition Values per 100g / 100ml				
			KCAL	PROT	CARB	FAT	FIBRE
RICE PUDDING,							
Everyday, Co-Op*	1 Can/396	333	84	3.4	15.5	0.9	0.1
GFY, Asda*	1 Pudding/119g	115	97	4.2	17.0	1.4	0.5
Libby's*	1 Serving/200g	180	90	3.3	16.2	1.6	0.2
Light, Mullerice, Muller*	1 Pot/100g	72	72	3.5	12.2	0.9	0.0
Low Fat, Budgens*	1 Can/425g	370	87	3.4	16.3	0.9	0.0
Low Fat, Canned, Ambrosia*	½ Can/200g	162	81	3.2	15.2	0.8	0.0
Low Fat, Co-Op*	1 Sm Can/170g	145	85	3.0	16.0	0.8	0.0
Low Fat, Good Intentions, Somerfield*	½ Can/212g	164	77	3.0	15.1	0.6	0.2
Low Fat, Healthy Selection, Somerfield*	1 Pot/213g	173	81	4.0	15.0	1.0	0.0
Low Fat, No Added Sugar, Weight Watchers*	½ Can/212g	155	73	3.7	11.4	1.5	0.0
Low Fat, Pot, Ambrosia*	1 Pot/150g	129	86	3.3	16.1	0.9	0.0
Luxury Rice, Llangadog Creamery*	1 Serving/220g	310	141	3.1	15.2	7.7	0.0
Milk, Economy, Sainsbury's*	½ Can/198g	139	70	3.2	12.6	0.8	0.2
Organic, Ambrosia*	1 Can/425g	455	107	3.4	15.1	3.7	0.0
Organic, Co-Op*	1 Can/425g	446	105	3.0	16.0	3.0	0.2
Original, 99% Fat Free, Mullerice, Muller*	1 Pot/150g	108	72	3.9	11.8	1.0	0.0
Original, Mullerice, Muller*	1 Pot/200g	232	116	3.7	19.1	2.7	0.0
Raisin & Nutmeg, Muller*	1 Pot/200g	244	122	3.3	22.0	2.3	0.0
Raspberry, Muller*	1 Pot/200g	228	114	3.4	20.0	2.3	0.0
Sainsbury's*	1 Serving/100g	102	102	3.8	14.5	3.2	0.2
Strawberry, 99% Fat Free, Muller*	1 Serving/150g	116	77	3.5	13.6	0.9	0.0
Strawberry, Muller*	1 Pot/150g	173	115	3.4	20.0	2.4	0.0
Thick & Creamy, Co-Op*	1 Can/425g	531	125	3.0	16.0	6.0	0.0
Thick & Creamy, Nestle*	1 Can/425g	527	124	3.1	15.4	5.6	0.2
Toffee, 99% Fat Free, Muller*	1 Tub/150g	119	79	3.3	14.3	1.0	0.0
Value, Tesco*	½ Can/212g	178	84	3.3	15.5	0.9	0.2
Vanilla Custard, Mullerice, Muller*	1 Pot/200g	250	125	3.3	22.1	2.6	0.0
Venetian, Cafe Culture, Marks & Spencer*	1 Serving/120g	300	250	3.4	21.8	16.4	0.2
With Cream, Sainsbury's*	1 Can/229.5g	242	105	3.1	9.8	5.9	0.0
With Jam, Kosy Shack, Costcutters*	1 Serving/150g	173	115	3.5	19.8	2.5	0.9
With Sultanas & Nutmeg, Ambrosia*	1 Pack/425g	446	105	3.2	16.6	2.9	0.1
With Sultanas & Nutmeg, Co-Op*	1 Can/425g	446	105	3.0	18.0	3.0	0.1
RICE SALAD, Average	1oz/28g	46	166	3.1	23.1	7.5	0.7
RIGATONI,							
Asda*	1 Serving/25g	87	346	12.0	71.0	1.5	3.0
Carbonara, Tesco*	1 Serving/205g	236	115	5.2	10.6	5.8	1.2
Cooked, Asda*	1 Serving/185g	242	131	4.4	27.0	0.6	1.1
Italian, Sainsbury's*	1 Serving/75g	281	375	12.3	73.1	1.7	2.5
Spicy Vegetable, HP*	1 Can/400g	230	58	1.8	9.2	1.5	0.9
Tomato & Cheese, Perfectly Balanced, Waitrose*	1 Pack/400g	664	166	7.6	28.6	2.3	2.3
RISOTTO,							
Balls, Mushroom, Occasions, Sainsbury's*	1 Ball/25g	76	304	3.8	41.2	13.8	1.7
Balls, Sun Dried Tomato, Occasions, Sainsbury's*	1 Ball/25g	71	285	6.8	30.8	15.0	2.9
Beef, For 1, Vesta*	1 Risotto/95g	329	346	15.3	57.8	5.9	5.6
Caramelised Onion & Gruyere Cheese, Marks & Spencer*	1 Pack/200g	350	175	3.0	17.8	10.3	1.7
Chargrilled Chicken, Ready Meal, Marks & Spencer*	1 Pack/365g	493	135	6.4	11.6	6.9	0.7
Cherry Tomato, COU, Marks & Spencer*	1 Pack/400g	320	80	1.9	16.6	0.9	1.8
Chicken & Asparagus, Eat Smart, Safeway*	1 Pack/380g	418	110	6.2	16.8	1.5	0.6
Chicken & Bacon, Italiano, Tesco*	1 Pack/450g	653	145	5.9	20.2	4.5	1.5
Chicken & Lemon, Weight Watchers*	1 Pack/330g	317	96	5.9	12.3	2.6	0.5
Chicken & Mushroom, Finest, Tesco*	1 Pack/400g	496	124	7.4	17.2	2.8	0.5
Chicken & Mushroom, Good Intentions, Somerfield*	1 Pack/300g	345	115	5.7	19.0	1.8	0.3
Chicken & Sun Dried Tomato, Waitrose*	1 Pack/350g	385	110	6.0	7.2	6.3	0.3

	Measure	per Measure	Nutrition Values per 100g / 100ml				
	INFO/WEIGHT	KCAL	KCAL	PROT	CARB	FAT	FIBRE
RISOTTO,							
Chicken, BGTY, Sainsbury's*	1 Pack/327g	356	109	7.5	15.5	1.9	1.0
Chicken, Co-Op*	1 Pack/340g	442	130	6.0	16.0	5.0	2.0
Chicken, Enjoy, Bird's Eye*	1 Pack/500g	735	147	8.5	14.0	6.3	0.5
Chicken, Ready Meal, Marks & Spencer*	1 Pack/360g	450	125	6.7	14.4	4.4	0.9
Haddock & Mushroom, COU, Marks & Spencer*	1 Pack/400g	320	80	6.4	12.1	0.8	2.0
Hot Smoked Salmon & Spinach, Marks & Spencer*	½ Pack/300g	420	140	6.4	11.0	8.0	0.6
Italian Red Wine With Creamed Spinach, Sainsbury's*	1 Pack/400g	596	149	2.4	19.3	6.9	0.4
King Prawn & Snow Crab, Marks & Spencer*	1 Pack/365g	402	110	4.1	12.7	4.5	0.5
King Prawn, Pea & Mint, Marks & Spencer*	½ Pack/300g	405	135	3.8	15.9	6.2	0.9
Lemon & Mint, Perfectly Balanced, Waitrose*	1 Pack/350g	462	132	3.9	20.7	3.7	1.0
Mushroom, Asda*	1 Pack/340g	340	100	2.3	15.0	3.4	0.6
Mushroom, BGTY, Sainsbury's*	1 Pack/400g	320	80	2.6	15.6	0.8	0.6
Mushroom, COU, Marks & Spencer*	1 Pack/330g	314	95	2.9	15.3	2.3	1.0
Mushroom, Finest, Tesco*	1 Pack/350g	550	157	3.1	16.4	8.8	1.2
Mushroom, Healthy Living, Tesco*	1 Pack/400g	320	80	2.6	15.6	0.8	0.6
Mushroom, Italiano, Tesco*	1 Pack/340g	367	108	2.4	20.0	2.0	4.6
Mushroom, Ready Meals, Marks & Spencer*	1 Pack/360g	450	125	2.8	16.9	4.9	1.0
Mushroom, Safeway*	1 Pack/350g	406	116	2.7	19.0	3.2	2.9
Mushroom, Somerfield*	1 Pack/300g	333	111	2.0	16.0	4.0	0.0
Mushroom, Waitrose*	1 Pack/350g	277	79	1.9	6.9	4.9	0.5
Roasted Vegetable & Sunblush Tomato, Finest, Tesco*	½ Pack/200g	306	153	3.7	14.5	9.0	1.4
Roasted Vegetables, Stir-in, Uncle Ben's*	½ Pack/75g	86	115	1.7	5.0	9.7	0.0
Seafood, Youngs*	1 Pack/350g	424	121	4.5	17.4	3.7	0.1
Spring Vegetable, Marks & Spencer*	1 Serving/330g	330	100	2.0	14.2	4.0	0.9
Tomato & Cheese, Good For You, Asda*	1 Pack/400g	428	107	3.1	17.0	3.0	0.7
Tomato & Mascarpone, Marks & Spencer*	1 Pack/360g	468	130	2.7	17.5	5.3	0.9
Wild Mushroom & Garlic, Tesco*	1 Pack/320g	522	163	3.6	27.2	4.4	1.6
RISPINOS,							
Apple & Cinnamon, Uncle Ben's*	1 Bag/60g	230	383	4.7	90.0	0.5	0.0
Barbecue, Uncle Ben's*	1 Pack/50g	182	363	8.4	82.0	0.2	0.0
Caramel, Uncle Ben's*	1 Pack/60g	229	382	5.1	89.0	0.7	0.0
Cheese & Onion, Uncle Ben's*	1 Pack/50g	181	361	8.4	81.0	0.4	0.0
Chocolate, Uncle Ben's*	1oz/28g	108	385	5.3	89.0	1.1	0.0
Coconut, Uncle Ben's*	1oz/28g	111	396	6.7	86.0	2.8	0.0
Pizza, Uncle Ben's*	1 Pack/50g	182	363	8.4	82.0	0.2	0.0
Vanilla, Uncle Ben's	1oz/28g	107	383	7.7	87.0	0.5	0.0
RISSOLES, Lentil, Fried in Vegetable Oil	1oz/28g	59	211	8.9	22.0	10.5	3.6
ROAST, Vegetarian, Chicken Style, Tesco*	1 Serving/113g	214	189	22.1	4.8	9.0	1.7
ROCKET,							
Wild, Sainsbury's*	1oz/28g	8	28	3.9	2.6	0.2	0.6
Wild, Tesco*	1 Bag/50g	9	18	3.3	0.6	0.3	1.7
ROCKET SOLO, Waitrose*	1 Serving/50g	8	15	0.8	1.7	0.5	0.9
ROCKY, Fox's*	1 Bar/25g	129	516	8.2	58.8	27.5	1.4
ROE,							
Cod, Hard, Coated in Batter, Fried	1oz/28g	53	189	12.4	8.9	11.8	0.2
Cod, Hard, Fried in Blended Oil	1oz/28g	57	202	20.9	3.0	11.9	0.1
Cod, Hard, Raw	1oz/28g	29	104	21.7	0.0	1.9	0.0
Cod, Pressed, John West*	1 Can/200g	198	99	17.6	1.4	2.6	0.1
Cod, Soft, John West*	1 Can/100g	84	84	12.0	0.0	4.0	0.0
Herring, Soft, Fried in Blended Oil	1oz/28g	74	265	26.3	4.7	15.8	0.2
Herring, Soft, Raw	1oz/28g	25	91	16.8	0.0	2.6	0.0
Soft Herring, in Brine, Sainsbury's*	1 Can/86g	105	122	22.2	0.1	3.7	0.0

R

	Measure	per Measure	Nutrition Values per 100g / 100ml				
	INFO/WEIGHT	KCAL	KCAL	PROT	CARB	FAT	FIBRE
ROGAN JOSH,							
Chicken & Rice, Sainsbury's*	1 Pack/500g	730	146	7.9	16.6	5.3	1.3
Chicken, With Pilau Rice, Farmfoods*	1 Pack/325g	354	109	5.3	17.1	2.1	0.4
Lamb With Basmati Rice, Eat Smart, Safeway*	1 Pack/380g	380	100	6.9	14.0	1.5	1.9
Lamb, Marks & Spencer*	1 Pack/300g	360	120	14.4	3.9	5.1	1.2
Lamb, Sainsbury's*	1 Pack/400g	660	165	11.3	4.9	11.1	1.9
Lamb, Tesco*	1 Pack/350g	504	144	12.2	6.7	7.6	2.4
Lamb, Waitrose*	1 Serving/60g	79	131	12.3	3.0	7.8	1.3
Lamb, With Pilau Rice, Eastern Classics*	1 Pack/400g	604	151	5.6	19.9	5.4	1.0
Prawn & Pilau Rice, BGTY, Sainsbury's*	1 Pack/401g	353	88	4.8	15.3	0.8	1.9
Prawn, COU, Marks & Spencer*	1 Pack/400g	360	90	4.9	16.2	0.6	0.8
ROLL,							
All Day Breakfast, Asda*	1 Roll/220g	581	264	10.0	29.0	12.0	0.0
Bacon With Brown Sauce, McDonald's*	1 Roll/118g	289	245	12.8	31.2	8.4	1.4
Bacon, Marks & Spencer*	2 Rolls/18g	40	220	14.2	0.4	18.3	0.0
Beef, Weight Watchers*	1 Roll/174g	276	159	10.8	23.1	2.5	1.0
Brie & Grapes, Marks & Spencer*	1 Roll/57g	174	306	11.1	24.5	18.2	1.4
Brown, Roast Chicken & Mayonnaise, Big, Sainsbury's*	1 Pack/185g	479	259	9.6	21.8	14.8	0.0
Cheese & Onion, Co-Op*	1 Roll/66g	195	295	7.0	26.0	18.0	2.0
Cheese & Onion, Iceland*	1 Roll/66.9g	222	332	7.5	29.6	20.4	1.5
Cheese & Onion, Sainsbury's*	1 Roll/67g	205	306	8.0	22.9	20.3	1.9
Cheese & Onion, Somerfield*	1 Roll/70g	242	345	8.0	28.0	22.0	0.0
Cheese & Pickle, Sainsbury's*	1 Roll/136g	359	264	10.6	35.1	10.0	0.0
Cheese & Tomato, Benjys*	1 Pack/263g	742	282	12.2	29.8	12.7	0.0
Cheese Ploughman's, Malted Wheat, BGTY, Sainsbury's*	1 Roll/171.7g	310	180	10.9	29.3	2.1	3.8
Chicken & Herb, Shapers, Boots*	1 Roll/167.6g	291	173	12.0	25.0	2.8	1.7
Chicken & Sun Dried Tomato, Weight Watchers*	1 Pack/170g	272	160	12.9	22.7	1.9	1.2
Chicken Salad, Healthy Eating, Tesco*	1 Serving/224g	289	129	10.3	16.0	2.6	1.1
Chunky Cheese & Mustard, Finest, Tesco*	1 Roll/88g	260	295	10.9	40.0	10.2	2.4
Chunky Herbes de Provence, Finest, Tesco*	1 Roll/82g	196	239	7.4	45.2	3.2	2.6
Egg & Tomato, Shapers, Boots*	1 Roll/166.3g	300	181	8.0	30.0	3.2	2.6
Ham & Pineapple, Eat Smart, Safeway*	1 Serving/180g	225	125	11.2	17.2	1.1	2.6
Ham Salad, BGTY, Sainsbury's*	1 Roll/178g	292	164	10.0	23.3	3.4	0.0
Ham Salad, Good Intentions, Somerfield*	1 Pack/213.8g	325	152	8.7	24.3	2.2	1.6
Leicester Ham & Cheese, Sub, Waitrose*	1 Pack/206.4ml	581	282	12.6	24.0	15.1	13.0
Mushroom & Bacon, Crusty, Marks & Spencer*	1 Roll/160g	424	265	8.7	29.0	12.6	2.3
Oak Smoked Salmon, Marks & Spencer*	1 Roll/55g	139	252	14.6	23.1	11.3	1.2
Prawn Mayo & Chicken Salad, Shapers, Boots*	1 Serving/100g	274	274	15.0	44.0	4.2	2.3
Roast Pork, Stuffing & Apple Sauce, Boots*	1 Roll/218.1g	602	276	10.0	32.0	12.0	1.8
Spicy Chicken, Crusty, Marks & Spencer*	1 Roll/150g	383	255	12.8	25.8	11.1	2.0
Steak & Onion, Marks & Spencer*	1 Serving/150g	308	205	11.0	24.5	7.0	3.8
Taiko California, Waitrose*	4 Pieces/120g	196	163	4.4	26.8	4.1	1.5
Tuna & Sweetcorn With Mayonnaise, Shell*	1 Pack/180g	536	298	13.1	28.6	14.6	0.0
Turkey Salad, Northern Bites*	1 Roll/230.7g	323	140	8.6	19.6	3.6	3.0
Turkey, Stuffed, Good for You, Asda*	½ Pack/225g	320	142	14.0	12.0	4.2	0.8
White, Cheese & Onion, Shell*	1 Roll/178g	554	311	14.5	30.2	14.8	0.0
ROLLMOPS, Tesco*	1 Serving/130g	181	139	7.8	8.6	8.2	0.4
ROLO,							
Giant, Nestle*	1 Rolo/5g	24	468	3.2	70.0	19.5	0.0
Minis, Nestle*	1 Pack/26g	124	473	3.5	69.1	20.3	0.0
Nestle*	1 Rolo/9g	43	473	3.5	69.1	20.3	0.0
ROLY POLY,							
Jam & Custard, Safeway*	1 Serving/112g	299	267	3.8	43.0	8.9	0.8
Jam & Custard, Sainsbury's*	1 Pack/205g	521	254	3.3	34.1	11.6	0.5

	Measure INFO/WEIGHT	per Measure KCAL	Nutrition Values per 100g / 100ml				
			KCAL	PROT	CARB	FAT	FIBRE
ROLY POLY,							
Jam, & Custard, Co-Op*	¼ Pack/100g	235	235	4.0	36.0	8.0	0.7
Jam, Tesco*	1 Serving/82g	308	375	4.7	51.5	16.7	1.2
Syrup, With Fresh Custard, Sainsbury's*	1 Pack/225g	524	233	3.4	29.9	11.1	0.4
ROOT BEER, Average	1 Can/330ml	135	41	0.0	10.6	0.0	0.0
ROSEMARY,							
Dried	1 Tsp/1g	3	331	4.9	46.4	15.2	0.0
Fresh	1oz/28g	28	99	1.4	13.5	4.4	0.0
ROSES, Cadbury's*	1oz/28g	136	485	4.8	60.9	24.8	0.0
ROSTI,							
Garlic & Mushroom, Finest, Tesco*	1 Serving/200g	346	173	5.7	15.4	9.8	1.7
Oven Baked, McCain*	1 Rosti/95g	234	246	3.7	29.7	12.8	0.0
Peppered Steak, British Classics, Tesco*	1 Pack/450g	599	133	9.0	10.7	6.2	1.7
Potato & Leek, Sainsbury's*	½ Pack/190g	296	156	4.5	9.8	11.0	0.3
Potato & Root Vegetable, COU, Marks & Spencer*	1 Cake/100g	85	85	1.6	13.3	2.7	1.5
Potato Cakes, Marks & Spencer*	1 Cake/100g	100	100	1.7	13.8	4.5	3.3
Potato, Fresh, Safeway*	1 Rost/100g	138	138	2.8	19.2	5.5	2.8
Potato, McCain*	1 Rosti/95g	161	169	2.2	19.6	9.1	0.0
Potato, Mini, Party Range, Tesco*	1 Rosti/16.7g	33	193	2.1	20.6	11.4	3.3
Potato, Onion & Gruyere, Finest, Tesco*	1 Pack/350g	403	115	3.5	11.9	5.9	1.4
Vegetable, Waitrose*	1 Pack/400g	248	62	1.4	8.8	2.3	1.3
ROUGHY, Orange, Raw	1oz/28g	35	126	14.7	0.0	7.0	0.0
ROULADE,							
Chocolate, Finest, Tesco*	1 Serving/80g	222	277	3.4	53.2	5.6	2.3
Lemon Meringue, Marks & Spencer	1 Serving/74g	230	311	3.2	46.6	12.5	0.3
Lemon, Asda*	1 Serving/100g	343	343	2.7	56.0	12.0	0.0
Orange & Lemon Meringue, Co-Op*	1 Serving/82g	287	350	3.0	57.0	12.0	0.3
Salmon & Spinach, Tesco*	1 serving/60g	155	258	9.5	1.7	23.7	0.2
RUBY BREAKFAST JUICE, Tropicana*	1 Glass/200ml	86	43	0.7	9.0	0.0	0.5
RUBY ORANGE JUICE, Marks & Spencer*	1 Bottle/250ml	125	50	0.7	11.5	0.0	0.2
RUM,							
37.5% Volume	1 Shot/25ml	52	207	0.0	0.0	0.0	0.0
40% Volume	1 Shot/25ml	56	222	0.0	0.0	0.0	0.0
RYVITA BREAKS, Ryvita*	1 Slice/14.4g	47	333	8.0	69.5	2.5	12.0

R

INFO/WEIGHT	Measure per Measure KCAL	Nutrition Values per 100g / 100ml KCAL	PROT	CARB	FAT	FIBRE
SAAG,						
Aloo, Canned, Tesco*	½ Can/200g	124	62	1.8	9.3	1.9	2.0
Aloo, Fresh, Sainsbury's*	1 Pack/400g	388	97	2.0	14.7	3.3	4.8
Aloo, Sainsbury's*	½ Pack/150g	177	118	2.4	9.0	8.0	1.6
Aloo, Tesco*	1 Serving/200g	144	72	2.1	8.0	3.5	2.0
Chicken, Marks & Spencer*	1 Pack/300g	435	145	11.1	4.0	9.4	1.9
Chicken, Safeway*	1 Pack/350g	504	144	11.6	5.4	8.4	1.4
Gobi Aloo, Indian Takeaway, Sainsbury's*	1 Pack/334g	164	49	1.7	8.0	1.1	1.5
Gobi Aloo, Marks & Spencer*	1 Pack/225g	270	120	1.9	9.3	8.5	2.4
Gobi Aloo, Tesco*	1 Servings/175g	182	104	2.3	7.3	7.3	1.4
Paneer, Sainsbury's*	½ Pack/200g	380	190	8.5	4.5	15.3	1.2
SACCHETINI, Italian Meat & Cheese, Tesco*	½ Pack/125g	323	258	13.8	34.4	7.2	2.1
SAFFRON, Average	1 Tsp/0.7g	3	310	11.4	61.5	5.9	0.0
SAGE,						
Dried, Ground	1 Tsp/1g	3	315	10.6	42.7	12.7	0.0
Fresh	1oz/28g	33	119	3.9	15.6	4.6	0.0
SALAD,						
Alfresco Style, Tesco*	1 Serving/200g	40	20	0.9	3.3	0.3	1.4
All Seasons, Sainsbury's*	1oz/28g	3	12	1.0	1.5	0.2	1.2
American Ranch, Asda*	1 Serving/220g	253	115	2.5	6.0	9.0	2.0
American Style, Morrisons*	1 Serving/25g	5	22	1.1	3.9	0.3	2.3
Aromatic Herb, Waitrose*	¼ Pack/27g	4	15	0.9	1.7	0.5	1.0
Assorted, Asda*	1 Serving/100g	22	22	2.4	1.7	0.6	0.0
Avocado, Spinach & Cherry Tomato, Marks & Spencer*	1 Pack/320g	416	130	8.7	2.4	10.7	0.0
Baby Leaf With Watercress, Tesco*	¼ Bag/25g	5	19	2.0	1.3	0.7	1.4
Baby Leaf, Fully Prepared, Sainsbury's*	½ Bag/63g	10	16	1.3	1.9	0.4	1.5
Baby Spinach & Red Mustard, Marks & Spencer*	1 Pack/170g	264	155	1.7	1.1	15.7	0.1
Baby Tomato, Tesco*	1 Pack/205g	35	17	0.8	2.8	0.3	0.9
Bacon Caesar, Marks & Spencer*	1oz/28g	48	170	5.5	5.7	14.0	1.2
Bacon Caesar, Sainsburys*	1 Pack/256g	415	162	4.7	7.3	12.7	1.4
Bean & Chorizo, Tapas Selection, Sainsbury's*	1 Serving/22g	29	132	8.1	10.7	6.3	1.9
Bean & Sweetcorn, Side, Marks & Spencer*	1 Serving/125g	131	105	2.5	7.0	7.2	1.3
Bean, & Mexican Rice, COU, Marks & Spencer*	1 Serving/250g	250	100	6.0	15.6	1.4	1.2
Bean, Marks & Spencer*	1 Serving/80g	72	90	6.4	14.3	0.9	3.9
Bean, Mint & Coriander, Somerfield*	1 Pack/250g	288	115	7.0	19.4	1.1	4.7
Bean, Three, Marks & Spencer*	1 Pack/225g	225	100	5.8	16.7	1.3	3.9
Bean, Vinaigrette Mixed, Tesco*	1 Can/400g	280	70	3.2	13.1	0.5	1.9
Beetroot & Carrot, Continental, Iceland*	1 Serving/100g	24	24	1.2	4.3	0.2	2.1
Beetroot, 1% Fat, Marks & Spencer*	1 Serving/225g	131	58	1.1	7.7	2.7	1.7
Beetroot, Co-Op*	1 Pack/250g	100	40	0.9	8.0	0.3	2.0
Beetroot, Good For You, Asda*	1 Serving/84g	46	55	1.0	12.0	0.3	1.8
Beetroot, Healthy Eating, Tesco*	1 Tub/200g	204	102	1.4	22.6	0.6	1.4
Beetroot, Sainsbury's*	1 Tub/200g	160	80	0.9	11.7	3.3	2.1
Bistro, Asda*	1 Serving/180g	29	16	1.4	2.7	0.0	2.5
Bistro, Morrisons*	1 Serving/20g	5	23	1.2	4.2	0.2	2.0
Bistro, Sainsbury's*	1 Pack/150g	33	22	1.1	3.6	0.4	1.3
Bistro, Washed Ready To Eat, Tesco*	1 Pack/140g	22	16	1.1	1.7	0.5	1.0
Bowl, French Style, Way to Five, Sainsbury's*	1 Pack/264g	103	39	0.7	4.2	2.2	2.2
Bowl, Large, Sainsbury's*	1 Pack/300g	51	17	1.1	2.9	0.2	2.3
Burger King*	1 Serving/165g	34	21	1.2	3.5	0.2	2.6
Cabbage & Leek, Crunchy Mix, Sainsbury's*	½ Pack/126.3g	24	19	1.2	2.1	0.6	1.9
Caesar Kit, New Improved, Tesco*	½ Pack/138g	279	202	4.7	4.5	18.3	1.3
Caesar Kit, Safeway*	2 Servings/295g	504	171	3.8	4.9	15.1	1.1
Caesar, BGTY, Sainsbury's*	½ Bag/127g	168	132	3.6	8.6	9.9	1.7

SALAD,	Measure INFO/WEIGHT	per Measure KCAL	KCAL	PROT	CARB	FAT	FIBRE
Caesar, Bistro, Waitrose*	½ Pack/112.5g	172	152	6.4	6.3	11.2	7.6
Caesar, Co-Op*	¼ Pack/50g	88	175	3.0	6.0	15.0	2.0
Caesar, Finest, Tesco*	1 Lge Bowl/220g	532	242	5.2	4.7	22.5	0.9
Caesar, Good For You, Asda*	½ Pack/87.4g	76	87	8.0	7.0	3.0	1.5
Caesar, Healthy Eating, Tesco*	1 Serving/100g	101	101	3.2	8.0	6.2	0.7
Caesar, Improved Recipe, Marks & Spencer*	1 Pack/290g	551	190	5.0	1.3	18.1	1.3
Caesar, Kit, Asda*	½ Pack/113g	154	136	5.0	11.0	8.0	1.4
Caesar, Kit, Tesco*	½ Pack/150g	237	158	3.2	6.7	13.2	0.7
Caesar, Lower Fat, BGTY, Sainsbury's*	½ Pack/126.9g	132	104	3.6	9.8	5.6	1.7
Caesar, Marks & Spencer*	1 Serving/100g	151	151	2.6	8.0	12.1	0.7
Caesar, Morrisons*	1 Serving/115g	179	156	3.4	9.5	12.8	0.3
Caesar, Sainsbury's*	½ Bag/128g	227	177	3.6	6.7	15.1	1.0
Caesar, Somerfield*	1 Pack/255g	339	133	4.6	5.1	10.5	1.3
Caesar, Waitrose*	1 Serving/115g	175	152	6.4	6.3	11.2	0.8
Caesar, Washed & Ready to Eat, Somerfield*	½ Bag/125g	155	124	5.0	6.5	8.7	0.8
Cajun Chicken, David Lloyd Leisure*	1 Pack/300g	429	143	11.7	17.7	3.3	1.0
Californian Crunch, GFY, Asda*	1 Pack/160g	75	47	0.9	8.0	1.3	1.8
Cannelini Bean & Chorizo, Sainsbury's*	1 Pack/250g	228	91	5.3	10.2	3.2	1.6
Carrot & Sultana, Healthy Living, Tesco*	1 Tub/225g	142	63	1.2	13.2	0.6	2.5
Carrot, Orange & Ginger, Good Intentions, Somerfield*	1 Serving/250g	275	110	2.0	22.4	1.4	1.4
Carrot, Peanut & Sultana, Asda*	1 Serving/20g	54	272	8.0	15.0	20.0	4.5
Ceasar, Bacon, Marks & Spencer*	1 Serving/250g	400	160	7.1	4.1	12.5	1.3
Celery, Nut & Sultana, Asda*	1oz/28g	76	272	2.9	11.2	23.9	1.9
Celery, Nut & Sultana, Waitrose*	1oz/28g	54	192	2.8	8.4	16.4	1.0
Chargrilled Chicken Tesco*	1 Serving/300g	384	128	6.1	15.0	4.8	2.4
Chargrilled Chicken Wholefood, Marks & Spencer*	1 Pot/219g	230	105	10.1	11.6	1.9	4.8
Chargrilled Chicken, Safeway*	1 Serving/200g	280	140	8.9	17.9	3.6	1.4
Chargrilled Pepper With Cous Cous, Asda*	1 Pack/325.2g	426	131	4.3	21.0	3.3	0.0
Chargrilled Vegetable Tortellini, Snack, Tesco*	1 Serving/300g	492	164	5.1	18.7	7.7	1.7
Cheddar Cheese & Pasta, Tesco*	1 Pot/215g	546	254	5.7	12.0	20.4	0.8
Cheese Layered, Marks & Spencer*	1 Pack/450g	923	205	4.3	9.0	17.0	0.7
Cheese Layered, Tesco*	1 Serving/165g	264	160	4.4	9.9	11.4	1.0
Chick Pea & Cous Cous, Tesco*	1 Serving/250g	245	98	3.2	15.5	2.6	0.0
Chick Pea & Spinach, Marks & Spencer*	1 Serving/260g	299	115	7.3	12.5	4.1	2.7
Chicken & Bacon, Asda*	1 Pack/381.0g	480	126	7.0	11.0	6.0	0.0
Chicken & Caesar, Boots*	1 Serving/200g	144	72	4.9	2.8	4.6	1.4
Chicken & Rice, Safeway*	1 Serving/200g	220	110	6.4	17.6	1.3	1.4
Chicken Caesar Bistro, Marks & Spencer*	½ Pack/135g	189	140	5.0	6.5	10.6	0.6
Chicken Caesar, Menu, Boots*	1 Serving/171g	145	85	5.8	3.3	5.4	1.6
Chicken Caesar, Pizza Express*	1 Serving/100g	519	519	32.0	39.0	29.0	0.0
Chicken Caesar, Shapers, Boots*	1 Serving/200g	316	158	6.6	19.0	6.2	1.1
Chicken Caesar, Simply, Boots*	1 Pack/162g	196	121	12.0	4.8	6.0	1.3
Chicken Caesar, Snack, Sainsbury's*	1 Pack/182.2g	164	90	5.9	5.3	5.0	1.0
Chicken Caesar, TTD, Sainsbury's*	1 Serving/190g	308	162	11.1	1.6	12.3	1.5
Chicken Caesar, Tesco*	1 Pack/300g	330	110	6.8	10.6	4.5	0.8
Chicken Ceasar, Marks & Spencer*	½ Pack/140g	266	190	6.7	8.7	14.3	0.8
Chicken Tikka & Rice, COU, Marks & Spencer*	1 Pack/390g	410	105	5.1	18.7	1.0	0.6
Chicken With Mayonnaise, Waitrose*	1 Pack/208g	406	195	10.3	17.1	9.5	2.5
Chicken, Healthy Eating, Tesco*	1 Salad/216g	296	137	8.4	22.6	1.4	1.2
Chicken, Healthy Option, Mattessons*	1 Pack/200g	344	172	11.1	20.0	5.3	2.9
Chicken, Safeway*	1 Serving/200g	279	140	8.9	17.9	3.6	1.4
Chicken, Sweetcorn & Pasta, Safeway*	1 Serving/200g	230	115	7.5	16.3	1.8	1.0
Chicken, Tesco*	1 Serving/300g	348	116	5.3	7.0	7.4	1.0

S

SALAD,

INFO/WEIGHT	Measure per Measure KCAL	Nutrition Values per 100g / 100ml KCAL	PROT	CARB	FAT	FIBRE
Chilli Chicken & Spicy Cous Cous, Healthy Eating, Tesco*	1 Serving/190g	251	132	6.5	21.1	2.4	1.5
Chilli, Tomato, Chick Pea & Butterbean, Tesco*	1 Pack/130g	146	112	3.4	14.3	4.6	0.5
Chunky, Somerfield*	1 Serving/250g	40	16	1.0	3.0	0.0	0.9
Classic Caesar, Marks & Spencer*	½ Pack/112g	174	155	2.9	6.8	12.7	0.5
Classic Caesar, Reduced Fat, Marks & Spencer*	1 Serving/115g	132	115	4.8	12.7	4.9	0.5
Club, Safeway*	1 Serving/215g	226	105	1.3	6.0	8.4	1.3
Coleslaw, Layered, Asda*	1 Pack/440g	810	184	1.1	4.5	18.0	0.0
Complete Hot Greek, Sainsbury's*	1 Pack/299g	287	96	4.3	2.9	7.5	1.7
Continental Style, Co-Op*	1 Bag/100g	15	15	1.0	2.0	0.3	0.5
Coronation Chicken, Sainsbury's*	1 Serving/62.4g	180	290	6.3	14.4	23.0	1.4
Coronation Chicken, Salad Bar, Asda*	1oz/28g	82	293	5.7	16.4	22.7	0.7
Coronation Rice, Tesco*	1 Serving/50g	104	207	2.0	15.9	15.1	0.8
Cous Cous With Chargrilled Chicken, Sainsbury's*	1 Pack/240g	446	186	7.4	19.6	8.7	0.0
Cous Cous, Better For You, Morrisons*	½ Pot/113g	164	145	4.6	23.8	3.5	0.5
Cous Cous, Tesco*	1 Serving/25g	35	141	4.8	26.9	1.6	0.6
Cous Cous, With Mixed Peppers & Cucumber, GFY, Asda*	¼ Pot/56g	66	117	3.9	25.0	0.2	1.5
Couton & Mediterranean Herb, Rochelle*	1 Serving/15g	77	510	8.5	62.7	25.0	2.5
Crayfish, Pret A Manger*	1 Av Pack/320g	200	63	3.0	0.8	5.2	0.3
Creamy Potato With Onion & Chives, Sainsbury's*	¼ Pot/62.5g	96	153	1.3	9.0	12.4	2.7
Crisp & Cruncy With French Dressing, GFY, Asda*	1/3 Pack/116g	26	22	0.8	3.3	0.6	1.4
Crisp & Light, Marks & Spencer*	1 Serving/170g	51	30	0.5	5.4	0.8	1.0
Crisp & Sweet, Asda*	1 Serving/100g	19	19	0.9	3.1	0.3	1.7
Crisp Mixed, Tesco*	1 Pack/200g	38	19	1.1	2.8	0.3	1.5
Crispy Duck & Herb, Marks & Spencer*	½ Pack/140g	378	270	20.7	3.7	18.3	1.4
Crispy Green, Safeway*	1 Bag/165g	21	13	1.0	1.6	0.3	1.1
Crispy Green, Sainsbury's*	1 Serving/70g	8	12	0.9	1.6	0.2	0.8
Crispy Leaf, Asda*	1oz/28g	4	14	0.8	1.6	0.5	0.9
Crispy Leaf, Sainsbury's*	½ Pack/75g	9	12	1.0	1.2	0.4	1.5
Crispy Medley, Waitrose*	1 Serving/50g	8	15	0.8	1.7	0.5	0.9
Crispy, Somerfield*	1 Pack/140g	17	12	1.0	2.0	0.0	0.0
Crispy, Tesco*	1oz/28g	6	20	1.2	3.0	0.3	1.6
Crunchy Coleslaw Bowl, Marks & Spencer*	1 Pack/325g	455	140	1.0	2.5	13.8	2.0
Crunchy Layered, Tesco*	1 Serving/54g	15	27	1.1	4.9	0.3	1.7
Crunchy Mix, Co-Op*	1oz/28g	7	25	1.0	4.0	0.3	2.0
Crunchy Shredded, Safeway*	1 Serving/50g	10	19	1.2	2.9	0.3	1.5
Crunchy Spring, Side, Marks & Spencer*	1 Serving/160g	32	20	0.9	4.1	0.2	1.3
Crunchy, Marks & Spencer*	1oz/28g	6	21	1.1	3.5	0.3	1.4
Crunchy, Waitrose*	½ Pack100g	18	18	1.0	2.6	0.4	1.5
Egg & Coleslaw, Boots*	1 Pot/233g	405	174	3.0	4.6	16.0	1.0
Egg & Potato, Fresh, Marks & Spencer*	1 Serving/250g	150	60	3.0	4.6	2.9	0.9
Egg & Potato, Good For You, Asda*	1 Serving/290g	206	71	2.6	5.0	4.5	0.0
Egg Layered Bowl, Tesco*	1 Pack/410g	726	177	4.2	8.4	14.1	1.3
Endive & Radicchio, Somerfield*	1 Pack/150g	20	13	2.0	1.0	0.0	0.0
English Garden, Tesco*	1 Serving/180g	22	12	0.7	1.8	0.2	0.7
Family, Somerfield*	1 Serving/67g	12	18	0.8	2.9	0.4	1.3
Feta Cheese & Sunblushed Tomato, Marks & Spencer*	1 Serving/190g	361	190	5.5	17.2	11.1	2.1
Feta Cheese &Pasta, McDonald's*	1 Pack/250g	240	96	3.8	11.2	3.9	0.9
Fine Noodle With Duck Breast, COU, Marks & Spencer*	1 Pack/280g	294	105	5.5	18.9	1.1	1.1
Free Range Egg & Baby Spinach, Waitrose*	1 Pack/215g	168	78	3.5	1.8	6.3	1.0
French Goat's Cheese, Extra Fine, Asda*	1 Pack/185g	463	250	8.4	11.4	19.0	0.8
French Style, Waitrose*	½ Pack/82g	149	182	5.1	7.2	14.8	1.8
Garden With Watercress, Marks & Spencer*	1 Salad/80g	10	12	1.5	1.4	0.1	1.4
Garden With Yoghurt & Mint Dressing, GFY, Asda*	1 Serving/195g	51	26	1.1	3.2	1.0	0.0

SALAD,	INFO/WEIGHT	KCAL	KCAL	PROT	CARB	FAT	FIBRE
Garden, Fresh, Safeway*	½ Pack/105g	27	26	1.1	4.8	0.3	1.1
Garden, Shapers, Boots*	1 Pack/237.3g	159	67	1.5	8.8	2.9	1.5
Goats Cheese & Roasted Pepper, Gourmet, Benjy's*	1 Pack/400g	412	103	3.4	12.4	3.8	0.0
Gourmet Nicoise, Marks & Spencer*	1 Serving/500g	575	115	4.8	3.9	8.9	0.0
Gourmet Caesar, Marks & Spencer*	1 Serving/100g	155	155	4.1	7.1	12.1	0.8
Gourmet Continental, Waitrose*	1 Serving/150g	23	15	0.8	1.6	0.5	0.9
Grapefruit, Tesco*	1 Serving/100g	42	42	0.6	10.0	0.0	0.4
Greek Layered, Perfectly Balanced, Waitrose*	½ Pack/140g	67	48	2.4	3.2	2.8	0.7
Greek Style Collection, Marks & Spencer*	1 Pack/328.6g	461	140	4.4	8.8	9.9	1.2
Greek Style Feta, Marks & Spencer*	½ Pack/130g	195	150	3.2	5.7	12.9	0.6
Greek Style Feta, Wth Herbed Bulgar Wheat, M&S*	1 Pack/345g	380	110	3.7	6.5	7.8	1.8
Greek Style Layered, Perfectly Balanced, Waitrose*	1 Serving/280g	134	48	2.4	3.2	2.8	0.7
Greek Style, Delphi*	1 Serving/220g	306	139	3.7	3.5	12.3	0.9
Greek, BGTY, Sainsbury's*	1 Serving/198.5g	133	67	2.0	9.0	2.5	0.8
Green Side With Salad Cream Dressing, M&S*	1 Serving/200g	210	105	0.9	1.9	10.5	0.7
Green Side, Marks & Spencer*	1 Serving/200g	30	15	0.9	2.5	0.2	0.0
Green Side, Sainsbury's*	1 Pack/200g	28	14	0.8	2.1	0.3	0.8
Green Side, Tesco*	1 Serving/100g	12	12	0.7	1.6	0.3	1.3
Green With Chives, Tesco*	½ Pack/90g	13	14	1.0	1.6	0.4	1.7
Green With Honey & Mustard Dressing, Marks & Spencer*	1 Pack/200g	120	60	0.9	2.7	4.8	0.8
Green With Sweetcorn & Radish, Fresh, Safeway*	1 Pack/210g	55	26	1.1	4.8	0.3	1.1
Green, Fresh, Safeway*	½ Pack/98g	14	14	0.9	1.9	0.3	0.8
Herb, Marks & Spencer*	1 Pack/100g	20	20	2.9	1.4	0.4	1.9
Hot Smoked Salmon & Rice, Deli Meal, Marks & Spencer*	1 Pack/380g	570	150	6.5	15.1	6.9	0.2
Iceberg & Cabbage, Asda*	½ Pack/125g	24	19	1.0	3.1	0.3	1.5
Italian Rice & Roasted Portobello Mushroom, M&S*	½ Pack/130g	130	100	2.8	21.2	0.5	0.6
Italian Style Pasta, Iceland*	1 Serving/75g	97	129	2.6	16.2	6.0	1.6
Italian Style Side, Waitrose*	1 Serving/160g	32	20	1.1	3.1	0.3	2.6
Italian Style, Sainsbury's*	1/3 Pack/60g	80	134	2.1	8.0	10.9	1.1
Italian Wild Rocket & Parmesan, Sainsbury's*	1 Serving/50g	89	177	7.5	3.4	14.8	0.5
Italian, Complete, Sainsbury's*	1 Pack/160g	203	127	3.6	9.0	8.5	1.5
King Prawn & Pasta, COU, Marks & Spencer*	1 Pack/270g	284	105	5.9	15.1	2.4	2.7
King Prawn, Thai Style, Marks & Spencer*	1 Pack/295g	266	90	4.4	12.6	2.5	1.3
Layered Tuna, Tesco*	1 Serving/370g	466	126	4.4	9.4	7.9	1.0
Layered With Egg, Somerfield*	1 Pot/300g	543	181	3.0	3.0	18.0	0.0
Layered With Tuna, Somerfield*	1 Pot/255g	599	235	5.0	5.0	22.0	0.0
Lemon Chicken, Snack, Good Intentions, Somerfield*	1 Pot/200.8g	249	124	8.0	17.0	2.7	1.3
Lemon Cous Cous & Roasted Pepper, COU, M&S*	1 Pack/340g	306	90	3.2	14.6	2.3	1.8
Luxury Potato, Asda*	1 Serving/50g	119	237	1.0	11.0	21.0	0.0
Marinated Seafood, Waitrose*	1 Tub/160g	331	207	15.7	3.1	14.6	0.0
Mediterranean Style Side, Way to Five, Sainsbury's*	1 Serving/244g	61	25	0.9	3.0	1.0	0.0
Mediterranean Style, Asda*	½ Pack/135g	22	16	1.0	3.0	0.0	0.0
Mediterranean Style, Morrisons*	1 Serving/90g	13	14	1.5	1.9	0.2	0.0
Mediterranean Style, Safeway*	1 Serving/25g	5	20	1.7	1.9	0.6	2.0
Mediterranean Tuna, John West*	1oz/28g	30	106	8.0	5.0	6.0	2.0
Mexican Style Bean & Cheese, Marks & Spencer*	½ Pot/150g	150	100	6.1	11.2	3.5	4.8
Mixed Bean With Onions & Peppers, Safeway*	½ Can/210g	141	67	4.0	11.4	0.6	2.7
Mixed Bean, Asda*	½ Can/145g	129	89	5.8	13.7	1.2	6.3
Mixed Bean, Tesco*	1 Serving/70g	49	70	3.2	13.1	0.5	1.9
Mixed Bean, Waitrose*	1 Serving/210g	229	109	8.7	13.6	2.2	4.6
Mixed Bean, Way To Five, Sainsbury's*	1 Can/270g	227	84	5.4	13.5	0.9	3.8
Mixed Leaf Medley, Waitrose*	1 Serving/25g	4	15	0.8	1.7	0.5	0.9
Mixed Leaf With Olive Oil Dressing, Pizza Express*	1 Pack/240g	326	136	0.9	2.1	14.1	0.7

S

SALAD,

INFO/WEIGHT	Measure	per Measure KCAL	KCAL	PROT	CARB	FAT	FIBRE
Mixed Leaf, Asda*	1 Serving/100g	21	21	1.5	3.2	0.2	2.1
Mixed Leaf, Tomato & Olive, Tesco*	1 Serving/170g	150	88	1.0	3.4	7.8	0.0
Mixed Leaf, Tomato, Feta, Boots*	1 Pack/179g	218	122	3.7	5.4	9.5	1.0
Mixed Leaves, Somerfield*	1 Pack/140g	17	12	1.0	2.0	0.0	0.0
Mixed Leaves, Tesco*	1 Serving/20g	3	14	0.9	1.6	0.4	0.9
Mixed Pepper, Asda*	½ Pack/100g	24	24	1.0	4.3	0.3	1.7
Mixed With Peppers & Iceberg Lettuce, Somerfield*	1 Pack/200g	50	25	1.0	5.0	0.0	0.0
Mixed, Sainsbury's*	1 Serving/100g	21	21	1.4	3.4	0.2	2.1
Mixed, Sweet & Crispy, Tesco*	1 Serving/200g	48	24	1.0	4.2	0.3	2.0
Moroccan Style Cous Cous, Marks & Spencer*	½ Pack/100g	160	160	5.0	32.8	1.2	4.8
Mozarella & Cherry Tomato, Shapers, Boots*	1 Bowl/194g	184	95	4.1	3.3	7.3	0.9
Nantaise, Waitrose*	1 Pack/160g	34	21	1.5	2.9	0.4	2.0
New Potato & Egg With Salad Cream, Marks & Spencer*	1 Pack/305g	183	60	3.0	4.6	2.9	0.9
New Potato & Egg, Way To Five, Sainsbury's*	1 Serving/315g	192	61	2.5	5.0	3.4	0.6
New Potato & Free Range Egg, Marks & Spencer*	1 Pack/305g	214	70	2.5	7.0	3.8	0.8
New Potato & King Prawn, Marks & Spencer*	1 Pack/210g	221	105	5.6	10.2	4.5	1.7
New Potato & Sweet Chilli Prawn, Marks & Spencer*	1 Pack/210g	147	70	2.8	14.0	0.5	0.7
New Potato, Less Than 3% Fat, Marks & Spencer*	1 Pot/190g	143	75	1.7	14.4	1.3	1.2
New Potato, Marks & Spencer*	1oz/28g	55	195	1.9	10.4	16.2	0.7
New Potatoe, Co-Op*	1 Serving/50g	98	195	1.0	16.0	16.0	2.0
Nicoise Style, Layered, Waitrose*	1 Bowl/275g	129	47	2.7	5.8	1.4	1.0
Nicoise, FTG, Marks & Spencer*	1 Pack/350g	473	135	5.9	7.5	9.0	0.5
Nicoise, Lunch Pot, Marks & Spencer*	1 Pot/330g	330	100	5.6	4.9	6.7	1.0
Nicoise, Pizza Express*	1 Salad/400g	729	182	10.0	16.3	9.3	0.0
Noodle & King Prawn, Perfectly Balanced, Waitrose*	1 Pack/225g	272	121	4.3	17.3	3.9	1.1
Noodle With Thai Style Chicken, Marks & Spencer*	½ Pot/145g	160	110	5.2	11.6	4.9	1.4
Pasta & Cheese, Asda*	1 Serving/125g	365	292	6.0	13.0	24.0	0.6
Pasta & Cheese, Somerfield*	½ Pack/225g	342	152	3.6	11.8	10.4	1.5
Pasta & Chesse, Safeway*	1 Serving/225g	554	246	4.8	15.2	18.4	0.0
Pasta & Garlic, Iceland*	1 Serving/75g	149	199	2.2	15.4	14.3	1.6
Pasta & Ham, Safeway*	1 Pot/225g	284	126	4.5	16.9	4.5	0.3
Pasta & Mushroom, Waitrose*	1 Pack/200g	320	160	4.1	14.0	9.7	0.6
Pasta & Pepper Side, Tesco*	1 Pack/230g	278	121	2.4	13.0	6.6	1.3
Pasta & Sweetcorn, Less Than 3% Fat, Marks & Spencer*	½ Pack/100g	85	85	2.8	14.7	1.4	1.5
Pasta & Tomato, GFY, Asda*	1 Pack/300g	348	116	3.0	19.0	3.1	1.6
Pasta & Tuna, McDonald's*	1 Pack/244g	217	89	4.5	12.5	2.2	0.9
Pasta, Spinach & Pinenut, Safeway*	1 Serving/200g	295	148	5.3	15.2	7.2	1.7
Pesto Pasta, Pret A Manger*	1 Pack/320g	442	138	4.0	7.7	10.3	1.1
Pollo, Pizza Express*	1 Serving/100g	572	572	41.2	32.5	31.8	0.0
Potato & Cheese, Pasta & Mixed Leaf, Waitrose*	1 Serving/205g	267	130	3.2	10.1	8.5	1.1
Potato & Egg Side, Tesco*	1 Pack/300g	192	64	2.5	4.2	4.1	1.1
Potato & Egg, Fresh, Safeway*	1 Serving/105g	84	80	8.4	3.0	3.6	1.6
Potato & Egg, Somerfield*	½ Pack/157.9g	90	57	2.5	5.1	3.0	1.2
Potato Baby, With Mint, TTD, Sainsbury's*	1 Serving/100g	204	204	2.0	10.8	17.0	0.7
Potato Layered, Tesco*	1 Pack/350g	284	81	1.3	7.8	4.9	1.3
Potato, 50% Less Fat, Asda*	½ Pot/62g	47	76	1.6	11.2	2.7	1.5
Potato, Asda*	¼ Pot/57g	67	117	0.9	12.5	7.0	1.1
Potato, Creamy, Asda*	1oz/28g	61	219	1.0	11.9	18.6	0.7
Potato, Eat Smart, Safeway*	½ Pack/121g	85	70	1.7	10.2	2.0	1.9
Potato, Good For You, Asda*	½ Pack/125g	145	116	1.3	12.0	7.0	0.0
Potato, Good Intentions, Somerfield*	1 Serving/50g	50	100	1.2	14.0	4.4	1.0
Potato, Healthy Eating, Tesco*	1 Pot/250g	218	87	2.2	12.0	3.4	0.9
Potato, Heinz*	½ Can/97g	137	141	1.4	14.8	8.5	0.8

S

SALAD,

INFO/WEIGHT	KCAL	KCAL	PROT	CARB	FAT	FIBRE
Potato, Iceland* — 1 Serving/75g	162	216	1.1	8.9	19.6	0.6
Potato, Kentucky Fried Chicken* — 1 Portion/160g	229	143	2.5	14.3	8.7	1.8
Potato, Less Than 4% Fat, Safeway* — 1 Serving/250g	213	85	2.1	13.1	2.7	0.9
Potato, Less Than 5% Fat, Somerfield* — 1oz/28g	24	86	2.0	11.0	4.0	0.0
Potato, Marks & Spencer* — 1oz/28g	55	195	1.2	8.5	17.3	1.3
Potato, Perfectly Balanced, Waitrose* — ½ Pot/125g	99	79	2.4	10.5	3.0	1.0
Potato, Reduced Calorie, Waitrose* — 1oz/28g	22	77	2.2	10.4	2.9	0.9
Potato, Reduced Fat, Sainsbury's* — 1oz/28g	34	121	1.0	11.8	7.3	1.6
Potato, Salad Bar, Asda* — 1oz/28g	52	187	0.6	11.6	15.4	1.1
Potato, Tesco* — 1 Pot/125g	219	175	1.5	12.2	13.3	0.9
Prawn & Egg, Leaf, Shapers, Boots* — 1 Pack/182g	193	106	6.7	2.1	7.9	1.0
Prawn Cocktail, Boots* — 1 Pack/202g	234	116	4.4	2.1	10.0	1.2
Prawn Cocktail, Tesco* — 1 Pack/300g	360	120	5.7	10.9	6.0	0.8
Prawn Layered, Asda* — 1 Sm Box/190g	265	139	3.6	11.0	9.0	0.0
Prawn Layered, Food To Go, Marks & Spencer* — 1 Pack/220g	176	80	4.8	9.6	2.4	1.1
Prawn Layered, Marks & Spencer* — 1 Pack/450g	338	75	4.1	10.0	2.3	0.7
Prawn Satay & Noodle, Tesco* — 1 Serving/250g	320	128	7.1	9.5	6.8	1.2
Primavera, Finest, Tesco* — 1 Pack/100g	25	25	2.4	2.4	0.6	1.3
Red Leaf & Rocket, Sainsbury's* — 1 Serving/50g	11	21	3.5	1.6	0.1	1.7
Red Thai Chicken With Noodles, Tesco* — 1 Pack/300g	342	114	7.2	20.2	0.5	1.4
Rice, Courgette & Pine Nut, BGTY, Sainsbury's* — 1/3 Pot/65g	68	105	2.7	20.0	1.6	1.5
Rice, Lentil & Roast Aubergine, Marks & Spencer* — 1 Serving/270g	405	150	4.6	18.2	6.8	1.7
Roast Chicken & Coleslaw, Boots* — 1 Serving/245g	392	160	4.5	3.9	14.0	1.3
Roast Chicken, Snack, Tesco* — 1 Pack/300g	324	108	6.0	4.8	7.2	1.9
Roast Chicken, Tesco* — 1 Salad/300g	348	116	5.3	7.0	7.4	1.0
Roasted Vegetables & Cous Cous, Sainsbury's* — 1 Pot/225g	349	155	5.5	26.3	3.1	0.0
Simply Chicken, Ginsters* — 1 Pack/186g	316	170	11.4	22.7	3.7	0.0
Skipjack Tuna, John West* — 1 Can/192g	190	99	7.3	3.7	6.1	0.0
Smoked Ham, Weight Watchers* — 1 Pack/181g	233	129	11.0	16.6	2.0	3.0
Spanish Style Rice, Marks & Spencer* — 1 Serving/220g	319	145	5.8	17.4	5.8	0.5
Spicy Bean, Tesco* — 1 Serving/125g	111	89	4.9	12.1	2.3	2.5
Spicy Rice, Waitrose* — 1 Serving/200g	318	159	3.2	21.7	6.6	0.9
Spinach, Watercress & Rocket, Safeway* — 1 Serving/60g	14	24	3.0	1.5	0.7	1.8
Super Club, Pret A Manger* — 1 Av Pack/200g	213	107	10.8	1.6	6.3	0.6
Sweet & Crispy, Side, Sainsbury's* — 1 Serving/74g	32	43	1.3	8.2	0.5	1.3
Sweet & Crispy, Somerfield* — 1 Pack/100g	25	25	1.0	5.0	0.0	0.0
Sweet & Crunchy, Sainsbury's* — 1 Serving/125g	21	17	0.8	2.9	0.2	1.3
Sweet & Crunchy, Tesco* — 1 Pack/285g	51	18	0.8	3.0	0.3	1.7
Sweet & Sour Prawn Noodle, Healthy Eating, Tesco* — 1 Pack/190g	122	64	5.0	9.4	0.7	0.4
Sweet Carrot, 3% Fat, Marks & Spencer* — 1oz/28g	21	75	1.3	16.7	1.2	1.4
Sweet Chilli Chicken Noodle, COU, Marks & Spencer* — 1 Pack/340g	408	120	6.8	17.4	2.3	1.2
Sweet Pepper Side, Tesco* — 1 Serving/54g	22	41	1.3	8.0	0.4	2.1
Sweet Pepper With Corn, Tesco* — 1 Pack/270g	103	38	1.3	7.2	0.5	1.5
Sweet Pepper, Medley, Waitrose* — ½ Pack/100g	22	22	0.9	3.8	0.4	1.5
Sweet, Layered, Tesco* — 1 Serving/285g	117	41	1.9	7.4	0.5	2.1
Tabbouleh Feta, Finest Tesco* — 1 Serving/100g	118	118	4.2	13.7	5.2	0.6
Tabbouleh Style, Perfectly Balanced, Waitrose* — 1 Pack/225g	234	104	2.8	14.3	3.9	2.6
Thai Prawn, Snack, Good Intentions, Somerfield* — 1 Serving/215g	230	107	5.0	17.9	1.7	1.1
Thai Style Chicken, Marks & Spencer* — 1 Serving/195g	205	105	6.7	15.1	1.9	1.9
Thai Style Noodle With King Prawns, Marks & Spencer* — 1 Pack/425g	446	105	4.6	19.8	0.7	1.1
Three Bean, Sainsbury's* — 1 Serving/125g	108	86	4.2	6.0	5.0	0.0
Three Bean, Tesco* — 1 Can/300g	330	110	7.7	17.6	1.0	5.3
Tiger Prawn & Pasta, Good For You, Asda* — 1 Serving/200g	250	125	4.6	20.0	2.9	2.0

S

	Measure INFO/WEIGHT	per Measure KCAL	KCAL	PROT	CARB	FAT	FIBRE
SALAD,							
Tomato & Mozarella, Marks & Spencer*	1oz/28g	49	175	10.6	2.6	13.3	0.5
Tomato & Mozarella, Starter, Pizza Express*	1 Serving/100g	288	288	15.6	5.9	22.4	0.0
Tomato, Pasta & Mozarella, Waitrose*	1 Serving/100g	169	169	4.3	10.0	12.4	0.6
Tuna & Pasta, Snack, BGTY, Sainsbury's*	1 Pack/260g	255	98	5.7	13.9	2.2	1.3
Tuna & Sweetcorn, Snack, Good Intentions, Somerfield*	1 Pot/215g	219	102	6.6	12.7	2.8	0.9
Tuna & Tomato, Boots*	1 Pack/171g	150	88	6.5	2.0	6.0	1.0
Tuna In a Tomato & Herb Dressing, John West*	1 Can/192g	190	99	7.3	3.7	6.1	0.0
Tuna Layered, COU, Marks & Spencer*	1 Tub/450g	360	80	6.7	8.3	2.0	0.8
Tuna Layered, Waitrose*	1 Bowl/300g	636	212	4.0	4.8	19.6	1.0
Tuna Nicoise, BGTY, Sainsbury's*	1 Pack/300g	315	105	6.3	15.5	2.0	2.5
Tuna Nicoise, Finest, Tesco*	1 Serving/250g	430	172	8.5	13.3	9.4	0.8
Tuna Nicoise, Marks & Spencer*	½ Pack/255g	306	120	6.0	3.7	8.8	0.2
Tuna Nicoise, No Mayonnaise, Shapers, Boots*	1 Pack/276.4g	152	55	4.5	6.4	1.3	1.4
Tuna Nicoise, Pret A Manger*	1 Av Pack/300g	194	65	8.9	1.0	2.8	1.0
Tuna Nicoise, Sainsbury's*	1 Pack/183g	234	128	11.3	1.8	8.4	0.0
Tuna Snack, Health Living, Tesco*	1 Serving/300g	252	84	7.6	11.5	0.9	0.9
Tuna, Healthy Eating, Tesco*	1 Serving/300g	399	133	6.2	10.5	7.3	0.9
Tuscan Style Bean & Sunblush Tomato, Waitrose*	1 Pot/225g	308	137	5.6	17.9	4.8	1.0
Vegetable, Heinz*	1 Can/195g	259	133	1.5	12.6	8.5	1.3
Waldorf, Waitrose*	1 Serving/50g	161	321	2.6	7.6	31.1	1.3
Watercress & Spinach, Asda*	1 Serving/50g	8	16	2.1	1.7	0.1	1.7
Watercress, Morrisons*	1 Bag/100g	17	17	1.7	1.2	0.7	0.0
Watercress, Spinach & Rocket, Sainsbury's*	1oz/28g	7	25	3.0	1.2	0.9	1.7
Watercress, Spinach & Rocket, Tesco*	1 Serving/30g	7	22	3.0	0.8	0.8	1.9
Watercress, Spinach & Rocket, Waitrose*	1 Bag/135g	28	21	2.2	1.2	0.8	1.5
Wheat With Roasted Vegetables, Sainsbury's*	1 Pack/220g	339	154	3.3	17.0	8.3	4.5
SALAD BOWL,							
Avocado & Tomato, Sainsbury's*	1 Pack/180g	97	54	1.0	6.7	2.6	1.3
Coleslaw, Budgens*	1 Pack/162.5g	221	135	1.5	7.1	11.2	1.4
Coleslaw, Marks & Spencer*	1 Pack/325g	293	90	1.3	4.9	7.4	1.3
Coleslaw, Somerfield*	½ Pack/162.6g	227	139	1.2	6.6	12.0	1.8
Coleslaw, Tesco*	1 Bowl/300g	327	109	1.0	3.4	10.1	1.3
Crispy, Marks & Spencer*	1 Serving/250g	88	35	1.3	6.6	0.5	1.2
Fruit Crunch, Marks & Spencer*	½ Pack/120g	174	145	3.1	25.5	3.4	0.6
Greek Style, Marks & Spencer*	1 Bowl/255g	242	95	2.5	2.4	8.2	0.7
Greek Style, Somerfield*	1 Bowl/225g	178	79	2.2	3.5	6.2	1.1
Italian Avocado & Tomato, Sainsbury's*	1 Bowl/180g	97	54	1.0	6.7	2.6	1.3
Large, Sainsbury's*	1/6 Pack/52g	12	23	0.9	4.3	0.3	1.1
Mozzarella & Sweet Plum Tomato, WTF, Sainsbury's*	1 Pack/153g	193	126	5.9	2.3	10.3	1.1
New Potato, Tuna & Egg, Marks & Spencer*	1 Pack/340g	255	75	3.8	6.7	3.8	0.7
Pasta With Sun Dried Tomato Dressing, WTF, Sainsbury's*	1 Bowl/320g	470	147	3.2	20.0	6.0	1.5
Pasta, Somerfield*	1 Pack/320g	541	169	3.3	20.8	8.1	1.5
Red Cheddar & Edam, Way to Five, Sainsbury's*	½ Pack/224g	240	107	4.4	12.8	4.2	1.1
Tomato & Basil, Marks & Spencer*	1 Serving/245g	233	95	0.8	4.4	8.4	0.7
Tomato, Sainsbury's*	½ Bowl/150g	93	62	0.9	4.4	4.5	1.6
Tuna, Fresh, Asda*	1 Serving/160g	184	115	8.0	5.0	7.0	0.0
SALAD CREAM,							
60% Less Fat, Asda*	1 Serving/10g	14	138	0.8	11.0	10.0	0.0
BGTY, Sainsbury's*	1 Tbsp/15g	21	140	0.8	10.8	9.9	0.3
Heinz*	1 Tbsp/10g	33	331	1.4	20.3	26.7	0.0
Light, Heinz*	1 Tbsp/10g	24	244	1.8	13.5	19.9	0.0
Morrisons*	1 Tsp/5g	16	312	1.4	19.0	25.0	0.0
Reduced Calorie	1 Serving/30g	58	194	1.0	9.4	17.2	0.0

	Measure INFO/WEIGHT	per Measure KCAL	Nutrition Values per 100g / 100ml				
			KCAL	PROT	CARB	FAT	FIBRE
SALAD CREAM,							
Reduced Fat, Safeway*	1 Serving/25g	33	130	0.6	13.1	8.4	0.0
Sainsbury's*	1 Tbsp/15g	50	333	2.7	17.0	27.7	0.0
Somerfield*	1 Serving/30g	104	348	1.0	20.0	29.0	0.0
Tesco*	1 Tbsp/25g	85	338	2.4	18.5	27.7	0.4
Waistline, Crosse & Blackwell*	1 Tbsp/10g	12	120	1.0	14.4	6.4	0.2
Weight Watchers*	1 Serving/14g	16	115	1.5	16.2	4.4	0.0
SALAMI,							
Ardennes Pepper, Waitrose*	2 Slices/14g	60	429	18.6	1.9	38.5	1.1
Campagnolo, Asda*	1 Slice/5g	18	360	30.0	0.0	26.0	0.0
Continental Peppered, Marks & Spencer*	1 Slice/8.3g	33	415	21.6	3.0	34.9	0.0
Danish, Asda*	1 Slice/8g	43	540	13.0	0.5	54.0	0.0
Danish, Sainsbury's*	1 Serving/100g	540	540	13.0	0.5	54.0	0.1
Danish, Tesco*	1 Serving/17g	83	491	13.7	2.8	47.2	0.0
German Pepper, Waitrose*	3 Slices/25g	78	313	22.0	2.0	24.5	0.3
German Peppered, Safeway*	1 Slice/8g	26	331	22.0	1.0	26.6	0.7
German Peppered, Tesco*	1 Serving/50g	175	349	21.8	2.5	28.0	0.0
German, Asda*	1 Slice/8g	29	367	19.0	2.9	31.0	0.0
German, Somerfield*	1 Pack/100g	322	322	22.0	1.0	26.0	0.0
Healthy Eating, Tesco*	4 Slices/25g	55	218	25.1	0.4	12.9	0.0
Milano, Antipasti, Marks & Spencer*	1 Serving/5g	20	394	25.0	0.0	33.0	0.0
Milano, Finest, Tesco*	1 Serving/70g	251	358	27.0	1.0	27.3	0.0
Milano, Sainsbury's*	1 Slice/6g	23	391	25.9	0.1	31.9	0.1
Milano, Waitrose*	1 Slice/5g	21	417	27.6	0.0	34.0	0.0
Milanoi, Asda*	1 Slice/5g	21	425	24.0	3.4	35.0	0.0
Napoli Piccante, Asda*	1 Slice/5g	17	340	30.0	0.0	24.0	0.0
Napolii, Sainsbury's*	1 Slice/8g	27	343	24.2	1.5	27.0	0.1
Pepper, German, Sainsbury's*	1 Slice/10g	33	326	22.0	1.0	26.0	0.3
Peppered, German, Asda*	1 Slice/20g	79	394	21.5	4.3	32.3	0.0
Peppered, German, Somerfield*	1 Pack/100g	341	341	24.0	4.0	25.0	0.0
Wafer Thin, Sainsbury's*	1 Serving/100g	223	223	19.6	0.9	15.7	0.1
SALMON,							
Appetisers, Smoked, Tesco*	1 Pack/100g	224	224	15.1	0.7	17.9	1.7
Canned, Aldi*	1 Serving/100g	168	168	24.0	0.0	7.0	0.0
Crusted, Mediterranean Style Crusted, Sainsbury's*	1 Serving/166g	322	194	18.0	5.3	11.5	0.8
Dill & Sauce, Youngs*	1 Pack/435g	265	61	6.1	4.2	2.3	0.1
En Croute, Iceland*	1 Serving/150g	407	271	12.0	19.3	16.2	0.9
En Croute, Sainsbury's*	1 Serving/179g	533	298	9.7	18.4	20.0	1.2
En Croute, Tesco*	1 Serving/205g	568	277	9.7	15.4	19.6	0.6
Fillets, & Butter, Marks & Spencer*	1oz/28g	64	230	16.7	0.0	18.0	0.0
Fillets, Boneless, Tesco*	1 Serving/150g	270	180	20.2	0.0	11.0	0.0
Fillets, Cajun, Waitrose*	1 Serving/150g	215	143	20.6	0.4	6.5	0.0
Fillets, Chargrilled, Sainsbury's*	1 Serving/270 g	270	243	20.9	0.2	17.6	0.0
Fillets, Creamy Watercress Sauce, Scottish, Seafresh*	1 Pack 300g	528	176	13.7	1.2	12.9	0.1
Fillets, Foil Baked, Tesco*	1 Fillet/130g	234	180	20.2	0.0	11.0	0.0
Fillets, Fresh, Smartprice, Asda*	1 Serving/150g	320	213	24.0	0.0	13.0	0.0
Fillets, Fresh, Somerfield*	1 Serving/150g	290	193	23.8	0.0	10.9	0.0
Fillets, Frozen, Safeway*	1 Fillet/110g	237	215	24.2	0.0	13.1	0.0
Fillets, Iceland*	1 Fillet/150g	293	195	22.3	0.0	11.7	0.0
Fillets, In Creme Fraiche & Red Pepper Sauce, Sainsbury's*	1 Serving/168g	227	135	13.8	2.0	8.0	0.0
Fillets, In Asparagus & Dill Sauce, PB, Waitrose*	1 Pack/370g	400	108	6.7	12.5	3.5	0.9
Fillets, In Brine, John West*	1oz/28g	52	187	22.0	0.0	11.0	0.0
Fillets, In Creamy Watercress Sauce, Sainsbury's*	1 Serving/180g	292	162	13.0	2.2	11.3	0.4
Fillets, Lightly Smoked, Scottish, Sainsbury's*	1 Fillet/130g	278	214	19.4	0.2	15.1	0.0

S

SALMON,

INFO/WEIGHT	Measure per Measure KCAL	KCAL	PROT	CARB	FAT	FIBRE
Fillets, Lime & Coriander Marinade, Pacific, Sainsbury's*	1 Serving/100g 139	139	24.4	1.3	4.1	0.9
Fillets, Marks & Spencer*	1 Serving/150g 203	135	20.2	0.2	5.8	0.0
Fillets, Moroccan Style, Asda*	1 Serving/240g 454	189	19.0	1.3	12.0	0.0
Fillets, Organic, Sainsbury's*	1 Fillet, Grilled/79g 134	170	23.0	0.3	8.6	0.0
Fillets, Poached, Marks & Spencer*	1oz/28g 56	200	21.7	0.1	12.7	0.0
Fillets, Scottish Caledonian, Marks & Spencer*	1 Fillet/130g 260	200	20.3	0.1	13.4	0.0
Fillets, Scottish Poached, Tesco*	1 Serving/112g 216	193	20.5	0.6	12.1	0.6
Fillets, Shetland Isles, Tesco*	1 Serving/130g 265	204	20.0	0.0	13.8	0.0
Fillets, Skinless & Boneless, Asda*	1 Fillet/130g 280	215	24.2	0.0	13.1	0.0
Fillets, Skinless & Boneless, Tesco*	1 Serving/130g 234	180	20.2	0.0	11.0	0.0
Fillets, Waitrose*	1 Serving/160g 285	178	20.7	0.0	10.5	0.0
Fillets, With Herb, Lemon & Paprika Butter, M&S*	½ Pack/147.6g 311	210	18.5	0.2	15.3	1.2
Fillets, With Lemon & Herb Butter, Asda*	1 Fillet/125g 305	244	20.0	0.4	18.0	0.0
Fillets, With Tarragon, BGTY, Sainsbury's*	1 Pack/402g 350	87	6.9	9.1	2.6	1.0
Fillets, With a Cream Sauce, Scottish, Marks & Spencer*	1 Serving/200g 360	180	13.8	1.0	13.0	0.1
Fillets, Youngs*	1 Serving/125g 266	213	24.0	0.0	13.0	0.0
Fillets, in Creamy Dill Sauce, Bird's Eye*	1 Pack/340g 333	98	5.6	8.7	4.5	1.3
Fillets, in Lime & Coriander, Good Choice, Iceland*	½ Pack/150g 189	126	19.8	5.1	2.9	0.8
Fillets, in Tomato & Mascarpone Sauce, Asda*	½ Pack/181.0g 219	121	13.0	1.4	7.0	0.0
Fillets, in White Wine & Parsley Dressing, Tesco*	1 Fillet/150g 291	194	17.5	0.3	13.6	0.6
Flakes, Honey Roast, Marks & Spencer*	1oz/28g 56	200	27.6	3.2	8.8	0.0
Flakes, Honey Roast, Sainsbury's*	1 Serving/100g 169	169	23.8	0.5	8.0	0.1
Flakes, Honey Roasted, Tesco*	1 Serving/100g 211	211	21.5	2.3	12.9	0.0
Flakes, Hot Smoked, Prime Scottish, Waitrose*	1 Pack/100g 238	238	22.6	0.0	16.4	0.0
Flakes, Poached, Marks & Spencer*	1oz/28g 53	190	24.0	0.0	10.5	0.0
Florentine, Asda*	1 Serving/190g 306	161	16.0	1.8	10.0	0.0
Fresh, Waitrose*	1 Fillet/163g 290	178	20.7	0.0	10.5	3.3
Frozen, Iceland*	1 Steak/150g 293	195	22.3	0.0	11.7	0.0
Grilled	1oz/28g 60	215	24.2	0.0	13.1	0.0
Grills, Tesco*	1 Serving/100g 165	165	20.3	1.1	8.8	1.3
Hot Smoked, Arbroath, Scottish, Spink & Sons*	1 Serving/50g 81	161	22.9	1.1	7.2	0.1
Hot Smoked, Side, The Best, Safeway*	1 Serving/100g 175	175	27.1	0.6	7.1	0.0
In Crust, Wild Alaska, Youngs*	1 Serving/160g 224	140	19.5	7.2	3.6	0.2
In Watercress Sauce, Somerfield*	1 Serving/212g 585	276	14.1	3.2	23.3	0.5
In a Watercress Sauce, Marks & Spencer*	1 Pack/400g 480	120	7.1	8.1	6.8	1.7
Lightly Smoked, Scottish, Marks & Spencer*	1 Portion/141g 228	162	19.5	0.1	8.8	0.2
Lunchbox, COU, Marks & Spencer*	1 Pack/235g 200	85	5.1	13.1	1.4	0.9
Mild Oak, Smoked, John West*	1 Serving/50g 93	185	22.2	0.5	10.5	0.0
Mild Oak, Smoked, Tesco*	1 Serving/100g 179	179	22.9	0.0	9.7	0.0
Minted Potatoes & Vegetables, Steam Cuisine, M&S*	1 Pack/400g 470	118	7.7	6.2	7.4	1.3
Mornay, With Broccoli, Weight Watchers*	1 Pack/290g 261	90	9.6	9.0	1.7	0.7
Oak, Smoked, Marks & Spencer*	1oz/28g 52	185	22.4	0.0	10.8	0.0
Oat Smoked, Wild Pacific, Marks & Spencer*	1 Serving/50g 55	110	24.6	0.0	1.1	0.3
Pepperonata, BGTY, Sainsbury's*	1 Pack/380g 300	79	5.8	8.8	2.3	0.9
Pink, Canned in Brine, Flesh & Bones, Drained	1oz/28g 43	153	23.5	0.0	6.6	0.0
Pink, Canned in Brine, Flesh Only, Drained	1oz/28g 43	153	23.5	0.0	6.6	0.0
Pink, John West*	½ Can/87g 135	155	23.0	0.0	7.0	0.0
Pink, Skinless & Boneless, John West*	1oz/28g 35	124	22.0	0.0	4.0	0.0
Pink, Skinless & Boneless, Sainsbury's*	1 Can/125g 173	138	21.5	0.1	6.0	0.1
Pink, Skinless & Boneless, Tesco*	½ Can/90g 125	139	19.0	0.0	7.0	0.0
Pink, SmartPrice, Asda*	½ Can/78g 121	155	23.0	0.0	7.0	0.0
Pink, Tin, Sainsbury's*	1 Tin/212g 280	132	16.3	0.1	7.4	0.1
Pink, Wild, Princes*	1 Serving/50g 62	124	18.3	0.0	5.6	0.0

S

SALMON,	Measure INFO/WEIGHT	per Measure KCAL	KCAL	PROT	CARB	FAT	FIBRE
Platter, GFY, Asda*	1 Pack/400g	376	94	7.0	8.0	3.8	1.4
Poached, Finest, Tesco*	1 Pack/200g	465	233	13.3	20.9	10.6	1.2
Potatoes & Vegetables, Scottish, Marks & Spencer*	1 Pack/400g	460	115	7.9	5.8	6.9	0.9
Potted, Marks & Spencer*	1 Serving/75g	184	245	17.1	0.5	19.4	1.2
Raw	1oz/28g	50	180	20.2	0.0	11.0	0.0
Red, Canned in Brine, Flesh & Bones, Drained	1oz/28g	43	153	23.5	0.0	6.6	0.0
Red, Canned in Brine, Flesh Only, Drained	1oz/28g	47	167	21.6	0.0	9.0	0.0
Red, Medium, John West*	½ Can/89g	142	160	22.0	0.0	8.0	0.0
Red, Pacific, Tesco*	1 Can/212g	335	158	16.8	0.0	10.1	0.0
Red, Sainsbury's*	1 Serving/106g	169	159	16.8	0.1	10.1	0.1
Red, Skinless & Boneless, Canadian, Marks & Spencer*	1 Serving/100g	160	160	19.0	0.0	9.1	0.0
Red, Skinless & Boneless, John West*	1oz/28g	40	142	22.0	0.0	6.0	0.0
Red, Skinless & Boneless, Tesco*	1 Serving/180g	302	168	22.5	0.0	8.7	0.0
Red, Wild Pacific, Safeway*	1 Can/213g	328	154	23.5	0.0	6.6	0.0
Red, Wild, Princes*	1 Can/200g	332	166	18.9	0.0	10.0	0.0
Rillettes, John West*	½ Can/62g	169	272	14.9	0.1	23.5	0.0
Scottish Poached Side, Somerfield*	1 Serving/90.2g	166	184	23.3	0.2	10.0	0.3
Scottish, Organic, Waitrose*	1oz/28g	50	180	20.2	0.0	11.0	0.0
Slices, Smoked, Marks & Spencer*	1oz/28g	52	185	22.4	0.0	10.8	0.0
Slices, Smoked, Tesco*	1oz/28g	50	179	22.9	0.0	9.7	0.0
Smoked	1oz/28g	40	142	25.4	0.0	4.5	0.0
Smoked & Poached, Slices, Sainsbury's*	1 Slice/20g	33	163	21.0	3.7	7.3	0.3
Smoked Trimmings, Value, Tesco*	1 Serving/50g	89	178	22.1	0.2	9.9	0.0
Smoked, For Sandwiches, Tesco*	1 Serving/50g	88	176	22.9	0.0	9.4	0.6
Smoked, Hot, Sainsbury's*	1 Serving/62g	100	161	22.0	1.1	7.2	0.1
Smoked, Irish, Marks & Spencer*	1oz/28g	38	136	23.3	0.0	4.8	0.0
Smoked, Organic, Scottish, Sainsbury's*	1 Serving/100g	186	186	22.7	1.6	9.9	0.1
Smoked, Pink, John West*	1oz/28g	43	155	23.0	0.0	7.0	0.0
Smoked, Ribbons, Marks & Spencer*	1 Serving/100g	165	165	22.3	0.8	8.2	0.0
Smoked, Rings, Marks & Spencer*	1 Ring/8.8g	26	285	10.6	3.4	25.2	0.0
Smoked, Scottish, Asda*	1 Slice/26g	46	182	23.0	0.0	10.0	0.0
Smoked, Scottish, Safeway*	½ Pack/50g	77	153	24.0	0.0	6.1	0.0
Smoked, Scottish, Sainsbury's*	1oz/28g	48	172	23.3	0.1	8.8	0.1
Smoked, Scottish, Somerfield*	1oz/28g	45	161	22.0	1.0	8.0	0.0
Smoked, Scottish, Waitrose*	1 Serving/70g	143	204	23.0	0.1	12.4	0.0
Smoked, Spey Valley, The Best, Safeway*	½ Pack/75g	140	186	23.6	0.1	10.1	0.0
Smoked, Thinly Sliced, Sainsbury's*	1 Slice/20g	31	157	23.6	0.1	7.0	0.1
Smoked, Triangles, Marks & Spencer*	1 Triangle/10.3g	20	195	13.7	1.9	14.9	0.0
Smoked, Waitrose*	1 Serving/100g	176	176	22.9	0.0	9.4	0.6
Steaks, Asda*	1oz/28g	60	215	24.2	0.0	13.1	0.0
Steaks, Marks & Spencer*	1 Serving/150g	308	205	19.1	0.5	14.2	0.0
Steaks, Somerfield*	1oz/28g	50	180	20.0	0.0	11.0	0.0
Steaks, Tesco*	1 Steak/175g	315	180	20.2	0.0	11.0	0.0
Steamed	1oz/28g	55	197	20.1	0.0	13.0	0.0
Strips, Smoked, Scottish, Tesco*	½ Pack/100g	179	179	22.9	0.0	9.7	0.0
Tail Joint, Lemon & Herb Butter, Marks & Spencer*	1 Pack/480g	864	180	18.8	0.8	11.4	0.2
Thai Noodles, Healthy Eating, Tesco*	1 Pack/350g	231	66	6.7	7.1	1.2	1.5
Wafer Thin, Scottish, Marks & Spencer*	1oz/28g	52	187	22.4	0.0	10.8	0.0
With Herb Vegetables, Healthy Eating, Tesco*	1 Pack/350g	228	65	6.6	3.8	2.6	0.9
With Sicilian Citrus Glaze, Sainsbury's*	1 Fillet/144.9g	371	256	21.9	2.3	17.8	0.0
With Spinach & Cheese, Atlantic, Bird's Eye*	1 Serving/241g	415	172	9.8	4.2	12.9	0.1
SALMON &, Pasta, Youngs*	1 Pack/300g	411	137	7.8	16.6	4.4	1.2
SALMON - GOUJONS, Tesco*	1 Pack/150g	305	203	19.2	5.9	11.4	0.6

S

	Measure INFO/WEIGHT	per Measure KCAL	Nutrition Values per 100g / 100ml				
			KCAL	PROT	CARB	FAT	FIBRE
SALSA,							
Chicken, Morrisons*	½ Sm Pot/85g	89	105	9.0	11.2	3.0	0.0
Chunky Tomato & Avocado, COU, Marks & Spencer*	½ Pot/85g	30	35	0.8	5.4	1.4	1.4
Chunky, Marks & Spencer*	½ Jar/132g	92	70	1.2	12.0	2.4	1.5
Cool, Sainsbury's*	1 Serving/100g	31	31	1.0	6.1	0.3	1.2
Cool, Tesco*	1oz/28g	11	38	0.9	7.1	0.3	0.8
Extra Hot, Fresh, Somerfield*	1oz/28g	13	47	1.0	8.0	1.0	0.0
Fire Roasted Pepper, Somerfield*	1 Pot/120g	50	42	1.2	8.1	0.5	1.3
Fresh, Asda*	1oz/28g	10	35	1.2	6.2	0.6	2.0
Fresh, Sainsbury's*	1oz/28g	15	54	1.7	7.0	2.1	0.9
Fresh, Somerfield*	1oz/28g	12	44	1.0	7.0	1.0	0.0
Fresh, Waitrose*	1oz/28g	16	57	1.2	6.9	2.7	1.0
Good For You, Asda*	½ Pot/236g	85	36	1.0	7.0	0.4	2.0
Hot, Fresh, Tesco*	1oz/28g	17	62	1.8	7.9	2.6	0.9
Hot, Primula*	1oz/28g	10	35	1.8	6.6	0.2	0.0
Hot, Tesco*	1 Serving/75g	24	32	1.0	6.1	0.4	1.3
King Prawn, Marks & Spencer*	1 Pack/160g	176	110	12.2	1.0	6.4	1.3
Medium Hot, Discovery*	1oz/28g	16	58	1.1	8.1	2.4	2.1
Mild, Amigos, Safeway*	1oz/28g	10	34	1.0	6.1	0.3	0.0
Red Onion & Tomato, Tapas Selection, Sainsbury's*	1 Serving/22g	17	77	3.0	6.0	4.5	0.9
Red Pepper, Sainsbury's*	1 Serving/85g	31	37	1.7	3.8	1.7	1.5
Smokey BBQ, Weight Watchers*	1 Serving/56g	20	36	1.1	7.6	0.1	2.3
Spicy, Less Than 3% Fat, Marks & Spencer*	½ Pot/85g	30	35	1.3	5.6	0.8	0.8
Spicy, Marks & Spencer*	1oz/28g	17	60	1.3	7.2	2.7	1.2
Taco, Old El Paso*	¼ Pack/29g	13	46	1.5	10.0	0.0	0.0
Tomato & Avocado, Marks & Spencer*	½ Pack/85.7g	30	35	0.8	5.4	1.4	1.4
Tomato, Chunky, Tesco*	1 Pot/170g	68	40	1.1	5.9	1.3	1.1
Tomato, Chunky, Tex Mex, Tesco*	1 Serving/50g	26	52	1.0	6.4	2.5	1.0
Tomato, Reduced Fat, Waitrose*	1 Serving/1g	0	27	1.5	4.7	0.2	1.4
Tomato, Spicy, Worldwide, Aldi*	1 Serving/25g	8	30	1.2	5.9	0.2	1.2
Tomato, Waitrose*	1 Serving/50g	24	47	1.5	5.0	2.3	1.7
SALT, Sea, Organic, Marks & Spencer*	1oz/28g	132	472	5.3	54.2	24.0	7.0
SAMBAL OELEK WOK, Findus*	½ Bag/300g	255	85	3.0	17.0	0.4	0.0
SAMOSAS,							
Chicken Tikka, Sainsbury's*	2 Samosas/100g	239	239	8.3	22.5	12.9	3.1
Chicken, Mumtaz*	1 Serving/105g	177	169	19.6	4.9	7.9	0.0
Dim Sum Selection, Sainsbury's*	1 Samosas/12g	24	196	3.4	28.6	7.6	2.8
Lamb, Morrisons*	1 Samosa/50g	144	288	9.8	27.0	15.7	1.5
Mini, Sainsbury's*	1 Serving/28g	82	294	6.9	33.2	14.8	2.7
Vegetable	1oz/28g	132	472	3.1	22.3	41.8	1.8
Vegetable, Marks & Spencer*	1 Samosa/45g	115	255	5.1	24.8	15.3	2.8
Vegetable, Mini, Indian Snack Selection, Sainsbury's*	1 Samosa/24.8g	65	258	5.8	25.6	14.6	2.5
Vegetable, Mini, Waitrose*	2 Samosas/59g	146	244	4.5	28.7	12.4	2.8
Vegetable, Northern Indian, Sainsbury's*	1 Samosa/50g	126	252	5.8	30.6	11.8	2.6
Vegetable, Tesco*	1 Samosa/50g	126	252	5.0	28.4	13.2	2.7
Vegetable, Waitrose*	1 Samosas/50g	107	214	3.3	26.3	10.6	0.8
SANDWICH,							
Aberdeen Angus With Pate & Shallot Relish, M&S*	1 Pack/187.9g	310	165	11.2	21.6	3.9	2.4
All Day Breakfast, Eat Smart, Safeway*	1 Pack/157g	236	150	10.0	21.6	2.1	2.2
All Day Breakfast, Finest, Tesco*	1 Pack/275g	660	240	9.7	16.4	15.1	1.6
All Day Breakfast, Ginsters*	1 Pack/241.3g	537	223	10.8	20.3	11.0	0.0
All Day Breakfast, Healthy Living, Tesco*	1 Pack/223.1g	328	147	11.9	16.8	3.6	2.7
All Day Breakfast, The Big Eat Street, Safeway*	1 Pack/213.1g	584	274	12.1	23.1	14.8	2.1
All Day Breakfast, Walls*	1 Pack/225.1g	610	271	9.2	24.3	15.4	1.4

	Measure INFO/WEIGHT	per Measure KCAL	Nutrition Values per 100g / 100ml				
			KCAL	PROT	CARB	FAT	FIBRE
Apple, Cheese & Celery, Asda*	1 Pack/173.0g	244	141	8.0	21.0	2.8	2.7
Avocado & Alfalfa Sprout, Pret A Manger*	1 Av Pack/250g	329	132	3.4	11.6	8.0	2.4
Avocado & Italian Matured Cheese, Pret A Manger*	1 Av Pack/250g	438	175	3.8	11.3	12.8	3.0
Avocado, Mozzarella & Tomato, Marks & Spencer*	1 Pack/272.9g	655	240	8.8	21.7	13.2	2.3
BBQ Chicken & Flamed Veg, CC, Northern Bites*	1 Pack/163g	287	176	13.3	18.4	5.5	2.1
BBQ Chicken & Ranch Coleslaw, Big, Sainsbury's*	1 Pack/276.6g	474	171	9.2	22.7	4.8	0.0
BBQ Chicken On Malted Bread, Fresh Bite*	1 Pack/225.8g	341	151	9.0	23.4	2.4	0.0
BBQ Chicken Wedge, Tesco*	1 Pack/195g	321	165	10.2	27.4	1.6	1.0
BBQ Rib, Rustlers*	1 Pack/170g	444	261	14.6	23.8	11.9	0.0
BLT, Eat Smart, Safeway*	1 Pack/165g	231	140	9.8	21.8	1.4	2.4
Bacon Lettuce & Tomato, Daily Bread*	1 Pack/171.1g	344	201	9.1	21.6	11.0	0.0
Bacon Lettuce & Tomato, Ginsters*	1 Pack/192g	516	269	15.6	21.2	15.6	0.0
Bacon Lettuce & Tomato, Safeway*	1 Pack/230g	529	230	15.9	35.4	2.3	3.9
Bacon, Chicken & Avocado, Ultimate, Marks & Spencer*	1 Pack/241g	552	229	10.7	17.9	12.7	2.8
Bacon, Chicken, Cheese Triple, BGTY, Sainsbury's*	1 Pack/263g	534	203	11.7	19.4	7.6	4.4
Bacon, Chicken, Cheese, Big, Sainsbury's*	1 Pack/254g	734	289	11.7	18.0	17.9	0.0
Bacon, Lettuce & Tomato & Chicken Salad, Co-Op*	1 Pack/230g	472	205	10.0	21.0	9.0	2.0
Bacon, Lettuce & Tomato, Asda*	1 Pack/262g	618	236	12.2	20.3	12.0	3.0
Bacon, Lettuce & Tomato, BGTY, Sainsbury's*	1 Pack/180g	268	149	10.8	20.8	2.5	1.6
Bacon, Lettuce & Tomato, COU, Marks & Spencer*	1 Pack/174g	270	155	11.0	22.4	2.3	2.4
Bacon, Lettuce & Tomato, Deep Filled, Asda*	1 Pack/206g	606	294	13.3	21.8	17.0	3.0
Bacon, Lettuce & Tomato, Good For You, Asda*	1 Pack/171g	294	172	9.0	26.0	3.5	1.6
Bacon, Lettuce & Tomato, Healthy Eating, Tesco*	1 Pack/165g	221	134	10.3	19.8	1.5	2.0
Bacon, Lettuce & Tomato, Healthy Living, Tesco*	1 Pack/190g	287	151	10.1	24.5	1.4	1.6
Bacon, Lettuce & Tomato, Healthy Selection, Budgens*	1 Pack/183g	388	212	10.1	21.3	9.6	2.8
Bacon, Lettuce & Tomato, Marks & Spencer*	1 Pack/194g	631	325	11.7	21.2	21.1	1.3
Bacon, Lettuce & Tomato, Shapers, Boots*	1 Pack/171g	328	192	10.0	22.0	7.1	2.3
Bacon, Lettuce & Tomato, Starbucks*	1 Pack/190g	437	230	7.7	28.3	9.6	0.0
Bacon, Lettuce & Tomato, Sutherland*	1 Pack/216g	654	303	10.6	27.3	16.8	0.0
Bacon, Lettuce & Tomato, Tesco*	1 Pack/203g	629	310	8.0	18.4	22.7	1.4
Bacon, Lettuce & Tomato, Waitrose*	1 Pack/210g	578	275	9.3	25.6	15.0	2.3
Bacon, Lettuce & Tomato, Weight Watchers*	1 Pack/171g	274	160	9.8	23.9	2.8	2.4
Bacon, Lettuce & Tomato, With Mayo, Safeway*	1 Pack/168g	462	275	10.4	20.7	16.7	2.3
Bap, Cheese & Coleslaw, Eat Smart, Safeway*	1 Bap/200g	624	312	9.9	24.4	19.8	2.6
Bap, Malted, Chargrilled Chicken, Co-Op*	1 Bap/201g	492	245	9.0	23.0	13.0	2.0
Bap, Malted, Tuna & Sweetcorn, Co-Op*	1 Bap/212g	530	250	9.0	24.0	13.0	2.0
Barm, White, Corned Beef & Onion, Open Choice Foods*	1 Roll/144g	331	230	12.7	30.7	6.1	0.0
Beef & Horseradish Mayonnaise, Shapers, Boots*	1 Pack/159.3g	266	167	12.0	25.0	2.1	2.6
Beef & Horseradish, Deep Filled, BGTY, Sainsbury's*	1 Pack/202g	313	155	11.4	22.0	2.4	2.4
Beef & Horseradish, Pret A Manger*	1 Av Pack/250g	382	153	11.2	17.7	4.4	2.5
Beef & Onion Sub, Marks & Spencer*	1 Pack/207g	611	295	13.3	25.6	15.3	1.5
Beef & Onion, American Style, The Big One, Sainsbury's*	1 Pack/386g	737	191	11.7	21.2	6.6	0.0
Beef & Pate, Marks & Spencer*	1 Pack/187.9g	310	165	11.2	21.6	3.9	2.4
Beef & Roast Onion, Healthy Living, Tesco*	1 Pack/185.3g	278	150	13.3	20.0	1.9	2.7
Beef Salad, Gibsons*	1 Pack/185g	348	188	10.6	23.5	5.7	0.0
Bloomer, Honey & Mustard Chicken, BGTY, Sainsbury's*	1 Pack/162g	288	178	12.0	25.0	3.3	0.0
Breakfast Special On Softgrain, Taste*	1 Pack/205.1g	439	214	9.6	23.3	9.2	2.1
Breakfast, Mega Triple, Co-Op*	1 Pack/267g	750	281	11.6	25.5	15.0	3.4
Breast of Chicken, Millers*	1 Pack/162g	343	212	13.8	19.3	8.9	0.0
Brie & Bacon, Asda*	1 Pack/181g	603	333	13.3	22.9	21.1	1.3
Brie & Grape, Finest, Tesco*	1 Pack/209g	527	252	8.5	20.6	15.1	1.5
Brie With Apple & Grapes, Sainsbury's*	1 Pack/220g	515	234	8.4	21.7	13.6	0.0
British Ham & Salad, COU, Marks & Spencer*	1 Pack/185g	259	140	8.8	21.4	1.9	3.5

S

	Measure INFO/WEIGHT	per Measure KCAL	Nutrition Values per 100g / 100ml				
			KCAL	PROT	CARB	FAT	FIBRE
Brunch, Eat Smart, Safeway*	1 Pack/250g	363	145	9.4	21.6	1.9	2.9
Brunch, St Ivel*	1 Pack/225g	581	258	10.2	26.0	12.6	0.0
Chargrill Chicken With Honey Mustard Mayo, Spar*	1 Pack/168g	428	255	13.1	25.0	11.4	0.0
Chargrilled Chicken & Tomato Relish, Shapers, Boots*	1 Pack/190g	295	155	12.0	20.0	3.0	3.1
Chargrilled Chicken & Watercress, BGTY, Sainsbury's*	1 Pack/172g	318	185	14.5	24.1	3.4	0.0
Chargrilled Chicken & Watercress, Marks & Spencer*	1 Pack/173g	285	165	12.8	23.9	1.7	2.1
Chargrilled Chicken Caesar, Big, Sainsbury's*	1 Pack/216g	657	304	12.2	25.3	17.1	0.0
Chargrilled Chicken Salad, Weight Watchers*	1 Pack/186g	296	159	9.9	20.4	4.2	1.9
Chargrilled Chicken Salsa, BGTY, Sainsbury's*	1 Pack/225g	306	136	10.6	19.9	1.6	2.9
Chargrilled Chicken With Mango, TTD, Sainsbury's*	1 Pack/217g	352	162	11.0	22.2	3.2	0.0
Chargrilled Chicken With Salad, Debenhams*	1 Pack/250g	325	130	7.6	18.0	3.6	0.0
Chargrilled Chicken, Budgens*	1 Pack/192.8g	483	250	10.3	24.9	12.1	1.8
Chargrilled Chicken, Ginsters*	1 Pack/209g	431	206	11.3	21.6	8.3	0.0
Chargrilled Chicken, Salsa Dressing, PB, Waitrose*	1 Pack/200g	296	148	11.1	19.9	2.6	3.5
Chargrilled Vegetable, Eat Smart, Safeway*	1 Pack/183g	265	145	7.4	23.4	2.3	2.8
Cheddar Cheese Ploughman's, Deep Fill, Asda*	1 Pack/228.6g	472	206	9.0	20.0	10.0	4.3
Cheddar Cheese Ploughman's, Marks & Spencer*	1 Pack/185g	435	235	9.6	23.7	12.4	2.5
Cheese & Celery, Marks & Spencer*	1 Pack/180g	466	259	10.8	14.7	17.4	2.9
Cheese & Coleslaw, Asda*	1 Pack/262g	799	305	10.1	22.1	19.6	3.3
Cheese & Coleslaw, Eat Smart, Safeway*	1 Pack/169.0g	245	145	10.1	20.7	2.2	4.0
Cheese & Coleslaw, Safeway*	1 Pack/187g	501	268	8.4	22.9	17.1	0.5
Cheese & Coleslaw, Shapers, Boots*	1 Pack/224g	338	151	11.0	22.0	2.1	3.2
Cheese & Coleslaw, Sutherland*	1 Pack/185g	376	203	10.7	29.9	4.5	0.0
Cheese & Marmite, No Mayonnaise, Boots*	1 Pack/156g	420	269	12.2	26.3	12.8	1.7
Cheese & Onion, GFY, Asda*	1 Pack/156g	253	162	13.0	23.0	2.0	0.0
Cheese & Onion, Healthy Living, Tesco	1 Pack/168g	314	187	10.3	23.2	5.9	1.7
Cheese & Onion, Heinz*	1 Pack/197g	563	286	11.2	24.0	16.1	3.2
Cheese & Onion, Tesco*	1 Pack/178g	621	349	11.5	17.1	26.1	2.2
Cheese & Onion, Waitrose*	1 Pack/176g	579	329	12.5	20.2	22.0	2.8
Cheese & Pickle, BHS*	1 Pack/177.7g	504	283	12.5	29.6	12.7	1.8
Cheese & Pickle, Shapers, Boots*	1 Pack/165g	342	207	9.8	31.0	4.9	2.3
Cheese & Salad, COU, Marks & Spencer*	1 Pack/188g	244	130	12.1	17.0	1.6	2.4
Cheese & Spring Onion, Asda*	1 Pack/172g	635	369	11.6	22.6	25.8	3.1
Cheese & Spring Onion, Co-Op*	1 Pack/164g	607	370	12.0	21.0	26.0	3.0
Cheese & Tomato, Asda*	1 Pack/154g	388	252	11.0	23.2	12.8	3.7
Cheese & Tomato, Co-Op*	1 Pack/161g	394	245	10.0	23.0	12.0	2.0
Cheese & Tomato, Freshmans*	1 Pack/111g	248	223	11.0	8.0	16.8	0.0
Cheese & Tomato, On Malted Brown, Oldfields*	1 Pack/198.2g	325	164	8.6	25.4	3.1	2.3
Cheese & Tomato, Organic, Marks & Spencer*	1 Pack/165g	559	339	11.8	24.8	21.4	1.9
Cheese & Tomato, Spar*	1 Pack/124g	294	237	11.1	24.4	10.5	0.0
Cheese & Tomato, Tesco*	1 Pack/182g	582	320	9.2	22.6	21.4	1.1
Cheese Coleslaw, Marks & Spencer*	1 Pack/186g	498	268	10.2	17.6	17.4	3.2
Cheese Ploughman's, BGTY, Sainsbury's*	1 Pack/216.7g	365	168	9.7	24.5	3.5	0.0
Cheese Ploughman's, Boots*	1 Pack/260g	640	246	7.8	20.0	15.0	1.9
Cheese Ploughman's, Deep Fill, Sutherland*	1 Pack/219.6g	528	240	10.1	22.6	12.1	0.0
Cheese Ploughman's, Deep Filled, Safeway*	1 Pack/231.4g	589	255	11.4	20.7	14.1	2.8
Cheese Ploughman's, Healthy Living, Tesco*	1 Pack/186g	279	150	11.2	22.3	1.8	0.9
Cheese Ploughman's, Marks & Spencer*	1 Pack/192.3g	499	260	9.1	25.1	13.4	3.0
Cheese Salad, Bugdens*	1 Pack/168.9g	250	148	10.9	21.9	1.8	1.6
Cheese Salad, Shapers, Boots*	1 Pack/205g	308	150	9.7	22.0	2.5	2.2
Cheese Tomato Spring Onion, Shapers, Boots*	1 Pack/179g	344	192	11.0	22.0	6.7	3.3
Cheese, Apple & Grape, COU, Marks & Spencer*	1 Pack/186.2g	270	145	8.5	24.9	1.2	2.0
Cheese, Asda*	1 Pack/262g	618	236	12.2	20.3	12.0	3.0

S

SANDWICH,

	Measure	per Measure		Nutrition Values per 100g / 100ml			
	INFO/WEIGHT	KCAL	KCAL	PROT	CARB	FAT	FIBRE
Cheese, Ham BLT Triple Pack, Asda*	1 Pack/260g	614	236	12.2	20.3	12.0	3.0
Cheese, Pickle & Tomato, Somerfield*	1 Pack/166.5g	317	191	12.5	25.6	4.3	3.5
Cheese, Salad & Mayonnaise, Reduced Fat, Waitrose*	1 Pack/180g	301	167	9.8	20.8	5.0	3.1
Cheese, Tomato & Apple Chutney, Half Fat, Starbucks*	1 Pack/200g	318	159	8.8	21.3	4.2	0.0
Cheese, Tomato & Spring Onion, Shapers, Boots*	1 Pack/178.2g	319	179	12.0	24.0	3.9	1.5
Chicken & Avocado, Pret A Manger*	1 Av Pack/250g	523	209	8.4	15.9	12.4	3.4
Chicken & Bacon, COU, Marks & Spencer*	1 Pack/181g	244	135	12.2	17.1	2.2	3.8
Chicken & Bacon, Club, Starbucks*	1 Pack/252g	590	234	11.5	12.8	15.3	0.0
Chicken & Bacon, Deep Filled, Co-Op*	1 Pack/166g	556	335	16.0	23.0	20.0	3.0
Chicken & Bacon, Good Intentions, Somerfield*	1 Pack/168g	282	168	10.7	24.9	2.9	2.3
Chicken & Bacon, Healthy Eating, Tesco*	1 Pack/155g	240	155	10.4	24.6	1.7	1.7
Chicken & Bacon, Marks & Spencer*	1 Pack/173g	450	260	14.1	23.8	12.1	3.4
Chicken & Bacon, Mattessons*	1 Pack/190g	604	318	13.3	26.0	17.9	1.1
Chicken & Bacon, Shapers, Boots*	1 Pack/179g	317	177	14.0	19.0	5.0	3.1
Chicken & Bacon, Tesco*	1 Pack/195g	538	276	11.2	18.7	17.4	1.3
Chicken & Basil, Safeway*	1 Pack/179g	303	169	12.3	20.7	4.9	1.7
Chicken & Pepperonata, COU, Marks & Spencer*	1 Pack/171.4g	239	140	10.4	20.9	1.7	1.3
Chicken & Roast Ham, Tesco*	1 Pack/228g	561	246	13.3	16.6	14.0	1.2
Chicken & Roast Tomatoes, COU, Marks & Spencer*	1 Pack/195g	273	140	12.0	21.7	2.1	4.2
Chicken & Salad, COU, Cafe, Marks & Spencer*	1 Pack/193g	261	135	9.8	19.0	1.9	1.6
Chicken & Salad, Low Fat, Waitrose*	1 Pack/188g	291	155	10.4	18.6	4.3	2.1
Chicken & Salad, Marks & Spencer*	1 Pack/200g	408	204	9.2	17.6	10.8	1.5
Chicken & Stuffing, Marks & Spencer*	1 Pack/166g	412	248	12.2	20.1	13.2	2.9
Chicken & Stuffing, Sutherland*	1 Pack/201.2g	505	251	11.9	22.1	12.8	3.0
Chicken & Stuffing, Waitrose*	1 Pack/183g	450	246	12.8	25.6	10.3	1.5
Chicken & Sweetcorn, Marks & Spencer*	1 Pack/186g	394	212	10.9	19.8	10.0	2.0
Chicken & Sweetcorn, Shapers, Boots*	1 Pack/180g	324	180	12.0	25.0	3.5	2.0
Chicken & Sweetcorn, Tesco*	1 Pack/194g	433	223	9.4	22.1	10.8	1.7
Chicken & Watercress, BGTY, Sainsbury's*	1 Pack/170g	284	167	14.2	22.9	2.1	2.0
Chicken & Watercress, Healthy Eating, Tesco*	1 Pack/160g	253	158	13.8	21.7	1.8	1.7
Chicken Breast, Bacon & Lettuce, Tesco*	1 Pack/195g	515	264	15.4	16.0	15.4	1.6
Chicken Caesar Salad, Sainsbury's*	1 Pack/186g	299	161	11.2	20.4	3.8	0.0
Chicken Caesar Style Salad, Good For You, Asda*	1 Pack/163g	289	177	11.0	27.0	2.8	2.1
Chicken Caesar, Boots*	1 Pack/226g	531	235	9.8	22.0	12.0	1.7
Chicken Caesar, COU, Marks & Spencer*	1 Pack/181g	244	135	12.2	19.9	2.4	4.3
Chicken Caesar, Finest, Tesco*	1 Pack/199g	454	228	15.4	19.2	10.0	1.4
Chicken Club, Burger King*	1 Pack/242g	620	256	12.3	22.3	13.2	1.6
Chicken Harvester, Tastel*	1 Pack/200g	295	148	7.7	20.3	4.0	0.0
Chicken Jalfrezi Naan, Ready To Go, Marks & Spencer*	1 Pack/288g	576	200	9.8	26.3	6.3	2.9
Chicken Kashmir, French Cuisiniers*	1 Pack/145g	204	141	12.9	20.3	1.6	2.9
Chicken Mayonnaise, Country Harvest*	1 Pack/120.2g	268	223	13.1	27.6	7.5	0.0
Chicken No Mayo, Marks & Spencer*	1 Pack/142g	220	155	15.0	17.5	3.0	3.1
Chicken Pesto With Rocket, Woolworths*	1 Pack/195g	326	167	5.0	16.9	8.8	0.0
Chicken Salad On Malted Bread With Mayo, Safeway*	1 Pack/195g	392	201	10.9	18.7	9.2	2.1
Chicken Salad Wedge, Tesco*	1 Pack/220g	458	208	9.4	18.2	10.8	1.2
Chicken Salad With Mayo. BGTY, Sainsbury's*	1 Serving/200g	314	157	12.0	21.9	2.4	0.0
Chicken Salad, BGTY, Sainsbury's*	1 Pack/197g	278	141	10.3	18.6	3.0	0.0
Chicken Salad, Baxter & Platts*	1 Pack/165g	254	154	11.4	17.8	4.2	2.8
Chicken Salad, Bernard Mathews*	1 Pack/162g	269	166	7.0	22.7	5.2	0.0
Chicken Salad, Big Fill, Somerfield*	1 Pack/247.8g	513	207	11.5	20.4	8.8	2.0
Chicken Salad, Big, Marks & Spencer*	1 Pack/283g	509	180	9.8	19.4	7.3	1.5
Chicken Salad, COU, Marks & Spencer*	1 Pack/194g	256	132	9.8	19.0	1.9	1.6
Chicken Salad, Co-Op*	1 Pack/195g	429	220	10.0	20.0	11.0	3.0

SANDWICH,	Measure INFO/WEIGHT	per Measure KCAL	KCAL	PROT	CARB	FAT	FIBRE
Chicken Salad, Deep Filled, Asda*	1 Pack/247g	551	223	18.1	22.2	7.4	1.3
Chicken Salad, Deep Filled, Co-Op*	1 Pack/213g	437	205	10.0	20.0	9.0	1.0
Chicken Salad, Deep Filled, Safeway*	1 Pack/211.9g	445	210	11.0	21.1	8.8	3.7
Chicken Salad, Deepfill, Woolworths*	1 Pack/180g	284	158	9.6	22.4	3.4	0.0
Chicken Salad, Eat Smart, Safeway*	1 Pack/183g	265	145	13.7	17.1	2.3	0.8
Chicken Salad, GFY, Asda*	1 Pack/194g	239	123	11.0	19.0	0.9	2.8
Chicken Salad, Ginsters*	1 Pack/186.5g	316	170	11.4	22.7	3.7	0.0
Chicken Salad, Good Intentions, Somerfield*	1 Pack/186g	294	158	10.4	23.5	2.5	1.5
Chicken Salad, Healthy Choice, Safeway*	1 Pack/185g	287	155	10.7	20.5	3.4	1.9
Chicken Salad, Healthy Eating, Tesco*	1 Pack/195g	255	131	10.6	16.6	2.5	3.9
Chicken Salad, Healthy Living, Co-Op*	1 Pack/180g	297	165	10.0	23.0	4.0	3.0
Chicken Salad, Heinz*	1 Pack/165.5g	246	148	11.8	22.3	1.3	5.3
Chicken Salad, Low Fat, Healthy, Spar*	1 Pack/191g	300	157	7.9	21.2	4.5	0.0
Chicken Salad, Mattesons*	1 Pack/193g	313	162	11.2	18.8	4.7	2.8
Chicken Salad, Millers*	1 Pack/200g	310	155	11.3	16.3	4.9	0.0
Chicken Salad, Montagu's*	1 Pack/162g	275	170	10.5	20.9	5.3	0.0
Chicken Salad, Prawn Mayo, Egg & Bacon, Waitrose*	1 Pack/246g	608	247	9.8	17.8	15.2	2.4
Chicken Salad, Scottish Slimmers*	1 Pack/168.7g	275	163	9.5	22.8	3.8	1.8
Chicken Salad, Shell*	1 Pack/201.0g	404	201	8.7	19.4	9.8	0.0
Chicken Salad, Superdrug*	1 Pack/181g	257	142	10.1	18.7	2.6	68.6
Chicken Salad, Sutherland*	1 Pack/181g	302	167	10.3	23.1	3.7	0.0
Chicken Salad, Waitrose*	1 Pack/208g	406	195	10.3	17.1	9.5	2.5
Chicken Tandoori, Waitrose*	1 Pack/181g	302	167	11.6	23.0	3.1	4.1
Chicken Tikka & Salad Pack, COU, Marks & Spencer*	1 Pack/253g	215	85	9.7	9.6	1.0	3.2
Chicken Tikka Masala, GO Foods Wonderfill*	1 Pack/136g	343	252	11.4	23.5	12.8	0.0
Chicken Tikka Naan, Ready To Go, Marks & Spencer*	1 Pack/298g	641	215	9.9	26.5	7.8	4.0
Chicken Tikka, Asda*	1 Pack/186g	316	170	11.0	21.0	4.7	1.5
Chicken Tikka, COU, Marks & Spencer*	1 Pack/185g	268	145	12.1	20.5	1.8	3.2
Chicken Tikka, Eat Smart, Safeway*	1 Pack/159g	240	151	11.8	21.6	1.9	2.5
Chicken Tikka, Garlic & Herb Bread Pocket, Somerfield*	1 Pack/168g	341	203	11.0	30.0	4.3	2.0
Chicken Tikka, Healthy Eating, Tesco*	1 Pack/159g	270	170	14.5	21.9	2.7	1.8
Chicken Tikka, Improved Recipe, COU, Marks & Spencer*	1 Pack/186g	270	145	12.1	20.5	1.8	3.2
Chicken Tikka, Marks & Spencer*	1 Pack/180g	391	217	10.4	19.5	10.9	2.0
Chicken Tikka, Open, COU, Marks & Spencer*	1 Pack/190g	260	137	9.6	21.8	1.2	2.2
Chicken Tikka, Sayers*	1 Pack/203g	315	155	10.8	19.8	3.7	2.8
Chicken Tikka, Taste!*	1 Pack/195.7g	368	188	11.7	21.7	6.0	0.0
Chicken Tikka, Thai Style, Korma, Big, Sainsbury's*	1 Pack/268g	581	217	11.9	20.5	9.7	0.0
Chicken Tikka, Weight Watchers*	1 Pack/158g	289	183	12.8	23.4	4.3	1.6
Chicken With Sour Cream, Malted Bread, Weight Watchers*	1 Pack/143g	265	185	14.7	25.8	2.6	2.0
Chicken, Bacon & Sweet Chilli, Feel Good, Shell*	1 Pack/173.5g	365	211	14.1	29.2	5.0	0.0
Chicken, Bacon & Tomato, BGTY, Sainsbury's*	1 Pack/190g	270	142	11.4	19.0	2.3	0.0
Chicken, Burger King*	1 Pack/224g	659	294	11.2	23.6	17.4	1.3
Chicken, Eat Smart, Safeway*	1 Pack/141g	240	170	14.9	22.2	2.0	0.6
Chicken, Healthier Choice, Ginsters*	1 Pack/183g	247	135	10.2	20.5	1.4	0.0
Chicken, Lightly Spiced, Starbucks*	1 Pack/200g	286	143	11.2	18.2	2.4	0.0
Chicken, Lime & Coriander, BP*	1 Pack/154.5g	291	189	12.5	25.2	4.2	0.0
Chicken, No Mayo, Cafe Revive, Marks & Spencer*	1 Pack/153g	230	150	14.1	17.9	2.4	3.1
Chicken, No Mayo, Daily Bread*	1 Pack/160.3g	278	174	8.6	23.8	4.4	0.0
Chicken, Prawn Mayo, Mixed, Shapers, Boots*	1 Pack/220g	416	189	12.0	20.0	6.8	2.8
Chicken, Prawn, Ham Salad Triple, HE, Tesco*	1 Pack/248g	350	141	10.4	20.8	1.8	2.1
Chicken, Rustlers*	1 Pack/150g	347	231	16.3	20.1	9.5	0.0
Chicken, Safeway*	1 Serving/200g	350	175	10.7	20.6	5.6	2.5
Chicken, Shell*	1 Pack/121g	334	276	13.9	25.9	13.0	0.0

S

SANDWICH,	Measure INFO/WEIGHT	per Measure KCAL	KCAL	PROT	CARB	FAT	FIBRE
Chicken, Sutherland*	1 Pack/220g	465	211	10.4	22.9	8.7	0.0
Chicken, Tikka, Coronation, Thai Style, Somerfield*	1 Pack/230g	614	267	12.6	27.4	11.9	3.4
Chicken, Triple, Good For You, Asda*	1 Pack/230g	453	197	13.0	25.0	5.0	1.6
Chicken, Triple, Shapers, Boots*	1 Serving/228g	440	193	13.0	23.0	5.4	2.3
Chicken, Woolworths*	1 Pack/120g	331	276	13.9	25.9	13.0	0.0
Chinese Chicken, Esso*	1 Pack/177.8g	409	230	13.0	22.8	9.0	4.0
Chinese Chicken, Low Calorie, Tesco*	1 Pack/169g	270	160	11.8	22.6	2.5	2.0
Chinese Chicken, Malted Brown Bread, Waitrose*	1 Pack/164g	333	203	13.5	21.9	6.8	3.3
Christmas Cheddar, Pret A Manger*	1 Av Pack/270g	671	249	8.8	18.3	15.5	2.0
Christmas, Shell*	1 Pack/182.7g	414	226	11.1	25.5	8.2	2.1
Ciabatta, Chicken & Herb, Shapers, Boots*	1 Pack/168g	290	173	11.9	25.0	2.8	1.7
Classic, Triple Pack, Somerfield*	1 Serving/250g	653	261	10.2	22.1	14.6	2.5
Club, Pret A Manger*	1 Av Pack/250g	542	217	12.8	18.7	10.1	2.3
Corned Beef With Onion & Tomato, The Salad Garden*	1 Pack/137g	338	247	14.2	23.0	10.8	0.0
Coronation Chicken, Marks & Spencer*	1 Pack/210g	420	200	11.2	20.2	9.7	3.1
Coronation Chicken, Pret A Manger*	1 Av Pack/250g	415	166	7.9	21.2	5.4	0.2
Cottage Cheese & Tomato, Shapers, Boots*	1 Pack/150g	219	146	7.8	18.0	4.8	2.4
Crab Marie Rose, Brown Bread, Royal London Hospital*	1 Pack/158g	293	185	9.7	22.0	7.1	0.0
Crayfish & Lemon Mayonnaise, Daily Bread*	1 Pack/173.0g	391	226	9.5	31.0	6.6	0.0
Crayfish & Rocket, Pret A Manger	1 Av Pack/250g	435	174	9.4	16.7	7.8	1.5
Cream Cheese & Cucumber, Gourmet Express*	1 Pack/104g	267	257	8.9	39.5	7.0	0.0
Cream Cheese & Peppers, Taste!*	1 Pack/154.2g	296	192	7.3	25.5	6.8	0.0
Cream Cheese Salad, The Sandwich Box*	1 Pack/138g	250	181	5.6	26.3	5.8	0.0
Cream Cheese, Red Pepper & Spinach, Daily Bread*	1 Pack/156g	273	175	7.4	24.0	5.2	0.0
Creole Chicken & Italian Leaves, Northern Bites*	1 Pack/189.8g	298	157	13.1	22.1	2.4	2.4
Crunchy Salad, Pesto Mayo, Tomato & Herb Bread, BP*	1 Pack/200g	246	123	4.4	19.0	3.3	3.0
Danish Ham Salad, COU, Marks & Spencer*	1 Pack/138g	181	131	9.3	17.4	2.7	1.9
Danish Ham Salad, Lean, COU, Marks & Spencer*	1 Pack/192g	250	130	10.6	19.5	0.9	1.4
Edam Cheese, Oldfields*	1 Pack/175g	326	186	9.8	23.9	5.7	0.0
Egg & Bacon, Bacon & Tomato, Sausage & Egg, Tesco*	1 Pack/256g	778	304	9.7	19.4	20.8	1.2
Egg & Bacon, Boots*	1 Pack/179g	480	268	12.0	19.0	16.0	1.4
Egg & Bacon, Burger King*	1 Pack/139g	296	213	11.1	21.7	9.1	1.9
Egg & Bacon, Co-Op*	1 Pack/188g	536	285	13.0	20.0	17.0	2.0
Egg & Bacon, Deep Fill, Ginsters*	1 Pack/210g	590	281	11.5	18.8	18.2	0.0
Egg & Bacon, Deep Fill, Spar*	1 Pack/191g	579	303	12.2	18.7	19.9	0.0
Egg & Bacon, Felix Van Den Berghe*	1 Pack/137.9g	382	277	8.9	22.2	17.0	0.0
Egg & Bacon, Ginsters*	1 Pack/210g	523	249	13.2	22.0	11.6	0.0
Egg & Bacon, Marks & Spencer*	1 Pack/215g	525	244	13.4	15.8	14.2	2.1
Egg & Bacon, Scottish Slimmers, Tesco*	1 Pack/139g	279	201	13.6	26.3	4.6	1.2
Egg & Bacon, Shell*	1 Pack/191g	579	303	12.2	18.7	19.9	0.0
Egg & Bacon, Taste!*	1 Pack/186.8g	496	265	12.8	19.1	15.3	0.0
Egg & Bacon, Tesco*	1 Pack/179g	530	298	10.6	20.2	19.4	1.3
Egg & Cress, BGTY, Sainsbury's*	1 Pack/166g	317	191	9.6	26.0	5.4	0.0
Egg & Cress, COU, Marks & Spencer*	1 Pack/192g	240	125	9.8	15.5	2.7	2.8
Egg & Cress, Co-Op*	1 Pack/159g	398	250	9.0	21.0	15.0	2.0
Egg & Cress, Free Range, Marks & Spencer*	1 Pack/192g	374	195	9.7	16.7	10.1	1.5
Egg & Cress, Free Range, Safeway*	1 Pack/190.4g	473	249	9.4	19.5	14.9	2.1
Egg & Cress, Free Range, Tesco*	1 Pack/195g	402	206	10.4	12.9	12.5	3.0
Egg & Cress, Heinz*	1 Pack/162g	241	149	9.6	22.7	2.2	5.4
Egg & Cress, Marks & Spencer*	1 Pack/182g	331	182	10.1	13.6	9.7	3.2
Egg & Cress, On Wholegrain Bread, Café Life*	1 Pack/154.7g	250	162	6.2	15.4	8.3	1.2
Egg & Cress, Organic, Marks & Spencer*	1 Pack/185g	444	240	9.6	18.0	14.2	3.6
Egg & Cress, Reduced Fat, Waitrose*	1 Pack/162g	262	162	9.7	16.5	6.4	6.4

S

SANDWICH,	Measure INFO/WEIGHT	per Measure KCAL	Nutrition Values per 100g / 100ml				
			KCAL	PROT	CARB	FAT	FIBRE
Egg & Cress, Sainsbury's*	1 Pack/170g	357	210	9.2	22.1	9.5	0.0
Egg & Cress, Tesco*	1 Pack/174g	445	256	10.0	20.3	15.0	1.7
Egg & Tomato, On Softgrain Bread, Daily Bread*	1 Pack/160.3g	278	174	8.6	23.8	4.4	0.0
Egg & Tomato, Organic, Waitrose*	1 Pack/192g	359	187	9.7	15.3	9.7	4.0
Egg & Tomato, Tesco*	1 Pack/172g	341	198	8.8	22.0	8.3	1.9
Egg & Tomato, With Salad Cream, Big, Sainsbury's*	1 Pack/266g	463	174	9.1	21.3	5.8	0.0
Egg & Watercress, Free Range, Marks & Spencer*	1 Pack/191.9g	355	185	9.2	18.1	8.2	2.9
Egg Mayo & Cress, Starbucks*	1 Pack/202g	450	223	9.5	18.5	12.3	0.0
Egg Mayonnaise & Cress, Co-Op*	1 Pack/159g	405	255	8.8	20.8	15.1	1.9
Egg Mayonnaise & Cress, Go Simple, Asda*	1 Pack/169g	370	219	10.0	20.0	11.0	1.7
Egg Mayonnaise & Cress, Millers*	1 Pack/166g	369	222	9.4	18.8	12.2	0.0
Egg Mayonnaise & Cress, Shapers, Boots*	1 Pack/161g	304	189	9.4	24.0	6.1	0.0
Egg Mayonnaise & Cress, Wheatgerm Bread, Asda*	1 Pack/158g	371	235	9.7	21.3	12.4	1.9
Egg Mayonnaise & Cress, Wheatgerm, Tesco*	1 Pack/146g	368	252	9.8	18.4	15.5	1.3
Egg Mayonnaise & Cress, Wholemeal Bread, Oldfields*	1 Pack/128g	301	235	9.7	24.0	11.2	3.6
Egg Mayonnaise & Salad, Superdrug*	1 Pack/169g	286	169	7.6	18.3	7.3	2.4
Egg Mayonnaise With Cress, Reduced Fat, Waitrose*	1 Pack/162g	300	185	10.4	18.1	7.9	3.4
Egg Mayonnaise, Boots*	1 Pack/183.6g	449	244	9.7	22.0	13.0	2.3
Egg Mayonnaise, Healthy Living, Tesco*	1 Pack/162.2g	253	156	9.3	21.4	3.7	2.8
Egg Mayonnaise, On Hi Bran Bread, Ginsters*	1 Pack/143g	343	240	10.7	17.6	15.2	0.0
Egg Mayonnaise, Pret A Manger*	1 Av Pack/250g	394	158	6.5	15.1	7.9	1.5
Egg Mayonnaise, Shell*	1 Pack/189g	522	276	9.8	24.7	15.4	0.0
Egg Mayonnaise, Snack & Shop, Esso*	1 Pack/240g	624	260	9.4	25.5	13.4	0.0
Egg Mayonnaise, Sub, Daily Bread*	1 Pack/165.2g	441	267	9.6	29.6	13.5	0.0
Egg Mayonnaise, Waitrose*	1 Pack/180g	396	220	10.1	19.1	11.4	3.4
Egg Salad With Mayonnaise Wholemeal, Waitrose*	1 Pack/180g	257	143	8.3	16.5	4.9	3.6
Egg Salad, Co-Op*	1 Pack/190g	285	150	7.0	22.0	4.0	4.0
Egg Salad, Deep Filled, Asda*	1 Pack/231g	404	175	7.3	18.5	7.9	1.3
Egg Salad, Free Range, Good Intentions, Somerfield*	1 Pack/173g	260	150	7.2	21.6	3.9	2.9
Egg Salad, Free Range, Sainsbury's*	1 Pack/224.5g	450	200	8.5	24.5	7.5	0.0
Egg Salad, Free Range, Waitrose*	1 Pack/180g	257	143	8.3	16.5	4.9	3.6
Egg Salad, Good for You, Asda*	1 Pack/156.8g	229	146	8.0	22.0	2.9	2.9
Egg Salad, Healthy Eating, Tesco*	1 Pack/169g	279	165	7.6	22.5	4.9	2.0
Egg Salad, Healthy Living, Tesco*	1 Pack/182g	264	145	7.2	18.6	4.2	1.8
Egg Salad, Malted Brown Bread, Healthy Eating, Tesco*	1 Pack/182g	264	145	7.2	19.6	4.2	1.8
Egg Salad, Shapers, Boots*	1 Pack/184g	304	165	6.9	24.0	4.6	1.1
Egg Salad, Weight Watchers*	1 Pack/171.6g	255	148	7.5	22.8	3.0	1.4
Egg, Co-Op*	1 Pack/190g	285	150	6.8	22.1	3.7	3.7
Egg, Delilite*	1 Pack/179.7g	337	187	8.0	22.0	7.2	3.0
Fire Roasted Red Pepper & Herbed Soft Cheese, M&S*	1 Pack/148.9g	335	225	7.0	24.6	10.7	2.7
Flame Grilled Chicken, Rustlers*	1 Pack/150g	347	231	16.3	20.1	9.5	0.0
Fresh Salad & Salad Cream, Fulfilled*	1 Pack/172g	244	142	4.9	21.5	4.1	0.0
Gammon & Egg, Safeway*	1 Pack/233.3g	489	210	12.9	20.4	8.0	0.0
Gourmet Prawn, Pret A Manger*	1 Av Pack/250g	454	182	7.8	15.2	10.2	1.8
Grilled Chicken & Watercress, COU, Marks & Spencer*	1 Pack/164g	266	162	12.8	23.9	1.7	2.1
Grilled Vegetable, Safeway*	1 Pack/150g	236	157	5.6	24.9	3.9	2.4
Ham & Cheddar, Marks & Spencer*	1 Pack/165g	396	240	15.1	20.0	11.3	1.7
Ham & Cheese Toasted, Coffee Republic*	1 Pack/160g	429	268	15.7	24.4	12.7	0.0
Ham & Cheese, Baxter & Platts*	1 Pack/168g	408	243	11.3	20.5	13.0	1.7
Ham & Cheese, Eat Smart, Safeway*	1 Pack/230g	311	135	11.3	19.3	1.3	3.2
Ham & Chicken, Healthy Living, Co-Op*	1 Pack/150g	285	190	12.0	28.0	4.0	3.0
Ham & Cream Cheese, Tesco*	1 Pack/212g	655	309	11.0	27.2	17.3	1.2
Ham & Dijon Mustard, Healthy Selection, Budgens*	1 Pack/120g	190	158	9.7	21.9	2.5	2.0

S

SANDWICH,	INFO/WEIGHT	KCAL	KCAL	PROT	CARB	FAT	FIBRE
Ham & Egg, Asda*	1 Pack/262g	590	225	10.4	16.8	12.8	2.1
Ham & Mustard, Eat Smart, Safeway*	1 Pack/139g	250	180	13.7	26.3	2.2	2.0
Ham & Mustard, Tesco*	1 Pack/147g	437	297	10.6	20.8	19.0	1.2
Ham & Swiss Cheese, BIG, Sainsbury's*	1 Pack/218g	652	299	11.6	25.4	16.7	0.5
Ham & Swiss Cheese, Marks & Spencer*	1 Pack/159g	393	247	14.7	18.9	12.6	3.3
Ham & Swiss Cheese, Safeway*	1 Pack/201.1g	533	265	14.5	19.7	14.3	1.5
Ham & Tomato, GFY, Asda*	1 Pack/173g	254	147	10.0	23.0	1.7	1.4
Ham & Turkey Salad, Co-Op*	1 Pack/188g	263	140	9.0	21.0	3.0	2.0
Ham & Turkey, Asda*	1 Pack/190g	393	207	12.9	15.8	10.2	2.3
Ham Cheese & Pickle, Sutherland*	1 Pack/230g	727	316	11.3	20.6	20.9	0.0
Ham Salad Wedge, Healthy Eating, Tesco*	1 Pack/198g	269	136	7.1	23.0	1.7	1.0
Ham Salad, Big Fill, Somerfield*	1 Pack/222g	515	232	9.4	22.9	11.4	2.3
Ham Salad, Co-Op*	1 Pack/193g	299	155	9.0	19.0	5.0	1.0
Ham Salad, Coffee Republic*	1 Pack/224g	309	138	8.6	19.9	2.7	0.0
Ham Salad, Ginsters*	1 Pack/179g	220	123	8.8	16.4	2.5	0.0
Ham Salad, Good Intentions, Somerfield*	1 Pack/178g	287	161	9.5	23.8	3.1	1.1
Ham Salad, Healthy Eating, Tesco*	1 Pack/163g	215	132	10.6	17.5	2.2	2.0
Ham Salad, Healthy Options, Oldfields*	1 Pack/156g	229	147	8.7	24.0	1.9	0.0
Ham Salad, Prawn Mayo & Chicken, HE, Tesco*	1 Pack/248g	350	141	10.4	20.8	1.8	2.1
Ham Salad, Safeway*	1 Pack/272g	403	148	8.3	24.5	1.8	1.9
Ham Salad, Snack & Shop*	1 Pack/191.2g	304	159	9.2	22.9	3.4	5.0
Ham Salad, Woolworths*	1 Pack/181g	286	158	8.4	22.7	3.7	0.0
Ham, Asda*	1 Pack/262g	618	236	12.2	20.3	12.0	3.0
Ham, Cheese & Pickle, Healthy Choice, Sutherland*	1 Pack/185g	368	199	13.4	27.4	4.0	0.0
Ham, Cheese & Pickle, Healthy Living, Co-Op*	1 Pack/185g	370	200	13.0	27.0	4.0	3.0
Ham, Cheese & Pickle, Marks & Spencer*	1 Pack/197g	459	233	13.0	15.9	13.1	2.4
Ham, Cheese & Pickle, Pret A Manger*	1 Av Pack/250g	592	237	11.9	25.0	11.0	2.4
Ham, Emmental Cheese & Mustard Mayonnaise, Classic*	1 Pack/163.8g	444	271	19.5	21.4	14.2	0.0
Ham, Marks & Spencer*	1 Pack/200g	220	110	17.2	3.2	2.6	0.0
Ham, Subway*	1 6" Pack/223g	288	129	8.1	20.6	2.3	1.8
Honey & Mustard Chicken, BGTY, Sainsbury's*	1 Pack/171g	296	173	13.1	24.0	2.7	0.0
Houmous & Crunchy Salad, Oldfields*	1 Pack/180g	256	142	6.3	20.0	4.2	0.0
Houmous With Crunchy Vegetables, Starbucks*	1 Pack/218.9g	359	164	4.7	26.4	4.4	2.9
Houmous With Mixed Leaves & Carrot, BGTY, Sainsbury's*	1 Pack/175g	275	157	6.1	26.7	2.9	0.0
Houmous, Costa*	1 Pack/165g	263	160	6.4	25.9	2.8	0.0
Italian Roast Vegetables & Cheddar Cheese, Starbucks*	1 Pack/223g	553	248	5.3	25.8	13.7	0.0
Italian Style Mozzarella, Taste*	1 Pack/183.1g	390	213	9.2	20.1	10.6	2.0
Lean Danish Ham & Salad, COU, Marks & Spencer*	1 Pack/182g	255	140	10.6	18.7	2.4	1.9
Leicester Ham, Cheese & Pickle, Waitrose*	1 Pack/205g	513	250	11.9	23.7	11.9	2.1
Lemon & Mint Chicken, Delilite*	1 Pack/178.6g	326	182	12.3	23.1	3.6	1.7
Lemon Chicken & Relish, Perfectly Balanced, Waitrose*	1 Pack/151g	243	161	12.3	21.4	2.9	3.5
Lime & Coriander Chicken, BGTY, Sainsbury's*	1 Pack/168g	282	168	10.6	23.5	3.5	0.0
Maple Flavoured Ham & Pineapple Salsa, Waitrose*	1 Pack/193.5g	330	170	8.4	23.8	4.6	3.1
Mature Cheddar & Pickle, Sainsbury's*	1 Pack/171g	588	344	14.3	38.7	15.8	7.0
Mature Cheddar Cheese & Tomato, Big, Sainsbury's*	1 Pack/233g	596	256	12.9	26.3	11.0	0.0
Mature Cheddar Cheese Salad, Upper Crust*	1 Pack/225.1g	466	207	9.5	20.3	9.8	0.0
Mature Cheddar, Soft Cheese & Celery, Sainsbury's*	1 Pack/183g	576	315	10.2	21.8	19.3	0.0
McChicken Sandwich, New, McDonald's*	1 Sandwich/100g	375	375	16.5	38.6	17.2	3.8
Mediterranean Style, Triple, Good For You, Asda*	1 Pack/211g	352	167	11.0	26.0	2.1	2.3
Mediterranean Tuna Salad, Waitrose*	1 Pack/207g	253	122	7.2	17.1	2.8	2.6
Mediterranean Tuna, COU, Marks & Spencer*	1 Pack/260g	364	140	10.3	19.6	2.2	1.6
Mediterranean Tuna, Scottish Slimmers*	1 Pack/147.2g	259	176	8.5	27.8	3.6	3.2
Mixed Seafood, Tesco*	1 Pack/184g	502	273	7.3	23.2	16.8	0.8

S

SANDWICH,	Measure INFO/WEIGHT	per Measure KCAL	Nutrition Values per 100g / 100ml				
			KCAL	PROT	CARB	FAT	FIBRE
Mozzarella & Salad, Coffee Republic*	1 Pack/242g	477	197	8.6	14.4	11.8	0.0
Mozzarella, Tomato & Basil, Healthy Options, Oldfields*	1 Pack/175g	285	163	8.1	22.1	4.8	3.3
Mozzarrella & Tomato Calzone, Waitrose*	1 Pack/175g	410	234	10.8	22.7	11.1	2.2
New York Deli, Boots*	1 Pack/245g	603	246	11.0	19.0	14.0	2.2
Oriental Chicken Triple, Shapers, Boots*	1 Pack/215g	398	185	12.0	22.0	5.4	2.6
Paprika Chicken, Bacon & Tomato, Shapers, Boots*	1 Pack/184g	296	161	11.0	19.0	4.6	2.3
Parmesan & Rocket, Egg, Cheese & Tomato, Boots*	1 Pack/241g	422	175	8.7	23.0	5.4	2.1
Pastrami & Gherkin, BGTY, Sainsbury's*	1 Pack/230g	357	155	9.8	23.1	2.6	3.0
Peking Duck no Mayo, Boots*	1 Pack/221.7g	400	180	7.7	27.0	4.6	1.7
Philadelphia Salad, The Classic Sandwich Co*	1 Pack/135g	264	196	6.2	22.1	9.1	0.0
Pitta Pocket, Chargrilled Chicken, Marks & Spencer*	1 Pack/208g	279	134	11.2	14.5	3.5	1.6
Plain Salad, Northern Bites*	1 Pack/210g	193	92	4.1	15.3	2.0	3.0
Ploughman's Wedge, Tesco*	1 Pack/269.1g	705	262	10.5	26.9	12.5	1.4
Ploughman's, Cheese, Marks & Spencer*	1 Pack/185g	451	244	9.3	21.5	13.4	1.5
Ploughman's, Deep Fill, Ginsters*	1 Pack/232g	636	274	9.6	20.8	17.6	0.0
Ploughman's, Deep Filled, Asda*	1 Pack/254g	650	256	10.3	21.3	14.5	2.9
Ploughman's, Healthy Eating, Tesco*	1 Pack/180g	261	145	11.6	21.0	1.6	2.0
Ploughman's, Shell*	1 Pack/225.9g	540	239	9.0	19.4	13.9	1.0
Poached Salmon & Cucumber, CC, Northern Bites*	1 Pack/148g	296	199	12.7	28.2	3.9	1.4
Poached Salmon & Rocket, Marks & Spencer*	1 Pack/180g	495	275	13.5	21.2	14.9	2.1
Poached Salmon & Rocket, Pret A Manger*	1 Av Pack/260g	516	198	10.3	14.9	10.7	1.9
Poached Salmon & Spinach, Shapers, Boots*	1 Pack/168.0g	284	169	9.2	23.0	4.5	3.1
Poached Salmon With Salad On Oatmeal, Costa*	1 Pack/151g	224	148	7.7	22.9	2.8	0.0
Poached Salmon, Coffee Republic*	1 Pack/191g	350	183	10.3	18.4	7.6	0.0
Poached Salmon, Marks & Spencer*	1 Pack/171g	397	232	12.9	16.2	12.8	2.6
Poached Salmon, Prawn & Rocket, Waitrose*	1 Pack/165.6g	309	186	11.2	23.5	5.2	2.1
Prawn & Egg, Deep Filled, Asda*	1 Pack/250g	570	228	12.0	17.0	12.0	2.3
Prawn & Egg, Safeway*	1 Pack/216g	400	185	9.4	18.8	8.0	1.0
Prawn & Mayonnaise, BGTY, Sainsbury's*	1 Pack/165g	312	189	10.4	20.3	7.3	3.1
Prawn & Mayonnaise, COU, Marks & Spencer*	1 Pack/141g	254	180	11.9	20.3	2.7	1.7
Prawn & Mayonnaise, Healthy Selection, Budgens*	1 Pack/143g	296	207	11.0	22.0	8.3	1.8
Prawn & Mayonnaise, Oatmeal Bread, Big, Sainsbury's*	1 Pack/259g	686	265	10.1	21.1	15.6	0.0
Prawn & Mayonnaise, Reduced Fat, Waitrose*	1 Pack/146g	276	189	9.2	24.1	6.2	2.5
Prawn & Mayonnaise, Safeway*	1 Pack/168g	402	239	9.0	21.1	13.2	3.1
Prawn & Rocket, Pret A Manger*	1 Pack/280g	435	155	8.4	14.9	6.9	1.3
Prawn & Salmon, Waitrose*	1 Pack/154g	345	224	12.5	22.0	9.5	2.8
Prawn Cocktail Salad, Shapers, Boots*	1 Pack/167g	296	177	10.0	18.0	7.2	2.9
Prawn Cocktail, Classic, Heinz*	1 Pack/193g	409	212	8.4	25.0	8.7	2.5
Prawn Cocktail, Healthy Eating, Tesco*	1 Pack/154g	245	159	11.0	22.0	2.7	1.8
Prawn Cocktail, Weight Watchers*	1 Pack/168g	252	150	8.9	18.1	4.6	2.8
Prawn Marie Rose, Fulfilled*	1 Pack/149g	292	196	13.4	26.3	4.1	0.0
Prawn Marie Rose, Waitrose*	1 Pack/164g	303	185	9.4	17.3	8.7	2.7
Prawn Mayo, Chicken Salad, Ham Salad, HL, Tesco*	1 Pack/250.7g	341	136	12.9	17.5	1.6	1.4
Prawn Mayo, Egg & Cress, Chicken, BGTY, Sainsbury's*	1 Pack/268g	501	187	9.9	24.8	5.3	0.0
Prawn Mayo, Ham Salad Triple Pack, Sutherland*	1 Pack/253g	620	245	9.8	24.8	11.9	0.3
Prawn Mayonaise, Healthy Living, Tesco*	1 Pack/157g	245	156	10.2	21.8	3.1	0.5
Prawn Mayonnaise Oatmeal Bread, Co-Op*	1 Pack/159g	445	280	11.0	28.0	14.0	2.0
Prawn Mayonnaise On Oatmeal Bread, Weight Watchers*	1 Pack/158g	254	161	10.4	23.7	2.7	2.3
Prawn Mayonnaise, BGTY, Sainsbury's*	1 Pack/175g	275	157	12.3	21.1	2.6	0.0
Prawn Mayonnaise, Co-Op*	1 Pack/154g	285	185	9.7	27.3	3.9	3.2
Prawn Mayonnaise, Daily Bread*	1 Pack/156.5g	373	239	11.9	23.0	11.0	0.0
Prawn Mayonnaise, Eat Smart, Safeway*	1 Pack/165g	256	155	10.4	23.0	2.3	2.0
Prawn Mayonnaise, Ginsters*	1 Pack/152g	415	273	12.4	17.8	17.8	0.0

S

SANDWICH,

INFO/WEIGHT	KCAL	KCAL	PROT	CARB	FAT	FIBRE
Prawn Mayonnaise, Good For You, Asda* 1 Pack/160g	270	169	10.0	22.0	4.6	2.1
Prawn Mayonnaise, Healthy Eating, Tesco* 1 Pack/154g	270	175	11.9	22.7	4.1	1.9
Prawn Mayonnaise, Heinz* 1 Pack/180g	493	274	8.9	24.0	15.8	2.5
Prawn Mayonnaise, Marks & Spencer* 1 Pack/156g	382	245	10.5	20.2	13.5	2.7
Prawn Mayonnaise, Oatmeal Bread, Waitrose* 1 Pack/180g	463	257	10.2	20.4	15.0	3.2
Prawn Mayonnaise, Reduced Fat, Waitrose* 1 Pack/155g	284	183	8.9	20.0	7.5	2.8
Prawn Mayonnaise, Shapers, Boots* 1 Pack/161g	291	181	10.0	25.0	4.6	1.9
Prawn Mayonnaise, Upper Crust* 1 Pack/207.9g	343	165	9.2	20.9	5.0	0.0
Prawn Mayonnaise, Woolworths* 1 Pack/144g	321	223	12.6	24.3	8.3	0.0
Prawn With Citrus Mango, Healthy Options, Oldfields* 1 Pack/220g	275	125	9.0	18.5	1.8	0.0
Rare Roast Beef & Horseradish, Marks & Spencer* 1 Pack/168g	311	185	14.8	21.1	4.3	2.4
Red Salmon & Cucumber, 2 Pack, Tesco* 1 Pack/144g	284	197	11.1	23.8	6.4	1.9
Red Salmon & Cucumber, BGTY, Sainsbury's* 1 Pack/178.1g	276	155	10.9	22.7	2.3	0.0
Red Salmon & Cucumber, Healthy Choice, Asda* 1 Pack/149g	285	191	10.6	19.9	7.7	2.1
Red Salmon & Cucumber, Marks & Spencer* 1 Pack/183g	375	205	11.1	18.5	9.3	1.4
Red Salmon & Cucumber, Tesco* 1 Pack/144g	251	174	11.3	24.2	3.5	1.9
Red Thai Chicken, Lettuce & Mayonnaise, Woolworths* 1 Pack/160g	328	205	11.5	26.1	6.0	0.0
Reformed Ham & Salad on Oatmeal Bread, Woolworths* 1 Pack/187g	286	153	9.1	18.4	4.8	0.0
Roast Beef & Onion, Deep Filled, Asda* 1 Pack/258g	550	213	11.3	22.6	10.8	1.1
Roast Beef On White, No Cheese or Sauce, Subway* 1 Pack/222g	289	130	8.5	20.0	2.3	1.8
Roast Beef With Cheese, Subway* 6" Sub/222g	291	131	8.6	20.3	2.3	1.8
Roast Beef With Horseradish Mayonnaise, Finest, Tesco* 1 Pack/222.8g	439	197	12.5	20.7	7.1	1.6
Roast Beef, Daily Bread* 1 Pack/199.3g	281	141	8.7	20.0	2.7	0.0
Roast Beef, Deep Fill, Woolworths* 1 Pack/191g	283	148	10.5	17.9	3.9	0.0
Roast Beef, English Mustard Mayonnaise, Oldfields* 1 Pack/150g	405	270	16.0	29.0	11.9	0.0
Roast Beef, Feel Good, Shell* 1 Pack/153g	390	255	17.6	24.2	9.7	0.0
Roast Beef, Healthy, Woolworths* 1 Pack/191g	283	148	10.5	17.9	3.9	0.0
Roast Chicken & Bacon, Boots* 1 Pack/250g	599	240	11.6	16.8	14.0	1.4
Roast Chicken & Bacon, Sainsbury's* 1 Pack/167g	433	259	14.1	18.6	14.2	0.0
Roast Chicken & Coleslaw, Sainsbury's* 1 Pack/186g	348	187	11.4	21.0	7.9	0.0
Roast Chicken & Ham, Ginsters* 1 Pack/180g	425	236	11.2	18.5	13.6	0.0
Roast Chicken & Oak Smoked Ham, Big, Sainsbury's* 1 Pack/244g	461	189	12.3	18.8	7.2	0.0
Roast Chicken & Salad With Mayo, Big, Sainsbury's* 1 Pack/268.8g	560	208	11.0	20.9	8.9	9.0
Roast Chicken & Salad, COU, Marks & Spencer* 1 Pack/196g	265	135	10.2	17.8	2.1	3.5
Roast Chicken & Salad, Marks & Spencer* 1 Pack/200g	430	215	10.0	20.3	11.0	1.7
Roast Chicken & Stuffing, Marks & Spencer* 1 Pack/182g	519	285	13.2	23.4	15.3	3.0
Roast Chicken & Stuffing, Tesco* 1 Pack/164g	313	191	14.6	20.3	5.7	1.7
Roast Chicken Breast, BGTY, Sainsbury's* 1 Pack/161.0g	277	172	14.9	22.2	2.6	0.0
Roast Chicken Salad, Luxury, Boots* 1 Pack/288g	697	242	10.0	19.0	14.0	2.3
Roast Chicken Salad, Marks & Spencer* 1 Pack/221g	420	190	10.4	23.4	6.3	1.1
Roast Chicken Salad, Shapers, Boots* 1 Pack/193g	284	147	11.0	19.0	3.0	2.3
Roast Chicken Salad, Weight Watchers* 1 Pack/186g	266	143	10.3	15.8	4.3	2.8
Roast Chicken Triple, Perfectly Balanced, Waitrose* 1 Pack/254g	356	140	8.7	19.2	3.2	2.8
Roast Chicken With Black Pepper Mayo, Boots* 1 Pack/160g	296	185	15.0	20.0	5.0	1.8
Roast Chicken, Bacon & Salad, Big, Sainsbury's* 1 Pack/249g	610	245	11.1	21.7	12.7	0.0
Roast Chicken, No Mayo, COU, Marks & Spencer* 1 Serving/147g	250	170	14.5	21.1	2.6	1.4
Roast Chicken, Prawn Mayo, BLT, Shapers, Boots* 1 Pack/221g	402	182	12.0	22.0	5.1	2.9
Roast Chicken, Prawn, Triple Pack, BLT, Waitrose* 1 Pack/241g	653	271	9.2	18.8	17.7	1.6
Roast Chicken, Shapers, Boots* 1 Pack/163g	289	177	15.0	19.0	4.6	1.5
Roast Peppers & Goats Cheese Focaccia, Finest, Tesco* 1 Focaccia/150g	419	279	7.0	21.5	18.3	1.7
Roasted Vegetable & Chilli Bean, Marks & Spencer* 1 Pack/200g	340	170	5.2	24.5	5.7	2.1
Roasted Vegetable Open, COU Marks & Spencer* 1 Pack/150g	260	173	8.4	31.3	1.5	4.4
Salad & Pepper Salsa, Hackens* 1 Pack/157.0g	197	126	5.1	21.8	2.0	0.0

S

SANDWICH,

	Measure INFO/WEIGHT	per Measure KCAL	KCAL	PROT	CARB	FAT	FIBRE
Salmon & Cucumber, Brown Bread, Waitrose*	1 Pack/150g	296	197	10.5	22.7	7.1	1.4
Salmon & Cucumber, Healthly Choice, Sutherland*	1 Pack/164g	321	196	9.8	26.6	5.6	0.0
Salmon & Cucumber, Healthy Living, Co-Op*	1 Pack/159g	286	180	10.0	24.0	5.0	2.0
Salmon & Cucumber, Marks & Spencer*	1 Pack/168g	329	196	11.0	19.5	8.3	2.6
Salmon & Cucumber, Shapers, Boots*	1 Pack/164.9g	310	188	12.0	23.0	5.3	3.4
Salmon & Cucumber, White Bread, Waitrose*	1 Pack/161.4g	304	189	9.8	25.5	5.3	1.7
Salmon & Soft Cheese, Feel Good, Shell*	1 Pack/174.1g	404	232	13.5	28.0	7.4	1.0
Salt Beef, Gherkins & Mustard Mayo, Sainsbury's*	1 Pack/242g	486	201	9.3	24.1	7.5	3.1
Sausage & Egg Wedge, Tesco*	1 Pack/269g	699	260	9.1	23.6	14.4	1.1
Sausage, Bacon & Egg, Burger King*	1 Pack/182g	430	236	13.2	17.5	12.7	1.7
Sausage, Egg & Bacon, Boots*	1 Pack/325g	887	273	9.3	23.0	16.0	2.2
Sausage, Onion Chutney & Tomato, Daily Bread*	1 Pack/166.5g	359	215	7.0	26.6	9.7	0.0
Sausage, Triple Pack, GFY, Asda*	1 Pack/215g	424	197	9.0	30.0	4.5	2.3
Seafood Cocktail, Asda*	1 Pack/190g	486	256	6.7	21.3	15.8	1.6
Seafood Cocktail, Waitrose*	1 Pack/210.2g	267	127	7.3	17.6	3.0	8.1
Seafood Medley, Marks & Spencer*	1 Pack/227g	468	206	7.2	16.3	12.4	3.5
Simply Cheddar Cheese & Coleslaw, Boots*	1 Pack/185g	538	291	9.2	23.0	18.0	1.8
Simply Cheese Ploughman's, Boots*	1 Pack/260g	640	246	7.8	20.0	15.0	1.9
Simply Chicken, Eat Smart, Safeway*	1 Pack/147g	250	170	14.5	23.0	2.2	1.4
Simply Egg Mayonnaise, Boots*	1 Pack/181g	449	248	9.2	19.0	15.0	2.9
Simply Egg Mayonnaise, Ginsters*	1 Pack/161g	309	192	8.5	24.1	6.8	0.0
Simply Prawn Mayonnaise, Boots*	1 Pack/261g	736	282	11.0	19.0	18.0	2.2
Simply Salad, Shapers, Boots*	1 Pack/216g	300	139	5.2	23.0	2.9	1.8
Simply Smoked Ham, Cheese & Pickle, Boots*	1 Pack/225g	551	245	11.0	21.0	13.0	2.4
Simply Tuna Mayonnaise & Cucumber, Boots*	1 Pack/200g	498	249	12.0	21.0	13.0	2.4
Smoked Ham & Cheddar Cheese Pickle, Finest, Tesco*	1 Pack/217.1g	532	245	11.9	23.7	11.4	3.9
Smoked Ham & Cheese, Ciabatta Style, Shapers, Boots*	1 Pack/179.3g	329	184	13.0	25.0	3.6	1.6
Smoked Ham & Cheese, Co-Op*	1 Pack/167g	334	200	15.0	24.0	5.0	2.0
Smoked Ham & Cheese, Tesco*	1 Pack/204g	620	304	14.1	19.7	18.7	1.6
Smoked Ham & Cream Cheese, HS, Budgens*	1 Pack/136g	269	197	11.4	25.7	5.5	3.4
Smoked Ham & Edam, Shapers, Boots*	1 Pack/183g	315	172	9.3	19.0	6.5	2.7
Smoked Ham & Mustard, Marks & Spencer*	1 Pack/149g	347	233	10.1	18.8	13.0	2.0
Smoked Ham & Mustard, Sainsbury's*	1 Pack/175g	406	232	10.6	21.9	11.3	0.0
Smoked Ham Salad, Weight Watchers*	1 Pack/181g	244	135	10.9	16.5	2.8	2.8
Smoked Ham, Cheese & Pickle, COU, Marks & Spencer*	1 Pack/174g	270	155	14.4	20.0	1.8	3.7
Smoked Ham, Cheese & Pickle, Shapers, Boots*	1 Pack/172g	296	172	13.0	19.0	4.9	2.9
Smoked Salmon & Black Pepper, Fulfilled*	1 Pack/120g	293	244	13.8	29.0	8.6	0.0
Smoked Salmon & Cream Cheese, Marks & Spencer*	1 Pack/162g	437	270	11.7	19.3	16.2	2.5
Smoked Salmon & Prawn, CC, Northern Bites*	1 Pack/148g	296	199	19.0	28.2	3.9	1.4
Smoked Salmon Creme Fraiche, Safeway*	1 Pack/171.4g	359	210	11.0	23.6	7.8	2.5
Smoked Salmon With Soft Cheese, Waitrose*	1 Pack/154g	300	195	14.8	19.2	6.5	4.2
Smoked Salmon, Daily Bread*	1 Pack/121.8g	296	243	13.5	28.0	8.7	0.0
Smoked Salmon, Felix Van Den Berghe*	1 Pack/118.8g	292	245	13.9	29.4	6.2	0.0
Smoked Salmon, Luxury, Marks & Spencer*	1 Pack/137g	333	243	15.0	19.0	11.9	1.8
Smoked Salmon, Pret A Manger*	1 Av Pack/250g	370	148	3.8	20.3	5.8	1.8
Smoked Turkey Summer Salad, Starbucks*	1 Pack/198g	303	153	10.8	22.3	2.4	1.5
Smokey Chicken, BGTY, Sainsbury's*	1 Pack/178g	276	155	11.1	25.6	1.0	0.0
Soft Cheese & Roast Tomato, Extra Light, Starbucks*	1 Pack/186g	283	152	8.0	24.0	2.7	3.1
Soft Cheese & Roasted Pepper, Weight Watchers*	1 Pack/158g	289	183	9.4	27.7	3.8	1.5
Southern Spiced Chicken, Marks & Spencer*	1 Pack/179g	421	235	11.2	21.7	13.0	3.1
Spicy Aubergine & Soft Cheese, Pret A Manger*	1 Av Pack/250g	319	128	4.6	21.2	2.7	2.8
Spicy Cajun Vegetable, Sandwich King*	1 Pack/140.5g	287	205	6.0	30.3	6.7	0.0
Spicy Chicken, Deep Filled, Co-Op*	1 Pack/216g	421	195	10.0	24.0	7.0	3.0

SANDWICH,	Measure INFO/WEIGHT	per Measure KCAL	Nutrition Values per 100g / 100ml				
			KCAL	PROT	CARB	FAT	FIBRE
Sub, Chargrilled Chicken Caesar, Sainsbury's*	1 Pack/216g	611	283	13.4	25.6	14.1	0.0
Sub, Chicken & Stuffing, Safeway*	1 Roll/275g	605	220	10.3	21.3	10.4	4.2
Sub, Chicken Salad, Asda*	1 Sub/200g	460	230	9.4	17.4	13.6	0.9
Sub, Meatball With Cheese & Salad, Subway*	1 Pack/286g	526	184	8.4	18.5	9.1	2.1
Sub, Nacho Style Chicken Sub, Global, Somerfield*	1 Roll/226g	513	227	7.4	30.8	8.3	4.2
Sub, The Big Chicken & Bacon, Marks & Spencer*	1 Pack/218g	545	250	15.6	24.9	10.0	1.4
Tandoori Chicken, Finest, Tesco*	1 Pack/224g	421	188	10.8	19.2	7.5	1.4
Tangy Lime & Ginger Chicken, Shapers, Boots*	1 Pack/168g	319	190	12.0	21.0	6.4	5.1
Thai Chicken, Tesco*	1 Pack/244g	634	260	8.5	21.1	15.7	1.5
Three Cheese & Onion, New Style, Weight Watchers*	1 Pack/148g	275	186	14.8	26.2	2.4	1.4
Three Cheese & Spring Onion, Shell*	1 Pack/168g	672	400	11.1	20.8	30.3	0.0
Tiger Prawn & Thai Dressing, Waitrose*	1 Pack/200g	342	171	9.6	23.6	4.3	2.2
Tomato & Basil Chicken, Healthy Eating, Tesco*	1 Pack/176g	266	151	11.5	21.1	2.3	2.0
Tomato, Parmesan & Rocket, Shapers, Boots*	1 Pack/164g	303	185	7.5	24.0	6.6	1.7
Tuna & Celery, Perfectly Balanced, Waitrose*	1 Pack/172g	272	158	11.7	20.5	3.2	3.9
Tuna & Chargrilled Vegetables, BGTY, Sainsbury's*	1 Pack/196g	329	168	10.7	21.5	4.4	0.0
Tuna & Cucumber, BGTY, Sainsbury's*	1 Pack/164g	275	169	12.0	21.6	3.9	3.0
Tuna & Cucumber, Ginsters*	1 Pack/171g	238	139	9.9	19.4	3.2	0.0
Tuna & Cucumber, Healthy Choice, Asda*	1 Pack/164g	315	192	10.9	22.3	6.6	1.1
Tuna & Cucumber, Healthy Choice, Sutherlands*	1 Pack/179g	344	192	12.2	22.0	6.2	0.0
Tuna & Cucumber, Healthy Living, Co-Op*	1 Pack/186.8g	355	190	12.0	25.0	5.0	2.0
Tuna & Cucumber, Heinz*	1 Pack/183.4g	276	151	12.3	21.6	1.6	6.8
Tuna & Cucumber, Marks & Spencer*	1 Pack/170g	430	253	12.0	18.0	14.8	2.4
Tuna & Cucumber, Red Cal Mayo, BGTY, Sainsbury's*	1 Pack/182g	288	158	12.2	22.5	2.3	0.0
Tuna & Cucumber, Shapers, Boots*	1 Pack/179g	322	180	11.0	24.0	4.4	1.7
Tuna & Cucumber, Shell*	1 Pack/188g	431	229	12.3	21.9	10.2	0.0
Tuna & Cucumber, on Malted Wheatgrain, Ginsters*	1 Pack/175g	319	182	14.1	21.8	4.3	0.0
Tuna & Green Pesto, BGTY, Sainsbury's*	1 Pack/211.4g	279	132	11.0	17.0	2.2	0.0
Tuna & Lemon Mayo, Shapers, Boots*	1 Pack/206g	318	154	10.0	18.0	4.7	1.7
Tuna & Peppers, Virgin Train*	1 Pack/177.5g	338	191	9.9	26.5	5.0	0.0
Tuna & Sweetcorn, Asda*	1 Pack/205g	592	289	11.5	21.8	17.2	2.7
Tuna & Sweetcorn, COU, Marks & Spencer*	1 Pack/180g	270	150	12.6	19.0	2.4	3.8
Tuna & Sweetcorn, Eat Smart, Safeway*	1 Pack/152g	251	165	13.4	21.9	2.5	2.8
Tuna & Sweetcorn, Ginsters*	1 Pack/163.3g	306	188	10.5	25.2	5.0	0.0
Tuna & Sweetcorn, Healthy Eating, Tesco*	1 Pack/154g	263	171	11.4	25.6	2.5	2.1
Tuna & Sweetcorn, Heinz*	1 Pack/208g	528	254	10.4	23.5	13.2	1.6
Tuna & Sweetcorn, Marks & Spencer*	1 Pack/185g	453	245	11.0	20.9	13.0	2.1
Tuna & Sweetcorn, New Recipe, Healthy Living, Tesco*	1 Pack/209.6g	330	157	13.0	22.5	1.7	2.3
Tuna & Sweetcorn, Safeway*	1 Pack/154.5g	256	165	12.8	23.2	1.8	1.7
Tuna & Sweetcorn, Sainsbury's*	1 Pack/183g	441	241	10.6	23.2	11.7	0.0
Tuna & Sweetcorn, Shapers, Boots*	1 Pack/170g	306	180	12.0	27.0	2.7	2.1
Tuna & Sweetcorn, Tesco*	1 Pack/174g	432	248	11.3	24.4	11.7	1.8
Tuna Creme Fraiche & Spring Onion, Oldfields*	1 Pack/185.2g	287	155	9.0	20.4	4.2	3.0
Tuna Crunch, Healthy Living, Tesco*	1 Pack/180g	261	145	11.0	19.9	2.4	0.5
Tuna Crunch, Shapers, Boots*	1 Pack/200g	290	145	9.1	20.0	3.2	3.2
Tuna Mayo, Pret A Manger*	1 Av Pack/250g	622	249	11.7	24.4	11.6	1.6
Tuna Mayonnaise With Spring Onions, Starbucks*	1 Pack/209g	318	152	9.0	19.9	4.0	1.5
Tuna Mayonnaise, White Bread, Open Choice Foods*	1 Pack/120g	298	248	12.0	29.6	8.4	0.0
Tuna Melt, Swedish Bread, Shapers, Boots*	1 Pack/163g	254	156	14.0	20.0	2.2	2.1
Tuna Pepper & Sweetcorn Salad, Shapers, Boots*	1 Pack/204g	345	169	9.2	24.0	4.0	1.9
Tuna Salad Wedge, Tesco*	1 Pack/204.9g	291	142	8.1	23.9	1.5	0.8
Tuna Salad With Sour Cream Dressing, Weight Watchers*	1 Pack/201g	260	129	9.8	17.7	2.1	2.8
Tuna Salad, Marks & Spencer*	1 Pack/250g	575	230	12.5	16.8	12.6	2.1

SANDWICH,	INFO/WEIGHT	KCAL	KCAL	PROT	CARB	FAT	FIBRE
Tuna Salad, On White, Tesco*	1 Pack/190g	352	185	9.8	20.8	7.0	1.1
Tuna Salad, Tesco*	1 Pack/197g	427	217	9.5	20.9	10.6	1.1
Tuna Salad, Weight Watchers*	1 Pack/191g	248	130	10.6	15.8	2.7	2.6
Tuna With Salad, Debenhams*	1 Pack/249g	309	124	7.7	16.9	3.4	0.0
Tuna, Healthy Options, Spar*	1 Pack/150g	269	179	14.3	24.9	2.4	0.0
Tuna, Tomato & Onion, COU, Marks & Spencer*	1 Pack/177g	250	141	11.1	18.8	2.4	2.2
Turkey & Coleslaw, Cafe, Asda*	1 Pack/193g	457	237	10.0	20.0	13.0	0.0
Turkey & Cranberry, COU, Marks & Spencer*	1 Pack/180g	279	155	12.1	22.8	1.7	2.9
Turkey & Ham Salad, Sutherland*	1 Pack/185g	303	164	9.8	25.2	2.6	0.0
Turkey & Stuffing, Marks & Spencer*	1 Pack/190g	352	185	12.3	23.1	4.9	1.9
Turkey Breast & Ham Sandwich, Subway*	1 Pack/235g	294	125	8.5	19.6	2.1	1.7
Turkey, Lettuce & Tomato, Shapers, Boots*	1 Pack/217g	310	143	9.8	21.0	2.2	2.9
Turkey, Pork & Herb, Starbucks*	1 Pack/198g	465	235	11.7	22.6	10.8	2.1
Turkey, Stuffing & Cranberry Sauce, Shapers, Boots*	1 Pack/167g	316	189	10.0	26.0	5.0	1.5
Two Cheese & Pickle, Heinz*	1 Pack/178g	543	305	13.8	28.4	15.1	3.8
Veggie Delite, Subway*	1 Pack/166g	226	136	5.4	26.5	1.8	2.4
Wensleydale & Carrot, Marks & Spencer*	1 Pack/183g	430	235	9.9	21.4	12.3	2.8
York Ham, Starbucks*	1 Pack/208g	341	164	10.4	21.2	4.2	2.9
SANDWICH FILLER,							
Chargrilled Vegetable, Sainsbury's*	½ Pot/85g	192	226	3.4	2.2	22.7	0.6
Cheese & Onion, Safeway*	1 Serving/50g	260	520	10.6	2.6	51.4	1.3
Cheese & Onion, Sainsbury's*	1 Serving/85g	463	545	10.8	1.1	55.3	0.4
Cheese & Spring Onion, Healthy Eating, Tesco*	1 Serving/85g	185	218	13.2	6.8	15.4	0.6
Cheese & Spring Onion, Marks & Spencer*	1 Serving/56g	199	355	8.5	5.0	33.6	0.2
Cheese & Spring Onion, Morrisons*	1 Serving/28g	119	426	12.8	3.1	44.6	0.0
Chicken & Bacon With Sweetcorn, Sainsbury's*	1 Serving/60g	187	312	13.2	2.6	27.6	1.1
Chicken & Sweetcorn, Deli, Marks & Spencer*	1 Pot/170g	306	180	11.6	4.2	12.9	1.5
Chicken Tikka & Citrus Raita, COU, Marks & Spencer*	½ Pot/85g	77	90	12.6	4.9	2.0	0.9
Chicken Tikka, BGTY, Sainsbury's*	½ Pot/85g	99	117	16.5	6.0	3.0	1.0
Chicken Tikka, Healthy Eating, Tesco*	1 Serving/100g	110	110	7.1	12.4	3.6	1.0
Chicken Tikka, Mild, Heinz*	1 Serving/52g	102	196	5.2	12.3	14.0	0.7
Chicken With Salad Vegetables, Heinz*	1 Filling/56g	114	203	5.1	11.7	15.1	0.5
Chicken, Stuffing & Bacon, COU, Marks & Spencer*	1 Pack/170g	170	100	13.1	6.2	2.2	1.3
Chicken, Sweetcorn & Sage, Healthy Eating, Tesco*	1 Serving/125g	105	84	9.4	8.8	1.3	1.3
Chicken, Tomato & Sweetcure Bacon, Marks & Spencer*	1 Pot/170g	502	295	11.4	2.8	26.4	0.7
Chunky Egg & Smoked Ham, Tesco*	1 Serving/100g	234	234	11.8	0.2	20.7	0.3
Chunky Seafood Cocktail, Tesco*	1 Serving/100g	347	347	5.6	3.3	34.6	1.7
Coronation Chicken, Somerfield*	1 Serving/85g	326	383	8.4	9.7	34.5	0.8
Coronation Chicken, Tesco*	1 Tbsp/30g	84	279	14.7	6.1	21.8	0.7
SANDWICH FILLER,							
Egg & Bacon, Fresh, Tesco*	1 Serving/45g	112	248	12.7	4.2	20.1	0.6
Egg Mayonaise, Better for You, Morrisons*	1 Spread/50g	71	142	10.0	1.7	10.6	0.0
Egg Mayonnaise & Bacon, Free Range, Co-Op*	1 Pot/200g	500	250	13.0	0.9	22.0	0.6
Egg Mayonnaise, BGTY, Sainsbury's*	1 Serving/85g	102	120	10.9	0.9	7.1	1.2
Egg Mayonnaise, Chunky Free Range, Tesco*	1 Serving/50g	104	208	12.3	0.2	17.6	0.3
Egg Mayonnaise, Deli, Somerfield*	1 Serving/40g	120	301	9.7	0.2	29.2	0.0
Egg Mayonnaise, Marks & Spencer*	1oz/28g	62	220	10.1	0.8	19.7	1.1
Egg Mayonnaise, Sainsbury's*	1 Serving/50g	138	275	10.1	1.1	25.6	0.5
Egg Mayonnaise, Tesco*	1 Serving/50g	122	243	10.5	2.5	21.2	0.8
Ham & Salad Vegetables, Heinz*	1oz/28g	57	204	5.3	10.0	15.9	0.4
Poached Salmon & Cucumber, Deli, Marks & Spencer*	1 Pot/170g	349	205	14.0	1.0	16.3	0.5
Prawn Mayonnaise, GFY, Asda*	1 Serving/57g	101	177	12.0	3.0	13.0	0.1
Prawn Mayonnaise, Marks & Spencer*	1oz/28g	91	325	8.7	0.7	31.7	0.8

S

INFO/WEIGHT	Measure per Measure KCAL		Nutrition Values per 100g / 100ml				
			KCAL	PROT	CARB	FAT	FIBRE
SANDWICH FILLER,							
Prawn Mayonnaise, Waitrose*	1 Pot/170g	537	316	8.9	0.2	31.1	0.0
Seafood Cocktail, Marks & Spencer*	1oz/28g	76	272	6.4	8.2	23.8	0.2
Seafood, BGTY, Sainsbury's*	1oz/28g	36	128	8.7	7.6	7.0	0.5
Smoked Salmon & Soft Cheese, Marks & Spencer*	1 Pack/170g	451	265	11.1	4.9	23.9	0.0
Tex-Mex Chicken, Tesco*	1 Pack/250g	255	102	12.3	11.2	0.9	1.2
Tuna & Sweetcorn With Salad Vegetables, Heinz*	1oz/28g	53	191	5.8	12.1	13.2	0.7
Tuna & Sweetcorn, COU, Marks & Spencer*	½ Pot/85g	77	90	11.6	5.7	2.0	1.3
Tuna & Sweetcorn, Marks & Spencer*	1oz/28g	70	250	14.2	2.3	20.7	1.3
SANDWICH FILLING,							
Cheese & Onion, Asda*	1 Serving/56g	288	515	9.8	4.4	50.9	0.3
Cheese & Onion, Co-Op*	1 Serving/56g	269	480	10.0	4.0	47.0	0.5
Cheese & Spring Onion, Better For You, Morrisons*	½ Pot/85g	216	254	10.4	7.0	20.0	2.2
Chicken & Sweetcorn, Asda*	1 Serving/60g	187	312	11.0	4.0	28.0	2.0
Chicken & Sweetcorn, Low Fat, Morrisons*	1 Serving/56g	101	180	8.8	8.5	12.3	1.6
Chicken Tikka, Less Than 5% Fat, Asda*	1 Serving/56g	65	116	11.0	7.3	4.7	1.3
Crab, BGTY, Sainsbury's*	1oz/28g	36	128	8.7	7.6	7.0	0.5
Egg Mayonnaise With Chives, Asda*	1oz/28g	92	327	9.1	1.1	31.8	0.0
Egg Mayonnaise, Asda*	1oz/28g	72	258	10.3	1.9	23.3	0.7
Egg Mayonnaise, Co-Op*	1oz/28g	69	245	11.0	3.0	21.0	0.8
Houmous & Vegetable, Asda*	1/3 tub/57g	133	233	8.0	12.0	17.0	3.5
Prawns With Seafood Sauce, Asda*	1oz/28g	107	382	11.7	1.4	36.8	0.0
Tuna & Sweetcorn With Mayonnaise, Morrisons*	1 Serving/25g	72	289	13.1	5.9	23.7	0.6
Tuna & Sweetcorn, Asda*	1oz/28g	83	295	8.2	6.0	26.5	0.6
Tuna & Sweetcorn, Good For You, Asda*	1/3 Pot/57g	73	128	11.0	12.0	4.0	0.3
Tuna & Sweetcorn, Reduced Fat, Co-Op*	1 Serving/50g	103	205	13.0	7.0	14.0	0.9
Tuna & Sweetcorn, Reduced Fat, Morrisons*	1oz/28g	50	178	13.0	7.8	10.5	1.2
Tuna & Sweetcorn, Tesco*	1 Serving/60g	172	287	9.4	10.0	23.3	0.9
SANDWICH SPREAD,							
Chicken Tikka, Asda*	1 Serving/50g	77	154	7.0	9.0	10.0	0.2
Cucumber, Heinz*	1oz/28g	46	164	1.7	12.7	11.6	0.6
Original, Heinz*	1oz/28g	66	237	1.7	15.2	18.6	0.7
SARDINES,							
Boneless, John West*	1 Can/62g	102	164	17.0	1.5	10.0	0.0
Canned in Brine, Drained	1oz/28g	48	172	21.5	0.0	9.6	0.0
Canned in Oil, Drained	1oz/28g	62	220	23.3	0.0	14.1	0.0
Canned in Tomato Sauce	1oz/28g	45	162	17.0	1.4	9.9	0.0
Grilled	1oz/28g	55	195	25.3	0.0	10.4	0.0
Headless, Somerfield*	1oz/28g	46	165	21.0	0.0	9.0	0.0
In Barbecue Sauce, Princes*	1 Can/120g	182	152	15.1	5.0	8.0	0.0
In Brine, John West*	1 Can/90g	156	173	23.0	0.0	9.0	0.0
In Brine, Portuguese, Sainsbury's*	1 Can/90g	165	183	22.4	0.1	10.3	0.1
In Brine, Tesco*	½ Can/42g	79	189	22.8	0.0	10.9	0.0
In Brine, Waitrose*	1 Can/120g	170	142	20.2	0.0	6.8	0.0
In Extra Virgin Olive Oil, Princes*, Drained	1 Can/90g	203	226	24.2	0.0	13.9	0.0
In Olive Oil, John West*	1 Can/96g	243	253	25.0	0.0	17.0	0.0
In Olive Oil, Portuguese, Marks & Spencer*	1 Can/90g	176	195	23.0	0.0	11.3	0.0
In Olive Oil, Portuguese, Sainsbury's*	1 Can/90g	194	216	25.5	0.1	12.6	0.3
In Smoky Barbecue Sauce, Princes*	1 Can/120g	182	152	15.1	5.0	8.0	0.0
In Sunflower Oil, John West*	1 Can/96g	209	218	23.0	0.0	14.0	0.0
In Sunflower Oil, Portuguese, Sainsbury's*	1 Can/90g	175	194	25.1	0.1	10.3	0.1
In Sunflower Oil, Princes*, Drained	1 Can/90g	189	210	22.0	0.0	13.9	0.0
In Tomato Sauce, Asda*	1 Can/120g	218	182	18.0	0.5	12.0	0.0
In Tomato Sauce, John West*	1oz/28g	46	164	17.0	1.5	10.0	0.0

S

	Measure INFO/WEIGHT	per Measure KCAL	Nutrition Values per 100g / 100ml				
			KCAL	PROT	CARB	FAT	FIBRE
SARDINES,							
In Tomato Sauce, Ocean Rise*	1 Can/120g	194	162	17.0	1.4	9.9	0.0
In Tomato Sauce, Portuguese, Marks & Spencer*	1 Can/120g	160	133	19.4	1.2	5.6	0.2
In Tomato Sauce, Portuguese, Sainsbury's*	1 Can/120g	212	177	17.4	2.2	11.0	0.4
In Tomato Sauce, Princes*	1 Can/120g	228	190	19.0	1.6	11.9	0.0
In Tomato Sauce, Skinless & Boneless, Sainsbury's*	1 Can/120g	143	119	22.1	1.0	3.0	0.1
In Tomato Sauce, Tesco*	1 Can/120g	214	178	17.8	0.5	11.6	0.0
Raw	1oz/28g	46	165	20.6	0.0	9.2	0.0
SATAY,							
Chicken & Turkey, Co-Op*	1 Pack/120g	264	220	20.0	4.0	14.0	0.1
Chicken & Turkey, Sainsbury's*	1 Stick/20g	44	222	20.0	4.0	14.0	1.9
Chicken, A Taste of Indonesia*	1 Serving/160g	232	145	22.0	3.0	5.0	0.0
Chicken, Marks & Spencer*	1 Satay/43g	90	210	19.1	4.4	12.7	0.7
Chicken, Mini, Iceland*	1 Satay/8g	19	236	23.0	4.5	14.0	0.7
Chicken, Morrisons*	1 Satay/10g	17	171	23.5	3.5	7.0	0.7
Chicken, Occasions, Sainsbury's*	1 Satay/10g	15	150	22.0	2.0	6.0	0.7
Chicken, Sticks, Asda*	1 Stick/20g	43	216	18.0	4.5	14.0	0.0
Chicken, Taste Original*	1 Serving/20g	33	164	23.0	2.5	6.5	0.7
Chicken, Tesco*	1 Serving/350g	483	138	13.4	5.1	7.1	0.7
Szechuan Style, Occasions, Sainsbury's*	1 Satay/10g	20	196	22.8	6.4	8.8	0.5
SATAY MIX, Thai Chicken, Schwartz*	1 Serving/9g	29	321	3.8	72.5	1.8	0.8
SATSUMAS,							
Fresh, Raw	1oz/28g	10	36	0.9	8.5	0.1	1.3
Weighed With Peel	1 Med/80g	21	26	0.6	6.0	0.1	0.9
SAUCE, APPLE,							
Baxters*	1 Tsp/15g	7	49	0.1	11.1	0.4	0.7
Bramley, Asda*	1 Tsp/15g	14	94	0.2	23.0	0.1	0.9
Bramley, Colman's*	1 Tsp/15ml	16	108	0.2	26.0	0.0	0.0
Bramley, Morrisons*	1 Tsp/15g	21	139	0.2	34.5	0.0	1.2
Bramley, Sainsbury's*	1 Tsp/15g	17	111	0.2	27.2	0.1	1.8
Heinz*	1 Tsp/15g	8	56	0.3	13.4	0.2	1.5
Shoprite*	1 Pot/113g	57	50	0.0	12.0	0.0	0.0
SAUCE, APRICOT & ALMOND Tagine, Sainsbury's*	1/3 Jar/120g	98	82	2.0	17.9	1.6	2.5
SAUCE, AROMATIC CANTONESE, Express, Uncle Ben's*	1 Serving/170g	172	101	0.6	24.6	0.1	0.0
SAUCE, ARRABIATA,							
Don Pomodoro*	½ Pot/185g	231	125	0.5	6.0	11.0	0.0
Italiano, Tesco*	1 Serving/175g	93	53	1.3	6.2	2.6	1.0
Lazio, Sainsbury's*	1/3 Jar/113g	154	136	2.2	7.2	10.9	0.0
Safeway*	½ Pot/175g	250	143	2.9	14.1	8.3	2.9
SAUCE, BBQ							
Original, Heinz*	1 Serving/9.5g	12	137	1.3	31.0	0.3	0.3
HP*	1 Serving/20ml	29	143	0.8	33.1	0.2	0.0
Smokey Tomato, HP*	1oz/28g	40	143	0.8	33.1	0.2	0.0
Spicy Mayhem, HP*	1 Serving/2g	3	156	0.9	36.7	0.1	0.0
Tesco*	1 Serving/50g	63	125	1.3	29.7	0.1	0.7
SAUCE, BALTI,							
97% Fat Free, Homepride*	1 Serving/230g	133	58	1.1	9.1	1.9	1.8
Cooking, BGTY, Sainsbury's*	¼ Jar/129g	98	76	1.1	10.9	3.1	0.6
Cooking, Eat Smart, Safeway*	1 Serving/88g	66	75	1.1	10.0	2.9	0.8
Cooking, Organic, Perfectly Balanced, Waitrose*	1 Jar/450g	257	57	0.9	7.6	2.6	0.9
Cooking, Organic, Sainsbury's*	1 Serving/225g	158	70	2.2	10.0	2.3	0.5
Cooking, Sharwood's*	1 Jar/420g	370	88	1.1	9.1	5.2	0.5
Cooking, Shere Khan*	1 Jar/425g	261	61	0.9	3.9	4.7	0.0
Cooking, Tesco*	1 Serving/500g	575	115	2.3	8.6	7.8	1.6

S

INFO/WEIGHT	Measure	per Measure KCAL	Nutrition Values per 100g / 100ml				
			KCAL	PROT	CARB	FAT	FIBRE
SAUCE, BALTI,							
Curry, Asda*	¼ Jar/125g	155	124	1.6	7.0	10.0	1.7
Curry, Loyd Grossman*	1 Serving/212g	346	163	1.7	8.8	13.4	1.4
Deliciously Good, Homepride*	1/3 Jar/153g	89	58	1.1	9.1	1.9	0.6
Indian Style, Iceland*	1 Serving/220g	154	70	1.6	10.1	2.6	0.5
Sizzle & Stir, Chicken Tonight*	1/3 Jar/168g	195	116	1.3	6.3	9.5	2.9
Tomato & Coriander, Patak's*	1 Serving/70g	58	83	0.8	6.5	6.0	1.2
SAUCE, BARBECUE,							
Asda*	1 Serving/135g	128	95	1.2	22.0	0.2	0.6
Chicken Tonight*	¼ Jar/125g	76	61	2.0	12.4	0.4	0.9
Cooking, BGTY, Sainsbury's*	¼ Jar/124g	46	37	0.4	8.4	0.2	0.7
SAUCE, BARBEQUE							
Cook In, Homepride*	1 Serving/130g	96	74	0.8	14.0	1.6	0.0
McDonald's*	1 Portion/32g	55	173	2.2	38.3	1.2	0.0
Simply Sausages Ranch, Colman's*	1 Serving/130g	96	74	1.8	16.6	0.1	1.1
SAUCE, BHUNA							
Cooking, Shere Khan*	1 Jar/425g	244	57	1.3	4.5	3.8	0.0
Sharwood's*	1 Jar/420g	361	86	0.8	8.4	5.4	0.6
SAUCE, BLACK BEAN,							
Amoy*	1oz/28g	42	150	10.0	23.0	2.0	0.0
Asda*	1 Serving/55g	55	100	2.9	19.0	1.4	0.0
Cantonese, Sainsbury's*	1 Serving/50ml	83	166	2.6	33.4	2.4	2.6
Finest, Tesco*	1 Jar/350g	252	72	0.8	16.1	0.5	0.8
Fresh, Sainsbury's*	1 Sachet/50ml	78	156	6.7	27.5	2.6	1.7
Iceland*	¼ Jar/125g	131	105	1.3	15.3	4.2	0.7
Sharwood's*	1 Serving/97.5g	98	100	2.0	20.3	1.2	0.6
Stir Fry, Amoy*	1oz/28g	29	104	1.8	12.0	5.6	0.0
Stir Fry, Asda*	1 Serving/50ml	54	108	2.9	21.0	1.4	0.0
Stir Fry, Fresh Ideas, Tesco*	½ Sachet/25g	33	132	4.2	22.6	2.8	0.8
Stir Fry, Marks & Spencer*	1 Serving/60g	108	180	6.3	20.0	8.0	2.0
Stir Fry, Morrisons*	½ Jar/237g	135	57	1.7	11.2	0.6	0.0
Stir Fry, Safeway*	1/3 Pack/33g	43	129	3.7	20.2	3.7	0.9
Stir Fry, Sainsbury's*	1 Serving/70ml	107	153	6.7	25.8	2.6	1.7
Stir Fry, Sharwood's*	1 Jar/160g	149	93	0.3	19.9	1.3	1.2
Stir Fry, Straight To Wok, Amoy*	1 Pack/220g	411	187	2.7	42.7	0.6	0.0
Stir Fry, Tesco*	½ Jar/220g	216	98	2.3	17.9	1.6	0.7
Uncle Ben's*	1 Serving/125g	89	71	2.0	12.8	1.3	0.0
SAUCE, BLACK PEPPER,							
Amoy*	1 Serving/60g	151	251	1.9	49.4	5.1	0.0
Hong Kong, Straight To Wok*	1oz/28g	40	142	2.2	20.5	5.7	0.0
Stir Fry, Blue Dragon*	½ Sachet/60g	47	79	1.6	8.4	4.4	0.1
SAUCE, BOLOGNESE,							
Fresh, Safeway*	½ Pot/153g	182	119	7.3	6.3	7.2	1.6
Lloyd Grossman*	¼ Jar/106g	80	75	2.0	10.2	2.9	1.4
Original, Deliciously Good, Homepride*	¼ Jar/112g	39	35	1.3	7.1	0.2	0.8
Original, Dolmio*	1 Serving/250g	130	52	1.7	8.8	1.1	0.0
Waitrose*	1 Serving/175g	151	86	5.4	5.3	4.9	2.0
SAUCE, BREAD,							
Made With Semi-Skimmed Milk	1 Serving/45g	42	93	4.3	12.8	3.1	0.3
Marks & Spencer*	1 Serving/85g	153	180	3.1	8.7	14.6	0.2
SAUCE, BROWN,							
Bottled	1 Tsp/6g	6	99	1.1	25.2	0.0	0.7
Daddies Favourite, HP*	1 Tsp/6g	6	102	0.9	24.3	0.1	0.0
Tesco*	1 Tsp/10g	10	104	0.7	25.1	0.1	0.6

S

	Measure INFO/WEIGHT	per Measure KCAL	Nutrition Values per 100g / 100ml				
			KCAL	PROT	CARB	FAT	FIBRE
SAUCE, BUTTER &							
Tarragon, Chicken Tonight*	1oz/28g	30	106	1.0	2.1	10.4	0.7
SAUCE, CAJUN, Sizzle & Stir, Chicken Tonight*	1/3 Jar/150g	189	126	0.8	12.0	8.3	0.0
SAUCE, CANTONESE,							
Sizzling, Uncle Ben's*	½ Jar/270g	416	154	0.7	24.0	6.1	0.0
SAUCE, CARBONARA,							
BGTY, Sainsbury's*	1 Serving/150g	110	73	3.5	4.5	4.5	0.5
Creamy, Loyd Grossman*	1oz/28g	52	186	3.8	8.9	15.0	0.3
Creamy, Microwaveable, Dolmio*	1 Serving/75g	116	155	3.3	4.0	13.5	0.0
Fresh, Safeway*	1 Serving/175g	285	163	7.1	5.2	12.6	0.5
Fresh, Sainsbury's*	½ Pot/150g	333	222	5.9	2.2	21.1	0.8
Good For You, Asda,*	1 Serving/170g	167	98	5.0	6.0	6.0	0.0
Healthy Eating, Tesco*	1 Serving/175g	121	69	5.2	6.2	2.6	0.0
Italiano, Tesco*	1 Serving/125g	388	310	7.8	8.7	27.0	0.0
Less Than 5% Fat, Safeway*	1 Serving/175g	130	74	4.1	4.8	4.2	0.2
Perfectly Balanced, Waitrose*	½ Pot/175g	154	88	7.8	6.0	3.6	1.2
Stir In, Dolmio*	1 Serving/75g	140	186	6.5	3.7	15.8	0.0
SAUCE, CARMELISED ONION & Red Wine, M&S*	1 Serving/52g	31	60	1.9	6.7	3.1	0.6
SAUCE, CHASSEUR,							
Cook In, Homepride*	1 Can/390g	156	40	0.7	9.2	0.1	0.0
Classic, Chicken Tonight*	1 Serving/100g	45	45	0.7	3.9	2.9	1.3
SAUCE, CHEESE,							
Cheddar, Dry, Colman's*	1 Pack/40g	156	389	19.0	46.0	14.0	0.0
Fresh, Italiano, Tesco*	½ Tub/175g	236	135	6.8	6.2	9.2	0.0
Fresh, Waitrose*	1 Pot/350g	459	131	5.1	5.7	9.8	0.0
Granules, Made Up, Bisto*	1floz/30ml	30	100	1.2	6.4	7.6	0.0
Italian Style, Finest, Tesco*	½ Pot/175g	355	203	10.1	14.0	11.9	0.0
Italiano, Tesco*	1 Pot/350g	368	105	5.3	8.0	5.7	0.0
Made With Semi-Skimmed Milk	1 Serving/60g	107	179	8.1	9.1	12.6	0.2
Made With Whole Milk	1 Serving/60g	118	197	8.0	9.0	14.6	0.2
SAUCE, CHILLI & GARLIC,							
Lea & Perrins*	1 Tsp/6g	4	60	1.0	14.9	0.0	0.0
Stir Fry, Marks & Spencer*	½ Jar/125g	188	150	1.5	35.2	0.4	1.2
SAUCE, CHILLI CON CARNE,							
2 Step Season, Discovery*	½ Jar/185g	176	95	3.8	17.6	1.2	3.1
Cook In, Homepride*	1 Can/390g	234	60	2.5	11.2	0.6	0.0
Cooking, BGTY, Sainsbury's*	1 Jar/500g	190	38	0.8	8.2	0.2	0.6
Hot, Sainsbury's*	1 Serving/116g	66	57	2.4	11.3	0.2	1.6
SAUCE, CHILLI,							
Amoy*	1 Tsp/6g	2	25	1.0	5.2	0.0	1.0
Cooking, SmartPrice, Asda*	1 Serving/140g	80	57	2.5	11.0	0.3	1.1
HP*	1 Tsp/6g	8	134	1.2	32.3	0.1	0.0
Hot, Co-Op*	1 Jar/440g	242	55	2.0	10.0	0.5	2.0
Iceland*	1 Serving/115g	75	65	2.7	12.0	0.7	1.6
Medium, Deliciously Good, Homepride*	1 Jar/460g	258	56	2.3	10.4	0.5	1.2
Mild, Healthy Eating, Asda*	½ Jar/250g	173	69	2.1	10.0	2.3	1.7
Mild, Safeway*	1 Serving/250g	188	75	2.4	11.3	2.2	1.2
Seeds Of Change*	1 Jar/400g	408	102	4.0	18.2	1.5	2.2
SAUCE, CHINESE							
Orange, Honey & Ginger, Cooking, Sainsbury's*	1 Serving/125g	91	73	0.3	17.2	0.3	0.3
Style, Stir Fry, Fresh, Asda*	½ Sachet/50ml	93	186	1.5	18.0	12.0	0.0
Sweet & Sour, Cooking, Sainsbury's*	¼ Jar/125g	109	87	0.7	20.1	0.1	0.7
SAUCE, CHINESE,							
Curry, Farmfoods*	1 Sachet/200g	220	110	0.6	7.1	8.8	0.7

S

INFO/WEIGHT	Measure per Measure KCAL		Nutrition Values per 100g / 100ml				
			KCAL	PROT	CARB	FAT	FIBRE
SAUCE, CHINESE,							
Stir Fry, Sachet, Fresh, Sainsbury's*	½ Sachet/51ml	83	163	1.7	14.1	11.1	1.8
Stir Fry, Tesco*	1 Pack/50g	170	340	0.8	17.3	29.7	0.0
SAUCE, CHIP SHOP Curry, Dry, Bisto*	1 Serving/10.7g	51	468	4.3	72.6	17.8	2.7
SAUCE, CHOCOLATE FLAVOUR, Lyles*	1 Serving/10g	31	305	1.0	74.0	0.5	0.0
SAUCE, CHOCOLATE, Sainsbury's*	1 Serving/30g	108	360	1.3	62.8	11.6	0.9
SAUCE, CHOP SUEY,							
Blue Dragon*	½ Sachet/60g	34	57	0.5	8.3	2.4	0.5
Cooking, Asda*	1 Serving/240g	214	89	0.6	17.0	2.1	0.2
Stir Fry, Sharwood's*	1 Jar/160g	120	75	0.7	14.6	1.5	0.2
SAUCE, CHOW MEIN,							
Sainsbury's*	1 Serving/50g	36	71	1.8	10.5	2.4	0.0
Stir Fry, Asda*	½ Jar/97.5g	97	99	1.6	21.0	1.0	0.1
Stir Fry, Blue Dragon*	1 Sachet/120g	110	92	1.1	15.4	2.9	0.4
SAUCE, COCONUT, Chilli & Lime, Cook-In, Homepride*	1 Serving/115g	110	96	1.1	5.9	7.5	0.0
SAUCE, CORONATION Chicken, Cook In, Homepride*	1 Serving/250g	233	93	0.8	13.2	4.2	0.0
SAUCE, COUNTRY FRENCH,							
Chicken Tonight*	¼ Jar/125g	123	98	0.7	3.3	9.1	0.7
Low Fat, Chicken Tonight*	1 Serving/125g	58	46	0.9	4.2	2.8	0.7
SAUCE, COUNTRY MUSHROOM, Ragu*	¼ Jar/129g	88	68	2.0	9.5	2.1	1.2
SAUCE, COWBOY JOE BBQ, Eazy Squirt, Heinz*	1 Serving/10ml	11	114	0.5	27.4	0.2	0.2
SAUCE, CRACKED BLACK PEPPER, Marks & Spencer*	1 Jar/300g	345	115	2.7	6.7	8.9	0.4
SAUCE, CRANBERRY,							
& Port, Marks & Spencer*	1 Serving/75g	71	95	2.3	20.2	0.4	2.1
& Red Onion, Sizzling, Homepride*	1 Serving/100g	83	83	0.5	17.7	1.0	0.0
Jelly, Baxters*	1 Tsp/15g	40	268	0.0	67.0	0.0	0.0
Safeway*	1 Tsp/15g	25	168	0.2	41.0	0.3	1.3
Sainsbury's*	1 Tsp/15g	23	154	0.8	37.1	0.3	1.3
Tesco*	1 Tsp/15g	23	156	0.1	38.8	0.0	0.9
SAUCE, CREOLE							
Recipe, Discovery*	¼ Jar/66g	62	94	0.9	17.9	1.8	0.7
Style, Aldi*	1 Serving/160g	158	99	1.3	18.6	2.2	0.0
SAUCE, CUMBERLAND SAUSAGE, Colman's*	¼ Jar/126g	43	34	0.7	7.4	0.2	0.8
SAUCE, CURRY,							
98% Fat Free, Homepride*	1oz/28g	15	54	1.4	9.2	1.5	0.6
Bettabuy, Morrisons*	1 Jar/440g	295	67	0.7	10.8	2.3	1.0
Cook In, Homepride*	½ Can/250g	270	108	0.7	9.1	7.6	0.6
Cooking, Savers, Safeway*	1 Jar/440g	295	67	1.4	7.4	3.5	0.9
Deliciously Good, Homepride*	1/3 Jar/149g	91	61	1.1	10.0	1.8	0.5
Medium, Uncle Ben's*	1 Serving/100g	66	66	0.9	11.1	2.0	0.0
Mild, Tesco*	1 Jar/500g	420	84	1.1	13.4	2.8	0.8
SmartPrice, Asda*	¼ Jar/110g	58	53	0.7	9.0	1.6	0.6
Sweet	1oz/28g	25	91	1.2	9.6	5.6	1.4
Sweet, McDonald's*	1 Portion/32g	61	192	1.2	41.1	2.5	0.0
SAUCE, DARK SOYA, Amoy*	1 Serving/10g	9	85	1.2	20.0	0.0	0.0
SAUCE, DHANSAK,							
Medium, Sharwood's*	1 Jar/420g	370	88	3.6	11.1	3.2	1.0
Sharwood's*	1 Jar/445g	668	150	4.7	15.2	7.8	1.4
SAUCE, DIANE, Safeway*	½ Pot/85g	40	47	0.8	3.3	3.5	0.3
SAUCE, DIPPING For Dim Sum, Amoy*	1 Tbsp/15ml	29	190	0.0	48.0	0.0	0.0
SAUCE, DOPIAZA, Patak's*	1 Serving/212g	235	111	1.7	9.1	7.6	1.3
SAUCE, ENCHILADA, Medium, Old El Paso*	1 Can/270g	92	34	0.0	5.0	1.7	0.0
SAUCE, FAJITA,							
Asda*	¼ Jar/125g	79	63	1.0	5.0	4.3	1.0

S

	Measure INFO/WEIGHT	per Measure KCAL	Nutrition Values per 100g / 100ml				
			KCAL	PROT	CARB	FAT	FIBRE
SAUCE, FAJITA,							
Marks & Spencer*	1oz/28g	24	85	1.3	6.4	6.1	2.2
SAUCE, FOR BOLOGNESE,							
Extra Onion & Garlic, Dolmio*	1 Serving/125g	66	53	1.7	9.0	1.0	0.0
Light, Original, Ragu*	1 Jar/515g	196	38	1.4	8.2	0.1	1.2
Original, Ragu*	1 Jar/515g	242	47	1.4	8.2	0.9	1.2
SAUCE, FOR LASAGNE,							
Tomato, Ragu*	1 Jar/515g	191	37	1.5	7.4	0.2	1.0
White, Dolmio*	1 Serving/140g	154	110	2.1	3.7	9.6	0.0
White, Light, Ragu*	¼ Jar/122g	88	72	0.5	6.3	5.0	0.2
White, Ragu	¼ Jar/123g	205	167	0.5	4.7	16.3	0.3
SAUCE, FOUR CHEESE,							
Less Than 5% Fat, Safeway*	½ Pot/175g	140	80	4.9	5.8	4.1	0.2
Safeway*	1 Serving/175g	261	149	5.7	6.4	11.2	0.5
SAUCE, FRUITY, HP*	1 Tsp/6g	8	141	1.2	35.1	0.1	0.0
SAUCE, GARLIC,							
Heinz*	1 Serving/10ml	32	323	1.0	12.1	29.9	1.2
Lea & Perrins*	1 Tsp/6g	20	337	1.8	17.8	29.0	0.0
SAUCE, GREEN							
Peppercorn, Sainsbury's*	1 Tbsp/15ml	68	455	0.4	3.8	48.5	0.1
Tandoori, Marks & Spencer*	1 Jar/385g	501	130	3.6	6.8	9.9	1.5
Thai, Curry, Asda*	1 Jar/340g	309	91	0.5	4.3	8.0	0.2
Thai, Loyd Grossman*	½ Jar/175g	228	130	2.3	10.1	9.0	1.2
Thai, So Good, Somerfield*	1 Jar/350g	413	118	1.2	7.0	9.5	0.5
Thai, Stir Fry, Fresh Ideas, Tesco*	1 Pack/50g	91	182	2.1	6.2	16.6	0.1
SAUCE, HP*	1oz/28g	33	119	0.9	27.5	0.2	0.0
SAUCE, HAM &							
Mushroom For Pasta, Stir & Serve, Homepride*	1 Serving/100g	95	95	1.5	1.3	9.3	0.0
Mushroom, Safeway*	½ Pot/154g	149	97	6.5	6.5	5.0	0.7
SAUCE, HOI SIN							
& Plum, Chinatown, Knorr*	¼ Jar/131g	96	73	0.8	15.8	0.7	1.2
& Plum, Finest, Tesco*	1 Serving/50g	78	156	2.3	35.3	0.6	1.4
& Plum, Sweet & Fruity Stir Fry, Sharwood's*	1 Serving/136g	126	93	0.9	19.3	1.3	0.7
& Spring Onion, Stir Fry, Sharwood's*	1 Jar/165g	223	135	2.6	27.8	1.5	0.9
Marks & Spencer*	½ Pot/50ml	80	160	3.2	31.8	2.0	2.2
Sharwood's*	1 Tbsp/20g	42	211	2.7	49.5	0.3	0.6
SAUCE, HOLLANDAISE,							
Colman's*	1 Pack/27g	102	379	10.0	54.0	13.0	0.0
Full Fat, Marks & Spencer*	1 Tbsp/20g	67	336	1.1	4.5	34.9	0.1
Maille*	1 Serving/30g	149	495	1.0	10.8	50.6	0.0
Marks & Spencer*	1oz/28g	56	200	1.6	2.4	20.5	0.1
Pour Over, Knorr*	1oz/28g	44	158	0.0	7.0	14.0	0.0
Schwartz*, Dry	1 Pack/25g	98	392	11.3	61.5	11.2	0.0
SAUCE, HONEY							
& Coriander, Stir Fry, Blue Dragon*	1 Pack/120g	115	96	0.5	22.1	0.6	0.3
& Mustard, COU, Marks & Spencer*	½ Jar/160g	112	70	2.3	9.2	2.9	0.7
& Mustard, Chicken Tonight*	¼ Jar/130g	139	107	1.6	13.5	5.2	1.3
& Mustard, For Cooking, Asda*	1 Serving/200g	234	117	0.6	13.0	7.0	0.0
n Chilli, Stir Fry, Discovery*	½ Pack/75g	123	164	1.1	37.3	1.1	1.9
SAUCE, HONG KONG Curry, Loyd Grossman*	1 Jar/350g	371	106	1.3	7.8	7.7	0.8
SAUCE, HORSERADISH,							
Asda*	1oz/28g	38	135	2.2	14.0	7.0	2.0
Creamed, Colman's*	1 Tsp/16g	37	229	4.3	21.4	13.3	0.0
Creamed, Marks & Spencer*	1 Tsp/5g	16	325	2.4	12.1	29.3	2.5

S

	Measure INFO/WEIGHT	per Measure KCAL	Nutrition Values per 100g / 100ml				
			KCAL	PROT	CARB	FAT	FIBRE
SAUCE, HORSERADISH,							
Creamed, Safeway*	1 Serving/10g	18	184	2.4	19.6	9.8	2.3
Creamed, Tesco*	1 Serving/15g	30	202	2.4	23.0	10.3	1.9
Creamed, Waitrose*	1 Tbsp/16g	30	185	2.4	19.6	9.9	2.3
Hot, Colman's*	1 Tbsp/15ml	16	105	1.8	9.7	5.7	0.0
Hot, Tesco*	1 Serving/10g	15	150	1.8	20.1	6.0	3.3
Mustard, Sainsbury's*	1 Tsp/5g	4	82	5.3	2.3	5.8	0.0
Sainsbury's*	1 Dtsp/10g	15	145	1.5	17.8	6.6	2.4
SAUCE, HOT CHILLI,							
Asda*	¼ Jar/126g	82	65	2.0	8.0	2.8	1.2
Deliciously Good, Homepride*	1 Serving/120g	62	52	1.3	10.6	0.5	1.1
Sharwood's*	1fl oz/30ml	36	120	0.5	29.4	0.6	1.3
Uncle Ben's*	1 Jar/500g	250	50	2.0	9.6	0.4	0.0
SAUCE, HOT ONION, TTD Sainsbury's*	1 Serving/10g	17	167	0.2	41.0	0.1	0.1
SAUCE, INDIAN TIKKA, Chicken Tonight*	1 Serving/250g	320	128	1.3	10.0	9.2	1.2
SAUCE, ITALIAN							
Hot Chili, Dolmio*	½ Pack/150g	104	69	1.3	7.1	3.9	0.0
Onion & Garlic, Sainsbury's*	1 Jar/500g	375	75	2.2	12.1	2.0	1.7
Tomato & Herb, For Pasta, BGTY, Sainsbury's*	½ Jar/250g	138	55	2.1	10.9	0.3	0.0
Tomato & Herb, Sainsbury's*	¼ Jar/126g	88	70	2.0	11.1	2.0	1.4
With Onion, Garlic & Herb, Safeway*	1 Serving/210g	143	68	2.1	11.5	1.6	1.8
SAUCE, JALFREZI							
Hot, Cooking, Sharwood's*	1 Jar/440g	264	60	1.4	7.8	2.6	1.5
Cooking, Asda*	1 Jar/500g	470	94	1.0	9.0	6.0	0.7
Cooking, Shere Khan*	1 Jar/425g	202	48	0.8	3.9	3.2	0.0
Cooking, Tesco*	¼ Jar/125g	144	115	2.6	11.4	6.5	1.6
Curry, Patak's*	1 Serving/135g	157	116	1.7	11.3	7.0	1.4
Hot, Tesco*	1 Serving/220g	125	57	1.1	8.3	2.1	0.8
Marks & Spencer*	1 Jar/385g	308	80	1.7	6.6	5.2	1.9
Mild, Sharwood's*	1 Jar/445g	347	78	1.4	10.6	3.3	1.3
Stir Fry, Patak's*	1 Jar/250g	260	104	1.4	7.6	7.5	1.4
SAUCE, KORMA,							
Asda*	1 Serving/225g	434	193	2.5	12.0	15.0	2.2
Coconut & Cream, Patak's*	1 Serving/135g	235	174	1.3	9.1	14.7	0.8
Cooking, BGTY, Sainsbury's*	¼ Jar/129g	119	92	1.1	10.8	4.9	1.4
Cooking, Healthy Eating, Tesco*	¼ Jar/125g	120	96	1.9	7.4	6.4	0.6
Cooking, Sainsbury's*	¼ Jar/125g	159	127	1.4	8.0	9.9	1.0
Deliciously Good, Homepride*	1 Jar/450g	396	88	1.4	10.6	4.4	1.4
Good For You, Asda*	1 Serving/240g	312	130	3.0	7.0	10.0	1.6
Homepride*	1 Serving/160g	110	69	1.3	11.6	2.0	0.0
Indian Style, Iceland*	¼ Jar/112g	150	134	1.5	11.4	9.1	1.0
Indian, Marks & Spencer*	1oz/28g	60	215	3.8	11.7	17.3	0.9
Loyd Grossman*	½ Jar/222g	542	244	3.6	19.1	17.0	0.6
Mild Curry, Better For You, Morrisons*	¼ Jar/118g	150	127	1.3	16.8	6.1	1.5
Organic, Patak's*	¼ Jar/106g	148	140	1.9	5.9	12.0	0.9
Patak's*	1 Jar/540g	751	139	2.4	11.4	9.4	1.0
Seeds of Change*	½ Jar/175g	231	132	1.2	12.8	8.4	1.3
Sharwood's*	1 Serving/105g	150	143	1.4	12.2	9.8	1.8
Sizzle & Stir, Knorr*	1 Serving/152g	365	240	1.2	11.2	21.2	2.7
Tesco*	1 Serving/125g	230	184	2.4	10.2	14.7	0.6
Tin, Patak's*	1 Can/283g	478	169	3.6	8.5	13.4	2.3
Uncle Ben's*	1 Jar/500g	625	125	1.2	11.4	7.8	0.0
SAUCE, LEMON							
& Ginger, Stir Fry, Asda*	1 Serving/107g	184	172	0.4	42.0	0.3	0.5

INFO/WEIGHT	Measure	per Measure KCAL	Nutrition Values per 100g / 100ml				
			KCAL	PROT	CARB	FAT	FIBRE
SAUCE, LEMON							
& Ginger, Stir Fry, Safeway*	1 Serving/110g	182	165	0.2	40.7	0.2	0.2
& Sesame, Sharwood's*	1 Serving/100g	118	118	0.2	28.9	0.2	0.1
Butter, Schwartz*	1 Serving/9g	35	388	10.2	61.4	11.3	0.0
Pepper, Stir It Up, Chicken Tonight*	1 Jar/80g	527	659	5.2	26.1	59.3	2.7
Stir Fry, Straight to Wok, Amoy*	½ Sachet/50g	81	162	0.3	40.0	0.2	0.0
Stir Fry, Tesco*	1 Jar/450g	369	82	0.1	19.3	0.2	0.1
SAUCE, LIME Honey & Ginger, Stir Fry, Sharwood's*	1 Serving/50g	35	69	0.3	16.6	0.1	0.2
SAUCE, MADRAS,							
Aldi*	1 Serving/113g	68	60	1.5	9.0	2.0	0.0
Cooking, Asda*	¼ Jar/141.6g	109	77	1.3	8.0	4.4	1.0
Cooking, Sharwood's*	1 Tsp/2g	2	86	1.5	6.9	5.8	1.3
Curry, Sharwood's*	1 Jar/420g	521	124	1.7	8.9	9.1	1.4
Curry, Somerfield*	1 Serving/110g	106	96	1.7	8.3	6.1	0.7
SAUCE, MEDITERRANEAN							
Chargrilled Red Pepper, Stir in For Pasta, Sainsbury's*	1 Serving/75g	62	82	1.9	9.0	4.3	1.4
Vegetable, Roasted, Sainsbury's*	½ Pot/150g	102	68	1.6	6.7	3.9	0.4
Vegetable, Waitrose*	1/3 Pot/120g	60	50	1.3	4.5	3.0	1.6
Vegetables, Stir In, BGTY, Sainsbury's*	1 Jar/150g	123	82	1.9	9.0	4.3	1.4
SAUCE, MEXICAN							
Recipe, Discovery*	1 Jar/265g	355	134	1.5	18.2	5.5	1.4
Style, Cooking, Eat Smart, Safeway*	1 Serving/178g	134	75	1.3	15.8	0.6	1.2
SAUCE, MINT							
Baxters*	1oz/28g	17	62	1.7	13.2	0.3	0.0
Classic, Colman's*	1 Serving/5ml	6	122	0.8	26.0	0.1	0.0
Garden, Fresh, Tesco*	1 Tsp/5g	2	40	2.6	3.6	0.4	1.5
Jelly, Sweet, Colman's*	1 Serving/14ml	35	249	0.2	61.0	0.0	0.0
Raita, Patak's*	1 Jar/270g	340	126	3.9	13.6	5.5	0.1
Sainsbury's*	1 Dtsp/10g	13	126	2.5	28.7	0.1	4.0
SmartPrice, Asda*	1 Serving/5g	3	52	0.1	13.0	0.0	1.2
SAUCE, MOROCCAN							
Seven Vegetable Cous Cous, Sainsbury's*	1 Serving/50g	89	178	2.6	5.9	16.0	0.0
Tagine, Pan Fry, Loyd Grossman*	1oz/28g	15	53	0.9	5.4	3.1	0.4
SAUCE, MORROCAN							
Chicken, Chicken Tonight*	1 Jar/500g	365	73	0.4	14.7	1.3	1.4
SAUCE, MUSHROOM							
& Garlic, 95% Fat Free, Homepride*	1 Serving/220g	154	70	0.9	7.0	4.2	0.3
& Herb, Cooking, BGTY, Sainsbury's*	¼ Jar/125g	68	54	1.8	6.6	2.3	0.5
& White Wine, Knorr*	1 Serving/100ml	99	99	1.0	4.0	8.0	0.6
Creamy, Tesco*	½ Pot/175g	128	73	1.3	6.4	4.7	0.4
For Pasta, Organic, Safeway*	1 Serving/220g	130	59	1.4	7.8	2.5	1.2
TTD, Sainsbury's*	1 Serving/150g	251	167	2.6	3.5	15.8	1.4
SAUCE, MUSTARD							
& Dill, Marks & Spencer*	1oz/28g	113	405	2.9	17.0	36.6	0.1
Mild, McDonald's*	1 Portion/30g	64	212	1.0	24.8	12.1	0.0
SAUCE, NAPOLETANA,							
Fresh, Sainsbury's*	½ Pot/150g	95	63	1.7	7.3	3.0	2.3
Italiano, New Improved Recipe, Tesco*	½ Pot/175g	126	72	1.6	8.7	3.4	1.1
Safeway*	1 Serving/175g	107	61	1.3	6.1	3.5	1.4
Tesco*	¼ Lge Tub/125g	90	72	1.6	8.7	3.4	1.1
Waitrose*	½ Pot/175g	88	50	1.2	5.2	2.7	1.8
SAUCE, OLIVE & Tomato, Stir Through, Sacla*	½ Jar/95g	189	199	2.1	4.1	19.4	0.0
SAUCE, ONION,							
Colman's*	1 Sachet/35g	111	316	8.3	68.0	1.0	0.0

S

INFO/WEIGHT	Measure per Measure KCAL		Nutrition Values per 100g / 100ml				
			KCAL	PROT	CARB	FAT	FIBRE
SAUCE, ONION,							
Made With Semi-Skimmed Milk	1 Serving/60g	52	86	2.9	8.4	5.0	0.4
Made With Skimmed Milk	1 Serving/60g	46	77	2.9	8.4	4.0	0.4
SAUCE, ORANGE & Green Ginger, Blue Dragon*	1 Pack/120g	118	98	0.5	20.4	1.6	0.5
SAUCE, ORIENTAL							
Orange & Ginger, Homepride*	1 Serving/100g	68	68	0.7	15.9	0.1	0.0
Sweet & Sour, Express, Uncle Ben's*	1 Serving/170g	221	130	0.8	27.5	1.9	0.0
SAUCE, OYSTER							
& Garlic, Stir Fry, Straight To Wok, Amoy*	½ Pack/50g	98	195	4.9	37.0	3.0	0.0
& Spring Onion, Stir Fry, Blue Dragon*	1 Serving/80g	74	92	1.6	19.9	0.7	1.1
Flavoured, Amoy*	1 Tsp/5ml	5	108	2.0	25.0	0.0	0.0
Stir Fry, Sainsbury's	1 Tbsp/15g	9	61	1.6	13.3	0.1	0.2
SAUCE, PARSLEY,							
Colman's*	1 Sachet/20g	64	320	10.4	66.0	1.7	0.0
Fresh, Sainsbury's*	½ Pot/150g	183	122	2.5	7.0	9.3	1.3
Instant, Asda*	1 Serving/23g	82	355	7.0	66.0	7.0	4.4
Made Up, Semi Skim Milk, Sainsbury's*	¼ Sachet/51ml	34	67	3.5	8.6	2.1	0.1
SAUCE, PASANDA, Almond & Yogurt, Patak's*	1 Jar/420g	634	151	2.2	8.5	12.0	0.5
SAUCE, PASSATA,							
Basil, Del Monte*	1 Jar/500g	160	32	1.4	5.9	0.2	0.0
Classic Italian With Onion & Garlic, Sainsbury's*	1oz/28g	10	37	1.4	7.7	0.1	1.3
Italian, Sainsbury's*	¼ Jar/175g	51	29	1.1	6.0	0.1	0.8
Italian, Tesco*	1 Pack/500g	170	34	1.1	6.4	0.2	1.0
Onion Garlic & Herbs, Safeway*	1 Serving/138g	47	34	1.4	5.7	0.6	1.2
SmartPrice, Asda*	1 Serving/15g	4	25	1.4	4.5	0.1	0.2
Traditional, Del Monte*	1 Jar/500g	155	31	1.4	5.5	0.1	0.0
Valfrutta*	1 Serving/50g	13	25	1.4	4.5	0.1	0.0
With Garlic & Italian Herbs, Tesco*	1 Serving/165g	53	32	1.2	6.4	0.2	1.1
SAUCE, PEKING							
Lemon, Stir Fry, Blue Dragon*	1 Serving/35g	58	166	0.3	36.8	1.9	0.1
Sizzle & Stir, Chicken Tonight*	1 Jar/510g	617	121	0.8	9.4	8.9	1.6
SAUCE, PEPPER							
& Brandy, Pour Over, Knorr*	1oz/28g	29	104	1.0	4.0	9.0	0.0
Creamy, Colman's*	1 Pack/25g	88	352	13.0	50.0	11.0	0.0
Creamy, Schwartz*	1 Serving/25g	92	368	17.6	61.0	5.9	0.0
SAUCE, PEPPERCORN,							
Creamy, Chicken Tonight*	¼ Jar/125g	100	80	1.0	3.8	6.7	0.5
Marks & Spencer*	1oz/28g	38	135	1.8	7.1	10.8	0.2
SAUCE, PESTO							
Average	1oz/28g	145	517	20.4	2.0	47.5	0.0
Basil, Stir In, Waitrose*	½ Bottle/85g	394	463	12.8	8.2	42.1	1.4
Bertolli*	1 Serving/20g	78	391	5.6	4.4	39.0	1.4
Black Olive, Sacla*	1oz/28g	115	409	2.9	4.3	42.2	0.0
Chargrilled Aubergine, Sacla' *	1 Serving/47.6g	79	164	1.9	3.5	16.0	0.0
Classic Green, Sacla' *	1oz/28g	142	507	4.1	8.5	50.7	0.0
Classsic, Sacla*	1 Serving/45g	209	465	5.5	5.6	46.7	0.0
Fresh, Waitrose*	1 Tbsp/26g	120	463	12.8	8.2	42.1	1.4
Green, Asda*	1 Tsp/5g	21	429	4.7	3.5	44.0	1.4
Green, BGTY, Sainsbury's*	1 Hpd Tsp/20g	60	299	13.0	5.9	24.8	0.1
Green, Bertolli*	1 Serving/47g	202	429	5.4	4.2	43.0	1.3
Green, Free From, Sainsbury's*	1/3 Jar/70g	298	425	4.1	5.4	43.0	2.8
Green, Fresh, Tesco*	1oz/28g	141	505	6.5	12.2	48.0	0.1
Green, Half the Fat, Grandissimo*	1 Serving/48g	85	177	4.4	2.2	16.7	0.0
Green, Italian, Safeway*	¼ Jar/50g	215	429	5.4	4.2	43.4	1.3

S

	Measure	per Measure	Nutrition Values per 100g / 100ml				
	INFO/WEIGHT	KCAL	KCAL	PROT	CARB	FAT	FIBRE
SAUCE, PESTO							
Green, Morrisons*	1 Serving/50g	255	510	10.7	4.7	49.8	0.0
Green, Sainsbury's*	1oz/28g	120	430	5.4	8.3	41.7	0.0
Marks & Spencer*	1oz/28g	115	411	3.2	3.5	43.3	3.9
Red Pepper, Barilla*	1 Serving/25g	91	364	2.8	22.9	29.0	0.0
Red, BGTY, Sainsbury's*	1 Serving/30ml	26	85	2.9	13.3	2.3	1.4
Red, Marks & Spencer*	1oz/28g	93	331	3.6	6.9	33.2	3.5
Red, Sacla*	1 Serving/25g	82	327	4.3	8.9	30.4	0.0
Red, Sainsbury's*	1 Serving/60g	242	404	4.8	17.0	35.5	0.8
Rich Tomato With Basil, Dolmio*	1 Jar/170g	146	86	2.0	6.2	5.9	0.0
Roasted Pepper, Sacla' *	1 Serving/47.6g	115	239	4.5	6.0	23.0	0.0
Spinach & Parmesan, Sainsbury's*	½ Heap Tsp/16g	63	396	5.6	3.4	40.0	0.0
SAUCE, PLUM							
& Ginger, Stir Fry, Asda*	½ Jar/97g	94	97	0.7	22.0	0.7	0.3
& Sesame, Stir Fry, Marks & Spencer*	½ Jar/115g	138	120	0.9	29.0	0.1	1.8
Sharwood's*	1 Serving/50g	121	241	0.5	59.4	0.2	0.6
SAUCE, PRAWN Cocktail, Frank Cooper*	1 Tbsp/15g	47	316	0.8	18.3	26.7	0.1
SAUCE, PRIMAVERA, Loyd Grossman*	¼ Jar/88g	86	98	1.4	6.3	7.4	0.9
SAUCE, PUTTANESCA, Fresh, Waitrose*	½ Pot/176.1g	118	67	1.8	6.2	4.4	1.2
SAUCE, RED THAI,							
Cooking, Perfectly Balanced, Waitrose*	1 Jar/430g	267	62	1.1	6.2	3.6	1.6
Curry, Worldwide Sauces*	1 Jar/450g	630	140	1.5	10.9	10.0	0.0
Loyd Grossman*	1oz/28g	34	123	2.6	11.7	7.3	1.1
SAUCE, RED WINE							
& Herb, Safeway*	1 Jar/680g	347	51	1.1	8.3	1.5	0.5
& Herbs, Ragu*	¼ Jar/130g	81	62	2.1	8.8	2.0	1.1
& Onion, Rich, Simply Sausages, Colman's*	¼ Jar/125g	49	39	0.9	8.5	0.2	1.3
Cook In, Homepride*	¼ Can/98g	47	48	0.5	10.1	0.6	0.0
Cooking, BGTY, Sainsbury's*	1 Serving/125g	53	42	0.5	8.8	0.5	0.8
SAUCE, REDCURRANT, Colman's*	1 Tsp/12g	44	368	0.7	90.0	0.0	0.0
SAUCE, ROASTED VEGETABLE,							
Finest, Tesco*	1 Serving/175g	102	58	1.4	7.8	2.4	1.0
Stir In, Dolmio*	1oz/28g	38	135	1.5	9.1	10.3	0.0
SAUCE, ROGAN JOSH,							
99% Fat Free, Homepride*	1/3 Jar/153g	92	60	1.8	11.6	0.7	2.0
Asda*	¼ Jar/125g	135	108	0.9	8.0	8.0	0.6
Loyd Grossman*	½ Jar/212.5g	413	194	2.4	10.5	15.8	1.5
Medium, Sharwood's*	½ Jar/210g	151	72	1.4	8.6	3.6	0.5
Patak's*	1 Serving/270g	192	71	1.8	9.4	2.9	0.0
Tesco*	½ Can/220g	130	59	1.5	11.5	0.6	0.9
Worldwide, Aldi*	1 Serving/150g	92	61	1.5	12.4	0.6	0.9
SAUCE, SATAY,							
Amoy*	1 Tsp/5ml	10	198	10.2	11.6	12.3	0.0
Indonesian, Sharwood's*	1oz/28g	31	112	2.8	11.8	6.0	0.6
SAUCE, SEAFOOD,							
25% Less Fat, Tesco*	1 Tsp/5g	17	344	2.7	18.2	28.5	0.3
Asda*	1 Serving/10g	47	474	1.2	16.0	45.0	0.0
BGTY, Sainsbury's*	1 Serving/15ml	23	150	0.8	15.1	9.3	0.1
Baxters*	1oz/28g	149	533	1.5	9.9	54.2	0.7
Colman's*	1 Serving/14ml	47	335	0.9	20.0	28.0	0.0
Good For You, Asda*	1 Dstp/10ml	31	313	0.6	17.0	27.0	0.0
Sainsbury's*	1 Tbsp/15g	50	330	0.7	17.6	28.2	·0.1
Somerfield*	1oz/28g	97	345	2.0	12.0	32.0	0.0

S

	Measure INFO/WEIGHT	per Measure KCAL	Nutrition Values per 100g / 100ml				
			KCAL	PROT	CARB	FAT	FIBRE
SAUCE, SMOKEY							
Bacon & Tomato, Stir In, Dolmio*	1 Pot/150g	248	165	5.5	6.9	12.8	0.0
Texan, Sizzle & Stir, Chicken Tonight*	1 Serving/150g	149	99	1.1	5.8	7.9	1.8
SAUCE, SOY							
Average	1 Tsp/5ml	3	64	8.7	8.3	0.0	0.0
Dark, Amoy*	1 Tsp/5ml	4	73	1.9	16.3	0.0	0.0
Ginger & Garlic, Stir Fry, Asda*	1 Pack/100ml	82	82	0.8	19.0	0.3	0.0
Light, Amoy*	1 Tsp/5ml	3	55	3.2	11.5	0.0	0.0
Light, Asda*	1 Tbsp/15ml	7	47	0.8	11.0	0.0	0.0
Reduced Salt, Amoy*	1 Tsp/5ml	3	56	4.0	10.0	0.0	0.0
Rich, Sharwood's*	1 Tsp/5ml	2	48	4.6	7.5	0.0	0.3
Superior Dark, Amoy*	1 Tsp/5ml	3	63	1.9	16.3	0.0	0.0
SAUCE, SPICY							
Bolognese, Cooking, Ragu*	1 Jar/510g	326	64	1.6	9.3	2.3	1.2
Durban, New World, Knorr*	1 Pack/500g	305	61	0.6	8.7	2.7	0.4
Peanut, Sharwood's*	1oz/28g	29	103	2.5	12.1	5.0	0.6
Pepper & Tomato, Stir Through, Marks & Spencer*	½ Jar/95g	166	175	1.6	7.5	15.4	0.0
Pepper, Eat Smart, Safeway*	1 Serving/84g	42	50	1.4	7.0	1.7	1.3
Red Pepper & Roasted Vegetable, For Pasta, Asda*	1 Serving/175g	140	80	1.2	9.0	4.4	1.0
Red Pepper & Roasted Vegetable, Sainsbury's*	1 Pot/302g	220	73	1.5	8.9	3.4	1.0
Sweet & Sour, Sharwood's*	1 Serving/138g	142	103	0.7	23.8	0.5	0.4
Szechuan Tomato, Stir Fry, Sharwood's*	1/3 Jar/140g	73	52	1.1	10.2	0.8	0.9
Tikka, Cooking, Sharwood's*	1oz/28g	27	95	1.3	9.4	5.9	0.8
Tomato & Pesto, COU, Marks & Spencer*	1 Serving/100g	60	60	2.2	6.8	2.5	1.3
Tomato & Red Pepper, Fresh, PB, Waitrose*	½ Pot/175g	65	37	1.4	5.7	0.8	0.8
Tomato, Fresh, Somerfield*	1/3 Pot/100g	41	41	0.8	6.4	1.3	1.1
SAUCE, SPINACH & Ricotta, Fresh, PB, Waitrose*	½ Pot/175g	103	59	2.7	4.9	3.1	1.0
SAUCE, STROGANOFF,							
Asda*	1 Serving/285g	305	107	1.5	5.0	9.0	0.3
Marks & Spencer*	1oz/28g	30	107	3.8	4.9	8.0	0.6
SAUCE, SUN DRIED TOMATO							
& Basil, Free From, Sainsbury's*	1 Serving/175g	126	72	2.9	8.7	2.8	1.5
& Basil, Seeds Of Change*	1 Serving/100g	169	169	1.8	9.3	13.2	0.0
For Pasta, Stir & Serve, Homepride*	1 Serving/100g	62	62	1.0	7.6	3.0	0.0
Heinz*	1 Serving/10ml	7	73	1.5	14.9	0.6	0.9
Mozzarella & Basil, Safeway*	½ Pot/159.1g	175	110	3.5	8.7	6.7	1.4
Stir In, Light, Dolmio*	1 Serving/75g	62	83	1.7	9.8	4.7	0.0
Stir-In, Dolmio*	1 Serving/75g	124	165	1.5	9.3	14.0	0.0
With Vodka & Chilli, TTD, Sainsbury's*	½ Pot/150g	99	66	1.7	6.9	3.5	0.5
SAUCE, SWEDISH Mustard & Dill, Safeway*	1 Serving/20g	32	162	17.1	1.5	9.8	0.2
SAUCE, SWEET & SOUR,							
Colman's*	1 Pack/40g	134	334	3.4	78.0	0.1	0.0
Cook In, NEW, Homepride*	1 Serving/125g	115	92	0.3	22.5	0.1	1.0
Cooking, Good For You, Asda*	1 Jar/500g	310	62	0.9	14.0	0.3	0.6
Cooking, Healthy Choice, Asda*	1 Jar/500g	175	35	0.6	8.0	0.1	0.5
Cooking, Organic, Sainsbury's*	1/3 Jar/150g	150	100	0.8	22.1	0.9	0.5
Extra Pineapple, Chinatown, Knorr*	1 Jar/525g	436	83	0.3	20.3	0.1	1.0
Extra Pineapple, Uncle Ben's*	1 Serving/165g	144	87	0.3	21.4	0.0	0.0
Fresh Ideas, Tesco*	1 Serving/50ml	77	154	1.1	34.3	1.4	0.5
Fresh, Safeway*	1 Sachet/50g	101	201	0.9	37.8	5.1	0.3
Fresh, Sainsbury's*	1 Sachet/50ml	103	205	0.8	31.2	8.6	0.3
Homepride*	1 Serving/195g	193	99	0.4	24.4	0.1	0.0
Light, Uncle Ben's*	1 Serving/200g	128	64	0.5	15.5	0.0	0.0
McDonald's*	1 Portion/32g	59	183	0.4	43.5	0.8	0.0

S

INFO/WEIGHT	per Measure KCAL	Nutrition Values per 100g / 100ml				
		KCAL	PROT	CARB	FAT	FIBRE
SAUCE, SWEET & SOUR,						
Oriental, Chicken Tonight*	¼ Jar/125g	115	92	0.6	20.9	0.7	0.9
Original, Uncle Ben's*	1 Pack/300g	264	88	0.5	21.7	0.0	0.0
Peking Style, Safeway*	1 Jar/340g	214	63	0.6	14.9	0.1	0.9
Seeds Of Change*	1 Serving/200g	174	87	0.3	21.3	0.0	0.7
Sizzle & Stir, Chicken Tonight*	1 Jar/465g	693	149	0.6	19.5	7.7	1.6
Sizzle & Stir, Knorr*	1 Serving/460g	676	147	0.6	15.6	9.0	0.2
Sizzling, Homepride*	¼ Jar/125g	88	70	0.4	16.8	0.1	0.0
Spicy, Uncle Ben's*	1 Jar/400g	364	91	0.6	22.1	0.1	0.0
Stir Fry, Asda*	1 Serving/63g	146	232	0.8	46.0	5.0	0.0
Stir Fry, Blue Dragon*	1 Serving/120g	150	125	0.7	23.3	3.2	0.9
Stir Fry, Good For You, Asda*	½ Pack/51ml	43	85	0.9	11.0	4.1	3.4
Stir Fry, Healthy Eating, Tesco*	1 Jar/440g	167	38	0.6	8.0	0.1	0.8
Stir Fry, Sharwood's*	1 Jar 160g	160	100	0.8	24.1	0.1	1.0
Stir Fry, Straight To Wok, Amoy*	1 Pack/220g	486	221	0.5	54.6	0.2	0.0
Stir Fry, Tesco*	½ Jar/222g	164	74	0.6	17.0	0.2	0.4
Straight To Wok*	1oz/28g	52	186	0.3	45.5	0.3	0.0
Take-Away	1oz/28g	44	157	0.2	32.8	3.4	0.0
Two Stage, Uncle Ben's*	½ Jar/200g	314	157	1.0	18.1	9.1	0.0
Uncle Ben's*	1 Serving/200g	168	84	0.4	21.7	0.0	0.0
SAUCE, SWEET BARBECUE,						
97% Fat Free, Homepride*	1 Serving/230g	166	72	1.4	11.7	2.7	2.3
Deliciously Good, Homepride*	1/3 Jar/149g	110	74	1.4	12.0	2.2	1.2
SAUCE, SWEET CHILLI						
& Coriander, Sharwood's*	1 Pack/370g	407	110	0.3	24.4	1.2	0.1
& Coriander, Sizzling, Homepride*	1 Serving/100g	51	51	0.7	11.5	0.2	0.0
& Garlic Noodle, Sharwood's*	1oz/28g	30	107	0.9	18.9	3.1	0.4
& Garlic, Stir Fry & Dipping, Tesco*	½ Jar/95ml	78	82	0.3	20.1	0.0	0.1
& Ginger, Stir Fry, Marks & Spencer*	1 Serving/60ml	207	345	0.5	44.9	18.1	0.6
& Lemon Grass, Sharwood's*	1 Serving/155g	119	77	0.4	18.3	0.2	0.3
& Lime, Chinatown, Knorr*	1 Jar/525g	635	121	0.6	22.0	3.3	0.5
& Red Pepper, Sharwood*	1 Serving/250g	178	71	0.8	16.4	0.2	1.1
Dipping, Blue Dragon*	1 Tsp/5ml	12	230	0.0	56.0	0.0	0.0
Dipping, Marks & Spencer*	1 Tbsp/15g	37	245	0.2	61.1	0.1	0.5
SAUCE, SZECHUAN						
Hot n Spicy, Safeway*	1 Jar/225g	281	125	1.2	17.9	5.4	0.9
Spicy Tomato, Stir Fry, Blue Dragon*	1 Sachet/120g	151	126	1.3	17.6	5.6	2.0
Stir Fry, Sharwood's*	1 Jar/150g	126	84	3.0	15.5	1.1	0.4
Stir Fry, Tesco*	½ Jar/220g	205	93	1.0	14.7	3.2	0.9
Style, Stir Fry, Fresh Ideas, Tesco*	1 Sachet/50g	114	228	1.9	33.4	9.7	0.1
SAUCE, TARTARE,						
Baxters*	1oz/28g	144	515	1.0	8.0	53.3	0.3
Colman's*	1 Serving/14ml	37	263	1.1	14.0	21.7	0.0
Sainsbury's*	1 Serving/20ml	94	469	0.4	5.8	49.0	1.0
Tesco*	1 Tbsp/15g	43	287	1.5	19.6	21.8	0.3
With Olives, EPC*	1 Tbsp/15g	64	425	2.2	5.7	43.7	0.7
SAUCE, TERIYAKI,						
Asda*	1 Serving/98g	99	101	2.1	23.0	0.1	0.0
Blue Dragon*	½ Pack/60g	104	173	2.0	28.6	0.0	0.0
Stir Fry, Fresh Ideas, Tesco*	1 Serving/25g	33	133	1.1	26.9	2.3	0.0
Stir Fry, Sharwood's*	1 Jar/150g	137	91	0.9	19.7	1.0	0.3
SAUCE, THAI						
Chilli, Dipping, Sainsbury's*	1 Tbsp/15g	30	201	0.2	49.8	0.0	5.0
Chilli, Sharwood's*	1 Serving/10g	16	164	1.8	39.1	0.0	0.3

	Measure INFO/WEIGHT	per Measure KCAL	Nutrition Values per 100g / 100ml				
			KCAL	PROT	CARB	FAT	FIBRE
SAUCE, THAI							
Fish, Amoy*	1 Tbsp/15ml	12	80	13.4	6.7	0.0	0.0
Green, Barts*	½ Pack/150ml	210	140	2.0	6.0	12.0	0.0
Green, Curry, Express, Uncle Ben's*	1 Pack/170g	131	77	1.1	5.4	5.8	0.0
Green, Curry, Stir Fry, Blue Dragon*	1 Sachet/120g	98	82	1.6	6.5	5.5	2.8
Green, Sainsbury's*	¼ Pack/125g	170	136	1.8	10.8	9.5	2.1
Green, Sharwood's*	1oz/28g	30	107	1.1	8.4	7.6	0.1
Panang, Sainsbury's*	1/3 Pack/166g	229	138	1.4	6.6	11.8	1.4
Red, Curry, Sainsbury's*	½ Pouch/250g	390	156	1.7	5.0	14.3	1.5
Red, Curry, Sharwood's*	1 Serving/138g	150	109	1.2	7.9	8.0	0.2
Red, Curry, Stir Fry, Blue Dragon*	1 Serving/60g	55	91	1.0	7.3	6.4	1.2
Sweet Chilli, Sizzle & Stir, Chicken Tonight*	1 Jar/510g	694	136	0.6	7.5	11.4	2.9
SAUCE, TIKKA BHUNA, Sizzle & Stir, Chicken Tonight*	1 Jar/460g	561	122	1.1	7.2	9.9	2.7
SAUCE, TIKKA MASALA							
For One, Express, Uncle Ben's*	1 Sachet/170g	168	99	1.5	9.0	6.3	0.0
Lemon & Coriander, Patak's*	1 Jar/270g	265	98	2.6	10.8	4.9	0.0
SAUCE, TIKKA MASALA,							
25% Fat Reduced, Asda*	1 Jar/500g	380	76	2.9	9.0	3.2	0.5
98% Fat Free, Homepride*	1oz/28g	14	49	1.4	7.9	1.7	0.8
Cooking, BGTY, Sainsbury's*	1 Jar/516g	516	100	1.5	12.1	4.9	1.3
Cooking, Budgens*	1oz/28g	27	96	1.6	10.1	5.5	0.2
Cooking, Eat Smart, Safeway*	½ Jar/180g	117	65	1.9	9.9	1.7	1.1
Cooking, Healthy Eating, Tesco*	1 Serving/250g	220	88	2.1	8.1	5.1	0.8
Cooking, Sharwood's*	1 Tsp/2g	2	122	1.2	11.9	7.8	0.9
Cooking, Tesco*	1 Jar/735g	1095	149	2.0	9.6	11.2	0.7
Deliciously Good, Homepride*	¼ Jar/149g	121	81	2.1	10.0	3.6	1.5
Fresh, Somerfield*	1 Pack/250g	308	123	3.0	10.0	8.0	0.0
Good For You, Asda*	½ Jar/250g	190	76	2.9	9.0	3.2	0.5
Jar, Sharwood's*	1 Jar/435g	492	113	1.4	9.6	7.6	1.4
Lemon & Coriander, Cooking, Patak's*	1 Serving/70g	119	170	2.8	10.3	13.0	1.6
Lemon & Corriander, Original, Patak's*	1 Serving/125g	111	89	1.2	6.2	6.6	0.5
Organic, Seeds Of Change*	1 Jar/385g	343	89	1.7	9.1	5.5	0.7
Organic, Tesco*	½ Jar/220g	229	104	1.9	9.4	6.2	0.8
Sizzle & Stir, Chicken Tonight*	1/3 Jar/168g	336	200	2.0	8.4	17.3	2.6
Uncle Ben's*	1 Serving/200g	212	106	1.3	8.7	7.3	0.0
SAUCE, TIKKA,							
Better for You, Morrisons*	½ Jar/237.5g	259	109	2.3	17.2	3.4	1.3
Creamy, Chicken Tonight*	1oz/28g	36	129	1.7	12.1	8.2	0.7
Indian Style, Iceland*	1 Serving/225g	284	126	1.7	12.9	7.5	2.2
SAUCE, TOFFEE, Good For You, Asda*	1 Serving/5g	15	306	2.2	68.0	2.8	0.0
SAUCE, TOMATO							
& Basil For Pasta Stir & Serve, Homepride*	1 Jar/480g	278	58	1.2	6.7	2.9	0.0
& Basil, Cooking, Marks & Spencer*	1 Serving/130g	78	60	1.4	5.7	3.4	1.2
& Basil, Eat Smart, Safeway*	1 Serving/250g	150	60	1.7	7.4	2.5	1.4
& Basil, Fresh, Organic, Waitrose*	¼ Pot/175g	77	44	1.0	6.2	1.7	0.8
& Basil, Sun-Ripened, Microwaveable, Dolmio*	1 Sachet/170g	95	56	1.4	7.9	2.1	0.0
& Basil, Tesco*	½ Jar/175g	84	48	0.7	3.8	3.3	0.8
& Chilli, Loyd Grossman*	½ Jar/175g	154	88	1.7	7.3	5.7	0.9
& Garlic, For Pasta, Asda*	¼ Jar/125g	80	64	2.7	8.0	2.3	1.1
& Herb, Fresh, Perfectly Balanced, Waitrose*	1 Pot/353g	173	49	1.2	5.3	2.6	0.9
& Herb, Somerfield*	1oz/28g	11	41	1.0	6.0	1.0	0.0
& Herbs, Italienne, Stir It Up, Chicken Tonight*	1/3 Pot/26g	164	632	4.8	18.3	60.0	4.4
& Marscapone, Italiano, Tesco*	1 Serving/175g	194	111	2.8	5.4	8.7	0.6
& Mascarpone, BGTY, Sainsbury's*	1 Pot/300g	150	50	2.0	3.6	3.0	3.6

S

	Measure INFO/WEIGHT	per Measure KCAL	Nutrition Values per 100g / 100ml				
			KCAL	PROT	CARB	FAT	FIBRE
SAUCE, TOMATO							
& Mascarpone, Fresh, Sainsbury's*	1/3 Pot/100g	118	118	2.2	4.2	10.3	1.1
& Mascarpone, Fresh, Tesco*	½ Pot/175g	207	118	2.8	7.1	8.7	0.6
& Mascarpone, Safeway*	½ Pot/175g	258	147	2.0	7.3	12.3	1.0
& Mozarella, Finest, Tesco*	1 Serving/175g	89	51	1.6	4.1	3.2	0.6
& Onion, Cook In, Homepride*	1 Can/390g	183	47	0.9	9.8	0.5	0.0
& Roasted Garlic, Stir In, Dolmio*	½ Pack/75g	94	125	1.2	7.7	10.2	0.0
& Wild Mushroom, Organic, Fresh, Sainsbury's*	1 Serving/152g	102	67	1.9	3.9	4.9	1.7
& Worcester, Table, Lea & Perrins*	1 Serving/10g	10	102	0.8	23.0	0.5	0.7
Fresh, Marks & Spencer*	1oz/28g	11	40	1.4	6.5	0.6	0.8
Indian, Sizzling, Homepride*	1 Serving/240g	82	34	0.9	7.0	0.2	0.0
Mozarella & Wild Rocket, Bistro, Waitrose*	½ Pot/175g	96	55	1.6	7.0	2.9	1.5
Organic, Heinz*	1 Tsp/5g	5	105	1.3	24.0	0.1	0.9
Parmesan & Dill, Tesco*	1 Serving/70g	81	115	3.1	4.8	9.2	0.7
Roasted Garlic & Mushroom, Bertolli*	¼ Jar/125g	68	54	1.9	6.4	2.0	1.5
Value, Tesco*	1 Serving/10g	14	139	2.3	32.2	0.1	1.4
SAUCE, VEGETABLE & Garlic, For Pasta, Dolmio*	1 Serving/150g	108	72	1.3	7.4	4.1	0.0
SAUCE, VODKA & Chilli, Finest, Tesco*	1 Serving/350g	343	98	2.2	9.4	5.7	2.1
SAUCE, WATERCRESS,							
Marks & Spencer*	1oz/28g	32	115	3.4	6.5	8.2	0.7
TTD, Sainsbury's*	1 Serving/100g	82	82	2.3	2.7	6.9	4.4
SAUCE, WHITE WINE							
& Cream, Homepride*	1 Jar/500g	405	81	1.1	9.0	4.5	0.0
& Herb, Creamy, Deliciously Good, Homepride*	1/3 Jar/150g	102	68	0.6	6.3	4.5	0.3
& Mushroom, BGTY, Sainsbury's*	1 Serving/166g	93	56	1.2	4.9	3.5	0.5
Mushroom & Herb, 98% Fat Free, Homepride*	1 Jar/450g	180	40	0.8	7.0	1.2	0.5
Cooking, Iceland*	1 Serving/220g	198	90	1.1	8.3	5.8	0.2
SAUCE, WHITE,							
Granules, Sauce In Seconds Asda*	1 Pack/57g	237	415	3.7	73.0	12.0	0.9
Savoury, Colman's*	1 Pack/25g	93	371	11.0	58.0	9.9	0.0
Savoury, Made With Semi-Skimmed Milk	1oz/28g	36	128	4.2	11.1	7.8	0.2
Savoury, Made With Whole Milk	1oz/28g	42	150	4.1	10.9	10.3	0.2
SAUCE, WILD Mushroom, Finest, Tesco*	½ Pack/175g	158	90	1.9	5.2	6.8	0.4
SAUCE, WORCESTERSHIRE,							
Average	1 Tsp/5g	3	65	1.4	15.5	0.1	0.0
Lea & Perrins*	1 Tsp/5ml	4	88	1.1	22.0	0.0	0.0
SAUCE, YELLOW BEAN,							
& Cashew Nut, Asda*	1 Serving/50g	60	119	2.7	21.0	2.7	0.9
& Cashew, Tesco*	½ Jar/210g	170	81	1.6	11.9	2.9	0.3
Sharwood's*	1 Jar/160g	211	132	0.3	28.9	1.7	1.5
Stir Fry, Sainsbury's*	½ Jar/100g	126	126	1.8	26.7	1.3	0.8
Stir Fry, Sharwood's*	1 Jar/195g	156	80	0.3	19.2	0.2	0.3
Stir Fry, Straight To Wok, Amoy*	1oz/28g	44	159	1.6	36.9	0.5	0.0
SAUCE MIX,							
Beef Stroganoff, Colman's*	1 Pack/40g	160	399	12.4	48.4	17.3	6.4
Bread, Colman's*	1 Pack/40g	130	325	12.0	66.0	1.3	0.0
Bread, Knorr*	½ Pint/40g	177	442	7.9	49.9	23.3	2.1
Cheddar Cheese, Colman's*	1 Serving/40g	158	394	19.7	45.2	14.9	1.5
Cheddar Cheese, Lidl*	1 Pack/40g	140	350	18.6	43.0	11.5	0.0
Cheese, Instant, Safeway*	1 Pack/54g	202	374	4.1	62.0	12.2	8.5
Cheese, Knorr*	1 Pack/58g	132	227	7.8	38.0	4.9	1.8
Cheese, Made Up With Skimmed Milk	1 Serving/60g	47	78	5.4	9.5	2.3	0.0
Chicken Chasseur, Colman's*	1 Pack/45g	123	273	12.0	53.0	1.0	0.0
Chicken Chasseur, Schwartz*	½ Pack/20g	64	322	9.1	64.5	3.1	0.0

S

	Measure	per Measure	Nutrition Values per 100g / 100ml				
	INFO/WEIGHT	KCAL	KCAL	PROT	CARB	FAT	FIBRE
SAUCE MIX,							
Chicken Korma, Colman's*	½ Pack/50g	230	459	6.6	38.8	30.8	13.2
Chicken Supreme, Colman's*	½ Pack/20g	72	362	12.1	53.2	11.2	6.5
Chilli Con Carne, Colman's*	1 Serving/13g	40	305	7.5	58.4	4.6	7.7
Chilli Con Carne, Schwartz*	1 Serving/10g	31	308	8.2	64.6	1.9	0.5
Coq Au Vin, Colman's*	1 Pack/50g	141	281	7.5	59.0	1.0	0.0
Creamy Cheese & Bacon, For Pasta, Colman's*	1 Pack/50g	197	394	16.6	44.6	16.6	5.7
Four Cheese, Colman's*	1 Pack/35g	145	414	17.8	40.5	20.1	3.8
Garlic Mushrooms, Creamy, Schwartz*	1 Pack/35g	109	310	7.1	60.1	4.6	0.0
Lamb Hot Pot, Colman's*	1 Serving/13.5g	37	282	7.3	59.8	1.5	2.7
Mushroom Stroganoff, Schwartz*	1 Pack/35g	41	117	3.3	21.7	1.9	0.0
Parsley, Colman's*	1 Serving/20g	61	307	8.1	65.3	1.5	3.7
Parsley, Instant, Made Up, Sainsbury's*	¼ Sachet/75ml	42	56	1.2	11.1	0.8	0.1
Parsley, Knorr*	1 Sachet/48g	210	437	4.2	50.6	24.2	0.8
Parsley, Somerfield*	1 Sachet/24g	17	72	4.0	9.0	2.0	0.0
Pepper, Instant, Safeway*	1 Serving/22g	77	348	3.2	66.3	7.5	4.1
Pork Casserole, Morrisons*	1 Pack/36g	118	327	8.1	70.6	1.4	0.0
Spaghetti Bolognese, Knorr*	1 Serving/15g	17	111	3.7	9.7	6.4	0.0
Spaghetti Bolognese, Schwartz*	1 Serving/40g	122	306	10.0	63.0	1.0	0.0
Tuna & Mushroom Pasta Melt, Schwartz*	1 Pack/40g	138	344	8.4	54.8	10.1	0.0
Tuna & Pasta Bake, Colman's*	1 Pack/45g	144	319	10.4	57.1	5.4	5.2
Tuna Napolitana, Schwartz*	1 Sachet/29g	107	368	9.7	53.0	13.0	0.0
White, Instant, Sainsbury's*	1 Serving/90ml	65	72	0.8	10.9	2.8	0.1
White, Made Up With Semi-Skimmed Milk	1oz/28g	20	73	4.0	9.6	2.4	0.0
White, Made Up With Skimmed Milk	1oz/28g	17	59	4.0	9.6	0.9	0.0
White, Savoury, Knorr*	½ Pint Pack/16g	46	290	7.8	52.2	5.6	5.2
SAUERKRAUT,							
Average	1oz/28g	3	9	1.1	1.1	0.0	2.2
Mildessa*	1 Pack/400g	68	17	1.5	2.7	0.1	0.0
SAUSAGE,							
3% Fat, Healthy Eating, Tesco*	1 Sausage/56g	66	117	14.2	8.5	2.9	0.9
Aberdeen Angus Beef, Asda*	1 Sausage/77g	203	263	16.0	7.0	19.0	0.5
Aberdeen Angus, Safeway	1 Sausage/55.9g	142	254	18.1	6.1	17.5	1.2
Aberdeenshire Beef, Safeway*	1 Sausage/48g	126	262	15.9	10.5	17.4	0.9
Aberdeenshire, Butchers Choice, Tesco*	1 Sausage/57g	168	294	9.6	8.5	24.6	2.1
BGTY, Sainsbury's*	1 Sausage/50g	95	189	16.9	10.9	8.6	0.5
Bangers & Cabbage Mash, Eat Smart, Safeway*	1 Pack/400g	340	85	6.4	9.0	2.5	1.3
Barbecue, Selection, Tesco*	1 Sausage/76g	206	271	12.0	10.1	20.3	1.0
Beef, Premium, Morrisons*	1 Sausage/67g	164	245	15.5	4.6	18.3	1.0
Beef, Somerfield*	1 Sausage/51g	122	240	13.0	10.0	17.0	0.0
Beef, Thick, Butchers Choice, Tesco*	1 Sausage/57g	171	300	10.7	6.3	25.8	1.0
Beef, With Onion & Red Wine, Finest, Tesco*	1 Sausage/63g	117	185	13.2	8.5	10.9	1.2
Best Olde English, Safeway*	1 Sausage/53g	164	310	15.8	8.3	23.8	1.3
Bockwurst German, Princes*	1 Sausage/45g	113	251	10.5	0.5	23.0	0.0
Bockwurst, In Brine, Ye Olde Oak*	1 Sausage/40.5g	105	255	11.0	1.0	23.0	0.0
Cambridge Gluten Free, Waitrose*	1 Sausage/121g	258	213	14.6	1.9	16.3	1.3
Chicken & Tarragon, Butchers Choice, Sainsbury's*	1 Sausage/47g	106	225	18.1	5.8	14.4	0.2
Chicken, Manor Farm*	1 Sausage/65g	126	194	13.7	6.6	12.5	1.2
Chilli Beef, Boston Style, Waitrose*	1 Sausage/66.5g	136	203	14.7	3.4	14.6	0.9
Chipolata, Basics, Somerfield*	1 Sausage/28g	76	271	10.0	14.0	20.0	0.0
Chipolata, Cumberland, Asda*	1 Sausage/33g	84	255	13.0	17.0	15.0	1.5
Chipolata, Cumberland, Finest, Tesco*	1 Chipolata/28g	66	235	15.6	3.1	17.8	0.7
Chipolata, Cumberland, TTD, Sainsbury's*	1 Grilled/46g	138	299	19.5	4.8	22.1	1.2
Chipolata, Finest Cumberland, Tesco*	1 Sausage/37g	99	267	12.9	4.0	22.2	0.3

S

	Measure INFO/WEIGHT	per Measure KCAL	Nutrition Values per 100g / 100ml				
			KCAL	PROT	CARB	FAT	FIBRE
Chipolata, Lamb & Rosemary, Tesco*	1 Sausage/31.6g	69	218	11.3	8.3	15.5	0.0
Chipolata, Pork & Tomato, Organic, Tesco*	1 Chipolata/28g	79	283	12.2	4.3	24.1	0.9
Chipolata, Pork, Extra Lean, BGTY, Sainsbury's*	1 Chipolata	46	189	16.9	10.9	8.6	0.5
Chipolata, Pork, Finest, Tesco*	1 Sausage/28g	78	280	13.7	3.9	23.3	0.2
Chipolata, Pork, Organic, Waitrose*	1 Serving/80g	162	202	14.4	2.2	15.1	0.9
Chipolata, Pork, Premium, Waitrose*	1 Chipolata/28.5g	70	242	14.6	1.4	19.8	1.5
Chipolata, Pork, Safeway*	1 Sausage/25.2g	61	242	12.8	10.0	16.8	1.2
Chipolata, Pork, Somerfield*	1 Chipolata/28g	80	286	12.0	10.0	22.0	0.0
Chipolata, Pork, Ultimate, TTD, Sainsbury's*	1 Sausage/45g	112	248	17.6	5.3	17.4	1.2
Chipolata, Value, Tesco*	1 Sausage/28.3g	82	292	8.4	11.6	23.6	2.4
Choice Pork, Co-Op*	1 Sausage/57g	200	350	10.0	9.0	31.0	2.0
Chorizo, Bites, Mini, Sainsbury's*	½ Pack/32.6g	141	426	25.5	2.3	35.0	0.7
Chorizo, Marks & Spencer*	1 Sausage/57g	140	245	14.4	7.0	18.3	1.7
Chorizo, Sliced, Tesco*	1 Serving/80g	234	292	26.3	1.4	20.1	0.0
Chorizo, Spanish Slices, Tesco*	1 Slice/20g	59	297	26.8	2.6	19.9	0.0
Chorizo, Spanish, Sainsbury's*	1 Serving/23g	70	304	20.0	2.0	24.0	0.1
Chorizo, Spanish, Waitrose*	1 Slice/5g	15	304	20.0	2.0	24.0	0.0
Chorizo, Spicy, Marks & Spencer*	1 Sausage/67g	154	230	13.0	10.3	15.6	0.9
Chorizo, Tapas Selection, Sainsbury's*	1 Slice/5g	15	304	20.0	2.0	24.0	0.2
Chorizo, Tesco*	1 Sausage/53g	161	303	11.7	4.4	26.5	0.9
Classic Sicilian Style, TTD, Sainsbury's*	1 Sausage/49g	135	275	16.8	0.5	22.5	0.9
Classic Toulouse, TTD, Sainsbury's*	1 Sausage/44.5g	138	310	23.2	2.1	23.3	0.9
Cocktail, Budgens*	1 Sausage/14g	44	309	10.5	9.0	25.7	0.0
Cocktail, Garnish Selection, Marks & Spencer*	2 Sausages/31g	110	355	10.6	5.4	32.5	1.5
Cocktail, Occasions, Sainsbury's*	1 Sausage/9g	31	353	12.1	9.8	29.5	0.3
Cumberland Pork, Butcher's Choice, Sainsbury's*	1 Sausage/57g	148	260	19.8	4.3	18.2	0.1
Cumberland Pork, Safeway*	1 Sausage/57g	156	273	14.2	10.0	19.6	1.0
Cumberland Pork, Waitrose*	1 Sausage/112g	317	283	13.3	5.8	23.0	2.0
Cumberland Ring, Finest, Tesco*	1 Ring/227g	606	267	12.9	4.0	22.2	0.3
Cumberland Ring, TTD, Sainsbury's*	1 Sausage/142g	410	289	17.7	6.2	21.5	0.8
Cumberland, Butchers Choice, Tesco*	1 Sausage/56g	180	321	11.1	7.6	27.4	1.8
Cumberland, Good For You, Asda*	1 Sausage/49g	72	147	17.0	10.0	4.3	0.7
Cumberland, Grilled, Cauldron Foods*	1 Sausage/50g	80	160	12.6	12.3	6.7	2.4
Cumberland, Sainsbury's*	1 Serving/53g	148	279	15.5	10.1	19.6	0.3
Cumberland, Waitrose*	1 Sausage/50g	80	160	12.6	12.3	6.7	2.4
Cumberland. Less Than 5% Fat, Safeway*	1 Sausage/57g	78	137	17.8	8.0	3.8	1.1
Extra Lean, Grilled, BGTY, Sainsbury's*	1 Sausage/49g	96	196	16.7	13.9	8.2	0.6
Extra Lean, Marks & Spencer*	1 Sausage/55g	61	110	15.3	7.2	3.3	2.9
Extra Special Toulouse, Asda*	1 Sausage/65g	212	326	15.0	8.0	26.0	0.6
French Garlic, Sainsbury's*	1 Slice/13g	30	228	16.6	0.4	17.8	0.0
French Saucisson, Tesco*	1 Slice/5g	19	379	26.7	4.1	28.4	0.0
Frozen, SmartPrice, Asda*	1 Sausage/40g	116	291	8.0	13.0	23.0	0.9
Frozen, Value, Tesco*	1 Sausage/38g	110	290	8.9	11.1	23.3	1.1
Garlic, Mild, Co-Op*	1 Slice/10g	24	235	17.0	0.7	19.0	0.0
Garlic, Strong, Asda*	1 Slice/11g	24	217	15.0	1.0	17.0	0.0
Garlic, Tesco*	1 Slice/12g	22	183	17.7	3.0	11.1	0.0
German Extrawurst, Waitrose*	1 Slice/12.5g	39	303	13.8	0.8	27.2	0.0
Glamorgan With Cheese & Leek, TTD, Sainsbury's*	1 Sausage/53g	171	323	18.9	3.3	26.0	0.6
Glamorgan, Organic, Waitrose*	1 Sausage/41.8g	81	194	14.5	11.2	10.1	1.7
Great British Banger Lincolnshire, 5% Fat, Asda*	1 Sausage/42g	96	229	15.0	13.0	13.0	1.2
Grilled, Healthy Eating, Tesco*	1 Sausage/46g	82	178	15.0	13.0	7.0	1.0
Honey Roasted Pepper & Dijon Mustard, Cauldron Foods*	1 Sausage/50g	67	133	8.4	12.0	5.7	2.2
Hot & Spicy Pork Cocktail, Cooked, Asda*	1 Sausage/10g	31	312	13.0	11.0	24.0	1.3

	Measure	per Measure	Nutrition Values per 100g / 100ml				
	INFO/WEIGHT	KCAL	KCAL	PROT	CARB	FAT	FIBRE
SAUSAGE,							
Hot Dog, Princes*	1 Sausage/50g	128	255	11.0	1.0	23.0	0.0
Hot Mustard Porker, Tesco*	1 Sausage/52g	143	275	16.1	8.1	19.8	3.1
In an Onion Gravy, Farmfoods*	1 Pack/180g	333	185	9.2	16.3	9.2	0.1
Irish Recipe, Morrisons*	1 Serving/50g	176	351	8.7	28.1	22.6	1.0
Irish Recipe, Sainsbury's*	1 Sausage/40g	111	277	12.2	18.8	17.2	0.6
Irish Recipe, Tesco*	1 Sausage/52g	146	281	10.9	11.0	21.5	0.2
Irish, Frozen, Tesco*	1 Sausage/46g	129	281	10.9	11.0	21.5	1.1
Leek & Cheese, Organic, Cauldron Foods*	1 Sausage/41g	80	194	14.5	11.2	5.2	1.7
Leek & Pork, Style Flavour, Quorn*	1 Sausage/44g	56	127	13.3	7.5	4.9	2.1
Lincolnshire Pork, Butcher's Choice, Sainsbury's*	1 Sausage/47g	146	310	18.3	5.5	23.9	0.2
Lincolnshire Pork, Tesco*	1 Sausage/46g	161	349	9.7	10.6	29.8	0.5
Lincolnshire, BGTY, Sainsbury's*	1 Sausage/48.0g	94	196	17.1	11.1	9.2	0.4
Lincolnshire, Cauldron Foods*	1 Sausage/50g	106	212	14.7	14.5	10.6	2.2
Lincolnshire, Good For You, Asda*	1 Sausage/50g	74	147	17.0	10.0	4.3	1.0
Lincolnshire, Somerfield*	1 Sausage/28.5g	79	281	13.0	8.0	22.0	0.0
Lincolnshire, TTD, Sainsbury's*	1 Sausage/59g	150	258	19.8	6.1	17.1	0.8
Lincolnshire, Tesco*	1 Sausage/60g	177	295	11.4	5.3	25.4	0.0
Lincolnshire, Tesco*	1 Sausage/50g	106	212	14.7	14.5	10.6	2.2
Lincolnshire, Thick, Asda*	1 Sausage/41.6g	90	214	16.0	15.0	10.0	1.6
Lincolnshire, Thick, Premium, Sainsbury's*	1 Sausage/48g	147	306	14.1	12.3	22.3	0.3
Lincolnshire, Waitrose*	1 Sausage/48g	91	189	13.3	6.0	12.4	0.9
Lorne, Hall's*	1 Sausage/25g	75	299	11.2	14.6	22.1	0.0
Lorne, Marks & Spencer*	1 Sausage/75g	240	320	11.2	14.3	25.2	1.8
Meat Free, Asda*	1 Sausage/43g	81	189	20.0	7.0	9.0	2.9
Meat Free, Premium, Realeat*	1 Sausage/50g	71	142	14.8	3.7	7.5	3.0
Mediterranean Style Paprika, Waitrose*	1 Sausage/67g	190	283	12.1	4.6	24.0	1.9
Mediterranean Style, 95% Fat Free, Bowyers*	1 Sausage/50g	60	120	13.9	8.9	3.2	0.0
Micro, Wall's*	1 Sausage/45g	149	330	12.2	13.4	25.3	2.3
Mini, Skinless, Asda*	1 Sausage/8g	22	279	10.0	17.0	19.0	0.3
Mushroom & Herb, Waitrose*	1 Sausage/50g	62	123	10.2	8.1	5.4	0.5
Mushroom & Tarragon, Wicken Fenn*	1 Sausage/47g	82	175	10.1	17.0	7.4	2.4
Pistachio, Waitrose*	1 Slice/12g	32	267	14.0	1.0	23.0	0.1
Pork & Apple, Finest, Tesco*	1 Sausage/75g	180	240	12.4	7.3	17.9	1.9
Pork & Apple, Lean Recipe, Wall's*	1 Sausage/57g	79	139	14.5	9.4	4.5	2.4
Pork & Apple, Marks & Spencer*	1 Sausage/57g	125	220	12.1	8.8	15.9	2.2
Pork & Apple, Sainsbury's*	1 Sausage/67g	184	275	18.4	7.8	18.9	1.7
Pork & Beef, Farmfoods*	1 Sausage/45g	125	277	9.3	7.9	23.1	0.9
Pork & Beef, Freshbake*	1 Sausage/45g	114	253	8.7	14.3	17.9	1.9
Pork & Beef, Somerfield*	1 Sausage/57g	164	288	8.0	14.0	22.0	0.0
Pork & Beef, Thick, Iceland*	1 Sausage/53g	165	312	10.4	12.1	24.7	0.6
Pork & Beef, Thick, Tesco*	1 Sausage/46g	139	302	6.7	18.7	22.3	0.5
Pork & Beef, Thin, Tesco*	1 Sausage/20g	60	302	6.7	18.7	22.3	0.5
Pork & Herb, BGTY, Sainsbury's*	1 Sausage/50.3g	72	143	16.9	12.6	2.8	1.3
Pork & Herb, COU, Marks & Spencer*	1 Sausage/59g	65	110	15.2	8.9	2.0	0.9
Pork & Herb, Finest, Tesco*	1 Sausage/75g	224	298	13.4	2.9	25.9	0.2
Pork & Leek, Extra Special, Asda*	1 Sausage/70g	179	255	8.0	13.0	19.0	2.4
Pork & Leek, Finest, Tesco*	1 Sausage/75.6g	194	255	11.8	7.5	19.8	0.7
Pork & Leek, TTD, Sainsbury's*	1 Sausage/44g	125	284	23.0	2.2	20.4	1.2
Pork & Leek, Tesco*	1 Sausage/75g	226	301	10.0	6.8	26.0	0.4
Pork & Leek, The Best, Safeway*	1 Sausage/52g	133	256	14.4	5.4	19.7	1.1
Pork & Onion, Asda*	1 Sausage/42g	108	257	20.0	6.0	17.0	1.8
Pork & Stilton Cheese, Budgens*	1 Sausage/57g	175	308	13.1	7.0	25.3	0.0
Pork & Stilton, Finest, Tesco*	1 Sausage/75g	244	325	13.3	4.7	28.1	0.6

S

SAUSAGE,

INFO/WEIGHT	Measure per Measure KCAL	KCAL	PROT	CARB	FAT	FIBRE
Pork & Sun Dried Tomato, Shire*	1 Sausage/67g 183	273	12.8	7.6	21.3	0.2
Pork & Tomato, Somerfield*	1 Sausage/57g 157	275	13.0	6.0	22.0	0.0
Pork Cocktail , Tesco*	1 Sausage/14g 39	279	12.1	9.2	21.5	1.1
Pork Cocktail, Cooked, Asda*	1 Sausage/10g 31	312	13.0	11.0	24.0	1.3
Pork Cocktail, Marks & Spencer*	1 Sausage/50g 170	340	12.6	10.7	27.5	0.9
Pork With Bramley Apple, Safeway*	1 Serving/100g 287	287	15.1	6.2	22.5	1.7
Pork With Mozzarella, Italian Style, Tesco*	1 Sausage/75.6g 206	271	12.0	10.1	20.3	1.0
Pork, 95% Fat Free, Bowyers*	1 Sausage/52g 55	105	15.3	7.0	2.4	0.0
Pork, Apricot & Lovage, Waitrose*	1 Sausage/67g 165	246	11.2	12.9	16.6	1.3
Pork, Bacon & Cheese, Asda*	¼ Pack/114g 329	289	18.0	7.0	21.0	0.4
Pork, Breakfast, Sainsbury's*	1 Sausage/20g 46	230	17.9	14.7	11.1	0.8
Pork, Butchers Choice, Tesco*	1 Sausage/57g 166	292	11.7	6.3	24.5	2.1
Pork, COU, Marks & Spencer*	1 Sausage/57g 66	115	15.6	9.5	2.1	1.4
Pork, Chilled, Grilled	1 Sausage/35g 103	294	14.5	9.8	22.1	0.7
Pork, Chilli & Coriander, Grilled, Sainsbury's*	1 Sausage/54g 123	228	18.9	3.5	15.4	1.8
Pork, Cocktail, Cooked, Geo Adams*	1 Sausage/8.9g 30	336	13.2	10.6	26.8	0.3
Pork, Cocktail, Cooked, Sainsbury's*	1 Sausage/10g 30	302	13.0	9.5	23.6	1.1
Pork, Eat Smart, Grilled, Safeway*	2 Sausages/91g 120	132	22.7	7.3	1.3	1.2
Pork, Economy, Sainsbury's*	1 Sausage/40g 116	289	12.6	16.8	19.0	0.5
Pork, Extra Lean Premium, Waitrose*	1 Serving/57g 89	156	17.2	2.7	8.5	1.8
Pork, Extra Lean, BGTY, Grilled, Sainsbury's*	1 Sausage/50g 95	189	16.9	10.9	8.6	0.5
Pork, Extra Lean, Better For You, Morrisons*	1 Sausage/54g 63	116	16.0	5.0	3.6	0.2
Pork, Extra Lean, Butchers Choice, Sainsbury's*	1 Sausage/50g 91	181	20.7	4.1	9.1	0.1
Pork, Extra Lean, GFY, Asda*	1 Sausage/57g 89	156	17.5	5.2	7.2	0.4
Pork, Farmfoods*	1 Sausage/45g 151	336	11.5	8.8	28.3	1.0
Pork, Finest, Tesco*	1 Sausage/76g 214	282	13.2	3.0	24.1	0.9
Pork, Free Range, Waitrose*	1 Sausage/57g 144	252	16.2	2.4	19.7	0.3
Pork, Fried	1 Sausage/35g 108	308	13.9	9.9	23.9	0.7
Pork, Frozen, Tesco*	2 Sausages/85g 244	287	11.1	8.9	23.0	0.6
Pork, Garlic & Herb, Speciality, Waitrose*	1 Sausage/67g 185	276	12.7	2.2	24.0	1.1
Pork, Garlic & Herb, Tesco*	1 Sausage/75.6g 198	261	11.3	9.7	19.7	1.2
Pork, Good Intentions, Somerfield*	1 Sausage/57g 116	203	17.3	9.7	10.6	0.7
Pork, Ham & Asparagus, Tesco*	1 Sausage/75.7g 173	228	14.9	3.8	17.0	1.1
Pork, Healthy Eating, Tesco*	1 Sausage/46g 117	254	11.7	24.1	12.3	0.5
Pork, Honey Roast, Westaways*	1 Sausage/75g 183	244	13.1	12.8	15.6	0.0
Pork, Jumbo, Asda*	1 Sausage/74g 155	209	17.0	15.0	9.0	1.0
Pork, Jumbo, Budgens*	1 Sausage/113g 351	309	10.5	9.0	25.7	0.0
Pork, Less Than 5% Fat, Safeway*	2 Sausages/106g 149	141	17.2	8.6	4.2	1.1
Pork, Low Fat, 95% Fat Free, Asda*	1 Sausage/50g 73	145	17.3	10.5	4.3	1.0
Pork, Olde English Style, Safeway*	1 Sausage/53g 155	293	13.9	10.4	21.7	1.5
Pork, Organic, Sainsbury's*	1 Sausage/40g 127	312	18.5	0.9	26.0	1.1
Pork, Organic, Tesco*	1 Sausage/50g 116	231	14.8	6.5	16.2	0.7
Pork, Ready Cooked, Iceland*	1 Sausage/24g 68	284	13.4	12.3	20.1	0.3
Pork, Reduced Fat, Chilled, Frozen, Raw	1 Sausage/35g 63	180	13.0	8.7	10.6	1.2
Pork, Roasted Pepper & Chilli, COU, Marks & Spencer*	1 Sausage/57g 57	100	15.2	7.1	2.0	2.1
Pork, Sainsbury's*	1 Sausage/49g 141	287	12.6	12.4	20.8	0.3
Pork, Skinless, Sainsbury's*	1 Sausage/26.2g 72	275	13.9	9.5	20.2	0.3
Pork, Skinless, Somerfield*	2 Sausages/57g 170	299	10.0	7.0	26.0	0.0
Pork, Skinless, Wall's*	1 Sausage/30g 94	313	11.4	11.6	24.6	1.0
Pork, Somerfield*	1 Sausage/124g 340	274	15.3	8.3	20.0	1.8
Pork, Special Value, Budgens*	1 Sausage/57g 176	309	11.8	5.2	26.8	0.0
Pork, Thick, Chef's Selection, Wall's*	1 Sausage/56g 181	323	11.8	8.7	26.5	0.8
Pork, Thick, Co-Op*	1 Sausage/57g 168	295	11.0	8.0	24.0	1.0

SAUSAGE,	INFO/WEIGHT	KCAL	KCAL	PROT	CARB	FAT	FIBRE
Pork, Thick, Good Choice, Iceland*	1 Sausage/50g	94	188	16.2	12.2	8.2	0.6
Pork, Thick, Half Fat, Butchers Choice, Tesco*	1 Sausage/57g	112	196	13.5	9.1	11.5	1.6
Pork, Thick, Healthy Eating, Tesco*	1 Sausage/52g	61	117	14.2	8.5	2.9	0.9
Pork, Thick, Lean Recipe, Wall's*	1 Sausage/57g	75	132	15.4	8.5	4.1	2.1
Pork, Thick, Low Fat, Iceland*	1 Sausage/50g	95	189	12.3	19.4	6.9	0.0
Pork, Thick, Premium, Sainsbury's	1 Sausage/49g	147	301	15.1	7.7	23.3	0.2
Pork, Thick, Somerfield*	1 Sausage/44.9g	123	274	15.3	8.3	20.0	1.8
Pork, Thick, Wall's*	1 Sausage/45g	154	343	11.9	11.4	27.4	0.9
Pork, Thin Link, Tesco*	1 Sausage/25g	68	272	14.8	19.2	15.2	1.2
Pork, Thin, Co-Op*	1 Sausage/28.3g	83	295	11.0	8.0	24.0	1.0
Pork, Thin, Economy, Sainsbury's*	1 Sausage/33g	95	288	13.5	18.7	17.7	0.6
Pork, Traditionally Made, Finest, Tesco*	1 Sausage/75g	210	280	13.7	3.9	23.3	0.2
Pork, Ultimate, TTD, Sainsbury's*	1 Sausage/54g	136	252	17.1	5.2	18.1	1.0
Pork, Value, Sainsbury's*	1 Sausage/37g	109	294	11.6	17.3	19.8	0.7
Premium Pork, Asda*	1 Sausage/75g	179	239	18.0	3.5	17.0	1.0
Premium Pork, Somerfield*	1 Sausage/57g	147	258	12.0	8.0	20.0	0.0
Red Thai & Lemon Grass, Extra Special, Asda*	1 Grilled/65.3g	159	245	18.0	5.0	17.0	1.3
Rich Venison & Redcurrant, Grilled, TTD, Sainsbury's*	1 Sausage/46g	138	299	21.2	3.0	22.5	1.8
Roasted Garlic & Oregano, Cauldron Foods*	1 Sausage/50g	90	179	13.1	9.0	10.1	2.1
Scottish Lorne, Somerfield*	1 Sausage/53g	168	317	10.0	19.0	22.0	0.0
Skinless, Tesco*	1 Sausage/27g	68	252	16.0	10.0	18.4	1.2
Sliced, Farmfoods*	1 Sausage/71g	175	247	9.7	12.5	17.6	1.0
Smoked Paprika & Chilli, Cauldron Foods*	1 Sausage/50g	76	152	7.8	11.8	8.2	2.6
Smoked Pork, Original, Mattessons*	1 Serving/113g	362	320	13.0	0.5	30.0	0.9
Smoked Pork, Reduced Fat, Mattessons*	1 Sausage/75g	191	255	14.0	7.0	19.0	0.9
Smoked, Sainsbury's*	1 Serving/250g	700	280	13.0	5.0	25.0	0.1
Smokey Barbeque Chunky Pork, Waitrose*	1 Sausage/174g	459	264	14.1	2.0	22.2	1.3
Smoky Cajun, TTD, Sainsbury's*	1 Sausage/46.4g	115	250	24.2	1.6	16.3	0.9
Snack Size, Tesco*	1 Sausage/10g	23	234	14.8	11.9	14.1	2.0
Spanish, Wafer Thin, Asda*	1 Slice/4g	12	298	25.4	4.1	20.0	0.0
Spicy Pork, Polenta & Sun Dried Tomato, Waitrose*	1 Sausage/67g	165	247	11.8	9.8	17.8	0.9
Spinach, Leek & Cheese, Gourmet, Wicken Fen*	1 Sausage/46g	92	201	10.3	17.0	10.2	1.9
Sun Dried Tomato & Herb, Linda McCartney*	1 Sausage/35g	93	266	21.8	10.1	15.4	1.7
Toulouse, Marks & Spencer*	1 Sausage/57g	123	215	12.4	5.8	15.6	1.3
Tuna & Herb, Sainsbury's*	1 Sausage/47g	109	231	19.6	10.0	12.5	1.5
Tuna & Smoked Salmon, Healthy Living, Tesco*	1 Sausage/67g	90	134	17.9	2.8	5.7	2.0
Tuna, Mediterranean Style, Sainsbury's*	1 Serving/50g	102	204	15.1	14.7	9.5	1.2
Turkey & Chicken, Butcher's Choice, Tesco*	1 Sausage/56.7g	110	193	13.8	8.3	11.6	1.0
Turkey & Pork, Bernard Matthews*	1 Sausage/55g	137	249	10.2	13.1	17.3	0.0
Turkey, Asda*	1 Serving/56g	98	175	14.0	5.0	11.0	0.0
Turkey, Premium, Somerfield*	1 Sausage/57g	76	134	18.0	7.0	4.0	0.0
Turkey, Somerfield*	1 Sausage/114g	186	163	15.0	7.0	9.0	0.0
Tuscan, Marks & Spencer*	1 Sausage/66g	145	220	14.9	4.6	16.0	0.6
Vegetable, Granose*	1oz/28g	63	226	8.5	17.5	13.5	0.0
Vegetarian, Hot Dog, Tesco*	2 Sausages/60g	163	271	19.0	6.0	19.0	2.0
Vegetarian, Linda McCartney*	1 Sausage/35g	88	252	23.2	8.6	13.8	1.2
Vegetarian, Quorn*	1 Sausage/42g	47	111	13.4	5.9	3.8	2.6
Vegetarian, Safeway*	2 Sausages/89g	149	165	17.2	2.0	9.8	8.1
With Onion, Gravy & Potato Crush, BGTY, Sainsbury's*	1 Pack/450g	401	89	5.7	10.4	2.7	1.4
SAUSAGE & BEANS, Sainsbury's*	1 Sm Can/219g	258	118	5.7	13.9	4.4	3.4
SAUSAGE & MASH,							
Asda*	1 Pack/400g	324	81	3.5	11.0	2.6	2.9
British Classic, Tesco*	1 Pack/450g	648	144	4.6	14.3	7.6	1.1

S

	Measure INFO/WEIGHT	per Measure KCAL	Nutrition Values per 100g / 100ml				
			KCAL	PROT	CARB	FAT	FIBRE
SAUSAGE & MASH,							
Eat Smart, Safeway*	1 Pack/400g	340	85	4.6	12.4	1.8	1.3
Healthy Living, Tesco*	1 Pack/450g	369	82	4.6	11.3	2.1	1.0
Iceland*	1 Pack/440g	484	110	3.8	10.4	5.9	1.6
Onion, Marks & Spencer*	1 Pack/300g	315	105	4.1	9.0	5.7	1.5
Quorn, Sainsbury's*	1 Pack/394g	339	86	3.8	11.0	3.0	0.7
Quorn, Tesco*	1 Pack/400g	292	73	4.1	8.8	2.4	1.3
Vegetarian, GFY, Asda*	1 Pack/400g	292	73	4.2	9.0	2.2	2.1
Vegetarian, Safeway*	1 Pack/450g	450	100	5.5	8.9	4.7	1.8
SAUSAGE & MASH,							
Vegetarian, Tesco*	1 Pack/410g	435	106	4.4	10.0	5.4	2.0
With Onion Gravy, Healthy Eating, Tesco*	1 Pack/450g	369	82	4.6	11.3	2.1	1.0
With Onion Gravy, Tesco*	1 Pack/500g	525	105	3.0	11.1	5.4	1.6
SAUSAGE & ONION, Puff Pastry Plait, Sainsbury's*	1/3 Plait/120g	451	376	9.9	18.6	29.1	4.3
SAUSAGE MEAT,							
Marks & Spencer*	1oz/28g	98	350	9.8	11.3	29.9	1.3
Pork, Somerfield*	1oz/28g	95	338	10.0	9.0	29.0	0.0
SAUSAGE ROLL,							
Asda*	1 Roll/64g	248	388	8.0	26.0	28.0	1.0
BGTY, Sainsburys*	1 Roll/65g	200	308	9.6	27.9	17.6	1.4
Basics, Party Size, Somerfield*	1 Roll/13g	45	343	7.0	29.0	22.0	0.0
Buffet, Healthy Eating, Tesco*	1 Roll/30g	83	278	9.6	31.2	12.8	1.5
Co-Op*	1 Roll/66g	244	370	8.0	25.0	27.0	2.0
Cocktail, Sainsbury's*	1 Roll/15g	57	381	8.2	26.4	27.0	1.0
Ginsters*	1 Roll/140g	753	538	13.0	33.7	39.1	2.2
Healthy Eating, Tesco*	1 Roll/70g	195	278	9.6	31.2	12.8	1.5
Kingsize, Pork Farms*	½ Roll/49.9g	242	483	10.5	39.9	31.8	0.0
Large, Sainsbury's*	1 Roll/43g	164	382	7.3	28.1	26.7	1.2
Lincolnshire, COU, Marks & Spencer*	1 Roll/175g	280	160	10.0	23.2	2.7	2.6
Lincolnshire, Geo Adams*	1 Serving/130g	475	365	8.3	28.2	24.3	1.1
Marks & Spencer*	1 Roll/32g	130	405	9.2	21.4	31.2	0.9
Mini, Marks & Spencer*	1oz/28g	122	435	9.8	29.6	30.9	1.8
Mini, Tesco*	1 Roll/15g	53	356	9.0	23.9	24.9	1.5
Party Size, Tesco*	1 Roll/12g	39	327	6.2	26.2	21.9	1.3
Party, Sainsbury's*	1 Roll/12g	54	422	8.7	26.7	31.1	1.2
Pork Farms*	1 Roll/54g	213	395	9.6	21.6	30.0	0.0
Pork, Large, Marks & Spencer*	1 Roll/63g	236	375	9.0	22.5	27.9	0.7
Pork, Morrisons*	1 Roll/70g	195	278	9.6	31.2	12.8	1.5
Puff Pastry, Large, Marks & Spencer*	1 Roll/63g	236	375	9.0	22.5	27.9	0.7
Puff Pastry, Sainsbury's*	1 Roll/65g	250	384	8.3	25.0	27.9	0.9
Snack Size, Safeway*	1 Roll/25g	86	344	8.4	24.1	23.8	0.9
Snack, GFY, Asda*	1 Roll/34g	112	329	9.4	26.5	20.6	0.9
Snack, Sainsbury's*	1 Roll/33g	125	378	7.5	25.5	27.3	1.0
Somerfield*	1 Roll/35g	149	426	9.0	32.0	29.0	0.0
Tesco*	1 Roll/67g	221	330	9.1	23.8	22.0	2.6
Vegetarian, Linda McCartney*	1 Roll/51g	133	260	10.9	23.1	14.5	1.6
Waitrose*	1 Roll/75g	287	383	10.1	27.0	26.1	1.3
SAVELOY, Unbattered, Takeaway	1 Saveloy/65g	192	296	13.8	10.8	22.3	0.8
SAVOURY EGGS,							
Mini, Asda*	1 Egg/19g	58	303	10.3	17.7	21.2	1.5
Mini, New Improved Recipe, Tesco*	1 Egg/20g	65	323	12.5	18.3	22.2	1.3
SCALLOPS,							
King, Marks & Spencer*	1 Serving/100g	70	70	15.0	1.3	0.8	0.0
Lemon Grass & Ginger, Tesco*	½ Pack/112g	90	80	15.2	2.5	1.0	0.6

	Measure INFO/WEIGHT	per Measure KCAL	Nutrition Values per 100g / 100ml				
			KCAL	PROT	CARB	FAT	FIBRE
SCALLOPS,							
Meat, Asda*	1oz/28g	33	118	23.2	1.4	1.4	0.0
Queen, Kintyre*	1 Serving/100g	105	105	23.2	0.1	1.4	0.1
Steamed	1oz/28g	33	118	23.2	3.4	1.4	0.0
Thai Style Breaded With Plum Sauce, Finest, Tesco*	1 Serving/210g	401	191	11.5	20.6	7.0	0.8
SCAMPI,							
& Chips, Tesco*	1 Serving/450g	689	153	5.1	22.4	4.8	1.6
& Chips, Youngs*	1oz/28g	42	150	5.0	20.3	5.4	1.7
Breaded, Asda*	1 Serving/70g	181	258	14.0	19.0	14.0	1.3
Breaded, Farmfoods*	1oz/28g	35	124	8.5	22.1	0.2	1.2
Breaded, Safeway*	1 Pack/340g	755	222	10.4	21.8	10.4	1.6
Breaded, Scottish, Sainsbury's*	1oz/28g	61	219	11.0	17.4	11.7	1.4
Breaded, Wholetail, Tesco*	½ Pack/85g	193	227	9.7	23.6	10.4	1.1
Golden in Ovencrisp Breadcrumbs, Tesco*	1oz/28g	49	175	10.0	16.0	7.9	1.0
Scottish Whole Tail, in Oven Crisp Crumb, Morrisons*	1 Pack/170g	393	231	9.7	24.7	10.4	1.1
Whole, Marks & Spencer*	1oz/28g	64	229	11.1	18.5	12.2	0.8
Whole, Scottish Island, Youngs*	1oz/28g	50	179	9.7	15.8	8.5	0.7
in Breadcrumbs, Frozen, Fried in Blended Oil	1oz/28g	66	237	9.4	20.5	13.6	0.0
in Breadcrumbs, Whole, Marks & Spencer*	1oz/28g	56	199	11.4	15.5	10.2	0.7
SCONE,							
3% Fat, Marks & Spencer*	1 Scone/65g	179	275	7.2	55.1	2.5	2.3
All Butter, Tesco*	1 Scone/41g	126	308	7.2	52.3	7.8	1.6
Blueberry, Starbucks*	1 Serving/128g	460	359	3.9	53.1	14.1	2.3
Cheese	1 Scone/40g	145	363	10.1	43.2	17.8	1.6
Cheese, Finest, Tesco*	1 Scone/70g	250	357	11.3	41.5	16.2	1.2
Cheese, Marks & Spencer*	1 Scone/60g	237	395	10.3	38.9	21.9	1.6
Cherry, Marks & Spencer*	1 Scone/60g	202	337	6.9	49.7	12.2	1.9
Cream, Sainsbury's*	1 Scone/50g	173	345	4.6	42.5	17.4	3.1
Derby, Asda*	1 Scone/59g	202	342	7.0	56.0	10.0	0.0
Derby, Mothers Pride*	1 Scone/60g	208	347	5.2	49.8	14.0	1.5
Derby, Somerfield*	1 Scone/60g	208	347	5.3	49.9	14.0	1.9
Devon, Sainsbury's*	1 Scone/54g	201	372	7.1	51.1	15.5	1.6
Devon, Waitrose*	1 Scone/71.8g	269	373	7.5	56.0	13.2	2.3
Fresh Cream, Tesco*	1 Scone/79.5g	244	304	15.8	32.3	12.5	0.9
Fruit	1 Scone/40g	126	316	7.3	52.9	9.8	0.0
Fruit, Economy, Sainsbury's*	1 Scone/34g	111	326	7.9	52.5	9.4	1.7
Fruit, SmartPrice, Asda*	1 Scone/41g	139	338	7.0	55.0	10.0	3.0
Fruit, Somerfield*	1 Scone/35g	116	332	8.0	53.0	10.0	0.0
Plain	1 Scone/40g	145	362	7.2	53.8	14.6	1.9
Potato	1 Scone/40g	118	296	5.1	39.1	14.3	1.6
Strawberry, Fresh Cream, BGTY, Sainsbury's*	1 Scone/50g	155	309	5.1	47.0	11.2	1.1
Strawberry, Marks & Spencer*	1 Scone/55g	132	240	3.2	23.0	14.9	0.7
Sultana, BGTY, Sainsbury's*	1 Scone/63g	178	283	7.7	56.7	2.8	2.4
Sultana, Finest, Tesco*	1 Scone/70g	225	321	8.9	46.7	10.9	2.1
Sultana, Less Than 5% Fat, Asda*	1 Scone/60g	198	330	7.0	62.0	6.0	1.8
Sultana, Low Fat, Marks & Spencer*	1 Scone/65g	179	275	7.2	55.1	2.5	2.3
Sultana, Marks & Spencer*	1 Scone/60g	235	392	7.0	58.7	13.8	2.8
Sultana, Reduced Fat, Waitrose*	1 Scone/65g	187	287	6.6	53.2	5.3	2.6
Sultana, Somerfield*	1 Scone/34g	108	318	5.7	55.4	8.2	0.0
Sultana, Tesco*	1 Scone/70g	215	307	6.8	53.8	7.2	2.0
Wholemeal	1 Scone/40g	130	326	8.7	43.1	14.4	5.2
Wholemeal, Fruit	1 Scone/40g	130	324	8.1	47.2	12.8	4.9
SCONE MIX, Fruit, Asda	1 Scone/47.5g	144	301	7.0	57.0	5.0	3.7

S

	Measure INFO/WEIGHT	per Measure KCAL	Nutrition Values per 100g / 100ml				
			KCAL	PROT	CARB	FAT	FIBRE
SCOTCH EGGS,							
Asda*	1 Egg/114g	286	251	11.2	13.7	16.8	1.4
Bar, Ginsters*	1 Bar/90g	256	284	11.8	20.1	17.4	1.7
Ginsters*	1 Egg/95g	228	240	15.3	9.7	15.9	0.6
Marks & Spencer*	1 Egg/125g	344	275	11.7	15.0	18.7	0.5
Mini, Sainsbury's*	1 Egg/12.2g	39	329	10.9	18.9	23.3	1.0
Retail	1 Egg/120g	301	251	12.0	13.1	17.1	0.0
Sainsbury's*	1 Egg/116g	287	247	11.4	13.2	16.5	0.6
Tesco*	1 Egg/114g	309	271	11.5	17.0	17.4	0.9
SEAFOOD COCKTAIL,							
Asda*	1oz/28g	26	92	14.0	5.7	1.5	0.1
Average	1oz/28g	24	87	15.6	2.9	1.5	0.0
Somerfield*	1oz/28g	23	81	14.0	2.0	2.0	0.0
SEAFOOD COLLECTION, Premium, Frozen, Tesco*	1 Serving/100g	70	70	12.2	2.4	1.3	0.0
SEAFOOD MEDLEY, Steam Cuisine, Marks & Spencer*	1 Pack/400g	320	80	8.5	4.5	3.1	1.3
SEAFOOD SELECTION,							
Healthy Eating, Tesco*	1 Pack/250g	175	70	12.2	2.4	1.3	0.0
Luxury, Safeway*	1 Pack/250g	215	86	13.8	3.1	2.0	0.0
Sainsbury's*	½ Pack/125g	125	100	18.6	2.2	1.9	0.1
SEAFOOD STICKS,							
Healthy Choice, Asda*	1 Stick/12g	14	113	7.0	21.0	0.1	0.1
Morrisons*	1 Stick/15g	16	108	7.0	19.8	0.1	0.0
Sainsbury's*	1 Stick/16g	17	107	7.0	21.0	0.1	0.1
Somerfield*	1 Stick/15.0g	17	113	8.6	18.8	0.4	0.0
Tesco*	1 Stick/16g	15	96	5.7	15.9	1.1	0.0
Value, Tesco*	1 Stick/15.6g	18	113	7.2	20.2	0.4	0.6
With Cocktail Dip, Asda*	1 Pot/95g	126	133	6.0	16.0	5.0	0.1
With Garlic & Lemon Dip, Asda*	1 Pot/97.9g	184	188	7.0	13.0	12.0	0.0
SEASONING, Aromat, Knorr*	1oz/28g	46	164	12.4	20.5	3.6	1.0
SEASONING CUBES,							
For Rice, Pilau, Knorr*	1 Cube/10g	31	305	11.4	13.9	22.6	1.4
For Rice, Saffron, Knorr*	1 Cube/10g	29	291	13.8	17.5	18.4	2.2
For Stir Fry, Oriental Spices, Knorr*	1 Cube/10g	41	414	9.7	25.0	30.6	1.1
Oriental Spice, Knorr*	1 Cube/10g	41	409	9.5	23.7	30.7	0.0
Perfect Pasta, Knorr*	1 Cube/10g	28	278	10.3	5.2	24.0	0.0
Wild Mushroom, Knorr*	1 Cube/10g	37	365	10.3	21.3	26.5	0.2
SEASONING MIX,							
Beef Taco, Colman's*	1 Pack/30g	76	252	9.1	26.9	12.0	14.0
Fajita, Chicken, Colmans*	1 Pack/40g	149	373	10.8	13.3	30.7	13.8
Fajita, Old El Paso*	1oz/28g	88	313	11.0	56.0	5.0	0.0
Garlic & Herb Potato Wedge, Schwartz*	½ Serving/337g	546	162	3.4	26.4	4.7	0.0
Mediterranean Roast Vegetable, Schwartz*	1oz/28g	92	330	7.0	65.6	4.4	0.0
Shepherd's Pie, Colman's*	1 Pack/50g	129	257	14.0	47.0	0.9	0.0
Shepherd's Pie, Schwartz*	1 Pack/38g	110	289	9.3	58.5	2.0	0.0
Taco, Old El Paso*	¼ Pack/9g	30	334	5.5	69.0	4.0	0.0
Wholegrain Mustard & Herb Potato Mash, Colman's*	1 Pack/30g	153	510	9.7	19.1	44.1	0.0
SEAWEED,							
Crispy, Blue Dragon*	1 packet/55g	345	628	6.2	19.2	58.0	8.9
Crispy, Budgens*	1 Serving/50g	304	608	7.0	14.2	58.1	6.4
Crispy, Marks & Spencer*	1oz/28g	168	600	6.5	16.8	56.1	6.3
Crispy, Sainsbury's*	½ Pack/35g	253	724	10.5	19.1	67.3	5.1
Irish Moss, Raw	1oz/28g	2	8	1.5	0.0	0.2	12.3
Kombu, Dried, Raw	1oz/28g	12	43	7.1	0.0	1.6	58.7
Nori, Dried, Raw	1oz/28g	38	136	30.7	0.0	1.5	44.4

S

	Measure INFO/WEIGHT	per Measure KCAL	Nutrition Values per 100g / 100ml				
			KCAL	PROT	CARB	FAT	FIBRE
SEAWEED,							
Wakame, Dried, Raw	1oz/28g	20	71	12.4	0.0	2.4	47.1
SEMOLINA,							
Co-Op*	1oz/28g	97	345	11.7	70.5	1.8	2.1
Flemings*	1oz/28g	98	350	10.7	77.5	1.8	2.1
Raw	1oz/28g	98	350	10.7	77.5	1.8	2.1
SEMOLINA PUDDING,							
Creamed, Ambrosia*	1 Can/425g	344	81	3.3	13.1	1.7	0.2
Creamed, Co-Op*	1 Can/425g	383	90	4.0	15.0	2.0	0.0
SESAME SEEDS,							
Average	1oz/28g	167	598	18.2	0.9	58.0	7.9
Organic, Evernat*	1oz/28g	174	623	26.4	6.4	54.8	7.6
SHALLOTS, Raw	1oz/28g	6	20	1.5	3.3	0.2	1.4
SHANDY,							
Bitter, Original, Ben Shaws*	1 Can/330ml	89	27	0.0	6.0	0.0	0.0
Homemade	1 Pint/568ml	148	26	0.2	2.9	0.0	0.0
Lemonade, Traditional Style, Tesco*	1 Can/330ml	63	19	0.0	4.7	0.0	0.0
SHARK, Raw	1oz/28g	29	102	23.0	0.0	1.1	0.0
SHARON FRUIT, Average	1oz/28g	20	73	0.8	18.6	0.0	1.6
SHERBET LEMONS, Marks & Spencer*	1oz/28g	107	382	0.0	93.9	0.0	0.0
SHERRY,							
Dry	1 Serving/50ml	58	116	0.2	1.4	0.0	0.0
Medium	1 Serving/50ml	58	116	0.1	5.9	0.0	0.0
Sweet	1 Serving/50ml	68	136	0.3	6.9	0.0	0.0
SHORTBREAD,							
All Butter Thins, Marks & Spencer*	1 Biscuit/10.3g	49	485	5.8	68.4	21.1	3.5
All Butter, Deans*	1 Biscuits/15g	77	511	4.9	65.7	25.4	1.2
All Butter, McVitie's*	Twin Finger/40g	216	541	6.3	62.6	29.5	1.9
All Butter, Royal Edinburgh, Asda*	1 Finger/18g	93	519	5.8	60.3	28.3	1.8
Average	1oz/28g	139	498	5.9	63.9	26.1	1.9
Chocolate & Caramel, TTD, Sainsbury's*	1 Serving/55g	245	446	4.7	45.0	27.7	1.3
Chocolate Chip, Jacob's*	1 Biscuit/17g	87	513	5.2	61.2	27.5	1.8
Clotted Cream, Finest, Tesco*	1 Biscuit/20g	109	543	5.2	58.0	32.2	1.7
Crawfords*	1 Biscuit/12.5g	64	533	6.6	65.0	27.4	2.0
Farmhouse, TTD, Sainsbury's*	1 Finger/20g	106	528	5.1	61.6	29.0	1.7
Fingers, All Butter, Royal Edinburgh Bakery*	1 Biscuit/17g	88	519	5.8	60.3	28.3	1.8
Fingers, All Butter, Tesco*	1 Finger/13g	67	519	5.8	60.3	28.3	1.8
Fingers, Asda*	1 Finger/18g	93	519	5.8	60.3	28.3	18.0
Fingers, Highland, Sainsbury's*	1 Finger/20g	106	528	5.6	57.8	30.5	1.9
Fingers, Safeway*	1 Finger/21g	109	520	5.8	58.5	29.2	18.9
Highland Demerara Rounds, Sainsbury's*	1 Biscuit/20g	113	565	5.5	70.5	29.0	2.0
Petticoat Tails, Sainsbury's*	1 Segment/13g	68	520	5.4	60.5	28.5	1.8
Pure Butter, Jacob's*	1 Biscuit/20g	105	525	5.7	58.6	29.7	1.8
Rounds, Safeway*	1 Biscuit/19.9g	108	538	5.9	59.2	31.1	1.6
Rounds, TTD, Sainsbury's*	1 Biscuit/20g	108	538	5.0	59.5	31.1	1.6
St. Clements Farmhouse Style, TTD, Sainsbury's*	1 Biscuit/20.2g	105	526	4.8	58.4	30.3	2.0
SHOTS, Cadbury's*	1 Pack/160g	752	470	5.9	59.7	23.2	0.0
SHRIMPS,							
Boiled	1oz/28g	33	117	23.8	0.0	2.4	0.0
Canned in Brine, Drained	1oz/28g	26	94	20.8	0.0	1.2	0.0
Dried	1oz/28g	69	245	55.8	0.0	2.4	0.0
Frozen	1oz/28g	20	73	16.5	0.0	0.8	0.0
SKATE,							
Grilled	1oz/28g	22	79	18.9	0.0	0.5	0.0

S

INFO/WEIGHT	Measure	per Measure KCAL	Nutrition Values per 100g / 100ml				
			KCAL	PROT	CARB	FAT	FIBRE
SKATE,							
Raw	1oz/28g	18	64	15.1	0.0	0.4	0.0
In Batter, Fried in Blended Oil	1oz/28g	47	168	14.7	4.9	10.1	0.2
SKIPS,							
Bacon, KP*	1 Pack/17.1g	81	474	6.5	62.1	22.2	2.3
Buzzboltz Bacon Flavour, KP*	1 Bag/17g	81	474	6.5	62.1	22.2	2.3
Easy Cheesy, KP*	1 Bag/19g	100	525	3.9	59.5	30.1	0.9
Pickled Onion, KP*	1 Pack/13.1g	67	512	3.4	56.4	30.3	1.4
Prawn Cocktail, KP*	1 Bag/17g	88	516	3.4	59.9	29.2	1.4
Tangy Tomato, KP*	1 Bag/17g	88	517	3.2	59.6	29.5	1.2
SKITTLES,							
Fruits, Mars*	1 Pack/18g	72	399	0.0	90.4	4.2	0.0
Mars*	1 Pack/55g	220	400	0.0	90.5	4.2	0.0
SLICES,							
Bacon & Cheese, Savoury, Somerfield*	1 Slice/165.0g	490	297	7.4	21.2	20.3	1.5
Beef, Minced Steak & Onion, Tesco*	1 Slice/150g	425	283	8.7	21.3	18.1	1.6
Beef, Minced With Onion, Sainsbury's*	1 Slice/120g	328	273	6.8	24.5	16.4	1.1
Beef, Pepper Steak, Ginsters*	1 Slice/155g	415	268	9.9	21.5	15.8	1.9
Cheese & Garlic, Safeway*	1 Slice/31g	123	398	11.4	44.1	19.5	2.2
Cheese & Ham, Sainsbury's*	1 Slice/112g	313	280	6.6	25.3	16.9	1.5
Cheese & Ham, Savoury, Somerfield*	1 Slice/150g	399	266	7.0	23.0	16.0	0.0
Cheese & Onion, Tesco*	1 Slice/150g	503	335	8.0	20.1	24.7	1.4
Chicken & Mushroom, Asda*	1 Slice/165g	474	287	8.0	21.0	19.0	1.2
Chicken & Mushroom, Ginsters*	1 Slice/155g	420	271	6.6	21.8	17.5	1.7
Chicken & Mushroom, Tesco*	1 Slice/165g	457	277	9.2	20.6	17.5	0.9
Ham & Cheese, Ginsters*	1 Slice/155g	625	403	9.8	31.9	28.2	4.2
Ham & Cheese, Sainsbury's*	1 Slice/118g	352	298	7.8	22.5	19.7	1.8
Spicy Chicken, Deep Fill, Ginsters*	1 Slice/180g	499	277	9.2	21.8	17.0	1.4
SLIMFAST,							
Banana Deluxe Meal Replacement Drink, SlimFast*	1 Serving/325ml	215	66	4.2	11.3	0.8	1.4
Bars, Caramel, Snack, SlimFast*	1 Bar/26g	94	360	3.1	66.3	11.2	0.0
Bars, Chocolate Caramel, SlimFast*	1 Bar/26g	99	382	3.0	72.0	12.0	1.2
Bars, Chocolate Chip, SlimFast*	1 Bar/26g	98	378	4.9	70.4	11.4	1.8
Bars, Chocolate Meal Replacement, SlimFast*	1 Bar/39g	122	314	19.9	46.2	9.4	5.5
Bars, Chocolate Muesli, SlimFast*	1 Bar/26g	97	373	4.6	53.8	14.2	6.5
Bars, Chocolate Peanut, SlimFast*	1 Bar/26g	97	373	5.4	63.1	12.7	1.2
Bars, Chocolate, SlimFast*	1 Bar/39g	107	274	20.6	35.3	9.0	5.5
Bars, Toffee, SlimFast*	1 Bar/39g	122	314	19.7	47.1	8.5	5.6
Chocolate Chip Snack Bar, SlimFast*	1 Bar/26g	99	382	4.9	70.4	11.4	1.8
Chocolate Muesli Snack Bar, SlimFast*	1 Bar/26g	99	379	4.7	64.5	13.3	6.5
Chocolate Royale, Ready To Drink, Ultra SlimFast*	1 Serving/11floz	220	71	3.2	12.8	0.9	1.6
Chocolate Shake, Dry Weight, SlimFast*	1 Serving/35g	123	351	13.6	54.3	9.3	17.1
Coffee Mocha, Ready to Drink, SlimFast*	1 Shake/325ml	215	66	4.2	10.6	0.8	1.5
French Vanilla, Ready To Drink, SlimFast*	1 Can/325ml	215	66	4.2	10.6	0.8	1.5
Pasta Carbonara With Cheese & Bacon, SlimFast*	1 Serving/70g	240	343	22.7	48.9	6.3	5.7
Pasta Florentina With Broccoli & Spinach, SlimFast*	1 Serving/71g	239	336	23.0	50.5	4.6	5.8
Pasta Pomodoro With Tomato & Herbs, SlimFast*	1 Serving/71g	235	331	21.5	51.5	4.3	6.0
Peach Shake, SlimFast*	1 Can/325ml	215	66	4.2	10.6	0.8	1.5
Soup, Chicken With Sweetcorn & Croutons, SlimFast*	1 Pack/60g	211	351	23.7	36.8	10.6	9.7
Soup, Mediterranean Tomato, SlimFast*	1 Sachet/62g	213	343	22.6	39.8	9.0	10.7
Soup, Wild Mushroom, Slim Fast*	1 Pack/60g	209	349	23.3	37.5	10.2	10.4
Strawberry Supreme, Ready To Drink, SlimFast*	1 Can/325ml	215	66	4.2	10.6	0.8	1.5
Toffee Delight Meal Replacement Bar, SlimFast*	1 Bar/78g	248	318	20.6	45.3	9.6	5.9
Vanilla Shake, Ready to Drink, SlimFast*	1 Can/325ml	215	66	4.2	10.6	0.8	1.5

S

	Measure INFO/WEIGHT	per Measure KCAL	Nutrition Values per 100g / 100ml				
			KCAL	PROT	CARB	FAT	FIBRE
SMARTIES,							
Biscuits, Nestle*	1 Biscuit/5g	26	519	7.7	57.6	28.6	0.0
Giants, Nestle*	1 Pack/186g	882	474	4.6	70.4	19.3	0.7
Mini Cones, Nestle*	1 Serving/44g	145	330	4.5	45.0	13.1	0.0
Mini Eggs, Nestle*	1 Lge Pack/112g	533	476	4.7	69.4	19.9	0.7
Minis, Nestle*	1 Serving/14.8g	69	458	4.1	73.5	16.4	0.6
Nestle*	1oz/28g	129	459	5.4	71.1	17.0	0.0
SMASH, With Smoked Bacon, Smash*	1 Serving/169g	137	81	1.7	13.6	2.2	0.6
SMOOTHIE,							
Apple, Grapes & Blackcurrant, P & J*	1 Bottle/250ml	125	50	0.8	11.1	0.3	0.7
Apple, Raspberries & Banana, P & J*	1 Bottle/330ml	188	57	0.7	12.2	0.3	0.0
Apricot & Peach, COU, Marks & Spencer*	1 Serving/250ml	100	40	0.9	8.3	0.4	0.4
Banana, Marks & Spencer*	1 Bottle/500ml	270	54	1.7	12.2	0.1	0.8
Banana, Measure Up, Dry, Asda*	1 Serving/61g	203	333	17.0	55.0	5.0	14.0
Blackberry & Blueberry, Innocent*	1 Bottle/250ml	120	48	0.6	11.5	0.1	0.0
Boysenberry & Raspberry, Fruit, Sainsbury's*	1 Bottle/250ml	108	43	0.7	10.0	0.1	1.6
Cranberries & Rasperries, Pure Fruit, Innocent*	1 Serving/250ml	103	41	0.5	9.5	0.2	0.0
Cranberries & Strawberries, Innocent*	1 Serving/250ml	103	41	0.5	9.5	0.2	0.0
Daily Detox, P & J*	1 Bottle/250ml	143	57	0.8	13.1	0.2	0.0
Ginseng & Ace Vitamins, Marks & Spencer*	1 Bottle/250ml	138	55	0.7	13.0	0.2	0.9
It's Alive, P & J*	1 Bottle/250ml	150	60	0.7	13.6	0.3	0.0
Mango & Passion Fruit, Innocent*	1 Bottle/250ml	138	55	0.4	12.8	0.2	0.0
Mango & West Indian Cherry, Plus, Tesco*	1 Serving/250ml	133	53	0.6	12.2	0.2	0.5
Mango, Pineapple & Passion Fruit, Eat Smart, Safeway*	1 Bottle/250ml	135	54	0.5	12.6	0.0	1.1
Mango, Pineapple & Passionfruit, Marks & Spencer*	1 Bottle/500ml	290	58	0.7	12.1	0.5	0.9
Orange & Mango, Safeway*	1 Bottle/250ml	130	52	0.5	12.1	0.2	0.7
Orange, Mango & Apricot, COU, Marks & Spencer*	1 Bottle/250ml	130	52	0.6	11.0	0.6	0.6
Orange, Strawberry & Guava, Sainsbury's*	1 Serving/300ml	159	53	0.3	12.0	0.2	0.8
Oranges & Mangos, Get Your Vits, P & J*	1 Bottle/250ml	128	51	0.6	11.6	0.2	0.0
Oranges Mangos & Bananas, P & J*	1 Bottle/330ml	195	59	0.9	13.6	0.2	0.7
Peach, Mild & Fruity, Campina*	1 Bottle/330ml	211	64	2.7	13.1	0.0	0.0
Peaches & Bananas, P & J*	1 Bottle/330ml	188	57	0.7	13.6	0.3	0.0
Pineapple, Banana & Coconut, P & J*	1 Bottle/330ml	234	71	0.8	12.3	1.4	0.0
Pineapple, Banana & Mango Fruit, Finest, Tesco*	1 Glass/200ml	94	47	0.1	11.2	0.2	0.0
Pineapple, Banana & Pear, Asda*	1 Bottle/250ml	147	59	0.5	13.6	0.1	0.3
Pineapple, Banana & Pear, Princes*	1 Bottle/250ml	153	61	0.5	13.9	0.2	0.5
Pineapple, Mango & Lime, Way To Five, Sainsbury's*	1 Bottle/250g	120	48	0.4	11.3	0.1	0.3
Pineapple, Mango & Passionfruit, 100% Fruit, Sainsbury's*	1 Bottle/250ml	163	65	0.7	15.2	0.1	1.0
Pineapple, Strawberries & Passion Fruit, P & J*	1 Bottle/330ml	152	46	0.6	10.8	0.1	1.3
Raspberry & Blueberry, Plus, Tesco*	1 Serving/100ml	59	59	2.6	11.6	0.3	0.5
Raspberry, Banana & Peach, Sainsbury's*	1 Bottle/250.9ml	138	55	0.8	12.8	0.1	1.5
Raspberry, Marks & Spencer*	1 Serving/250ml	138	55	1.7	12.2	0.6	1.9
Strawberries & Bananas, Innocent*	1 Bottle/250ml	118	47	0.4	10.7	0.2	0.0
Strawberries & Bananas, P & J*	1 Bottle/330ml	172	52	0.9	11.5	0.3	0.0
Strawberry & Banana Fruit, Finest, Tesco*	1 Bottle/250ml	135	54	0.3	12.5	0.3	0.5
Strawberry & Cherry, Organic, Marks & Spencer*	1 Bottle/250ml	138	55	0.8	12.3	0.3	0.4
Strawberry & Raspberry, Shapers, Boots*	1 Bottle/250ml	110	44	0.6	10.0	0.2	0.6
Strawberry & Raspberry, The Best Safeway*	1fl oz/30ml	15	49	0.6	10.2	0.2	0.6
Strawberry & White Chocolate, Marks & Spencer*	1 Serving/250ml	100	40	2.5	5.5	1.0	0.1
Strawberry Dairy, Shapers, Boots*	1 Bottle/250ml	120	48	1.7	9.7	0.3	0.5
Strawberry, Raspberry, Bio Yoghurt, Eat Smart, Safeway*	1 Bottle/250ml	163	65	2.0	12.5	0.6	0.6
Strawberry, Wild Orchard*	1 Bottle/250ml	120	48	0.6	11.8	0.0	1.4
Vanilla & Honey, Sainsbury's*	1 Bottle/250ml	238	95	3.2	14.8	2.4	0.3
Vanilla Bean, Marks & Spencer*	1 Bottle/500ml	450	90	3.3	13.9	2.6	0.0

S

Measure INFO/WEIGHT	per Measure KCAL	Nutrition Values per 100g / 100ml				
		KCAL	PROT	CARB	FAT	FIBRE
SNACK SALAD,						
Cheese Layered, Sainsbury's*	1 Pack/190g	397	209	5.4	12.4	15.3	0.0
Chicken & Bacon, Tesco*	1 Pack/300g	501	167	7.2	10.9	10.5	3.2
Chicken Noodle, Sainsburys*	1 Snack/240g	278	116	5.2	12.4	5.1	1.4
Chicken, Sun Dried Tomato & Basil, HL, Tesco*	1 Pack/300g	429	143	10.6	21.0	1.8	1.0
Greek Style, BGTY, Sainsbury's*	1 Pack/198.5g	133	67	2.0	9.0	2.5	0.8
Ham & Mushroom, Tesco*	1 Pot/300g	600	200	4.7	21.2	10.7	1.4
Hoi Sin Chicken & Noodle, TTD, Sainsburys*	1 Pack/230g	214	93	4.7	15.2	1.5	1.8
Honey & Mustard Chicken, Tesco*	1 Pot/300g	585	195	8.4	20.4	8.9	1.1
Pasta & Tuna, BGTY, Sainsbury's*	1 Pack/260g	218	84	6.0	11.5	1.6	2.3
Pasta & Tuna, Healthy Living, Co-Op.*	1 Tub/225g	146	65	5.0	10.0	0.4	1.0
Pasta & Tuna, Healthy Selection, Somerfield*	1 pot/190g	194	102	6.5	13.0	2.7	1.1
Pasta, Cheese, Somerfield*	1 Salad/200g	422	211	8.0	14.0	14.0	0.0
Pasta, Egg Mayo, Asda*	1 Serving/180g	364	202	4.0	12.8	15.0	0.3
Pasta, Tuna, Asda*	1 Serving/180g	196	109	5.5	13.2	3.8	0.9
Pasta, Tuna, Sainsbury's*	1 Pot/260g	218	84	6.0	11.5	1.6	2.3
Salmon & Dill, Tesco*	1 Pack/300g	600	200	7.7	13.4	12.8	0.8
Tuna, Tesco*	1 Pack/300g	252	84	7.6	11.5	0.9	0.9
SNACK STOP,						
Chicken & Mushroom Flavour Pasta, Crosse & Blackwell*	1 Pot/60g	251	418	10.3	74.3	8.8	0.0
Creamy Cheese Pasta, Crosse & Blackwell*	1 Pot/218.3g	251	115	3.0	19.2	2.9	0.0
Creamy Chicken Pasta, Crosse & Blackwell*	1 Pot/247g	210	85	2.7	15.7	1.6	0.0
Macaroni Cheese, Light, Crosse & Blackwell*	1 Pack/248g	260	105	3.2	16.4	3.0	0.9
Melting Cheese & Pepperoni, Crosse & Blackwell*	1 Pack/237g	237	100	2.9	13.3	4.1	0.0
Mushroom Pasta Twirls, Crosse & Blackwell*	1 Pot/248g	248	100	3.1	15.9	2.7	0.9
Roast Onion & Potato, Crosse and Blackwell*	1 Pot/210g	210	100	1.7	14.4	3.7	0.0
Roast Parsnip & Potato, Crosse & Blackwell*	1 Pot/210g	200	95	1.7	13.6	3.6	0.0
Spicy Tomato Pasta, Crosse & Blackwell*	1 Pot/412g	358	87	2.4	15.9	1.5	0.0
Sun Ripened Tomato & Herb, Crosse & Blackwell*	1 Pot/ 237g	201	85	2.6	16.1	1.1	0.0
SNACK-A-JACKS,						
Apple & Cinnamon Flavour, Quaker*	1 Jumbo/10g	38	376	6.2	83.1	2.2	3.9
Apple Danish Flavour, Quaker*	1 Jumbo/13g	51	390	5.0	87.0	2.5	1.0
Barbecue Flavour, Jumbo, Quaker*	1 Serving/10g	38	376	7.0	80.0	2.5	1.0
Barbecue Flavour, Quaker*	1 Pack/30g	126	421	6.5	77.0	10.0	1.0
Barbecue, Invidual Bag, Quaker*	1 Bag/30g	122	407	7.0	79.0	6.5	1.0
Caramel Flavour, Jumbo, Quaker*	1 Cake/13g	52	397	5.0	87.0	2.5	1.0
Caramel, Quaker*	1 Bag/35g	140	401	5.5	86.0	3.5	0.5
Cheddar Cheese Flavour, Jumbo, Quaker*	1 Cake/10g	40	399	8.5	81.0	4.0	1.0
Cheddar Cheese Flavour, Quaker*	1 Bag/30g	128	427	8.0	73.0	10.0	1.0
Chocolate Flavour, Quaker*	1 Cake/14g	57	406	5.5	85.0	4.5	1.0
Chocolate, Jumbo, Quaker*	1 Cake/12g	49	406	5.5	85.0	4.5	1.0
Chocolate, Quaker*	1 Bag/35g	144	410	5.0	85.0	4.5	1.0
Creamy Lemon Flavour, Quaker*	1 Pack/35g	137	390	5.0	87.0	2.5	1.0
Crispy Cheese, Quaker*	1 Pack/30g	122	407	8.0	78.0	6.5	1.0
Crispy Chocolate Flavour, Snack-A-Jacks, Quaker*	1 Pack/30g	122	407	5.5	85.0	4.5	1.0
Salt & Vinegar, Quaker*	1 Bag/30g	123	410	6.5	77.5	8.0	1.0
Savoury Salted, Quaker*	1 Bag/30g	124	414	7.5	77.0	8.0	1.0
Sour Cream & Chive, Quakers*	1 Pack/30g	123	410	7.5	77.0	8.0	1.0
Spudz, Oriental Barbecue, Quaker*	1 Bag/20g	79	395	6.0	73.0	8.5	1.5
Spudz, Smoked Bacon & Cheese, Quaker*	1 Bag/20g	80	398	7.5	76.5	10.0	1.5
Spudz, Sour Cream & Sweet Chilli, Quaker*	¼ Pack/30g	118	394	6.5	75.0	7.5	2.0
SNAPPER,						
Red, Fried in Blended Oil	1oz/28g	35	126	24.5	0.0	3.1	0.0
Red, Raw	1oz/28g	25	90	19.6	0.0	1.3	0.0

S

	Measure INFO/WEIGHT	per Measure KCAL	Nutrition Values per 100g / 100ml				
			KCAL	PROT	CARB	FAT	FIBRE
SNICKERS,							
Cruncher, Mars*	1 Bar/40g	209	523	9.0	57.0	30.0	2.3
Mars*	1 Standard/61g	311	510	10.2	55.3	27.6	0.0
SNOW FLAKE, Cadbury's*	1 Bar/36g	198	550	7.2	60.1	30.9	0.0
SODA, Orange & Strawberry, Freekee, Britvic*	1 Bottle/330ml	20	6	0.0	1.0	0.0	0.0
SOFTMINTS, Trebor*	1 Tube/40g	156	391	0.0	93.3	2.0	0.0
SOLERO, Exotic, Wall's*	1 Solero/95ml	115	121	1.6	20.6	3.3	0.4
SORBET,							
A Really Lemon, The Real Ice Cream Company*	1 Serving/100g	117	117	0.1	29.1	0.1	0.4
Blackcurrant, Del Monte*	1oz/28g	30	106	0.4	27.1	0.1	0.0
Blackcurrant, Iceland*	¼ Pot/100g	100	100	0.0	25.0	0.0	0.0
Kiwi & Papaya, World Fruit, Del Monte*	1 Lolly/90ml	61	68	0.2	16.2	0.3	0.0
Lemon	1 Scoop/60g	79	131	0.9	34.2	0.0	0.0
Lemon Harmony, Haagen-Dazs*	1 Serving/90ml	214	238	1.5	32.5	11.3	0.0
Lemon, Del Monte*	1 Sorbet/500g	570	114	0.1	29.2	0.1	0.0
Lemon, Tesco*	1 Serving/75g	80	106	0.0	26.2	0.0	0.4
Mango, Del Monte*	1 Sorbet/500g	575	115	0.2	29.6	0.1	0.0
Mango, Sainsbury's*	¼ Pot/88.9g	104	117	0.2	28.9	0.1	0.7
Mango, Tropicale, Haagen-Dazs*	1oz/28g	32	116	0.2	28.6	0.1	0.0
Mango, Waitrose*	1 Pot/100g	90	90	0.1	22.1	0.0	0.6
Orange, Del Monte*	1 Sorbet/500g	625	125	0.2	32.1	0.1	0.0
Passion Fruit, Fat Free, Marks & Spencer*	1 Sorbet/125g	129	103	0.4	25.0	0.0	0.4
Peach & Strawberry, Haagen-Dazs*	1oz/28g	30	108	0.0	27.0	0.0	0.0
Peach & Vanilla Fruit Swirl, Healthy Living, Tesco*	1 Pot/73g	93	127	1.1	28.9	0.8	0.5
Pear, Organic, Evernat*	1oz/28g	33	119	0.0	28.3	0.6	0.0
Pineapple, Del Monte*	1 Sorbet/500g	600	120	0.3	30.6	0.1	0.0
Raspberry & Blackberry, Fat Free, Marks & Spencer*	1 Sorbet/125g	140	112	0.4	27.5	0.0	0.6
Raspberry, Häagen-Dazs*	½ Cup/105g	120	114	0.0	28.6	0.0	1.9
Raspberry, Select, Safeway*	½ Cup/105g	100	95	0.0	27.6	0.0	1.0
Raspberry, Sticks, Haagen-Dazs*	1oz/28g	28	99	0.2	24.2	0.1	0.0
Raspberry, Tesco*	1 Serving/70ml	97	138	0.5	34.0	0.0	0.0
Strawberry & Champagne, Sainsbury's*	¼ Pot/89g	95	107	0.2	25.5	0.0	0.6
Strawberry, Fruit Ice, Starburst, Mars*	1 Stick/93ml	99	106	0.1	26.7	0.1	0.0
Strawberry, Marks & Spencer*	1oz/28g	27	95	0.3	23.4	0.1	0.5
Summer Berry, Swirl, Asda*	¼ Pack/89g	97	109	3.0	26.0	0.4	0.0
Swirl, Raspberry & Blackcurrant, Safeway*	1 Serving/50g	58	115	0.6	27.0	0.0	1.6
Tropical, Really Fruity, Asda*	1 Scoop/75g	90	120	0.1	30.0	0.0	0.3
Zesty Lemon, Haagen-Dazs*	1 Serving/125ml	120	96	0.0	24.8	0.0	1.0
SORBET CONE,							
Raspberry, Yoghurt & Sorbet, BGTY, Sainsbury's*	1 Cone/69g	151	219	2.6	37.5	6.5	1.3
Sorbet, Sainsbury's*	1 Serving/70g	153	219	2.6	37.5	6.5	1.3
SOSMIX,							
Direct Foods*	1oz/28g	124	443	18.5	27.0	29.0	0.0
Organic*	1oz/28g	122	435	20.0	37.0	23.0	0.0
SOUFFLE,							
Cheese	1oz/28g	71	253	11.4	9.3	19.2	0.3
Lemon, Finest, Tesco*	1 Pot/80g	270	338	2.9	24.1	25.6	0.2
Plain	1oz/28g	56	201	7.6	10.4	14.7	0.3
Raspberry & Amaretto, Marks & Spencer*	1oz/28g	83	298	2.8	33.1	16.7	0.1
Strawberry, Marks & Spencer*	1 Serving/95g	171	180	1.6	19.5	10.6	0.9
SOUP,							
Asparagus & Chicken, Waitrose*	1 Can/415g	166	40	2.1	5.3	1.1	0.7
Asparagus With Croutons, In a Cup, Sainsbury's*	1 Serving/200ml	103	52	1.0	6.4	2.5	1.7
Asparagus, Batchelors*	1 Serving/223g	143	64	0.5	9.2	2.8	0.4

SOUP,

INFO/WEIGHT	Measure	per Measure KCAL	KCAL	PROT	CARB	FAT	FIBRE
Asparagus, Fresh, New Covent Garden Soup Co*	1 Carton/600g	324	54	2.1	1.8	4.3	0.9
Asparagus, Knorr*	1 Serving/300ml	114	38	0.7	4.8	1.7	0.1
Asparagus, Less Than 60 Cals, Waitrose*	1 Serving/204ml	51	25	0.4	4.3	0.7	0.7
Asparagus, Marks & Spencer*	1 Serving/300g	180	60	1.1	3.3	4.5	0.7
Asparagus, New Covent Garden Soup Co*	½ Carton/300g	162	54	2.1	1.8	4.3	0.9
Aubergine & Red Pepper, New Covent Garden Soup Co*	½ Pint/296ml	71	24	0.9	4.8	0.1	0.4
Autumn Vegetable, Baxters*	1 Can/425g	170	40	1.8	8.0	0.2	1.5
Autumn Vegetable, Vie Country, Knorr*	1 Pack/500ml	190	38	0.7	4.3	2.0	0.7
Bean, Italian Style, Tesco*	1 Can/300g	153	51	2.8	7.3	1.2	1.1
Beef & Tomato Cup a Soup, Batchelors*	1 Serving/215g	71	33	0.6	7.3	0.2	0.5
Beef & Vegetable Big, Heinz*	½ Can/200g	90	45	2.4	7.3	0.7	0.9
Beef & Vegetable Mighty, Asda*	½ Can/81g	32	40	2.3	6.0	0.8	0.6
Beef & Vegetable, Tesco*	1 Serving/410g	312	76	2.0	5.3	4.8	0.6
Beef Broth Big, Heinz*	½ Can/200g	82	41	2.0	6.8	0.6	0.7
Beef Chilli Baked Potato Big, Heinz*	1 Can/400g	232	58	3.4	9.1	0.9	1.3
Beef Consomme, Sainsbury's*	1 Can/415g	46	11	2.0	0.7	0.0	0.0
Beef, Big, Heinz*	1 Can/400g	180	45	2.4	7.2	0.7	0.9
Beetroot & Rosemary, New Covent Garden Soup Co*	1 Pack/600g	138	23	1.3	4.0	0.2	1.2
Blended Autumn Vegetable, Heinz*	½ Can/200g	114	57	1.2	6.4	3.0	0.7
Blended Carrot & Coriander, Heinz*	½ Can/200g	104	52	0.7	6.2	2.7	0.6
Blended Leek & Bacon, Heinz*	½ Can/200g	108	54	1.9	5.0	2.9	0.5
Blended Red Pepper With Tomato, Heinz*	½ Can/200g	102	51	0.8	5.2	2.9	0.7
Blended Sweetcorn & Yellow Pepper, Heinz*	½ Can/200g	98	49	0.9	6.6	2.1	0.6
Broccoli & Blue Stilton, New Covent Garden Soup Co*	1 Carton/600g	378	63	3.5	2.9	4.2	0.0
Broccoli & Cauliflower, Cup, Better For You, Morrisons*	1 Sachet/15g	56	376	4.9	57.2	14.2	4.9
Broccoli & Cauliflower, Slim A Soup, Batchelors*	1 Serving/203g	59	29	0.5	4.9	0.8	0.4
Broccoli & Cheddar, Heinz*	1 Can/430g	340	79	2.6	4.4	5.6	0.6
Broccoli & Dolcelatte Cheese, Soupreme, Aldi*	½ Carton/250g	60	24	3.3	1.1	1.0	1.0
Broccoli & Melton Mowbray Stilton, Marks & Spencer*	½ Pot/300g	240	80	2.8	3.3	6.4	0.9
Broccoli & Potato, Organic, Baxters*	1 Can/425g	132	31	1.3	5.8	0.3	0.7
Broccoli & Stilton, Asda*	1 Pack/302g	172	57	2.2	6.0	2.7	0.0
Broccoli & Stilton, Canned, Sainsbury's*	½ Can/207g	126	61	1.7	4.8	3.9	0.4
Broccoli & Stilton, Canned, Tesco*	1 Can/400g	224	56	1.8	4.2	3.5	0.3
Broccoli & Stilton, Fresh, Safeway*	1 Serving/250g	133	53	2.4	3.5	3.3	0.5
Broccoli & Stilton, Fresh, Sainsbury's*	½ Bottle/300ml	156	52	2.1	3.9	3.1	0.9
Broccoli & Stilton, Fresh, Tesco*	½ Pot/300g	219	73	3.3	5.0	4.4	0.7
Broccoli & Stilton, Homestyle, Somerfield*	1 Pack/500g	350	70	2.0	5.0	4.0	0.0
Broccoli & Stilton, Special Recipe, Sainsbury's*	½ Can/208g	127	61	1.7	4.8	3.9	0.4
Broccoli & Stilton, Tesco*	1 Pack/600g	564	94	2.9	2.5	8.1	0.7
Broccoli With Mustard, New Covent Garden Soup Co*	1 Carton/568g	204	36	1.3	3.3	1.9	1.2
Broccoli With Stilton, New Covent Garden Soup Co*	1floz/30ml	14	47	2.0	2.5	3.2	1.0
Broccoli, Baxters*	1 Can/425g	191	45	1.3	5.9	1.8	0.4
Broccoli, Leek & Horseradish, NCGSC*	1 Serving/284g	97	34	1.6	3.9	1.3	0.2
Brocoli & Stilton, Fresh, Safeway*	1 Serving/500g	290	58	3.5	4.8	2.8	0.7
Butternut Squash & Red Pepper, Baxters*	1 Can/425g	153	36	0.7	6.1	1.0	0.6
Butternut Squash With Parmesan, EAT*	1 Can/400ml	127	32	1.9	1.7	2.0	0.5
Butternut Squash, Apricot & Ginger, NCGSC*	½ Pack/300g	138	46	1.0	5.2	2.4	0.8
Cajun Spicy Vegetable, Slim A Soup, Batchelors*	1 Serving/211g	57	27	0.8	5.0	0.5	0.6
Cantonese Chicken & Sweetcorn, Fresh, Sainsbury's*	½ Bottle/300ml	135	45	2.1	7.9	0.5	0.5
Cantonese Hot & Sour Noodle, Baxters*	1 Serving/215g	133	62	1.4	11.1	1.3	0.5
Carrot & Butterbean, Baxters*	1 Can/425g	234	55	1.6	7.9	1.9	1.7
Carrot & Coriander, 'a' Meal, Feeling Great, Findus*	1 Serving/371g	130	35	1.5	5.5	1.0	1.5
Carrot & Coriander, Asda*	1 Pack/297g	92	31	1.0	6.0	0.3	0.0

SOUP,	INFO/WEIGHT	KCAL	KCAL	PROT	CARB	FAT	FIBRE
Carrot & Coriander, BGTY, Sainsbury's*	½ Can/200g	48	24	0.3	4.8	0.4	0.1
Carrot & Coriander, Baxters*	1 Can/425g	162	38	0.8	5.5	1.4	0.8
Carrot & Coriander, COU, Marks & Spencer*	1oz/28g	7	25	0.4	4.3	0.7	0.5
Carrot & Coriander, Carton, Campbell's*	1 Serving/250ml	110	44	0.7	5.4	2.2	0.0
Carrot & Coriander, Classic Homestyle, Marks & Spencer*	1 Can/425g	170	40	0.6	5.6	2.0	0.7
Carrot & Coriander, Fresh, Improved, Sainsbury's*	½ Bottle/300ml	84	28	0.5	3.0	1.6	2.6
Carrot & Coriander, Fresh, Marks & Spencer*	½ Pot/300g	90	30	0.4	4.2	1.5	0.5
Carrot & Coriander, Fresh, Organic, Simply Organic*	1 Serving/250g	83	33	0.6	3.3	2.0	1.0
Carrot & Coriander, Fresh, Sainsbury's*	½ Bottle/300ml	150	50	1.4	4.1	3.1	0.6
Carrot & Coriander, Fresh, Tesco*	1 Pack/600g	270	45	0.6	5.9	2.1	0.9
Carrot & Coriander, Fresh, Waitrose*	½ Pot/300g	117	39	0.5	5.4	1.7	0.9
Carrot & Coriander, Good For You, Asda*	½ Pot/251g	88	35	1.2	4.0	1.6	0.4
Carrot & Coriander, Heinz*	1 Can/400g	208	52	0.7	6.2	2.7	0.6
Carrot & Coriander, Less Than 5% Fat, Asda	1 Serving/300g	96	32	1.0	6.0	0.3	0.8
Carrot & Coriander, New Covent Garden Soup Co*	1floz/30ml	13	42	0.8	3.9	2.6	0.6
Carrot & Coriander, Packet, Sainsbury's*	1oz/28g	7	24	0.7	3.9	0.6	0.7
Carrot & Coriander, Perfectly Balanced, Waitrose*	1 Can/413ml	66	16	0.5	3.1	0.2	1.0
Carrot & Coriander, Sainsbury's*	½ Bottle/300ml	84	28	0.5	3.0	1.6	2.6
Carrot & Coriander, Seeds Of Change*	1 Pack/500g	210	42	0.5	5.7	1.9	0.9
Carrot & Coriander, Selection, Campbell's*	1 Carton/500ml	185	37	0.6	6.4	1.0	0.6
Carrot & Coriander, Somerfield*	1 Pack/450g	212	47	1.0	3.0	4.0	0.0
Carrot & Coriander, Soup-A-Cup, Asda*	1 Sachet/26g	102	392	4.6	62.0	14.0	4.5
Carrot & Coriander, Special Recipe, Sainsbury's*	1 Can/415g	170	41	0.7	4.7	2.1	0.7
Carrot & Coriander, Tesco*	½ Can/210g	92	44	0.7	5.4	2.2	0.8
Carrot & Coriander, Vie Country, Knorr*	1 Pack/500ml	190	38	0.6	3.9	2.2	1.0
Carrot & Ginger, Perfectly Balanced, Waitrose*	½ Pot/300g	66	22	0.4	3.1	0.9	1.0
Carrot & Lentil, Microwave, Heinz*	1 Can/303.2g	94	31	1.5	6.1	0.1	0.8
Carrot & Lentil, Weight Watchers*	1 Can/295g	91	31	1.4	6.0	0.1	0.7
Carrot & Orange, Pouch, Heinz*	½ Pack/300g	165	55	0.6	8.3	2.2	1.0
Carrot & Parsnip, Marks & Spencer*	1oz/28g	9	32	0.5	4.9	1.2	0.9
Carrot Potato & Coriander, Weight Watchers*	1 Can/295g	74	25	0.5	5.5	0.1	0.6
Carrot With Creme Fraiche, Baxters*	1 Can/415g	166	40	0.6	5.8	1.7	0.7
Carrot, Eat Smart, Safeway*	½ Pot/225g	79	35	0.6	5.5	1.3	0.4
Carrot, Honey & Ginger, EAT*	1 Serving/474ml	268	57	0.7	4.7	3.9	1.0
Carrot, Onion & Chick Pea, Healthy Choice, Baxters*	1 Can/425g	145	34	1.7	7.1	0.1	1.5
Carrot, Orange & Coriander, COU, Marks & Spencer*	1 Pack/415g	145	35	0.6	6.9	0.6	1.2
Carrot, Parsnip & Nutmeg, Organic, Baxters*	1 Can/425g	115	27	0.7	5.7	0.2	1.0
Cauliflower Cheddar & Dijon, NCGSC*	1 Pack/284ml	287	101	2.3	10.7	5.4	0.5
Cauliflower Cheese, Somerfield*	1 Pack/500g	345	69	3.0	3.0	5.0	0.0
Celeriac & Bacon, New Covent Garden Soup Co*	1 Serving/300g	228	76	1.1	3.0	7.1	1.6
Cheese, Leek & Bacon, Somerfield*	1 Carton/300g	441	147	5.0	5.0	12.0	0.0
Chestnut Mushroom, Rosehip & English Parsley, NCGSC*	1 Carton/600g	144	24	2.1	2.8	0.5	0.0
Chicken & Asparagus, Eat Smart, Safeway*	1 Pack/450g	248	55	3.3	3.2	2.7	0.7
Chicken & Broccoli Cup A Soup, Asda*	1 Serving/16g	55	341	7.0	58.0	9.0	6.0
Chicken & Broccoli, Soup a Cups, GFY, Asda*	1 Cup/226.1ml	52	23	0.5	4.0	0.6	0.4
Chicken & Broccoli, Soup-a-Slim, Asda*	1 Sachet/16g	55	341	7.0	58.0	9.0	6.0
Chicken & Golden Sweetcorn, Microwaveable, Heinz*	1 Cup/275ml	149	54	1.4	5.6	3.0	0.2
Chicken & Ham, Big, Heinz*	½ Can/200g	92	46	2.3	6.9	1.0	0.7
Chicken & King Prawn Noodle, Tesco*	1 Pot/400g	180	45	4.7	5.5	0.4	0.4
Chicken & Leek, Big, Heinz*	½ Can/200g	118	59	2.3	7.8	2.0	0.5
Chicken & Leek, Cup A Soup, Batchelors*	1 Sachet/213g	77	36	0.6	6.7	0.9	0.3
Chicken & Leek, In A Mug, Slim Choice, Safeway*	1 Sachet/12g	53	439	7.2	55.9	20.7	10.0
Chicken & Leek, In a Cup, Symingtons*	1 Serving/224.5ml	110	49	0.5	6.0	2.5	1.2

S

SOUP,

	Measure	per Measure	Nutrition Values per 100g / 100ml				
	INFO/WEIGHT	KCAL	KCAL	PROT	CARB	FAT	FIBRE
Chicken & Leek, TTD, Sainsbury's*	½ Bottle/300ml	177	59	4.7	2.1	3.5	0.3
Chicken & Mushroom In A Cup, Sainsbury's*	1 Sachet/223ml	107	48	0.7	7.1	1.9	0.1
Chicken & Mushroom In A Cup, Tesco*	1 Sachet/15g	9	57	1.4	8.5	2.0	0.2
Chicken & Mushroom With Pasta Cupa Soup, Batchelors*	1 Serving/250g	115	46	1.3	7.1	1.4	0.5
Chicken & Mushroom, Better For You, Morrisons*	1 Serving/14g	47	337	16.0	54.8	6.1	2.5
Chicken & Mushroom, Slim A Soup, Batchelors*	1 Sachet/203g	59	29	0.7	4.1	1.1	0.3
Chicken & Mushroom, Soup-a-Slim, Asda*	1 Sachet/14g	51	362	10.0	58.0	10.0	4.2
Chicken & Pasta Big, Heinz*	½ Can/200g	68	34	1.8	5.9	0.4	0.8
Chicken & Red Pepper Noodle, Fresh, Tesco*	1 Serving/400ml	200	50	3.6	8.5	0.3	0.4
Chicken & Sweet Corn, Cup, Morrisons*	1 Serving/14g	48	341	14.0	57.5	6.1	2.5
Chicken & Sweetcorn, BGTY, Sainsbury's*	1 Serving/200g	42	21	1.2	3.5	0.2	0.1
Chicken & Sweetcorn, Baxters*	1 Can/425g	166	39	1.6	6.2	0.9	0.6
Chicken & Sweetcorn, Fresh, Asda*	1 Pack/500g	260	52	2.6	6.0	1.9	0.0
Chicken & Sweetcorn, Fresh, Morrisons*	1 Pot/500g	205	41	2.1	6.7	0.6	0.2
Chicken & Sweetcorn, Fresh, Sainsbury's*	½ Bottle/300ml	135	45	2.1	7.9	0.5	0.5
Chicken & Sweetcorn, Good For You, Asda*	1 Can/400g	108	27	1.5	4.2	0.5	0.2
Chicken & Sweetcorn, Healthy Eating, Tesco*	1 Serving/200ml	64	32	1.5	5.3	0.5	0.2
Chicken & Sweetcorn, In A Cup, BGTY, Sainsbury's*	1 Sachet/200ml	50	25	0.7	3.8	0.8	0.6
Chicken & Sweetcorn, In A Mug, Tesco*	1 Sachet/28g	122	434	4.8	63.4	17.9	1.1
Chicken & Sweetcorn, Slim A Soup, Batchelors*	1 Sachet/203g	59	29	0.6	4.5	0.9	0.1
Chicken & Sweetcorn, Slim Choice, Safeway*	1 Sachet/13g	47	363	12.2	48.8	13.2	5.1
Chicken & Sweetcorn, Tesco*	1 Can/400ml	128	32	1.5	5.3	0.5	0.2
Chicken & Tarragon, Thick & Creamy, Batchelors*	1 Sachet/281g	118	42	0.8	5.7	2.3	0.3
Chicken & Vegetable Broth, Morrisons*	1 Serving/200g	50	25	1.2	4.5	0.2	0.5
Chicken & Vegetable, Big, Heinz*	1 Can/400g	188	47	2.4	7.3	1.0	0.9
Chicken & Vegetable, Cup A Soup, Batchelors*	1 Sachet/30g	131	437	4.8	62.7	18.6	1.1
Chicken & Vegetable, Cup, Tesco*	1 Sachet/29ml	122	422	5.6	61.3	17.1	0.5
Chicken & Vegetable, Fresh, Somerfield*	½ Pot/300g	177	59	2.9	5.6	2.8	3.0
Chicken & Vegetable, Healthy Choice, Baxters*	1 Can/426g	132	31	1.3	5.6	0.5	1.6
Chicken & Vegetable, Marks & Spencer*	1oz/28g	17	59	5.3	5.7	1.7	1.1
Chicken & Vegetable, Mighty, Asda*	1 Can/410g	176	43	2.5	6.8	1.3	0.7
Chicken & Vegetable, Perfectly Balanced, Waitrose*	1 Can/68g	23	34	1.8	5.4	0.6	1.0
Chicken & Vegetable, Simply, Kwik Save*	1 Serving/22g	83	379	4.6	56.4	15.0	7.8
Chicken & Vegetable, Thick, Heinz*	1 Can/400g	152	38	1.2	6.2	0.9	0.6
Chicken & White Wine, Campbell's*	1 Serving/295g	145	49	1.0	4.0	3.3	0.0
Chicken Broth, Baxters*	1 Can/425g	145	34	1.2	5.3	0.9	0.6
Chicken Broth, Fresh, Baxters*	1 Serving/300g	117	39	4.9	2.1	1.2	0.7
Chicken Broth, Traditional, Baxters*	½ Can/207g	62	30	1.2	5.3	0.4	0.6
Chicken Flavour, Calorie Counter, Co-Op*	1 Serving/10g	32	320	6.0	49.0	11.0	7.0
Chicken Fusion, Fresh, New Covent Garden Co*	½ Carton/300g	162	54	2.6	4.8	2.7	0.4
Chicken Mulligatawny, Asda*	1 Serving/300g	150	50	3.8	7.0	0.8	0.8
Chicken Mulligatawny, Perfectly Balanced, Waitrose*	1 Serving/300g	138	46	1.7	5.3	2.0	0.4
Chicken Mulligatawny, Tesco*	1 Pack/600g	570	95	3.6	5.4	6.6	0.4
Chicken Noodle & Vegetable, Slim A Soup, Batchelors*	1 Serving/203g	59	29	0.8	4.9	0.7	0.3
Chicken Noodle, Asda*	1 Can/410g	107	26	1.6	4.0	0.4	0.1
Chicken Noodle, Batchelors*	1 Pack/284g	71	25	1.6	4.2	0.2	0.3
Chicken Noodle, Cup A Soup, Batchelors*	1 Serving/217g	89	41	1.7	7.4	0.6	0.2
Chicken Noodle, Cup, Asda*	1 Sachet/13g	40	305	9.0	63.0	1.9	3.6
Chicken Noodle, Healthy Eating, Tesco*	1 Pack/500g	215	43	1.6	6.6	1.1	0.4
Chicken Noodle, Heinz*	1oz/28g	8	27	1.1	4.9	0.3	0.2
Chicken Noodle, In a Mug, Safeway*	1 Sachet/100g	325	325	8.4	69.5	1.5	0.0
Chicken Noodle, Morrisons*	1oz/28g	11	39	1.7	7.4	0.3	0.7
Chicken Noodle, Old Fashioned, EAT*	1 Can/400ml	240	60	6.0	5.5	1.6	0.6

SOUP,

INFO/WEIGHT	Measure	per Measure KCAL	Nutrition Values per 100g / 100ml KCAL	PROT	CARB	FAT	FIBRE
Chicken Noodle, Safeway*	1 Can/425g	111	26	1.4	3.5	0.7	0.3
Chicken Noodle, Sainsbury's*	1 Sachet/600ml	102	17	0.8	3.0	0.2	0.1
Chicken Noodle, Symingtons*	½ Pack/15g	48	318	8.6	65.4	2.4	2.4
Chicken Noodle, Weight Watchers*	1 Can/295g	50	17	0.7	3.1	0.1	0.2
Chicken, Campbell's*	1 Can/295g	142	48	1.1	3.5	3.6	0.0
Chicken, Coconut & Lemon Grass, Fresh, Waitrose*	½ Pot/300g	303	101	2.6	4.1	8.3	0.8
Chicken, Coconut & Sweet Potato, EAT*	1 Pack/343g	235	69	2.0	7.0	3.8	1.1
Chicken, Condensed, 99% Fat Free, Campbell's*	1 Can/295g	100	34	1.6	5.0	0.9	0.0
Chicken, Cream of Canned	1oz/28g	16	58	1.7	4.5	3.8	0.0
Chicken, Cup A Soup, Batchelors*	1 Serving/213g	98	46	0.7	5.8	2.2	0.3
Chicken, Cup, Calorie Counter, Co-Op*	1 Sachet/12.5g	42	320	6.0	49.0	11.0	7.0
Chicken, Cupa, Original, Batchelors*	1 Pack/213g	98	46	0.7	5.8	2.2	0.3
Chicken, In A Cup, Symingtons*	1 Serving/22g	93	424	7.0	57.7	18.4	11.7
Chicken, In a Cup, Sainsbury's*	1 Serving/221ml	86	39	0.7	5.3	1.7	0.1
Chicken, Leek & White Wine, Finest,Tesco*	1 Pack/300g	216	72	2.8	5.7	4.2	0.3
Chicken, Marks & Spencer*	1 Pack/213g	196	92	1.6	5.5	7.2	0.2
Chicken, Mushroom & Pasta Cup A Soup, Batchelors*	1 Serving/286g	132	46	1.3	7.1	1.4	0.5
Chicken, Mushroom & Potato, Big, Heinz*	½ Can/200g	122	61	2.9	7.3	2.2	0.4
Chicken, Mushroom & Rice, Chilled, Marks & Spencer*	½ Pot/300g	240	80	3.4	8.6	3.8	0.6
Chicken, Our Best, New Covent Garden Soup Co*	1 Carton/600ml	804	134	4.7	12.2	7.4	0.9
Chicken, Sainsbury's*	1 Serving/300g	126	42	2.3	3.2	2.2	0.7
Chicken, Sweetcorn & Potato, Heinz*	1 Can/400g	204	51	1.2	5.5	2.8	0.3
Chicken, Weight Watchers*	1 Can/295g	89	30	1.2	4.1	1.0	0.1
Chicken, Windsor Jubilee, New Covent Garden Soup Co*	1 Can/284g	159	56	3.5	3.5	3.1	0.5
Chilli Bean, Marks & Spencer*	½ Carton/300g	150	50	2.5	4.7	2.5	2.7
Chilli Pumpkin, Sainsbury's*	1 Serving/300g	120	40	0.6	4.0	2.4	1.3
Chilli Tomato & Pasta, COU, Marks & Spencer*	1 Serving/300g	150	50	1.3	7.2	1.9	0.9
Chinese Chicken Noodle, Knorr*	1 Pack/45g	138	307	15.1	51.8	4.4	2.9
Chorizo & Tomato With Vegetables, Sainsbury's*	1 Pack/400g	228	57	2.6	4.9	3.0	0.3
Chunky Chicken & Vegetable Meal, Tesco*	1 Can/410g	176	43	2.3	7.2	0.5	0.7
Chunky Chicken & Vegetable, Marks & Spencer*	1 Can/425g	276	65	5.2	6.6	1.8	0.6
Chunky Chicken & Vegetable, Sainsbury's*	1 Can/400g	188	47	3.3	6.9	0.7	0.0
Chunky Chicken Noodle, Campbell's*	½ Can/200g	86	43	2.8	6.5	0.6	0.0
Chunky Chicken, Leek & Potato, Heinz*	1 Can/400g	236	59	2.3	7.8	2.0	0.5
Chunky Minestrone Meal, Tesco*	½ Can/205g	78	38	1.3	6.8	0.6	0.9
Chunky Roasted Vegetable, Marks & Spencer*	1 Can/400g	140	35	1.3	5.8	0.6	1.1
Chunky Tomato, New Covent Garden Soup Co*	½ Pack/300g	135	45	1.8	5.3	1.8	1.1
Chunky Tuscan Style Bean & Sausage, Marks & Spencer*	1 Can/415g	249	60	2.4	7.7	2.2	1.0
Chunky Vegetable & Lentil, Good Intentions, Somerfield*	1 Pack/22.5g	77	333	7.1	61.8	6.7	8.0
Chunky Vegetable, Big, Heinz*	1 Serving/400g	208	52	1.5	8.7	1.3	1.2
Chunky Vegetable, Eat Smart, Safeway*	1 Can/415g	95	23	0.7	4.6	0.2	1.2
Chunky Vegetable, Fresh, Baxters*	1 Serving/300ml	117	39	1.6	7.8	0.2	1.1
Chunky Vegetable, Fresh, Sainsbury's*	½ Bottle/296ml	77	26	0.5	4.8	0.5	1.2
Chunky Vegetable, Fresh, Tesco*	1 Serving/300g	123	41	0.6	5.5	1.9	1.0
Chunky Winter Vegetable, Marks & Spencer*	1 Can/415ml	166	40	1.5	7.5	0.3	0.4
Chunky With Pasta Minestrone, Co-Op*	1 Pack/400g	140	35	1.0	6.0	0.6	0.7
Classic Tomato, Pret A Manger*	1 Serving/336g	179	53	0.9	7.5	2.1	0.7
Cock-a-Leekie Traditional, Baxters*	1 Can/425g	98	23	1.0	4.1	0.3	0.3
Country Garden, Baxters*	1 Can/425g	149	35	0.9	6.5	0.6	0.7
Country Mixture, Sainsbury's*	1 Serving/75g	83	110	6.6	20.1	0.4	3.9
Country Mushroom, Baxters*	1 Pot/600g	360	60	0.9	5.4	3.9	0.3
Country Mushroom, Selection, Campbell's*	1 Serving/250ml	80	32	0.6	3.4	1.8	0.5
Country Vegetable, Chilled, Marks & Spencer*	½ Pot/300g	105	35	0.5	3.2	2.1	1.0

S

SOUP,

INFO/WEIGHT	per Measure KCAL	KCAL	PROT	CARB	FAT	FIBRE
Country Vegetable, Fresh, Asda*	1 Carton/500g	195	39	1.9	7.0	0.4	0.0
Country Vegetable, Fresh, Chilled, Marks & Spencer*	1 Pot/600g	210	35	0.5	3.2	2.1	1.0
Country Vegetable, Fresh, Morrisons*	½ Pot/250g	108	43	1.0	6.3	1.5	1.2
Country Vegetable, Fresh, Somerfield*	½ Pack/300g	123	41	1.1	4.6	2.0	1.2
Country Vegetable, Fresh, Waitrose*	1 Serving/300g	165	55	2.1	7.1	2.0	1.6
Country Vegetable, Slim Choice, Safeway*	1 Serving/16.5g	59	345	6.7	63.6	7.3	9.1
Country Vegetable, Thick, Asda*	1 Pack/410g	164	40	1.6	7.0	0.6	1.2
Country Vegetable, Vie Knorr*	1 Pack/500ml	160	32	0.9	5.5	0.7	1.2
Country Vegetable, Weight Watchers*	1 Can/295g	89	30	1.1	5.9	0.2	1.0
Courgette & Parmesan, Sainsbury's*	1 Pack/300ml	198	66	1.5	2.5	5.6	0.4
Courgette, Parmesan & Bacon, Somerfield*	1 Pack/500g	255	51	2.0	2.0	4.0	0.0
Cream Of Asparagus, Campbell's*	½ Can/150g	68	45	0.5	4.6	2.8	0.0
Cream Of Celery, Campbell's*	1 Serving/150g	71	47	0.6	3.2	3.4	0.0
Cream Of Chicken & Mushroom, Sainsbury's*	1 Can/400g	232	58	1.1	5.1	3.7	0.1
Cream Of Chicken, Asda*	1 Can/410g	209	51	1.2	4.0	3.4	0.1
Cream Of Chicken, Cambell's*	1 Can/590g	295	50	3.7	1.0	3.5	0.0
Cream Of Chicken, Fresh, Waitrose*	1 Serving/300g	180	60	2.6	3.7	3.9	0.2
Cream Of Chicken, Sainsbury's*	½ Can/200g	130	65	1.5	6.2	3.8	0.1
Cream Of Mushroom Cup a Soup, Batchelors*	1 Serving/219g	125	57	0.6	7.5	2.8	0.4
Cream Of Mushroom In A Bottle, Homepride*	¼ Bottle/250ml	110	44	0.5	3.5	3.1	0.0
Cream Of Mushroom, Good For You, Asda*	1 Serving/250g	93	37	2.1	6.0	0.5	0.3
Cream Of Mushroom, Tesco*	1 Serving/200g	108	54	0.9	4.6	3.5	0.1
Cream Of Sweetcorn, Condensed, Campbell's*	1 Can/295g	150	51	0.6	6.2	2.7	0.0
Cream Of Tomato, Asda*	½ Can/205g	150	73	0.8	9.0	3.7	0.5
Cream Of Tomato, Fresh, Waitrose*	½ Pot/300g	210	70	1.0	4.9	5.1	0.5
Cream Of Tomato, Homepride*	¼ Bottle/250ml	138	55	0.9	7.7	2.6	0.0
Cream Of Tomato, Improves, Tesco*	½ Can/200g	142	71	0.9	8.7	3.6	0.5
Cream Of Tomato, SmartPrice, Asda*	1 Can/408g	290	71	0.7	9.0	3.6	0.0
Cream of Asparagus In Seconds, Knorr*	1 Pack/61g	320	524	6.5	42.2	36.6	1.1
Cream of Asparagus Soup in a Cup, Sainsbury's*	1 Serving/230ml	129	56	0.7	8.2	2.3	0.1
Cream of Asparagus, Baxters*	1 Can/415g	266	64	1.2	5.3	4.2	0.2
Cream of Asparagus, Cup A Soup, Batchelors*	1 Sachet/223g	143	64	0.5	9.2	2.8	0.4
Cream of Asparagus, Heinz*	1oz/28g	13	46	1.1	4.5	2.6	0.2
Cream of Asparagus, Soup-a-Cup, Asda*	1 Pack/112g	491	438	6.0	54.0	22.0	4.1
Cream of Celery, Asda*	1 Can/410g	189	46	0.6	4.8	2.7	0.2
Cream of Chicken & Mushroom, Campbell's*	1 Can/250g	108	43	0.5	3.5	3.1	0.0
Cream of Chicken & Mushroom, Heinz*	1oz/28g	14	49	1.3	4.6	2.9	0.1
Cream of Chicken, Batchelors*	1 Pack/289g	165	57	1.1	5.6	3.3	0.3
Cream of Chicken, Baxters*	½ Can/209g	144	69	1.8	6.1	4.2	0.1
Cream of Chicken, Co-Op*	½ Can/200g	120	60	0.8	5.0	4.0	0.1
Cream of Chicken, Fresh, Somerfield*	1 Carton/450g	234	52	2.0	4.0	3.0	0.0
Cream of Chicken, Fresh, Tesco*	1 Serving/300g	294	98	3.3	6.3	6.6	0.2
Cream of Chicken, Heinz*	1oz/28g	14	51	1.3	4.4	3.2	0.1
Cream of Chicken, Homepride*	¼ Bottle/250ml	113	45	1.3	4.0	2.9	0.0
Cream of Chicken, In Seconds, Knorr*	1 Pack/58g	300	518	11.2	36.0	36.6	0.3
Cream of Chicken, Simmer, Sainsbury's*	1 Pack/500ml	182	36	0.8	4.9	1.5	0.8
Cream of Chicken, Somerfield*	1 Serving/215g	129	60	1.5	4.4	4.1	0.1
Cream of Corn, EAT*	1 Pack/343g	316	92	1.7	8.4	5.8	0.8
Cream of Leek In Seconds, Knorr*	1 Pack/64g	326	509	5.9	45.2	33.8	1.4
Cream of Leek, Traditional, Baxters*	1 Can/425g	196	46	0.7	5.2	2.5	0.4
Cream of Mushroom, Asda*	1 Can/410g	258	63	1.0	6.0	3.9	0.3
Cream of Mushroom, Co-Op*	1 Pack/400g	240	60	1.0	5.0	4.0	0.0
Cream of Mushroom, Condensed, 99% FF, Campbell's*	1 Can/295g	71	24	0.6	3.5	0.9	0.0

S

INFO/WEIGHT	Measure	per Measure KCAL	Nutrition Values per 100g / 100ml				
			KCAL	PROT	CARB	FAT	FIBRE
Cream of Mushroom, Condensed, Campbell's*	1 Can/295ml	204	69	1.7	5.3	4.5	0.0
Cream of Mushroom, Fresh, Tesco*	½ Pot/250g	108	43	1.0	4.0	2.6	0.2
Cream of Mushroom, Fresh, Waitrose*	½ Pot/300g	210	70	1.3	3.7	5.5	0.5
Cream of Mushroom, Heinz*	1oz/28g	14	51	1.4	5.1	2.7	0.1
Cream of Mushroom, Knorr*	1 Serving/25g	125	500	5.2	47.8	31.8	1.0
Cream of Mushroom, Sainsbury's*	1 Can/400g	220	55	0.6	1.4	5.2	0.1
Cream of Potato & Leek, Sainsbury's*	½ Can/200g	116	58	0.9	6.8	3.0	0.4
Cream of Scottish Smoked Salmon, Baxters*	1 Can/415g	241	58	1.5	5.7	3.2	0.5
Cream of Tomato & Basil, Somerfield*	1 Pack/450g	279	62	1.0	5.0	4.0	0.0
Cream of Tomato, Campbell's*	1 Can/295g	195	66	0.7	7.6	3.6	0.0
Cream of Tomato, EAT*	1 Can/400ml	247	62	1.5	3.9	4.3	0.9
Cream of Tomato, For One, Heinz*	1 Can/300g	192	64	0.9	7.1	3.6	0.4
Cream of Tomato, Fresh, Sainsbury's*	½ Bottle/300ml	126	42	0.9	7.0	1.2	0.6
Cream of Tomato, Heinz*	1oz/28g	18	64	0.9	7.1	3.6	0.4
Cream of Tomato, Knorr*	1 Pack/90g	392	435	4.3	51.3	23.6	3.3
Cream of Tomato, Lidl*	1oz/28g	19	69	1.2	9.4	3.0	0.6
Cream of Tomato, Microwave, Heinz*	1oz/28g	19	68	0.9	7.5	3.8	0.4
Cream of Tomato, Morrisons*	1 Serving/205g	141	69	1.2	9.4	3.0	0.6
Cream of Tomato, Organic, Heinz*	1 Can/400g	220	55	0.9	7.2	2.5	0.4
Cream of Tomato, Tesco*	1 Pack/600g	474	79	2.2	5.7	5.3	0.5
Cream of Tomato, Traditional, Baxters*	1 Can/425g	302	71	1.5	10.6	2.5	0.7
Cream of Vegetable Cup A Soup, Batchelors*	1 Sachet/33g	134	406	5.8	59.8	16.0	6.2
Creamed Asparagus, Asda*	1 Sachet/30g	131	451	6.0	55.0	23.0	1.1
Creamed Tomato, In A Cup, Sainsbury's*	1 Sachet/233ml	112	48	0.7	9.3	0.9	0.1
Creamed Vegetable, In A Mug, Safeway*	1 Sachet/29g	117	405	5.6	57.9	16.8	3.2
Creamy Carrot, In a Mug, Thick, Safeway*	1 Sachet/28g	105	375	2.9	60.7	13.6	5.4
Creamy Chicken & Vegetables, For One, Wattie's*	1 Can/300g	115	38	0.9	3.8	2.1	0.0
Creamy Leek With Croutons In A Cup, Sainsbury's*	1 Serving/228g	130	57	1.1	7.2	2.6	0.1
Creamy Mushroom, Safeway*	1 Pack/300ml	137	46	1.1	3.8	2.9	0.5
Creamy Mushroom, Somerfield*	1 Pack/450g	225	50	1.0	4.0	3.0	0.0
Creamy Potato & Leek, Cup-A-Soup, Batchelors*	1 Sachet/280ml	132	47	0.8	7.4	1.5	1.1
Creamy Potato, Bacon & Onion, Cup A Soup, Batchelors*	1 Sachet/280ml	106	38	0.9	7.3	1.0	0.5
Creamy Tomato, Seeds Of Change*	1 Pack/500g	320	64	1.1	10.9	1.8	0.5
Crofter's Thick Vegetable, Knorr*	1 Pack/66g	240	364	10.8	52.9	12.2	3.3
Cucumber Pea & Mint, New Covent Garden Soup Co*	1 Serving/200ml	90	45	1.8	4.7	2.1	0.6
Cullen Skink, Baxters*	1 Can/415g	369	89	6.1	7.7	3.7	0.3
Dutch Curry & Rice Cup A Soup, Continental*	1 Serving/250ml	125	50	0.7	8.8	1.3	0.0
English Asparagus, New Covent Garden Soup Co*	½ Pack/300g	114	38	0.7	5.5	1.5	0.1
English Broccoli & Stilton, Knorr*	1 Pack/65g	331	509	11.7	30.3	37.9	1.6
Extra Chinese Chicken Noodle Cup A Soup, Batchelors*	1 Sachet/281g	101	36	1.3	6.8	0.4	0.7
Extra Minestrone With Pasta, Cup A Soup, Batchelors*	1 Pack/286g	123	43	1.4	8.5	0.4	0.8
Extra Tangy Tomato With Pasta Cup A Soup, Batchelors*	1 Sachet/286g	132	46	1.3	8.5	0.8	0.8
Farmhouse Chicken Leek, Knorr*	1 Pack/54g	248	459	10.3	39.3	29.0	1.5
Farmhouse Vegetable, BGTY, Sainsbury's*	1 Serving/200ml	52	26	0.5	4.4	0.8	0.9
Farmhouse Vegetable, Thick, Co-Op*	1 Can/400g	140	35	1.0	7.0	0.4	0.3
Fire Flamed Tomato & Red Onion, Sainsbury's*	½ Bottle/300ml	129	43	0.8	5.0	2.2	1.0
Fire Roasted Tomato & Red Pepper, Asda*	½ Tub/265.1g	114	43	0.7	4.1	2.6	1.0
Florentine Pea, The Best, Safeway*	½ Pot/300g	165	55	2.5	4.9	2.5	1.4
Florida Spring Vegetable, Knorr*	1 Pack/36g	104	290	7.8	52.2	5.6	5.2
Forest Mushroom, Heinz*	1oz/28g	12	43	1.0	4.5	2.3	0.1
Four Mushroom, Loyd Grossman*	1 Pack/420g	202	48	0.8	2.5	3.9	0.2
French Onion & Cider, Waitrose*	1 Can/425g	94	22	0.5	4.8	0.1	0.4
French Onion & Croutons, Tesco*	1 Serving/30g	106	353	7.3	63.7	7.7	2.0

S

SOUP,

INFO/WEIGHT	Measure per Measure KCAL	KCAL	PROT	CARB	FAT	FIBRE
French Onion & Gruyere Cheese, Finest, Tesco*	½ Pot/300g	210	70	1.4	4.7	5.1	0.5
French Onion, Baxters*	1 Can/425g	94	22	0.7	4.2	0.2	0.4
French Onion, Chilled, Marks & Spencer*	½ Pot/300g	150	50	2.0	7.2	1.5	1.0
French Onion, Fresh, Morrisons*	1 Serving/500g	155	31	0.8	5.0	0.9	0.5
French Onion, Good For You, Asda*	½ Pot/253g	91	36	1.9	6.0	0.5	0.4
French Onion, Heinz*	1 Pack/400g	100	25	0.5	5.7	0.1	0.4
French Onion, Knorr*	1 Pack/40g	118	296	6.0	62.5	2.5	6.6
French Onion, Made Up, Sainsbury's*	1/3 Serving/205g	39	19	0.4	4.0	0.1	0.1
French Onion, Safeway*	½ Pot/250g	85	34	0.8	3.9	1.7	0.5
French Onion, Sainsbury's*	1 Serving/300ml	153	51	0.5	5.7	3.0	0.5
Garden Vegetable, Heinz*	1 Can/400g	160	40	0.9	7.2	0.8	0.9
Gazpacho, Fresh, New Covent Garden Soup Co*	1 Pack/284g	68	24	0.8	2.6	1.2	0.6
Gazpacho, Marks & Spencer*	½ Pack/390g	117	30	1.3	5.7	0.2	1.5
Giant Minestrone, Big, New Recipe, Heinz*	½ Can/200g	98	49	1.5	9.3	0.7	1.1
Goats Cheese & Rocket, Sainsbury's*	1 Serving/300g	180	60	2.0	3.2	4.4	0.3
Golden Vegetable With Croutons Cup Soup, Co-Op*	1 Sachet/25g	120	480	4.0	56.0	26.0	2.0
Golden Vegetable With Croutons, Instant, Morrisons*	1 Sachet/27g	118	438	5.3	60.7	19.3	0.0
Golden Vegetable, Asda*	1 Pack/300g	150	50	1.9	6.0	2.0	0.0
Golden Vegetable, Calorie Counter, Cup, Co-Op*	1 Sachet/12g	40	335	7.0	54.0	10.0	5.0
Golden Vegetable, Cup A Soup, Batchelors*	1 Serving/212g	70	33	0.5	7.3	0.2	0.4
Golden Vegetable, Cup, Calorie Counter, Co-Op*	1 Sachet/10.9g	35	320	7.0	50.0	10.0	9.0
Golden Vegetable, Instant, Tesco*	1 Sachet/17g	60	351	8.2	62.0	7.8	3.7
Golden Vegetable, Knorr*	1 Pack/76g	299	394	10.4	45.4	19.0	3.3
Golden Vegetable, Slim A Soup, Batchelors*	1 Sachet/207g	58	28	0.5	4.7	0.8	0.7
Golden Vegetable, Soup-A-Slim, Asda*	1 Sachet/15g	50	336	6.0	60.0	8.0	1.9
Green Thai Chicken, Waitrose*	1 Pack/400g	324	81	3.8	5.7	4.8	0.3
Haddock, Chowder, Smoked, Asda*	1 Serving/300g	135	45	2.4	6.0	1.3	0.7
Haggis Broth, Baxters*	1 Can/425g	221	52	1.9	6.8	1.9	0.7
Harvest Vegetable, In A Cup With Croutons, Sainsbury's*	1 Sachet/226.3ml	86	38	1.0	5.9	1.2	0.9
Hearty Vegetable, 99% Fat Free, Campbells*	1 Can/295g	91	31	0.8	6.1	0.4	0.0
Highlanders Broth, Baxters*	1 Can/425g	183	43	1.6	6.1	1.4	0.5
Italian Bean & Pasta, Baxters*	1 Can/425g	162	38	1.9	7.0	0.2	1.3
Italian Chicken & Pasta, Big, Heinz*	1oz/28g	15	55	2.4	9.7	0.7	0.8
Italian Chicken Broth, Healthy Choice, Baxters*	½ Can/210g	84	40	1.5	6.6	0.8	0.8
Italian Chunky, New Covent Garden Soup Co*	½ Carton/300g	135	45	1.8	5.3	1.8	1.1
Italian Plum Tomato & Basil, Perfectly Balanced, Waitrose*	½ Pot/300g	69	23	0.9	3.8	0.5	0.9
Italian Style Tomato & Basil, Co-Op*	1 Pack/500g	200	40	1.0	4.0	2.0	0.6
Italian Style Tomato & Chicken, BGTY, Sainsbury's*	1 Can/400g	148	37	3.1	5.5	0.3	0.4
Italian Style Tomato, Safeway*	½ Pot/248g	134	54	1.3	5.7	2.9	0.9
Italian Tomato With Basil, Baxters*	1 Can/425g	242	57	2.6	9.3	1.0	1.1
Jamaican Jerk Chicken & Pumpkin, Sainsbury's*	1 Pack/600g	282	47	2.7	5.1	1.7	0.2
Lamb & Vegetable, Big, Heinz*	1oz/28g	16	56	2.4	9.3	1.0	1.1
Lamb & Vegetable, Mega, Morrisons*	1 Pack/410g	172	42	1.9	6.3	1.0	0.8
Leek & Chicken, Knorr*	1 Serving/300ml	82	27	0.6	2.4	1.7	0.1
Leek & Potato, Chilled, Marks & Spencer*	1 Serving/300g	240	80	0.9	5.2	6.2	0.6
Leek & Potato, Cup A Soup, Batchelors*	1 Sachet/28g	121	432	5.2	63.2	17.6	1.8
Leek & Potato, Eat Smart, Safeway*	½ Pot/225g	113	50	1.1	6.0	2.4	0.6
Leek & Potato, Fresh, Morrisons*	½ Pot/250g	185	74	2.0	6.4	4.5	0.7
Leek & Potato, Fresh, Sainsbury's*	1 Bowl/300ml	189	63	1.1	3.9	4.8	0.5
Leek & Potato, Fresh, Tesco*	½ pack/300g	201	67	1.4	6.3	4.0	0.8
Leek & Potato, GFY, Asda*	1 Sachet/220g	55	25	0.3	5.0	0.4	0.3
Leek & Potato, In A Cup, BGTY, Sainsbury's*	1 Sachet/196ml	55	28	0.3	4.9	0.8	0.8
Leek & Potato, In A Cup, Tesco*	1 Sachet/15g	51	343	5.3	66.4	6.2	3.5

SOUP,

INFO/WEIGHT	Measure per Measure KCAL	KCAL	PROT	CARB	FAT	FIBRE
Leek & Potato, New Covent Garden Soup Co*	½ Carton/284g	105	37	1.2	7.1	1.5	0.8
Leek & Potato, Organic, Sainsbury's*	½ Can/200g	84	42	1.6	5.7	1.4	0.9
Leek & Potato, Reduced Calorie Quick, Waitrose*	1 Sachet/190ml	51	27	0.4	5.3	0.5	0.4
Leek & Potato, Slim A Soup, Batchelors*	1 Serving/204g	57	28	0.4	5.0	0.7	0.2
Leek & Potato, Tastebreaks, Knorr*	1 Pot/225g	162	72	1.1	9.1	3.4	0.5
Leek & Potato, Vie Country, Knorr*	1 Pack/500ml	155	31	0.9	4.8	0.9	1.0
Leek & Potato, Weight Watchers*	1 Sachet/214.8ml	58	27	0.5	5.1	0.5	0.1
Lentil & Bacon, Baxters*	1 Can/425g	255	60	2.7	7.9	1.9	0.8
Lentil & Bacon, Sainsbury's*	½ Can/200g	116	58	3.0	8.9	1.1	1.0
Lentil & Bacon, Tesco*	1 Serving/200g	96	48	3.2	7.2	0.7	0.5
Lentil & Chick Pea, Organic, Tesco*	1 Serving/300ml	117	39	1.9	6.1	0.8	0.5
Lentil & Tomato, New Covent Garden Soup Co*	½ Pack/284g	162	57	3.6	8.1	1.1	0.7
Lentil & Vegetable With Bacon, Organic, Baxters*	½ Can/211.4g	93	44	1.9	7.6	0.7	1.0
Lentil & Vegetable, Baxters*	1 Can/423g	144	34	1.9	6.8	0.1	1.5
Lentil & Winter, New Covent Garden Soup Co*	1 Serving/250ml	133	53	3.1	7.7	1.1	0.9
Lentil, Asda*	½ Can/202g	89	44	2.6	8.0	0.2	0.7
Lentil, Bacon & Mixed Bean, Low Fat, Aldi*	1 Meal/400g	260	65	4.7	9.5	0.9	1.6
Lentil, Campbell's*	1 Can/295g	139	47	2.6	7.7	0.6	0.0
Lentil, Canned	1 Serving/220g	86	39	3.1	6.5	0.2	1.2
Lentil, Carrot & Cumin, BGTY, Sainsbury's*	1 Pack/400g	204	51	2.3	8.4	0.9	0.1
Lentil, Farmfoods*	1 Can/225g	304	135	8.4	16.9	3.7	3.2
Lentil, Heinz*	1 Can/300g	117	39	2.3	7.1	0.2	1.0
Lobster Bisque, Baxters*	1 Can/415g	220	53	3.4	5.2	2.1	0.1
Luxury Game, Baxters*	1 Can/415g	187	45	3.7	5.9	0.7	0.5
Malaysian Chicken & Sweetcorn, Knorr*	1 Pack/57g	211	370	10.6	56.3	11.4	1.8
Manhattan Clam Chowder, EAT*	1 Can/400ml	262	66	5.2	5.5	2.6	1.0
Manhattan Prawn Chowder, Sainsbury's*	1 Pack/300ml	177	59	1.6	7.9	2.3	0.1
Mediteranean Vegetable, Homepride*	1 Serving/250ml	83	33	0.9	4.3	1.3	0.0
Mediterranean Fish, Waitrose*	½ Pot/300g	108	36	3.4	3.5	0.9	0.7
Mediterranean Minestrone, Campbell's*	½ Carton/250ml	95	38	0.9	6.1	1.1	0.6
Mediterranean Style Tomato, Healthy Eating, Tesco*	1 Serving/22g	78	353	9.7	64.3	6.3	3.0
Mediterranean Tomato & Vegetable, Weight Watchers*	1 Can/295g	47	16	0.4	3.0	0.3	0.4
Mediterranean Tomato, Baxters*	1 Can/425g	140	33	1.0	6.9	0.2	0.7
Mediterranean Tomato, COU, Marks & Spencer*	1 Pack/415g	104	25	0.7	4.8	0.5	0.6
Mediterranean Tomato, Campbell's*	1 Can/295g	83	28	0.6	6.4	0.0	0.0
Mediterranean Tomato, Chicken & Pasta, HE, Tesco*	1 Serving/400ml	160	40	1.5	7.3	0.5	0.3
Mediterranean Tomato, Fresh, Baxters*	1 Can/300g	171	57	2.2	8.1	1.8	1.4
Mediterranean Tomato, Fresh, Organic, Sainsbury's*	1 Serving/250ml	78	31	1.3	3.3	1.4	1.0
Mediterranean Tomato, In A Cup, BGTY, Sainsbury's*	1 Serving/200ml	60	30	0.7	5.7	0.4	0.7
Mediterranean Tomato, In A Cup, Sainsbury's*	1 Serving/214ml	60	28	0.7	5.3	0.4	0.2
Mediterranean Tomato, Reduced Calorie, Waitrose*	1 Serving/200ml	52	26	0.7	4.2	0.7	0.3
Mediterranean Tomato, Slim A Soup, Batchelors*	1 Serving/207g	54	26	0.5	4.7	0.6	0.4
Mediterranean Vegetable, Perfectly Balanced, Waitrose*	½ Pot/300g	57	19	0.8	2.8	0.8	0.8
Mediterranean Vegetable, Tesco*	½ Can/200g	76	38	0.6	6.8	0.9	0.5
Mediterraniean Vegetable, Aldi*	1 Serving/250g	78	31	5.2	2.0	0.2	0.9
Melon & Carrot, New Covent Garden Soup Co*	1 Serving/300g	60	20	0.6	3.6	0.4	0.6
Mexican Black Bean, Extra Special, Asda*	½ Pot/262.5g	195	74	2.3	7.0	4.1	1.7
Minestrone With Croutons, Soup in a Cup, Sainsbury's*	1 Sachet/225ml	72	32	0.9	6.3	0.4	0.5
Minestrone With Ribbon Noodles, Extra, Aldi*	1 Serving/34g	107	315	11.0	62.8	2.2	2.0
Minestrone With Wholemeal Pasta, Baxters*	1 Can/415g	133	32	0.9	6.7	0.2	1.0
Minestrone, Asda*	½ Can/200g	54	27	0.9	4.4	0.6	0.6
Minestrone, Batchelors*	1 Serving/296g	77	26	0.7	5.1	0.3	0.4
Minestrone, Baxters*	1 Can/425g	145	34	1.3	6.0	0.6	0.8

S

SOUP,

	Measure INFO/WEIGHT	per Measure KCAL	KCAL	PROT	CARB	FAT	FIBRE
Minestrone, Calorie Counter, Low Calorie Cup, Co-Op*	1 Sachet/13g	40	310	7.0	66.0	2.0	3.0
Minestrone, Chilled, Marks & Spencer*	½ Pot/300g	66	22	1.4	2.5	0.7	1.2
Minestrone, Cup A Soup, BGTY, Sainsbury's*	1 Serving/200ml	54	27	0.8	6.0	0.1	0.6
Minestrone, Cup A Soup, Batchelors*	1 Serving/217g	100	46	0.9	8.3	1.1	0.5
Minestrone, Delicious, Tesco*	1 Serving/300g	129	43	1.1	7.2	1.1	0.6
Minestrone, For One, Heinz*	1 Can/303g	97	32	1.4	5.2	0.7	0.7
Minestrone, Fresh, Baxters*	1 Box/568ml	233	41	1.8	6.2	1.0	0.6
Minestrone, Fresh, Morrisons*	1 Pot/506ml	182	36	1.9	6.4	0.4	0.2
Minestrone, Fresh, Safeway*	½ Pot/250g	83	33	1.0	6.2	0.5	0.8
Minestrone, Fresh, Sainsbury's*	½ Bottle/300ml	93	31	1.2	4.4	0.9	0.9
Minestrone, Fresh, Tesco*	1 Serving/300g	126	42	1.4	6.9	1.0	0.6
Minestrone, Fresh, Waitrose*	1 Pack/600g	240	40	1.1	5.8	1.4	0.8
Minestrone, Healthy Choice, Baxters*	½ Can/207.5g	67	32	0.9	6.7	0.2	1.2
Minestrone, Healthy Eating, Tesco*	1 Pack/500g	140	28	1.0	4.4	0.7	0.6
Minestrone, Heinz*	1 Can/300g	96	32	1.4	5.2	0.7	0.7
Minestrone, In a Cup, BGTY, Sainsbury's*	1 Serving/200ml	54	27	0.8	6.0	0.1	0.6
Minestrone, In a Mug, Healthy Eating, Tesco*	1 Sachet/21g	72	342	3.6	67.7	6.3	3.2
Minestrone, Instant With Croutons, Value, Tesco*	1 Sachet/21g	68	325	6.4	60.2	6.5	1.7
Minestrone, Instant, Under 60 Calories, Tesco*	1 Sachet/19g	58	307	7.3	63.6	2.6	2.3
Minestrone, Mighty, Asda*	1 Serving/38.2g	130	343	9.0	74.0	1.2	2.4
Minestrone, New Covent Garden Soup Co*	1 Serving/250ml	83	33	1.7	5.8	0.4	0.7
Minestrone, Organic, Marks & Spencer*	1 Pack/208g	83	40	1.4	8.9	0.5	1.1
Minestrone, Organic, Seeds of Change*	1 Sachet/500g	325	65	1.3	7.5	3.2	0.9
Minestrone, Packet, Knorr*	1 Pack/61g	178	292	9.2	53.9	4.4	6.5
Minestrone, Safeway*	1 Pack/425g	132	31	1.1	6.4	0.1	0.5
Minestrone, Simmer, Asda*	1 Pack/50g	131	262	6.0	57.0	1.1	15.0
Minestrone, Slim A Soup, Batchelors*	1 Serving/203g	53	26	0.7	4.5	0.6	0.6
Minestrone, Soup a Slim, Asda*	1 Serving/17g	53	311	6.0	69.0	1.2	4.5
Minestrone, Tesco*	1 Pack/600g	222	37	0.9	4.0	2.0	0.6
Minestrone, Weight Watchers*	1 Can/295g	59	20	0.8	3.3	0.4	0.5
Minestrone, With Pesto, EAT*	1 Pack/400ml	276	69	2.8	9.2	2.4	2.2
Minestrone, in a Cup, Sainsbury's*	1 Serving/227ml	84	37	1.4	6.3	0.7	0.2
Mixed Bean & Pepper, Organic, Marks & Spencer*	1 Pack/208g	94	45	2.3	7.7	0.3	1.8
Moroccan Chick Pea, Marks & Spencer*	1oz/28g	20	70	3.6	8.8	2.1	2.0
Moroccan Chicken, New Covent Garden Soup Co*	1 Serving/300g	108	36	2.1	2.7	1.9	0.4
Moroccan Lentil, Waitrose*	½ Pot/300g	153	51	3.5	8.2	0.5	3.4
Mulligatawny Beef Curry, Heinz*	1oz/28g	17	60	1.8	7.2	2.7	0.5
Mulligatawny, Asda*	1 Can/400g	172	43	2.2	6.0	1.1	0.3
Mulligatawny, In A Cup, Symingtons*	1 Serving/232ml	95	41	0.7	8.3	0.6	0.5
Mulligatawny, Tesco*	1 Can/400g	144	36	1.2	6.8	0.5	0.3
Mushroom & Chicken, Co-Op*	1 Pack/400g	220	55	0.9	5.0	4.0	0.0
Mushroom & Garlic, Slimming Cup A Soup, Tesco*	1 Serving/16g	58	360	5.8	61.1	10.3	3.2
Mushroom & Garlic, Tesco*	1 Sachet/16g	58	360	5.8	61.1	10.3	3.2
Mushroom & Mascarpone, TTD, Sainsbury's*	½ Bottle/300ml	108	36	0.6	2.8	2.5	0.4
Mushroom Creme Fraiche, Waistline, Crosse & Blackwell*	1 Carton/300g	69	23	1.2	2.8	0.8	0.3
Mushroom Potage, Baxters*	1 Can/415g	303	73	1.6	5.6	4.9	0.4
Mushroom, 98% Fat Free, Baxters*	1 Can/425g	170	40	0.9	5.6	1.6	0.3
Mushroom, Budgens*	1 Can/400g	284	71	1.2	6.6	4.5	0.1
Mushroom, Chilled, Marks & Spencer*	1 Pack/300g	135	45	1.9	3.3	2.6	0.5
Mushroom, Condensed, Campbell's*	1 Can/300g	207	69	1.7	5.3	4.5	0.0
Mushroom, Cream of, Canned	1 Serving/220g	101	46	1.1	3.9	3.0	0.1
Mushroom, Delicious, Tesco*	1 Serving/300g	111	37	1.2	3.1	2.2	0.4
Mushroom, For One, Heinz*	1 Tin/290g	148	51	1.4	5.1	2.7	0.1

S

INFO/WEIGHT	Measure	per Measure KCAL	Nutrition Values per 100g / 100ml KCAL	PROT	CARB	FAT	FIBRE

SOUP,

	Measure INFO/WEIGHT	per Measure KCAL	KCAL	PROT	CARB	FAT	FIBRE
Mushroom, Fresh, Sainsbury's*	1 Serving/300g	204	68	1.6	4.7	4.8	0.8
Mushroom, Morrisons*	1 Serving/500g	250	50	1.3	3.2	3.6	0.3
Mushroom, Quick, Knorr*	1 Serving/100g	85	85	2.0	8.5	4.5	0.0
Mushroom, Symingtons*	1 Serving/23g	80	348	17.8	48.4	9.2	6.7
Mushroom, Weight Watchers*	1 Can/295g	86	29	1.2	5.6	0.2	0.1
New England Clam Chowder, Select, Campbell's*	1 Cup/240ml	221	92	2.5	6.0	6.0	0.8
Oxtail, Canned	1 Serving/220g	97	44	2.4	5.1	1.7	0.1
Oxtail, Condensed, Classics, Diluted, Campbell's*	1 Can/590g	236	40	1.4	5.3	1.5	0.0
Oxtail, Cup A Soup, Batchelors*	1 Serving/211g	76	36	0.8	6.5	0.8	0.5
Oxtail, Cup Soup, Co-Op*	1 Sachet/19g	67	355	7.0	63.0	9.0	1.0
Oxtail, Sainsbury's*	½ Can/200g	66	33	2.3	5.1	0.4	0.2
Oxtail, Soup in A Cup, Sainsbury's*	1 Serving/223ml	69	31	1.0	5.7	0.5	0.2
Oxtail, Tesco*	1 Can/400g	152	38	2.0	5.9	0.7	0.3
Parsnip & Honey, Sainsbury's*	½ Bottle/300g	192	64	1.1	5.4	4.2	1.5
Parsnip, Fresh, Morrisons*	½ Pot/250g	100	40	0.9	5.8	1.5	1.4
Parsnip, Honey & Ginger, COU, Marks & Spencer*	1 Can/415g	125	30	0.7	5.3	0.6	0.7
Parsnip, Leek & Ginger, New Covent Garden Food Co*	1 Carton/600g	162	27	1.2	4.9	0.3	1.3
Pea & Ham, Asda*	½ Can/205g	107	52	2.6	9.0	0.6	0.6
Pea & Ham, Baxters*	1 Can/425g	247	58	2.9	8.1	1.6	1.2
Pea & Ham, Fresh, Sainsbury's*	½ Bottle/302ml	136	45	2.6	4.9	1.7	1.1
Pea & Ham, Morrisons*	1 Serving/250g	93	37	2.0	4.8	1.1	1.2
Pea & Ham, Tesco*	1 Serving/300g	207	69	3.4	6.6	3.2	1.0
Pea & Ham, Thick, Heinz*	1 Can/400g	204	51	3.2	8.7	0.4	1.0
Pea & Mint, Baxters*	1 Serving/300g	186	62	2.3	6.1	3.2	1.5
Pea & Mint, Fresh, Marks & Spencer*	1 Serving/164g	49	30	1.8	6.3	0.1	1.5
Pea & Mint, Fresh, Tesco*	1 Serving/300g	207	69	2.4	5.1	4.4	0.0
Pea & Mint, Tesco*	½ Pouch/250g	198	79	2.0	5.6	5.4	1.5
Pea, In a Cup, Symingtons*	1 Sachet/30.5g	97	311	7.2	54.1	7.2	6.9
Peking Shiitake Mushroom Noodle, Baxters*	1 Serving/215g	90	42	1.3	7.5	0.8	0.2
Pepper & Chorizo, Sainsbury's*	1 Bowl/400ml	172	43	7.0	2.0	1.0	0.0
Pepper & Tomato, Safeway*	½ Pot/100g	100	100	2.6	11.9	4.2	2.5
Plum Tomato & Creme Fraiche, NCGSC*	½ Carton/300g	141	47	1.0	3.6	3.2	0.9
Pork, Chinese Dumpling, New Cultural Revolution*	1 Serving/250ml	156	62	6.4	6.0	1.6	0.4
Potato & Leek With Peppers & Chicken, Stockmeyer*	½ Can/200g	118	59	2.6	6.7	2.4	0.8
Potato & Leek, Asda*	½ Pack/292ml	158	54	1.2	6.0	2.8	0.7
Potato & Leek, Baxters*	1 Can/425g	170	40	1.0	6.3	1.2	0.5
Potato & Leek, Fresh, Asda*	½ Pot/250g	98	39	1.2	7.0	0.7	0.0
Potato & Leek, Thick, Heinz*	1 Can/400g	136	34	0.7	6.5	0.6	0.5
Potato, Leek & Chicken, BGTY, Sainsbury's*	1 Can/400g	152	38	2.1	5.4	0.9	0.5
Provencal Vegetable, Marks & Spencer*	1 Serving/300g	150	50	1.0	6.0	2.5	1.1
Pumpkin & Bramley Apple, NCGSC*	½ Carton/300g	99	33	1.1	5.9	0.6	0.8
Pumpkin, New Covent Garden Soup Co*	½ Pint/296ml	95	32	1.1	4.8	0.9	1.0
Red Pepper & Tomato, Perfectly Balanced, Waitrose*	1 Can/415g	154	37	0.8	4.5	1.8	0.9
Red Pepper & Tomato, Vie Country, Knorr*	1 Pack/500ml	195	39	0.8	6.4	1.2	1.0
Red Pepper, Tomato & Basil, Marks & Spencer*	1 Can/415g	83	20	1.3	2.7	0.3	0.8
Rich Tomato & Basil, Batchelors*	1 Serving/280g	104	37	0.5	6.7	0.9	0.6
Rich Woodland Mushroom, Cup a Soup, Batchelors*	1 Pack/280g	123	44	0.6	5.8	1.9	0.5
Roast Pumpkin, EAT*	1 Can/400ml	260	65	1.1	5.9	4.2	0.8
Roasted Parsnip, Chunky Carrot & Sweet Potato, Baxters*	½ Pot/300g	186	62	0.9	8.5	2.7	1.4
Roasted Pepper, Eat Smart, Safeway*	½ Pot/225g	79	35	0.8	3.7	1.8	1.4
Roasted Red Pepper, Fresh, Waitrose*	1 Pack/600g	172	29	0.8	3.0	1.5	1.0
Roasted Vegetable, Eat Smart, Safeway*	1 Serving/450g	180	40	0.8	4.1	2.2	2.0
Roasted Vegetable, Fresh, Sainsbury's*	½ Pot/273ml	71	26	0.5	4.8	0.5	1.2

S

SOUP,

	Measure INFO/WEIGHT	per Measure KCAL	KCAL	PROT	CARB	FAT	FIBRE
Roasted Vegetable, TTD, Sainsbury's*	½ Pack/297.7g	128	43	0.5	3.4	3.0	1.0
Roasted Winter Vegetable, Sainsbury's*	1 Serving/300ml	129	43	0.5	3.4	3.0	1.0
San Marzano Tomato & Mascarpone, Marks & Spencer*	1 Serving/150g	98	65	1.4	5.7	4.3	2.0
Scotch Broth, Asda*	½ Can/205g	90	44	1.6	6.0	1.5	0.6
Scotch Broth, Baxters*	1 Can/425g	200	47	1.9	7.1	1.2	0.9
Scotch Broth, New Covent Garden Soup Co*	½ Pint/296ml	118	40	1.6	2.8	2.5	0.5
Scotch Broth, Sainsbury's*	½ Can/200g	108	54	1.9	8.2	1.5	0.8
Scotch Broth, Tesco*	1 Can/400g	152	38	1.5	6.7	0.6	0.8
Scotch Broth, Thick, Heinz*	½ Can/200g	94	47	2.1	8.1	0.7	0.9
Scotch Vegetable, Baxters*	1 Can/425g	183	43	1.9	7.4	0.6	1.3
Scottish Vegetable With Lentils & Beef, Heinz*	1 Can/403.8g	210	52	3.4	8.2	0.7	1.2
Sicilian Tomato, New Covent Garden Soup Co*	½ Pint/284ml	114	40	1.6	4.8	1.6	0.8
Smoked Bacon & Celeriac, NCGSC*	1 Serving/300g	228	76	1.1	2.0	7.1	1.6
Smoked Haddock Chowder, NCGSC*	½ Pint/284ml	142	50	2.2	8.1	1.0	0.5
Spiced Spinach & Green Lentil, Asda*	½ Pot/250g	123	49	2.7	5.0	2.0	0.0
Spicy Corn Chowder, New Covent Garden Soup Co*	½ Pint/284ml	133	47	1.4	5.9	2.0	0.9
Spicy Gumbo, Sainsbury's*	1 Carton/600ml	240	40	1.5	4.5	1.8	0.9
Spicy Lentil & Tomato, Soup A Slim, Asda*	1 Serving/17g	56	327	12.0	63.0	3.0	4.6
Spicy Lentil, COU, Marks & Spencer*	1 Pack/415g	187	45	2.6	6.7	0.9	1.2
Spicy Lentil, Seeds Of Change*	1 Pack/500g	345	69	2.8	9.4	2.2	0.8
Spicy Parsnip, BGTY, Sainsbury's*	1 Pack/400g	180	45	2.2	7.1	0.9	1.0
Spicy Parsnip, Baxters*	1 Can/425g	217	51	1.1	6.1	2.5	1.5
Spicy Parsnip, Fresh, Tesco*	1 Serving/300g	102	34	0.6	4.5	1.6	1.6
Spicy Parsnip, Perfectly Balanced, Waitrose*	1 Can/415g	125	30	1.0	4.8	0.7	1.1
Spicy Pumpkin, Sainsbury's*	½ Bottle/300ml	96	32	0.4	3.8	1.7	0.6
Spicy Red Lentil & Tomato, Marks & Spencer*	½ Pack/300g	150	50	2.7	8.0	0.8	1.1
Spicy Sausage & Bean Meal, Tesco*	1 Can/500g	265	53	2.8	6.4	1.4	1.2
Spicy Thai Chicken, Baxters*	1 Can/415g	278	67	1.8	7.1	3.5	0.3
Spicy Tomato & Lentil, Asda*	1 Can/410g	156	38	1.0	6.0	1.1	0.4
Spicy Tomato & Lentil, BGTY, Sainsbury's*	1 Can/400g	240	60	3.2	10.4	0.7	0.1
Spicy Tomato & Lentil, Tesco*	1 Can/400g	180	45	2.1	8.7	0.2	0.8
Spicy Tomato & Rice With Sweetcorn, Baxters*	½ Can/207g	93	45	1.3	9.2	0.3	0.6
Spicy Tomato, Cup A Soup, Batchelors*	1 Sachet/23g	74	322	7.6	65.8	3.2	3.2
Spicy Tomato, EAT*	1 Can/400ml	137	34	0.7	3.6	1.8	0.8
Spinach & Ricotta, EAT*	1 Pack/400ml	224	56	2.1	3.0	4.0	0.7
Spinach & Watercress, New Covent Garden Soup Co*	½ Carton/298g	60	20	1.3	2.8	0.4	0.8
Split Pea & Ham, Asda*	1 Serving/300g	129	43	3.5	6.9	0.2	0.7
Split Peas, Yellow, Simply Organic*	1 Pot/500g	270	54	3.5	9.7	0.2	2.5
Spring Vegetable, Condensed, Campbell's*	1 Can/295g	62	21	0.5	4.5	0.1	0.0
Spring Vegetable, Heinz*	1 Can/400g	124	31	0.8	6.2	0.4	0.7
Sugar Snap Pea & Mint, New Covent Garden Soup Co*	½ Pack/300g	87	29	1.7	3.0	1.1	1.4
Summer Minestrone With Basil Pesto, Marks & Spencer*	½ Pot/300g	240	80	1.9	5.7	5.4	1.2
Sun Dried Tomato & Basil, Heinz*	1 Serving/275ml	124	45	0.6	6.5	1.9	0.1
Super Chicken Noodle in Seconds, Knorr*	1 Pack/37g	111	299	17.9	46.1	4.7	0.3
Super Chicken Noodle, Knorr*	1 Pack/56g	182	325	14.3	56.0	4.9	1.8
Sweet Cherry Tomato, TTD, Sainsbury's*	1 Pack/300g	120	40	0.7	6.0	1.5	1.0
Sweetcorn & Chicken Chowder, Heinz*	1 Serving/200g	108	54	1.5	5.2	3.0	0.3
Sweetcorn & Chicken, Cup, Calorie Counter, Co-Op*	1 Sachet/11.1g	35	315	5.0	49.0	11.0	11.0
Sweetcorn Chowder, New Covent Garden Soup Co*	½ Carton/250ml	118	47	1.4	5.9	2.0	0.9
Sweetcorn, Carrot & Elderflower, New Covent Garden*	½ Carton/300g	126	42	1.0	5.0	2.0	0.9
Tangy Tomato, Slim A Soup, Batchelors*	1 Serving/230ml	81	35	1.1	6.7	0.4	0.5
Thai Chicken Fusion, New Covent Garden Soup Co.*	1 Carton/111g	59	54	2.6	4.8	2.7	0.4

S

SOUP,

	Measure INFO/WEIGHT	per Measure KCAL	Nutrition Values per 100g / 100ml				
			KCAL	PROT	CARB	FAT	FIBRE
Thai Chicken Noodle, Baxters*	1 Serving/430g	202	47	1.7	6.8	1.4	0.3
Thai Chicken, Good For You, Asda*	1 Serving/200g	85	43	1.7	5.5	1.5	0.5
Thai Chicken, Safeway*	1 Serving/200g	178	89	4.1	2.5	7.0	1.3
Thai Pumpkin Coconut, New Covent Garden Soup Co*	1 Carton/568ml	182	32	1.3	3.5	1.3	1.1
Thai Red Chicken, Fresh, Sainsbury's*	½ Pot/300ml	159	53	1.9	5.0	2.8	0.5
Thai Style Chicken, Morrisons*	1 Serving/250g	205	82	3.3	4.6	5.6	0.0
Thai Style Chicken, Sainsbury's*	½ Can/200g	106	53	2.9	5.5	2.1	0.7
Three Bean, Organic, Seeds of Change*	1 Pack/500g	285	57	1.7	9.9	1.2	1.1
Tomato & Basil With Onion, Waistline, Crosse & Blackwell*	1 Serving/300g	87	29	0.9	5.1	0.6	0.3
Tomato & Basil, 1% Fat, Marks & Spencer*	1 Can/400g	152	38	0.6	9.0	0.4	1.4
Tomato & Basil, 99% Fat Free, Baxters*	½ Can/207g	75	36	0.7	6.1	1.0	0.6
Tomato & Basil, Chilled, Marks & Spencer*	1 Serving/300g	105	35	0.9	6.2	0.7	0.7
Tomato & Basil, Delicious, Tesco*	1 Serving/300ml	150	50	1.0	7.4	1.9	0.7
Tomato & Basil, Finest, Tesco*	½ Pot/300g	204	68	1.0	4.1	5.2	0.6
Tomato & Basil, Fresh, Improved, Sainsbury's*	½ Bottle/300ml	105	35	1.4	4.1	1.4	0.6
Tomato & Basil, Fresh, Morrisons*	1 Serving/500g	210	42	2.5	4.9	1.4	0.0
Tomato & Basil, Fresh, Sainsbury's*	1 Pack/300ml	78	26	0.8	4.0	0.7	0.7
Tomato & Basil, Fresh, Tesco*	1 Pack/300g	129	43	1.0	5.7	1.8	0.7
Tomato & Basil, Good For You, Asda*	1 Serving/250ml	103	41	1.4	3.9	2.2	0.4
Tomato & Basil, New Covent Garden Soup Co*	1 Pack/568g	187	33	1.8	5.7	0.4	0.5
Tomato & Basil, Organic, Sainsbury's*	1 Serving/200g	96	48	0.4	7.0	2.0	0.3
Tomato & Basil, Safeway*	½ Pot/285g	137	48	0.8	5.9	2.3	0.8
Tomato & Basil, Soup-a-Slim, Asda*	1 Sachet/16g	52	326	7.0	70.0	2.0	3.9
Tomato & Basil, Thick & Creamy, Batchelors*	1 Serving/281g	104	37	0.5	6.7	0.9	0.6
Tomato & Basil, Vie Country, Knorr*	1 Pack/500ml	145	29	0.8	5.5	0.4	0.9
Tomato & Basil, Waitrose*	1 Serving/300ml	123	41	0.6	4.5	2.3	0.6
Tomato & Brown Lentil, Baxters*	1 Can/425g	166	39	2.4	8.7	0.1	1.5
Tomato & Butterbean, Baxters*	1 Can/425g	234	55	2.0	8.8	1.3	1.8
Tomato & Herb, Campbell's*	1 Carton/500ml	180	36	1.0	5.0	1.3	0.0
Tomato & Herb, Marks & Spencer*	1oz/28g	20	72	1.3	7.9	4.0	0.4
Tomato & Lentil, Heinz*	1 Can/400g	216	54	2.7	10.4	0.2	1.0
Tomato & Lentil, Marks & Spencer*	½ Can/211.1g	95	45	2.3	8.4	0.2	1.5
Tomato & Orange, Baxters*	1 Can/425g	183	43	1.1	8.4	0.5	0.5
Tomato & Orange, Healthy Eating, Tesco*	1 Pack/400g	132	33	0.6	7.1	0.2	0.4
Tomato & Red Pepper, Campbell's*	1 Can/590g	366	62	0.5	7.7	3.3	0.0
Tomato & Red Pepper, Soupreme*	1 Serving/250ml	90	36	1.1	5.7	1.0	1.7
Tomato & Red Pepper, Weight Watchers*	1 Serving/205g	25	12	0.4	2.5	0.1	0.4
Tomato & Spinach, Organic, Waitrose*	1 Serving/300g	126	42	1.4	4.9	1.9	0.7
Tomato & Three Bean, BGTY, Sainsbury's*	1 Can/400g	216	54	2.9	8.5	0.9	0.8
Tomato & Vegetable, Cup A Soup, Batchelors*	1 Serving/218g	107	49	1.1	8.5	1.2	0.6
Tomato & Vegetable, Cup, Soupreme*	1 Sachet/24g	87	361	6.0	64.6	8.7	1.4
Tomato, 99% Fat Free, Campbell's*	1 Can/200g	88	44	0.7	8.0	1.0	0.0
Tomato, Aubergine & Grilled Pepper, NCGSC*	½ Carton/300g	48	16	0.6	1.9	0.7	0.7
Tomato, Creme Fraiche & Basil, The Best, Safeway*	1/3 Pot/200g	130	65	1.0	5.0	4.2	1.0
Tomato, Cup A Soup, Batchelors*	1 Serving/212g	85	40	0.4	8.1	0.7	0.6
Tomato, Fresh Country, New Covent Garden Soup Co*	½ Pint/284ml	114	40	1.9	6.4	0.8	0.8
Tomato, Fresh, Tesco*	1 Serving/100g	44	44	0.7	5.2	2.3	0.4
Tomato, In A Cup, Tesco*	1 Serving/23g	75	328	6.4	68.5	3.2	0.1
Tomato, In a Cup, Symingtons*	1 Sachet/31.5g	99	308	3.5	62.0	5.0	3.8
Tomato, Mixed Bean & Vegetable, Chunky, Sainsbury's*	1 Can/400g	232	58	2.2	11.5	0.3	1.6
Tomato, Onion & Basil, GFY, Asda*	1 Can/400g	116	29	0.8	5.0	0.6	0.3
Tomato, Pasta & Basil Cup, Good Intentions, Somerfield*	1 Serving/26g	92	355	5.4	69.1	6.3	5.1
Tomato, Pepper & Basil, Safeway*	1 Can/415.4g	162	39	0.9	4.8	1.7	1.8

S

	Measure INFO/WEIGHT	per Measure KCAL	Nutrition Values per 100g / 100ml				
			KCAL	PROT	CARB	FAT	FIBRE
SOUP,							
Tomato, Weight Watchers*	1 Can/295g	74	25	0.7	4.6	0.5	0.3
Tuscan Bean, Good for You, Asda*	1 Carton/400ml	224	56	2.9	9.0	0.9	0.8
Tuscan Bean, New Covent Garden Soup Co*	½ Carton/300g	171	57	3.9	8.8	0.7	2.4
Tuscan Bean, Organic, Sainsbury's*	1 Pack/400g	148	37	2.2	5.2	0.8	1.3
Tuscan Bean, Perfectly Balanced, Waitrose*	½ Pot/300g	147	49	2.0	6.1	1.8	1.8
Vegetable & Beef, Sainsbury's*	1 Can/400g	260	65	2.1	8.5	2.5	1.3
Vegetable & Lentil, Fresh, Somerfield*	½ Pack/300g	183	61	2.7	8.4	1.9	1.5
Vegetable Broth, Healthy Eating, Tesco*	1 Can/400g	148	37	1.2	7.4	0.2	1.0
Vegetable Broth, Marks & Spencer*	1 Pack/213g	85	40	1.0	6.3	1.4	0.8
Vegetable Chowder, New Covent Garden Soup Co*	½ Carton/300g	159	53	2.9	6.6	1.7	1.1
Vegetable, 99% Fat Free, Watties*	1 Serving/105g	30	29	0.8	5.9	0.2	0.8
Vegetable, Bean & Pasta, Organic, Baxters*	1 Can/415g	212	51	2.2	8.7	0.8	1.4
Vegetable, Chunky, Simply Organic*	1 Pot/500g	200	40	1.6	5.3	1.4	1.4
Vegetable, Condensed, Campbell's*	1 Can/295g	103	35	0.8	6.2	0.8	0.0
Vegetable, Cup, Soupreme*	1 Sachet/26g	111	444	8.1	49.7	23.6	2.3
Vegetable, Extra Thick, Sainsbury's*	1 Can/400g	176	44	1.6	8.0	0.6	1.3
Vegetable, Fresh, Co-Op*	1 Pack/600g	150	25	0.6	4.0	1.0	1.0
Vegetable, Heinz*	1 Can/400g	188	47	1.4	8.4	0.9	1.1
Vegetable, In A Cup, BGTY, Sainsbury's*	1 Sachet/200g	52	26	0.5	4.4	0.8	0.9
Vegetable, In A Mug, Healthy Eating, Tesco*	1 Mug/18g	66	365	7.0	66.3	8.0	2.6
Vegetable, New Covent Garden Soup Co*	½ Pint/284ml	88	31	1.1	5.9	0.4	1.1
Vegetable, Safeway*	1 Can/295g	109	37	1.5	7.1	0.3	1.2
Vegetable, Sainsbury's*	1 Can/400g	184	46	1.5	8.3	0.7	1.2
Vegetable, Soup-a-Cups, Asda*	1 Sachet/200ml	59	30	0.7	5.5	0.6	0.5
Vegetable, Tesco*	½ Can/200g	88	44	1.3	9.3	0.2	1.0
Vegetable, Vie Country, Knorr*	1 Pack/500ml	160	32	0.9	5.5	0.7	1.2
Vegetable, Weight Watchers*	1 Serving/295ml	83	28	0.9	5.6	0.2	0.8
Wild Mushroom & Maderia, Finest, Tesco*	1 Serving/300g	156	52	1.4	5.0	2.9	0.3
Wild Mushroom & Porcini Pieces, BGTY, Sainsbury's*	1 Serving/196.4g	55	28	0.5	4.7	0.8	0.6
Wild Mushroom in a Cup, BGTY, Sainsbury's*	1 Serving/200ml	56	28	0.5	4.7	0.8	0.6
Wild Mushroom, Fresh, Tesco*	1 Serving/300g	159	53	1.3	4.7	3.2	0.3
Winter Vegetable & Lentil, New Covent Garden Soup Co*	1 Serving/300g	243	81	5.1	12.0	1.4	2.6
Winter Warmer, New Covent Garden Soup Co*	1 Serving/300g	180	60	2.5	10.5	0.9	2.3
Won Ton, Blue Dragon*	1 Can/410g	62	15	1.4	2.1	0.1	0.0
SOYA,							
Bolognese Style, Sainsbury's*	½ Pack/168g	113	67	3.1	13.9	0.7	2.7
Mince, Dry Weight, Sainsbury's*	1 Serving/50g	164	328	47.2	33.2	0.8	3.6
Mince, Granules	1oz/28g	74	263	43.2	11.0	5.4	0.0
Mince, Organic*	1oz/28g	101	359	46.0	28.0	7.0	0.0
Mince, Unflavoured, Nature's Harvest*	1 serving/100g	345	345	50.0	35.0	1.0	4.0
Protein Powder, Holland & Barrett*	1oz/28g	109	390	88.0	0.5	4.0	0.0
SPACE RAIDERS,							
Beef Flavour, Corn & Wheat Snacks, Space Raiders*	1 Pack/17g	82	482	8.3	61.0	22.7	2.6
Cheese, Space Raiders*	1 Bag/16g	76	473	7.1	61.6	22.0	3.1
Pickled Onion, Space Raiders*	1 Bag/16g	74	461	7.0	61.4	20.8	3.4
Salt & Vinegar, Space Raiders*	1 Bag/16.9g	81	478	6.9	61.7	22.6	2.2
SPAGHETTI,							
Authentic Italian, Tesco*	1 Serving/100g	345	345	13.2	68.5	2.0	2.9
Buitoni*	1 Serving/150g	543	362	12.2	74.4	1.7	0.0
Cooked, Sainsbury's	1 Serving/240g	322	134	4.6	27.4	0.6	1.0
Dried, Safeway*	1 Serving/60g	209	348	13.2	70.1	1.7	2.9
Dried, Spar*	1 Serving/100g	346	346	12.0	71.0	1.6	0.0
Durum Wheat, Seeds Of Change*	1 Serving/75g	263	350	11.5	75.0	0.3	0.0

	Measure INFO/WEIGHT	per Measure KCAL	Nutrition Values per 100g / 100ml KCAL	PROT	CARB	FAT	FIBRE
SPAGHETTI,							
Durum Wheat, Tesco*	1oz/28g	97	345	13.2	68.5	0.4	2.9
Egg, Fresh, Italiano, Tesco*	½ Pack/125g	360	288	11.9	51.8	3.7	1.5
Egg, Fresh, Waitrose*	¼ Pack/125g	361	289	11.4	53.1	3.4	2.1
Faster, Asda*	1 Serving/50g	173	346	12.0	71.0	1.5	3.0
Happy Shopper*	1 Serving/75g	259	345	12.0	72.0	1.0	3.0
In Tomato Sauce With Parsley, Weight Watchers*	1 Can/400g	196	49	1.8	10.0	0.2	0.6
In Tomato Sauce, Asda*	1 Serving/200g	122	61	1.7	13.0	0.2	0.5
In Tomato Sauce, HP*	1 Can/410g	247	60	1.5	13.1	0.2	0.4
In Tomato Sauce, Heinz*	1 Can/400g	244	61	1.7	13.0	0.2	0.5
In Tomato Sauce, Organic, Sainsbury's*	½ Can/205g	133	65	1.8	13.9	0.2	1.0
In Tomato Sauce, Sainsbury's*	1 Can/410g	262	64	1.9	13.3	0.4	0.5
In Tomato Sauce, Tesco*	1 Can/410g	246	60	1.6	12.9	0.2	0.5
In Tomato Sauce, Value, Tesco*	½ Can/205g	131	64	1.9	13.3	0.4	0.5
In Tomato Sauce, Wholewheat, Sainsbury's*	1 Serving/205g	125	61	2.0	11.9	0.6	1.1
Italian, Sainsbury's*	1 Serving/100g	357	357	12.3	73.1	1.7	2.5
Long, Buitoni*	1 Serving/50g	176	352	11.2	72.6	1.9	0.0
Quick Cook, Sainsbury's*	1 Serving/50g	179	357	12.3	73.1	1.7	2.5
Quick Cook, Tesco*	1 Serving/50g	173	345	13.2	68.5	2.0	2.9
Raw, Somerfield*	1 Serving/75g	261	348	12.5	69.9	2.0	3.5
Safeway*	1oz/28g	95	338	13.2	67.3	1.8	2.9
Sainsbury's*	1 Serving/92g	318	346	12.0	72.2	1.0	2.3
Short, Dry, Napolina*	1oz/28g	99	352	11.5	73.0	1.5	2.2
Strands, Tesco*	1oz/28g	97	345	13.2	68.5	2.0	2.9
Whole Wheat, Asda*	1 Serving/90g	291	323	14.0	60.0	3.0	10.0
Wholewheat, Co-Op*	1 Pack/500g	1600	320	14.0	60.0	3.0	8.0
Wholewheat, Dry, Safeway*	1 Serving/75g	241	321	14.4	60.2	2.5	8.4
Wholewheat, Italian, Sainsbury's*	1 Serving/100g	316	316	12.7	61.9	2.0	10.0
Wholewheat, Morrisons*	1 Serving/75g	272	362	12.5	71.2	2.5	0.0
Wholewheat, Organic, Sainsbury's*	1 Serving/90g	284	316	12.7	61.9	2.0	10.0
Wholewheat, Sainsbury's*	1oz/28g	92	330	13.3	61.9	3.2	9.3
Wholewheat, Tesco*	1oz/28g	90	321	14.4	60.2	2.5	8.4
With Sausages, Heinz*	1 Can/400g	328	82	3.7	11.0	2.6	0.5
With Tomato & Cheese, Tesco*	½ Pack/250g	280	112	4.0	18.1	2.6	1.1
SPAGHETTI & MEATBALLS,							
American, Superbowl, Asda*	1 Pack/453.4g	593	131	11.0	13.0	3.9	1.1
BGTY, Sainsbury's*	1 Pack/300g	249	83	5.9	12.7	0.9	3.1
Chicken in Tomato Sauce, Heinz*	1 Can/400g	352	88	4.1	11.0	3.0	0.5
Italian, Sainsbury's*	1 Pack/450g	495	110	5.0	11.9	4.7	2.7
Sainsbury's*	1 Serving/260g	226	87	5.7	12.6	1.5	1.5
Somerfield*	1 Pack/900g	1035	115	5.0	15.0	4.0	0.0
Vegetarian, Safeway*	1 Pack/350g	382	109	5.0	13.7	3.8	0.5
SPAGHETTI BOLOGNESE,							
Al Forno, Sainsbury's*	1 Pack/400g	460	115	7.8	10.0	4.9	1.1
Asda*	1 Pack/400g	388	97	5.0	17.0	1.0	0.9
BGTY, Sainsbury's*	1 Pack/450g	392	87	4.7	14.8	1.0	1.1
Bird's Eye*	1 Pack/362g	404	112	4.8	13.4	4.4	0.9
COU, Marks & Spencer*	1 Pack/359g	395	110	6.5	17.3	1.5	1.1
Canned, Asda*	½ Can/205g	174	85	4.2	10.7	2.8	0.6
Canned, Garlini, Aldi*	1 Can/410g	324	79	3.7	10.2	2.6	1.2
Co-Op*	1 Pack/300g	285	95	4.0	11.0	4.0	1.0
Cost Cutter*	1 Pack/600g	504	84	5.7	11.2	1.9	0.9
Eat Smart, Safeway*	1 Pack/393g	350	89	5.9	13.1	1.4	1.3
Finest, Tesco*	1 Pack/400g	548	137	9.5	12.3	5.5	1.2

S

INFO/WEIGHT	Measure	per Measure KCAL	Nutrition Values per 100g / 100ml				
			KCAL	PROT	CARB	FAT	FIBRE

SPAGHETTI BOLOGNESE,

	INFO/WEIGHT	KCAL	KCAL	PROT	CARB	FAT	FIBRE
Flavour, Sainsbury's*	1 Serving/233g	231	99	2.9	19.1	1.2	2.1
GFY, Asda*	1 Serving/250g	220	88	5.0	13.0	1.8	0.7
HP*	1 Pack/410g	312	76	3.8	11.3	1.9	0.7
Healthy Choice, Iceland*	1 Pack/400g	428	107	6.8	17.8	1.0	1.1
Healthy Eating, Tesco*	1 Pack/340g	326	96	5.3	13.7	2.2	1.5
Heinz*	1 Can/400g	344	86	3.4	12.8	2.3	0.7
In Tomato & Beef Sauce, Carlini, Aldi*	1 Can/410g	324	79	3.7	10.2	2.6	1.2
Italia, Marks & Spencer*	1 Pack/400g	600	150	8.8	14.0	6.3	1.1
Italiano, Pro-Cuisine*	1 Pack/600g	522	87	5.7	11.7	1.9	0.0
Italiano, Tesco*	1 Pack/340g	367	108	9.8	9.8	3.3	1.3
Lean Cuisine, Findus*	1 Pack/320g	275	86	4.5	11.5	2.3	1.1
Loved by Kids, Marks & Spencer*	½ Pack/200g	250	125	6.6	15.3	4.4	1.9
Meat Free, Heinz*	1 Serving/200g	162	81	3.3	13.1	1.7	0.6
Meat Free, Sainsbury's*	1 Can/400g	280	70	3.4	12.0	0.9	1.2
Morrisons*	1 Pack/300g	306	102	5.8	12.2	3.3	1.4
Perfectly Balanced, Waitrose*	1 Pack/350g	319	91	4.2	10.0	3.8	1.0
Quick Pasta, Sainsbury's*	1 Serving/63g	231	367	10.8	71.0	4.4	3.3
Quorn*	1 Pack/400g	292	73	5.7	9.4	1.4	2.4
Quorn, Sainsbury's*	1 Pack/450g	347	77	4.9	11.9	1.1	1.8
Ready Meals, Marks & Spencer*	1 Pack/360g	576	160	8.8	12.7	8.1	1.2
Safeway*	1 Pack/650g	780	120	9.5	13.1	3.3	1.7
Sainsbury's*	1 Pack/300g	237	79	4.9	10.5	1.9	0.9
Smartprice, Asda*	½ Can/205g	215	105	3.2	12.0	4.9	0.8
Somerfield*	1 Pack/300g	339	113	5.3	18.0	2.2	2.0
Spar*	1 Pack/500g	440	88	5.6	8.6	3.5	1.5
Tesco*	1 Pack/257g	339	132	6.5	14.1	5.5	1.2
Value, Tesco*	1 Pack/300g	294	98	5.2	11.8	3.3	0.5
Vegetarian, Tesco*	1 Pack/340g	374	110	5.1	13.7	3.9	1.2
Weight Watchers*	1 Pack/320g	301	94	5.8	14.6	1.3	1.0

SPAGHETTI CARBONARA,

	INFO/WEIGHT	KCAL	KCAL	PROT	CARB	FAT	FIBRE
COU, Marks & Spencer*	1 Pack/330g	347	105	5.7	15.5	2.0	1.8
Cappelletti, Balanced Lifestyle, Carlini, Aldi*	1 Can/400g	328	82	4.1	10.0	2.8	0.6
GFY, Asda*	1 Pack/365g	460	126	4.4	20.0	3.2	0.7
Good For You, Asda*	1 Pack/120g	151	126	4.4	20.0	3.2	0.7
Italian Express*	1 Pack/320g	310	97	4.3	11.6	3.7	1.1
Italiano, Tesco*	1 Pack/450g	702	156	6.9	14.8	7.7	1.7
Marks & Spencer*	1 Pack/360g	630	175	7.6	14.3	9.5	0.1
Quorn*	1 Pack/400g	460	115	5.0	9.1	6.5	1.1
Safeway*	1 Pack/360g	569	158	7.9	15.7	7.1	1.2
Sainsbury's*	1 Pack/450g	558	124	7.3	14.2	4.2	0.9
Tesco*	1 Pack/450g	612	136	5.9	15.2	5.7	1.3

SPAGHETTI HOOPS,

	INFO/WEIGHT	KCAL	KCAL	PROT	CARB	FAT	FIBRE
'N' Hot Dogs, Heinz*	1 Can/400g	304	76	2.8	11.0	2.4	0.4
In Tomato Sauce, Heinz*	1 Can/400g	224	56	1.9	11.7	0.2	0.6
Tesco*	½ Can/205g	123	60	1.6	12.9	0.2	0.5
SPAGHETTI LOOPS, SmartPrice Asda*	1 Serving/205g	127	62	1.7	13.0	0.3	0.4

SPARE RIBS,

	INFO/WEIGHT	KCAL	KCAL	PROT	CARB	FAT	FIBRE
American Style, Somerfield*	½ Pack/125g	303	242	18.8	15.6	11.6	1.8
Cantonese, Sainsbury's*	1 Serving/300g	633	211	18.1	10.3	10.8	0.4
Chinese Style, Asda*	1 Serving/300g	642	214	20.0	11.0	10.0	0.8
Chinese Style, Safeway*	½ Pack/285g	633	222	16.5	16.1	10.2	2.1
Chinese, Iceland*	1oz/28g	61	219	14.7	9.6	13.5	0.2
Chinese, Somerfield*	1oz/28g	70	251	14.0	13.0	16.0	0.0

INFO/WEIGHT	Measure	per Measure KCAL	KCAL	PROT	CARB	FAT	FIBRE
SPARE RIBS,							
Marks & Spencer*	1oz/28g	57	205	16.6	8.6	11.5	0.2
Mini, Ready Meals, Marks & Spencer*	1oz/28g	57	205	16.6	8.6	11.5	0.2
Raw, Lean & Fat	1oz/28g	55	195	18.7	0.0	13.4	0.0
Sweet Chinese Style, Co-Op*	1 Pack/250g	553	221	13.9	15.9	11.3	0.8
SPICE BLEND,							
Balti, Sharwood's*	1oz/28g	34	122	1.8	7.1	9.6	1.2
Thai, Sharwood's*	1 Pack 260g	424	163	1.8	12.0	11.9	1.0
Tikka, Sharwood's*	1 Pack/260g	263	101	2.7	10.2	5.4	1.7
SPICE MIX,							
Chicken Tikka Masala & Pilau Rice, Colman's*	1 Pack/85g	309	364	11.5	39.9	18.0	11.2
Chili Mix for Chilli, Schwartz*	1oz/28g	96	344	9.6	63.6	5.7	1.0
Chilli & Garlic Seed, The Food Doctor*	1 Serving/15g	88	584	30.5	3.7	49.7	11.0
Chilli Con Carne, Colman's*	1 Pack/50g	154	308	8.6	62.0	1.7	0.0
Chilli Con Carne, Hot, Schwartz*	1 Pack/41g	141	344	10.8	59.0	7.2	0.0
Green Thai Chicken Curry, Schwartz*	1 Pack/41g	137	334	11.3	67.6	3.2	0.3
Mexican Chili Potato Wedges, Schwartz*	1oz/28g	45	162	3.4	26.1	4.9	0.0
Nacho Cheese Wedges, Schwartz*	1 Serving/10g	15	153	3.6	20.8	6.2	2.0
SPINACH,							
& Carrot Pilau, Waitrose*	1oz/28g	44	158	5.8	22.9	5.8	0.0
Baby Leaf, Organic, Sainsbury's*	1 Serving/90g	23	25	2.8	1.6	0.8	2.1
Baby, Waitrose*	1 Serving/110g	28	25	2.8	1.6	0.8	2.1
Boiled in Salted Water	1oz/28g	5	19	2.2	0.8	0.8	2.1
Boiled in Unsalted Water	1oz/28g	5	19	2.2	0.8	0.8	2.1
Canned, Drained	1oz/28g	5	19	2.8	0.8	0.5	1.6
Chopped, Sainsbury's*	1 Serving/100g	22	22	3.1	0.5	0.8	2.1
Creamed, Marks & Spencer*	½ Pack/150g	270	180	2.8	5.4	16.2	2.4
Frozen, Boiled in Unsalted Water	1oz/28g	6	21	3.1	0.5	0.8	2.1
Leaf in Water, Salt Added, Tinned, Sainsbury's*, Drained	1 Can/185g	44	24	4.1	1.1	0.4	5.1
Leaf, Fresh, Frozen, Tesco*	1 Block/25g	6	24	2.8	1.5	0.8	2.1
Leaf, Fresh, Tesco*	1 Serving/75g	19	25	2.8	1.6	0.8	2.1
Leaf, Iceland*	1 Serving/100g	21	21	3.1	0.5	0.8	2.1
Leaf, In Brine, Tesco*	1 Can/265g	66	25	2.2	3.4	0.3	3.0
Raw	1oz/28g	7	25	2.8	1.6	0.8	2.1
Steamed, Tesco*	1oz/28g	7	25	2.8	1.6	0.8	2.1
SPIRA, Cadbury's*	2 Twists/40g	210	525	7.8	56.8	29.4	0.0
SPIRALI,							
Dried, Sainsbury's*	1 Serving/50g	179	357	12.3	73.1	1.7	2.5
Tubes, Bolognese, Fresh, Asda*	1 Serving/250g	265	106	4.7	12.0	4.4	0.6
SPIRALS,							
Co-Op*	1 Serving/100g	350	350	12.0	73.0	1.0	3.0
Glutenfree, Glutano*	1oz/28g	100	357	4.0	83.0	1.0	0.0
SPIRITS,							
37.5% Volume	1 Shot/25ml	48	207	0.0	0.0	0.0	0.0
40% Volume	1 Shot/25ml	51	222	0.0	0.0	0.0	0.0
SPLIT PEAS,							
Dried, Boiled in Unsalted Water	1oz/28g	35	126	8.3	22.7	0.9	2.7
Dried, Raw	1oz/28g	92	328	22.1	58.2	2.4	6.3
Yellow, Organic, Evernat*	1oz/28g	87	310	22.1	56.6	1.0	0.0
SPONGE FINGERS,							
Boudoir, Sainsbury's*	1 Biscuit/5g	20	396	8.1	82.8	3.6	0.4
Tesco*	1 Finger/5g	19	386	7.6	80.6	3.7	1.0
SPONGE PUDDING,							
Banoffee, Heinz*	¼ Can/78g	239	307	2.8	46.6	12.2	0.6

S

SPONGE PUDDING,

	Measure INFO/WEIGHT	per Measure KCAL	KCAL	PROT	CARB	FAT	FIBRE
Banoffee, Morrisons*	1 Pudding/109g	316	287	3.0	59.6	2.9	0.7
Blackberry & Apple, Healthy Eating, Tesco*	1 Pot/102.5g	159	155	3.1	32.6	1.4	0.7
Blackcurrant, BGTY, Sainsbury's*	1 Serving/110g	277	252	2.8	50.0	4.5	1.4
Blackcurrant, Low Fat, Iceland*	1 Pudding/90g	159	177	2.2	39.5	1.1	1.6
Canned	1 Portion/75g	214	285	3.1	45.4	11.4	0.8
Caramel Chocolate, Heinz*	1 Serving/67g	255	381	3.5	52.3	16.9	0.6
Cherry & Almond Flavour, Sainsbury's*	¼ Pudding/110g	334	304	3.5	40.3	14.3	0.7
Cherry & Chocolate, Eat Smart, Safeway*	1 Serving/86g	151	175	2.7	35.6	2.4	0.8
Chocolate & Chocolate Sauce, Healthy Eating, Tesco*	1 Pudding/90g	186	207	3.9	38.7	4.1	2.1
Chocolate & Sauce, Co-Op*	1 Pack/225g	608	270	5.0	34.0	13.0	0.6
Chocolate Chip, Healthy Eating, Tesco*	1 Serving/103g	197	191	4.4	34.7	3.8	0.9
Chocolate Custard, Muller*	1 Pot/175g	305	174	3.4	31.0	4.0	0.0
Chocolate, Good For You, Asda*	1 Pudding/105g	252	240	5.0	46.0	4.0	2.3
Chocolate, Healthy Eating, Tesco*	1 Pudding/90g	184	204	4.2	45.4	0.6	1.3
Chocolate, Heinz*	1 Serving/50g	150	300	4.8	45.0	11.2	1.2
Chocolate, Marks & Spencer*	¼ Pudding/131g	524	400	6.1	38.6	24.6	1.8
Chocolate, Somerfield*	¼ Pudding/100g	369	369	5.0	35.0	23.0	0.0
Circus, & Custard, Weight Watchers*	1 Serving/140g	239	171	4.2	32.1	2.9	0.9
Citrus, BGTY, Sainsbury's*	1 Pudding/110g	230	209	3.5	39.7	4.0	0.7
Double Chocolate, BGTY, Sainsbury's*	1 Pot/110g	293	266	4.3	51.5	4.7	0.6
Fruit, Co-Op*	1 Can/300g	1110	370	3.0	53.0	16.0	2.0
Fruits Of The Forest, Asda*	1 Pudding/115g	323	281	2.8	59.0	3.8	1.3
Ginger, With Plum Sauce, Waitrose*	1 Pudding/120g	424	353	3.1	51.7	14.9	0.7
Ginger, With Vanilla Custard, PB, Waitrose*	1 Serving/120g	259	216	3.5	43.1	3.3	1.9
Golden Syrup, Co-Op*	1 Can/300g	945	315	2.0	47.0	13.0	0.6
Jam & Custard, Co-Op*	1 Pack/244g	598	245	3.0	37.0	9.0	0.3
Jam & Custard, Somerfield*	¼ Pudding/62g	143	231	3.0	38.0	8.0	0.0
Jam Custard, Muller*	1 Pot/175g	291	166	2.7	30.1	3.9	0.0
Jam, Safeway*	1 Serving/110g	396	360	3.6	55.6	13.7	2.3
Lemon Curd, Heinz*	¼ Can/78g	236	302	2.6	46.7	11.7	0.6
Lemon, COU, Marks & Spencer*	1 Pudding/100g	157	157	2.0	32.1	2.3	1.9
Lemon, Healthy Eating, Tesco*	1 Pudding/102g	195	191	3.7	40.1	2.0	0.5
Lemon, Marks & Spencer*	1 Pudding/105g	326	310	4.3	39.4	15.2	2.3
Lemon, Waitrose*	1 Serving/105g	212	202	3.4	41.7	2.4	1.4
St Clements, Good For You, Asda*	1 Pudding/116g	332	286	2.6	60.0	3.9	1.2
Sticky Toffee Custard, Muller*	1 Pot/175g	306	175	2.8	29.1	5.3	0.0
Sticky Toffee, COU, Marks & Spencer*	1 Pack/150g	240	160	2.4	33.7	1.7	1.6
Sticky Toffee, Heinz*	¼ Can/77g	235	305	3.1	45.2	12.5	0.7
Sticky Toffee, Mini, Somerfield*	1 Pudding/110g	349	349	3.0	54.0	13.0	0.0
Sticky Toffee, Somerfield*	1 Pudding/440g	1456	364	3.0	56.0	14.0	0.0
Strawberry Jam, Heinz*	¼ Can/82g	230	281	2.6	50.4	7.6	0.6
Strawberry, Co-Op*	1 Can/300g	960	320	2.0	48.0	13.0	0.8
Summer Fruits, BGTY, Sainsbury's*	1 Serving/110g	243	221	2.7	42.9	4.3	1.0
Syrup & Custard, Morrisons*	1 Serving/125g	290	232	3.4	39.1	6.9	0.8
Syrup, & Custard, Iceland*	1 Pudding/130g	410	315	3.6	38.8	16.2	0.4
Syrup, BGTY, Sainsbury's*	1 Pudding/110g	338	307	2.8	64.6	4.1	0.4
Syrup, Good For You, Asda*	1 Sponge/105g	256	244	3.0	50.0	3.6	0.6
Syrup, Sainsbury's*	¼ Pudding/110g	404	371	2.7	63.5	11.8	0.4
Treacle, With Custard, Farmfoods*	1 Serving/145g	539	372	3.2	38.4	22.8	0.8
Very Fruity Cherry, Marks & Spencer*	1 Pot/110g	286	260	3.5	38.6	10.3	1.8
SPOTTED DICK, Average	1oz/28g	92	327	4.2	42.7	16.7	1.0
SPRATS,							
Fried	1oz/28g	116	415	24.9	0.0	35.0	0.0

S

	Measure INFO/WEIGHT	per Measure KCAL	Nutrition Values per 100g / 100ml				
			KCAL	PROT	CARB	FAT	FIBRE
SPRATS,							
Raw	1oz/28g	48	172	18.3	0.0	11.0	0.0
SPREAD,							
63% Fat, Benecol*	1 Serving/12g	69	573	0.6	1.0	63.0	0.0
Blackcurrant, Weight Watchers*	1 Tsp/5.7g	6	106	0.2	26.3	0.0	0.9
Butter & Olive, Olivio*	Thin Spread/7g	38	536	0.5	0.7	59.0	0.0
Butterlicious, Sainsbury's*	Thin Spread/7g	44	628	0.6	1.1	69.0	0.1
Buttery Gold, Somerfield*	1 Tbsp/15g	94	627	0.5	1.0	69.0	0.0
Buttery Taste, Benecol*	1 Tsp/7g	40	573	0.6	1.0	63.0	0.0
Chocolate Hazelnut, Tesco*	1 Tsp/10g	54	542	7.0	50.8	34.5	3.7
Diet, Delight*	1oz/28g	64	228	3.6	1.6	23.0	0.0
Fat, Carapelli, St Ivel*	Thin Spread/7g	38	537	0.6	0.8	59.0	0.0
Flora Buttery, Flora*	Thin Spread/7g	45	637	1.1	0.5	70.0	0.0
Flora Diet Light, Flora*	1 Tbsp/10g	23	227	3.5	1.6	23.0	0.0
Flora Light, Flora*	1oz/28g	100	357	0.1	3.7	38.0	0.6
Flora Original, Flora*	1 Serving/10g	63	630	0.1	0.1	70.0	0.0
Flora Pro-Activ, Flora*	1 Serving/10g	33	328	0.1	3.2	35.0	0.3
Flora, Low Salt, Flora*	1oz/28g	176	630	0.1	0.1	70.0	0.0
From Soya, Kallo*	1 Tsp/7g	27	380	7.0	6.0	37.0	0.0
Gold, Low Fat, St Ivel*	Thin Spread/7g	26	365	2.1	2.9	38.0	0.0
Gold, Lowest, Low Fat, St Ivel*	Thin Spread/7g	18	259	0.7	3.3	27.0	0.0
Gold, Semi Skimmed, St Ivel*	1 Serving/5g	18	359	0.9	3.3	38.0	0.0
Gold, Unsalted, Low Fat, St Ivel*	Thin Spread/7g	25	360	0.7	3.9	38.0	0.0
Golden, Light, Healthy Eating, Tesco*	1 Serving/10g	35	354	1.5	1.5	38.0	0.0
Hazelnut & Chocolate, Organic, Green & Black's*	1 Serving/28g	155	553	5.9	53.0	35.0	0.0
Light, Benecol*	2 Tsp/12g	38	318	2.8	0.2	34.0	0.0
Light, Olivio*	Thin Soread/7g	34	486	0.0	0.0	55.0	0.0
Low Fat 32%, Benecol*	1 Serving/12g	36	300	2.8	0.2	32.0	0.0
Low-Fat	Thin Spread/7g	27	390	5.8	0.5	40.5	0.0
Morning Gold, Low Fat, Morrisons*	1 Tbsp/15g	56	372	7.5	0.0	38.0	0.0
Olive Gold, Reduced Fat, Co-Op*	1oz/28g	150	535	0.2	1.0	59.0	0.0
Olive Gold, With Olive Oil, Low Fat, Asda*	1 Serving/10g	54	537	0.2	1.2	59.0	0.0
Olive Light, Low Fat, BGTY, Sainsbury's*	Thin Spread/ 7g	25	356	2.0	1.5	38.0	0.0
Olive Light, Low Fat, Tesco*	1 Serving/15g	52	348	1.5	0.0	38.0	0.0
Olive Light, Safeway*	1 Tsp/10g	35	346	1.0	0.0	38.0	0.0
Olive Oil, 55% Reduced Fat, Benecol*	Thin Spread/7g	35	498	0.3	0.5	55.0	0.0
Olive Oil, 59% Reduced Fat, Safeway*	Thin Spread/7g	37	532	0.1	0.1	59.0	0.0
Olive Oil, 59% Vegetable Fat, Olivio*	Thin Spread/7g	38	536	0.2	1.0	59.0	0.0
Olive, BGTY, Sainsbury's*	1 Tsp/14g	50	356	2.0	1.5	38.0	0.0
Olive, Marks & Spencer*	Thin Soread/7g	38	536	0.2	1.2	59.0	0.0
Olive, Reduced Fat, Asda*	Thin Spread/7g	38	537	0.2	1.2	59.0	0.0
Olive, Reduced Fat, Morrisons*	Thin Spread/7g	38	537	0.9	0.0	59.3	0.3
Olive, Reduced Fat, Organic, Sainsbury's*	Thin Spread/7g	37	531	0.0	0.0	59.0	0.0
Olive, Reduced Fat, Sainsbury's*	1 Serving/10g	54	536	0.1	1.2	59.0	0.0
Olive, Tesco*	1 Serving/28g	150	537	0.2	1.2	59.0	0.0
Olivio, Van Den Bergh Foods Ltd*	Thin Spread/7g	38	536	0.2	1.0	59.0	0.0
Olivite, Low Fat, Weight Watchers*	Thin Spread/7g	25	351	0.0	0.2	38.9	0.0
Pure Gold, Good for You, Asda*	1 Serving/10g	35	353	1.7	1.0	38.0	0.0
Pure Gold, Light, 65% Less Fat, Asda*	1 Serving/10g	24	239	2.5	1.0	25.0	0.0
Soft, Dairy Free, Free From, Sainsbury's*	1 Serving/30g	89	296	2.5	4.0	30.0	0.0
Soft, Economy, Sainsbury's*	1oz/28g	126	450	0.2	1.0	50.0	0.0
Sunflower, Asda*	1 Serving/10g	64	635	0.2	1.0	70.0	0.0
Sunflower, Co-Op*	Thin Spread/7g	44	635	0.2	1.0	70.0	0.0
Sunflower, Light, 38% Less Fat, Asda*	Thin Spread/7g	24	342	0.0	0.0	38.0	0.0

S

	Measure INFO/WEIGHT	per Measure KCAL	Nutrition Values per 100g / 100ml KCAL	PROT	CARB	FAT	FIBRE
SPREAD,							
Sunflower, Light, BGTY, Sainsbury's*	1 Serving/10g	35	352	1.0	1.5	38.0	0.0
Sunflower, Light, Better For You, Morrisons*	1 Tsp/5g	17	342	0.0	0.0	38.0	0.0
Sunflower, Light, Good For You, Asda*	1 Serving/10g	35	351	0.0	0.0	39.0	0.0
Sunflower, Light, Healthy Eating, Tesco*	1 Serving/6g	21	347	0.3	1.0	38.0	0.0
Sunflower, Light, Summerlite, Aldi*	1 Serving/10g	34	344	0.2	0.3	38.0	0.0
Sunflower, Light, Tesco*	Thin Spread/7g	24	348	1.4	0.0	38.0	0.0
Sunflower, Low Fat, Good Intentions, Somerfield*	1 Serving/10g	35	347	0.0	0.0	38.6	0.0
Sunflower, Low Fat, Marks & Spencer*	1 Serving/14g	48	342	0.0	0.0	38.0	1.0
Sunflower, Low Fat, Somerfield*	1 Serving/10g	34	342	0.0	0.0	38.0	0.0
Sunflower, Lowest, Healthy Eating, Tesco*	Thin Spread/7g	8	109	2.0	14.0	5.0	10.0
Sunflower, Marks & Spencer*	Thin Spread/7g	44	635	0.2	1.0	70.0	0.0
Sunflower, Reduced Fat, Asda*	Thin Spread/7g	37	531	0.2	1.0	58.5	0.0
Sunflower, Reduced Fat, Suma*	1 Serving/25g	134	537	0.0	0.4	59.5	0.0
Sunflower, Sainsbury's*	Thin Spread/7g	44	631	0.2	0.1	70.0	0.1
Sunflower, Tesco*	1 Serving/15g	95	631	0.0	0.2	70.0	0.0
Sunflower, Value, Tesco*	Thin Spread/7g	31	439	0.1	0.4	48.6	0.0
Tuna & Mayonnaise, Shippam's*	1 Pot/75g	189	252	18.3	3.1	18.5	0.0
Vegetable, Dairy Free, Free From, Sainsbury's*	1 Serving/10g	63	630	0.0	0.0	70.0	3.0
Vegetable, Diet, Low Fat, Flora*	1 Serving/20g	45	227	3.5	1.6	23.0	0.0
Vegetable, Soft, Tesco*	1 Tbsp/15g	99	661	0.1	1.0	73.0	0.0
Vitalite, Lite, St Ivel*	Thin Spread/7g	24	348	1.5	0.0	38.0	0.0
Vitalite, St Ivel*	Thin Spread/7g	40	578	0.4	1.2	63.0	0.0
With Garlic & Herb, Soft, Free From, Sainsbury's*	1 Serving/30g	91	302	2.5	5.5	30.0	0.1
With Pure Olive Oil, Bertolli*	1 Serving/10g	54	536	0.2	1.0	59.0	0.0
SPRING GREENS,							
Boiled in Salted Water	1oz/28g	6	20	1.9	1.6	0.7	2.6
Boiled in Unsalted Water	1oz/28g	6	20	1.9	1.6	0.7	2.6
Raw	1oz/28g	9	33	3.0	3.1	1.0	3.4
SPRING ONIONS,							
Bulbs & Tops, Raw	1oz/28g	6	23	2.0	3.0	0.5	1.5
Bulbs Only, Raw	1oz/28g	10	35	0.9	8.5	0.0	1.7
Tesco*	1 Serving/4g	1	25	2.0	3.0	0.5	1.5
SPRING ROLLS,							
Cantonese Chicken & Chilli, Sainsbury's*	1 Roll/51g	85	166	9.7	19.4	5.5	0.6
Char Sui Pork & Bacon, Marks & Spencer*	1 Pack/220g	528	240	4.8	33.9	9.4	0.6
Chicken & Chilli, Sainsbury's*	1 Roll/50g	93	185	9.6	15.6	9.3	2.8
Chicken, Asda*	1 Roll/58g	115	199	4.6	25.0	9.0	3.4
Chicken, Tesco*	1 Roll/50g	116	231	8.1	24.5	11.2	1.5
Chinese Takeaway, Tesco*	1 Roll/50g	101	201	4.4	26.4	8.6	1.5
Dim Sum, Sainsbury's*	1 Spring Roll/12g	26	216	4.1	28.2	9.6	2.9
Marks & Spencer*	1 Pack/180g	333	185	3.5	24.2	8.4	2.3
Mini, Asda*	1 Roll/20g	35	175	3.5	33.6	3.0	1.9
Mini, Safeway*	1 Serving/30g	63	210	4.0	30.3	8.0	1.9
Mini, Sainsbury's	1 Roll/12g	27	221	4.2	28.7	9.9	1.6
Mini, Tesco*	1 Roll/18g	47	263	3.9	24.9	16.5	1.9
Prawn, Chinese, Sainsbury's*	1 Roll/30g	65	217	9.6	21.8	10.2	1.3
Prawn, Tesco*	3 Rolls/100g	211	211	8.7	22.8	9.4	1.4
Thai Prawn, Waitrose*	1 Roll/50g	110	219	8.0	25.4	9.5	2.4
Vegetable, Asda*	1 Roll/62g	126	203	3.5	27.0	9.0	2.7
Vegetable, Chinese Takeaway, Sainsbury's*	1Roll/59g	100	170	4.0	24.4	6.3	2.8
Vegetable, Chinese, Sainsbury's*	1 Roll/26g	69	193	4.1	26.9	7.7	1.4
Vegetable, Marks & Spencer*	1 Roll/29g	70	240	3.0	29.5	12.2	1.3
Vegetable, Mini, Nirvana, Aldi*	1 Roll/26g	54	208	3.5	25.1	10.4	1.7

	Measure	per Measure		Nutrition Values per 100g / 100ml				
	INFO/WEIGHT	KCAL		KCAL	PROT	CARB	FAT	FIBRE
SPRING ROLLS,								
Vegetable, Mini, Occasions, Sainsbury's*	1 Roll/24g	52		216	4.1	28.2	9.6	2.9
Vegetable, Mini, Party Food, Marks & Spencer*	1 Spring Roll/17g	35		205	3.5	26.3	9.7	2.0
Vegetable, Occasions, Sainsbury's*	1 Roll/25g	52		206	3.7	24.4	10.4	2.1
Vegetable, Safeway*	1 Serving/117g	242		207	3.5	27.1	9.4	2.7
Vegetable, Somerfield*	1 Roll/60g	107		179	3.8	26.1	6.6	1.6
Vegetable, Tempura, Marks & Spencer*	1 Pack/140g	280		200	2.8	27.9	8.6	1.8
Vegetable, Tesco*	1 Roll/60g	100		166	4.0	21.2	7.2	2.0
Vegetable, Waitrose*	1 Roll/57g	107		187	3.7	22.1	9.3	3.4
SQUARES,								
Rice Krispies, Chocolate Caramel, Kellogg's*	1 Bar/21g	90		430	4.5	74.0	13.0	0.5
Rice Krispies, Chocolate, Kellogg's*	1 Bar/18g	74		410	4.5	76.0	10.0	1.5
SQUASH,								
Acorn, Baked	1oz/28g	16		56	1.1	12.6	0.1	3.2
Acorn, Raw	1oz/28g	11		40	0.8	9.0	0.1	2.3
Apple & Strawberry High Juice, Sainsbury's*	1 Serving/250ml	83		33	0.1	8.2	0.1	0.1
Apple, Blackcurrant, Low Sugar, Sainsbury's*	1 Glass/250ml	5		2	0.1	0.2	0.1	0.1
Blackcurrant, High Juice, Marks & Spencer*	1 Glass/250ml	50		20	0.1	5.2	0.0	0.1
Butternut, Baked	1oz/28g	9		32	0.9	7.4	0.1	1.4
Butternut, Raw	1oz/28g	10		36	1.1	8.3	0.1	1.6
Lemon, High Juice, Sainsbury's*	1 Glass/250ml	98		39	0.1	9.1	0.1	0.1
Lemon, No Sugar, Asda*	1 Serving/200ml	5		3	0.1	0.3	0.1	0.1
Lemon, Whole, Low Sugar, Sainsbury's*	1 Glass/250ml	5		2	0.1	0.2	0.1	0.1
Mixed Fruit, Low Sugar, Sainsbury's*	1 Glass/250ml	5		2	0.1	0.2	0.1	0.1
Orange & Mango, Low Sugar, Sainsbury's*	1 Serving/250ml	5		2	0.1	0.2	0.1	0.1
Orange & Pineapple, Original, Robinson's*	1 Serving/250ml	138		55	1.0	13.0	0.0	0.0
Pink Grapefruit, High Juice, Sainsbury's*	1 Serving/250ml	103		41	0.1	9.9	0.1	0.1
Tropical Fruits, High Juice Sainsbury's*	1 Serving/250ml	95		38	0.1	9.3	0.1	0.1
SQUID,								
Dried	1oz/28g	88		313	63.3	4.8	4.6	0.0
Prepared, Asda*	1oz/28g	23		82	15.4	1.2	1.7	0.0
Raw	1oz/28g	23		81	15.4	1.2	1.7	0.0
Rings, Asda*	1oz/28g	23		81	15.4	1.2	1.7	0.0
in Batter, Fried in Blended Oil	1oz/28g	55		195	11.5	15.7	10.0	0.5
STARBAR, Cadbury's*	1 Bar/53g	286		540	9.1	55.0	31.6	0.0
STARBURST,								
Juicy Gums, Mars*	1 Pack/45g	139		309	5.9	71.0	4.1	0.0
Mars*	1 Pack/45g	185		411	0.3	85.3	7.6	0.0
Joosters, Mars*	1 Pack/45g	160		356	0.0	88.8	0.1	0.0
Tropical Fruit Chews, Mars*	1 Tube/45g	168		373	0.0	76.9	7.3	0.0
STEAMED PUDDING,								
Apple With Wild Berry Sauce, BGTY, Sainsburys*	1 Pudding/110g	308		280	2.6	59.7	3.4	1.4
Chocolate Fudge, Aunty's*	1 Pudding/110g	314		285	3.0	59.0	4.2	1.8
Chocolate, BGTY, Sainsbury's*	1 Pudding/110g	308		280	3.0	59.0	3.6	1.8
Golden Syrup, Aunty's*	1 Pudding/110g	366		333	2.6	69.0	5.0	2.3
Toffee & Date, Aunty's*	1 Serving/110g	320		291	2.6	59.1	4.6	1.1
STEW,								
Beef & Dumplings, Asda*	1 Pack/400g	392		98	6.0	11.0	3.3	0.8
Beef & Dumplings, Countryside*	1 Pack/300g	246		82	8.1	7.3	2.3	0.5
Beef & Dumplings, Eat Smart, Safeway*	1 Pack/394g	335		85	8.1	6.8	2.5	1.1
Beef & Dumplings, Farmfoods*	1 Pack/300g	312		104	4.0	12.0	4.4	1.1
Beef & Dumplings, Frozen, Asda*	1 Pack/400g	392		98	6.0	11.0	3.3	0.8
Beef & Dumplings, Traditional English Meals, Bird's Eye*	1 Pack/338g	355		105	6.7	11.5	3.6	0.0
Beef & Dumplings, Weight Watchers*	1 Pack/327g	262		80	5.2	10.0	2.1	0.8

S

	Measure INFO/WEIGHT	per Measure KCAL	Nutrition Values per 100g / 100ml				
			KCAL	PROT	CARB	FAT	FIBRE
STEW,							
Beef With Dumplings, COU, Marks & Spencer*	1 Pack/454g	431	95	8.9	9.1	2.6	0.8
Beef With Dumplings, Classic British, Sainsbury's*	1 Pack/450g	531	118	7.7	10.2	5.2	0.5
Beef With Dumplings, Morrisons*	1 Pack/700g	686	98	5.3	7.0	5.5	0.8
Beef With Dumplings, Tesco*	½ Pack/360g	641	178	5.7	14.0	12.1	0.8
Beef, Asda*	½ Can/196g	178	91	10.0	7.0	2.5	1.5
Beef, Meal for One, Marks & Spencer*	1 Pack/440g	350	80	7.0	8.7	1.9	2.0
Chicken & Dumplings, Bird's Eye*	1 Pack/320g	282	88	7.0	8.9	2.7	0.5
Chicken & Dumplings, Tesco*	1 Serving/300g	402	134	7.4	11.0	6.7	0.6
Chicken, Morrisons*	1 Pack/400g	492	123	17.6	8.9	1.9	0.5
Irish, Plumrose*	1 Can/392g	318	81	7.5	7.2	2.5	0.0
Irish, Sainsbury's*	1 Pack/450g	275	61	5.7	4.8	2.1	0.5
Irish, Smartprice, Asda*	1 Can/392g	298	76	3.0	8.0	3.6	0.9
Irish, Tesco*	1 Can/400g	308	77	7.0	5.9	2.8	0.8
Lentil & Winter Vegetable, Organic, Pure + Pronto*	1 Pack/400g	364	91	3.6	14.0	2.4	4.0
Mixed Vegetable Topped With Herb Dumplings, Tesco*	1 Pack/420g	508	121	1.9	14.5	6.2	1.3
Vegetable & Dumplings, Linda McCartney*	1 Pack/340g	384	113	2.5	13.7	1.8	0.5
STIR FRY,							
Bean Sprout & Vegetable, Asda*	½ Pack/175g	63	36	1.8	4.7	1.1	2.3
Bean Sprout & Vegetable, Tesco*	1 Serving/150g	47	31	2.1	4.8	0.4	1.9
Bean Sprout Mix, Safeway*	1 Serving/175g	123	70	2.5	4.6	4.6	1.9
Bean Sprout, Morrisons*	1 Serving/150g	47	31	2.0	4.8	0.4	1.8
Bean Sprout, Sainsbury's*	1 Pack/300g	144	48	1.9	5.1	2.8	1.5
Bean Sprouts & Vegetables, Asda*	½ Pack/173g	107	62	2.0	4.5	4.0	1.8
Bean Sprouts, Asda*	½ Pack/175g	56	32	2.9	4.0	0.5	1.5
Bean Sprouts, Safeway*	½ Pack/150g	83	55	2.3	4.4	3.1	1.9
Beef & Black Bean, Sizzling, Oriental Express*	1 Pack/400g	420	105	7.2	14.0	2.1	2.1
Beef, BGTY, Sainsbury's*	½ Pack/125g	156	125	22.0	0.1	4.1	0.0
Beef, Less Than 10% Fat, Asda*	1 Pack/227g	275	121	24.0	0.0	2.8	0.8
British Pork, Healthy Eating, Tesco*	½ Pack/150g	165	110	21.3	0.0	2.7	0.0
Cantonese Style Egg Fried Noodles, Sainsbury's*	¼ Pack/107g	110	104	3.4	10.7	5.3	1.1
Cantonese Vegetable, Sainsbury's*	1 Serving/150g	90	60	2.8	4.2	3.5	2.7
Chicken Chow Mein, Orient Express*	1 Pack/400g	384	96	7.3	10.7	2.7	2.2
Chicken, Safeway*	1 Serving/200g	204	102	22.0	0.0	1.6	0.0
Chinese Bean Sprout, Sainsbury's*	½ Pack/313g	150	48	1.9	5.1	2.8	1.5
Chinese Chicken, Iceland*	1 Pack/298g	262	88	6.2	12.7	1.4	2.9
Chinese Chicken, Sizzling , Oriental Express*	1 Pack/400g	400	100	6.6	13.8	2.0	1.7
Chinese Chop Suey Veg, Sharwood's*	1 Pack/310g	223	72	1.5	13.9	1.1	0.6
Chinese Exotic Vegetable, Sainsbury's*	1 Pack/350g	133	38	1.7	2.8	2.2	1.8
Chinese Mixed Vegetable, Sainsbury's*	1 Serving/150g	75	50	1.7	4.7	2.7	0.0
Chinese Mushroom, Sainsbury's*	1 Serving/175g	67	38	1.7	2.4	2.4	1.7
Chinese Prawn, Asda*	1 Serving/375g	345	92	3.6	18.0	0.6	1.8
Chinese Prawn, Iceland*	1 Pack/340g	235	69	3.1	11.1	1.3	2.1
Chinese Prawns, Sizzling, Oriental Express*	1 Pack/400g	384	96	3.9	14.7	2.4	1.6
Chinese Style Chicken & Noodle, Good For You, Asda*	1 Pack/330g	482	146	7.0	21.0	3.8	2.7
Chinese Style Chicken, GFY, Asda*	1 Pack/338.3g	362	107	6.0	17.0	1.7	1.5
Chinese Style Prawn, Good for You, Asda*	1 Pack/400g	324	81	3.6	13.0	1.6	1.6
Chinese Style Rice With Vegetables, Tesco*	1 Serving/550g	495	90	2.2	14.8	2.5	0.3
Chinese Vegetable & Oyster Sauce, Asda*	1 Serving/150g	93	62	1.9	8.0	2.5	0.0
Chinese Vegetables, Tesco*	1 Serving/175g	93	53	1.6	10.8	0.4	1.3
Chow Mein, Safeway*	1 Pack/400g	536	134	3.8	15.2	6.4	1.9
Creamy Coconut & Lime, The Best, Safeway*	½ Pack/165g	231	140	3.4	14.4	7.2	2.1
Crunchy Vegetable, Tesco*	1 Serving/100g	31	31	2.1	4.0	0.8	2.3
Family, Tesco*	1 Serving/150g	51	34	2.2	5.4	0.4	1.7

S

STIR FRY,	Measure INFO/WEIGHT	per Measure KCAL	Nutrition Values per 100g / 100ml				
			KCAL	PROT	CARB	FAT	FIBRE
Green Vegetable, Marks & Spencer*	1 Pack/220g	165	75	3.1	2.5	5.9	2.2
Lamb Strips, Tesco*	1 Serving/200g	212	106	13.9	6.8	2.6	0.8
Mange Tout Baby Corn & Vegetable, Asda*	1 Serving/100g	53	53	2.8	5.0	2.4	2.2
Mixed Pepper & Sweet Chilli Sauce, Asda*	1 Pack/300g	180	60	1.6	9.0	2.0	2.6
Mixed Pepper, Tesco*	½ Pack/170g	114	67	1.8	5.3	4.3	1.8
Mixed Vegetable, Safeway*	1 Serving/150g	105	70	2.1	6.2	3.6	2.5
Mixed Vegetables, Sainsbury's*	½ Pack/140g	70	50	1.7	7.7	2.7	3.0
Mushroom & Vegetables, Asda*	1oz/28g	19	68	2.2	3.8	4.9	0.0
Mushroom, Safeway*	1 Pack/500g	315	63	2.6	4.2	4.0	1.7
Mushroom, Sainsbury's*	1 Serving/175g	67	38	1.7	4.0	2.4	1.7
Mushroom, Somerfield*	1 Pack/350g	109	31	3.0	5.0	0.0	0.0
Mushroom, Tesco*	1 Pack/350g	102	29	2.4	4.0	0.4	1.7
Mushroom, Waitrose*	1oz/28g	8	28	1.8	4.9	0.3	1.8
Noodles & Bean Sprouts, Tesco*	1 Serving/125g	155	124	5.4	19.8	2.6	1.9
Oriental Style Pak Choi, Marks & Spencer*	1 Pack/220g	165	75	2.2	3.5	5.7	2.4
Oriental Style Vegetables, Sainsbury's*	1oz/28g	17	62	1.5	5.2	3.9	1.5
Oriental Vegetables, Frozen, Asda*	1 Serving/150g	116	77	2.1	7.0	4.5	1.7
Oriental Vegetables, Safeway*	1 Serving/175g	196	112	2.6	15.5	4.4	0.5
Pineapple, Safeway*	1 Pack/300g	237	79	3.6	4.7	5.1	0.5
Plum Hoisin Noodle, Tesco*	1 Carton/400g	392	98	3.6	17.5	1.5	1.8
Pork, BGTY, Sainsbury's*	¼ Pack/113g	104	92	21.4	0.1	0.7	0.1
Prawns, Chinese Sizzling, Oriental Express*	1 Pack/400g	384	96	3.9	14.7	2.4	1.6
Quorn, Spicy Chilli With Vegetables & Rice, Quorn*	½ Pack/170g	162	95	5.9	15.6	1.0	1.8
Singaporean Noodle, Sainsbury's*	½ Pack/160g	202	126	3.2	11.9	7.3	2.4
Spicy Oriental Vegetable, Sainsbury's*	½ Pack/175g	112	64	1.3	4.9	4.4	1.7
Spicy Thai Style Noodle, Tesco*	1 Pack/500g	335	67	2.6	8.4	2.6	1.3
Sweet & Sour Vegetable, Somerfield*	1 Pack/350g	249	71	2.0	14.0	1.0	0.0
Sweet & Sour, Marks & Spencer*	1oz/28g	19	68	1.1	15.2	0.3	0.5
Sweet & Sour, Tesco*	1 Pack/350g	161	46	1.8	9.1	0.3	1.3
Sweet Pepper, Marks & Spencer*	1 Pack/400g	160	40	2.3	3.5	1.8	0.6
Szechuan Spicy Oriental Vegetable, Sainsbury's*	1 Pack/350g	224	64	1.3	4.9	4.4	1.7
Thai Style, Tesco*	1 Pack/350g	322	92	3.8	8.4	4.8	1.8
Vegetable & Noodle, Asda*	1 Pack/330g	465	141	4.0	21.0	4.5	3.0
Vegetable & Noodle, Tesco*	1 Pack/300g	243	81	3.5	13.2	1.6	2.1
Vegetable & Sprouting Beans, Waitrose*	1 Pack/300g	213	71	4.8	10.4	1.1	2.7
Vegetable Mix, Fried in Vegetable Oil	1oz/28g	18	64	2.0	6.4	3.6	0.0
Vegetable Noodles, BGTY, Sainsbury's*	1 Pack/455g	391	86	3.2	14.0	2.0	1.4
Vegetable, Asda*	1 Pack/500g	220	44	1.6	4.2	2.3	3.1
Vegetable, Crispy, Oriental Inspired, Marks & Spencer*	1 Pack/300g	81	27	3.1	2.5	0.6	1.8
Vegetable, Premium, Sainsbury's*	½ Pack/150g	90	60	2.8	4.2	3.5	2.7
Vegetable, Safeway*	½ Pack/150g	68	45	1.1	3.2	3.1	1.6
Vegetable, Tesco*	1 Pack/300g	90	30	1.7	4.9	0.4	2.1
Vegetables & Bean Sprout, Marks & Spencer*	1 Pack/350g	105	30	1.8	4.6	0.4	2.0
Vegetables With Oyster Sauce, Asda*	1 Serving/150g	93	62	1.9	8.0	2.5	0.0
Vegetables, Amoy*	1 Can/250g	30	12	1.0	2.1	0.0	2.7
Vegetables, Asda*	1oz/28g	7	26	1.1	3.1	1.0	2.6
Vegetables, Cantonese Style, Tesco*	1 Serving/125g	40	32	2.0	4.1	0.9	1.4
Vegetables, Family Pack, Co-Op*	½ Pack/300g	90	30	2.0	5.0	0.4	5.0
Vegetables, Fresh, Asda*	½ Pack/150g	107	71	1.7	4.9	5.0	1.7
Vegetables, Somerfield*	1 Pack/300g	93	31	2.0	5.0	0.0	0.0
Vegetables, Tesco*	1oz/28g	8	27	1.7	4.4	0.3	1.9
Vegetable & Bean Sprout Mix, Safeway*	1 Serving/160g	96	60	2.3	4.6	3.4	2.3

S

	Measure INFO/WEIGHT	per Measure KCAL	Nutrition Values per 100g / 100ml				
			KCAL	PROT	CARB	FAT	FIBRE
STOCK,							
Chicken, Asda*	½ Pot/150g	26	17	1.8	0.7	0.9	0.2
Chicken, Concentrated, Marks & Spencer*	1 Serving/5g	16	315	25.6	12.2	18.1	0.8
Chicken, Fresh, Sainsbury's*	½ Pot/142ml	23	16	3.7	0.1	0.1	0.3
Chicken, Knorr*	1 Pack/150g	348	232	13.1	36.5	3.7	0.4
Chicken, Slowly Prepared, Sainsbury's*	1 Pot/300g	27	9	0.6	1.3	0.1	0.5
Vegetable, Campbell's*	1 Serving/250ml	38	15	0.3	2.0	0.7	0.0
Vegetable, Concentrated, Vecon*	1 Serving/5g	9	171	25.0	17.5	1.5	3.5
Vegetable, Knorr*	1 Serving/9g	18	199	8.5	39.9	0.6	0.9
Vegetable, Waitrose*	1 Serving/50g	3	6	0.4	1.2	0.0	0.0
STOCK CUBES,							
Beef, Dry, As Sold, Bovril*	1 Cube/5.9g	12	197	10.8	29.3	4.1	0.0
Beef, Dry, As Sold, Oxo*	1 Cube/5.8	15	265	17.3	38.4	4.7	1.5
Beef, Knorr*	1 Cube/10g	33	326	11.1	21.0	22.0	0.2
Beef, Value, Tesco*	1 Cube/10g	19	189	11.2	17.0	8.5	0.1
Chicken	1 Cube/6g	14	237	15.4	9.9	15.4	0.0
Chicken, Dry, As Sold, Oxo*	1 Cube/6g	15	243	15.6	36.6	3.4	1.4
Chicken, Just Bouillon, Kallo*	1 Cube/12g	30	247	11.8	26.1	10.6	1.0
Chicken, Knorr*	1 Cube/10g	30	301	10.1	23.6	18.5	0.2
Chinese, Dry, As Sold, Oxo*	1 Cube/6g	16	263	11.0	40.9	6.1	3.6
Fish, Knorr*	1 Cube/10g	32	321	18.9	15.9	20.2	0.7
Garlic, Dry, As Sold, Oxo*	1 Cube/6g	18	298	13.4	48.5	5.5	3.6
Ham, Knorr*	1 Cube/10g	31	313	11.8	24.4	18.7	0.0
Indian, Dry, As Sold, Oxo*	1 Cube/6g	17	291	11.5	43.9	7.7	6.7
Italian, Dry, As Sold, Oxo*	1 Cube/6g	19	309	11.9	48.9	7.3	4.6
Lamb, Knorr*	1 Cube/10g	30	301	14.7	12.9	21.2	0.2
Mexican, Dry, As Sold, Oxo*	1 Cube/6g	15	248	11.8	36.8	6.0	3.7
Pork, Knorr*	1 Cube/24g	8	34	1.2	1.8	2.5	0.0
Vegetable	1 Cube/7g	18	253	13.5	11.6	17.3	0.0
Vegetable, Dry, As Sold, Oxo*	1 Cube/6g	15	253	11.2	41.9	4.5	1.7
Vegetable, Knorr*	1 Pack/80g	246	308	11.9	21.7	19.3	1.3
STRAWBERRIES,							
Fresh, Raw	1oz/28g	8	27	0.8	6.0	0.1	1.1
In Apple Juice, Safeway*	1 Serving/145g	73	50	0.4	12.0	0.0	1.0
In Fruit Juice, Asda*	1 Serving/150g	75	50	0.4	12.0	0.0	0.7
In Fruit Juice, John West*	1 Can/410g	176	43	0.5	10.0	0.0	0.9
In Grape Juice, Somerfield*	1/3 Can/127g	47	37	0.5	8.8	0.0	1.3
In Grape Juice, Tesco*	1 Serving/100g	43	43	0.5	11.0	0.0	0.9
In Light Syrup, Sainsbury's*	1oz/28g	17	62	0.4	15.0	0.1	1.0
In Raspberry Sauce, WTF, Sainsbury's*	1 Serving/170g	111	65	0.7	15.3	0.1	2.3
Scottish, Safeway*	1oz/28g	8	28	0.8	6.0	0.1	0.0
Tesco*	1 Serving/227g	64	28	0.8	6.0	0.1	1.1
STRAWBERRY & CREAM, Thorntons*	1 Chocolate/12g	64	533	5.1	54.2	32.5	0.8
STRAWBERRY & KIWI, Fresh, Marks & Spencer*	1 Serving/200g	80	40	1.0	8.3	0.3	1.5
STRAWBERRY LACES,							
Co-Op*	1 Sweet/6g	21	345	7.0	79.0	0.0	1.0
Somerfield*	1 Pack/100g	374	374	3.0	86.0	0.0	0.0
STREAKY STRIPS, Meat Free, Morningstar Farms*	1 Strip/8g	28	348	11.5	13.4	27.6	3.9
STREUSEL, Baked Apple & Plum, Healthy Eating, Tesco*	1 Serving/120g	161	134	1.9	29.4	1.0	2.0
STROGANOFF,							
Beef, Asda*	1 Serving/120g	276	230	16.0	3.3	17.0	0.6
Beef, Sainsbury's*	1 Can/200g	232	116	12.5	3.0	6.0	0.2
Beef, TTD, Sainsbury's*	1 Pack/300g	491	164	11.9	5.2	10.6	0.4
Beef, The Best, Safeway*	1 Serving/250g	400	160	19.6	2.2	7.8	0.8

	Measure INFO/WEIGHT	per Measure KCAL	Nutrition Values per 100g / 100ml				
			KCAL	PROT	CARB	FAT	FIBRE
STROGANOFF,							
Beef, With Long Grain & Wild Rice, Somerfield*	1 Pack/400g	485	121	7.3	13.8	4.1	1.6
Beef, With Mixed Rice, Tesco*	1 Pack/450g	558	124	7.5	15.2	3.7	1.5
Beef, With Rice, Tesco*	1 Pack/475g	518	109	5.6	13.7	3.5	3.4
Chicken & Mushroom, COU, Marks & Spencer*	1 Pack/400g	340	85	8.6	9.0	1.5	1.0
Chicken, Healthy Living, Tesco*	1 Pack/450g	491	109	7.7	13.5	2.7	0.6
Mushroom With Rice, Eat Smart, Safeway*	1 Pack/400g	280	70	2.7	11.3	1.3	1.6
Mushroom With Rice, Healthy Eating, Tesco*	1 Pack/450g	396	88	3.8	13.3	2.2	1.2
Mushroom With Rice, Tesco*	1 Pack/450g	500	111	3.0	12.8	5.3	1.3
Mushroom, BGTY, Sainsbury's*	1 Pack/451g	392	87	3.2	17.4	0.5	0.5
Mushroom, Good For You, Asda*	1 Pack/450g	339	75	2.9	12.4	1.6	0.7
Pork With Rice, Healthy Eating, Tesco*	1 Pack/450g	482	107	7.0	15.8	1.8	0.5
STRUDEL,							
Apple & Mincemeat, Tesco*	1 Serving/100g	322	322	3.3	39.6	16.7	2.0
Apple, Safeway*	¼ Strudel/150g	414	276	3.1	35.7	14.4	2.4
Apple, Sainsbury's*	1/6 Portion/90g	269	299	3.6	36.4	15.4	1.9
Apple, Tesco*	1 Serving/150g	432	288	3.3	36.4	14.4	2.8
Wooland Fruit, Sainsbury's*	1/6 Strudel/95.2g	276	290	3.7	34.0	15.5	2.0
STUFFING,							
Chestnut & Pork, Marks & Spencer*	1oz/28g	67	240	6.6	16.3	16.7	2.9
Olde English Chestnut, Sainsbury's*	1 Serving/110g	216	196	9.4	13.5	11.6	2.1
Parsley & Thyme, Co-Op*	1 Serving/28g	95	340	10.0	67.0	3.0	6.0
Sage & Onion, Somerfield*	1oz/28g	100	358	6.0	74.0	5.0	0.0
Sausage Meat, Balls, Aunt Bessie's*	1 Ball (Baked)/26g	56	214	7.5	29.6	7.3	2.4
STUFFING MIX,							
Apple & Herb, Special Recipe, Sainsbury's*	1 Serving/41g	68	165	3.8	32.4	2.2	2.2
Apple Mustard & Herb, Paxo*	1 Serving/50g	83	166	4.2	32.8	2.0	4.0
Apricot & Walnut, Celebration, Paxo*	1 Serving/50g	81	161	4.3	28.0	3.5	2.8
Chestnut & Cranberry, Celebration, Paxo*	1 Serving/25g	35	141	4.0	26.7	2.0	2.4
Date, Walnut & Stilton, Special Recipe, Sainsbury's*	1 Serving/25g	49	196	5.2	25.0	8.4	2.0
Dried, Made Up	1oz/28g	27	97	2.8	19.3	1.5	1.3
Parsley, Thyme & Lemon, Sainsbury's*	1 Pack/170g	240	141	4.2	28.2	1.3	1.3
Sage & Onion, Asda*	1 Serving/27g	29	107	3.4	22.0	0.6	1.3
Sage & Onion, Balls, Aunt Bessie's*	1 Stuffing Ball/26g	56	214	7.5	29.6	7.3	2.4
Sage & Onion, Balls, Meat-Free, Aunt Bessie's*	1 Ball/28g	54	193	5.4	28.0	6.7	1.7
Sage & Onion, Made Up, Paxo*	1 Serving/50g	62	123	3.6	23.0	1.8	1.7
SUET,							
Beef, Tesco*	1 Serving/100g	854	854	0.6	6.2	91.9	0.1
Shredded Vegetable, Atora Light*	1oz/28g	197	704	3.8	28.5	63.9	1.2
Vegetable	1oz/28g	234	836	1.2	10.1	87.9	0.0
SUET PUDDING, Average	1oz/28g	94	335	4.4	40.5	18.3	0.9
SUGAR,							
Brown, Soft, Tesco*	1 Serving/40g	153	383	0.0	95.8	0.0	0.0
Caster, Silver Spoon*	1 Tsp/5g	20	400	0.0	100.0	0.0	0.0
Dark Brown Muscovado, Waitrose*	1 Tsp/7g	25	360	0.0	90.0	0.0	0.0
Dark Brown, Soft, Silver Spoon*	1 Tsp/5g	18	362	0.3	90.0	0.0	0.0
Demerara, Tesco*	1 Tsp/5g	17	339	0.5	99.3	0.0	0.0
For Making Jam, Silver Spoon*	1oz/28g	111	398	0.0	99.5	0.0	0.0
Golden Caster, Waitrose*	1 Serving/100g	398	398	0.0	99.6	0.0	0.0
Golden, Unrefined, Sainsbury's*	1 Serving/5g	20	400	0.0	100.0	0.0	0.0
Granulated, Morrisons*	1 Tsp/5g	20	394	0.0	99.9	0.0	0.0
Granulated, Silver Spoon*	1 Tsp/4g	16	400	0.0	100.0	0.0	0.0
Half Spoon Granuated, With Sweeteners, Silver Spoon*	1 Tsp/5g	20	398	0.0	99.5	0.0	0.0
Icing	1 Tsp/4g	16	393	0.0	104.9	0.0	0.0

S

	Measure INFO/WEIGHT	per Measure KCAL	Nutrition Values per 100g / 100ml				
			KCAL	PROT	CARB	FAT	FIBRE
SUGAR,							
Light Brown, Soft, Silver Spoon*	1 Serving/2g	8	386	0.1	96.4	0.0	0.0
Light Muscovado, Sainsbury's*	1oz/28g	108	384	0.1	96.0	0.0	0.0
Light, Silver Spoon*	1 Serving/18g	72	400	0.0	100.0	0.0	0.0
Organic, Marks & Spencer*	1 Tsp/4g	16	394	0.0	99.9	0.0	0.0
White	1 Tsp/4g	16	394	0.0	105.0	0.0	0.0
SUGOCASA							
With Herbs, TTD, Sainsbury's*	¼ Jar/175g	81	46	2.0	8.4	0.5	1.3
SULTANAS,							
Australian, Waitrose*	1oz/28g	82	292	2.7	69.4	0.4	2.0
Average	1oz/28g	77	275	2.7	69.4	0.4	2.0
Co-Op*	1 Serving/28g	81	290	3.0	69.0	0.4	4.0
Dried, Marks & Spencer*	1oz/28g	87	309	2.4	73.1	0.8	5.7
Organic, Waitrose*	1oz/28g	82	292	2.7	69.4	0.4	2.0
Safeway*	1 Serving/50g	146	292	2.7	69.4	0.4	0.0
Sainsbury's*	1 Serving/30g	88	292	2.7	69.4	0.4	2.0
Somerfield*	1oz/28g	82	292	3.0	69.0	0.0	0.0
Sun Dried, Organic, Crazy Jack*	1 Serving/100g	292	292	2.7	69.4	0.4	0.0
Value, Tesco*	1 Dtsp/30g	88	292	0.0	69.4	0.4	2.0
SUMMER FRUITS,							
Frozen, Asda*	1 Serving/100g	28	28	0.9	6.0	0.0	2.5
Frozen, Sainsbury's*	1 Serving/80g	26	33	0.9	7.4	0.1	2.4
In Syrup, Sainsbury's*	1 Pudding/289g	188	65	0.5	15.6	0.1	1.2
Mix, Marks & Spencer*	1oz/28g	9	33	1.0	6.7	0.3	2.5
Mix, Sainsbury's*	1 Serving/80g	26	32	0.9	7.4	0.0	2.4
Oasis*	1 Bottle/500ml	185	37	0.0	9.0	0.0	0.0
Shearway*	1oz/28g	10	34	0.9	6.9	0.1	0.0
SUNDAE,							
Blackcurrant, Marks & Spencer*	1 Sundae/49g	196	400	4.5	51.7	19.5	1.9
Chocolate & Orange, Weight Watchers*	1 Pot/102g	137	134	1.2	25.2	2.2	0.2
Chocolate & Vanilla Ice Cream, Tesco*	1 Sundae/70.2g	139	199	2.8	27.5	8.6	0.5
Chocolate Brownie, Finest, Tesco*	1 Serving/215g	808	376	3.1	30.1	27.0	0.4
Chocolate Mint, COU, Marks & Spencer*	1 Pot/90g	108	120	5.4	17.8	2.6	0.5
Chocolate Nut	1 Portion/70g	195	278	3.0	34.2	15.3	0.1
Chocolate, Eat Smart, Safeway*	1 Serving/97g	150	155	3.5	29.0	2.7	4.3
Chocolate, Healthy Eating, Tesco*	1 Serving/130g	199	153	4.5	24.9	3.9	0.6
Hot Caramel, McDonald's*	1 Sundae/189g	357	189	3.8	33.9	4.4	0.0
Hot Fudge, McDonald's*	1 Sundae/187g	352	188	4.5	30.0	5.7	0.0
No Topping, McDonald's*	1 Sundae/149g	219	147	4.2	21.6	5.1	0.0
Peach & Apricot, Perfectly Balanced, Waitrose*	1 Pot/175ml	142	81	1.7	17.7	0.4	0.0
Raspberry, Eat Smart, Safeway*	1 Serving/97g	150	155	3.0	30.9	2.1	2.8
Raspberry, Perfectly Balanced, Waitrose*	1 Pot/175ml	151	86	1.7	18.9	0.6	0.0
Strawberry & Vanilla Ice Cream, Tesco*	1 Serving/68g	120	177	2.0	29.5	5.7	0.1
Strawberry & Vanilla, Weight Watchers*	1 Pot/105g	148	141	1.2	29.1	2.1	0.3
Strawberry, Co-Op*	1 Pot/155g	279	180	3.0	24.0	8.0	0.5
Strawberry, Marks & Spencer*	1 Sundae/45g	173	385	3.4	53.3	17.8	1.0
Strawberry, McDonald's*	1 Sundae/186g	296	159	3.4	27.5	4.1	0.0
SUNFLOWER SEEDS,							
Average	1 Tbsp/14g	81	581	19.8	18.6	47.5	6.0
Evernat*	1oz/28g	171	609	26.8	6.3	52.9	6.1
SUNNY DELIGHT*							
Average	1 Glass/200ml	88	44	0.1	10.0	0.2	0.0
Apple & Kiwi Kick	1 Glass/200ml	15	7	0.2	1.3	0.2	0.2
Light	1 Glass/200ml	16	8	0.1	1.0	0.2	0.0

S

	Measure INFO/WEIGHT	per Measure KCAL	Nutrition Values per 100g / 100ml				
			KCAL	PROT	CARB	FAT	FIBRE
SUSHI,							
Advent, Medium, Tesco*	1 Serving/210g	307	146	3.8	25.7	3.1	0.9
Aya Set, Waitrose*	1 Pack/110g	200	182	5.4	31.7	3.9	1.5
California Roll Box, Marks & Spencer*	1 Box/230g	391	170	7.0	22.0	5.2	1.1
Californian, Fish Roll, Nigiri & Maki Selection, M&S*	1 Serving/200g	300	150	6.5	25.8	2.3	1.0
Californian, Yakatori, Marks & Spencer*	1 Serving/200g	340	170	6.4	25.0	4.7	1.0
Deluxe, Pret A Manger*	1 Pack/350g	522	149	5.8	26.2	2.4	0.9
Fish Nigiri, Adventurous, Tesco*	1 Med Pack/200g	270	135	7.1	21.7	2.2	0.5
Fish Selection Box, Marks & Spencer*	1 Serving/220g	396	180	6.6	27.1	4.5	0.9
Fish Selection, Marks & Spencer*	1 Serving/210g	315	150	6.5	25.8	2.3	1.0
Fish, Large Box, Tesco*	1 Box/290g	423	146	4.9	25.8	2.6	0.8
Fish, Medium Box, Tesco*	1 Box/195g	281	144	5.1	25.7	2.3	0.7
Fish, Small, Tesco*	1 Serving/105g	148	141	5.9	23.9	2.4	0.6
Fish, Tesco*	1 Pack/105g	155	148	6.2	25.1	2.5	0.6
Good For You, Asda*	1 Pack/220g	352	160	4.9	32.0	1.4	0.0
Hana Set, Waitrose*	1 Serving/175g	324	185	5.4	35.7	2.3	1.4
Komachi Set, Waitrose*	1 Box/235g	425	181	6.1	31.3	3.5	1.4
Large, Boots*	1 Pack/324g	480	148	5.0	28.0	1.8	0.7
Maki Selection, Shapers, Boots*	1 Pack/158g	225	142	3.5	29.0	1.3	1.1
Medium Box, Marks & Spencer*	1 Serving/215g	366	170	9.7	24.3	2.8	0.9
Medium Selection Pack, Tesco*	1 Pack/195g	312	160	5.6	27.9	2.9	1.4
Mini, Boots	1 Serving/182g	269	148	4.2	29.0	1.7	1.2
Mixed Box, Somerfield*	1 Pack/220g	339	154	4.6	31.4	1.1	0.0
Nigiri, Marks & Spencer*	1 Serving/190g	285	150	5.2	25.7	2.5	0.9
Oriental Fish Box, Marks & Spencer*	1 Box/205g	318	155	6.1	23.3	4.1	0.9
Prawn & Salmon Selection, Marks & Spencer*	1 Serving/150g	218	145	5.5	27.4	1.7	0.6
Prawn Feast, Marks & Spencer*	1 Box/219g	350	160	5.7	25.8	3.7	1.1
Salmon & Roll Set, Small. Sainsbury's*	1 Serving/101g	167	165	4.9	30.4	2.6	0.8
Salmon Feast Box, Marks & Spencer*	1 Pack/200g	330	165	5.6	27.0	2.9	1.0
Selection, Boots*	1 Pack/268g	434	162	5.5	27.0	3.6	1.6
Selection, Shapers, Boots*	1 Pack/189g	293	155	5.1	28.0	2.5	2.2
Taiko Hagi Set, Waitrose*	1 Box/370g	688	186	7.1	33.6	2.6	1.1
Taiko Vegetable Set, Waitrose*	1 Serving/135g	254	188	4.4	37.1	2.4	1.4
Tesco*	1 Pack/195g	285	146	5.1	25.9	2.3	0.7
Tokyo Set, Marks & Spencer*	1 Pack/150g	240	160	7.3	25.3	3.1	0.6
Trial Pack, Asda*	1 Pack/115g	186	162	4.1	31.0	2.4	0.0
Tuna, To Snack Selection, Food To Go, Marks & Spencer*	1 Serving/150g	225	150	5.2	26.4	2.6	2.3
Vegetarian, Marks & Spencer*	1 Pack/223g	290	130	4.1	25.5	1.5	1.3
Vegetarian, Tesco*	1 Pack/132g	185	140	3.1	27.2	2.1	0.9
Yo!, Bento Box, Sainsbury's*	1 Pack/208g	530	255	8.4	48.7	3.0	0.9
Yo!, Salmon Lunch Set, Sainsbury's*	1 Pack/150g	242	161	5.9	28.1	2.8	0.8
SWEDE,							
Boiled in Salted Water	1oz/28g	3	11	0.3	2.3	0.1	0.7
Boiled in Unsalted Water	1oz/28g	3	11	0.3	2.3	0.1	0.7
Mash, COU, Marks & Spencer*	1oz/28g	15	55	1.1	9.5	1.2	2.1
Raw	1oz/28g	7	24	0.7	5.0	0.3	1.9
SWEDE & CARROT,							
Cubes, Sainsbury's*	1 Serving/250g	43	17	0.4	3.5	0.2	1.5
For Mashing, Safeway*	½ Pack/250g	43	17	0.4	3.3	0.2	1.4
Mash, Asda*	1 Serving/150g	107	71	1.3	10.0	2.9	1.7
Mix, Tesco*	1 Serving/75g	23	30	0.7	6.2	0.3	2.2
SWEET & SOUR,							
Beef, Feeling Great, Findus*	1 Pack/350g	385	110	4.0	19.0	2.0	1.5
Beef, Feeling Great, New, Findus*	1 Pack/350g	420	120	4.5	20.0	2.5	1.3

S

INFO/WEIGHT	per Measure KCAL	KCAL	PROT	CARB	FAT	FIBRE

SWEET & SOUR,

	Measure INFO/WEIGHT	per Measure KCAL	KCAL	PROT	CARB	FAT	FIBRE
Chicken & Egg Fried Rice, BGTY, Sainsbury's*	1 Pack/450g	612	136	7.0	19.2	3.5	0.6
Chicken & Fried Rice, Good For You, Asda*	1 Pack/400g	580	145	6.0	23.0	3.2	1.1
Chicken & Noodles, BGTY, Sainsbury's*	1 Pack/400g	356	89	7.5	13.3	0.6	0.7
Chicken & Noodles, Chinese Takeaway, Tesco*	1 Pack/350g	350	100	5.7	18.8	0.2	0.2
Chicken & Rice, Mega Value, Tesco*	1 Pack/500g	675	135	4.4	25.0	1.9	1.9
Chicken & Rice, Morrisons*	1 Pack/400g	452	113	3.6	18.8	2.6	0.8
Chicken Cantonese, Sainsbury's*	1 Pack/350g	368	105	10.4	14.6	0.6	0.6
Chicken In Crispy Batter, Cantonese, Sainsbury's*	1 Pack/300g	546	182	9.0	21.4	6.7	1.1
Chicken With Egg Fried Rice, BGTY, Sainsbury's*	1 Pack/400g	396	99	6.5	16.8	0.6	0.7
Chicken With Egg Fried Rice, Healthy Eating, Tesco*	1 Pack/450g	468	104	7.4	15.5	1.4	1.2
Chicken With Egg Fried Rice, BGTY, Sainsbury's*	1 Pack/400g	424	106	5.4	17.3	1.7	1.0
Chicken With Egg Fried Rice, Somerfield*	1 Pack/400g	428	107	8.5	16.7	0.7	2.0
Chicken With Noodles, Healthy Eating, Tesco*	1 Pack/350g	277	79	8.3	10.4	0.4	0.8
Chicken With Noodles, Steamed, Healthy Eating, Tesco*	1 Pack/370g	289	78	8.3	10.8	0.2	0.6
Chicken With Noodles, Tesco*	1 Pack/350g	441	126	5.7	24.4	0.6	1.4
Chicken With Peppers & Egg Fried Rice, HE, Tesco*	1 Pack/450g	450	100	7.6	12.1	2.4	1.2
Chicken With Rice, Asda*	1 Pack/400g	440	110	4.7	22.0	0.3	0.6
Chicken With Rice, BGTY, Sainsbury's*	1 Pack/450g	675	150	8.1	21.1	3.7	0.9
Chicken With Rice, Eat Smart, Safeway*	1 Pack/390g	312	80	5.4	12.2	0.9	1.2
Chicken With Rice, Farmfoods*	1 Pack/300g	324	108	5.9	19.2	0.9	0.7
Chicken With Rice, Healthy Eating, Tesco*	1 Pack/450g	450	100	8.0	16.3	0.3	0.8
Chicken With Rice, Iceland*	1 Pack/400g	400	100	5.0	19.8	0.1	0.6
Chicken With Rice, Kwik Save*	1 Pack/500g	520	104	4.0	21.9	0.3	0.7
Chicken With Rice, Nisa, Heritage*	1 Pack/600g	606	101	6.0	17.4	0.8	0.4
Chicken With Rice, Oriental Express*	1 Pack/340g	350	103	4.4	21.3	0.6	0.7
Chicken With Rice, Perfectly Balanced, Waitrose*	1 Pack/100g	95	95	6.4	16.1	0.6	1.3
Chicken With Vegetable Rice, COU, Marks & Spencer*	1 Pack/400g	320	80	6.7	10.7	1.2	1.0
Chicken, Battered, Chinese, Sainsbury's*	1 Pack/350g	532	152	9.1	22.5	2.9	0.7
Chicken, Battered, Tesco*	1 Serving/100g	149	149	7.7	22.1	3.3	0.9
Chicken, Cantonese, Sainsbury's*	½ Pack/200g	176	88	8.2	11.8	0.9	0.8
Chicken, Chinese Takeaway, Sainsbury's*	1 Pack/264g	515	195	13.1	21.3	6.4	1.0
Chicken, Chinese Takeaway, Tesco*	1 Serving/100g	149	149	7.7	22.1	3.3	0.9
Chicken, Crispy, Iceland*	1 Serving/125g	221	177	18.3	14.2	5.2	1.2
Chicken, GFY, Asda*	1 Serving/165g	213	129	16.0	15.0	0.5	1.6
Chicken, Good Choice, Iceland*	1 Pack/400g	520	130	5.0	27.2	0.1	0.4
Chicken, Healthy Choice, Safeway*	1 Pack/400g	580	145	6.5	25.6	1.8	1.4
Chicken, Low Fat, Iceland*	1 Pack/400g	444	111	8.1	15.7	1.7	1.1
Chicken, Marks & Spencer*	1 Pack/300g	465	155	6.6	24.4	3.6	0.8
Chicken, Somerfield*	1 Serving/175g	156	89	9.5	12.6	0.1	0.6
Chicken, Take It Away, Marks & Spencer*	1 Pack/200g	200	100	9.4	13.2	0.8	1.2
Chicken, Tesco*	1 Pack/350g	319	91	6.4	12.9	1.5	4.0
Chicken, Weight Watchers*	1 Pack/320g	304	95	5.2	17.4	0.4	0.3
Pork, Battered, Sainsbury's*	½ Pack/175g	306	175	7.3	25.1	5.0	0.6
Pork, Cantonese, & Egg Fried Rice, Farmfoods*	1 Pack/327g	520	159	4.8	22.0	5.8	0.1
Pork, In Crispy Batter, Sainsbury's*	½ Pack/150g	293	195	10.0	20.0	8.3	1.1
Quick Snack, Rice, Sainsbury's*	1 Serving/237g	230	97	2.5	20.5	0.5	0.0
Roasted Vegetables, Cantonese, Sainsbury's*	1 Pack/348g	327	94	1.1	19.6	1.2	0.9
Vegetables With Rice, Waitrose*	1 Pack/400g	384	96	1.9	19.5	1.1	1.1

SWEET POTATO,

	Measure INFO/WEIGHT	per Measure KCAL	KCAL	PROT	CARB	FAT	FIBRE
Baked	1oz/28g	32	115	1.6	27.9	0.4	3.3
Boiled in Salted Water	1oz/28g	24	84	1.1	20.5	0.3	2.3
Raw	1oz/28g	24	87	1.2	21.3	0.3	2.4
Steamed	1oz/28g	24	84	1.1	20.4	0.3	2.3

S

INFO/WEIGHT	Measure	per Measure KCAL	Nutrition Values per 100g / 100ml				
			KCAL	PROT	CARB	FAT	FIBRE
SWEETBREAD,							
Lamb, Fried	1oz/28g	61	217	28.7	0.0	11.4	0.0
Lamb, Raw	1oz/28g	37	131	15.3	0.0	7.8	0.0
SWEETCORN,							
& Petit Pois, Marks & Spencer*	1oz/28g	20	73	4.6	10.8	1.3	3.6
American, In Water, Waitrose*	½ Can/80g	73	91	3.4	16.0	1.5	1.2
American, Organic, Waitrose*	½ Can/164.8g	150	91	3.4	16.0	1.5	1.2
Asda*	½ Can/71g	73	103	2.9	21.0	0.8	2.1
Extra Crisp, Green Giant*	1 Can/165g	116	70	2.7	13.3	0.7	2.7
Fritters With Chilli Dip, Sainsbury's*	1 Fritter/40g	60	151	3.0	27.0	3.4	3.0
Frozen, Asda*	1 Serving/75g	83	110	4.2	18.0	2.3	2.2
Frozen, Indiviual Portion, Tendafrost*	1 Sachet/115g	105	91	3.4	15.5	1.8	1.5
Frozen, Morrisons*	1 Serving/45g	42	93	3.4	17.0	1.8	1.5
Frozen, Organic, Tesco*	1 Serving/100g	98	98	3.4	17.0	1.8	2.2
Frozen, Safeway*	1 Serving/100g	116	116	4.2	19.6	2.3	2.2
Green Giant*	1 Can/200g	140	70	2.7	13.3	0.7	2.7
Healthy Eating, Tesco*	1 Serving/40g	33	82	2.4	15.5	1.1	2.2
In Brine, John West*	1oz/28g	30	107	3.3	23.1	0.2	2.2
In Water, Morrisons*	1 Serving/80g	71	89	2.0	18.0	1.0	0.0
In Water, No Added Sugar or Salt, Waitrose*	1 Serving/100g	89	89	3.4	15.7	1.4	1.2
In Water, No Salt & Sugar, Sainsbury's*	1 Serving/163g	166	102	2.9	20.1	1.1	1.8
In Water, Sugar & Salt Added, American, Waitrose*	½ Can/73g	62	85	3.2	14.2	1.4	1.1
In Water, Sugar & Salt Added, Sainsbury's*	½ Can/78g	85	109	2.9	21.8	1.1	1.8
In Water, Tesco*	1 Serving/130g	107	82	2.4	15.5	1.1	2.2
Kernels In Water With Salt & Sugar, SmartPrice, Asda*	¼ Can/72g	74	103	2.9	21.0	0.8	2.1
Kernels, Boiled in Salted Water	1oz/28g	31	111	4.2	19.6	2.3	2.2
Kernels, Boiled in Unsalted Water	1oz/28g	31	111	4.2	19.6	2.3	2.2
Kernels, Canned, Re-Heated, Drained	1oz/28g	34	122	2.9	26.6	1.2	1.4
Kernels, Raw	1oz/28g	26	93	3.4	17.0	1.8	1.5
Marks & Spencer*	1oz/28g	26	93	3.4	17.0	1.8	1.5
Naturally Sweet in Water, Sainsbury's*	1oz/28g	17	61	2.8	10.6	0.8	1.4
Niblets With Peppers, Green Giant*	1 Serving/165g	135	82	2.6	17.9	0.0	1.3
Niblets in Water, Sugar & Salt Added, Green Giant*	1oz/28g	28	100	2.7	20.8	0.7	1.2
Niblets, No Salt, No Sugar, Green Giant*	1 Serving/80g	62	77	2.6	16.7	0.0	2.6
Organic, Waitrose*	1oz/28g	26	93	3.4	17.0	1.8	1.5
Sainsbury's*	½ Can/70g	75	109	2.9	21.8	1.1	1.8
Smartprice, Asda*	1 Serving/113g	124	110	4.2	18.0	2.3	2.2
SWEETCORN,							
Supersweet, Frozen, Sainsbury's*	1 Serving/85g	99	116	4.2	19.6	2.3	2.2
Value, Tesco*	1 Serving/130g	107	82	2.4	15.5	1.1	2.2
Whole Kernel, Green Giant*	1 Can/270g	176	65	1.6	14.6	0.4	0.0
With Peppers, Canned, Asda*	1 Serving/50g	38	76	2.7	15.0	0.6	0.0
SWEETENER,							
Canderel*	1 Tsp/0.53	2	379	24.7	7.0	0.0	5.3
Canderel, Spoonful, Canderel*	2 Tsp/1g	4	384	2.9	93.0	0.0	0.0
Granulated, Asda*	1 Tsp/1g	4	400	3.0	97.0	0.0	0.0
Granulated, Safeway*	1 Tsp/1g	4	392	3.0	95.0	0.0	0.0
Granulated, Splenda*	1 Tsp/1g	4	391	0.0	97.7	0.0	0.0
Granulated, Tesco*	1 Tsp/1g	4	400	3.0	97.0	0.0	0.0
SlendaSweet, Sainsbury's*	1 Tsp/1g	4	395	1.8	97.0	0.0	0.1
Spoonfull, Low Calorie, SupaSweet*	1 Tsp/1g	4	392	3.0	95.0	0.0	0.0
Tablets, Splenda*	1 Tablet/0.1g	0	345	10.0	76.2	0.0	1.6
Tablets, Tesco*	5 Tablets/5g	1	20	2.0	2.0	0.5	0.0

S

	Measure INFO/WEIGHT	per Measure KCAL	Nutrition Values per 100g / 100ml				
			KCAL	PROT	CARB	FAT	FIBRE
SWEETS,							
Banana, Baby Foam, Marks & Spencer*	1/3 Pack/34g	131	385	4.1	92.7	0.0	0.0
Candy Butter, Werther's Original*	1 Sweet/5g	22	430	1.0	86.0	9.0	0.0
Chew	1oz/28g	107	381	1.0	87.0	5.6	1.0
Eclair, Marks & Spencer*	1 Sweet/14g	65	465	3.3	69.8	19.3	0.2
Fizzy Lemon Fish, Asda*	1 Sweet/4.3g	13	325	5.0	76.0	0.1	0.0
Fruit Gums & Jellies	1 Tube/33g	107	324	6.5	79.5	0.0	0.0
Kisses, Hershey*	1 Kiss/5g	28	561	7.0	59.0	32.0	0.0
Lances, Fizzy, Strawberry, Somerfield*	1 Lance/3.7g	14	362	2.8	79.8	2.7	1.5
Sherbert Cocktails, Sainsbury's*	1 Sweet/9g	36	400	0.0	83.1	7.5	0.0
Sweetshop Favourites, Bassett's*	1 Sweet/5g	17	340	0.0	84.3	0.0	0.0
SWORDFISH,							
Grilled	1oz/28g	39	139	22.9	0.0	5.2	0.0
Loins, Asda*	1oz/28g	41	147	25.5	0.0	5.1	0.0
Raw	1oz/28g	31	109	18.0	0.0	4.1	0.0
SYRUP,							
Coffee, Caramel, Lyle's*	2 Tsps/10ml	33	329	0.0	83.0	0.0	0.0
Corn, Dark	1 Tbsp/20g	56	282	0.0	76.6	0.0	0.0
Golden	1 Tbsp/20g	60	298	0.3	79.0	0.0	0.0
Hazelnut Flavoured, Starbucks*	1 Pump/10g	20	200	0.0	50.0	0.0	0.0
Maple	1 Tbsp/20g	52	262	0.0	67.2	0.2	0.0

S

	Measure INFO/WEIGHT	per Measure KCAL	Nutrition Values per 100g / 100ml				
			KCAL	PROT	CARB	FAT	FIBRE
TABOULEH,							
Average	1oz/28g	33	119	2.6	17.2	4.6	0.0
Share The Taste, Marks & Spencer*	1oz/28g	31	110	3.4	15.1	4.0	2.0
TACO,							
Mixed Beans, Tesco*	1 Serving/140g	108	77	4.7	13.5	0.5	3.9
Shells, Old El Paso*	1 Taco/12g	57	478	7.4	60.8	22.8	0.0
TAGLIATELLE,							
Barilla*	1 Serving/100g	360	360	14.0	68.1	3.5	0.0
Basil, Marks & Spencer*	1 Serving/100g	365	365	15.1	69.0	2.8	4.0
Bicolore, Asda*	¼ Pack/125g	203	162	7.0	28.0	2.4	1.4
Carbonara, Frozen, Tesco*	1 Pack/400g	408	102	3.9	13.5	4.1	0.5
Carbonara, Italiano, Tesco*	1 Serving/325g	757	233	8.6	23.8	11.5	1.2
Carbonara, Low Fat, Bertorelli*	1 Pack/350g	301	86	5.3	12.0	2.2	0.9
Carbonara, Naturally Less 5% Fat, Asda*	1 Pack/400g	440	110	4.2	18.0	2.4	0.8
Carbonara, Perfectly Balanced, Waitrose*	1 Pack/350g	357	102	5.3	12.1	3.6	0.7
Carbonara, Reduced Fat, Waitrose*	1 Pack/350g	399	114	5.0	12.1	5.1	0.6
Carbonara, Safeway*	1 Serving/298g	277	93	3.7	13.2	2.8	0.6
Chicken & Mushroom, GFY, Asda*	1 Pack/400g	359	90	7.3	11.3	1.8	0.7
Chicken & Tomato, Eat Smart, Safeway*	1 Pack/400g	360	90	7.5	10.8	1.4	1.1
Chicken, Italia, Marks & Spencer*	1 Pack/360g	342	95	8.1	12.1	1.8	1.2
Egg & Spinach, Safeway*	1 Serving/125g	435	348	13.2	67.3	2.9	2.9
Egg, Dried, Sainsbury's*	1 Serving/90g	332	369	14.0	71.2	3.1	2.0
Egg, Dry, Tesco*	1 Serving/75g	266	355	14.5	66.4	3.5	2.6
Egg, Fresh, Tesco*	¼ Pack/125g	360	288	11.9	51.8	3.7	1.5
Fresh, Morrisons*	½ Pack/125g	364	291	11.3	54.0	3.3	2.5
Garlic & Herb, Fresh, Tesco*	1 Serving/125g	361	289	12.0	51.8	3.7	1.5
Garlic & Herb, Fresh, Waitrose*	1 Serving/125g	353	282	11.9	49.8	3.9	2.1
Garlic & Herbs, Cooked, Pasta Reale*	1 Pack/250g	390	156	6.2	30.4	1.1	1.0
Garlic Mushroom, BGTY, Sainsbury's*	1 Pack/450g	369	82	3.6	12.3	2.0	1.0
Garlic Mushroom, Italiano, Tesco*	1 Pack/450g	738	164	5.2	15.2	9.1	0.6
Ham & Mushroom, Asda*	1 Pack/340g	469	138	6.0	20.0	3.8	0.2
Ham & Mushroom, BGTY, Sainsbury's*	1 Pack/450g	486	108	5.3	14.5	3.2	0.8
Ham & Mushroom, Better For You, Morrisons*	1 Pack/350g	326	93	5.3	9.4	3.8	0.8
Ham & Mushroom, Co-Op*	1 Pack/300g	270	90	6.0	10.0	3.0	2.0
Ham & Mushroom, Eat Smart, Safeway*	1 Pack/400g	380	95	5.0	13.0	2.5	1.2
Ham & Mushroom, Good For You, Asda*	1 Pack/400g	304	76	3.8	9.0	2.7	0.4
Ham & Mushroom, Good Intentions, Somerfield*	1 Serving/300g	333	111	5.6	15.6	2.9	0.3
Ham & Mushroom, Healthy Choice, Safeway*	1 Pack/400g	400	100	5.5	12.1	3.3	0.3
Ham & Mushroom, Healthy Eating, Tesco*	1 Meal/340g	306	90	4.3	13.6	2.0	0.9
Ham & Mushroom, Italiano, Tesco*	1 Pack/340g	445	131	5.4	18.0	4.2	1.0
Ham & Mushroom, Morrisons*	1 Pack/350g	462	132	5.1	9.6	8.4	0.1
Ham, Ready Meals, Marks & Spencer*	1 Pack/360g	414	115	5.8	10.5	5.7	1.0
Meditarranean Style Chicken, Eat Smart Safeway*	1 Pack/400g	320	80	5.6	8.7	2.5	1.4
Mushroom & Tomato, Asda*	1 Pack/340g	211	62	2.5	10.0	1.3	1.2
Red Pepper, Organic, Sainsbury's*	½ Bag/125g	183	146	5.4	27.8	1.5	1.4
Ribbon Noodles, Waitrose*	1 Serving/125g	471	377	10.8	82.8	0.3	0.0
Salmon & Prawn, Perfectly Balanced, Waitrose*	1 Pack/401.2g	341	85	6.8	7.1	3.3	1.1
Seeds of Change*	1 Serving/100g	350	350	11.5	75.0	0.3	0.0
Smoked Salmon, Ready Meals, Marks & Spencer*	1 Pack/360g	612	170	6.2	10.6	11.2	0.9
Tomato & Basil Chicken, Weight Watchers*	1 Pack/330g	254	77	5.9	11.8	0.6	0.8
Tricolore, Waitrose*	½ Pack/125g	351	281	12.0	51.6	2.9	1.6
Verdi, Barilla*	1 Serving/150g	555	370	14.0	70.5	3.5	0.0
Verdi, Fresh, Sainsbury's*	1 Serving/240g	353	147	6.4	26.4	1.8	1.8
Verdi, Fresh, Tesco*	1 Serving/125g	163	130	5.2	25.1	1.0	2.0

T

	Measure INFO/WEIGHT	per Measure KCAL	Nutrition Values per 100g / 100ml				
			KCAL	PROT	CARB	FAT	FIBRE
TAGLIATELLE,							
With Chicken, Garlic & Lemon, BGTY, Sainsbury's*	1 Pack/450g	410	91	7.8	14.2	0.3	1.7
With Chicken, Garlic & Lemon, New, BGTY, Sainsbury's*	1 Pack/300g	324	108	9.2	15.1	1.2	1.7
With Ham & Mushroom, New, BGTY, Sainsbury's*	1 Pack/450g	401	89	5.3	11.8	2.3	1.4
With Roasted Vegetables, Good Intentions, Somerfield*	1 Pack/340g	349	103	3.7	16.6	2.4	1.7
Wth Ham, COU, Marks & Spencer*	1 Pack/357.9g	340	95	5.4	13.1	2.3	1.1
TAHINI PASTE, Average	1 Tsp/19g	115	607	18.5	0.9	58.9	8.0
TAMARILLOS, Average	1oz/28g	8	28	2.0	4.7	0.3	0.0
TAMARIND,							
Average	1oz/28g	67	238	2.3	56.5	0.3	0.0
Leaves, Fresh	1oz/28g	32	115	5.8	18.2	2.1	0.0
Pulp	1oz/28g	76	273	3.2	64.5	0.3	0.0
TANDOORI CHICKEN,							
GFY, Asda*	1 Pack/420g	420	100	9.0	8.0	3.6	1.4
Healthy Choice, McCain*	1 Pack/270g	297	110	7.5	17.5	1.0	0.0
Masala, Asda*	1 Pack/400g	580	145	7.0	18.0	5.0	1.3
Sizzler, Sainsbury's*	1 Pack/400g	536	134	12.8	4.3	7.3	1.7
Sizzler, Tesco*	1 Serving/175g	243	139	10.0	10.0	6.6	1.0
Safeway*	1 Pack/350g	595	170	13.7	5.7	10.3	1.3
Tesco*	1 Serving/175g	198	113	10.6	6.7	4.9	1.0
With Spicy Potatoes & Dip, Healthy Eating, Tesco*	1 Pack/370g	322	87	9.7	10.3	0.8	1.3
TANGERINES,							
Fresh, Raw	1oz/28g	10	35	0.9	8.0	0.1	1.3
Weighed With Peel & Pips	1 Med/70g	18	25	0.7	5.8	0.1	0.9
TAPAS, Pequillo Peppers, Sainsbury's*	½ Can/115g	110	96	3.6	8.6	5.2	1.8
TAPENADE,							
Green Olive, Best, Safeway*	1 Tsp/15g	71	470	1.6	10.2	47.0	1.7
Olive With Capers & Anchovy, Safeway*	1 Tbsp/20g	103	513	2.1	1.0	55.6	2.2
TAPIOCA, Raw	1oz/28g	101	359	0.4	95.0	0.1	0.4
TARAMASALATA,							
Average	1oz/28g	141	504	3.2	4.1	52.9	0.0
Fresh, BGTY, Sainsbury's*	1oz/28g	71	253	4.3	13.5	20.2	0.7
Fresh, Healthy Eating, Tesco*	1 Pot/170g	430	253	4.3	13.5	20.2	0.7
Fresh, Safeway*	1 Pot/170g	797	469	3.4	8.7	46.7	0.0
Marks & Spencer*	1oz/28g	140	500	3.9	5.5	51.2	1.7
Tesco*	1 Serving/50g	220	440	7.4	8.8	41.7	0.3
Reduced Fat, Waitrose*	1 Pot/170g	598	352	4.2	9.6	33.0	0.6
TARRAGON,							
Dried, Ground	1 Tsp/1.6g	6	295	22.8	42.8	7.2	0.0
Fresh	1oz/28g	14	49	3.4	6.3	1.1	0.0
TART,							
Apricot Lattice, Sainsbury's*	1 Slice/125g	321	257	3.4	35.3	11.4	2.6
Bakewell, Marks & Spencer*	¼ Tart/75g	345	460	7.5	48.1	26.7	2.1
Bakewell, Somerfield*	¼ Tart/80g	296	370	5.0	45.0	19.0	0.0
Cherry Tomato Mascarpone, Asda*	1 Tart/160g	290	181	4.4	15.6	11.3	1.1
Chocolate, Co-Op*	1 Tart/22g	102	465	4.0	42.0	31.0	0.7
Coconut & Cherry, Asda*	1 Serving/50g	215	430	4.4	58.0	20.0	4.0
Coconut, Marks & Spencer*	1 Tart/53g	220	415	5.8	57.8	18.1	3.6
Congress, Morrisons*	1 Tart/38g	149	393	6.0	59.7	14.4	2.4
Custard, Individual	1 Tart/94g	260	277	6.3	32.4	14.5	1.2
Egg Custard, Marks & Spencer*	1 Tart/85g	243	286	6.3	34.7	14.5	0.7
Egg Custard, Safeway*	1 Tart/85g	225	265	5.3	33.3	12.6	0.8
Egg Custard, Sainsbury's	1 Tart/85g	230	270	6.1	30.1	14.1	0.7
Egg Custard, Somerfield*	1 Tart/85g	206	242	5.1	29.9	11.3	0.7

	Measure	per Measure	Nutrition Values per 100g / 100ml				
	INFO/WEIGHT	KCAL	KCAL	PROT	CARB	FAT	FIBRE
TART,							
Egg Custard, Tesco*	1 Cake/82g	214	261	6.2	31.5	12.2	1.1
Feta Cheese & Spinach, Puff Pastry, Tesco*	1 Tart/108g	306	283	7.1	23.5	17.8	0.9
Filo Asparagus Tartlette, Marks & Spencer*	1 Serving/15g	45	300	4.4	25.2	20.4	2.1
Fruit, Safeway*	1 Tart/180g	425	236	2.7	30.6	11.4	0.0
Goats Cheese & Onion, Marks & Spencer*	1 Serving/161g	451	280	5.8	22.4	18.7	1.5
Italian Lemon & Almond, Sainsbury's*	1 Slice/49g	182	371	7.4	31.9	23.7	4.1
Jam	1 Slice/90g	342	380	3.3	62.0	14.9	1.6
Jam, Assorted, Tesco*	1 Tart/35g	123	351	3.4	51.9	14.4	1.2
Jam, Farmfoods*	1 Tart/34g	132	387	3.6	60.5	14.5	2.8
Jam, Real Fruit, Mr Kipling*	1 Tart/35g	136	389	3.5	61.0	14.5	0.0
Jam, Real Fruit, Sainsbury's*	1 Tart/37g	142	383	3.4	60.9	14.0	1.4
Leek & Stilton, Morrisons*	1 Serving/125g	393	314	6.9	23.1	21.5	0.3
Lemon & Raspberry, Finest, Tesco*	1 Tart/120g	360	300	5.2	38.4	14.0	2.9
Lemon Curd, Lyons*	1 Tart/30g	122	406	3.7	59.3	17.0	0.0
Lemon, Marks & Spencer*	1/6 Tart/50g	208	415	5.0	32.7	29.3	0.9
Manchester, Marks & Spencer*	1oz/28g	104	370	4.1	36.0	23.5	1.1
Mixed Fruit, Marks & Spencer*	1oz/28g	59	210	2.8	26.9	10.4	0.8
Pear & Chocolate With Brandy, TTD, Sainsbury's*	1/6 Tart/90g	261	290	3.5	32.0	16.4	1.4
Raspberry Flavoured, Value, Tesco*	1 Tart/29.0g	113	389	3.8	56.6	16.4	1.6
Raspberry, Reduced Sugar, Asda*	1 Tart/34g	129	380	4.6	67.5	10.1	1.2
Roasted Vegetable & Goats Cheese Filo, M&S*	1 Tart/120g	276	230	7.4	16.6	14.8	1.3
Roasted Vegetable, Finest, Tesco*	1 Serving/130g	250	192	3.0	19.6	11.3	1.2
Strawberry & Fresh Cream, Finest, Tesco*	1 Tart/129g	350	271	3.3	31.1	14.8	1.2
Strawberry Sundae, Asda*	1 Tart/46g	187	407	3.3	58.0	18.0	1.3
Strawberry, Reduced Sugar, Asda*	1 Tart/37g	141	380	4.6	67.5	10.1	1.2
Toffee Apple, Co-Op*	1 Tart/20g	69	345	3.0	47.0	16.0	0.7
Toffee Pecan, Marks & Spencer*	1 Tart/91g	414	455	6.0	48.5	26.5	2.0
Tomato, Mozzarella & Basil Puff, Sainsbury's	1/3 Tart/120g	318	265	9.2	10.2	20.8	0.9
Treacle Lattice, Mr Kipling*	1/6 Tart/70g	256	365	4.4	59.8	12.1	1.1
Treacle, Somerfield*	1/6 Tart/59g	232	394	5.0	64.0	14.0	0.0
Treacle, Teatime Selection, Safeway*	1 Tart/45g	171	380	4.2	63.9	12.0	1.1
TARTE,							
Aux Fruits, Finest, Tesco*	1 Tart/147g	345	235	3.0	33.4	9.9	1.1
Creme Fraiche, Roast Onion & Brie, TTD, Sainsbury's*	1/3 Tart/72g	201	279	4.9	17.9	20.9	0.8
Goats Cheese & Spinach Flambe, Sainsbury's*	1/3 Tart/76.8g	223	289	7.4	15.9	21.8	0.9
Normande, French Style, Marks & Spencer*	1/6 Tarte/84.5g	244	290	3.3	26.8	19.0	0.7
Tatin, Sainsbury's*	1 Serving/120g	244	203	2.9	32.8	6.7	1.9
au Chocolat, Finest, Tesco*	1/6 Tarte/85g	421	495	5.1	44.0	33.2	1.6
au Citron, TTD, Sainsburys*	1 serving/105g	360	343	3.7	36.6	20.2	0.6
TARTLETS,							
Caramelised Onion & Gruyere, Sainsbury's*	1 Tart/145g	381	263	5.8	17.3	19.0	1.3
Mushroom, Bacon & Spinach, Safeway*	1 Tartlet/120g	312	260	7.0	13.0	20.0	1.0
Onion, Caramelised, Creamy, Somerfield*	1 Tartlet/105g	310	295	4.0	21.0	22.0	0.0
Red Onion & Goats Cheese, Sainsbury's*	1 Tart/112.8g	336	297	7.0	23.7	19.3	1.5
Roast Pepper & Mascarpone, Sainsbury's*	1 Tart/100g	232	232	3.5	17.7	16.4	1.5
Sausage & Tomato, Sainsbury's*	1 Tartlet/135g	323	239	4.8	19.5	15.8	1.6
TARTLETTE, Cherry & Almond, Go Ahead, McVitie's*	1 Tartlette/46.0g	165	359	4.1	67.5	9.8	0.7
TARTUFO, Thorntons*	1 Chocolate/15g	77	513	7.4	40.0	36.0	3.3
TEA,							
Camomile Lemon, Herbal, Tetley*	1 Serving/175ml	3	2	0.1	0.1	0.0	0.0
Earl Grey, Iced, Twinings*	1fl oz/30ml	10	34	0.1	8.0	0.0	0.0
Fruit Punch, London Fruit & Herb Company*	1 Mug/200ml	4	2	0.0	0.5	0.0	0.0
Fruit, Whittards*	1fl oz/30ml	12	40	0.0	1.2	0.0	0.0

T

	Measure INFO/WEIGHT	per Measure KCAL	Nutrition Values per 100g / 100ml				
			KCAL	PROT	CARB	FAT	FIBRE
TEA,							
Green & Lemon, Iced, Twinings*	1 Serving/250ml	75	30	0.1	7.3	0.1	0.0
Green & Lemon, Twinings*	1 Serving/250ml	65	26	0.0	7.3	0.0	0.0
Herbal	1 Mug/227ml	2	1	0.0	0.2	0.0	0.0
Lemon Iced, Costa*	1 Bottle/275ml	91	33	0.0	8.0	0.0	0.0
Lemon, Instant Drink, Reduced Sweetness, Lift*	1 Serving/15g	53	352	0.0	87.0	0.0	0.0
Lemon, Original, Instant Drink, Lift*	1 Serving/15g	53	352	0.0	87.0	0.0	0.0
Made With Water With Semi-Skimmed Milk	1 Cup/200ml	14	7	0.4	0.5	0.4	0.0
Made With Water With Skimmed Milk	1 Mug/227ml	14	6	0.5	0.7	0.2	0.0
Made With Water With Whole Milk	1 Cup/200ml	22	11	1.2	1.5	0.2	0.0
Peach Flavour, Lift*	1 Cup/15g	58	384	0.3	95.6	0.0	0.0
Peach, Iced, Twinings*	1 Serving/200ml	60	30	0.1	7.3	0.1	0.0
Pure Peppermint, Herbal, Tetley*	1 Serving/175ml	3	2	0.1	0.2	0.0	0.0
UHT Skimmed Milk, McDonald's*	1 Cup/14ml	10	74	3.7	5.4	4.1	0.0
TEACAKES,							
Chocolate, Marks & Spencer*	1 Cake/17g	73	430	5.0	65.4	16.7	1.0
Chocolate, Tunnocks*	1 Cake/22g	91	413	5.3	61.0	18.1	0.0
Fruit, Lidl*	1 Cake/62g	166	267	10.6	46.3	4.4	2.2
Fruited, Co-Op*	1 Cake/62g	160	258	9.7	46.8	3.2	3.2
Fruited, Marks & Spencer*	1 Cake/60g	156	260	8.9	53.4	1.0	2.0
Fruited, Warburton's*	1 Cake/62g	162	261	9.7	48.0	3.4	2.7
Jam, Burton's*	1 Cake/10g	43	429	3.6	66.0	16.7	1.0
Mallow, Tesco*	1 Cake/14g	63	450	4.1	65.4	19.1	1.0
Reduced Fat, Marks & Spencer*	1 Cake/17g	68	401	5.0	69.1	11.7	0.9
Richly Fruited, Waitrose*	1 Cake/72g	205	285	7.8	55.0	3.7	2.2
Sainsbury's*	1 Cake/70g	171	244	8.0	45.0	3.6	2.6
Tesco*	1 Cake/61g	163	267	7.8	51.1	3.5	2.4
Tunnock's*	1 Cake/22g	91	413	5.3	61.0	18.1	0.0
With Fruit, Morning Fresh, Aldi*	1 Cake/65g	155	239	7.4	44.6	3.4	2.3
TEMPEH, Average	1oz/28g	46	166	20.7	6.4	6.4	4.3
TERIYAKI CHICKEN, Asda*	1 Pack/360g	299	83	9.1	8.6	1.4	0.8
TERRINE,							
Lobster & Prawn, Slices, Marks & Spencer*	1 Serving/55g	107	195	18.2	0.7	13.4	0.7
Poached Salmon, Tesco*	1 Pack/113g	349	309	15.5	0.8	27.1	0.0
Prawn, TTD, Sainsbury's*	1 Pot/60g	115	192	9.0	3.7	15.7	0.4
Salmon & Asparagus, Cooked, Tesco*	1 Serving/60g	118	196	9.9	2.7	16.2	0.3
Salmon & Crayfish, Slice, Finest, Tesco*	1 Slice/110g	149	135	21.9	0.1	5.2	0.1
Salmon & King Prawn, Waitrose*	1 Serving/75g	98	130	19.3	1.3	5.3	0.0
Salmon, Reduced Fat, Tesco*	1 Serving/56g	100	179	15.5	1.1	12.5	3.5
Salmon, Three, Marks & Spencer*	1 Serving/80g	168	210	17.6	0.8	15.3	0.9
Salmon, With Prawn & Lobster, Marks & Spencer*	1 Serving/55g	107	195	18.2	0.7	13.4	0.7
Scottish Smoked Salmon, Tesco*	1 Slice/25g	56	225	13.9	4.9	16.6	0.5
TEX MEX PLATTER, Marks & Spencer*	1 Pack/415g	934	225	12.6	10.5	14.6	0.9
THAI BITES,							
Lightly Salted, Jacob's*	1 Pack/25g	94	375	6.9	79.7	3.2	0.1
Oriental Spice, Jacob's*	1 Pack/25g	93	373	7.1	78.0	3.6	0.2
Seaweed Flavour, Jacob's*	1 Pack/25g	94	377	7.1	80.0	3.2	0.5
Sweet Herb, Jacob's*	1 Pack/25g	93	372	7.1	78.8	3.2	0.2
THYME,							
Dried, Ground	1 Tsp/1.2g	3	276	9.1	45.3	7.4	0.0
Fresh	1 Tsp/0.8g	1	95	3.0	15.1	2.5	0.0
TIA, MARIA	1 Serving/25ml	75	300	0.0	0.0	0.0	0.0
TIC TAC,							
Fresh Mint, Ferrero*	2 Tic Tacs/1g	4	390	0.0	97.5	0.0	0.0

T

INFO/WEIGHT	Measure per Measure	KCAL	Nutrition Values per 100g / 100ml KCAL	PROT	CARB	FAT	FIBRE
TIC TAC,							
Lime & Orange, Ferrero*	2 Tic Tacs/1g	4	386	0.0	95.5	0.0	0.0
Orange, Ferrero*	2 Tic Tacs/1g	4	385	0.0	95.5	0.0	0.0
Spearmint, Ferrero*	1 Box/16g	62	390	0.0	97.5	0.0	0.0
TIKKA MASALA,							
Chicken & Basmati Rice, Patak's*	1 Pack/400g	580	145	9.9	15.1	5.0	0.2
Chicken & Pilau Rice, Asda*	1 Pack/400g	548	137	7.0	16.0	5.0	1.6
Chicken & Pilau Rice, GFY, Asda*	1 Pack/400g	596	149	8.0	19.0	4.6	1.1
Chicken & Pilau Rice, Safeway*	1 Pack/399g	654	164	7.5	16.5	7.5	1.4
Chicken & Rice, COU, Marks & Spencer*	1 Pack/400g	420	105	7.8	14.6	1.6	2.1
Chicken & Rice, Healthy Living, Tesco*	1 Pack/420g	483	115	7.6	16.2	2.3	1.6
Chicken & Rice, Takeaway, Tesco*	1 Pack/350g	525	150	4.4	20.3	5.7	1.2
Chicken With Basmati Rice, Eat Smart, Safeway*	1 Pack/363g	290	80	6.4	9.6	1.4	0.7
Chicken With Pilau Rice, BGTY, Sainsbury's*	1 Pack/450g	428	95	7.8	12.7	1.4	0.9
Chicken With Pilau Rice, Co-Op*	1 Pack/400g	560	140	7.0	12.0	7.0	1.0
Chicken With Pilau Rice, Eat Smart, Safeway*	1 Pack/400g	396	99	5.7	14.3	2.1	1.6
Chicken With Pilau Rice, New, BGTY, Sainsbury's*	1 Pack/400g	416	104	8.0	16.0	0.9	1.8
Chicken With Pilau Rice, Perfectly Balanced, Waitrose*	1 Pack/400g	520	130	7.7	16.9	3.5	1.1
Chicken With Rice, GFY, Asda*	1 Pack/400g	504	126	6.0	19.0	2.9	0.7
Chicken With Rice, Healthy Eating, Tesco*	1 Pack/400g	472	118	6.1	17.0	2.8	1.8
Chicken With Rice, Patak's*	1 Carton/350g	571	163	5.1	21.8	6.1	4.4
Chicken With Tumeric Rice, BGTY, Sainsbury's*	1 Pack/369g	446	121	6.7	20.5	1.3	0.4
Chicken With White Rice, BGTY, Sainsbury's*	1 Pack/400g	436	109	5.8	16.1	2.4	0.7
Chicken, BGTY, Sainsbury's*	1 Pack/450g	513	114	8.6	17.0	1.3	1.1
Chicken, Boiled Rice & Nan, Meal For One, GFY, Asda*	1 Pack/605g	823	136	6.0	21.0	3.1	0.0
Chicken, COU, Marks & Spencer*	1 Pack/300g	300	100	12.1	6.0	2.8	1.3
Chicken, Feeling Great, Findus*	1 Pack/350g	420	120	5.5	17.0	3.5	2.0
Chicken, Good Choice, Iceland*	1 Pack/398g	486	122	6.6	20.4	1.5	0.6
Chicken, Good Intentions, Somerfield*	1 Pack/400g	612	153	7.6	26.0	2.1	1.7
Chicken, Healthy Choice, Iceland*	1 Pack/399g	431	108	6.5	18.0	1.1	0.9
Chicken, Healthy Eating, Tesco*	1 Pack/350g	333	95	12.3	6.6	2.2	0.8
Chicken, Hot, Sainsbury's*	1 Pack/400g	604	151	13.2	3.6	9.3	1.5
Chicken, Indian Takeaway, Iceland*	1 Pack/400g	316	79	7.5	6.9	2.4	1.2
Chicken, Indian, Medium, Sainsbury's*	1 Pack/400g	848	212	13.2	5.3	15.3	0.1
Chicken, Low Fat, Iceland*	1 Pack/400g	360	90	7.8	12.5	1.0	0.5
Chicken, Marks & Spencer*	1 Pack/300g	585	195	12.2	5.3	13.8	1.5
Chicken, Medium, Tesco*	1 Pack/350g	532	152	11.2	4.9	9.8	0.6
Chicken, Microwave Meal, Good Choice, Iceland*	1 Pack/400g	488	122	6.6	20.4	1.5	0.6
Chicken, Morrisons*	1 Pack/340g	388	114	11.9	5.4	5.0	0.0
Chicken, Sainsbury's*	1 Pack/400g	736	184	12.8	4.6	12.7	0.2
Chicken, Sharwood's*	1 Pack/375g	563	150	7.2	15.1	6.7	0.8
Chicken, SmartPrice, Asda*	1 Pack/300g	405	135	7.0	17.0	4.3	0.3
Chicken, Somerfield*	1 Pack/350g	553	158	11.7	3.6	10.8	1.5
Chicken, Take Away Menu, BGTY, Sainsbury's	1 Pack/251g	226	90	13.4	4.2	2.2	1.3
Chicken, Tesco*	1 Pack/350g	511	146	11.1	4.3	9.4	1.5
Chicken, Tinned, Asda*	½ Can/200g	238	119	8.0	6.0	7.0	0.9
Chicken, Waitrose*	½ Pack/200g	298	149	12.8	2.6	9.7	1.6
Healthy Eating, Tesco*	1 Serving/220g	191	87	1.0	10.2	4.7	0.5
Quorn, & Rice, Tesco*	1 Pack/400g	364	91	3.4	13.9	2.4	1.7
Vegetable & Rice, Patak's*	1 Pack/370g	503	136	2.5	19.0	6.1	0.9
Vegetable, Aldi*	1 Can/400g	496	124	1.9	10.3	8.4	1.4
Vegetable, Asda*	½ Can/204g	190	93	2.0	10.0	5.0	2.0
Vegetable, Waitrose*	1 Can/200g	204	102	2.4	6.4	7.4	0.0
Vegetable, With Rice, Tesco*	1 Pack/450g	500	111	2.6	15.5	4.3	0.9

T

	Measure INFO/WEIGHT	per Measure KCAL	Nutrition Values per 100g / 100ml				
			KCAL	PROT	CARB	FAT	FIBRE
TIKKA MASALA,							
With Rice, Quorn*	1 Pack/400g	476	119	4.3	13.5	5.3	1.6
TIME OUT,							
Cadbury's*	2 Fingers/35g	189	540	5.4	61.8	29.9	0.0
Orange, Snack Size, Cadbury's*	1 Finger/11g	61	555	5.0	59.4	32.9	0.0
TIP TOP, Nestle*	1 Serving/40g	45	112	4.8	9.0	6.3	0.0
TIRAMISU,							
Asda*	1 Pot/100g	252	252	4.3	34.0	11.0	0.5
BGTY, Sainsbury's*	1 Pot/90g	140	156	4.5	28.3	2.7	0.3
COU, Marks & Spencer*	1 Serving/95g	138	145	3.7	26.9	2.7	0.6
Italian, Co-Op*	1 Pack/90g	230	255	5.0	37.0	10.0	0.4
Italian, Safeway*	1 Serving/125g	353	282	4.4	34.4	14.0	1.6
Morrisons*	1 Pot/90g	248	276	4.0	38.0	11.0	0.0
Raspberry, Marks & Spencer*	1 Serving/84g	197	235	3.8	22.9	14.4	0.2
Somerfield*	1 Pot/100g	286	286	5.0	39.0	11.0	0.0
Trifle, Sainsbury's*	1 Serving/100g	243	243	2.3	23.2	15.7	0.6
Waitrose*	1 Pot/90g	221	246	6.4	27.2	12.4	0.0
TOAD IN THE HOLE,							
Large, Great Value, Asda*	¼ Pack/81.2g	237	293	10.0	25.0	17.0	2.3
Sainsbury's*	1 Serving/144g	449	312	11.5	23.4	19.2	0.9
Vegetarian, Aunt Bessie's*	1 Pack/190g	481	253	13.1	19.9	13.6	1.2
Vegetarian, Tesco*	1 Pack/190g	471	248	13.1	26.5	10.0	2.8
With Three Sausages, Asda*	1 Pack/150g	435	290	10.0	22.0	18.0	1.0
Co-Op*	1 Pack/170g	366	215	7.8	12.3	14.9	2.6
Vegetarian, Meat Free, Asda*	1 Toad/173g	407	235	9.0	25.0	11.0	3.1
Vegetarian, Linda McCartney*	1 Pack/190g	359	189	13.6	13.9	8.8	1.1
TOAST TOPPERS,							
Chicken & Mushroom, Heinz*	1 Serving/56g	31	56	5.1	5.7	1.4	0.2
Mushroom & Bacon, Heinz*	1 Serving/56g	53	94	6.9	6.6	4.4	0.3
TOASTIES,							
Cheese & Ham, Tayto*	1 Serving/50g	260	519	6.8	58.0	29.7	0.0
Cheese & Onion, Warburton's*	1 Toastie/42g	120	286	7.5	33.1	13.7	0.0
TOBLERONE, Milk, Toblerone*	1oz/28g	147	525	5.3	60.7	29.0	2.7
TOFFEE,							
Assorted, Sainsbury's*	1 Sweet/8g	37	457	2.2	76.5	15.8	0.2
Chocolate Coated, Thorntons*	1 Bag/100g	521	521	3.5	57.9	30.7	0.3
Devon Butter, Thorntons*	1 Sweet/9g	40	444	1.7	72.2	16.7	0.0
Double Devon, Marks & Spencer*	1 Sweet/8g	37	460	1.8	73.1	19.9	0.0
English Butter, Co-Op*	1 Toffee/8g	38	470	2.0	71.0	20.0	0.0
Liquorice, Thorntons*	1 Bag/100g	506	506	1.9	58.8	29.4	0.0
Mixed	1oz/28g	119	426	2.2	66.7	18.6	0.0
Original, Thorntons*	1 Bag/100g	514	514	1.8	59.3	30.1	0.0
Vanilla Flavour, Diabetic, Thorntons*	1oz/28g	124	442	2.0	60.9	31.4	0.0
TOFFEE CRISP,							
Mini, Nestle*	1 Bar/18g	92	507	4.1	60.8	27.5	0.0
Nestle*	1 Bar/48g	237	494	4.1	62.1	25.5	0.0
TOFU,							
Marinated Organic Pieces, Cauldron Foods*	1oz/28g	64	230	19.3	2.4	15.9	0.7
Natural, Organic, Evernat*	1oz/28g	34	120	14.4	1.8	6.2	0.0
Organic, Cauldron Foods*	1oz/28g	33	118	12.9	1.2	6.8	0.2
Smoked, Organic, Evernat*	1oz/28g	36	127	16.3	0.8	6.6	0.0
Soya Bean, Fu Juk	1oz/28g	108	387	45.1	23.3	16.2	0.0
Soya Bean, Steamed	1oz/28g	20	73	8.1	0.7	4.2	0.0
Soya Bean, Steamed, Fried	1oz/28g	73	261	23.5	2.0	17.7	0.0

T

	Measure INFO/WEIGHT	per Measure KCAL	Nutrition Values per 100g / 100ml				
			KCAL	PROT	CARB	FAT	FIBRE
TOMATO FRITO,							
Heinz*	1oz/28g	20	73	1.3	7.7	4.1	0.8
TOMATO JUICE,							
Del Monte*	1 Glass/200ml	38	19	0.8	3.5	0.0	0.0
Fresh Pressed, Tesco*	1 Glass/200ml	42	21	0.6	4.6	0.0	0.6
Sainsbury's*	1 Glass/250ml	55	22	1.1	3.9	0.1	0.4
Tesco	1 Glass/200ml	34	17	0.8	3.1	0.0	0.6
TOMATO PASTE, Sun Dried, Sainsbury's*	1 Heaped Tsp/10g	37	373	3.4	14.8	33.3	0.0
TOMATO PUREE,							
Double Concentrate, Safeway*	1oz/28g	20	71	4.4	12.9	0.2	2.8
Double Concentrate, Tesco*	1 Sm Can/142g	131	92	4.8	18.1	0.0	2.5
Double Concentrated, Morrisons*	1 Serving/5g	3	68	4.5	12.9	0.2	0.0
Heinz*	1 Des Sp/11g	6	57	3.7	10.1	0.2	2.3
Italian, Princes*	1 Serving/25g	22	86	6.0	15.0	0.2	3.0
Napolina*	1oz/28g	28	99	3.9	20.0	0.4	2.0
Sainsbury's*	1 Tbsp/16g	13	82	4.7	14.9	0.4	2.0
Smartprice, Asda*	1 Tbsp/15g	10	66	3.6	13.0	0.3	2.5
Tesco*	1oz/28g	26	92	4.8	18.1	0.0	2.5
Tinned, Sharwood's*	1oz/28g	15	55	4.1	9.5	0.4	2.3
Tube, Sharwood's*	1oz/28g	20	72	5.3	12.3	0.5	3.0
Value, Tesco*	1 Tbsp/16g	11	66	3.6	13.0	0.0	2.6
TOMATOES,							
Baby Plum, Tesco*	1 Serving/50g	9	18	0.7	3.1	0.3	1.0
Canned, Whole Contents	1 Can/410g	66	16	1.0	3.0	0.1	0.7
Cherry, Asda*	1oz/28g	5	19	0.8	3.0	0.4	1.0
Cherry, Canned, Waitrose*	1 Can/395g	83	21	1.1	4.0	0.1	0.9
Cherry, On the Vine, Finest, Tesco*	1 Serving/50g	10	19	0.8	3.0	0.4	1.0
Cherry, On the Vine, Speciality, Waitrose*	1 Pack/300g	54	18	0.7	3.1	0.3	1.1
Cherry, Organic, Tesco*	1 Serving/100g	19	19	0.8	3.2	0.4	2.4
Cherry, Raw, Fresh	1oz/28g	5	18	0.8	3.0	0.4	1.0
Cherry, Safeway*	1 Serving/73g	12	16	0.7	3.0	0.3	0.0
Cherry, Somerfield*	1 Pack/100g	18	18	0.8	3.0	0.4	1.0
Cherry, Tesco*	1 serving/75g	14	19	0.8	3.0	0.4	1.0
Chopped & Garlic, Asda*	1 Can/400g	92	23	1.0	4.0	0.3	0.0
Chopped, Ardmona*	1 Can/415g	91	22	0.9	4.3	0.1	1.0
Chopped, Asda*	1 Can/410g	86	21	1.2	3.8	0.1	0.8
Chopped, Canned, For Bolognese, Napolina*	1 Can/400g	120	30	1.3	5.7	0.2	0.7
Chopped, Chunky, Tesco*	½ Can/200g	62	31	1.5	5.8	0.2	0.9
Chopped, Economy, Sainsbury's*	1 Serving/100g	20	20	1.2	3.5	0.1	0.9
Chopped, In Rich Tomato Juice, Premium, Safeway*	½ Can/200g	42	21	1.2	3.8	0.1	0.8
Chopped, In Rich Tomato Sauce, Heinz*	1 Serving/130g	21	16	0.7	2.9	0.2	0.9
Chopped, Italian, Organic, Waitrose*	½ can/200g	40	20	1.1	4.0	0.0	0.9
Chopped, Italian, Tesco*	1oz/28g	6	23	1.4	4.0	0.2	0.9
Chopped, Italian, Waitrose*	1 Can/227g	45	20	1.1	4.0	0.0	0.9
Chopped, Italian, With Olive Oil & Garlic, Waitrose*	1 Serving/100g	33	33	1.1	3.6	1.6	0.0
Chopped, Italian, With Olives, Waitrose*	1 Can/400g	184	46	1.4	6.0	1.8	0.8
Chopped, Itlalian, With Herbs, Tesco*	1 Can/400g	116	29	1.1	5.7	0.2	0.7
Chopped, Marks & Spencer*	1oz/28g	6	20	1.2	3.5	0.1	0.9
Chopped, Napolina*	1 Sm Can/227g	50	22	1.1	3.5	0.4	0.3
Chopped, Napolina*	1 Serving/100g	22	22	1.1	3.5	0.4	0.0
Chopped, Organic, Biona*	½ Can/200g	37	19	1.1	2.9	0.4	0.0
Chopped, Organic, Tesco*	1 Can/400g	112	28	1.1	5.7	0.1	0.7
Chopped, Princes*	1 Can/400g	68	17	1.1	3.0	0.1	0.7
Chopped, Safeway*	1 Can/230g	44	19	1.1	3.5	0.1	0.8

T

TOMATOES,	Measure INFO/WEIGHT	per Measure KCAL	KCAL	PROT	CARB	FAT	FIBRE
Chopped, Safeway*	1 Can/400g	124	31	1.5	5.8	0.2	0.9
Chopped, Sainsbury's*	1 Can/400g	80	20	1.2	3.5	0.1	0.9
Chopped, Sugocasa, Premium, Sainsbury's*	¼ Jar/172g	59	34	1.6	6.5	0.2	0.9
Chopped, Thick, Asda*	1oz/28g	8	29	1.2	5.8	0.1	0.9
Chopped, Value, Tesco*	1 Can/400g	68	17	1.0	2.9	0.1	0.7
Chopped, With Chilli & Peppers, Asda*	1 Pack/400g	92	23	1.0	4.0	0.3	0.0
Chopped, With Chilli, Sainsbury's*	½ Can/200g	44	22	1.0	3.5	0.5	0.9
Chopped, With Garlic, Sainsbury's*	½ Can/200g	40	20	1.2	3.5	0.1	0.9
Chopped, With Herbs In Tomato Juice, Co-Op*	1 Serving/110g	19	17	1.0	2.9	0.1	0.7
Chopped, With Herbs, Carlini*	½ Can/200g	48	24	1.2	4.6	0.1	0.9
Chopped, With Herbs, Heinz*	1 Serving/100g	17	17	0.8	3.0	0.2	0.9
Chopped, With Herbs, Napolina*	1 Can/400g	100	25	1.0	5.1	0.1	0.4
Chopped, With Herbs, Sainsbury's*	½ Can/200g	40	20	1.2	3.5	0.1	0.9
Chopped, With Onion & Herbs, Napolina*	1 Can/400g	84	21	1.0	4.0	0.1	0.4
Chopped, With Peppers & Onions, Sainsbury's*	½ Can/200g	40	20	1.2	3.5	0.1	0.9
Creamed, Sainsbury's*	1 Carton/500g	150	30	1.1	6.0	0.1	0.8
Fresh, Raw	1 Med/85g	14	17	0.7	3.1	0.3	1.0
Fried in Blended Oil	1 Av Tomato/85g	77	91	0.7	5.0	7.7	1.3
Grilled	1oz/28g	14	49	2.0	8.9	0.9	2.9
Italian Cherry, Waitrose*	1 Serving/100g	21	21	1.1	4.0	0.1	0.9
Italian, Tesco*	1 Serving/100g	36	36	1.4	6.2	0.6	0.0
Organic, Marks & Spencer*	1oz/28g	6	20	1.4	3.5	0.2	1.4
Plum, Asda*	1 Serving/100g	23	23	1.3	4.0	0.2	0.9
Plum, Canned, Marks & Spencer*	1oz/28g	6	20	1.2	3.5	0.1	0.9
Plum, In Tomato Juice, Value, Tesco*	1 Can/400g	64	16	0.7	3.4	0.0	0.0
Plum, Peeled, Carlini, Aldi*	1 Can/240g	41	17	1.0	3.0	0.1	0.0
Plum, Peeled, Economy, Sainsbury's*	½ Can/200g	42	21	1.0	4.0	0.1	0.8
Plum, Peeled, Italian, Tesco*	1oz/28g	7	24	1.3	4.0	0.2	0.9
Plum, Peeled, Napolina*	1oz/28g	6	23	1.2	3.5	0.5	0.3
Plum, Peeled, Premium, Safeway*	½ Can/200g	38	19	1.1	3.5	0.1	1.8
Plum, Peeled, Premium, Sainsbury's*	1 Can/400g	148	37	2.2	7.0	0.1	1.6
Plum, Peeled, SmartPrice, Asda*	½ Can/200g	32	16	1.0	3.0	0.0	0.8
Plum, Peeled, Somerfield*	1oz/28g	4	16	1.0	3.0	0.0	0.0
Plum, Tinned, Sainsbury's*	1 Can/233g	42	18	1.1	3.5	0.1	0.8
Ripened On The Vine, Safeway*	1 Serving/100g	18	18	0.7	3.0	0.3	0.0
Selected, Merevale, Aldi*	1oz/28g	5	17	0.7	3.1	0.3	1.0
Sun Blush, Sainsbury's*	1 Serving/65g	79	121	2.9	13.6	7.4	4.3
Sun Dried	1oz/28g	139	495	3.3	5.4	51.3	0.0
Sun Dried, Marinated, Waitrose*	1 Serving/100g	126	126	2.4	8.0	9.4	1.2
Sun Dried, Marks & Spencer*	1oz/28g	65	232	4.7	15.5	16.8	6.6
Sun Dried, Sacla*	3 pieces/20g	39	195	4.7	10.4	15.0	0.0
Sweet Vine, Asda*	1 Serving/100g	18	18	0.7	3.0	0.3	1.0
Tesco*	1 Serving/100g	17	17	0.7	3.1	0.3	1.0
Tinned, Bettabuy, Morrisons*	1 Serving/200g	34	17	1.0	2.9	0.1	0.7
Vine Ripened, Finest, Tesco*	1 Pack/135g	24	18	0.7	3.1	0.3	1.0
Whole, Peeled, Heinz*	1 Serving/240g	38	16	0.7	2.9	0.2	0.8
TONDO'S, SALSA Flavour, Ryvita*	1 Serving/25g	99	395	7.1	84.8	3.0	0.9
TONGUE,							
Lunch, John West*	1oz/28g	48	173	19.5	3.0	10.4	0.0
Ox, Wafer Thin, Traditional, Marks & Spencer*	1oz/28g	64	230	22.3	0.0	15.5	0.0
Slices	1oz/28g	56	201	18.7	0.0	14.0	0.0
TONIC WATER,							
Average	1 Glass/250ml	83	33	0.0	8.8	0.0	0.0

T

	Measure INFO/WEIGHT	per Measure KCAL	Nutrition Values per 100g / 100ml				
			KCAL	PROT	CARB	FAT	FIBRE
TONIC WATER,							
Diet, Asda*	1 Glass/200ml	2	1	0.0	0.0	0.0	0.0
Indian, Low Calorie, Tesco*	1 Serving/200ml	2	1	0.0	0.0	0.0	0.0
Indian, Slimline, Schweppes*	1 Serving/188ml	3	2	0.4	0.1	0.0	0.0
Marks & Spencer*	1 Bottle/500ml	100	20	0.0	4.8	0.0	0.0
TOOTY FROOTIES, Rowntree's*	1oz/28g	113	402	0.4	92.1	3.6	0.0
TOPIC, Mars*	1 Bar/47g	232	493	6.0	58.1	26.3	0.0
TOPPING,							
Bruschetta, Safeway*	1 Serving/100g	26	26	1.2	3.6	0.8	0.0
Bruschetta, Sainsbury's*	1 Sm Tin/230g	60	26	1.2	3.6	0.8	1.1
Mediterranean, For Cod, Schwartz*	½ Jar/147g	128	87	1.7	9.5	4.7	0.0
Pizza, Italian Tomato & Herb, Sainsbury's*	1/5 Jar/50g	19	38	1.6	7.1	0.4	1.1
Pizza, Tomato With Cheese & Onion, Napolina*	1 Jar/250g	195	78	2.9	7.0	4.0	0.8
Pizza, Traditional Tomato With Basil, Napolina*	1 Jar/250g	153	61	1.2	7.8	2.6	0.7
TORTE,							
Chocolate, Safeway*	1/6 Torte/55g	122	221	4.1	27.6	10.5	1.5
Chocolate, Tesco*	1 Serving/50g	126	251	3.6	32.3	11.9	1.0
Lemon & Mango, Waitrose*	1 Serving/80g	142	177	3.9	33.6	3.0	0.6
Lemon, Farmfoods*	1/6 Cake/70g	137	195	4.3	21.9	10.0	0.5
Lemon, Somerfield*	1 Serving/45g	71	157	0.8	32.6	2.6	0.8
Raspberry, Safeway*	1/6 Serving/54g	93	172	1.2	25.1	7.4	1.5
TORTELLINI,							
3 Cheese, Sainsbury's*	1 Serving/50g	196	391	14.4	63.8	8.7	3.0
Aubergine & Pecorino, Sainsbury's*	½ Pack/150g	354	236	8.9	40.3	4.3	3.2
Beef & Red Wine, Italian, Asda*	½ Pack/150.3g	242	161	9.0	25.0	2.8	0.0
Cheese & Tomato, Marks & Spencer*	1 Meal/125g	238	190	10.0	29.1	3.6	1.8
Cheese, Weight Watchers*	1 Can/395g	233	59	2.1	8.5	1.8	0.5
Four Cheese & Tomato, Italian, Asda*	1 Serving/150g	249	166	8.0	25.0	3.8	0.0
Four Cheese with Tomato & Basil Sauce, Tesco*	1 pack/400g	500	125	6.1	16.9	3.7	0.6
Four Cheese, Asda*	1 Serving/150g	201	134	6.0	20.0	3.3	0.0
Four Cheese, Tesco*	1 Serving/125g	351	281	12.0	38.7	8.7	2.2
Garlic & Herb, Fresh, Sainsbury's*	½ Pack/150g	365	243	11.1	32.2	7.8	1.8
Garlic, Basil & Ricotta, Asda*	1 Serving/150g	227	151	6.0	24.0	3.4	0.0
Ham & Cheese, Asda*	1 Serving/125g	191	153	7.0	20.0	5.0	1.8
Ham & Cheese, Fresh, Asda*	½ Pack/150g	198	132	6.0	20.0	3.1	0.0
Ham & Cheese, Tesco*	1 Serving/225g	578	257	13.5	38.1	5.6	1.8
Italian Meat, Tesco*	1 Serving/125g	333	266	10.6	38.9	7.6	2.3
Italiana, Weight Watchers*	1 Can/395g	237	60	2.1	8.5	1.9	0.5
Mushroom, Asda*	1 Serving/125g	218	174	6.0	28.0	4.2	2.3
Mushroom, BGTY, Sainsbury's*	½ Can/200g	180	90	2.2	13.2	3.1	0.7
Mushroom, Perfectly Balanced, Waitrose*	1 Pack/250g	573	229	9.4	39.8	3.6	2.4
Pepperoni, Italian, Asda*	½ Pack/150g	250	167	6.7	26.0	4.0	0.0
Pork & Beef, BGTY, Sainsbury's*	½ Can/200g	142	71	2.3	11.9	1.6	1.2
Ricotta & Spinach, Somerfield*	1 Can/250g	283	113	12.0	4.0	6.0	0.0
Smoked Bacon & Tomato, Asda*	1 Pack/300g	591	197	9.0	29.0	5.0	0.0
Spicy Pepperoni, Asda*	½ Pack/150g	252	168	7.0	26.0	4.0	0.0
Spicy Pepperoni, Fresh, Asda*	½ Pack/150g	249	166	7.0	26.0	4.0	0.0
Spinach & Ricotta, Fresh, Sainsbury's*	½ Pack/125g	269	215	10.0	31.3	5.5	3.7
Spinach & Ricotta, Italian, Asda*	½ Pack/150g	189	126	5.0	21.0	2.4	0.0
Spinach & Ricotta, Pasta Reale*	½ Pack/125g	314	251	10.4	44.5	5.1	3.7
Spinach & Ricotta, Tesco*	1 Serving/125g	323	258	11.9	36.2	7.3	1.9
Spinach & Ricotta, Verdi, Asda*	1 Serving/125g	186	149	6.0	21.0	4.5	2.4
Tomato & Mozzarella, Fresh, Asda*	½ Pack/150g	236	157	8.0	25.0	2.8	0.0
Trio, Fresh, Tesco*	½ Pack/125g	323	258	12.8	35.8	7.1	2.0

T

INFO/WEIGHT	Measure	per Measure KCAL	Nutrition Values per 100g / 100ml				
			KCAL	PROT	CARB	FAT	FIBRE
TORTELLONI,							
Carbonara, Sainsbury's*	1 Serving/154g	416	270	13.1	27.7	12.6	2.5
Cheese & Ham, Co-Op*	1 Serving/125g	344	275	12.0	42.0	7.0	3.0
Cheese & Pesto, Somerfield*	1 Pack/250g	788	315	12.0	40.0	12.0	0.0
Cheese & Sun Dried Tomato, Fresh, Safeway*	½ Pack/199g	364	183	7.7	24.2	6.2	2.7
Five Cheese, Safeway*	1 Serving/150g	275	183	7.8	24.2	6.2	2.7
Four Cheese, Waitrose*	½ Pack/125g	298	238	10.3	34.2	6.7	1.6
Garlic & Herb, Cooked, Pasta Reale*	1 Pack/300g	546	182	6.7	30.1	3.9	0.9
Garlic Mushroom & Onion, Eat Smart, Safeway*	1 Serving/125g	231	185	9.3	31.4	2.0	1.4
Goats Cheese & Pesto, Sainsbury's*	1 Pack/250g	518	207	8.9	24.6	8.1	2.6
Meat & Cheese, Fresh, Sainsbury's*	½ Pack/125g	304	243	13.5	28.3	8.4	2.6
Mushroom, Perfectly Balanced, Waitrose*	½ Pack/125g	286	229	9.4	39.8	3.6	2.4
Porcini & Pancetta, TTD, Sainsbury's*	1 Serving/175g	294	168	7.1	20.8	6.3	3.4
Potato & Rosemary, Fresh, Sainsbury's*	½ Pack/175g	364	208	5.7	26.6	8.8	2.3
Ricotta & Spinach, Waitrose*	½ Pack/125g	328	262	11.3	38.4	7.0	2.4
Scamorza Cheese & Sun Dried Tomato, Sainsbury's*	½ Pack/125g	249	199	9.8	20.6	8.6	2.3
Spinach & Ricotta, Fresh, Safeway*	½ Pack/202g	341	169	7.4	24.0	4.8	2.4
Spinach & Ricotta, Fresh, Sainsbury's*	½ Pack/150g	323	215	10.0	31.3	5.5	3.7
Leek, Fresh, Sainsbury's*	½ Pack/175g	450	257	9.7	38.8	7.1	2.6
Walnut & Gorgonzola, Fresh, Sainsbury's*	½ Pack/175g	345	197	8.4	27.8	5.8	2.4
TORTIGLIONI,							
Buitoni*	1 Serving/75g	272	362	12.2	74.4	1.7	0.0
Tubes, Dried, Safeway*	1oz/28g	95	338	13.2	67.3	1.8	2.9
TORTILLA CHIPS,							
Blazing BBQ, Sainsbury's*	1 Serving/50g	237	474	6.8	58.9	23.5	4.6
Chilli Flavour, Somerfield*	1 Serving/50g	242	484	6.8	60.1	24.1	5.3
Cool, Salted, Sainsbury's*	1 Serving/50g	253	506	6.5	58.6	27.3	4.3
Cool, Tesco*	1 Serving/50g	246	492	7.4	58.9	25.2	4.6
Easy Cheesy!, Sainsbury's*	1 Serving/50g	249	498	7.1	58.7	26.1	4.5
Lightly Salted, Marks & Spencer*	1 Serving/20g	99	495	7.0	62.2	25.0	4.0
Lightly Salted, Waitrose*	1 Bag/40g	188	471	6.5	58.6	23.4	4.3
Nacho Cheese Flavour, Marks & Spencer*	1 Serving/25g	126	505	8.0	57.5	26.8	3.0
Waitrose*	1 Serving/25g	128	510	7.9	65.5	24.0	4.5
TORTILLAS,							
Asda*	1 Tortilla/34g	106	311	8.0	54.0	7.0	2.5
Flour, Asda*	1 Tortilla/34g	106	311	8.0	54.0	7.0	2.5
Flour, Mexican Style, Morrisons*	1 Tortilla/33g	103	313	8.6	53.9	7.0	2.5
Flour, Old El Paso*	2 Tortillas/81g	277	342	10.0	60.0	6.6	0.0
Flour, Tex "n" Mex 12, Sainsbury's*	1 Tortilla/26g	85	326	8.6	53.9	9.6	2.5
Plain Flour, Tesco*	1 Serving/63g	171	272	6.9	48.2	5.7	2.0
Plain Wheat, Waitrose*	1 Tortilla/43g	134	311	8.1	51.5	8.1	3.0
Plain, Wheat Flour, Sainsbury's*	1 Tortilla/56g	175	313	8.6	53.9	7.0	2.5
Soft Flour, Discovery*	1 Serving/39g	122	313	8.6	53.9	7.0	2.5
Wheat Flour, Waitrose*	1 Wrap/62g	203	327	8.5	51.5	9.8	0.0
Wrap, Bueno, Aldi*	1 Tortilla/62.9g	171	272	6.9	48.2	5.7	2.0
Wrap, Marks & Spencer*	1 Wrap/44g	134	305	8.1	51.8	8.4	2.9
Wrap, Morrisons*	1 Serving/35g	84	240	6.8	45.8	3.8	1.9
Wrap, Spicy Tomato, Tesco*	1 Wrap/63g	175	278	7.8	49.2	5.6	2.4
Wrap, Tomato & Herb, Tesco*	1 Serving/63g	165	262	7.9	45.1	5.5	2.1
Wrap, Tomato & Herbs, Sainsbury's**	1 Tortilla/52g	157	302	7.8	54.1	6.0	2.4
TRAIL MIX, Average	1oz/28g	121	432	9.1	37.2	28.5	4.3
TREACLE, Black	1 Tbsp/20g	51	257	1.2	67.2	0.0	0.0
TRIFLE,							
Banana & Mandarin, Co-Op*	¼ Trifle/125g	238	190	2.0	21.0	11.0	0.1

T

	Measure INFO/WEIGHT	per Measure KCAL	Nutrition Values per 100g / 100ml				
			KCAL	PROT	CARB	FAT	FIBRE
TRIFLE,							
Blackforest, BGTY, Sainsburyy's*	1 Pot/125g	171	137	2.1	21.9	4.5	1.6
Caramel, Galaxy, Mars*	1 Pot/100g	255	255	4.5	30.0	13.0	1.0
Cherry & Almond, Somerfield*	1 Trifle/125g	230	184	2.0	23.0	9.0	0.0
Chocolate, Healthy Living, Tesco*	1 Serving/150g	189	126	4.0	21.4	2.7	4.6
Chocolate, Light Milk, Cadbury's*	1 Pot/90g	171	190	5.6	25.5	7.3	0.0
Chocolate, Tesco*	1 Serving/125g	313	250	4.3	24.0	15.2	0.7
Cream Mandarin, Good For You, Asda*	1 Serving/113g	151	134	1.6	27.0	4.4	0.2
Fruit Cocktail, Co-Op*	1 Trifle/125g	213	170	2.0	23.0	8.0	0.2
Fruit Cocktail, Individual, Shape*	1 Trifle/115g	136	118	3.2	19.6	2.7	1.6
Fruit Cocktail, Individual,Tesco*	1 Pot/113g	175	155	1.7	19.6	7.8	0.6
Fruit Cocktail, Luxury Devonshire, St Ivel*	1 Trifle/125g	211	169	1.9	22.6	7.9	0.2
Fruit Cocktail, Somerfield*	1 Trifle/125g	211	169	2.0	23.0	8.0	0.0
Fruit, Marks & Spencer*	1 Trifle/50g	83	166	1.9	19.0	9.1	0.4
Fruit, Sainsbury's*	1 Serving/125g	233	186	2.3	21.7	10.0	0.3
Peach & Zabaglione, COU, Marks & Spencer*	1 Glass/130g	150	115	2.8	20.6	2.3	0.8
Raspberry, Asda*	1 Serving/100g	175	175	1.8	24.0	8.0	0.1
Raspberry, Co-Op*	1 Trifle/125g	206	165	2.0	22.0	8.0	0.3
Raspberry, Individual, Safeway*	1 Pot/125g	259	207	2.7	26.2	10.2	0.0
Raspberry, Sainsbury's*	1 Pot/125g	204	163	1.7	21.5	7.8	0.6
Raspberry, Somerfield*	1 Trifle/125g	208	166	2.0	22.0	8.0	0.0
Raspberry, Tesco*	1 Pot/150g	210	140	1.7	18.5	6.5	1.0
Sherry Sainsbury's*	1 Serving/132g	215	162	2.4	20.1	7.5	0.3
Strawberry, COU, Marks & Spencer*	1 Serving/142g	170	120	3.0	21.8	2.3	0.3
Strawberry, Co-Op*	1 Serving/123g	234	190	2.0	21.0	11.0	0.2
Strawberry, Healthy Eating, Tesco*	1 Serving/113g	114	101	1.7	18.5	2.2	0.6
Strawberry, Healthy Living, Tesco*	1 Pot/150g	161	107	2.3	19.3	2.3	2.7
Strawberry, Individual, Shape*	1 Pot/115g	137	119	3.3	19.8	2.7	1.6
Strawberry, Individual, Somerfield*	1 Trifle/125g	208	166	2.0	22.0	8.0	0.0
Strawberry, Luxury Devonshire, St Ivel*	1 Trifle/125g	208	166	2.0	21.7	7.9	0.2
Strawberry, Marks & Spencer*	1 Trifle/50g	81	161	2.0	17.7	9.2	0.6
Strawberry, Sainsbury's*	¼ Trifle/125g	232	186	2.2	21.7	10.0	0.2
Strawberry, Somerfield*	¼ Trifle/125g	235	188	2.0	21.0	11.0	0.0
Strawberry, St Ivel*	1 Trifle/113g	194	172	2.4	21.0	8.7	0.2
Strawberry, Tesco*	1 Serving/83g	140	169	1.6	17.7	10.2	0.7
Summerfruit, BGTY, Sainsbury's*	1 Trifle/125g	151	121	1.2	19.2	4.4	0.5
Triple Chocolate, Farmfoods*	¼ Trifle/86.25g	223	259	2.1	21.6	18.2	1.2
TRIFLE SPONGES,							
Safeway*	1 Sponge/23g	73	318	5.3	70.8	1.5	1.1
Somerfield*	1 Sponge/24g	81	339	5.0	76.0	2.0	0.0
Tesco*	1 Sponge/24g	78	325	5.4	72.2	1.6	1.1
TRIPE & ONIONS,							
Stewed	1oz/28g	26	93	8.3	9.5	2.7	0.7
TROMPRETTI,							
Sainsbury's*	1 Serving/75g	268	357	12.3	73.1	1.7	2.5
Tricolour, Fresh, Tesco*	1 Pack/250g	675	270	11.2	48.6	3.4	4.0
TROPICAL FRUIT,							
Drink, Tesco*	1 Glass/250ml	125	50	0.1	12.1	0.0	0.0
Drink, Waitrose*	1 Glass/250ml	118	47	0.2	11.2	0.0	0.0
Fresh, Marks and Spencer*	1 Pack/425g	213	50	0.7	11.8	0.3	2.0
Juice Drink, Safeway*	1 Glass/250ml	118	47	0.2	11.2	0.0	0.0
Juice Drink, Somerfield*	1 Glass/250ml	130	52	0.0	12.0	0.0	0.0
Juice, Plenty*	1 Glass/200ml	120	60	0.5	13.7	0.1	0.0
Mixed, Fruit Express, Del Monte*	1 Pot/185g	89	48	0.2	11.2	0.1	1.2

T

	Measure INFO/WEIGHT	per Measure KCAL	Nutrition Values per 100g / 100ml				
			KCAL	PROT	CARB	FAT	FIBRE
TROPICAL JUICE,							
No Added Sugar, Safeway*	1 Glass/200ml	10	5	0.1	0.9	0.0	0.0
Pure, Sainsbury's*	1 Glass/200ml	104	52	0.5	12.0	0.1	0.1
TROPICAL MIX,							
Sainsbury's*	1 Serving/50g	203	406	3.6	54.8	19.2	6.4
Somerfield*	1 Bag/50g	306	611	71.1	68.4	5.9	3.7
TROPICAL TUNES, Mars*	1 Pack/37g	143	387	0.0	96.6	0.0	0.0
TROTTOLE, Pasta, Sainsbury's*	1 Serving/90g	321	357	12.3	73.1	1.7	2.5
TROUT,							
Brown, Raw	1oz/28g	31	112	19.4	0.0	3.8	0.0
Brown, Steamed	1oz/28g	38	135	23.5	0.0	4.5	0.0
Fillets, Boneless, Grilled, Sainsbury's*	1 Serving/100g	132	132	22.9	0.0	4.5	0.0
Fillets, Chunky, Sainsbury's*	1 Serving/150g	257	171	19.1	0.0	9.5	0.1
Fillets, Fresh, Loch Etive, Waitrose*	1 Serving/125g	156	125	19.6	0.0	5.2	0.0
Fillets, Hot Smoked, Scottish, Tesco*	1 Serving/125g	183	146	23.0	0.1	6.0	0.1
Fillets, Scottish Loch, Tesco*	1 Fillet/115g	144	125	19.6	0.0	5.2	0.0
Fillets, Smoked, Organic, Waitrose*	2 Fillets/135g	219	162	26.5	0.0	6.2	0.0
Fillets, Smoked, Waitrose*	1 Fillet/65g	87	134	21.5	0.0	4.8	0.2
Rainbow, Fillets, Fresh, Safeway*, Grilled	1 Fillet/150g	203	135	21.5	0.0	5.4	0.0
Rainbow, Fillets, With Lemon & Rosemary Butter, M&S*	1 Serving/230g	460	200	17.5	1.4	13.9	0.5
Rainbow, Grilled	1oz/28g	38	135	21.5	0.0	5.4	0.0
Rainbow, Raw	1oz/28g	35	125	19.6	0.0	5.2	0.0
Rainbow, Sainsbury's*	1 Trout/265g	358	135	21.5	0.0	5.4	0.0
Rainbow, Smoked, Marks & Spencer*	1 Pack/135g	169	125	20.1	0.1	5.0	0.0
Rainbow, Whole, Asda*	1 Trout/130g	163	125	20.0	0.0	5.0	0.0
Rainbow, Whole, Tesco*	1 Fish/286g	358	125	19.6	0.0	5.2	0.0
Rosemary Crusted, Finest, Tesco*	1 Trout/150g	264	176	16.2	12.2	6.9	1.0
Smoked, Marks & Spencer*	1oz/28g	34	120	20.2	0.0	4.5	0.0
Whole, Somerfield*	1oz/28g	35	125	20.0	0.0	5.0	0.0
TRUFFLE, Mint, Marks & Spencer*	1 Bar/35g	190	543	6.8	55.9	32.4	1.2
TUNA,							
Canned in Brine, Drained	1oz/28g	28	99	23.5	0.0	0.6	0.0
Canned in Oil, Drained	1oz/28g	53	189	27.1	0.0	9.0	0.0
Chunks, Bettabuy, Morrisons*	1 Serving/60g	64	107	24.9	0.0	0.8	0.0
Chunks, In Brine, Canned, Sailor*	½ Can/92g	104	113	27.0	0.0	0.6	0.0
Chunks, In Brine, Drained, Osprey*	1 Serving/100g	99	99	23.5	0.0	0.6	0.0
Chunks, In Brine, Drained, SmartPrice Asda*	1 Can/129g	128	99	23.0	0.0	0.6	0.0
Chunks, In Brine, Marks & Spencer*	1 Can/139g	146	105	25.0	0.0	0.5	0.0
Chunks, In Brine, Skipjack, Waitrose*	¼ Can/70g	77	110	26.1	0.0	0.6	0.0
Chunks, In Brine, Tesco*	1 Serving/80g	83	104	25.9	0.0	0.6	0.0
Chunks, In Spring Water, Asda*	½ Can/77g	82	106	26.0	0.0	0.2	0.0
Chunks, In Spring Water, Princes*	1 Can/139g	147	106	26.0	0.0	0.2	0.0
Chunks, In Spring Water, Skipjack, BFY, Morrisons*	1 Can/130g	139	107	24.9	0.0	0.8	0.4
Chunks, SmartPrice, Asda*	1 Can/130g	138	106	26.0	0.0	0.2	0.0
Chunks, in Brine, Aldi*	1 Can/130g	147	113	27.0	0.1	0.5	0.0
Chunks, in Brine, Asda*	1oz/28g	30	106	26.0	0.0	0.2	0.0
Chunks, in Brine, Heinz*	1oz/28g	28	99	23.5	0.0	0.6	0.0
Chunks, in Brine, John West*	1oz/28g	32	113	27.0	0.0	0.5	0.0
Chunks, in Brine, Ocean Rise*	1 Serving/100g	101	101	23.6	0.0	0.6	0.0
Chunks, in Brine, Princes*	1oz/28g	29	105	25.0	0.0	0.5	0.0
Chunks, in Brine, Safeway*	1oz/28g	28	99	23.5	0.0	0.6	0.0
Chunks, in Brine, Sainsbury's*	¼ Can/71g	80	113	27.0	0.1	0.5	0.0
Chunks, in Brine, Skipjack, Morrisons*	1 Can/138g	135	98	23.3	0.0	0.5	0.0
Chunks, in Brine, Skipjack, Safeway*	1oz/28g	28	99	23.5	0.0	0.6	0.0

TUNA,

	Measure INFO/WEIGHT	per Measure KCAL	Nutrition Values per 100g / 100ml				
			KCAL	PROT	CARB	FAT	FIBRE
Chunks, in Brine, Somerfield*	1oz/28g	28	99	24.0	0.0	1.0	0.0
Chunks, in Brine, Value, Tesco*	1oz/28g	28	101	23.8	0.0	0.6	0.0
Chunks, in Oil, Somerfield*	1oz/28g	53	189	27.0	0.0	9.0	0.0
Chunks, in Spring Water, John West*	1oz/28g	32	113	27.0	0.0	0.5	0.0
Chunks, in Sunflower Oil, John West*	1oz/28g	53	189	27.0	0.0	9.0	0.0
Chunks, in Sunflower Oil, Princes*	1 Can/60g	117	195	25.0	0.0	10.5	0.0
Chunks, in Sunflower Oil, Drained, Sainsbury's*	1 Can/138g	250	181	27.0	0.1	8.1	0.0
Chunks, in Sunflower Oil, Tesco*	½ Can/92g	174	189	27.1	0.0	9.0	0.0
Chunks, in Water, Sainsbury's*	1oz/28g	35	125	26.2	0.1	2.2	0.0
Coronation Style, Weight Watchers*	1 Can/80g	122	152	10.2	6.5	9.5	0.6
Coronation, John West*	1 Can/80g	122	152	10.2	6.5	9.5	0.6
Fillets, In Tomato Sauce, Princes*	1 Can/120g	131	109	19.0	2.5	2.5	0.0
Flakes, In Brine, Value, Tesco*	1oz/28g	28	101	23.8	0.0	0.6	0.0
Flakes, SmartPrice, Asda*	½ Can/59g	53	90	22.0	0.0	0.2	0.0
Flakes, in Brine, Osprey*	1 Serving/100g	95	95	22.5	0.0	0.5	0.0
In Brine, Lidl*	1 Tin/150g	170	113	27.0	0.0	0.5	0.0
In Light Lemon Mayonnaise, Princes*	1 Can/80g	99	124	16.8	3.5	4.8	0.0
In Olive Oil, Waitrose*	1 Can/75g	142	189	27.1	0.0	9.0	0.0
In Olive Oil, Yellowfin, Princes*	1 Can/56g	116	207	24.5	0.0	12.1	0.0
In Salted Water, Ready To Go, Princes*	1 Pack/85g	89	105	25.0	0.0	0.5	0.0
In Spring Water, Albacore, Sainsbury's*	1 Serving/85g	93	109	25.0	0.1	1.0	0.0
In Spring Water, John West*	½ Can/93g	92	99	23.5	0.0	0.6	0.0
In Spring Water, Marks & Spencer*	1 Can/180g	189	105	25.0	0.0	0.5	0.0
In Spring Water, Yellowfin, Princes*	1 Can/56g	61	109	25.0	0.0	1.0	0.0
In Sweet & Sour Sauce, Safeway*	1 Can/185g	148	80	10.9	5.6	1.6	1.0
In Water, Canned, Bumble Bee*	1 Serving/56g	70	125	26.7	0.0	1.8	0.0
In Water, Canned, Clover Leaf*	1 Serving/120g	108	90	20.0	0.0	0.6	0.0
In a Red Chilli & Lime Dressing, Princes*	1 Sachet/85g	102	120	21.5	1.0	3.3	0.0
In a Tikka Dressing, Princes*	1 Sachet/85g	116	137	18.6	5.5	4.5	0.0
Light Lunch, French Style, John West*	1 Pack/250g	208	83	7.8	7.6	2.4	1.0
Light Lunch, Mediterranean, John West*	1 Pack/250g	180	72	8.0	7.5	1.1	1.1
Light Lunch, Nicoise Style, John West*	1 Pack/250g	241	96	10.4	8.9	2.1	2.8
Light Lunch, Tomato Salsa, John West*	1 Serving/250g	180	72	8.0	7.5	1.1	1.1
Lime & Black Pepper, John West*	1 Serving/85g	133	156	15.6	2.8	9.2	0.0
Loins, Asda*	1oz/28g	37	132	24.0	0.0	4.0	0.0
Mayonnaise With Sweetcorn, John West*	½ Can/92g	231	251	12.0	4.5	20.6	0.2
Mayonnaise, Weight Watchers*	1 Can/80g	114	142	11.5	6.2	7.9	0.1
Pasta, Eat Smart, Safeway*	1 Serving/210g	210	100	8.0	12.2	1.6	0.5
Raw	1oz/28g	38	136	23.7	0.0	4.6	0.0
Steaks, Chargrilled, Italian, Sainsbury's*	1 Serving/125g	199	159	25.1	0.2	6.4	0.5
Steaks, Finest, Tesco*	1 Serving/120g	138	115	26.0	0.6	0.9	0.0
Steaks, Fresh, Asda*	1 Steak/96g	118	123	29.0	0.0	0.8	0.0
Steaks, Fresh, Marks & Spencer*	1 Steak/120g	156	130	23.1	0.0	3.9	0.0
Steaks, Fresh, Sainsbury's*	1 Serving/100g	117	117	28.9	0.0	0.4	0.0
Steaks, Frozen, Iceland*	1 Steak/150g	201	134	32.0	0.0	0.6	0.0
Steaks, Frozen, Marks & Spencer*	1 Serving/140g	160	114	24.8	0.0	1.8	0.0
Steaks, Frozen, Sainsbury's*	1 Steak/150g	210	140	34.8	0.1	0.1	1.1
Steaks, In Brine, Skipjack, Waitrose*	½ Tin/75g	82	109	26.0	0.0	0.6	0.0
Steaks, In Brine, Tesco*	1 Can/149g	155	104	25.9	0.0	0.6	0.0
Steaks, In Olive Oil, Albacore, Antonio Alonso*	1 Serving/111g	203	183	24.7	0.0	9.3	0.0
Steaks, In Olive Oil, Palacio de Oriente*	1 Can/111g	203	183	24.7	0.0	9.3	0.0
Steaks, In Spring Water, Sainsbury's*	1 Sm Can/75g	85	113	27.0	0.0	0.5	0.0
Steaks, In Spring Water, Waitrose*	1 Serving/200g	198	99	23.5	0.0	0.6	0.0

T

	Measure INFO/WEIGHT	per Measure KCAL	Nutrition Values per 100g / 100ml				
			KCAL	PROT	CARB	FAT	FIBRE
TUNA,							
Steaks, In Sunflower Oil, John West*	½ Can/75g	142	189	27.0	0.0	9.0	0.0
Steaks, In Sunflower Oil, Sainsbury's*	1 Can/75g	136	181	27.0	0.1	8.1	0.0
Steaks, Marinated, Sainsbury's*	1 Serving/100g	153	153	25.1	1.3	5.3	0.5
Steaks, Skinless & Boneless, Fresh From The Sea, Marr*	1 Steak/105g	147	140	34.8	0.1	0.1	1.1
Steaks, Somerfield*	1 Serving/50g	81	161	28.4	0.0	5.3	0.0
Steaks, With Lime & Coriander Dressing, Tesco*	1 Serving/150g	156	104	21.6	3.6	0.4	0.6
Steaks, With Sweet Red Pepper Glaze, Sainsbury's*	1 Steak/100g	135	135	28.5	5.0	0.1	0.1
Steaks, in Brine, Co-Op*	1 Sm Can/99g	99	100	24.0	0.0	0.1	0.0
Steaks, in Brine, John West*	1 Can/150g	170	113	27.0	0.0	0.5	0.0
Steaks, in Brine, Princes*	1oz/28g	29	105	25.0	0.0	0.5	0.0
Steaks, in Brine, Sainsbury's*	1oz/28g	32	115	26.2	0.1	1.1	0.0
Steaks, in Brine, Skipjack, Morrisons*	½ Can/75g	65	86	20.4	0.0	0.5	0.0
Steaks, in Cajun Marinade, Sainsbury's*	1 Steak/100g	141	141	29.8	0.0	2.4	0.0
Steaks, in Mineral Water, John West*	½ Can/75g	74	99	23.5	0.1	0.0	0.0
Steaks, in Oil, Somerfield*	1oz/28g	53	189	27.0	0.0	9.0	0.0
Steaks, in Olive Oil, John West*	1 Serving/112g	212	189	27.0	0.1	9.0	0.1
Steaks, in Olive Oil, Sainsbury's*	1oz/28g	53	189	26.9	0.0	9.0	0.0
Steaks, in Oriental Sauce, Good Choice, Iceland*	1 Pack/260g	333	128	22.3	8.1	0.7	0.4
Steaks, in Spring Water, John West*	1 Can/80g	90	113	27.0	0.0	0.5	0.0
Steaks, in Sunflower Oil, Skipjack, Waitrose*	1 Serving/100g	181	181	26.4	0.0	8.4	0.0
Steaks, in Vegetable Oil, Heinz*	1oz/28g	53	189	27.1	0.0	9.0	0.0
Tomato & Herb, Weight Watchers*	1 Can/80g	79	99	11.6	5.1	3.6	0.5
Twists, Italian, Weight Watchers*	1 Can/385g	239	62	4.3	8.2	1.4	0.6
Whitemeat, In Spring Water, Albacore, Kingfisher*	½ Can/133g	132	99	23.5	0.0	0.6	0.0
With A Twist, Touch Of Water, John West*	1 Serving/85g	87	102	23.4	0.8	0.6	0.0
With Basil Butter, Microwave Easy Steam, Sainsbury's*	1 Pack/170g	292	172	23.3	0.5	8.5	0.1
With Light Mayonnaise, Princes*	1 Sachet/100g	112	112	20.5	3.0	2.0	0.0
With Onion, John West*	1oz/28g	33	118	19.0	6.0	2.0	0.0
With Salsa Verde, Sainsbury's*	1 Serving/125g	310	248	25.5	0.6	16.0	0.0
With a Twist, French Dressing, John West*	1 Pack/85g	135	159	15.2	2.8	9.7	0.1
With a Twist, Lime & Black Pepper Dressing, John West*	1 Pack/85g	133	156	15.6	2.8	9.2	0.0
With a Twist, Oven Dried Tomato & Herb, John West*	1 Pack/85g	129	152	16.1	3.9	8.0	0.1
TUNA SNACK POT,							
Italian, Weight Watchers*	1 Pot/240g	245	102	9.1	8.5	3.6	0.5
Oriental, Weight Watchers*	1 Pot/240g	269	112	9.0	12.6	2.9	0.3
Provencale, Weight Watchers*	1 Pot/240g	266	111	9.8	10.2	3.4	0.5
TURBOT,							
Grilled	1oz/28g	34	122	22.7	0.0	3.5	0.0
Raw	1oz/28g	27	95	17.7	0.0	2.7	0.0
TURKEY,							
Boneless Breast Joint, Basted, Healthy Eating, Tesco*	1 Serving/125g	124	99	20.5	0.8	1.5	1.2
Breast Fillet Strips, Fresh, Sainsbury's*	1 Serving/100g	143	143	30.8	0.1	2.1	0.1
Breast Joint With Cranberry & Orange Glaze, Sainsbury's*	1 Serving/180g	281	156	29.6	3.0	2.9	1.0
Breast Joint, Butter Basted, Boneless, Tesco*	1 Serving/100g	136	136	18.6	4.0	5.1	0.4
Breast Joint, Lemon & Pepper Basted, Tesco*	¼ Pack/132g	238	180	19.7	0.0	11.2	0.0
Breast Joint, Marks & Spencer*	¼ Pack/130g	143	110	19.6	0.2	3.3	0.0
Breast Joint, Sage & Onion, Glazed, Good For You, Asda*	1 Serving/100g	101	101	19.0	2.5	1.7	1.0
Breast Roll, Cooked, Bernard Matthews*	1 Slice/10g	9	92	17.6	3.5	0.8	0.0
Breast Roll, Norfolk, Cooked, Bernard Matthews*	1 Slice/10g	9	92	17.6	3.5	0.8	0.0
Breast Strips, Chinese Style, Sainsbury's*	1 Pack/650g	1274	196	26.4	12.5	4.5	0.5
Breast, Butter Basted, Sainsbury's*	1 Serving/100g	179	179	29.5	0.1	6.7	0.8
Breast, Carvery, Morrisons*	1 Slice/32g	34	105	24.9	0.1	0.6	0.5
Breast, Cooked With Stuffing, Somerfield*	1oz/28g	29	104	17.0	6.0	2.0	0.0

	Measure INFO/WEIGHT	per Measure KCAL	KCAL	PROT	CARB	FAT	FIBRE
Breast, Cooked, Low Fat, Safeway*	1 Slice/14.1g	15	104	19.7	1.8	2.0	0.0
Breast, Diced, Asda*	1/3 Pack/150g	216	144	32.0	0.5	1.5	0.9
Breast, Diced, BGTY, Sainsbury's*	½ Pack/225g	252	112	24.5	0.1	1.5	0.1
Breast, Fillet, Raw, Asda*	1 Serving/150g	155	103	24.0	0.0	0.8	0.0
Breast, Fillet, Y Cut, Non Breaded, Bernard Matthews*	1oz/28g	29	105	23.8	0.1	1.0	0.0
Breast, Golden Roasted, Bernard Matthews*	1 Piece/38g	43	113	24.3	0.4	1.6	0.0
Breast, Hand Carved, Butter Basted, TTD, Sainsbury's*	1oz/28g	40	142	24.7	1.2	4.1	0.3
Breast, Honey Roast, Bernard Matthews*	1 Serving/50g	54	107	23.5	1.1	1.0	0.0
Breast, Honey Roast, Wafer Thin, Bernard Matthews*	1 Serving/50g	48	96	18.6	4.4	0.4	0.0
Breast, Marks & Spencer*	1oz/28g	39	140	24.5	0.0	4.4	0.0
Breast, Norfolk, Premium, Bernard Mathews*	1 Serving/40g	40	100	19.7	2.5	1.2	0.0
Breast, Organic, Waitrose*	1 Serving/25g	30	118	25.7	0.0	1.7	0.0
Breast, Premium, Smoked, Bernard Matthews*	1 Slice/20g	19	97	20.8	1.4	0.9	0.0
Breast, Roast, Bernard Matthews*	1oz/28g	30	106	18.5	1.3	3.2	0.4
Breast, Roast, Premium, Sainsbury's*	1 Slice/20g	25	127	28.5	0.8	1.2	0.2
Breast, Roast, Somerfield*	1oz/28g	27	98	21.0	2.0	1.0	0.0
Breast, Roasted, Less Than 5% Fat, Asda*	1oz/28g	32	116	25.6	0.2	1.4	0.2
Breast, Sage & Onion Style, Premium, Bernard Matthews*	1 Slice/20g	21	104	19.6	2.2	2.0	0.0
Breast, Sainsbury's*	1 Serving/170g	318	187	25.8	0.1	9.3	0.2
Breast, Slices, Bernard Matthews*	1 Serving/100g	100	100	19.0	2.7	1.2	0.0
Breast, Smoked, Somerfield*	1oz/28g	36	129	26.0	0.0	3.0	0.0
Breast, Somerfield*	1oz/28g	34	122	20.0	0.0	5.0	0.0
Breast, Spicy Tikka Flavoured, Safeway*	1 Pack/450g	698	155	28.8	5.4	1.7	1.2
Breast, Steaks & Pieces, SmartPrice, Asda*	1 Serving/100g	105	105	24.0	0.0	1.0	0.1
Breast, Steaks, Asda*	1 Steak/100g	103	103	24.0	0.0	0.8	0.0
Breast, Steaks, Bernard Matthews*	1 Steak/76.3g	182	240	12.4	15.1	14.4	0.0
Breast, Steaks, Family Value, Bernard Matthews*	1 Steak/115g	370	322	11.2	15.3	24.0	0.0
Breast, Steaks, Fresh, Co-Op*	1 Serving/112g	118	105	23.0	0.0	1.0	0.0
Breast, Steaks, Fresh, Waitrose*	1oz/28g	29	105	24.4	0.0	0.8	0.0
Breast, Steaks, Healthy Eating, Tesco*	1 Serving/200g	206	103	23.2	0.0	1.1	0.0
Breast, Steaks, Sainsbury's*	1oz/28g	37	133	30.0	0.0	1.4	0.0
Breast, Steaks, Thai, Bernard Matthews*	1 Serving/175g	280	160	29.4	4.6	2.7	0.0
Breast, Wafer Thin, Chinese Style, Bernard Matthews*	1 Pack/100g	110	110	18.0	6.1	1.5	0.0
Chargrilled, Finely Sliced, No Added Water, Sainsbury's*	1 Slice/16g	17	106	24.8	0.9	0.4	0.5
Cooked Roll, Dinosaur, Bernard Matthews*	1 Slice/10g	17	170	13.6	6.0	10.2	1.1
Cooked, Sainsbury's	1 Slice/20g	20	98	19.8	2.1	1.1	0.7
Cooked, Tesco*	1 Slice/20g	23	114	22.6	1.4	2.0	0.4
Dark Meat, Raw	1oz/28g	29	104	20.4	0.0	2.5	0.0
Dark Meat, Roasted	1oz/28g	50	177	29.4	0.0	6.6	0.0
Diced Breast, British, Healthy Eating, Tesco*	1 Serving/100g	103	103	23.2	0.0	1.1	0.0
Diced Thigh, British, Tesco*	1 Pack/300g	342	114	20.3	0.0	3.6	0.0
Drumsticks, Tesco*	1 Serving/200g	272	136	19.9	0.0	6.3	0.0
Fillets, Chinese Marinated, Bernard Matthews*	1 Pack/200g	304	152	23.4	7.2	3.3	0.0
Fillets, Marinated, Lidl*	1 Serving/250g	238	95	19.0	2.5	1.0	0.0
Fillets, Tikka Marinated, Bernard Matthews*	1 Pack/200g	310	155	21.8	5.2	5.2	1.6
Golden Drummers, Bernard Matthews*	1 Drummer/57g	146	256	12.2	10.1	18.6	0.9
Honey Roast, Slices, Tesco*	1 Slice/20g	24	122	24.5	2.1	1.7	0.5
Honey Roast, Wafer Thin, Asda*	1oz/28g	33	119	19.6	4.7	2.4	0.0
Honey Roast, Wafer Thin, Safeway*	1 Serving/50g	57	114	19.7	3.9	2.2	0.0
Honey Roast, Wafer Thin, Sainsbury's*	1 Serving/100g	107	107	18.8	3.7	1.9	0.7
Leg Roast, Uncooked, Bernard Matthews*	1 Serving/283g	317	112	15.4	0.5	5.4	0.0
Light Meat, Raw	1oz/28g	29	105	24.4	0.0	0.8	0.0
Light Meat, Roasted	1oz/28g	43	153	33.7	0.0	2.0	0.0

T

	Measure INFO/WEIGHT	per Measure KCAL	Nutrition Values per 100g / 100ml				
			KCAL	PROT	CARB	FAT	FIBRE
TURKEY,							
Meat For Casseroles, Bernard Matthews*	1oz/28g	33	118	19.3	0.0	4.5	0.0
Mince, Asda*	1 Serving/120g	173	144	18.0	0.0	8.0	0.0
Mince, BGTY, Sainsbury's*	1 Serving/100g	113	113	21.9	0.1	2.8	0.0
Mince, Extra Lean, Iceland*	1 Serving/100g	122	122	19.0	0.0	5.1	0.0
Mince, Frozen, Asda*	1 Serving/100g	147	147	21.0	0.0	7.0	0.0
Mince, Healthy Eating, Tesco*	1 Serving/175g	217	124	18.0	0.0	5.8	0.0
Mince, Safeway*	1 Serving/150g	264	176	28.5	0.0	6.8	0.0
Mince, Sainsbury's*	½ Pack/250g	495	198	28.6	0.0	9.6	0.0
Mince, Value, Tesco*	1 Serving/100g	124	124	18.0	0.0	5.8	0.0
On The Bone, Honey Roast, Somerfield*	1oz/28g	42	149	26.0	0.0	5.0	0.0
Rashers Lightly Smoked, Healthy Eating, Tesco*	1 Serving/75g	76	101	19.8	1.5	1.8	0.0
Rashers, Bernard Matthews*	1 Slice/25g	26	105	18.0	3.7	2.0	0.0
Rashers, Healthy Choice, Safeway*	1 Rasher/27g	27	99	20.0	2.4	1.0	0.0
Rashers, Lightly Smoked, Tesco*	1 Serving/75g	76	101	19.8	1.5	1.8	0.0
Rashers, Original, Unsmoked, Mattesons*	1 Rasher/26g	26	99	19.3	1.8	1.6	0.0
Rashers, Smoked, Mattessons*	1 Rasher/26g	26	99	19.3	1.8	1.6	0.0
Rashers, Unsmoked, Co-Op*	1 Rasher/25g	26	105	19.0	2.0	2.0	0.0
Ready to Roast, Marks & Spencer*	½ Joint/253.6g	356	140	18.7	1.6	6.5	0.0
Roast Dinner, Bird's Eye*	1 Pack/359g	330	92	6.7	9.5	3.0	1.4
Roast, Frozen, Cooked	1oz/28g	48	170	26.7	0.0	7.0	0.0
Roast, Mattessons*	1 Slice/25g	36	143	29.2	3.0	1.9	0.6
Roast, Meat & Skin	1oz/28g	48	171	28.0	0.0	6.5	0.0
Roast, Thin Sliced, Asda*	1 Slice/13g	15	112	20.0	3.6	2.0	0.0
Schnitzel, Lidl*	1 Schnitzel/115g	210	183	19.0	11.0	7.0	0.0
Sliced, Marks & Spencer*	1 Pack/240g	314	131	29.0	0.2	1.6	0.5
Slices	1oz/28g	32	114	23.0	1.2	1.9	0.0
Slices, 97% Fat Free, Bernard Matthews*	1 Slice/37g	42	113	24.3	0.4	1.6	0.0
Smoked, Wafer Thin, Aldi*	1 Slice/10g	15	147	16.5	5.0	6.8	0.0
Smoked, Wafer Thin, Tesco*	1 Serving/50g	58	116	19.1	3.6	2.8	0.0
Wafer Thin, Bernard Matthews*	1oz/28g	27	98	13.6	3.5	3.3	0.0
Wafer Thin, Smoked, Bernard Matthews*	1oz/28g	26	93	18.6	2.1	1.5	0.0
TURKEY - ESCALOPE,							
Asda*	1 Serving/140g	399	285	13.0	20.0	17.0	0.6
Bernard Matthews*	1 Escalope/143g	380	266	10.7	18.4	16.6	0.0
Breaded, Tesco*	1 Escalope/138g	298	216	13.7	13.4	11.9	1.6
Breast, Safeway*	1 Serving/141g	304	217	13.9	18.8	9.6	0.9
In Pepper Sauce, Bernard Matthews*	1 Escalope/143g	350	245	9.4	18.2	15.0	1.5
Lemon & Pepper, Bernard Matthews*	1 Escalope/143g	362	253	11.2	17.2	15.5	0.0
Lemon & Pepper, Tesco*	1 Escalope/137g	367	266	14.0	16.2	16.1	0.9
Southern Fried, Somerfield*	1 Pack/280g	700	250	16.0	13.0	15.0	0.0
Spicy Mango, Bernard Matthews*	1 Escalope/136g	354	260	11.6	24.6	12.8	0.0
With a Cheese & Leek Sauce, Bernard Matthews*	1 Portion/134g	340	254	9.2	17.6	16.3	0.0
TURKEY - GOUJONS, Bernard Matthews*	1 Goujon/32g	78	245	11.3	18.1	14.1	0.0
TURKEY DINNER, Roast Dinner, New, Bird's Eye*	1 Pack/340g	320	94	6.7	10.0	3.2	1.2
TURKISH DELIGHT,							
Bar, Marks & Spencer*	1 Bar/55g	219	399	1.6	79.0	8.5	0.0
Cadbury's*	1 Bar/51g	186	365	2.0	73.3	7.2	0.0
Dark, Thorntons*	1 Chocolate/10g	39	390	2.7	69.0	11.0	2.0
Fry's*	1 Bar/51g	186	365	2.0	73.3	7.2	0.0
Plain, Without Nuts	1oz/28g	83	295	0.6	77.9	0.0	0.0
TURMERIC, Powder	1 Tsp/3g	11	354	7.8	58.2	9.9	0.0
TURNIP,							
Boiled in Salted Water	1oz/28g	3	12	0.6	2.0	0.2	1.9

T

	Measure INFO/WEIGHT	per Measure KCAL	Nutrition Values per 100g / 100ml				
			KCAL	PROT	CARB	FAT	FIBRE
TURNIP,							
Boiled in Unsalted Water	1oz/28g	3	12	0.6	2.0	0.2	1.9
Raw	1oz/28g	6	23	0.9	4.7	0.3	2.4
TURNOVER,							
Apple, Co-Op*	1 Turnover/77g	308	400	4.0	35.0	27.0	1.0
Apple, Dutch, Sainsbury's*	1 Serving/33g	130	393	3.6	56.9	16.8	1.4
Apple, Tesco*	1 Turnover/88g	294	334	3.2	29.8	22.4	0.9
TWIGLETS,							
Curry, Jacob's*	1 Bag/30g	134	448	8.0	55.7	21.5	6.0
Original, Jacob's*	1 Bag/30g	117	390	12.0	61.3	10.8	6.8
TWIGLETS,							
Original, Tub, Jacob's*	1 Tub/200g	802	401	11.8	60.1	12.6	6.7
Tangy, Jacob's*	1 Bag/30g	136	454	8.1	55.9	22.0	5.4
TWIRL, Cadbury's*	1 Finger/22g	116	525	8.1	55.9	30.1	0.0
TWIRLS,							
Prawn Cocktail, Bobby's*	1 Pack/26g	116	445	3.4	65.9	18.6	0.0
Salt & Vinegar, Tesco*	1 Bag/80g	349	436	3.9	65.8	17.5	2.4
TWISTER, Kentucky Fried Chicken*	1 Twister/240g	600	250	9.1	21.6	14.1	1.6
TWISTS,							
Tomato & Herb, Shapers, Boots*	1 Pack/20g	94	468	3.7	66.0	21.0	3.9
With Tuna, Balanced Lifestyle, Aldi*	1 Can/400g	264	66	4.8	7.8	1.7	1.7
TWIX,							
Fingers, Mars*	1 Bar/29g	143	494	4.6	64.8	24.1	0.0
TWIXELS, Mars*	1 Finger/6g	31	513	5.0	64.0	26.1	0.0
TZATZIKI,							
Fresh, Sainsbury's*	1oz/28g	35	126	4.0	3.7	10.6	0.3
Marks & Spencer*	1oz/28g	41	145	5.6	5.9	10.9	0.4
Tesco*	1 Serving/85g	121	142	5.1	4.1	11.7	1.0
Total*	1oz/28g	27	98	4.9	4.1	7.0	0.0
Waitrose*	1 Serving/50g	57	113	6.8	5.0	7.3	0.7

T

	Measure INFO/WEIGHT	per Measure KCAL	Nutrition Values per 100g / 100ml				
			KCAL	PROT	CARB	FAT	FIBRE
VEAL,							
Mince, Raw	1oz/28g	40	144	20.3	0.0	7.0	0.0
Escalope, Fried	1oz/28g	55	196	33.7	0.0	6.8	0.0
VEGE ROAST, Chicken Style, Realeat*	1 Pack/454g	844	186	23.0	3.2	9.0	0.0
VEGEMITE,							
Australian, Kraft*	1 Tsp/5g	9	173	23.5	19.7	0.0	0.0
Kraft*	Thin Spread/1g	2	180	30.0	14.0	0.0	0.0
VEGETABLE - ESCALOPE, Italian Style, Dalepak*	1 Escalope/163g	355	218	4.3	26.5	11.9	1.0
VEGETABLE - ROAST,							
Arrabbiata, Healthy Eating, Tesco*	1 Pack/450g	437	97	3.3	18.4	1.1	1.1
Lavash, Ready Meals, Waitrose*	1oz/28g	67	239	4.7	28.9	11.6	1.8
VEGETABLE BAKE,							
Marks & Spencer*	½ Pack/225g	203	90	1.8	10.0	4.8	3.1
Potato & Vegetable, Co-Op*	1 Bake/340g	425	125	4.0	11.0	8.0	1.0
Vegetable & Lentil, Somerfield*	1 Pack/350g	319	91	4.9	13.8	1.8	2.5
VEGETABLE FINGERS,							
Crispy Crunchy, Dalepak*	1 Finger/28g	78	277	4.1	25.8	17.5	8.7
Crispy, Birds Eye*	1 Finger/29g	50	171	3.8	21.0	8.0	1.2
VEGETABLE JUICE, Organic, Evernat*	1 Glass/200ml	36	18	0.9	3.5	0.1	0.2
VEGETABLE MASALA,							
Somerfield*	1 Pack/350g	406	116	2.7	11.0	6.8	3.0
With Rice, Feeling Great, Findus*	1 Pack/350g	350	100	3.0	18.0	2.0	1.7
VEGETABLE MEDLEY,							
& Carrot, Waitrose*	½ Pack/100g	28	28	1.5	4.7	0.4	2.2
Asda*	1 Serving/150g	39	26	1.9	3.0	0.7	0.0
Asparagus Tips, Perfectly Balanced, Waitrose*	1 Serving/225g	122	54	1.3	4.6	3.4	1.4
Basil & Oregano Butter, Waitrose*	1 Serving/113g	59	52	1.7	3.7	3.4	1.9
Crunchy, Marks & Spencer*	1 Pack/250g	75	30	3.3	2.7	0.8	2.9
Green, Marks & Spencer*	1 Serving/250g	63	25	3.0	1.8	0.5	1.8
Green, Sainsbury's*	1 Pack/220g	178	81	3.0	2.5	6.5	2.9
Marks & Spencer*	½ Pack/250g	88	35	2.9	3.9	0.7	3.5
Tesco*	1 Serving/200g	52	26	1.8	3.6	0.5	2.4
Winter, Safeway*	1 Serving/250g	68	27	1.4	3.6	0.8	2.4
With Ginger & Coriander Butter, PB, Waitrose*	1 Pack/225g	115	51	1.5	4.0	3.2	2.0
With Herby Butter, Marks & Spencer*	1 Pack/300g	180	60	1.4	5.2	3.6	1.5
VEGETABLE MIX, Baby, Iceland*	1 Serving/100g	20	20	1.2	3.9	0.0	2.7
VEGETABLE SELECTION,							
Casserole, Somerfield*	1 Pack/600g	174	29	1.0	5.7	0.3	1.4
Chefs, Marks & Spencer*	1 Pack/250g	75	30	2.7	3.8	0.6	2.4
Country, Way To Five, Sainsbury's*	½ Pack/125g	36	29	2.1	3.7	0.6	2.2
Garden, Tesco*	1 Pack/275g	124	45	1.2	2.7	3.3	1.2
Green, Fresh, Finest, Tesco*	1 Pack/250g	138	55	3.3	4.8	2.5	2.3
Winter, Marks & Spencer*	1 Bag/400g	80	20	2.2	3.2	0.0	3.1
Winter, Ready to Roast, Safeway*	½ Pack/175g	140	80	0.8	12.4	2.7	3.5
With Herb Butter, Waitrose*	1 Pack/300g	270	90	1.9	8.1	5.6	2.1
VEGETABLES,							
& Feta Cheese, Roasted, BGTY, Sainsbury's*	1 Pack/200g	264	132	6.4	21.7	2.2	0.0
Chargrilled With Tomato Sauce, GFY, Asda*	1 Serving/260g	164	63	1.4	8.0	2.8	0.0
Chargrilled, Deli Filler, Sainsbury's*	½ Pot/85g	251	295	2.3	3.8	29.7	0.8
Chinese Inspired, Crisp, Marks & Spencer*	1 Pack/250g	63	25	1.7	4.6	0.3	1.9
Chinese Water, Amoy*	1 Pack/200g	46	23	1.8	3.7	0.3	1.5
Country, Way To Five, Sainsbury's*	1 Serving/250g	73	29	2.1	3.7	0.6	2.2
Crispy, Tesco*	1 Pack/200g	54	27	1.9	3.9	0.4	2.3
Crudite Selection, Prepared, Marks & Spencer*	1 Serving/250g	75	30	1.4	5.8	0.4	2.0

INFO/WEIGHT	Measure	per Measure KCAL	Nutrition Values per 100g / 100ml KCAL	PROT	CARB	FAT	FIBRE
VEGETABLES,							
Mediterranean Style, Asda*	½ Pack/205g	172	84	1.4	6.0	6.0	2.8
Mediterranean Style, Finest, Tesco*	1 Serving/150g	153	102	1.9	7.3	7.2	1.2
Mediterranean Style, Marks & Spencer*	1 Serving/100g	50	50	1.1	4.4	2.8	0.7
Mediterranean Style, Ready to Roast, Sainsbury's*	1 Serving/200g	268	134	3.1	6.2	10.8	1.0
Mediterranean Style, Roasting, Tesco*	1 Serving/200g	72	36	1.1	5.7	1.0	1.3
Mediterranean Style, Safeway*	½ Pack/205g	111	54	1.7	7.4	1.9	2.4
Mediterranean Style, Somerfield*	1 Serving/200g	50	25	1.2	4.5	0.3	1.5
Mixed, in Salt Water, Tesco*	1/3 Can/65g	34	53	2.6	9.2	0.6	2.7
Oriental Inspired, Marks & Spencer*	1 Pack/260g	78	30	1.9	4.6	0.5	2.7
Oven Roasted, Somerfield*	1oz/28g	36	129	1.0	19.0	5.0	0.0
Roast, Marks & Spencer*	1 Pack/420g	273	65	1.4	4.9	4.2	0.4
Roasted Root, Extra Special, Asda*	½ Pack/205g	160	78	1.1	15.0	1.5	6.0
Roasted Winter, Tesco*	1 Serving/200g	170	85	2.2	10.0	4.0	2.0
Roasted, Italian, Marks & Spencer*	1 Serving/95g	219	230	1.8	7.1	21.0	1.7
Root, Ready to Roast, Sainsbury's*	½ Pack/200g	188	94	1.3	13.0	4.3	2.2
Special Mix, Sainsbury's*	1 Serving/80g	54	68	3.4	9.7	1.7	3.2
Special Mixed, Freshly Frozen, Morrisons*	1 Serving/100g	48	48	3.2	7.2	0.8	0.0
Steam Fresh, Bird's Eye*	1 Bag/121.2g	40	33	2.0	5.0	0.5	2.2
Sweet & Crunchy, Safeway*	1 Bag/200g	86	43	2.3	7.0	0.6	2.4
Winter Crunchy, Marks & Spencer*	½ Pack/125g	31	25	2.0	3.1	0.8	2.7
Winter, Fresh, Asda*	1 Bag/250g	75	30	3.0	2.2	1.0	2.3
Winter, Ready to Roast, Fresh, Sainsbury's*	1 Pack/272g	226	83	1.2	13.2	2.8	0.0
Winter, Tesco*	1 Pack/250g	73	29	2.0	3.3	0.8	2.6
With Sun Dried Tomato, Roasted, Finest, Tesco*	½ Pack/150g	153	102	1.9	7.3	7.2	1.2
VEGETABLES & COUS COUS, Chargrilled, Sainsbury's*	1 Serving/56g	88	158	5.2	23.7	4.7	3.4
VEGETARIAN MINCE,							
Meat Free, Asda*	1oz/28g	49	176	27.0	7.0	4.4	4.1
Vegemince, Realeat*	1 Serving/125g	220	176	15.5	6.0	10.0	2.0
Easy Cook, Linda McCartney*	1oz/28g	35	126	21.4	9.3	0.4	1.7
VENISON,							
Grill Steak, Finest, Tesco*	1 Steak/170g	202	119	19.0	5.0	2.5	1.9
Raw	1oz/28g	29	103	22.2	0.0	1.6	0.0
Roasted	1oz/28g	46	165	35.6	0.0	2.5	0.0
VENISON - ESCALOPE, Prime, Finest, Tesco*	1 Serving/112g	123	110	23.1	0.0	2.0	0.0
VENISON STEAKS, Prime, Tesco*	1 Steak/140g	154	110	23.0	0.0	2.0	0.0
VERMICELLI,							
Dry	1oz/28g	99	355	8.7	78.3	0.4	0.0
Egg, Cooked, Asda*	1 Serving/185g	239	129	5.0	24.0	1.4	1.0
Egg, Sainsbury's*	1 Serving/260g	335	129	5.0	24.0	1.4	1.0
VERMOUTH,							
Dry	1 Shot/50ml	55	109	0.1	3.0	0.0	0.0
Sweet	1 Shot/50ml	76	151	0.0	15.9	0.0	0.0
VIMTO*							
Average	1 Can/330ml	147	45	0.0	11.0	0.0	0.0
Cordial	1 Serving/10ml	3	30	0.0	7.4	0.0	0.0
Grape Blackcurrant & Raspberry Juice Drink	1 Bottle/500ml	223	45	0.0	11.0	0.0	0.0
Ice Lolly, Vimto*	1 Lolly/73.0ml	84	115	1.3	18.2	4.1	0.1
Light	1 Can/330ml	17	5	0.0	1.2	0.0	0.0
VINAIGRETTE,							
BGTY, Sainsbury's*	1fl oz/30ml	23	78	0.6	8.4	4.7	0.7
Balsamic Vinegar & Pistachio, Finest, Tesco*	1 Tbsp/15ml	56	370	0.2	2.8	39.2	0.0
Finest, Tesco*	1 Serving/50ml	248	495	0.9	13.2	48.7	0.5
Frank Cooper*	1 Pot/28g	46	163	1.0	14.1	11.4	0.3

V

	Measure INFO/WEIGHT	per Measure KCAL	Nutrition Values per 100g / 100ml				
			KCAL	PROT	CARB	FAT	FIBRE
VINAIGRETTE,							
French Style, Finest, Tesco*	1 Tbsp/15ml	69	461	0.8	5.9	47.4	0.2
French, Full Flavoured, Fat Free, Kraft*	1 Tbsp/15ml	7	47	0.1	10.5	0.0	0.3
Luxury French, Hellmann's*	1 Tsp/5ml	15	305	0.8	16.0	26.1	0.4
Newman's Own*	½ Tbsp/5g	17	333	0.5	3.9	35.0	0.0
Oil Free, Tesco*	1 Tbsp/15ml	5	30	0.3	6.0	0.1	1.4
Perfectly Balanced, Waitrose*	1 Tsp/5ml	4	89	0.4	20.9	0.4	0.5
Portuguese, Nando's*	1 Tbsp/15g	61	409	1.0	2.1	44.0	0.3
Waistline, 99% Fat Free, Crosse & Blackwell*	1 Tbsp/15ml	1	9	1.0	0.7	0.2	0.2
VINE LEAVES,							
Preserved in Brine	1oz/28g	4	15	3.6	0.2	0.0	0.0
Stuffed With Rice & Mixed Herbs, Sainsbury's*	1 Leaf/36.7g	44	120	2.6	16.3	4.9	1.2
Stuffed, Marks & Spencer*	1oz/28g	31	110	3.8	13.1	4.4	2.2
VINEGAR,							
Cider, Tesco*	1 Tbsp/15ml	3	19	0.4	0.6	0.0	0.0
Malt, Frank Cooper*	1 Sachet/8g	0	4	0.4	0.6	0.0	0.0
Malt, Heinz*	1 Tsp/5ml	1	18	0.2	0.6	0.0	0.0
Red Wine, Tesco*	1 Tsp/5ml	1	22	0.4	0.6	0.0	0.0
Rice, White, Amoy*	1 Tsp/5ml	0	4	0.0	1.0	0.0	0.0
Wine, White, Heinz*	1 Tsp/5ml	1	21	0.1	0.6	0.0	0.0
VODKA,							
37.5% Volume	1 Shot/25ml	52	207	0.0	0.0	0.0	0.0
40% Volume	1 Shot/25ml	56	222	0.0	0.0	0.0	0.0
Blue Original WKD, (Caculated Estimate)	1 Bottle/330ml	244	74	0.3	5.1	0.0	0.0
VOL AU VENTS,							
Chicken & Mushroom, Marks & Spencer*	1oz/28g	98	350	7.7	25.2	24.3	2.1
Mushroom, Sainsbury's*	1 Vol Au Vent/14g	49	350	6.9	30.8	22.1	1.4
Party Seafood, Youngs*	1 Vol Au Vent/17g	60	354	8.3	26.0	24.8	1.0
Prawn, Marks & Spencer*	1oz/28g	101	360	8.0	26.2	24.7	1.9

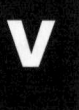

WAFERS,

	Measure INFO/WEIGHT	per Measure KCAL	KCAL	PROT	CARB	FAT	FIBRE
Cafe Curls, Rolled, Askeys*	1 Curl/5g	21	422	5.8	80.3	8.6	0.0
Caramel, Dark Chocolate, Tunnock's*	1 Wafer/26g	128	492	5.2	60.7	25.4	0.0
Caramel, Tunnock's*	1 Biscuit/26g	118	454	4.6	68.0	20.1	0.0
Chocolate Curl, Mini, Marks & Spencer*	1 Biscuit/5g	28	550	5.8	56.0	33.6	1.5
Ice Cream, Askeys*	2 Wafers/3g	11	380	11.0	79.0	2.5	0.0
Milk Chocolate Caramel, Farmfoods*	1 Biscuit/22g	105	475	5.9	61.9	22.8	3.1
Milk Chocolate, Sainsbury's*	1 Biscuit/10g	51	506	6.2	60.5	26.7	1.4
Pink, Crawfords*	1 Biscuit/7g	36	521	2.5	68.6	26.5	1.1

WAFFLES,

	Measure INFO/WEIGHT	per Measure KCAL	KCAL	PROT	CARB	FAT	FIBRE
Bacon Flavour, Better For You, Morrisons*	1 Bag/12g	41	344	5.6	76.3	1.8	1.5
Barbecue Flavour, American Style, Shapers, Boots*	1 Pack/20g	95	476	4.5	65.0	22.0	3.7
Caramel, Starbucks*	1 Waffle/30g	140	467	4.3	66.7	20.3	1.3
Caramel, The Big Cereal Company*	1 Serving/23g	84	367	7.5	80.1	1.9	2.8
Ready Salted, Marks & Spencer*	1 Bag/40g	194	485	2.1	65.6	23.6	1.6
Smokey Bacon, BGTY, Sainsbury's*	1 Bag/12g	41	344	5.6	76.3	1.8	1.5
Toasting, McVitie's*	1 Waffle/23g	108	469	5.9	53.9	25.6	0.9
WAGON WHEEL, Burton's*	1 Wheel/36g	159	441	4.9	67.3	16.9	1.3

WALNUT WHIP,

	Measure INFO/WEIGHT	per Measure KCAL	KCAL	PROT	CARB	FAT	FIBRE
The Classic, Marks & Spencer*	1 Whip/26g	127	490	7.2	54.9	27.4	1.1
Vanilla, Nestle*	1 Whip/34g	160	486	5.7	60.5	24.6	0.0

WALNUTS,

	Measure INFO/WEIGHT	per Measure KCAL	KCAL	PROT	CARB	FAT	FIBRE
Average	6 Halves/20g	138	688	14.7	3.3	68.5	3.5
Halves, Organic, Evernat*	1oz/28g	193	689	14.7	3.3	68.5	3.5
Halves, Somerfield*	1oz/28g	193	688	15.0	3.0	69.0	0.0
Organic Shelled, Waitrose*	1oz/28g	195	698	17.3	3.1	68.5	3.5
Pieces, Asda*	1 Serving/10g	69	694	15.0	3.3	69.0	3.5
Safeway*	1oz/28g	83	295	6.3	1.4	29.4	1.5
Sainsbury's*	1 Nut/3g	21	688	14.7	3.3	68.5	3.5

WATER,

	Measure INFO/WEIGHT	per Measure KCAL	KCAL	PROT	CARB	FAT	FIBRE
Black Cherry Flavoured, Abbey Well*	1 Glass/200ml	1	1	0.0	0.1	0.0	0.0
Blackcurrant Flavour, Still, Danone'*	1 Serving/120ml	25	21	0.0	5.0	0.0	0.0
Grapefruit Flavoured, Balanced Lifestyle, Aldi*	1 Serving/100ml	2	2	0.1	0.4	0.0	0.1
Lemon & Elderflower, Slightly Sparkling, Tesco*	1 Glass/200ml	2	1	0.0	0.1	0.0	0.0
Lemon & Lime Flavoured, Marks & Spencer*	1 Glass/250ml	13	5	0.0	1.0	0.0	0.0
Mandarin & Cranberry, Still, Marks & Spencer*	1 Bottle/500ml	100	20	0.0	5.0	0.0	0.0
Mineral Or Tap	1 Glass/200ml	0	0	0.0	0.0	0.0	0.0
Mineral, Touch of Fruit, Still, Volvic*	1fl oz/30ml	7	23	0.0	5.5	0.0	0.0
Orange & Peach, Touch of Fruit, Volvic*	1 Bottle/400ml	93	23	0.0	5.5	0.0	0.0
Peach & Lemon, Still, Marks & Spencer*	1 Bottle/500ml	100	20	0.0	5.0	0.0	0.0
Peach, Perfectly Clear, Silver Spring Mineral Water Co*	1 Bottle/500ml	4	1	0.0	0.0	0.0	0.0
Spring Peach, Safeway*	1 Bottle/500ml	10	2	0.1	0.2	0.1	0.1
Spring, Apple & Blackcurrant, Hadrian*	1 Bottle/365ml	3	1	0.1	0.1	0.0	0.0
Spring, Apple & Cherry Flavoured, Sparkling, Sainsbury's*	1 Glass/250ml	5	2	0.1	0.2	0.1	0.1
Spring, Apple & Raspberry Flavoured, Sainsbury's*	1fl oz/30ml	1	2	0.1	0.1	0.1	0.1
Spring, Boysenberry, Shapers, Boots*	1 Bottle/700ml	7	1	0.0	0.1	0.0	0.0
Spring, Peach Flavour, Shapers, Boots*	1 Bottle/500ml	5	1	0.0	0.0	0.0	0.0
Spring, Peach Flavoured, No Added Sugar, Asda*	1 Glass/200ml	4	2	0.0	0.2	0.0	0.0
Spring, Peach Flavoured, Sainsbury's*	1 Glass/250ml	5	2	0.1	0.2	0.1	0.1
Spring, Raspberry & Mango, Shapers, Boots*	1 Bottle/500ml	7	1	0.0	0.1	0.0	0.0
Spring, Stawberry & Vanilla, Sainsbury's*	1 Glass/250ml	5	2	0.1	0.2	0.1	0.1
Spring, White Grape & Blackberry, Tesco*	1 Glass/200ml	4	2	0.0	0.3	0.0	0.0
Spring, White Grape & Jasmine, Marks & Spencer*	1 Bottle/500ml	5	1	0.0	0.2	0.0	0.0
White Grape & Blackberry, Sparkling, Tesco*	1 Glass/200ml	4	2	0.0	0.5	0.0	0.0

W

INFO/WEIGHT	Measure per Measure KCAL	KCAL	Nutrition Values per 100g / 100ml PROT	CARB	FAT	FIBRE
WATER CHESNUTS,						
Whole, Crunchy, Sainsbury's*	1 Can/140g	46	33	0.9	7.4	0.1	2.3
Amoy*	1oz/28g	12	42	0.9	10.1	0.0	0.0
Canned, Drained	1oz/28g	9	31	0.9	7.4	0.0	0.0
Raw	1oz/28g	13	46	1.4	10.4	0.2	0.0
WATER ICE,						
Fruit, Iceland*	1 Lolly/75ml	74	98	0.2	24.4	0.0	0.2
Orange, Iceland*	1 Ice/75ml	73	98	0.2	24.4	0.0	0.2
Pineapple, Iceland*	1 Ice/75ml	65	86	0.0	21.5	0.0	0.2
Raspberry, Iceland*	1 Ice/75ml	67	89	0.0	22.2	0.0	0.2
WATERCRESS,						
Fresh, Asda*	1 Serving/5g	1	23	3.0	0.4	1.0	1.5
Raw	1oz/28g	6	22	3.0	0.4	1.0	1.5
WATERMELON,						
Cantaloupe Style*	1 Segment/100g	19	19	0.6	4.2	0.1	1.0
Fresh, Marks & Spencer*	1 Serving/240g	72	30	0.5	7.1	0.3	0.1
Slices, Marks & Spencer*	1 pack/240g	72	30	0.4	7.0	0.3	0.5
WHEAT, Ebly*	1oz/28g	98	351	12.1	71.9	1.7	5.4
WHEAT CRUNCHIES,						
Bacon, Crispy, Golden Wonder*	1 Bag/35g	172	491	11.1	55.9	24.9	2.8
Golden Wonder*	1 Pack/35g	172	491	11.1	55.9	24.8	0.0
Salt & Vinegar, Golden Wonder*	1 Bag/34g	165	484	10.5	54.5	24.9	2.8
Spicy Tomato, Golden Wonder*	1 Bag/35g	171	488	10.7	55.5	24.8	3.0
Worcester Sauce, Golden Wonder*	1 Bag/35g	170	487	10.7	54.9	24.9	3.0
WHEATGERM, Average	1oz/28g	100	357	26.7	44.7	9.2	15.6
WHELKS, Boiled	1oz/28g	25	89	19.5	0.0	1.2	0.0
WHIPS, Double Chocolate, Marks & Spencer*	1 Whip/28.9g	141	485	6.6	57.8	25.3	1.0
WHISKEY,						
37.5% Volume	1 Shot/25ml	52	207	0.0	0.0	0.0	0.0
40% Volume	1 Shot/25ml	56	222	0.0	0.0	0.0	0.0
Jack Daniels*	1 Shot/25ml	56	222	0.0	0.0	0.0	0.0
Scotch, 37.5% Volume	1 Shot/25ml	52	207	0.0	0.0	0.0	0.0
Scotch, 40% Volume	1 Shot/25ml	56	222	0.0	0.0	0.0	0.0
Teacher's*	1 Shot/25ml	56	222	0.0	0.0	0.0	0.0
WHITE GRAPE & Peach Juice Drink, Sainsbury's*	1 Glass/250ml	95	38	0.2	9.0	0.1	0.1
WHITE GRAPE JUICE, Sparkling, Sainsbury's*	1 Glass/200ml	120	60	0.1	14.5	0.1	0.1
WHITE PUDDING, Average	1oz/28g	126	450	7.0	36.3	31.8	0.0
WHITEBAIT, in Flour, Fried	1oz/28g	147	525	19.5	5.3	47.5	0.2
WHITECURRANTS, Raw	1oz/28g	7	26	1.3	5.6	0.0	3.4
WHITING,						
Raw	1oz/28g	23	81	18.7	0.0	0.7	0.0
Steamed	1 Serving/85g	78	92	20.9	0.0	0.9	0.0
in Crumbs, Fried in Blended Oil	1 Serving/180g	344	191	18.1	7.0	10.3	0.2
WIENER SCHNITZEL, Average	1oz/28g	62	223	20.9	13.1	10.0	0.4
WINDERS, Real Fruit, Kellogg's*	1 Serving/18g	67	370	0.5	77.0	7.0	3.0
WINE,						
Mulled, Homemade	1 Glass/120ml	227	196	0.1	25.2	0.0	0.0
Red	1 Glass/120ml	80	68	0.1	0.2	0.0	0.0
Rose, Medium	1 Glass/120ml	83	71	0.1	2.5	0.0	0.0
Strong Ale Barley	1 Can/440ml	290	66	0.7	6.1	0.0	0.0
White, Dry	1 Glass/120ml	77	66	0.1	0.6	0.0	0.0
White, Medium	1 Glass/120ml	87	74	0.1	3.0	0.0	0.0
White, Non Alcoholic, Ame*	1 Glass/120ml	46	38	0.0	9.5	0.0	0.0
White, Sparkling	1 Glass/120ml	87	74	0.3	5.1	0.0	0.0

	Measure	per Measure	Nutrition Values per 100g / 100ml				
	INFO/WEIGHT	KCAL	KCAL	PROT	CARB	FAT	FIBRE
WINE,							
White, Sweet	1 Glass/120ml	110	94	0.2	5.9	0.0	0.0
WINE GUMS,							
Co-Op*	1 Sweet/6g	20	337	3.5	80.8	0.0	0.0
Iceland*	1oz/28g	85	302	6.7	67.8	0.4	0.0
Marks & Spencer*	1oz/28g	94	335	3.9	78.5	0.1	0.0
Maynards*	1 Sweet/5g	17	331	6.0	76.6	0.0	0.0
Mini, Co-Op*	1 Sweet/2g	7	330	6.0	76.0	0.1	0.0
Sour, Bassett's*	¼ Bag/50g	160	319	3.7	78.0	0.0	0.0
WINKLES, Boiled	1oz/28g	20	72	15.4	0.0	1.2	0.0
WISPA,							
Bite, With Biscuit In Caramel, Cadbury's*	1 Bar/47g	240	510	6.4	56.9	28.6	0.0
Cadbury's*	1 Treatsize/15g	83	550	7.1	53.9	34.2	0.0
Gold, Cadbury's*	1 Bar/52g	263	505	5.7	57.0	28.0	0.0
Mint, Cadbury's*	1 Bar/50g	275	550	7.0	54.7	33.6	0.0
WONTON,							
Chicken, Asda*	1 Wonton/15g	46	306	14.0	18.0	20.0	1.9
Chinese Prawn, Sainsbury's*	1 Wonton/16g	38	252	11.9	16.5	15.4	1.2
Prawn, Dim Sum Selection, Sainsbury's*	1 Wonton/10g	26	259	11.3	26.8	11.8	1.3
WOTSITS,							
BBQ, Walkers*	1 Bag/21g	109	521	7.2	55.8	29.9	1.2
Cheesy Wafflers, Walkersr*	1 Bag/31g	168	542	5.8	54.1	33.6	1.5
Cheesy, Walkers*	1 Pack/19g	104	545	8.0	54.0	33.0	1.0
Prawn Cocktail, Walkers*	1 Pack/21g	109	520	5.5	55.0	31.0	1.1
WRAP,							
All Day Breakfast, Marks & Spencer*	1 Pack/196g	529	270	10.8	21.2	16.0	1.4
American Deli, Shapers, Boots*	1 Pack/171.7g	249	145	9.5	21.0	2.6	2.0
Aromatic Duck, Safeway*	1 Pack/180g	376	209	9.1	21.3	9.7	1.6
Avocado & Salad, Pret a Manger*	1 Serving/200g	605	303	5.3	18.1	23.3	2.9
BBQ Steak, Marks & Spencer*	1 Pack/253g	506	200	10.6	24.8	6.8	1.8
Bean & Cheese, Tesco*	1 Pack/105g	258	246	5.5	28.5	12.3	1.0
Beef in Black Bean, Marks & Spencer*	1 Pack/150g	338	225	10.2	20.5	11.4	1.6
Brie & Cranberry, Marks & Spencer*	1 Pack/224.5g	549	245	6.1	27.3	12.4	1.7
Cajun Chicken Louisiana Style, Sainsbury's*	1 Pack/190g	395	209	11.1	23.9	7.6	0.0
Cajun, Good For You, Asda*	1 Pack/176.3g	231	131	9.0	21.0	1.2	0.9
Chargrilled Chicken, Perfectly Balanced, Waitrose*	1 Pack/230g	361	157	10.3	22.7	2.9	2.9
Cheese & Bean, Tesco*	1 Pack/209.8g	470	224	7.0	28.6	9.0	1.0
Cheestring & Ham, Attack-a-Snak, Golden Vale*	1 Pack/109.9g	266	242	13.4	28.0	8.2	1.4
Chicken & Bacon Caesar Salad, Asda*	1 Pack/160g	565	353	18.0	20.8	22.0	0.9
Chicken & Bacon, Simple Solutions, Tesco*	1 Serving/300g	474	158	20.7	1.2	7.8	0.5
Chicken & Cous Cous, BGTY, Sainsbury's*	1 Pack/230g	359	156	8.8	21.5	3.9	0.0
Chicken Caesar, Boots*	1 Pack/160.4g	254	159	13.0	22.0	2.1	2.0
Chicken Caesar, Good Intentions, Somerfield*	1 Pack/184g	357	194	13.0	25.7	4.3	1.1
Chicken Caesar, Healthy Eating, Tesco*	1 Pack/170g	296	174	12.0	26.2	2.4	2.6
Chicken Caesar, Marks & Spencer*	1 Pack/225g	675	300	11.9	20.5	19.1	1.4
Chicken Caesar, Tesco*	1 Pack/110g	252	229	9.8	25.0	10.0	0.1
Chicken Fajita Red, Yellow Peppers, Weight Watchers*	1 Pack/177g	297	168	9.0	24.7	3.7	1.7
Chicken Fajita, Asda*	1 Pack/180g	369	205	9.4	20.6	9.4	0.4
Chicken Fajita, Tesco*	1 Pack/220g	381	173	9.7	22.6	4.8	0.3
Chicken Fajita, Waitrose*	1 Pack/174g	279	160	8.3	21.2	4.7	2.0
Chicken Fillet With Cheese & Bacon, Asda*	1 Pack/164.1g	366	223	25.0	1.4	13.0	0.0
Chicken Jalfrezi, Boots*	1 Pack/215g	456	212	8.6	28.0	7.3	1.7
Chicken Korma, Patak's*	1 Pack/150g	294	196	7.6	20.0	9.5	0.0
Chicken Salad, Pret A Manger*	1 Av Pack/230g	323	140	7.4	13.6	6.4	0.7

W

WRAP,

INFO/WEIGHT	Measure per Measure KCAL	KCAL	PROT	CARB	FAT	FIBRE
Chicken Salad, Sainsbury's*	1 Pack/211.0g	519	246	10.2	21.6	13.2	0.0
Chicken Salsa, Healthy Eating, Tesco*	1 Pack/240g	348	145	8.3	22.0	2.6	0.5
Chicken Southern Style, Ginsters*	1 Pack/150g	435	290	14.3	37.7	9.6	2.1
Chicken Sweet & Sour, Ginsters*	1 Pack/150g	378	252	13.4	40.8	3.9	2.4
Chicken Thai Style, Boots*	1 Pack/156g	290	186	11.0	21.0	6.4	2.2
Chicken Tikka Masala, Patak's*	1 Pack/150g	252	168	7.8	19.3	6.6	0.0
Chicken Tikka, French Cuisiniers*	1 Pack/130.0g	185	142	15.4	18.3	1.3	1.5
Chicken Tikka, Ginsters*	1 Pack/150g	278	185	8.9	25.5	5.3	1.6
Chicken Tikka, Mattessons*	1 Pack/150g	284	189	9.8	21.5	7.0	3.2
Chicken With Stilton & Pear, Sainsbury's*	1 Serving/150g	264	176	25.4	2.1	7.3	0.1
Chicken, Eat Smart, Safeway*	1 Pack/153g	230	150	12.5	19.7	1.9	2.0
Chicken, Tandoori Style, Good Intentions, Somerfield*	1 Pack/175g	299	171	10.9	28.8	1.4	1.6
Chicken, Tasties*	1 Pack/148.6g	325	218	11.7	26.5	7.1	0.0
Chilli Beef, COU, Marks & Spencer*	1 Pack/179g	260	145	9.7	22.7	1.4	1.9
Chilli Beef, Co-Op*	1 Pack/163g	310	190	10.0	26.0	6.0	2.0
Chilli Chicken, BGTY, Sainsbury's*	1 Pack/180g	313	174	10.2	28.0	2.4	0.0
Chinese Chicken, Asda*	1 Pack/200g	404	202	9.0	28.0	6.0	0.0
Chinese Chicken, Marks & Spencer*	1 Pack/155g	239	154	14.0	22.3	1.0	2.0
Coronation Chicken, Waitrose*	1 Pack/163.6g	284	173	10.1	21.3	5.1	2.2
Dhansak Prawn, Marks & Spencer*	1 Pack/208.1g	385	185	7.1	23.3	7.2	2.4
Duck, Food To Go, Marks & Spencer*	1 Pack/257g	474	185	8.5	25.5	5.4	1.0
Egg Mayonnaise, Tomato & Cress, Sainsbury's*	1 Pack/255g	592	232	7.3	17.7	15.0	0.0
Feta Cheese Flat Bread, COU, Marks & Spencer*	1 Pack/180g	225	125	6.3	20.6	2.2	1.9
Feta Cheese, GFY, Asda*	1 Pack/165g	256	155	7.0	22.0	4.3	2.1
Fiery Mexican Cheese, Ginsters*	1 Pack/150g	437	291	11.1	37.5	10.9	2.7
Garlic & Coriander, Discovery*	1 Pack/55.9g	175	313	8.6	53.9	7.0	2.5
Goats Cheese & Tomato, TTD, Sainsbury's*	1 Pack/204g	420	206	7.0	25.6	8.4	0.0
Greek Salad, COU, Marks & Spencer*	1 Pack/180g	225	125	6.3	20.6	2.2	1.9
Green Thai Chicken, Sainsbury's*	1 Pack/212g	422	199	9.5	25.5	6.5	0.0
Gressingham Duck & Hoi Sin Sauce, TTD, Sainsbury's*	1 Pack/199g	354	178	9.3	24.8	4.6	0.0
Ham, Cheese & Pickle Tortilla, Weight Watchers*	1 Pack/170.1g	296	174	10.9	26.4	2.8	1.2
Ham, Cheese & Pickle, Sainsbury's*	1 Pack/234g	662	283	11.4	23.4	15.8	0.0
Hoisin Duck, Marks & Spencer*	1 Pack/232g	510	220	9.9	24.4	9.3	1.3
Houmous Salad, Pret A Manger*	1 Av Pack/230g	351	153	5.0	17.9	6.8	3.4
Houmous, Royal London Hospital*	1 Pack/200g	318	159	6.3	20.0	6.7	0.0
Italian Chicken, Just Cook, Sainsbury's*	1 Pack/225g	329	146	16.7	3.5	7.2	0.7
Italian Chicken, Sainsbury's*	½ Pack/211g	395	187	15.7	6.2	11.0	0.9
Louisiana Style Chicken, Good For You, Asda*	1 Pack/195g	355	182	11.0	31.0	1.5	2.0
Mediterranean Style, Sainsbury's*	1 Tortilla/56.0g	169	302	7.8	54.1	6.0	2.4
Meditter'anean Style Chicken, Waitrose*	1 Pack/182.7g	296	162	8.3	18.6	6.0	2.3
Mexican Bean & Potato In Spinach Tortilla, Daily Bread*	1 Pack/195.8g	329	168	4.9	25.0	5.4	0.0
Mexican Bean, Good for You, Asda*	1 Pack/173g	303	175	5.0	31.0	3.4	2.3
Mexican Chicken, Marks & Spencer*	1 Serving/218g	447	205	8.6	19.7	10.3	1.3
Mexican Style Chicken, Co-Op*	1 Pack/163g	367	225	11.0	26.0	9.0	3.0
Mexican Style Chicken, Good Intentions, Somerfield*	1 Pack/220g	387	176	8.3	26.0	4.3	1.4
Mexican Sweet Potato & Three Bean, Marks & Spencer*	1 Pack/222g	522	235	7.6	26.4	11.0	1.4
Mexican Three Bean, Marks & Spencer*	1 Pack/246.8g	580	235	7.6	26.4	11.0	1.4
Mexican Tortilla, Ainsley Harriott*	1 Pack/230g	421	183	7.1	22.4	7.5	0.0
Mild Chicken Curry, Patak's*	1 Pack/150g	239	159	8.1	21.3	6.0	2.8
Monterey Jack & Ham, Tesco*	1 Pack/200g	522	261	7.9	25.9	14.1	0.2
Moroccan Style Cous Cous, Tesco*	1 Serving/240g	370	154	5.3	27.3	2.7	1.3
Morrocan Chicken, Shapers, Boots*	1 Serving/154g	271	176	9.6	26.0	3.7	1.7
Nacho Chicken, COU, Marks & Spencer*	1 Pack/181.5g	244	135	9.6	19.7	2.1	1.4

W

INFO/WEIGHT	Measure	per Measure KCAL	Nutrition Values per 100g / 100ml				
			KCAL	PROT	CARB	FAT	FIBRE
WRAP,							
Original, Discovery*	1 Pack/55.9g	175	313	8.6	53.9	7.0	2.5
Parma Ham Chicken, Perfectly Balanced, Waitrose*	½ Pack/198g	212	107	20.1	2.5	1.8	0.9
Peking Duck, Asda*	1 Pack/172g	427	248	9.4	28.5	10.7	1.1
Peking Duck, Boots*	1 Pack/229g	440	192	8.3	30.0	4.3	2.6
Peking Duck, Finest, Tesco*	1 Pack/200g	378	189	8.4	29.5	4.2	0.3
Peking Duck, Shell*	1 Pack/173g	337	195	8.7	24.2	7.1	0.0
Peking Duck, Waitrose*	1 Pack/182g	319	175	10.0	25.9	3.5	1.6
Pepperoni, Tesco*	1 Pack/153g	271	177	6.4	26.9	4.9	1.4
Plain Tortilla, Morrisons*	1 Pack/35g	84	240	6.8	45.8	3.8	1.9
Pork Caribbean Spicy, Ginsters*	1 Pack/150g	396	264	11.3	34.1	9.1	2.3
Red Thai Chicken, BGTY, Sainsbury's*	1 Pack/194g	384	198	11.3	29.3	3.9	1.0
Roasted Vegetable & Feta, BGTY, Sainsbury's*	1 Serving/200g	318	159	5.8	25.0	4.0	0.0
Sushi Salmon & Cucumber, Waitrose*	1 Pack/180g	299	166	6.3	27.2	3.6	1.6
Sweet & Sour Prawn, Eat Smart, Safeway*	1 Pack/204g	275	135	6.4	24.0	1.2	1.4
Tandoori Chicken, Good For You, Asda*	1 Pack/167g	281	168	10.0	26.0	2.7	1.7
Thai Prawn, COU, Marks & Spencer*	1 Pack/181g	235	130	6.1	22.4	1.3	1.8
Tomato & Chilli, Discovery*	1 Pack/55.9g	161	288	7.9	53.5	5.9	2.5
Tortilla, Chicken Fajita, Sutherland*	1 Pack/158g	379	240	13.0	27.0	9.0	0.0
Tortilla, Chicken, Asda*	1 Pack/125g	253	202	9.6	36.9	1.8	3.3
Tortilla, Mediterranean Vegetable, Sainsbury's*	1 Pack/202g	267	133	4.0	26.3	1.3	2.1
Tortilla, Vegetable, Asda*	1 Pack/125g	245	196	6.8	37.2	2.2	0.8
Tuna Nicoise, BGTY, Sainsbury's*	1 Pack/181g	273	151	11.0	18.0	3.9	0.0
Tuna Nicoise, Healthy Eating, Tesco*	1 Pack/117g	160	137	8.3	20.6	2.3	0.5
Tuna Salsa, Healthy Eating, Wild Bean Cafe*	1 Pack/159g	245	154	11.3	23.5	1.7	1.5
Tuna, Sweetcorn & Red Pepper, BGTY, Sainsbury's*	1 Pack/178g	306	172	11.5	21.2	4.6	2.1
Tuna, Tomato & Pepper Salad, Weight Watchers*	1 Pack/182g	291	160	8.3	22.9	3.9	1.4
Turkey, Bacon & Cranberry, COU, Marks & Spencer*	1 Pack/143.8g	230	160	9.6	27.1	1.5	2.3
Twister, Kentucky Fried Chicken*	1 Twister/252g	670	266	10.7	21.8	15.1	1.2
WRAP KIT,							
Chapatis Bread, Tikka Masala, Patak's*	1 Bread/42.2g	121	287	7.5	53.1	6.4	3.2
Moroccan Style, Sainsbury's*	1 Wrap/63.7g	206	322	8.0	41.1	15.1	3.6

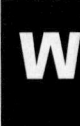

INFO/WEIGHT	Measure	per Measure KCAL	Nutrition Values per 100g / 100ml				
			KCAL	PROT	CARB	FAT	FIBRE
YAM,							
Baked	1oz/28g	43	153	2.1	37.5	0.4	1.7
Boiled in Salted Water	1oz/28g	37	133	1.7	33.0	0.3	1.4
Boiled in Unsalted Water	1oz/28g	37	133	1.7	33.0	0.3	1.4
Raw	1oz/28g	32	114	1.5	28.2	0.3	1.3
YEAST,							
Bakers, Compressed	1oz/28g	15	53	11.4	1.1	0.4	0.0
Dried	1oz/28g	47	169	35.6	3.5	1.5	0.0
Extract	1 Tsp/9g	16	180	40.7	3.5	0.4	0.0
YOGHURT, ADORE Vanilla With Choc Flakes, Ehrmann*	1 Pot/150g	215	143	3.1	17.0	7.0	0.0
YOGHURT, APPLE							
& Blackberry, Bio, Sainsbury's*	1 Pot/125g	134	107	4.1	16.6	2.7	0.2
& Blackberry, Custard Style, Co-Op*	1 Pot/150g	195	130	3.7	15.9	5.3	0.1
& Blackberry, Deep Fill Fruit, Ski*	1 Pot/160g	139	87	4.0	14.2	1.6	0.0
& Blackberry, Organic, Yeo Valley*	1 Pot/125g	121	97	4.3	12.5	3.3	0.1
& Blackberry, Perfectly Balanced, Waitrose*	1 Pot/125g	115	92	4.6	18.2	0.1	0.3
& Cinnamon Crumble, Ski*	1 Pot/125g	151	121	3.8	19.6	3.0	0.0
& Cinnamon, COU, Marks & Spencer*	1 Pot/150g	68	45	4.2	6.1	0.1	0.2
& Cranberry, Bio Fruit, Shape*	1 Pot/175g	135	77	3.9	13.2	0.9	0.0
& Custard, Low Fat, Sainsbury's*	1 Pot/125g	116	93	4.3	15.5	1.5	0.2
& Pear, Low Fat, Sainsbury's*	1 Pot/125g	115	92	4.3	15.2	1.5	0.2
& Prune, Fat Free, Yeo Valley*	1 Pot/125g	98	78	5.1	14.1	0.1	0.2
& Spice Bio, Virtually Fat Free, Shape*	1 Pot/120g	67	56	5.6	7.3	0.1	0.2
Cinnamon Crumble, Ski*	1 Pot/125g	151	121	3.8	19.6	3.0	0.0
Custard & Crumble, Muller*	1 Pot/190g	287	151	11.6	17.7	3.7	0.0
Danish Fruit Pudding Style, Healthy Eating, Tesco*	1 Pot/125g	99	79	4.1	14.1	0.7	0.2
YOGHURT, APPLE,							
99% Fat Free, Mullerice, Muller*	1 Pot/150g	125	83	3.5	15.3	0.9	0.0
Light, Muller*	1 Pot/200g	108	54	4.4	9.0	0.1	0.0
Mullerice, Muller*	1 Pot/200g	224	112	3.6	19.0	2.4	0.0
YOGHURT, APRICOT							
& Mango Tropical Fruit, Ski*	1 Pot/125g	126	101	4.9	16.3	1.8	0.0
& Mango, 25% Extra Fruit, Low Fat, Asda*	1 Pot/125g	120	96	4.6	17.0	1.1	0.0
& Mango, Best There Is, Yoplait*	1 Pot/125g	130	104	4.7	17.4	1.6	0.0
& Mango, Low Fat, Tesco*	1 Pot/125g	126	101	4.9	16.3	1.8	0.0
& Mango, Thick & Creamy, Sainsbury's*	1 Pot/150g	179	119	4.3	17.3	3.6	0.2
& Nectarine, Healthy Eating, Tesco*	1 Pot/175g	79	45	2.1	8.9	0.1	0.3
& Nectarine, Sunshine Selection, Sainsbury's*	1 Pot/125g	115	92	4.4	15.3	1.5	0.1
Bio, Healthy Eating, Tesco*	1 Pot/125g	58	46	4.2	7.1	0.1	0.0
YOGHURT, APRICOT,							
Bio-Live, Fat Free, Rachel's Organic*	1 Pot/142g	81	57	3.5	10.5	0.1	0.0
Custard Style, Shapers, Boots*	1 Pot/146g	82	56	3.9	8.3	0.8	0.2
French Style Smooth, Tesco*	1 Pot/125g	123	98	3.6	14.1	3.0	0.0
Healthy Living, Tesco*	1 Pot/125g	68	54	5.1	7.9	0.3	1.1
Jubileum, Tine*	1 Pot/135g	146	108	3.1	13.3	4.8	0.0
Low Fat, Benecol*	1 Pot/150g	119	79	3.7	14.6	0.6	0.0
Low Fat, Organic, Sainsbury's*	1 Pot/125g	103	82	5.3	13.0	1.0	0.1
Low Fat, Organic, Somerfield*	1 Pot/150g	153	102	6.0	17.0	2.0	0.0
Low Fat, Sainsbury's*	1 Pot/125g	115	92	4.3	15.2	1.5	0.1
Low Fat, Tesco*	1 Pot/125g	111	89	4.9	13.4	1.7	0.2
Organic, Low Fat, Tesco*	1 Pot/125g	111	89	5.3	14.6	1.0	0.2
Organic, Yeo Valley*	1 Pot/150g	146	97	4.3	12.4	3.3	0.1
Smooth Set French, Sainsbury's*	1 Pot/125g	100	80	3.5	13.6	1.2	0.0
Vitality, Muller*	1 Pot/200g	196	98	4.7	15.8	1.8	0.0

Y

	Measure INFO/WEIGHT	per Measure KCAL	Nutrition Values per 100g / 100ml				
			KCAL	PROT	CARB	FAT	FIBRE
YOGHURT, BANANA							
& Orange, Low Fat, 25% Extra Fruit, Asda*	1 Pot/125g	125	100	4.6	18.0	1.1	0.0
Childrens, Co-Op*	1 Pot/125g	124	99	3.7	15.1	2.6	0.2
Choco Flakes Corner, Muller*	1 Pot/150g	218	145	4.1	22.5	4.3	0.0
Custard Style, Asda*	1 Pot/150g	224	149	3.7	20.0	6.0	0.2
Light, Muller*	1 Pot/200g	106	53	4.4	8.7	0.1	0.0
Low Fat, Asda*	1 Pot/150g	149	99	4.6	18.0	1.0	0.1
Low Fat, Sainsbury's*	1 Pot/125g	116	93	4.4	15.4	1.5	0.1
Low Fat, Tesco*	1 Pot/125g	128	102	4.9	16.8	1.7	0.1
Müllermilch, Müller*	1 Pot/500ml	365	73	3.6	11.8	1.3	0.0
Smooth, Marks & Spencer	1 Pot/150g	165	110	4.8	19.3	1.7	0.2
Toffee, Low Fat, Somerfield*	1 Pot/125g	123	98	4.1	18.0	1.1	0.0
YOGHURT, BANOFFEE,							
Eat Smart, Safeway*	1 Pot/125g	68	54	4.7	8.5	0.1	0.0
Low Fat, Asda*	1 Pot/125g	126	101	4.6	18.2	1.2	1.0
Thick & Creamy, Safeway*	1 Pot/150g	189	126	4.3	18.2	4.0	0.1
YOGHURT, BERRY							
Crunch, McDonald's*	1 Serving/194.8g	224	115	3.5	18.9	2.6	1.2
YOGHURT, BIO							
Activia With Cereals, Danone*	1 Pot/125g	123	98	4.1	15.6	2.1	0.0
Activia With Prunes, Danone*	1 Pot/125g	124	99	3.3	15.2	2.8	0.0
Activia With Raspberry, Danone*	1 Pot/125g	113	90	3.6	13.0	2.8	0.0
Activia, With Strawberry, Danone*	1 Pot/125g	124	99	3.9	13.4	3.3	0.0
Fruits With Cherries, 0% Fat, Danone*	1 Pot/125g	65	52	3.6	9.1	0.1	0.0
YOGHURT, BLACK CHERRY							
Live Bio, Perfeclty Balanced, Waitrose*	1 Pot/125g	115	92	4.6	18.3	0.1	0.1
YOGHURT, BLACK CHERRY,							
BGTY, Sainsbury's*	1 Pot/125g	64	51	4.7	7.6	0.2	0.1
Best There Is, Yoplait*	1 Pot/125g	134	107	4.2	17.8	1.6	0.0
Bio, Waitrose*	1 Serving/170g	184	108	3.7	17.9	2.4	0.5
COU, Marks & Spencer*	1 Pot/150g	68	45	4.2	5.9	0.1	0.1
Economy, Tesco*	1 Pot/125g	85	68	3.0	11.9	1.0	0.1
Extra Fruit, Low Fat, Ski*	1 Pot/125g	120	96	3.4	17.2	1.5	0.1
Extra Fruity, Low Fat, Safeway*	1 Pot/150g	143	95	3.9	17.7	0.9	0.5
Extremely Fruity, Marks & Spencer*	1 Pot/200g	220	110	4.9	18.4	1.5	0.2
Fat Free, Safeway*	1 Pot/125g	75	60	5.2	9.2	0.0	0.1
Fat Free, Weight Watchers*	1 Pot/120g	55	46	4.2	7.0	0.1	0.1
Fayrefield*	1 Pot/140g	185	132	4.0	17.4	5.1	0.0
Frozen, Marks & Spencer*	1 Pot/125g	164	131	3.1	27.1	1.1	0.5
Healthy Living, Tesco*	1 Pot/200g	96	48	4.2	7.5	0.1	0.0
Live, Turner's Dairies*	1 Pot/125g	86	69	4.9	11.9	0.3	0.0
Low Fat, Asda*	1 Pot/150g	143	95	4.6	17.4	1.0	0.2
Low Fat, Co-Op*	1 Pot/150g	128	85	3.2	16.0	0.9	0.4
Low Fat, Sainsbury's*	1 Pot/125g	118	94	4.2	16.1	1.4	0.1
Low Fat, Somerfield*	1 Pot/150g	116	77	3.0	14.0	1.0	0.0
Low Fat, Tesco*	1 Pot/125g	124	99	4.9	16.0	1.7	0.1
Marks & Spencer*	1 Pot/150g	149	99	4.8	16.5	1.6	0.2
YOGHURT, BLACK CHERRY,							
So-Good*	1 Pot/120g	92	77	2.1	16.6	1.3	0.0
Thick & Fruity, Weight Watchers*	1 Pot/120.8g	58	48	4.2	7.5	0.1	0.1
Virtually Fat Free, Shapers, Boots*	1 Pot/125g	71	57	5.3	8.8	0.1	0.1
YOGHURT, BLACKBERRY							
& Apple, BGTY, Sainsbury's*	1 Pot/122g	61	50	4.7	7.2	0.2	0.3
& Apple, Best There Is, Yoplait	1 Pot/124g	133	107	4.7	18.0	1.6	0.0

Y

YOGHURT, BLACKBERRY

	Measure INFO/WEIGHT	per Measure KCAL	KCAL	PROT	CARB	FAT	FIBRE
& Apple, Healthy Living, Tesco*	1 Serving/176g	86	49	2.1	10.0	0.1	1.5
& Apple, Low Fat, Sainsbury's*	1 Pot/125g	116	93	4.3	15.5	1.5	0.2
& Raspberry Flip, Morrisons*	1 Pot/175g	207	118	3.4	15.8	4.6	0.5
& Raspberry, Fruit Corner, Muller*	1 Pot/175g	193	110	3.7	15.0	3.9	0.0
& Raspberry, Low Fat, Ski*	1 Pot/126g	67	53	5.7	7.2	0.0	2.0
& Raspberry, Simply Berries, Shape, Danone*	1 Pot/120g	61	51	4.4	8.1	0.1	1.2
BGTY, Sainsbury's*	1 Pot/150g	107	71	3.4	13.5	0.4	1.6
Boysenberry & William Pear, Marks & Spencer*	1 Pot/150g	188	125	4.0	13.6	6.5	2.4
Elderberry & Lavender, Biowild, Onken*	1 Pot/175g	159	91	4.4	14.7	1.6	0.4
Fat Free, BGTY, Sainsbury's*	1 Pot/150g	101	67	3.4	13.6	0.1	1.6
Sveltesse 0%, Nestle*	1 Pot/125g	63	50	4.3	7.9	0.1	0.0
Weight Watchers*	1 Pot/120g	49	41	4.2	5.8	0.1	0.3

YOGHURT, BLACKCHERRY,

	Measure INFO/WEIGHT	per Measure KCAL	KCAL	PROT	CARB	FAT	FIBRE
Everyday, Low Fat, Co-Op*	1 Pot/125g	88	70	3.0	13.0	0.7	0.0

YOGHURT, BLACKCURRANT

	Measure INFO/WEIGHT	per Measure KCAL	KCAL	PROT	CARB	FAT	FIBRE
& Loganberry, Cereal Topped, Bio, GFY, Asda*	1 Pot/190g	194	102	4.6	18.0	1.3	0.8
& Vanilla, TTD, Sainsbury's*	1 Pot/143g	136	95	3.6	13.6	2.9	1.0
BGTY, Sainsbury's*	1 Pot/200g	100	50	4.8	7.3	0.2	0.1
Bio Live, Rachel's Organic*	1 Serving/225g	167	74	3.6	11.0	1.7	0.0
Childrens, Co-Op*	1 Pot/125g	120	96	3.7	14.2	2.7	0.2
Low Fat, Sainsbury's*	1 Pot/125g	116	93	4.2	15.9	1.4	0.6
Low Fat, Tesco*	1 Pot/125g	110	88	4.9	13.2	1.7	0.4
Marks & Spencer*	1 Pot/150g	147	98	4.8	16.1	1.6	0.8
Smooth, Ski*	1 Pot/125g	129	103	5.0	16.4	1.9	0.0
Thick & Creamy, Sainsbury's*	1 Pot/150g	171	114	4.3	15.9	3.6	0.4
Vitually Fat Free, Morrisons*	1 Pot/200g	114	57	5.4	8.4	0.2	0.2
With Liquorice, Tesco*	1 Pot/150g	138	92	4.6	15.8	1.1	0.4

YOGHURT, BLUEBERRY

	Measure INFO/WEIGHT	per Measure KCAL	KCAL	PROT	CARB	FAT	FIBRE
Bio, Co-Op*	1 Pot/125g	141	113	4.5	16.5	2.8	0.4
Flip, Morrisons*	1 Pot/175g	201	115	3.1	15.1	4.6	0.5
Fruit Corner, Muller*	1 Pot/175g	196	112	3.7	15.5	3.9	0.0
Light, Muller*	1 Pot/200g	98	49	4.4	7.7	0.1	0.0
Low Fat, Somerfield*	1 Pot/150g	131	87	4.0	16.0	1.0	0.0
Marks & Spencer*	1 Pot/150g	141	94	4.7	15.8	1.6	0.4
Muffin, Eat Smart, Safeway*	1 Pot/125g	66	53	4.7	8.2	0.1	0.3
Starbucks*	1 Pot/130g	116	89	4.4	17.8	0.0	0.0
Wholemilk, Organic, Sainsbury's*	1 Pot/150g	123	82	3.5	9.2	3.5	0.1

YOGHURT, CAPPUCCINO,

	Measure INFO/WEIGHT	per Measure KCAL	KCAL	PROT	CARB	FAT	FIBRE
Thick & Creamy, Safeway*	1 Pot/150g	228	152	4.5	20.8	5.6	0.0

YOGHURT, CARAMEL

	Measure INFO/WEIGHT	per Measure KCAL	KCAL	PROT	CARB	FAT	FIBRE
& Praline, Indulgent Greek Style, Somerfield*	1 Pot/125g	245	196	4.0	28.0	8.0	0.0
Mullerice, Muller*	1 Pot/200g	210	105	3.5	17.4	2.4	0.0

YOGHURT, CHAMPAGNE RHUBARB

	Measure INFO/WEIGHT	per Measure KCAL	KCAL	PROT	CARB	FAT	FIBRE
& Vanilla, Marks & Spencer*	1 Pot/150g	195	130	3.8	15.7	5.8	0.8
Finest, Tesco*	1 Pot/150g	213	142	3.3	16.8	6.9	0.2

YOGHURT, CHERRY

	Measure INFO/WEIGHT	per Measure KCAL	KCAL	PROT	CARB	FAT	FIBRE
& Vanilla Flavour, Light, Brooklea*	1 Pot/200g	138	69	5.5	11.4	0.1	0.6
Bio, Co-Op*	1 Pot/125g	144	115	4.5	17.0	2.8	0.1
Flip, Better For You, Morrisons*	1 Pot/175g	93	53	3.9	8.7	0.3	0.4
Fruit Corner, Muller*	1 Pot/175g	193	110	3.7	15.0	3.9	0.0
Healthy Eating, Tesco*	1 Pot/200g	96	48	4.2	7.5	0.1	0.0
Light, Muller*	1 Pot/200g	100	50	4.4	7.9	0.1	0.0
Low Fat, Asda*	1 Pot/125g	120	96	4.6	17.0	1.1	0.0

Y

	Measure INFO/WEIGHT	per Measure KCAL	Nutrition Values per 100g / 100ml				
			KCAL	PROT	CARB	FAT	FIBRE
YOGHURT, CHERRY							
Low Fat, Benecol*	1 Pot/150g	122	81	3.8	15.2	0.6	0.0
Morello Bio, Tesco*	1 Pot/124g	51	41	4.4	5.4	0.2	0.9
Muller*	1 Pot/150g	177	118	3.3	17.0	3.7	0.0
Pie Layered, Custard Style, Healthy Eating,Tesco*	1 Pot/125g	99	79	4.1	13.9	0.8	0.2
Somerfield*	1 Pot/125g	61	49	5.0	7.0	0.0	0.0
Virtually Fat Free Bio, Morrisons*	1 Pot/200g	120	60	5.4	9.2	0.2	0.0
YOGHURT, CHOCOLATE							
& Orange, COU, Marks & Spencer*	1 Pot/200g	100	50	4.2	6.0	0.4	0.2
Chip, Dessert Recipes, Ski*	1 Pot/125g	163	130	3.8	19.3	4.2	0.0
Light, Muller*	1 Pot/200g	108	54	4.8	8.1	0.3	0.0
Mullerice, Muller*	1 Pot/200g	246	123	3.4	21.5	2.6	0.0
Seriously Smooth, Waitrose*	1 Pot/125g	158	126	6.0	20.1	2.4	0.1
Shape*	1 Pot/100g	111	111	4.9	17.4	2.0	0.2
Village Dairy*	1 Pot/125g	181	145	6.3	23.5	3.0	0.0
Vitaline*	1 Pot/125g	103	82	3.5	15.8	0.5	0.0
YOGHURT, CITRUS FRUIT,							
Fat Free, Weight Watchers*	1 Pot/120g	52	43	4.1	6.3	0.1	0.2
Tesco*	1 Serving/117g	53	45	4.2	6.5	0.1	0.1
YOGHURT, COCONUT,							
Greek Style, Bio Live, Rachel's*	1 Pot/450g	702	156	3.6	10.5	11.0	0.0
Muller*	1 Pot/150g	156	104	3.4	13.0	3.9	0.0
Ski*	1 Pot/125g	126	101	4.9	15.8	2.0	0.0
YOGHURT, CRANBERRY							
& Blackcurrant, Fat Free, Bio, Shape*	1 Pot/120g	54	45	4.6	5.7	0.1	0.3
& Blackcurrant, Low Fat Bio, Ocean Spray*	1 Pot/150g	147	98	4.6	17.4	1.1	0.0
& Blackcurrant, Shape, Danone*	1 Pot/120g	62	52	4.4	8.4	0.1	1.0
& Pink Grapefruit, Low Fat Bio, Ocean Spray*	1 Pot/125g	118	94	4.6	16.5	1.1	0.0
& Raspberry, Low Fat Bio, Ocean Spray*	1 Pot/150g	144	96	4.6	17.0	1.1	0.0
& Raspberry, Perfectly Balanced, Waitrose*	1 Pot/150g	135	90	4.5	17.8	0.1	0.6
Classic, Low Fat Bio, Ocean Spray*	1 Pot/150g	144	96	4.6	17.0	1.1	0.0
YOGHURT, DAIRY TOFFEE, Shape*	1 Pot/100g	99	99	4.6	15.4	1.8	0.0
YOGHURT, DEVON Toffee, Shape, Danone*	1 Pot/125g	129	103	4.9	16.2	2.0	1.0
YOGHURT, DIET, Yoplait*	1 Pot/125g	100	80	4.0	16.0	0.0	0.0
YOGHURT, FARMHOUSE							
Blackberry, BGTY, Sainsbury's*	1 Pot/150g	107	71	3.4	13.5	0.4	1.6
Natural, Virtually Fat Free, TTD, Sainsbury's*	1 Serving/100g	44	44	4.5	6.6	0.2	0.0
Peaches, BGTY, Sainsbury's*	1 Pot/150g	134	89	3.2	17.8	0.4	0.3
Raspberry, BGTY, Sainsbury's*	1 Pot/150g	107	71	3.3	13.6	0.4	2.0
Strawberries & Clotted Cream, TTD, Sainsbury's*	1 Pot/150g	155	103	3.6	12.5	4.5	0.3
Strawberry & Redcurrant, Ann Forshaw's*	1 Pot/150g	194	129	3.8	17.4	4.9	0.2
Strawberry, BGTY, Sainsbury's*	1 Pot/150g	107	71	3.2	13.7	0.4	0.5
YOGHURT, FOREST FRUITS							
French Set Wholemilk, Asda*	1 Pot/125g	125	100	3.6	14.1	3.2	0.0
Marks & Spencer*	1 Pot/150g	149	99	4.7	16.8	1.6	0.5
YOGHURT, FRENCH							
Set, Low Fat, Iceland*	1 Pot/125g	100	80	3.6	13.6	1.2	0.0
Set, Waitrose*	1 Pot/125g	120	96	3.5	13.4	3.1	0.0
Style, Tesco*	1 Pot/125g	123	98	3.6	14.1	3.0	0.0
YOGHURT, FRUIT							
& Nut Layer, Indulgent Greek Style, Somerfield*	1 Pot/125g	214	171	3.0	24.0	7.0	0.0
Bio, Low Fat, Sainsbury's*	1 Pot/150g	156	104	4.6	18.9	1.1	0.3
Deep Fill, Ski*	1 Pot/160g	138	86	4.0	13.8	1.6	0.0
Halo Strawberry & Vanilla, Light, Muller*	1 Pot/145g	116	80	3.6	15.8	0.3	0.0

Y

	Measure INFO/WEIGHT	per Measure KCAL	Nutrition Values per 100g / 100ml KCAL	PROT	CARB	FAT	FIBRE
YOGHURT, FRUIT							
Halo, Peach, Pineapple & Passion Fruit, Light, Muller*	1 Pot/145g	123	85	3.8	16.9	0.3	0.0
Halo, Raspberry, Light, Muller*	1 Pot/144.0g	121	84	3.7	16.5	0.3	0.0
Low Fat	1 Pot/120g	108	90	4.1	17.9	0.7	0.0
Low Fat, Light, Muller*	1 Pot/200g	100	50	4.4	7.9	0.1	0.0
Low Fat, Safeway*	1 Pot/125ml	88	70	2.1	13.7	0.8	0.0
Whole Milk	1 Pot/150g	158	105	5.1	15.7	2.8	0.0
YOGHURT, FRUITS OF THE FOREST,							
Smooth Set, Co-Op*	1 Pot/125g	95	76	3.7	12.5	0.9	0.0
Lite, Yoplait*	1 Pot/200g	184	92	5.0	15.9	0.9	0.0
YOGHURT, FUDGE							
Layer, Indulgent Greek Style, Somerfield*	1 Pot/125g	226	181	3.0	26.0	7.0	0.0
Thick & Creamy, Co-Op*	1 Pot/150g	197	131	3.8	17.6	5.0	0.0
Thick & Creamy, Marks & Spencer*	1 Pot/150g	195	130	4.4	17.3	5.0	0.7
Thick & Creamy, Waitrose*	1 Pot/150g	197	131	4.4	21.5	3.0	0.0
YOGHURT, GOATS Whole Milk	1 Carton/150g	95	63	3.5	3.9	3.8	0.0
YOGHURT, GOOSEBERRY,							
Custard Style, Co-Op*	1 Pot/150g	216	144	3.7	19.3	5.3	0.3
Custard Style, Shapers, Boots*	1 Pot/151g	106	70	3.9	12.0	0.7	0.2
Custard Style, Somerfield*	1 Pot/125g	151	121	3.0	17.0	5.0	0.0
Low Fat, Sainsbury's*	1 Pot/125g	113	90	4.4	14.6	1.5	0.2
Low Fat, Tesco*	1 Pot/125g	106	85	4.9	12.5	1.7	0.2
Seriously Fruity, Low Fat, Waitrose*	1 Pot/125g	111	89	4.4	15.7	1.0	0.6
YOGHURT, GREEK STYLE							
Luxury, Loseley*	1 Pot/175g	226	129	4.8	4.5	10.2	0.0
Sainsbury's*	1 Serving/200g	258	129	4.6	4.8	10.2	0.0
With Honey, Asda*	1 Pot/150g	225	150	4.0	13.9	8.7	0.0
With Honey, Somerfield*	1oz/28g	43	152	4.0	15.0	9.0	0.0
With Strawberries, Asda*	1 Pot/125g	159	127	3.2	13.6	6.6	0.2
With Strawberry, Morrisons*	1 Pot/125g	163	130	3.3	14.4	6.6	0.0
With Toffee & Hazelnuts, Asda*	1 Pot/125g	230	184	3.7	23.1	8.6	0.1
With Tropical Fruits, Asda*	1 Pot/125g	164	131	3.3	14.5	6.6	0.3
YOGHURT, GREEK,							
0% Fat, Total*	1 Pot/150g	84	56	10.0	4.0	0.0	0.0
Light, Total*	1 Pot/150g	120	80	6.0	3.0	5.0	0.0
Original, Total*	1oz/28g	36	130	6.0	4.0	10.0	0.0
Shape*	1 Serving/100g	108	108	7.1	12.7	2.7	0.0
YOGHURT, GUAVA							
& Orange, Fat Free, Organic, Yeo Valley*	1 Pot/125g	93	74	5.1	13.2	0.1	0.3
& Passion Fruit, Virtualy Fat Free, Tesco*	1 Pot/125g	56	45	4.2	6.7	0.2	1.2
YOGHURT, HAZELNUT,							
Low Fat, Asda*	1 Pot/125g	150	120	4.8	20.2	2.3	0.1
Low Fat, Co Op	1 Pot/125g	119	95	4.0	15.0	2.0	3.0
Low Fat, Safeway*	1 Pot/150g	179	119	4.9	19.3	2.5	0.2
Low Fat, Sainsbury's*	1 Pot/125g	135	108	4.5	16.4	2.7	0.2
Low Fat, Somerfield*	1 Pot/150g	126	84	4.0	15.0	1.0	0.0
Low Fat, Tesco*	1 Pot/150g	147	98	4.5	14.0	2.7	0.0
Praline, The Best, Safeway*	1 Pot/175g	302	173	3.7	20.3	8.5	0.2
Morrisons*	1 Pot/150g	159	106	3.9	16.9	2.6	0.0
Seriously Nutty, Waitrose*	1 Pot/150g	179	119	5.3	17.7	3.0	0.2
Yoplait*	1 Pot/125g	166	133	4.6	19.6	4.0	0.0
YOGHURT, HINT OF Coconut, Bio Activia, Danone*	1 Pot/125g	119	95	3.6	13.2	3.1	0.0
YOGHURT, HONEY							
& Ginger, Enhanced, Low Fat, Asda*	1 Pot/150g	150	100	4.6	18.0	1.1	0.0

Y

	Measure INFO/WEIGHT	per Measure KCAL	Nutrition Values per 100g / 100ml				
			KCAL	PROT	CARB	FAT	FIBRE
YOGHURT, HONEY							
& Ginger, Tesco*	1 Pot/150g	150	100	4.6	18.0	1.1	0.0
& Greek, Total*	1 Pot/150g	245	163	4.8	19.2	8.0	0.0
& Multigrain, Breakfast Selection, Sainsbury's*	1 Pot/125g	126	101	4.4	17.4	1.5	0.2
Greek Style, Boots*	1 Pot/140g	204	146	3.1	18.0	6.8	0.0
Greek Style, Co-Op*	1 Pot/150g	228	152	4.0	13.8	8.5	0.0
Low Fat, Asda*	1 Pot/125g	130	104	4.6	19.0	1.1	0.0
YOGHURT, JAFFA ORANGE,							
Low Fat, Co-Op*	1 Pot/150g	126	84	3.9	15.0	0.9	0.4
Morrisons*	1 Pot/150g	134	89	3.6	16.2	1.1	0.0
YOGHURT, JUBILEUM							
Kiwi, Tine*	1 Pot/135g	149	110	3.2	13.5	4.9	0.0
Raspberry, Tine*	1 Pot/135g	163	121	3.2	16.1	4.8	0.0
YOGHURT, KELLOGG'S							
Coco Pops Corner, Muller*	1 Pot/150g	180	120	4.0	19.0	3.1	0.0
Frosties Crunch Corner, Muller*	1 Pot/150g	185	123	4.0	20.1	2.9	0.0
With Rice Krispies, Muller*	1 Pot/150g	185	123	4.1	19.9	3.0	0.0
YOGHURT, LAYERED, Eat Smart, Safeway*	1 Pot/125g	81	65	4.1	11.3	0.1	0.4
YOGHURT, LEMON							
& Lime, Bio, Shape*	1 Pot/120g	54	45	5.7	5.7	0.1	0.1
& Lime, Fat Free, Shape*	1 Pot/120g	61	51	4.5	7.3	0.1	0.1
& Lime, Light, Muller*	1 Pot/200g	106	53	4.7	8.2	0.1	0.0
& Lime, Weight Watchers*	1 Pot/119ml	50	42	4.1	5.9	0.1	0.0
Amore Luxury, Muller*	1 Pot/150g	210	140	2.3	15.0	7.9	0.0
Cheesecake, Corner, Muller*	1 Pot/150g	224	149	3.7	23.9	4.3	0.0
Cheesecake, Sveltesse, Nestle*	1 Pot/125g	95	76	4.4	12.9	0.7	0.0
COU, Marks & Spencer*	1 Pot/200g	80	40	4.2	5.4	0.1	0.0
Curd, Channel Island, Marks & Spencer*	1 Pot/150g	225	150	5.4	20.2	5.1	0.1
Curd, Farmhouse, TTD, Sainsbury's*	1 Pot/149.6g	182	121	4.1	17.7	3.7	0.2
Curd, Farmhouse, Waitrose*	1 Pot/150g	245	163	4.3	18.7	7.9	0.2
Fat Free, Weight Watchers*	1 Pot/120g	49	41	4.0	5.8	0.1	0.0
Greek Style, GFY, Asda*	1 Pot/150g	125	83	4.1	10.0	2.9	0.1
Low Fat, Asda*	1 Pot/125g	130	104	4.6	19.0	1.1	0.0
Low Fat, Safeway*	1 Pot/150g	155	103	4.6	18.7	1.1	0.1
Meringue, Eat Smart, Safeway*	1 Pot/125g	68	54	4.7	8.6	0.1	0.0
Meringue, Sveltesse 0%, Nestle*	1 Pot/125g	60	48	4.1	7.7	0.1	0.0
Smooth Set, Co-Op*	1 Pot/125g	95	76	3.7	12.5	0.9	0.0
Smooth Set French, Low Fat, Sainsbury's*	1 Pot/125g	100	80	3.5	13.6	1.2	0.0
Summer, Biopot, Onken*	1 Pot/150g	155	103	3.9	15.9	2.6	0.1
Thick & Creamy, Channel Island, Marks & Spencer*	1 Pot/150g	195	130	4.2	17.6	5.1	1.0
Virtually Fat Free, Morrisons*	1 Pot/200g	118	59	5.4	8.9	0.2	0.0
YOGHURT, LOGANBERRY, Low Fat, Sainsbury's*	1 Pot/125g	111	89	4.2	14.5	1.5	0.2
YOGHURT, MANDARIN,							
Light, Muller*	1 Pot/200g	108	54	4.3	9.0	0.1	0.1
Longley Farm*	1 Pot/150g	161	107	4.9	13.3	3.8	0.0
Low Fat, Safeway*	1 Pot/150g	141	94	4.6	16.4	1.1	0.2
YOGHURT, MANGO							
& Guava, Fat Free, Weight Watchers*	1 Pot/120g	55	46	4.1	6.8	0.1	0.3
& Guava, Sunshine Selection, Sainsbury's*	1 Pot/125g	145	116	5.4	19.3	1.9	0.3
& Pineapple, BGTY, Sainsbury's*	1 Pot/124g	63	51	4.6	7.6	0.2	0.2
& Vanilla, Organic, Onken*	1 Serving/20g	20	102	3.9	13.5	3.3	0.0
BGTY, Sainsbury's*	1 Pot/125g	66	53	4.8	8.3	0.1	1.2
Bio, Healthy Eating, Tesco*	1 Pot/125g	59	47	4.7	6.8	0.1	0.2
Bio, Virtually Fat Free, Shape*	1 Pot/120g	60	50	4.7	6.8	0.1	0.2

Y

	Measure INFO/WEIGHT	per Measure KCAL	Nutrition Values per 100g / 100ml				
			KCAL	PROT	CARB	FAT	FIBRE
YOGHURT, MANGO							
Low Fat, Tesco*	1 Pot/125g	111	89	4.9	13.6	1.7	0.3
Papaya & Passion Fruit, Onken*	1 Serving/100g	101	101	3.9	15.6	2.6	0.2
Passion, D'lite, Ski*	1 Pot/200g	186	93	5.1	14.9	0.9	0.1
Passionfruit, D'lite 0.2 Ski, Nestle*	1 Pot/125g	103	82	4.6	15.7	0.1	0.1
Smooth, Marks & Spencer*	1 Pot/150g	158	105	4.7	18.0	1.6	0.5
Ski*	1 Pot/125g	125	100	4.9	15.8	1.9	0.1
Virtually Fat Free, Tesco*	1 Pot/125g	56	45	4.1	6.6	0.2	0.9
Weight Watchers*	1 Pot/120g	54	45	3.9	7.1	0.1	1.1
YOGHURT, MELON & Passion Fruit, Weight Watchers*	1 Pot/120g	54	45	4.0	7.0	0.1	0.0
YOGHURT, MISSISSIPPI MUD PIE							
Corner, Muller*	1 Pot/150g	254	169	4.1	26.3	5.3	0.0
Crunchable, Brooklea, Aldi*	1 Pot/140g	237	169	4.0	28.0	4.5	0.3
Shape St Ivel*	1 Pot/120g	166	138	3.8	24.5	2.8	0.8
YOGHURT, MIXED BERRY, Fat Free, Shape*	1 Pot/120g	62	52	4.4	8.2	0.1	1.0
YOGHURT, MORELLO CHERRY,							
Healthy Eating, Tesco*	1 Pot/125g	58	46	4.2	7.1	0.1	0.1
Seriously Fruity, Low Fat, Waitrose*	1 Pot/150g	146	97	4.4	17.5	1.0	0.3
YOGHURT, MUESLI NUT, Low Fat	1 Pot/120g	134	112	5.0	19.2	2.2	0.0
YOGHURT, NATURAL							
With Honey,Greek Style, Sainsbury's*	1 Sm Pot/150g	243	162	4.0	15.4	9.4	0.0
With Prunes, Bio Activia, Danone*	1 Pot/125g	124	99	3.3	15.2	2.8	0.0
Bio Activia, Low Fat, Danone*	1 Pot/125g	75	60	4.7	6.1	1.9	0.0
Bio, Ann Forshaws*	1 Pot/125g	53	42	5.0	5.5	0.1	0.0
Bio, Co-Op*	1 Pot/150g	117	78	4.8	5.5	3.6	0.0
Bio, Fat Free, Waitrose*	1 Pot/150g	90	60	6.1	8.6	0.1	0.0
Bio, Good For You, Asda*	1oz/28g	17	62	6.0	9.0	0.2	0.0
Bio Live, Organic, Yeo Valley*	1 Pot/100g	82	82	4.5	6.6	4.2	0.0
Biopot, Set, Onken*	1 Pot/150g	101	67	3.9	4.8	3.6	0.0
Bio Wholemilk, Waitrose*	1 Pot/125g	100	80	4.8	6.9	3.7	0.0
Danone*	1 Pot/125g	71	57	3.2	3.8	2.9	0.0
Fat Free, Organic, Rachel's Organic*	1 Pot/500g	180	36	3.9	4.8	0.1	0.0
Greek Style, Asda*	1oz/28g	36	129	4.6	4.8	10.8	0.0
Greek Style, BGTY, Sainsbury's*	1 Serving/50g	48	95	6.2	6.4	5.0	0.0
Greek Style, Bio-Live, Rachel's Organic*	1 Pot/450g	513	114	3.7	4.6	9.0	0.0
Greek Style, Healthy Eating, Tesco*	1oz/28g	22	79	6.5	4.0	4.1	0.0
Greek Style, Organic, Tesco*	1oz/28g	37	133	4.5	6.2	10.0	0.0
Greek Style, Somerfield*	1oz/28g	36	129	5.0	5.0	10.0	0.0
Greek Style, Waitrose*	1 Pot/150g	210	140	4.8	6.9	10.3	0.0
Greek Style, With Cow's Milk, Tesco*	1 Pot/150g	215	143	4.5	6.6	10.9	0.0
Low Fat, Asda*	1oz/28g	17	62	6.1	7.1	1.0	0.0
Low Fat, Bio, Co-Op*	1 Pot/150g	98	65	6.0	8.0	1.0	0.0
Low Fat, Bio, Sainsbury's*	1 Pot/125g	85	68	5.6	7.9	1.5	0.0
Low Fat, Budgens*	1 Serving/112g	65	58	5.1	7.5	0.8	0.0
Low Fat, Co-Op*	1 Pot/150g	93	62	5.6	6.3	1.0	0.0
Low Fat, Live, Waitrose*	1 Pot/175g	114	65	5.8	8.2	1.0	0.0
Low Fat, Morrisons*	1 Pot/150g	84	56	5.2	6.2	1.2	0.0
Low Fat, TTD, Sainsbury's*	1 Pot/125g	80	64	6.7	4.6	1.8	0.0
Low Fat, Tesco*	1 Pot/200g	112	56	5.6	5.8	1.1	0.0
Organic, Evernat*	1oz/28g	29	104	3.9	12.9	4.1	0.0
Organic, Fat Free, Yeo Valley*	1 Serving/100g	58	58	5.9	8.4	0.1	0.0
Organic, Low Fat, Sainsbury's*	1oz/28g	20	71	6.2	8.8	1.2	0.0
Organic, Yeo Valley*	1 Pot/150g	120	80	4.7	6.9	3.7	0.0
Set, Asda*	1oz/28g	16	57	5.1	6.8	1.0	0.0

Y

INFO/WEIGHT	Measure	per Measure KCAL	Nutrition Values per 100g / 100ml KCAL	PROT	CARB	FAT	FIBRE
YOGHURT, NATURAL							
Set, Low Fat, Waitrose*	1 Pot/150g	99	66	5.7	8.1	1.2	0.0
Unsweetened, Bio, Marks & Spencer*	1 Pot/225g	135	60	5.6	5.5	1.8	0.0
Very Low Fat Bio, Somerfield*	1 Pot/150g	98	65	7.0	9.0	0.0	0.0
Very Low Fat, Longley Farm*	1 Serving/80g	46	57	6.5	7.5	0.1	0.0
Virtually Fat Free, Bio, Safeway*	1 Pot/100g	65	65	6.4	9.4	0.2	0.0
Vitality Probiotic, Low Fat, Muller*	1 Serving/100g	67	67	5.5	6.9	1.9	0.0
Weight Watchers*	1 Serving/100g	44	44	4.8	5.3	0.1	1.6
Wholemilk, Organic, Sainsbury's*	1 Pot/125g	86	69	3.7	5.0	3.8	0.1
YOGHURT, NECTARINE							
& Apricot Bio, Virtually Fat Free, Shape*	1 Pot/120g	53	44	4.8	5.3	0.1	0.1
& Orange, Best There Is, Yoplait*	1 Pot/122g	131	107	4.7	18.0	1.6	0.0
& Orange, Channel Island, Marks & Spencer*	1 Pot/150g	158	105	4.5	14.7	3.3	0.3
& Orange, Marks & Spencer*	1 Pot/150g	147	98	4.9	16.0	1.6	0.3
& Orange, Virtually Fat Free, Shape*	1 Pot/120g	55	46	4.7	5.8	0.1	0.1
& Orange, Virtually Fat Free, Tesco*	1 Pot/125g	58	46	4.1	7.2	0.1	0.0
& Passion Fruit, BGTY, Sainsbury's*	1 Pot/151g	122	81	3.2	16.3	0.4	0.6
& Passion Fruit, Fat Free, Weight Watchers	1 Pot/120g	54	45	4.2	6.6	0.1	0.1
& Raspberry, Low Fat, Somerfield*	1 Pot/150g	134	89	4.0	17.0	1.0	0.0
& Raspberry, Very Low Fat, Somerfield*	1 Pot/125g	60	48	5.0	7.0	0.0	0.0
YOGHURT, ORANGE							
& Guava Tropical Fruit, Ski*	1 Pot/125g	128	102	4.9	16.3	1.9	0.0
& Lemon, BGTY, Sainsbury's*	1 Pot/125g	63	50	4.7	7.3	0.2	0.2
& Mango, COU, Marks & Spencer*	1 Serving/145g	65	45	4.3	6.0	0.1	0.2
& Nectarine, Weight Watchers*	1 Pot/120g	54	45	4.2	6.5	0.1	0.1
BGTY, Sainsbury's*	1 Pot/125g	66	53	4.8	8.1	0.1	1.2
Fat Free, Shape*	1 Pot/120g	61	51	4.5	8.7	0.2	0.1
Greek Style, Boots*	1 Pot/140g	207	148	3.7	14.0	8.6	0.2
Greek Style, Shape*	1 Pot/100g	105	105	7.7	9.4	3.6	0.1
Low Fat, Tesco*	1 Pot/125g	111	89	4.9	13.5	1.7	0.2
With Chocolate Flakes, Shape*	1 Pot/150g	140	93	4.6	11.8	2.8	0.2
With Grains, Good Intentions, Somerfield*	1 Pot/125g	91	73	5.9	11.6	0.3	0.1
YOGHURT, ORIGINAL,							
99% Fat Free, Mullerice, Muller*	1 Pot/150g	108	72	3.9	11.8	1.0	0.0
YOGHURT, PASSION FRUIT							
& Peach, Fruit Corner, Muller*	1 Pot/175g	186	106	3.7	14.1	3.9	0.0
With Elderflower Extract, Tesco*	1 Pot/150g	147	98	4.7	17.3	1.1	0.2
YOGHURT, PEACH							
& Apricot, COU, Marks & Spencer*	1 Pot/150g	68	45	4.2	5.7	0.1	0.2
& Apricot, Extremely Fruity, Marks & Spencer*	1 Pot/200g	194	97	4.8	15.8	1.6	0.4
& Apricot, Healthy Living, Tesco*	1 Pot/92g	42	46	4.1	7.1	0.1	0.0
& Apricot, Marks & Spencer*	1oz/28g	27	97	4.8	15.8	1.6	0.4
& Apricot, Shape*	1 Pot/120g	54	45	4.6	5.8	0.1	0.1
& Lemon Balm, Biowild, Onken*	1 Pot/175g	158	90	4.3	14.9	1.5	0.1
& Mango, Low Fat, Live, Aldi*	1 Pot/200g	162	81	4.6	12.4	1.4	0.0
& Maracuya, Light, Muller*	1 Pot/200g	100	50	4.4	7.9	0.1	0.0
& Papaya, Low Fat, Sunshine Selection, Sainsbury's*	1 Pot/125g	114	91	4.3	15.0	1.5	0.1
& Papaya, Waitrose*	1 Pot/150g	129	86	4.2	17.1	0.1	0.2
& Passion Fruit Flip, Morrisons*	1 Pot/175g	89	51	3.9	8.2	0.3	0.6
& Passion Fruit, Balanced Lifestyle, Aldi*	1 Serving/100g	49	49	4.3	7.3	0.3	0.5
& Passion Fruit, Eat Smart, Safeway*	1 Pot/125g	69	55	5.2	8.5	0.1	0.3
& Passion Fruit, Fruit Layered, Bio, GFY, Asda*	1 Pot/125g	76	61	4.0	11.0	0.1	0.0
& Passion Fruit, Lite Biopot, Onken*	1 Serving/100g	45	45	4.6	6.0	0.2	0.2
& Passion Fruit, Low Fat, Ski*	1 Pot/125g	129	103	5.0	16.4	1.9	0.0

Y

	Measure INFO/WEIGHT	per Measure KCAL	Nutrition Values per 100g / 100ml				
			KCAL	PROT	CARB	FAT	FIBRE
YOGHURT, PEACH,							
& Passion Fruit, Low Fat, Somerfield*	1 Pot/150g	132	88	4.0	16.0	1.0	0.0
& Passion Fruit, Organic, Muller*	1 Pot/150g	147	98	3.9	16.6	1.8	0.0
& Passion Fruit, Very Low Fat, Somerfield*	1 Pot/125g	61	49	5.0	7.0	0.0	0.0
& Pineapple, Fat Free, Weight Watchers*	1 Pot/120g	53	44	4.1	6.5	0.1	0.1
& Pineapple, Light, Ski*	1 Pot/125g	68	54	5.7	7.5	0.1	2.0
& Raspberry, Custard Style, Fat Free, Shape*	1 Pot/170g	77	45	4.1	6.3	0.1	0.2
& Raspberry, Marks & Spencer*	1 Pot/150g	144	96	4.8	15.7	1.6	0.4
& Vanilla Flip, Morrisons*	1 Pot/175g	212	121	3.4	16.5	4.6	0.6
& Vanilla, Healthy Eating, Tesco*	1 Pot/125g	55	44	4.8	6.0	0.1	0.1
& Vanilla, Thick & Creamy, Co-Op*	1 Pot/150g	180	120	3.6	16.0	4.6	0.1
BGTY, Sainsbury's*	1 Pot/125g	61	49	4.7	7.2	0.2	0.2
Bio Activia 0%, Danone*	1 Pot/125g	64	51	3.7	8.9	0.0	0.0
Bio, Virtually Fat Free, Shape*	1 Pot/120g	55	46	4.7	5.8	0.1	0.1
Custard Style, Low Fat, Sainsbury's*	1 Pot/125g	110	88	4.4	14.2	1.5	0.1
D'lite, Ski*	1 Pot/125g	100	80	4.6	15.2	0.1	0.2
Economy, Sainsbury's*	1 Pot/125g	93	74	2.8	14.7	0.4	0.0
Extra Fruit, Low Fat, Ski*	1 Pot/125g	114	91	3.5	15.7	1.5	0.1
Fat Free, Weight Watchers*	1 Pot/118g	53	45	4.2	6.7	0.1	0.2
Honey & Grain, Eat Smart, Safeway*	1 Serving/200g	120	60	4.7	9.4	0.2	0.3
Low Fat, Asda*	1 Pot/125g	119	95	4.6	17.4	1.0	0.2
Low Fat, Co-Op*	1 Pot/150g	122	81	3.7	14.6	0.8	0.4
Low Fat, Muller*	1 Pot/150g	152	101	4.8	16.1	1.9	0.0
Low Fat, Safeway*	1 Pot/150g	141	94	4.7	16.2	1.1	0.2
Low Fat, Sainsbury's*	1 Pot/125g	114	91	4.3	15.0	1.5	0.1
Low Fat, Ski*	1 Pot/125g	126	101	4.9	16.3	1.8	0.0
Low Fat, Yeo Valley*	1 Pot/125g	113	90	4.6	15.3	1.1	0.1
Melba, Everyday Low Fat, Co-Op*	1 Pot/125g	88	70	3.0	13.0	0.7	0.0
Melba, Low Fat, Tesco*	1 Pot/125g	80	64	2.7	11.7	0.7	0.1
Melba, Sveltesse 0%, Nestle*	1 Pot/125.5g	64	51	4.3	8.2	0.1	0.0
Pineapple Passion Fruit, Very Low Fat, Loseley*	1 Pot/140g	99	71	3.3	14.3	0.0	0.0
Shape*	1 Pot/120g	55	46	4.7	5.8	0.1	0.1
Smooth, Ski*	1 Pot/125g	128	102	4.9	16.3	1.9	0.0
Vitality Probiotic, Muller*	1 Pot/150g	113	75	2.6	13.0	1.4	0.0
Wholegrain, Biopot, Onken*	1 Serving/200g	226	113	4.2	17.9	2.7	0.3
YOGHURT, PEANUT Toffee, Low Fat, Somerfield*	1 Pot/150g	131	87	4.0	15.0	1.0	0.0
YOGHURT, PEAR							
& Butterscotch, Finest, Tesco*	1 Pot/150g	413	275	5.0	32.3	14.0	0.5
Rosehip & Marigold, Biowild, Onken*	1 Pot/175g	161	92	4.4	15.1	1.5	0.3
YOGHURT, PINEAPPLE							
& Coconut, Weight Watchers*	1 Pot/120g	56	47	3.9	7.4	0.1	0.1
& Papaya, Ski*	1 Pot/125g	126	101	4.9	16.3	1.8	0.0
& Passion Fruit, Low Fat, Marks & Spencer*	1 Pot/145g	65	45	4.3	5.7	0.1	0.2
& Passion Fruit, Sunshine Selection, Sainsbury's*	1 Pot/125g	115	92	4.3	15.2	1.5	0.1
& Peach, Virtually Fat Free, Light, Muller*	1 Pot/200g	106	53	4.4	8.7	0.1	0.0
BGTY, Sainsbury's*	1 Pot/125g	66	53	4.8	8.3	0.1	1.1
Channel Island, Marks & Spencer*	1 Pot/150g	165	110	4.3	15.9	3.3	0.3
D'Lite 0.2, Ski, Nestle*	1 Pot/125g	100	80	4.4	15.3	0.1	0.1
Eat Smart, Safeway*	1 Pot/125g	66	53	4.5	8.4	0.1	0.1
Extremely Fruity, Marks & Spencer*	1 Pot/200g	200	100	4.3	17.6	1.4	0.2
Finest, Tesco*	1 Pot/200g	220	110	3.5	17.5	2.9	0.2
Healthy Living, Tesco*	1 Pot/125g	69	55	5.1	8.1	0.3	1.1
Low Fat, Bio, Asda*	1 Pot/150g	144	96	4.6	17.0	1.1	0.1
Low Fat, Somerfield*	1 Pot/150g	134	89	4.0	17.0	1.0	0.0

YOGHURT, PINEAPPLE

	Measure INFO/WEIGHT	per Measure KCAL	KCAL	PROT	CARB	FAT	FIBRE
Low Fat, Tesco*	1 Pot/125g	111	89	4.6	13.4	1.7	0.0
Passion Fruit & Guava, Fat Free, Weight Watchers*	1 Pot/120g	54	45	4.1	6.6	0.1	0.1
Truly Fruity, Shape*	1 Pot/120g	61	51	4.5	7.3	0.1	0.1
Virtually Fat Free, Tesco*	1 Pot/125g	55	44	4.1	6.5	0.2	0.9
Weight Watchers*	1 Pot/120g	52	43	4.1	6.3	0.1	0.1
YOGHURT, PINK GRAPEFRUIT							
Fruit Corner, Muller*	1 Pot/175g	189	108	4.1	13.9	4.0	0.0
With Grains, Good Intentions, Somerfield*	1 Pot/125g	87	70	6.0	10.8	0.3	0.1
YOGHURT, PINK GRAPEFRUIT,							
Breakfast Selection, Sainsbury's*	1 Pot/117g	109	93	4.2	15.9	1.4	0.1
Weight Watchers*	1 Pot/120g	52	43	4.1	6.3	0.1	0.2
YOGHURT, PLAIN, Low Fat	1 Pot/120g	67	56	5.1	7.5	0.8	0.0
YOGHURT, PLUM							
& Hop, Biowild, Onken*	1 Pot/175g	158	90	4.3	14.9	1.5	0.3
Low Fat, Ski*	1 Pot/125g	126	101	4.8	16.4	1.8	0.0
YOGHURT, PRUNE, Breakfast Selection, Sainsbury's*	1 Pot/125g	119	95	4.2	16.3	1.4	0.2
YOGHURT, RASPBERRY							
& Black Cherry, Virtually Fat Free, Tesco*	1 Pot/125g	54	43	4.2	6.1	0.2	1.1
& Blackberry Bio, Fat Free, Shape*	1 Pot/120g	54	45	4.6	5.6	0.1	0.2
& Blackberry, Thick & Creamy, Co-Op*	1 Pot/150g	188	125	3.6	17.3	4.6	0.1
& Blackcurrant, Ski*	1 Pot/125g	129	103	4.4	14.6	3.0	0.0
& Cranberry, Light, Healthy Living, Tesco*	1 Pot/125g	55	44	4.2	6.3	0.2	1.1
& Cranberry, Light, Muller*	1 Pot/200g	104	52	4.4	8.3	0.1	0.0
& Cranberry, Low Fat, Bio Live, Rachel's*	1 Pot/125g	119	95	4.7	15.1	1.8	0.0
& Redcurrant, Low Fat, Sainsbury's*	1 Pot/125g	109	87	4.2	14.5	1.4	0.5
& Strawberry, Extremely Fruity, Marks & Spencer*	1 Pot/150g	165	110	4.7	18.9	1.5	0.4
BGTY, Sainsbury's*	1 Pot/125g	64	51	4.4	7.9	0.2	2.0
Bio Pot, Onken*	1 Pot/150g	153	102	4.4	15.1	2.7	0.0
Bio, Virtually Fat Free, Shape*	1 Pot/120g	56	47	4.7	6.1	0.1	0.2
COU, Marks & Spencer*	1 Pot/150g	68	45	4.2	5.5	0.1	0.3
D'lite 0.2%, Ski*	1 Pot/125g	99	79	4.6	14.9	0.1	0.6
Eat Smart, Safeway*	1 Pot/127g	70	55	5.2	8.5	0.1	0.7
Economy, Sainsbury's*	1 Pot/125g	85	68	3.0	11.9	1.0	0.0
Everyday, Low Fat, Co-Op*	1 Pot/125g	88	70	3.0	13.0	0.7	0.0
Extremely Fruity, Marks & Spencer*	1 Pot/200g	190	95	5.0	15.6	1.5	0.5
Fat Free, Bio Live, Organic, Yeo Valley*	1 Pot/125g	98	78	5.2	14.0	0.1	0.4
Fat Free, Farmhouse, BGTY, Sainsbury's*	1 Pot/150g	101	67	3.4	13.7	0.1	2.0
Fat Free, Weight Watchers*	1 Pot/120g	49	41	4.2	5.7	0.1	0.3
Fimbles, Marks & Spencer*	1 Pot/87.5g	70	80	3.6	11.1	2.6	0.6
French Set Wholemilk, Asda*	1 Pot/125g	125	100	3.6	14.1	3.2	0.0
Frozen, Orchard Maid*	1 Serving/80ml	89	111	2.8	19.9	2.1	0.0
Greek Style, Layered, GFY, Asda*	1 Pot/150g	123	82	4.3	10.0	2.7	1.3
Healthy Eating, Tesco*	1 Pot/125g	49	39	4.4	5.0	0.2	1.0
Healthy Living, Tesco*	1 Serving/175g	74	42	2.1	8.3	0.1	2.0
Light, Healthy Living, Tesco*	1 Pot/200g	76	38	3.7	5.7	0.1	0.0
Low Fat, Asda*	1 Pot/125g	121	97	4.7	17.0	1.1	0.0
Low Fat, Benecol*	1 Pot/125ml	100	80	3.8	14.5	0.7	0.0
Low Fat, Bio, Sainsbury's*	1 Pot/150g	146	97	4.7	17.0	1.1	0.7
Low Fat, Budgens*	1 Pot/125g	121	97	4.7	17.0	1.1	0.2
Low Fat, Co-Op*	1 Pot/150g	120	80	4.0	13.6	1.0	0.4
Low Fat, Muller*	1 Pot/150g	152	101	4.8	16.1	1.9	0.0
Low Fat, Organic, Marks & Spencer*	1 Pot/170g	162	95	4.4	16.1	1.4	0.4
Low Fat, Safeway*	1 Pot/150g	143	95	4.7	16.5	1.1	0.3

Y

	Measure INFO/WEIGHT	per Measure KCAL	Nutrition Values per 100g / 100ml				
			KCAL	PROT	CARB	FAT	FIBRE
YOGHURT, RASPBERRY							
Low Fat, Sainsbury's*	1 Pot/125g	115	92	4.4	15.2	1.5	0.2
Low Fat, Ski*	1 Pot/125g	125	100	4.9	15.9	1.9	0.0
Low Fat, Somerfield*	1 Pot/150g	128	85	4.0	16.0	1.0	0.0
Low Fat, Tesco*	1 Pot/125g	123	98	4.9	15.5	1.8	0.3
Marks & Spencer*	1 Pot/150g	144	96	4.9	15.4	1.6	0.6
Mullerice, Muller*	1 Pot/200g	228	114	3.4	20.0	2.3	0.0
Organic, Low Fat, Tesco*	1 Pot/125g	109	87	5.3	14.1	1.0	0.1
Organic, Yeo Valley*	1 Pot/150g	144	96	4.4	12.3	3.3	0.1
Pavlova, Corner, Muller*	1 Pot/150g	230	153	3.4	24.4	4.7	0.0
Seriously Fruity, Low Fat, Waitrose*	1 Pot/150g	149	99	4.8	16.2	1.7	0.3
Smooth Set, Co-Op*	1 Pot/125g	95	76	3.7	12.5	0.9	0.0
Smooth, Marks & Spencer*	1 Pot/150g	150	100	4.9	16.2	1.6	0.5
Thick & Creamy, Sainsbury's*	1 Pot/150g	179	119	4.4	17.2	3.7	0.2
Virtually Fat Free, Tesco*	1 Pot/125g	51	41	4.1	5.8	0.2	1.1
Way To Five, Sainsbury's*	1 Pot/151g	104	69	3.3	13.6	0.1	2.1
YOGHURT, RED BERRY, Blender, Pret A Manger*	1 Av Pack/125g	175	140	5.6	23.0	3.0	2.4
YOGHURT, RED CHERRIES, Bio Activia 0%, Danone*	1 Pot/125g	65	52	3.6	9.1	0.0	0.0
YOGHURT, RED CHERRY,							
Bio, Shape*	1 Pot/120g	58	48	4.6	6.4	0.1	0.1
D'lite, Ski*	1 Pot/125g	101	81	4.5	15.4	0.1	0.1
Fruit Layered, GFY, Asda*	1 Pot/125g	75	60	3.7	11.0	0.1	0.0
Light, 99.9% Fat Free, Ski*	1 Pot/125g	73	58	4.9	9.2	0.1	1.2
Simply Berries, Shape, Danone*	1 Pot/120g	64	53	4.4	8.7	0.1	7.4
Virtually Fat Free, Ski*	1 Pot/125g	64	51	4.5	7.7	0.2	2.0
YOGHURT, RED FRUITS, Crumble Style, Sveltesse, Nestle*	1 Pot/125g	58	46	4.2	7.1	0.1	0.0
YOGHURT, RHUBARB							
& Orange, Perfectly Balanced, Waitrose*	½ Pot/250ml	218	87	1.9	18.4	0.6	0.2
& Orange, Tesco*	1 Pot/150g	146	97	4.6	17.1	1.1	0.5
& Vanilla, Onken*	1 Serving/100g	106	106	3.8	16.9	2.6	0.3
Crumble Corner, Muller*	1 Pot/150g	222	148	3.3	21.7	5.3	0.0
Crumble, Layered Style, Healthy Eating, Tesco*	1 Pot/125g	93	74	4.1	12.9	0.7	0.2
Custard Style, Co-Op*	1 Pot/150g	203	135	3.7	17.2	5.3	0.3
Custard Style, Somerfield*	1 Pot/125g	149	119	3.0	16.0	5.0	0.0
Eat Smart, Safeway*	1 Pot/125g	69	55	5.1	7.8	0.1	0.2
Extremely Fruity, Marks & Spencer*	1 Pot/150g	158	105	4.5	18.2	1.4	0.4
Farmhouse, Sainsbury's*	1 Pot/150g	149	99	4.3	13.4	3.1	0.3
Fat Free, Bio Live, Summer Selection, Yeo Valley*	1 Pot/125g	89	71	5.2	12.3	0.1	0.2
Live Bio, Perfectly Balanced, Waitrose*	1 Pot/151g	131	87	4.6	17.0	0.1	0.2
Low Fat, Asda*	1 Pot/125g	110	88	4.6	15.0	1.1	0.0
Low Fat, Bio Live, Organic, Rachel's*	1 Pot/100g	73	73	3.5	11.0	1.7	0.0
Low Fat, Organic, Marks & Spencer*	1 Pot/170g	145	85	4.1	14.7	1.2	0.2
Low Fat, Safeway*	1 Pot/150g	137	91	4.6	15.7	1.1	0.1
Low Fat, Tesco*	1 Pot/125g	106	85	4.9	12.4	1.7	0.1
Marks & Spencer*	1 Pot/150g	149	99	4.4	17.4	1.4	0.3
Ski*	1 Pot/125g	121	97	4.8	15.5	1.8	0.0
Very Low Fat, Somerfield*	1 Pot/125g	58	46	5.0	6.0	0.0	0.0
YOGHURT, RUM Raisin Crunch Corner, Muller*	1 Pot/150g	219	146	4.2	22.0	4.6	0.0
YOGHURT, SOMERSET With Vanilla, TTD, Sainsbury's*	1 Pot/150g	222	148	4.0	18.1	6.6	0.0
YOGHURT, STICKY Toffee Pudding Corner, Muller*	1 Pot/150g	239	159	3.6	24.7	5.1	0.0
YOGHURT, STRAWBERRY							
& Cornish Clotted Cream, Marks & Spencer*	1 Pot/150g	218	145	3.2	15.4	7.7	0.5
& Multigrain, Low Fat, Breakfast Selection, Sainsbury's*	1 Pot/125g	126	101	4.4	17.4	1.5	0.3
& Orange Crunch Corner, Muller*	1 Pot/150g	218	145	4.1	22.5	4.3	0.0

Y

YOGHURT, STRAWBERRY

	Measure INFO/WEIGHT	per Measure KCAL	Nutrition Values per 100g / 100ml KCAL	PROT	CARB	FAT	FIBRE
& Raspberry, Bio Live Organic, Yeo Valley*	1 Pot/125g	125	100	4.2	12.0	3.9	0.1
& Raspberry, Bio, GFY, Asda*	1 Pot/125g	75	60	3.8	11.0	0.1	0.0
& Raspberry, Healthy Eating, Tesco*	1 Pot/125g	58	46	4.2	7.0	0.1	0.0
& Raspberry, Low Fat, Asda*	1 Pot/150g	143	95	4.6	17.4	1.0	0.2
& Raspberry, Low Fat, Sainsbury's*	1 Pot/125g	109	87	4.2	14.3	1.4	0.2
& Rhubarb, Channel Island, Marks & Spencer*	1 Pot/150g	158	105	3.9	15.4	3.0	0.0
& Rhubarb, Low Fat, Somerfield*	1 Pot/125g	108	86	4.1	15.6	0.8	0.1
& Rhubarb, Onken*	1 Serving/100g	85	85	4.6	16.2	0.1	0.4
& Vanilla, Low Fat, Somerfield*	1 Pot/125g	109	87	4.0	15.9	0.8	0.1
& Vanilla, Marks & Spencer*	1 Pot/150g	143	95	4.8	15.4	1.6	0.2
& Vanilla, Weight Watchers*	1 Pot/120g	54	45	4.2	6.8	0.1	0.1
& Wholegrain, Bio Break, Tesco*	1 Pot/175g	175	100	4.7	17.8	1.1	0.2
& Wild Strawberry, Sveltesse 0%, Nestle*	1 Pot/125g	58	46	4.3	7.0	0.1	0.0
& Wild Strawberry, Weight Watchers*	1 Pot/120g	49	41	4.2	5.8	0.1	0.1
99% Fat Free, Mullerice, Muller*	1 Pot/150g	107	71	3.5	12.2	0.9	0.0
BGTY, Sainsbury's*	1 Pot/123g	64	52	4.7	7.7	0.2	0.1
Balanced Lifestyle, Aldi*	1 Pot/150g	72	48	4.1	7.1	0.3	0.5
Bettabuy, Morrisons*	1 Pot/115g	91	79	4.4	12.8	1.3	0.3
Bio & Cereal Clusters, Rumblers*	1 Pot/168g	267	159	4.3	22.4	5.8	1.1
Bio Activia 0% Fat, Danone*	1 Pot/125g	63	50	3.8	8.4	0.0	0.0
Bio Virtually Fat Free, Tesco*	1 Pot/125g	50	40	4.4	5.3	0.2	0.9
Bio, Co-Op*	1 Pot/125g	143	114	4.5	16.7	2.8	0.1
Bio, Healthy Eating, Tesco*	1 Pot/125g	61	49	4.7	7.0	0.2	0.2
Bio-Live, Fat Free, Rachel's Organic*	1 Pot/142g	81	57	3.5	10.5	0.1	0.0
COU, Marks & Spencer*	1 Pot/125g	63	50	4.3	6.4	0.1	0.1
Childrens, Co-Op*	1 Pot/125g	121	97	3.5	14.9	2.7	0.2
Crumble Corner, Muller*	1 Pot/150g	222	148	3.3	21.7	5.3	0.0
Custard Style, Shapers, Boots*	1 Pot/150g	117	78	3.9	14.0	0.7	0.5
Custard Style, Somerfield*	1 Pot/125g	153	122	3.0	17.0	5.0	0.0
D'lite, Ski*	1 Pot/125g	99	79	4.5	14.7	0.1	0.2
Duo, Co-Op*	1 Pot/175g	219	125	3.0	17.0	5.0	0.7
Eat Smart, Safeway*	1 Pot/125g	69	55	5.1	8.3	0.1	0.3
Everyday Low Fat, Co-Op*	1 Pot/125g	88	70	3.0	13.0	0.7	0.0
Extra Light, 0.1% Fat, Muller*	1 Pot/200g	118	59	5.0	8.8	0.1	0.0
Extremely Fruity, Marks & Spencer*	1 Pot/200g	190	95	4.8	15.4	1.6	0.2
Fat Free, Waitrose*	1 Pot/150g	135	90	4.6	17.8	0.1	0.1
Fat Free, Weight Watchers*	1 Pot/120g	52	43	4.1	6.2	0.1	0.1
Frozen, Marks & Spencer*	1oz/28g	35	125	3.1	24.9	1.2	0.6
Fruit Corner, Muller*	1 Pot/175g	207	118	3.7	17.1	3.9	0.0
Fruit'n'Creamy, Ubley*	1 Pot/150.5g	167	111	4.3	16.9	2.9	0.3
Happy Shopper*	1 Pot/150g	131	87	3.0	18.5	0.3	0.0
Healthy Living, Tesco*	1 Pot/175g	70	40	2.1	7.7	0.1	0.3
Light & Refreshing, Campina*	1 Pot/125g	110	88	2.5	16.9	1.1	0.0
Light, 99.9% Fat Free, Ski*	1 Pot/125g	60	48	4.7	7.7	0.1	1.0
Light, Healthy Living, Tesco*	1 Pot/200g	96	48	4.1	7.6	0.1	0.0
Light, Muller*	1 Pot/200g	106	53	4.4	8.7	0.1	0.0
Lite, Onken*	1 Pot/235g	110	47	5.2	6.1	0.2	0.2
Live, Turner's Dairies*	1 Pot/125g	86	69	4.9	11.9	0.3	0.0
Low Fat, Asda*	1 Pot/125g	114	91	4.4	16.0	1.0	0.0
Low Fat, Benecol*	1 Pot/150g	119	79	3.7	14.8	0.6	0.0
Low Fat, Budgens*	1 Pot/125g	113	90	4.6	15.5	1.1	0.1
Low Fat, Co-Op*	1 Pot/150g	129	86	3.9	15.5	0.9	0.3
Low Fat, Lakeland*	1 Pot/125g	98	78	4.3	13.4	0.8	0.1

Y

	Measure INFO/WEIGHT	per Measure KCAL	Nutrition Values per 100g / 100ml				
			KCAL	PROT	CARB	FAT	FIBRE
YOGHURT, STRAWBERRY,							
Low Fat, Organic, Marks & Spencer*	1 Pot/170g	153	90	4.8	15.3	1.4	0.4
Low Fat, Organic, Muller*	1 Pot/150g	147	98	3.9	16.6	1.8	0.0
Low Fat, Organic, Sainsbury's*	1 Pot/125g	100	80	5.3	12.6	1.0	0.1
Low Fat, Organic, Somerfield*	1 Pot/150g	153	102	6.0	17.0	2.0	0.0
Low Fat, Safeway*	1 Pot/150g	138	92	4.6	16.0	1.1	0.1
Low Fat, Sainsbury's*	1 Pot/125g	115	92	4.3	15.2	1.5	0.1
Low Fat, Shape*	1 Pot/100g	56	56	4.9	5.9	1.1	0.1
Low Fat, Ski*	1 Pot/125g	124	99	4.8	15.8	1.8	0.0
Low Fat, SmartPrice, Asda*	1 Pot/125g	85	68	2.2	13.0	0.8	0.0
Low Fat, Spelga*	1 Pot/125g	129	103	4.5	18.0	1.8	0.0
Low Fat, Tesco*	1 Pot/125g	110	88	4.8	13.6	1.6	0.1
Low Fat, Value, Tesco*	1 Pot/125g	81	65	2.7	11.8	0.7	0.1
Marks & Spencer*	1 Pot/150g	143	95	4.8	15.4	1.6	0.2
Mullerice, Muller*	1 Pot/200g	230	115	3.4	20.0	2.4	0.0
Organic, Bio Live, Fat Free, Yeo Valley*	1 Pot/125g	98	78	5.1	14.3	0.1	0.1
Organic, Low Fat, Tesco*	1 Pot/125g	104	83	5.3	13.2	1.0	0.1
Organic, Yeo Valley*	1 Pot/150g	144	96	4.3	12.4	3.3	0.1
Perfectly Balanced, Waitrose*	1 Pot/150g	136	91	4.6	17.8	0.1	0.1
Seriously Fruity, Low Fat, Waitrose*	1 Pot/150g	152	101	4.8	16.6	1.7	0.2
Ski*	1 Pot/125g	111	89	3.4	15.3	1.5	0.9
Smooth Set French, Low Fat, Sainsbury's*	1 Pot/125g	100	80	3.5	13.6	1.2	0.0
Smooth Set, Co-Op*	1 Pot/125g	95	76	3.7	12.5	0.9	0.0
Smooth, Marks & Spencer*	1 Pot/150g	150	100	4.8	16.1	1.6	0.2
Smooth, Ski*	1 Pot/124g	123	99	4.9	15.7	1.9	0.2
Soyage, Granovita*	1 Pot/145g	112	77	1.8	16.5	0.4	0.0
Thick & Creamy, Channel Island, Marks & Spencer*	1 Pot/150g	135	90	3.4	13.6	3.0	1.4
Thick & Creamy, Co-Op*	1 Pot/150g	182	121	3.6	16.4	4.6	0.1
Very Low Fat, Bio, Somerfield*	1 Pot/200g	100	50	5.0	7.0	0.0	0.0
Very Low Fat, Loseley*	1 Pot/140g	92	66	3.3	13.0	0.1	0.0
Virtually Fat Free, Morrisons*	1 Pot/200g	114	57	5.4	8.4	0.2	0.0
Virtually Fat Free, Organic, Yeo Valley*	1 Pot/125g	98	78	5.1	14.3	0.1	0.1
Virtually Fat Free, Shapers, Boots*	1 Pot/125g	67	54	5.2	8.1	0.1	0.1
Virtually Fat Free, Ski*	1 Pot/127g	61	48	4.5	7.1	0.2	2.0
Virtually Fat Free, Tesco*	1 Pot/125g	53	42	4.1	6.0	0.2	1.0
Vitality Probiotic, Muller*	1 Pot/175g	138	79	2.6	14.1	1.4	0.0
Wholegrain, Biopot, Onken*	1 Serving/100g	109	109	4.7	16.5	2.7	0.0
Wholemilk, Organic, Sainsbury's*	1 Pot/150g	123	82	3.5	9.2	3.5	0.1
Yoplait*	1 Pot/125g	63	50	4.4	7.9	0.1	0.0
YOGHURT, TOFFEE							
Apple, COU, Marks & Spencer*	1 Pot/200g	90	45	4.2	6.3	0.2	0.2
Apple, Indulgent Greek Style, Somerfield*	1 Pot/125g	225	180	3.0	27.0	7.0	0.0
Benecol*	1 Pot/125g	124	99	3.8	19.3	0.7	0.0
Childrens, Co-Op*	1 Pot/125g	143	114	3.6	18.6	2.8	0.0
Economy, Sainsbury's*	1 Pot/126g	91	72	3.0	12.8	1.0	0.0
Fat Free, Eat Smart, Safeway*	1 Pot/200g	100	50	4.6	7.7	0.1	0.0
Light, Healthy Living, Tesco*	1 Pot/200g	74	37	3.6	5.4	0.1	0.0
Light, Muller*	1 Pot/200g	106	53	4.4	8.5	0.1	0.0
Light, Ski*	1 Pot/120g	60	50	4.6	7.7	0.2	0.6
Live Bio, Perfectly Balanced, Waitrose*	1 Pot/150g	156	104	4.2	21.1	0.3	0.0
Low Fat, Asda*	1 Pot/150g	174	116	4.6	22.0	1.1	0.0
Low Fat, Budgens*	1 Pot/125g	145	116	4.7	21.6	1.2	0.0
Low Fat, Co-Op*	1 Pot/150g	125	83	3.8	15.0	0.9	0.2
Low Fat, Safeway*	1 Pot/150g	174	116	4.7	21.6	1.2	0.0

Y

	Measure INFO/WEIGHT	per Measure KCAL	Nutrition Values per 100g / 100ml				
			KCAL	PROT	CARB	FAT	FIBRE
YOGHURT, TOFFEE							
Low Fat, SmartPrice, Asda*	1 Pot/125g	96	77	2.2	15.0	0.9	0.0
Low Fat, Somerfield*	1 Pot/150g	149	99	3.0	19.0	1.0	0.0
Low Fat, Tesco*	1 Pot/125g	158	126	5.0	22.3	1.9	0.0
Marks & Spencer*	1 Pot/150g	180	120	4.9	21.6	1.7	0.0
Seriously Smooth, Low Fat, Waitrose*	1 Pot/150g	156	104	4.7	16.5	2.1	0.1
Very Low Fat Bio, Somerfield*	1 Pot/200g	100	50	5.0	7.0	0.0	0.0
Virtually Fat Free, Boots*	1 Pot/125g	69	55	5.1	8.3	0.1	0.0
Weight Watchers*	1 Pot/120g	52	43	4.2	6.2	0.1	0.0
YOGHURT, TREACLE Toffee, Low Fat, Sainsbury's*	1 Pot/125g	145	116	4.3	20.7	1.8	0.0
YOGHURT, TROPICAL FRUIT, Greek Style, Asda*	1 Pot/125g	170	136	3.3	15.0	7.0	0.0
YOGHURT, VALENCIA							
Orange, Layered, Bio, GFY, Asda*	1 Pot/125g	80	64	3.7	12.0	0.1	0.0
Valencia Orange, Seriously Fruity, Waitrose*	1 Pot/150g	147	98	4.3	18.0	1.0	0.3
YOGHURT, VANILLA							
& Chocolate Flakes, Low Fat Bio, Shape*	1 Pot/150g	140	93	4.5	12.0	2.7	0.0
& Pineapple, Nestle*	1 Pot/125g	120	96	4.2	16.7	1.5	0.0
Bio-Live, Low Fat, Rachel's Organic*	1 Pot/142g	104	73	3.7	10.5	1.8	0.0
Blender, Pret a Manger*	1 Pot/250ml	230	92	4.5	12.8	2.7	0.0
Breakfast, Tesco*	1 Pot/150g	108	72	2.9	13.9	0.5	0.0
Channel Island, Marks & Spencer*	1 Pot/150g	173	115	4.5	16.5	3.5	0.0
Choco Balls, Crunch Corner, Muller*	1 Pot/150g	218	145	4.1	22.5	4.3	0.0
COU, Marks & Spencer*	1 Pot/200g	90	45	4.1	6.1	0.1	0.0
Creme, D'lite, Ski*	1 Pot/200g	192	96	5.1	15.8	0.8	0.0
Custard, Mullerice, Muller*	1 Pot/200g	250	125	3.3	22.1	2.6	0.0
Flavour, Healthy Living, Light, Tesco*	1 Pot/200g	72	36	3.6	5.2	0.1	0.0
Flavour, Organic, Low Fat, Tesco*	1 Pot/125g	114	91	5.3	15.3	1.0	0.0
French Set Wholemilk, Asda*	1 Pot/125g	125	100	3.6	14.1	3.2	0.0
Frozen, Less Than 5% Fat, Tesco*	1 Pot/120g	179	149	8.1	23.8	2.4	0.7
Light, Muller*	1 Pot/200g	106	53	4.6	8.2	0.1	0.0
Live Bio, Waitrose*	1 Pot/150g	132	88	4.6	17.3	0.1	0.0
Live, Bio, Green Dairy*	1 Bottle/250ml	263	105	2.5	17.7	2.9	0.0
Low Fat, Bio, Sainsbury's*	1 Pot/150g	147	98	4.8	17.2	1.1	0.0
Low Fat, Safeway*	1 Pot/150g	155	103	4.6	18.7	1.1	0.0
Low Fat, Tesco*	1 Pot/125g	125	100	4.9	16.3	1.7	0.0
Organic, Low Fat, Sainsbury's*	1 Pot/125g	114	91	5.3	15.3	1.0	0.0
Seriously Smooth, Low Fat, Waitrose	1 Pot/150g	149	99	4.7	16.3	1.7	0.0
Ski*	1 Pot/125g	123	98	5.0	15.5	1.9	0.0
Smooth Set, Co-Op*	1 Pot/125g	95	76	3.7	12.5	0.9	0.0
Thick & Creamy, Waitrose*	1 Pot/150g	188	125	4.2	20.6	2.9	0.0
Thickie, Innocent*	1 Bottle/250ml	200	80	2.4	12.2	2.0	0.0
Toffee, Low Fat, Sainsbury's*	1 Pot/125g	145	116	4.3	20.6	1.8	0.0
Very Low Fat Bio, Somerfield*	1 Pot/200g	98	49	5.0	7.0	0.0	0.0
Virtually Fat Free, Shapers, Boots*	1 Pot/125g	66	53	5.0	7.9	0.1	0.0
Virtually Fat Free, Ski*	1 Pot/120g	59	49	4.7	7.2	0.2	0.6
Virtually Fat Free, Yeo Valley*	1 Pot/150g	122	81	5.1	15.0	0.1	0.0
Weight Watchers*	1 Pot/120g	49	41	4.2	5.7	0.1	0.0
YOGHURT DRINK,							
Actimel, Orange, Danone*	1fl oz/30ml	26	88	2.7	16.0	1.5	0.0
Actimel, Original, 0% Fat, Danone*	1fl oz/30ml	10	33	2.8	4.9	0.1	1.9
Actimel, Original, Danone*	1fl oz/30ml	25	83	2.8	14.3	1.6	0.0
Blueberry & Blackcurrant, Orchard Maid*	1 Carton/250ml	148	59	1.6	13.6	0.0	0.0
Light, Yakult*	1 Pot/66ml	31	47	1.3	12.2	0.0	1.8
Raspberry & Passion Fruit, Everybody, Yoplait*	1 Bottle/90g	60	67	2.6	12.2	0.9	0.0

Y

	Measure INFO/WEIGHT	per Measure KCAL	Nutrition Values per 100g / 100ml				
			KCAL	PROT	CARB	FAT	FIBRE
YOGHURT DRINK,							
Yakult*	1 Pot/65ml	51	78	1.4	17.8	0.1	0.0
YORK FRUITS, Terry's*	1 Sweet/9g	30	328	0.0	81.4	0.0	1.0
YORKIE,							
Honeycomb, Nestle*	1 Bar/65g	331	509	5.7	63.6	25.8	0.0
Nestle*	1 Bar/24g	121	504	6.8	60.4	26.1	1.2
Original, Nestle*	1 Bar/70g	368	525	6.5	58.6	29.4	0.0
Raisin & Biscuit, Nestle	1 Bar/63g	307	487	5.9	60.5	24.6	0.0
YORKSHIRE PUDDING,							
4 Minute, Aunt Bessie's*	1 Pudding/18g	59	326	9.6	38.4	14.8	2.1
Asda*	1 Pudding/30g	97	322	10.0	39.0	14.0	0.5
Chicken & Vegetable, COU, Marks & Spencer*	1 Pudding/150g	195	130	12.2	14.3	2.2	1.3
Filled With Chicken & Roast Vegetables, ES, Safeway*	1 Pack/320g	400	125	7.6	17.8	2.2	1.8
Filled, Roast Chicken, COU, Marks & Spencer*	1 Pudding/150g	210	140	12.6	15.7	2.7	0.9
Filled, Steak & Red Wine, COU, Marks & Spencer*	1oz/28g	39	140	11.0	14.7	2.5	1.2
Four Minute, Aunt Bessie's*	1 Pudding/18g	59	326	9.6	38.4	14.8	2.1
Frozen, Ovenbaked, Iceland*	1 Pudding/12.4g	35	290	9.7	45.1	7.9	4.1
Fully Prepared, Marks & Spencer*	1 Pudding/22g	63	285	9.4	31.6	13.2	1.2
Giant, Aunt Bessie's*	1 Pudding/110g	290	264	8.5	37.4	9.0	2.0
Individual, Aunt Bessie's*	1 Pudding/18g	59	326	9.6	38.4	14.8	2.1
Large, Aunt Bessie's*	1 Pudding/39g	104	267	8.8	32.3	11.4	1.4
Large, Safeway*	1 Pudding/45g	123	273	8.5	41.1	8.3	2.5
Large, The Real Yorkshire Pudding Co*	1 Pudding/34g	103	304	11.5	37.3	12.1	2.5
Made From Batter Mix, Sainsbury's*	1 Pudding/100g	248	248	9.9	40.1	5.3	4.0
Mini, Asda*	1 Pudding/13g	34	260	10.0	37.0	8.0	2.8
Mini, Farmfoods*	1 Pudding/3g	8	281	9.6	43.2	7.7	1.9
Ready Baked, SmartPrice, Asda*	1 Pudding/12g	36	297	10.0	44.0	9.0	2.8
Ready To Bake, Aunt Bessie's*	1 Pudding/17g	42	246	8.5	35.1	8.0	1.7
Ready To Bake, Sainsbury's*	1 Pudding/18g	48	263	9.9	35.9	8.9	1.3
Safeway*	1 Serving/22g	58	265	8.4	38.9	8.4	2.5
Sausage & Onion Gravy Filled, Safeway*	1 Pudding/300g	540	180	6.2	18.0	9.2	1.2
Steak & Vegetable, COU, Marks & Spencer*	1 Pudding/150g	188	125	9.6	14.9	2.7	0.9
Traditional Style, Small, Asda*	1 Pudding/19g	49	259	10.0	39.0	7.0	2.1
Unbaked, Iceland*	1 Pudding/18g	47	263	9.9	35.9	8.9	1.3
With Beef in Gravy, Asda*	1 Serving/290g	406	140	7.0	20.0	3.5	0.7
3", Baked, Aunt Bessie's*	1 Pudding/36g	91	252	9.0	36.4	7.9	1.7
7", Baked, Aunt Bessie's*	1 Pudding/110g	290	264	8.5	37.4	9.0	2.0
YULE LOG,							
Chocolate, Sainsbury's*	1/8 Log/48g	186	382	5.1	46.5	19.6	0.7
Christmas Range, Tesco*	1 Serving/30g	131	442	4.9	56.8	21.7	2.8

Y

Feedback

If you have any comments or suggestions about the Calorie, Carb & Fat
Bible, or would like further information on Weight Loss Resources,
please call, email, or write to them:

Email: helpteam@weightlossresources.co.uk

Tel: 01733 345592

Address: Weight Loss Resources, FREEPOST ANG30222, PE2 9BR

About Weight Loss Resources

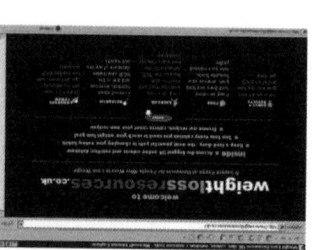

"What this does is put you in control with no guilt, no awful groups and no negativity! Fill in your food diary, get support on the boards and watch it fall off!"

LINDAB, Weight Loss Resources Member

How Does It Work?

You simply tap in your height, weight, age and basic activity level - set a weight loss goal, and the programme does all the necessary calculations.

What Does It Do?

The site enables you to keep a food diary which keeps running totals of calories, fat, fibre, carbs, proteins and portions of fruit and veg. You can also keep an exercise diary which adds the calories you use during exercise. At the end of a week, you update your weight and get reports and graphs on your progress.

How Will It Help?

You'll learn a great deal about how your eating and drinking habits affect your weight and how healthy they are. Using the diaries and other tools you'll be able to make changes that suit your tastes and your lifestyle. The result is weight loss totally tailored to your needs and preferences. A method you can stick with that will help you learn how to eat well for life!

Try It Free!

Go to **www.weightlossresources.co.uk** and take a completely free, no obligation, 3 day trial. If you like what you see you can sign up for membership from £7 per month.